Core Curriculum

CONTINENCE
MANAGEMENT

SECOND EDITION

Wound, Ostomy, and Continence Nurses Society™ (WOCN®)

Core Curriculum

CONTINENCE MANAGEMENT

SECOND EDITION

EDITED BY

JoAnn M. Ermer-Seltun, MS, RN, ARNP, FNP-BC, CWOCN, CFCN
President, Co-Director and Faculty
WEB WOC Nursing Education Programs
Minneapolis, Minnesota
MercyOne North Iowa Continence Clinic & Vascular and Wound Center
Mason City, Iowa

Sandra Engberg, PhD, CRNP, FAAN
Professor and Associate Dean for Graduate Clinical Education
University of Pittsburgh School of Nursing
Pittsburgh, Pennsylvania

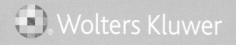

Philadelphia · Baltimore · New York · London
Buenos Aires · Hong Kong · Sydney · Tokyo

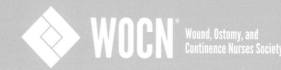

Acquisitions Editor: Jamie Blum
Development Editor: Maria M. McAvey
Editorial Coordinator: Anthony Gonzalez/Linda Christina
Senior Production Project Manager: Alicia Jackson
Design Coordinator: Teresa Mallon/Stephen Druding
Manufacturing Coordinator: Kathleen Brown/Beth Welsh
Marketing Manager: Linda Wetmore
Prepress Vendor: SPI Global

Second Edition

Cataloging-in-Publication Data available on request from the Publisher

ISBN: 978-1-9751-6453-9

shop.lww.com

PREVIOUS EDITION CONTRIBUTORS

Laurie L. Callan, MSN, ARNP, FNP, CWOCN

Michael Clark, DrNP, MSN, CRNP, DCC

Tamara Dickinson, BSN, CURN, CCCN, BCB-PMD

Dorothy B. Doughty, MN, RN, CWOCN, FAAN

Marcus John Drake, MA, DM, FRCS(Urol)

Sandra Engberg, PhD, RN, CRNP, FAAN

Mandy Fader, RN, PhD

Lynette Franklin, MSN, APRN-BC, CWOCN-AP

William Gibson, MBChB, MRCP(UK)

Mikel Gray, PhD, FNP, PNP, CUNP, CCCN, FAANP, FAAN

Claire Jungyoun Han, MSN, RN

Margaret Heitkemper, PhD, RN, FAAN

Anne Jinbo, PhD, MPH, CWOCN, CPNP

Darcie Kiddoo, MD, FRCSC, MPH

Katherine N. Moore, PhD, RN

Kelly Kruse Nelles, RN, MS, APRN-BC

Mary H. Palmer, PhD, RNC

Shiv Kumar Pandian, MBBS, MS, MD, FRCS(Ed), FRCS(Urol)

Joanne P. Robinson, PhD, RN, GCNS-BC, FAAN

JoAnn Ermer-Seltun, MS, RN, ARNP, FNP-BC, CWOCN

Susan E. Steele, PhD, RN, CWOCN

Adrian Wagg, MB, BS, FRCP, FRCP(E), FHEA, (MD)

Mary H. Wilde, RN, PhD

Midge Willson, BSN, MSN, CWOCN

The names and credentials are listed as they were printed during the time of the previous edition publication.

CONTRIBUTORS

Laurie Lonergan Callan, MSN, ARNP, CCCN, CWCN
Family Nurse Practitioner
Wound Center
MercyOne Clinton Medical Center
Clinton, Iowa

Tamara Dickinson, MSN, NP, CCCN
Nurse Practitioner
Radiation Oncology
University of Texas Southwestern Medical Center at
    Dallas
Dallas, Texas

Nicole L. Dugan, MPT, DPT, MSOD
Physical Therapy Clinical Specialist
Department of Rehabilitation Medicine
Thomas Jefferson University
Philadelphia, Pennsylvania

Sandra Engberg, PhD, CRNP, FAAN
Professor and Associate Dean for Graduate Clinical
    Education
University of Pittsburgh School of Nursing
Pittsburgh, Pennsylvania

**JoAnn M. Ermer-Seltun, MS, RN, ARNP, FNP-BC,
    CWOCN, CFCN**
President, Co-Director and Faculty
WEB WOC Nursing Education Programs
Minneapolis, Minnesota
MercyOne North Iowa Continence Clinic & Vascular and
    Wound Center
Mason City, Iowa

Kathleen Francis, DNP, FNP
Wound, Ostomy, and Continence Nurse Practitioner
WOC Series
NYU Langone Health
Brooklyn, New York

Dorothea Frederick, DNP, FNP-C, CNOR, RNFA
Assistant Professor of Nursing
College of Nursing
Thomas Jefferson University
Philadelphia, Pennsylvania

Susan Gallagher, PhD, MSN, MA
Senior Clinical Consultant
Clinical Services
The Celebration Institute
Sierra Madre, California

**Mikel Gray, PhD, RN, FNP, PNP, CUNP, CCCN,
    FAANP, FAAN**
Professor
Department of Urology
School of Medicine
Department of Acute & Specialty Care
School of Nursing
University of Virginia
Charlottesville, Virginia

Margaret Heitkemper, RN, PhD, FAAN
Professor
School of Nursing
University of Washington
Seattle, Washington

Leah Holderbaum, OTR, CBIS, ATP
Account Manager
Nu-Motion Medical Supply
Houston, Texas

Amy Hull, RNC, MSN, WHPN-BC
Assistant in OBGYN
OBGYN
Vanderbilt Health
Nashville, Tennessee

Kelly Jaszarowski, MSN, RN, CNS, CWOCN
Clinical Instructor
Nursing
Cleveland Clinic WOCNEP
Cleveland, Ohio

Anne Jinbo, PhD, MSN, MPH
Private Practice
Nursing
University of Hawai'i at Manoa Libraries
Honolulu, Hawaii

Kendra Kamp, PhD, RN
Post-doctoral Fellow
Division of Gastroenterology
School of Medicine
University of Washington
Seattle, Washington

Dea J. Kent, DNP, RN, NP-C, CWOCN
Director
Nurse Practitioner Program
School of Nursing
Indiana University Kokomo
Kokomo, Indiana

Rose W. Murphree, DNP, RN, CWOCN, CFCN
Assistant Professor
General
Emory University Nell Hodgson Woodruff School of
    Nursing
Atlanta, Georgia

Kelly Nelles, RN, APRN-BC, MS
Nurse Practitioner
Continence
Urogyn Consultations LLC
Blue Mounds, Wisconsin

Diane Kaschak Newman, ANP-BC, DNP
Adjunct Professor of Urology in Surgery
Surgery
University of Pennsylvania Perelman School of Medicine
Philadelphia, Pennsylvania

Denise Nix, MS, RN, CWOCN
Wound, Ostomy, Continence Nurse
WOC Nursing
M Health Fairview
Edina, Minnesota

Mary H. Palmer, PhD
Distinguished Professor
Nursing
University of North Carolina at Chapel Hill
Chapel Hill, North Carolina

Joanne P. Robinson, PhD, RN, CNE, FAAN
Associate Dean for Research and Innovation
College of Nursing
Thomas Jefferson University
Philadelphia, Pennsylvania

Margaret Mary Santos, MS (Nursing)
Clinical Nurse Specialist Perianesthesia
Perianesthesia
Phelps Hospital
Sleepy Hollow, New York

Phyllis Sheldon, MS, CUCNS, CNS-BC, RN-BC
Clinical Nursing Instructor
Nursing
Dominican College
Orangeburg, New York

Debra Thayer, MS, RN, CWOCN
Lead Technical Service Specialist
Medical Solutions Division Laboratory
3M
St. Paul, Minnesota

Donna L. Thompson, MSN, CRNP, FNP-BC, CCCN-AP
Nurse Practitioner
Division of Urogynecology
University of Pennsylvania Health System
Philadelphia, Pennsylvania

Valre Welch, MSN, CPNP
Nurse Practitioner
Pediatric Urology
VCU Health System
Richmond, Virginia

Leslie Sazsteinlt Wooldridge, GNP-BC
Consultant
Self-employed
Spring Lake, Michigan

FOREWORD

I t is an honor to be invited to write the foreword to the *Wound, Ostomy, and Continence Nurses Society™ (WOCN®) Core Curriculum*, 2nd edition. Having served 22 years as a Wound, Ostomy, and Continence (WOC) Nursing Program Director, I can attest as to how valuable a resource these books will be to students, faculty, preceptors, and all clinicians caring for people with wounds, ostomies, and incontinence.

Terms currently popular in health care refer to patient-centered and patient-focused care. For those of you entering the wonderful WOC nursing specialty, know this: the patient has always been the focus of WOC nursing! In fact, our specialty grew from a need identified by patients themselves. As colorectal and urologic surgeries advanced, so did the number of people living with ostomies. In 1958, Akron, Ohio, native Norma N. Gill joined her surgeon, Rupert B. Turnbull Jr, MD, in founding what was then coined by Dr. Turnbull as enterostomal therapy (ET).

Beginning in 1948, when she was a 28-year-old mother of two young children, Norma began a long odyssey battling mucosal ulcerative colitis. She manifested all the gastrointestinal symptoms, including massive bouts of bloody diarrhea associated with this disease, along with many of the extraintestinal manifestations, such as uveitis, iritis, and extensive pyoderma gangrenosum on her face, chest, abdomen, and legs. During a brief remission in 1951, much to the amazement of Norma and her husband Ted, she became pregnant. The pregnancy was fraught with complications, the need for numerous blood transfusions, and fear for the lives of both mother and child throughout. Despite all of these life-threatening occurrences, in June 1952, Norma gave birth to a healthy baby girl. The complications continued after her baby's birth, and Norma's response to treatment was spotty at best. In October 1954, she was admitted to the Cleveland Clinic, and there her life was saved, and history forever changed. Dr. Turnbull operated to remove Norma's colon and create an ileostomy. Her postoperative course after ileostomy was rocky, and she had to undergo some additional operations to remove her rectum and have plastic surgery performed on her face.

Despite all of this, Norma began to feel better—incredibly better. As she was resuming her role as a wife and mother, she felt the need, as we now say, to "pay it forward." Norma wanted to help others who were facing the same challenges she had endured and emerged stronger than she had been before her illness. Her journey began with the Akron physicians and hospital she had come to know well during her illness. Norma started from scratch and cobbled together an inventory of the limited equipment available at the time. Soon she had many referrals from the surgeons and knew she had found her calling. In 1958, during an appointment with Dr. Turnbull, she told him what she was doing in Akron to help people with new ostomies and fistulae. He was impressed and called her a couple of months later to offer her a job at the Cleveland Clinic.

August 1958 is when the seeds for the modern specialty of WOC nursing were planted. It was not long before the word was out, and surgeons began requesting that their staff come to train with Norma and Dr. Turnbull. The R.B. Turnbull Jr., School of Enterostomal Therapy (now WOC Nursing) was established. After her long work day in Cleveland, Norma would return to Akron and see patients in hospitals there before heading home to her family and doing it all again the next day.

There was a child in an Akron hospital born with exstrophy of the bladder after years of urinary incontinence, reflux, and renal stones whose family made the lifesaving decision to have her undergo a urinary diversion. She always remembered her first encounter with Norma. Here was a woman who commanded respect. The surgeon, head nurse, and staff nurses, as well as the girl's mom, crowded around the bed as Norma taught the proper way to care for a new ileal conduit. The equipment at that time was very primitive. Heavy stoma plates, rubber pouches with complex assembly secured with cement and a belt and a prayer! Norma never gave up attempting to help her patients and along with Dr. Turnbull urged industry to develop better, more secure pouching systems. Thanks to a great family and the one and only Norma Gill, the child in that Akron hospital grew up well adjusted to her new stoma, that child grew up to be me! I knew I wanted to "pay it forward" just like Norma. The baby who was predicted never to be born to Norma and Ted is Sally Gill-Thompson—one of my best friends and a famous ET practitioner in her own right.

After establishment of the formal program in Cleveland, other ET schools soon opened, and graduates from the United States and abroad spread the word across the globe. Professional organizations were established, and admission criteria became more stringent as health care became more complex. ET nurses became well respected for their skills and experience caring for people with complex ostomies and fistulae. It was a natural extension of our practice to embrace wound and continence care. In the 1990s, we bid good-bye to our ET designation and became known as WOC nurses to better reflect our practice. After 38 years, I have retired from clinical practice but my passion for WOC nursing is not diminished. As you embark on your studies of WOC nursing, take time to reflect and appreciate the wonderful legacy you are continuing with your specialty practice. Your actions will have an immeasurable impact improving the lives of your patients through direct care and advocacy, educating your colleagues, and expanding research to support our evidence-based practice. I know our future is in good hands.

Norma (and I) will be watching!

Paula Erwin-Toth, MSN, RN, FAAN

PREFACE

We are proud to support both wound, ostomy, and continence (WOC) nursing education and WOC nursing practice with this evidence-based *Continence Management* textbook, one of a set of three generously funded by the Wound, Ostomy, and Continence Nurses Society (WOCN®) to form the *Wound, Ostomy, and Continence Nurses Society™ Core Curriculum*. The continence field is growing, new research is informing practice, and practice is shifting with the new evidence. In this book, we address the fundamentals and the advances in both urinary and fecal incontinence in adults and children. The separate urinary and fecal sections begin with basic physiology and pathophysiology; subsequent chapters integrate pharmacology, include case studies, discuss the many complexities of conservative management of urinary and fecal incontinence, and highlight the unique aspects of care for the older patient. There is considerable emphasis on basic and advanced assessment. The fecal section includes an in-depth discussion of normal bowel function and defecation, followed by chapters on motility disorders, fecal incontinence, and bowel dysfunction in the pediatric population.

Unique features of this continence management book are chapters dedicated to the appropriate use of containment devices and absorptive products, and indwelling catheters. In this edition, we have added chapters on professional practice, the fundamentals of bladder and bowel management, advanced pelvic health considerations for the APRN continence nurse, the evaluation and management of incontinence in individuals with obesity, incontinence-associated dermatitis, and UTI prevention and management in adults. To assist the WOC nursing student, each chapter begins with curriculum objectives addressed in the specific chapter and a topic outline to give the reader a quick overview of the chapter content. Throughout each chapter, key points are embedded to highlight "take home" messages, and multiple illustrations, tables, and boxes facilitate understanding. Finally, there are questions and answers with rationale at the end of each chapter to support the individual's self-assessment of knowledge. Our goal was to present to both the novice and the advanced practitioner a set of logically progressive chapters, thoroughly researched and current, on a pervasive problem in the United States.

The chapters are written by expert clinicians "by continence clinicians, for continence clinicians." As editors, we wish to express our gratitude to the staff at Wolters Kluwer—Anthony Gonzales and Maria McAvey, and others behind the scenes who facilitated the organization and spearheaded the necessary planning to bring this series to publication. Finally, we express our sincere thanks to our extremely knowledgeable and committed contributors, and we thank each of them for saying "yes" to our request!

ACKNOWLEDGMENTS

The Wound, Ostomy, and Continence Nurses Society™ (WOCN®) wishes to thank all of the clinical experts who generously shared their time and expertise to create the second edition of this textbook. The Society would like to especially acknowledge the consulting editors, JoAnn Ermer-Seltun and Sandra Engberg, for their inspiration, knowledge, and unwavering commitment to the development of this resource and to the field of wound, ostomy, and continence nursing.

The WOCN Society would like to acknowledge Hollister Incorporated for providing a commercially supported educational grant for the development of this textbook.

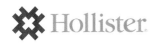

CONTENTS

CHAPTER 1

PROFESSIONAL PRACTICE FOR WOUND, OSTOMY, AND CONTINENCE NURSING

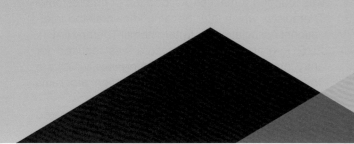

Rose W. Murphree and Kelly Jaszarowski

OBJECTIVES

1. Define the nursing specialty of wound, ostomy, and continence nursing and describe the key role components.
2. Identify the WOC nurse's specific scope of practice based upon licensure
   a. WOC registered nurse
   b. WOC graduate registered nurse
   c. Advanced practice (APRN)
3. Describe the tri-specialty role of WOC nursing.
4. Name the various populations served by the WOC nurse.
5. List the WOC nurse practice settings.

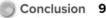
 ## WOUND, OSTOMY, AND CONTINENCE NURSING SPECIALTY

Wound, ostomy, and continence (WOC) nursing is a multifaceted, evidence-based practice that incorporates a unique body of knowledge to enable nurses to provide excellence in prevention of wound, ostomy, and/or continence problems and complications (WOCN, 2018). Also included in the scope of WOC nursing is health maintenance; therapeutic intervention; and rehabilitative and palliative nursing care to persons with select disorders of the gastrointestinal, genitourinary, and integumentary systems. The WOC nurse directs efforts at improving the quality of care, life, and health of health care consumers with wound, ostomy, and/or continence care needs. WOC nursing is a complex nursing specialty that encompasses the care of individuals of all ages, in all health care settings, and across the continuum of care.

 ## HISTORY AND EVOLUTION OF WOC NURSING

WOC nursing originated as a lay practice to address the unmet needs of health care consumers with an ostomy. During the 1940s and 1950s, surgical techniques developed rapidly with an increase in ostomy surgeries (WOCN, 2010). Stoma construction was often poor, there were few pouching systems available and hospitals lacked support systems to help the affected individuals deal with the life-altering surgeries. To fill the gap in ostomy care, one particular individual with an ostomy began the quest to improve ostomy care and services (WOCN, 2010). In 1955, Norma Gill Thompson had surgery at Cleveland Clinic (Ohio) with Dr. Rupert Turnbull, which resulted in the creation of an ileostomy. During one of her postop follow-up visits, she spoke with Dr. Turnbull about her rehabilitation with her ostomy care. He was impressed with her adaptation, willingness to help others, and attitude toward life with an ostomy that he asked her to become an ostomy technician (the role became known an enterostomal therapist) for Cleveland Clinic. In 1961, they opened the first formal Enterostomal Therapy School to provide rehabilitative care and psychological support to individuals with ostomies. The following chronology highlights, adapted from the WOCN Scope and Standards (2018) documents, some of the top defining moments in the history of WOC nursing.

- 1958: Norma Gill became the first "ostomy technician" at Cleveland Clinic.
- 1961: The first enterostomal therapy (ET) program was established at Cleveland Clinic.

- 1968: The first professional specialty organization was founded (American Association of Enterostomal Therapists), which later became known as the International Association for Enterostomal Therapy (IAET).
- 1976: Registered nurse licensure was required for entry into ET nursing education programs, which are now known as WOC nursing education programs (WOCNEPs).
- 1979: Certification in the specialty was first offered by the Enterostomal Therapy Nursing Certification Board, founded in 1978, which is a separate entity from the WOC nursing society, and is now known as the Wound, Ostomy and Continence Nursing Certification Board (WOCNCB).
- 1982: The scope of practice was expanded to include the care of individuals with wounds and urinary and fecal continence disorders.
- 1985: A baccalaureate degree was implemented as the minimum educational requirement for admission to the WOCNEPs and eligibility for certification in the specialty.
- 1992: The International Association of Enterostomal Therapy evolved into the Wound, Ostomy and Continence Nurses Society: An Association of ET Nurses, which is now known as the Wound, Ostomy and Continence Nurses Society™.
- 2010: WOC nursing was recognized as a nursing specialty by the American Nurses Association.

 ## KEY COMPONENTS OF THE WOC NURSE ROLE

Core values that guide the professional practice of the WOC nurse include integrity, leadership, and knowledge. These values are demonstrated by the following beliefs and behaviors (WOCN 2018):

- Integrity: WOC nurses are uncompromised in their dedication to being a trusted, unbiased, and credible source of evidence-based information, care, and expertise.
- Leadership: WOC nurses are stewards of excellence with a common passion for mutual respect, shared experiences, and lifelong learning.
- Knowledge: WOC nurses demonstrate a continued commitment to education and research to generate and disseminate knowledge that improves patient outcomes.

WOC nursing integrates art and science using creativity and innovation and assimilates evidence-based practices to manage patients with wounds, abdominal stomas, fistulas, percutaneous tubes/drains, and continence problems. WOC nurses are often called on to create new products, modify therapies, use innovative approaches for topical therapies or products, and orchestrate interdisciplinary resources to provide treatment plans for individuals or groups of health care consumers to achieve optimum health and independence (WOCN, 2018). In addition to providing unique and creative clinical skills, WOC nurses address other problems that patients experience such as limited access to supplies, lack of support and teaching family, caregivers, and staff. Essential to the practice of WOC nursing is the establishment of a relationship with the patient and their families/caregivers to gain trust, to help set goals, and to move the patient toward an optimal state of health.

PROFESSIONAL PRACTICE GOALS

Throughout the process of care, key goals for WOC nurses are to promote safe, patient-centered, quality, effective, equitable, efficient, timely, evidence-based, and cost-effective care for health care consumers (WOCN, 2018). WOC nurses contribute to achieving these goals through a variety of activities including, but not limited to, the following (WOCN, 2018):

- Collaborating with the health care consumer, family members, and other health care providers to develop individualized care plans and outcomes
- Implementing and marketing the role
- Providing evidence-based care to promote quality, effective and safe care and practice, and optimal outcomes for health care consumers who are culturally, socioeconomically, and geographically diverse
- Preventing complications and reducing readmissions
- Using proactive risk management strategies to reduce health care–acquired injuries such as the following: surgical site and wound infections, catheter-associated urinary tract infections, medical adhesive–related skin injuries, pressure injuries and medical device–related skin injuries, etc.
- Educating staff to improve the quality, effectiveness, and safety of care and staff productivity, competency, and efficiency
- Using advanced technology for prevention, diagnosis, and treatment of wound, ostomy and/or continence problems
- Coordinating care to promote continuity across health care settings
- Translating research into practice
- Developing metrics for quality outcomes
- Establishing standards for documentation and practice
- Developing formularies for supply management
- Developing protocols for cost-effective utilization of resources (e.g., pressure redistribution support surfaces, negative wound pressure therapy)

- Engaging in advocacy efforts for reimbursement of supplies and services
- Participating in/or conducting trials and evaluations of new products and treatments

 ## LEVELS OF THE WOC NURSING PRACTICE

WOC REGISTERED NURSE

The WOC nurse is a registered nurse with a baccalaureate degree or higher, with at least 1 year of clinical nursing experience following RN licensure. To attend an accredited WOC Nursing Educational Program, the applicant must have current clinical nursing experience within 5 years prior to applying to WOCNEP. Applicants can choose from several accredited WOCN Educational Programs and the structure of each program is diverse. Programs follow the curriculum blueprint that is part of the WOCN accreditation of the educational program; all programs contain a didactic and clinical component. Upon completion of the educational program in wound, ostomy, and/or continence, the nurse is awarded a certificate designating WOC nurse or specialty status, and the graduate is qualified to take national board examinations to become board certified in wound, ostomy, and/or continence care.

Those nurses not attending a WOCNEP have advanced their knowledge through additional studying in the specialty area(s) as well as through clinical practical experience. It is the inclusion of a clinical practicum with an approved certified Wound Ostomy Continence Nurse (CWOCN) preceptor, which sets the WOC nurse apart. Certification is through the WOCNCB®, an organization that is separate and distinct from the WOCN® Society.

WOC GRADUATE DEGREE REGISTERED NURSE

The WOC graduate degree RN is licensed as an RN within the state of practice and has a masters or doctoral degree but is not a graduate of an APRN educational program. They have attended an accredited WOCNEP or sought additional focused education and practical experience.

ADVANCED PRACTICE WOC REGISTERED NURSE

Advanced practice registered nurses (APRNs) have completed the educational requirements for licensure as an advanced practice nurse, either at the masters or doctoral level and are licensed in the state or states that they practice as APRNs. They have obtained education in one, two, or all three specialty areas through an accredited WOCNEP or through additional study focused in the specialty or specialties including focused practical experience. Certification is through the WOCNCB®. The WOC

APRN may practice independently or in collaboration with a physician, which depends on the state board of nursing, where the nurse practices.

THE TRI-SPECIALTY OF WOC NURSING

WOUND SPECIALTY

WOC nurses provide care to health care consumers across the continuum of care with varied types of acute or chronic wounds due to pressure; venous, arterial, or diabetes/neuropathic disease; trauma; thermal injury; surgery; and/or other disease processes (e.g., cancer, infection, vasculitis, sickle cell disease, calciphylaxis, etc.). Wounds can have devastating effects on the health care consumer with increased morbidity and mortality due to complications. Pain, bleeding, odor, drainage, necrosis, infection, sepsis, and limb loss are some of the complications associated with wounds. Throughout the process of care, WOC nurses collaborate and coordinate with other health care providers in developing and implementing wound treatment plans.

OSTOMY SPECIALTY

Health care consumers undergoing ostomy surgery require intensive physical and emotional care and continued support to return to their normal lives. For health care consumers with fecal or urinary diversions, fistulas, or percutaneous tubes/drains, WOC nurses (regardless of the practice setting) provide specialized care to maximize the individual's independence in self-care and adaptation to the life-altering changes in their body image and function. According to the American Society of Colon and Rectal Surgeons, "... all patients who have ostomies should have access to an ostomy nurse for follow-up care, as needed and wherever possible" (Hendren et al., 2015).

After ostomy surgery, individuals are faced with life-altering changes that can be overwhelming and devastating without proper care and education. The selection and fitting of an ostomy pouching system requires a specially educated nurse who is qualified and skilled to assess and determine the unique medical and physical needs of each individual.

The need for specialized ostomy care continues well beyond the immediate surgical period. WOC nurses are needed to provide long-term support and follow-up care to health care consumers with ostomies.

CONTINENCE SPECIALTY

Living with fecal or urinary dysfunction and incontinence places a great burden on affected individuals and their families or caregivers. Loss of continence can cause skin and wound care complications and may contribute to individuals being prematurely placed in long-term care facilities (WOCN, 2013b). Unfortunately, many individuals, family/caregivers, and health care providers do not intervene in continence issues believing that loss of continence is a normal part of the aging process (WOCN, 2016). Successful outcomes for individuals with continence problems require specialized care, and WOC nurses play an important role in the management of fecal and urinary continence issues.

COMPLEX PROBLEMS

A fistula is an abnormal tract that develops between a body cavity or organ or an organ and the skin (Bryant & Best, 2016). Some of the most difficult fistulas that WOC nurses care for are enterocutaneous fistulas that develop an opening from the small intestine to the skin, enteroatmospheric fistulas that open into the base of a wound, and multiple fistulas (Bryant & Best, 2016). An interdisciplinary team is required to manage an individual with a fistula, and WOC nurses are essential members of the team. WOC nurses utilize a variety of creative and adaptive techniques for both pouching and nonpouching modalities to achieve the goals for topical management of fistulas: skin protection, containment and accurate measurement of drainage, odor control, comfort and mobility of the individual, and cost containment (Bryant & Best, 2016).

WOC nurses are also often consulted to assist in management of complications due to percutaneous tubes/drains (i.e., gastrostomy, jejunostomy, nephrostomy, biliary). Percutaneous tubes/drains are placed to provide drainage; relieve an obstruction and maintain an opening into an organ; and/or for administration of fluids, medications, or feedings. Multiple complications occur with enteral tubes/drains that include irritant dermatitis from leakage around the tube, device-related pressure ulcers/injuries from inappropriate stabilization of the tube, fungal infections, cellulitis, and hypertrophic granulation tissue (Fellows & Rice, 2016).

WOC NURSE ROLES

WOC nurses serve in a variety of roles including clinician, educator, consultant, researcher, and administrator; they may engage in dual or multiple roles.

CLINICIAN

The WOC nurse provides care to individuals in multiple practice settings. The WOC nurse may also evaluate individuals and their care via telehealth services. To achieve optimal outcomes, the WOC nurse uses the nursing process when caring for health care consumers. Each plan of care is individualized to complement the developmental age of the health care consumer and their caregiver and achieve the best outcomes (ANA, 2010, 2015a).

EDUCATOR

Education is an integral component of every WOC nurse's role. The WOC nurse provides education directly to health care consumers, caregivers, nurses, clinical staff, and other health care providers. WOC nurses provide staff education through orientation, on the job training, in-service education, and development of protocols and/or guidelines (WOCN, 2013a).

WOC nurses may also provide formal education in academia or other organized continuing education programs that focus on one or more aspects of wound, ostomy, or continence care (WOCN, 2013a). Educational webinars are examples of some of the numerous continuing education programs provided by WOC nurses and the WOCN® Society. These programs extend the reach of the WOC nurse and the WOCN® Society to areas and settings that lack a WOC nurse.

CONSULTANT

In a direct consultant role, the WOC nurse partners with the health care consumer and other members of the health care team (WOCN, 2013a). The WOC specialty nurse has unique skills to coordinate individualized care based on assessment of the needs of the health care consumer, knowledge of current best practices, and an ongoing evaluation of outcomes. Collaboration with other health care providers and groups is also an essential part of the WOC nurses consultant's role. Some WOC nurses serve as independent consultants with contractual arrangements for the delivery of wound, ostomy, and/or continence care services in various settings. WOC nurses may also utilize their expertise in other practice areas such as legal nurse consulting.

RESEARCHER

In the role of researcher, the WOC nurse advances the science and art of wound, ostomy, and/or continence care. Varied types of research are conducted using different methodologies (e.g., applied research/clinical trials, problem-focused research, exploratory research, etc.). WOC nurse researchers are active in all settings where WOC nurses practice including academia, industry, and direct patient care areas (WOCN, 2013a). At the clinical level, WOC nurses assist in the translation of research and evidence-based guidelines into practice to enhance the delivery of quality care.

ADMINISTRATOR

The WOC nurse may also assume the role of an administrator. As an administrator, the WOC nurse's duties and responsibilities include management and oversight of clinical staff and the delivery of services across a broad spectrum of care (WOCN, 2013a). Other activities involved in administration include program development and efforts to ensure quality outcomes. The WOC nurse manager may be responsible for developing and overseeing operating budget for their department/unit.

PRECEPTOR

A WOC nurse can assume the role of preceptor for students. The most common role of preceptor is for either graduate nursing students (if the WOC nurse is an advanced degree nurse) or WOC nurse students. The WOCNEP have a clinical component of 40 hours per specialty, and a WOC nurse who has completed the WOC-NEP and is certified with an active practice can become a preceptor.

DUAL/MULTIPLE ROLES

Often WOC nurses assume dual or multiple roles, depending on their educational preparation and setting. In addition, WOC graduate-level prepared registered nurses and WOC APRNs contribute to the specialty and profession by delivering direct care as providers, examining systems, spearheading research, and providing clinical leadership in WOC nursing.

POPULATIONS SERVED BY WOC NURSES

Although the basic principles of wound, ostomy, and continence care are the same regardless of population or practice setting, certain populations may be at greater risk for wound, ostomy, and/or continence problems and complications. Also, they may require adaptation or modifications in their care to address their unique needs including, but not limited to, the following patient populations: pediatric patients (neonates, infants, children, adolescents), older adults, patients needing palliative or hospice care, and obese patients. WOC nurses have expertise in caring for individuals with wound, ostomy, and/or continence needs across the spectrum of ages and developmental stages, including those at end of life and others with unique or special needs.

PEDIATRIC POPULATION

Key concepts in effective management of the pediatric population include development of rapport with the patient, family, and caregivers; interdisciplinary collaboration and coordination of care; patient and family education; and ongoing follow-up, support, and positive reinforcement by the WOC nurse to promote cooperation and adherence to the treatment plan. Education must always be presented that is appropriate for the cognitive abilities of the child.

OLDER ADULTS

It is important for WOC nurses to collaborate and coordinate care with the patient, family and caregivers, and members of the interdisciplinary team to assess needs and provide appropriate, dignified care for the older adult with wound, ostomy, and/or continence needs. The assessment must include the preferences for care and personal goals of the older adult. Coordination of care with other disciplines (e.g., physical and occupational therapists, dieticians, social workers, etc.) is needed to provide comprehensive care to manage frail older adults and those with comorbid conditions.

PALLIATIVE/HOSPICE CARE

Increasing numbers of infants, children, adolescents, and adults are living with serious or critical illnesses or injuries (ANA & Hospice & Palliative Nurses Association [HPNA], 2017). Palliative care that includes hospice care is provided by an interdisciplinary team, and WOC nurses contribute in wound care (prevention or management of pressure injuries, malignant wounds), continence issues (fecal or urinary incontinence), and in management of fecal and urinary diversions.

 ## WOC NURSE PRACTICE SETTINGS

The majority of WOC nurses work in the acute care setting. In addition, WOC nurses have the opportunity to practice in other settings such as outpatient care, home health care, long-term care, nursing homes, industry, academia, private practice, etc. WOC nurses may practice in multiple clinical settings that are affiliated with/ or part of a large organization or health care system, or they may function as an independent consultant to several settings.

The following descriptions provide a brief overview of WOC nursing practice in some of the most common settings (WOCN, 2010).

ACUTE CARE

In the acute care setting, WOC nurses care for health care consumers with a wide variety of medical, surgical, and/or trauma diagnoses. The WOC nurse may provide services in one or more areas of the tri-specialty practice to health care consumers across the lifespan from newborns to the elderly. Health care consumers with wound, ostomy, and/or continence needs may be found in any level of care within the hospital setting including the emergency department, intensive/critical care units, operating room, and medical–surgical units.

OUTPATIENT CARE

WOC nurses may practice in outpatient care settings that include private practice settings, hospital-based outpatient clinics, and freestanding ambulatory care centers. WOC nurses may work in conjunction with physicians and surgeons (e.g., urologists, vascular specialists, colorectal surgeons) to optimize management of health care consumers with wound, ostomy, and/or continence disorders. WOC APRNs may also serve as providers within these practices.

HOME HEALTH CARE

In the home care setting, WOC nurses provide direct care and consultation to health care consumers with wound,

ostomy, and/or continence concerns. The prospective payment system in home care has fueled an increased demand for WOC nursing expertise to help streamline services, educate caregivers and staff, and contain costs. WOC nurses can develop protocols for care and product formularies to reduce costs while maintaining quality care. In addition to serving as a direct care provider, the WOC nurse's responsibilities often include educating other home health nurses and clinical staff to promote quality, evidence-based care for management of health care consumers with wound, ostomy, and/or continence needs. WOC nurses are integral members of interdisciplinary teams and work closely with rehabilitation staff to facilitate self-care and independence in the home environment. Additionally, the WOC nurse may serve as a case manager/care coordinator to facilitate care delivery.

LONG-TERM/EXTENDED CARE

In long-term care and extended care settings, WOC nurses may monitor, direct, or assist with care and/or provide education to facilitate care by other registered and/ or licensed practical/vocational nursing staff and nursing assistants. WOC nurses must be knowledgeable about the regulatory and risk management issues and assessment and documentation requirements that are unique to the setting. The WOC nurse may serve as an independent consultant or an employee of the facility.

REHABILITATION

Services in skilled nursing facilities focus on care that enables health care consumers to achieve maximum independence in self-care. WOC nurses, with their emphasis on optimizing self-care and strong educations skills, are able to meet the challenges posed by individuals who need rehabilitative services and have wound, ostomy, and/or continence issues. WOC APRNs who practice in this setting may be able to receive third-party reimbursement for their services.

INDUSTRY

WOC nurses may practice in one or more areas of the tri-specialty, depending on the industry's focus. The WOC nurse in this setting may function primarily as a researcher and/or educator to investigate and develop new products and teach the end-users. The WOC nurse in industry may serve as a resource to direct care providers and provide research evidence about the clinical effectiveness of products for wound, ostomy, and/or continence care and can offer guidance about the appropriate indications and use of products.

ACADEMIA

The WOC nurse in academia may function as an educator, researcher, administrator, or department head. The WOC nurse may provide formal education for one or more areas of the tri-specialty, or the content may be incorporated into other graduate or undergraduate courses. In addition to an academic appointment, a WOC nurse faculty member may have an active clinical practice as part of their role. Academic accreditation standards for nursing programs dictate faculty educational standards; therefore, the WOC nurse in this practice area will have an advanced degree.

RESEARCH CONSUMER AND EVIDENCE-BASED PRACTICE

Health care consumers and providers, including agencies such as the Centers for Medicare & Medicaid Services (CMS) and the health care insurance industry, expect care to be delivered based on the best available research and evidence. Many agencies and groups utilize and publish evidence-based clinical practice guidelines, including the WOCN Society. WOC nurses use all types of research and evidence to influence the quality of patient care that is provided while practicing in the full scope of WOC specialty nursing.

There are many roles for a WOC nurse in research and EBP, such as consumer and developer of EB guidelines and standards of care, investigator in a scientific research trial, as well as evaluator of products.

The WOC nurse can contribute to the development of evidence-based care in many ways without assuming the role (or responsibility) of a primary investigator such as by participating in the following activities:

Surveys or polls

Clinical trials or product evaluations (see section on product evaluation)

Data collection for pressure injury prevalence and incidence studies or continuous quality improvement projects/studies that relate to WOC care or foot and nail care

The components of EBP include a systematic search and appraisal of evidence to answer the clinical question(s), integration of the expertise and experience of the WOC nurse, as well as consideration of the patient's preference, values, and concerns. As part of the critical appraisal process, it is necessary to be able to discern the level and quality of the evidence. There are levels and criteria for rating research evidence utilized by the WOCN® Society in developing clinical practice guidelines.

CARE COORDINATION AND COLLABORATION BY WOC NURSE

The WOC nurse works collaboratively with other health care disciplines to provide comprehensive care. Successful collaboration between the WOC nurse, physicians, and other health care members increases member's awareness of each other's type of knowledge and skills that will lead to improvement in patients'

treatment plan and successful outcome. In order to coordinate individualize patient care, the WOC nurse should partner with members of the health care team, patient's families/caregivers, and other health care providers across the continuum of care (WOCN, 2018). Collaboration and coordinating of care requires skill to ensure the patient receives quality care.

The WOC nurse coordinates care for complex cases, utilizing their expertise, skills, and resources in various practice settings. The WOC APRN can provide additional services: order and interpret diagnostic and laboratory tests, prescribe pharmacological and nonpharmacological agents, and treatments for wound, ostomy, and continence complications (WOCN, 2018).

 HEALTH CARE REIMBURSEMENT

Health care reimbursement has a direct effect on the amount and type of care provided to patients by all health care providers, including WOC nurses. Payment for health care in the United States involves several mechanisms, including self-pay by the consumers, insurance companies, and government agencies. The federal government is the single largest payer through Medicare, Medicaid, and the Department of Veterans Affairs (Sherman, 2012). Medicare is a federally provided health insurance program that is administered by the US Department of Health and Human Services through CMS. Medicare provides coverage individuals over the age of 65, younger than 65 with disabilities, and with end-stage renal disease at any age.

Medicare Part A covers hospital and hospice visits, stays in skilled nursing facilities, and home health. Medicare Part B covers 80% of expenses incurred with outpatient visits/care, some home health, and durable medical equipment. Medicare Part C provides insurance coverage by private-run insurance companies. And Medicare Part D helps cover the cost of prescriptions. More information about Medicare can be found on the CMS Web site.

Medicaid is a joint state and federal health insurance program for low-income individuals. States establish and administer their own Medicaid programs and determine the type, amount, duration, and scope of services within broad federal guidelines. Medicaid provides health coverage to pregnant women, seniors and individuals with disabilities, and nonelderly, low-income parents, or caretaker relatives and varies from state to state.

The Wound, Ostomy and Continence Nurses Society has developed two fact sheets about reimbursement for its members and are available on the Web site (http://www.wocn.org) in the Public Policy and Advocacy section. The fact sheet, *Reimbursement of Advanced Practice Registered Nurse Services*, provides information about reimbursement opportunities and challenges for the advanced practice RN (WOCN® Society, 2019a).

In addition, the fact sheet, *Understanding Medicare Part B Incident to Billing*, provides some insight into cases where a nonadvanced practice WOC nurse might bill in the outpatient setting. "Incident to" is a billing mechanism for Medicare that allows services provided in an outpatient setting to be delivered by auxiliary personnel and billed under the provider's national provider identification (NPI). For example, under the incident to provision, a physician or APRN could develop the plan of care and a non-APRN could provide the care and bill under the provider's NPI (WOCN® Society, 2019b).

CONTINUOUS PROFESSIONAL DEVELOPMENT

Continued professional development is critical for the practicing WOC nurse. There are many opportunities through the WOCN® Society for the WOC nurse to maintain current, evidence-based practice. This can be accomplished by reading the *Journal of Wound Ostomy and Continence Nursing,* attending conferences, and working within the WOCN® Society as a volunteer. The WOCN offers an annual conference, which provides current research, topics related to the WOC practice. WOCN regions and affiliates offer on-site conferences. The WOCN® Society also provides live streaming/webcasts of sessions presented at the annual conference. Throughout the year, there are webinars available that provide continuing education credits. WOC nursing practice requires lifelong learning.

Involvement in professional activities can provide professional growth where opportunities are available to become a committee member to work on important projects, develop strategies to enhance care delivery, as well as opportunities to develop relationships with other WOC nurse specialists. Examples of organizations that are within the scope of WOC practice include WOCN® Society, World Council of Enterostomal Therapists, and National Pressure Injury Advisory Panel.

Certification

WOCNCB is a national certified organization that provides credentials based on valid and reliable testing process. The WOCNCB is a separate and distinct organization from the WOC Nursing Society. WOCNCB validates the specialized knowledge, skills, and expertise of nurses who meet the requirements for certification. Certification is voluntary, however, recommended as it provides assurance to patients and employers of a safe and competent practice. WOCN certification is granted for 5 years. Compliance must be demonstrated every 5 years by either re-examination or development of a professional growth program portfolio. Advance practice nursing certification in wound ostomy continence nursing is available through WOCNCB. (See **Table 1-1** on credentials.) For more information on WOCNCB and certification requirements, see their Web site: www. wocncb.org.

TABLE 1-1 WOCNCB'S WOUND, OSTOMY, AND CONTINENCE CERTIFICATION CREDENTIALS

CWOCN	Certified Wound Ostomy, and Continence Nurse
CWCN	Certified Wound Care Nurse
COCN	Certified Ostomy Care Nurse
CCCN	Certified Continence Care Nurse
CWON	Certified Wound Ostomy Nurse
Advanced Practice Certifications Credentials	
CWOCN-AP	Certified Wound Ostomy, and Continence Nurse–Advanced Practice
CWCN-AP	Certified Wound Care Nurse–Advanced Practice
COCN-AP	Certified Ostomy Care Nurse–Advanced Practice
CCCN-AP	Certified Continence Care Nurse–Advanced Practice
CWON-AP	Certified Wound Ostomy Nurse–Advanced Practice

ETHICS IN WOC NURSING

WOC nursing as a specialty practice embraces the provisions of the *Code of Ethics for Nurses with Interpretive Statements* (ANA, 2015b). WOC nurses are obligated to "adhere to standards of ethical practice established by the WOCN Society and to conduct themselves in a manner that upholds the highest professional standards" (WOCN, 2018). The *Code of Ethics for Nurses:*

Provision 1. The nurse practices with compassion and respect for the inherent dignity, worth, and unique attributes of every person.

Provision 2. The nurse's primary commitment is to the patient, whether an individual, family, group, community, or population.

Provision 3. The nurse promotes, advocates for, and protects the rights, health, and safety of the patient.

Provision 4. The nurse has authority, accountability, and responsibility for nursing practice; makes decisions; and takes action consistent with the obligation to promote health and to provide optimal care.

Provision 5. The nurse owes the same duties to self as to others, including the responsibility to promote health and safety, preserve wholeness of character and integrity, maintain competence, and continue personal and professional growth.

Provision 6. The nurse, through individual and collective effort, establishes, maintains, and improves the ethical environment of the work setting and conditions of employment that are conducive to safe, quality health care.

Provision 7. The nurse in all roles and settings advances the profession through research and scholarly inquiry, professional standards development, and the generation of both nursing and health policy.

Provision 8. The nurse collaborates with other health professionals and the public to protect human rights, promote health diplomacy, and reduce health disparities.

Provision 9. The profession of nursing, collectively through its professional organizations, must articulate nursing values, maintain the integrity of the profession, and integrate principles of social justice into nursing and health policy.

For interpretive statements specific to WOC nursing are available in the full scope and standards document (WOCN, 2018).

 ## CONCLUSION

WOC nurses are professionals dedicated to individuals with WOC care needs. It is the goal of the WOC nurse to enhance delivery of wound ostomy and continence care directly and indirectly to those persons in need of such care.

REFERENCES

American Nurses Association. (2010). *Nursing's social policy statement: The essence of the profession* (3rd ed.). Silver Spring, MD: Author.

American Nurses Association. (2015a). *Nursing: Scope and standards of practice* (3rd ed.). Silver Spring, MD: Author.

American Nurses Association. (2015b). *Code of ethics for nurses with interpretive statements*. Silver Spring, MD: Author.

American Nurses Association & Hospice and Palliative Nurses Association. (2017). Call for action: Nurses lead and transform palliative care. Retrieved August 21, 2017, from http://nursingworld.org/MainMenuCategories/ThePracticeofProfessionalNursing/Palliative-Care-Call-for-Action/Draft-PalliativeCare-ProfessionalIssues-Panel-CallforAction.pdf

Bryant, R., & Best, M. (2016). Management of draining wounds and fistulas. In R. Bryant & D. Nix (Eds.), *Acute & chronic wounds* (5th ed.). St. Louis, MO: Elsevier.

Fellows, J., & Rice, M. (2016). Nursing management of the patient with percutaneous tubes. In J. E. Carmel, J. C. Colwell, & M. T. Goldberg (Eds.), *Wound, Ostomy and Continence Nurses Society Core curriculum: Ostomy management* (pp. 220–230). Philadelphia, PA: Wolters Kluwer.

Hendren, S,. Hammond, K., Glasgow, S. C., et al. (2015). Clinical practice guidelines for Ostomy surgery. *Dis Colon Rectum*, 58(4): 375–387. doi: 10.1097/DCR.0000000000000347.

Sherman, R., & Bishop, M. (2012). The business of caring: What every nurse should know about cutting costs. *American Nurse Today*, 7(11):32–34.

Wound, Ostomy and Continence Nurses Society (WOCN) Society. (2010). *Wound, ostomy, and continence nursing: Scope & standards of practice*. Mt. Laurel, NJ: Author.

Wound, Ostomy and Continence Nurses Society. (2013a). *Professional practice manual* (4th ed.). Philadelphia, PA: Wolters Kluwer/Lippincott Williams & Wilkins. Retrieved April 11, 2020, from the Lippincott Nursing Center at http://www.nursingcenter.com/journalarticle

Wound, Ostomy and Continence Nurses Society. (2013b). A quick reference guide for managing fecal incontinence. Retrieved April 3, 2017, from http://www.wocn.org/?page=QuickRefGuide

Wound, Ostomy and Continence Nurses Society. (2016). Reversible causes of acute/transient urinary incontinence: Clinical resource guide. Retrieved April 3, 2017, from http://www.wocn.org/?page=RevAcuteTransientUI

Wound, Ostomy and Continence Nurses Society. (2018). *Wound, ostomy and continence nursing scope & standards of practice* (2nd ed.). Mt. Laurel, NJ: Author.

Wound, Ostomy and Continence Nurses Society. (2019a). *Reimbursement of advanced practice registered nurse services: A fact sheet*. Mt. Laurel, NJ: Author.

Wound, Ostomy and Continence Nurses Society. (2019b). *Understanding Medicare Part B incident to billing: A fact sheet*. Mt. Laurel, NJ: Author.

QUESTIONS

1. Medicare Part B covers
A. Hospice visits
B. Durable medical equipment
C. Prescriptions
D. Hospital visits

2. When designing and implementing a WOC nurse role, it is important to
A. Practice according to the WOCN® Scope and Standards.
B. Read the *Journal of WOC Nursing*.
C. Practice in all roles of the WOC nurse.
D. Provide annual reports to administration.

3. Completion of an accredited WOCNEP to become a WOC nurse requires
A. Didactic, special project, and passing final examination
B. Didactic and 40 hours of clinical experience
C. Didactic and acceptance of previous wound experience
D. Didactic and 120 clinical hours with an approved CWOCN preceptor

4. As an educator, the WOC nurse is responsible for
A. Providing staff nurse orientation
B. Conducting clinical trials of products
C. Develops protocols and guidelines
D. Collect data for quality improvement

5. Data collection for the WOC nurse should be
   A. Purposeful and outcome oriented
   B. Filled with everything the WOC nurse does
   C. Provided to administration annually
   D. Created by the WOC nurse only

6. As a research consumer, the role of the WOC nurse is
   A. Primary investigator for rigorous research studies
   B. Evaluator of WOC patient products
   C. Required to show proof of education in research
   D. Developer of evidence outside the scope of practice

7. The components of evidence-based practice include all of the following *except*
   A. Appraisal of evidence
   B. Systematic search of the literature
   C. Integration of the expertise of WOC nurse
   D. Work independently of others

8. Best practice documents provide which type of evidence?
   A. Randomized clinical trials
   B. Expert opinion
   C. Quasi-experimental studies
   D. Task force reviews

9. The first program for WOC nursing (previously enterostomal therapy) was located in
   A. Minneapolis
   B. New York City
   C. Cleveland
   D. Boston

10. Name two of the most common roles of the WOC nurse practices in acute care setting.
   A. Clinician and research
   B. Clinician and educator
   C. Educator and administrator
   D. Educator and preceptor

ANSWERS AND RATIONALES

1. B. Rationale: Medicare part B covers durable medical equipment. Medicare A covers hospice and hospitals and Medicare D covers prescriptions.

2. A. Rationale: The WOCN® Scope and Standards is the foundation to incorporate into the WOC nursing practice.

3. D. Rationale: Requirements to complete a WOCNEP are didactic and 120 clinical hours (40 hours each specialty: in wound, ostomy, and continence) with an approved CWOCN preceptor.

4. A. Rationale: As an educator, the WOC nurse has the responsibility to provide orientation to staff nurses. Conducting clinical trials of products and developing guidelines is an example of the role in research. In the role of a clinician, the WOC nurse is responsible for quality improvement projects related to the specialty.

5. A. Rationale: Data collection is important to the WOC nurse's practice. It should be purposeful and outcome oriented to validate the role and position of the WOC nurse.

6. B. Rationale: The WOC nurse can contribute to research by evaluating WOC products.

7. D. Rationale: The components of evidence-based practice does not include work independently of others.

8. B. Rationale: Best practice documents level of evidence is from expert opinion.

9. C. Rationale: Cleveland was the first site for an enterostomal therapy program (WOCN Program).

10. B. Rationale: Clinician and educator are the many roles of the WOC nurse in the acute care setting. The role of a consultant is also a major role for the WOC nurse.

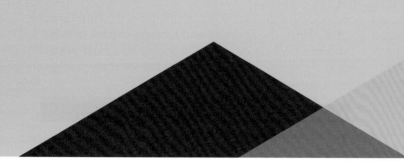

CHAPTER 2

VOIDING PHYSIOLOGY

JoAnn M. Ermer-Seltun

OBJECTIVES

1. Explain the physiology of normal voiding, to include the role of each of the following: cerebral cortex, pontine micturition center, spinal cord and nerve pathways, bladder, urethral sphincter mechanism, and pelvic floor.

2. Explain how kidney, bladder, and sphincter function change with aging and how these changes affect voiding patterns and continence.

The lower urinary tract (bladder, urethra, and sphincter) is responsible for low pressure storage and coordinated elimination of urine, with normal function characterized by cyclical filling and emptying. The ability to delay voiding until a time and place that is socially acceptable and the ability to empty the bladder effectively are important to quality of life for children past the age of toilet training, adolescents, and adults. Normal voiding and urinary continence are dependent on normal bladder and sphincter function, neural control, and intact cognition (Girard et al., 2017).

KEY POINT

Normal voiding and urinary continence are dependent on normal bladder and sphincter function, neural control, and intact cognition. In order to understand the pathology of voiding dysfunction and the various types of urinary incontinence, it is critical to understand normal function.

Voiding dysfunction and urinary incontinence are common disorders that have a major impact on quality of life; voiding dysfunction and neurogenic bladder dysfunction can also potentially affect upper tract function and overall health. In order to understand the pathology of voiding dysfunction and the various types of urinary incontinence, it is critical to understand normal function. That is the focus of this chapter.

 STRUCTURES AND FUNCTIONS CRITICAL TO NORMAL VOIDING AND CONTINENCE

The individual with normal lower urinary tract function never really thinks about the components of bladder control and effective voiding. The average adult with normal function voids approximately six to eight times daily (every 3 to 4 hours) (Lukacz et al., 2009, 2011; Zderic & Chacko, 2012). He/she is able to sense bladder filling, delay voiding if necessary (even if the bladder is quite full), and initiate voiding when a socially acceptable time and place are found. The individual with normal lower urinary tract function can also initiate urination even when there is very little urine in the bladder and no "need to void" should this be necessary (e.g., when a urine sample is requested) (Griffiths, 2015). These abilities are supported by an anatomically intact lower urinary tract (bladder, urethra, and sphincter) and pelvic floor, an intact and functional neural control system (brain, spinal cord, and nerve

pathways), and intact cognition (Birder et al., 2017; Girard et al., 2017). The structure and function of each of these structures will be discussed, followed by a brief discussion of changes in function across the life span.

KEY POINT

The child/adult with normal bladder function is able to sense bladder filling, delay voiding until a socially acceptable time and place are found (even if the bladder is quite full), and initiate voiding when desired (even if there is very little urine in the bladder and no sensation of "need to void").

STRUCTURE AND FUNCTION OF THE LOWER URINARY TRACT

The lower urinary tract consists of the bladder, urethra, and pelvic floor muscles. These structures work together as a unit to maintain continence through storage and elimination of urine at a desirable time (**Fig. 2-1**).

URINARY BLADDER

The urinary bladder is a hollow, muscular organ that has a fixed base and quite a dispensable body designed to fill with urine at low pressures, store approximately 300 to 600 mL in the healthy adult and eliminates urine. The bladder lies within the pelvic cavity and is located posterior to the symphysis pubis and inferior to the parietal peritoneum. In females, the anterior uterine wall and vagina come in contact with the bladder, while in males, the posterior bladder neighbors the rectum (Shier et al., 2019). The pressure of surrounding organs modifies the spherical shape of the bladder, but the size and shape of the bladder are dependent upon the amount of urine being stored. Often, anatomic drawings inaccurately depict an air bubble in the bladder; however, as the bladder empties, the walls collapse down upon the fixed base creating a tetrahedron (triangular pyramid)-like shape.

As the bladder fills, the superior surface expands upward into a dome; it pushes above the pubic crest if distended and near the umbilicus if greatly distended (Shier et al., 2019). The trigone is a triangular-shaped smooth muscle at the base of the bladder with the apex extending into the bladder neck in women and the verumontanum (an elevation in the floor of the prostrate where seminal ducts enter) in men. The trigone has an inlet at each of the angles that resemble a flap-like fold of the mucous membrane. This fold acts like a valve at the

Urinary Bladder, Anterior View

A Female

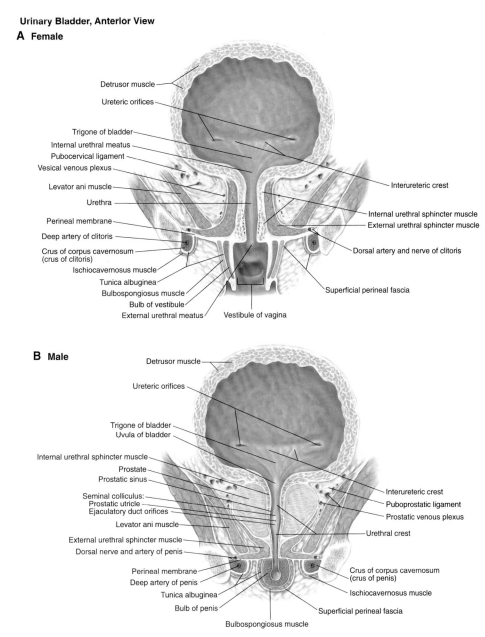

B Male

FIGURE 2-1. A, B. Female and male bladders. (From Tank, P. W., & Gest, T. R. (2009). *Lippincott Williams & Wilkins Atlas of anatomy.* Baltimore, MD: Wolters Kluwer Health.)

ureteral vesical junction (UVJ) that allows urine to enter the bladder but prevents backing up of urine from the bladder to the ureter even during coughing, sneezing, and physical exertion (Shier et al., 2019).

KEY POINT

The UVJ plays a pivotal role in promoting antegrade urine flow from the kidney into the bladder and preventing reflux (retrograde movement) from the bladder to the upper tracts.

The bladder has two critical and repetitive functions: to stretch and store moderate volumes of urine at low pressures and to contract effectively to empty. The ability to distend with urine while maintaining low intravesical pressures is a property known as compliance and is important both to preservation of upper tract (renal) health and to normal voiding intervals and quality of life (Chai & Birder, 2015). Maintenance of low filling pressures is essential to renal health because it permits continued delivery of urine from the kidneys to the bladder; once the intravesical pressure rises to a level greater than that exerted by the low-pressure ureters, delivery of urine ceases and there is resulting back pressure on the kidneys, which can eventually result in hydronephrosis (distention of the kidney). In addition, a rapid rise in intravesical (within bladder) pressure with low volumes of urine is associated with intense urgency in the patient who has normal sensation (because the bladder feels and acts "full" when there is a marked increase in intravesical pressure).

KEY POINT

The bladder's ability to distend with urine while maintaining low intravesical pressures is a property known as compliance and is important both to preservation of upper tract (renal) health and to normal voiding intervals and quality of life.

It is also important for the bladder to mount a strong and sustained contraction to effectively empty the urine. A weakly contractile bladder is associated with significant volumes of retained urine, which causes increased urinary frequency and urgency, nocturia, and increased risk of urinary tract infection (UTI).

The bladder is very well designed for alternate storage and expulsion of urine (see **Fig. 2-2**). Depending upon anatomy texts, multiple equivalent terms are used for the four layers of the bladder (mucosal, submucosal, muscular, and serous coat). It has three main microscopic layers (urothelium or mucosa; lamina propria, suburothelium or submucosal; muscularis or detrusor), each of which plays an important role in bladder filling, sensory inputs to the central nervous system (CNS) regarding state of filling, and effective emptying. In addition, it has an outer serosal coat or adventitia (Bolla & Jetti, 2019; Chai & Birder, 2015; Kurz & Guzzo, 2017; Shier et al., 2019).

Urothelium

The mucosa coat is composed of several thicknesses of the transitional epithelial cells or uroepithelium that are similar to the lining of the renal pelvis and ureters as well as the upper portion of the urethra. The thickness of this layer becomes reduced (only one to two cells deep) as the bladder fills and distends and returns to five to seven cells deep with urine elimination, thereby earning its "transitional" name. The apical or umbrella cell is the inner most urothelium layer that comes in contact with urine and microorganisms (Chai & Birder, 2015).

The uroepithelium is impermeable to the contents of the urine and coated with a thick, mucoid-like substance called glycosaminoglycans (GAG layer) that is thought to limit adherence of bacteria and penetration of urine irritants. Damage to this layer might permit penetration by noxious substances, bacterial adherence and infection, and/or abnormal release of inflammatory molecules by the urothelium, resulting in symptoms such as pain, urgency, and frequency. Recently, it is believed that proteins within the umbrella cell membranes (uroplakins) and tight junction proteins play a greater role in the impermeability and barrier function of the bladder urothelium (Chai & Birder, 2015).

The urothelium was previously conceptualized as a passive layer that primarily provided separation between the bladder wall and the constituents of the urine. However, it is now recognized that there are a number of ion channels and receptors located in the urothelial layer that detect mechanical, thermal, and chemical stimuli; in response to these stimuli, the urothelium secretes signaling molecules (such as ATP, ACh, and NO) that provide

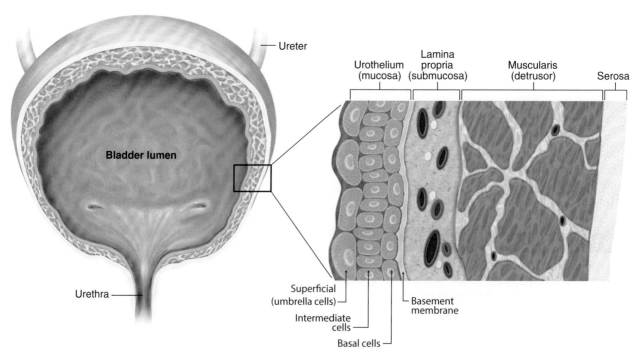

FIGURE 2-2. Layers of the Bladder.

input to the brain regarding bladder filling and messaging to the bladder muscle that help to modulate relaxation and contractility (Gonzalez et al., 2014a,b). For example, nitric oxide (NO) released by the urothelium may contribute to normal bladder filling via two mechanisms: (1) There is evidence that NO modulates and down-regulates activation of sensory pathways signaling bladder filling and (2) NO is known to contribute to detrusor muscle relaxation. There is also evidence that activation of stretch receptors in the bladder wall causes release of ATP by the urothelium, which stimulates the sensory pathways signaling bladder filling. Finally, emerging evidence suggests that, in the "normal" bladder, there is a balance between release of NO and ATP and that the ATP/NO ratio is one factor determining the frequency of bladder contractions (Chai & Birder, 2015; Fry & Vahabi, 2016). Disease, injury, stress, or inflammation may alter the urothelium's ability to release signaling molecules potentially contributing to bladder dysfunction (Girard et al., 2017).

KEY POINT

The bladder is lined with urothelium, which was previously thought to be a passive layer separating the bladder wall from the constituents of the urine; it is now recognized that the urothelium secretes signaling molecules that provide input to the brain regarding bladder filling and input to the bladder that modulates bladder relaxation and contractility.

Lamina Propria

The *lamina propria* is also known as the suburothelium and is the layer lying between the urothelium and the detrusor. It is often referred as the "functional center" of the bladder by coordinating detrusor muscle and uroepithelium activities (Chai & Birder, 2015). It includes interstitial cells called myofibroblasts that may have a pacemaker role, fibroblasts, blood vessels, and both afferent (sensory) and efferent (motor) nerves. This layer is thought to contribute to normal bladder distensibility (compliance) by maintaining a balance between type III and type I collagen (25% and 75%, respectively) and by production of the elastic fibers that allow the bladder to return to its normal shape following emptying (Andersson & McCloskey, 2014). Recent studies suggest that the lamina propria may also contribute to modulation and signaling related to bladder filling and contractility (Andersson & McCloskey, 2014; Gonzalez et al., 2014b).

Muscularis or Detrusor

The third layer consists of a complex meshwork of smooth muscle bundles (unlike the organized circular and longitudinal layers of the intestine) surrounded by an extracellular matrix known as the detrusor muscle. The muscle layer contains 50% collagen and 2% elastin to provide structural integrity to the bladder (Chai & Birder, 2015). The long

slender smooth muscle cells of the bladder are known as single unit smooth muscle, meaning that the ratio between muscle cells and nerve endings is almost 1:1; this rich innervation provides high-level neural control of bladder contractility (Chai & Birder, 2015). The smooth muscle cells of the bladder have length and tension properties that permit them to stretch slowly without inducing a contraction until emptying is initiated voluntarily or until capacity has been reached. In the event of rapid stretch (e.g., rapid bladder filling due to diuresis or rapid filling during cystometrogram), the muscle cells respond initially with a marked increase in tension that dissipates before a detrusor contraction is produced; this phenomenon is known as the stress relaxation response and is dependent in part on normal viscoelastic properties of the detrusor muscle and extracellular matrix (collagen). Excessive stretch on the detrusor muscle cells, as occurs with marked overdistention of the bladder, results in irreversible changes in the muscle; this explains why inadequate management of acute urinary retention can result in chronic urinary retention (Wyndaele et al., 2011; Zderic & Chacko, 2012).

Detrusor contraction occurs in response to parasympathetic stimulation and is normally characterized by a contraction of sufficient force and duration to expel all or most of the urine; normal contractility is dependent both on normal innervation and normal contractility (Chai & Birder, 2015).

KEY POINT

The inner layer of the bladder (detrusor muscle) is comprised of smooth muscle cells with length and tension properties that permit them to stretch slowly without inducing a contraction until emptying is initiated voluntarily or until capacity has been reached.

In addition to the myocytes (muscle cells), the detrusor contains stretch receptors that signal bladder filling. Further, there is some evidence for a motor–sensory system within the bladder that may increase sensory awareness of the need to void. Specifically, there are data suggesting that, as the bladder becomes progressively more distended with urine, there is increasing low-level muscle activity (localized low amplitude contractions, or "twitches," in the muscle); these low amplitude contractions in response to stretch do not produce voiding but are thought to contribute to the afferent "noise" produced by the distending bladder that signals the CNS regarding the need to void (Eastham & Gillespie, 2013).

Serosal Coat

The fourth and most outer layer of the bladder is the serosal coat or adventitia. It covers most of the bladder with fibroelastic connective tissue except the upper portion of the bladder where simple squamous epithelium covers the area along with a small amount of connective tissue. The primary role of the serosal/adventitia is to connect to surrounding tissues and protect the bladder from friction from adjacent organs. Perivesical fat covers beyond the serosa/adventitia (Bolla & Jetti, 2019; Girard et al., 2017).

Blood Supply to Bladder

The bladder receives its arterial blood supply via the superior, inferior, and medial vesical arteries, in addition to branches of the obturator, inferior gluteal, or internal iliac arteries. Females also receive arterial blood to the bladder from uterine and vaginal arteries. This profuse blood supply to the bladder accounts for blood in the urine (hematuria) that easily arises with UTIs, trauma, or surgery (Huether, 2019).

KEY POINT

The detrusor also contains stretch receptors that signal bladder filling as well as a rich blood supply.

URETHRA AND URETHRAL SPHINCTER MECHANISM

The urethra serves as a conduit for elimination of urine from the bladder (and for semen in men) and plays an important role in both effective bladder emptying and in maintenance of continence. Normally, the urethra functions synergistically with the bladder; during the storage cycle, the urethra remains closed to maintain continence (even during periods of increased abdominal pressure), and during voiding, the urethra funnels and opens to permit unobstructed flow. Normal function is dependent on structural integrity of the bladder neck, urethral sphincter mechanism, and pelvic floor as well as intact neural structures, pathways, and activity.

KEY POINT

Normally, the urethra functions synergistically with the bladder; during the storage phase, the urethra maintains closure, and during the emptying phase, the urethral funnels and opens to permit unobstructed flow.

Anatomic Features

Anatomically, the urethra is short and straight in women, averaging 4.0 cm (2.5 to 5.0 cm), and long and curved in men, averaging 20 cm (15.0 to 25.0 cm) (**Figs. 2-3 and 2-4**). The greater urethral length and curvature in men provides increased urethral resistance, and this anatomic difference between men and women is thought to be one factor contributing to the increased risk of

Sagittal section

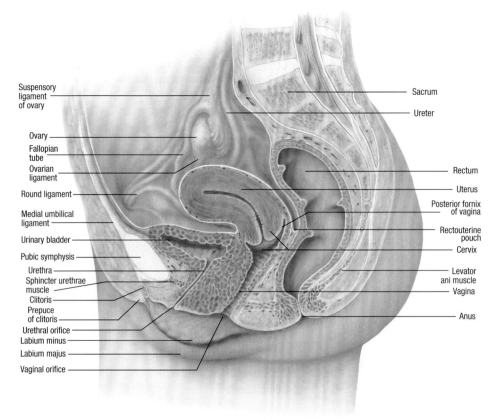

Suspensory ligament of ovary
Ovary
Fallopian tube
Ovarian ligament
Round ligament
Medial umbilical ligament
Urinary bladder
Pubic symphysis
Urethra
Sphincter urethrae muscle
Clitoris
Prepuce of clitoris
Urethral orifice
Labium minus
Labium majus
Vaginal orifice

Sacrum
Ureter
Rectum
Uterus
Posterior fornix of vagina
Rectouterine pouch
Cervix
Levator ani muscle
Vagina
Anus

FIGURE 2-3. Female Urethra. Asset provided by Anatomical Chart Co.

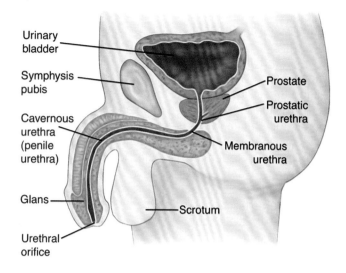

Urinary bladder

Symphysis pubis

Cavernous urethra (penile urethra)

Glans

Urethral orifice

Prostate

Prostatic urethra

Membranous urethra

Scrotum

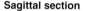
Sagittal section

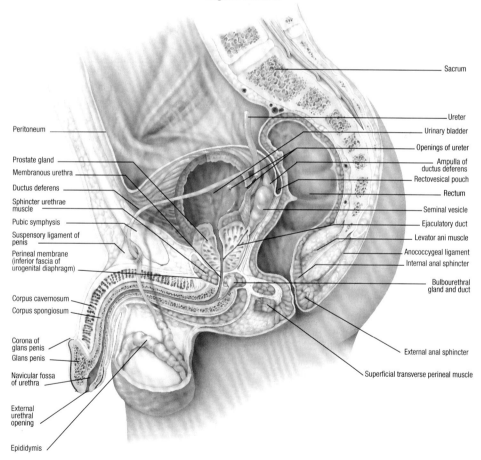

Peritoneum

Prostate gland

Membranous urethra

Ductus deferens

Sphincter urethrae muscle

Pubic symphysis

Suspensory ligament of penis

Perineal membrane (inferior fascia of urogenital diaphragm)

Corpus cavernosum

Corpus spongiosum

Corona of glans penis

Glans penis

Navicular fossa of urethra

External urethral opening

Epididymis

Sacrum

Ureter

Urinary bladder

Openings of ureter

Ampulla of ductus deferens

Rectovesical pouch

Rectum

Seminal vesicle

Ejaculatory duct

Levator ani muscle

Anococcygeal ligament

Internal anal sphincter

Bulbourethral gland and duct

External anal sphincter

Superficial transverse perineal muscle

FIGURE 2-4. Male Urethra. Asset provided by Anatomical Chart Co.

incontinence among women (Gill, 2019; Kurz & Guzzo, 2017). The male urethra can be subdivided into three sections: the prostatic urethra (the section surrounded by the prostate gland), the membranous urethra (the section involving the voluntary sphincter mechanism), and the penile urethra. Like the upper urinary tract and bladder, the urethra is composed of the same four histologi-cal layers (urothelium, lamina propria, muscularis, and serosa or adventitia) but differs in that it is composed of both smooth and specialized striated muscle that aids in maintaining continence. The smooth muscle maintains a level of tonic contraction that helps to maintain urethral closure during the filling cycle (Sadananda et al., 2011) while the specialized striated muscle that contains both fast-twitch and short-twitch muscle fibers aid in tone of the urethra during periods of sudden increase in abdominal pressure (i.e., cough) and prolong periods needed for continence between voids.

Additional support for continence is provided by a rich vascular plexus that is located in the subepithelial layer. This network of vessels acts as a fluid-filled sponge that provides compressive support to the urethra, which seems to be particularly important to continence in women (Sadananda et al., 2011). In addition, to promote female continence even further, the anterior vaginal wall is fused with the distal two thirds of the urethra and shares vascular components, muscular and endopelvic fascial support (Pradidarcheep et al., 2011; Sampselle & DeLancey, 1998; Siccardi & Valle, 2019). Finally, in women, anatomic support for continence is provided by coaptation of the urethral walls, which helps to maintain urethral closure and to resist leakage; coaptation is dependent on soft moist urethral tissue and may be adversely affected by estrogen deficiency (Alperin et al., 2019). In males, passive support is provided by the prostate gland as another contributing factor to continence although late in life, prostatic hypertrophy may result in outlet obstruction and urinary retention (Wagg et al., 2017).

KEY POINT

Anatomic features of the male urethra contributing to continence include the greater length and curvatures, which increases resistance, and support provided by the prostate gland. In women, the suburethral vascular plexus, anterior vaginal wall fusion to the distal urethra, and coaptation of the urethral walls seem to play an important role upholding continence.

Smooth Muscle (also known as *internal sphincter*)

The bladder neck is comprised of smooth muscle innervated by the autonomic nervous system (ANS) and controlled by descending nerve pathways from the pontine micturition center (PMC); the internal sphincter is tonically contracted throughout the filling phase and provides primary support for continence. As noted, neural control of the bladder neck and detrusor muscle assures synergistic response of the bladder and its outlet. Specifically, during the storage phase, sympathetic pathways are activated; sympathetic stimulation of the alpha-adrenergic receptors in the smooth muscle of the bladder neck causes increased urethral tone, while sympathetic stimulation of the beta-adrenergic receptors in the bladder wall causes detrusor relaxation. Conversely, during voiding, sympathetic stimulation to the bladder neck and detrusor is turned "off," causing relaxation of the bladder outlet, and parasympathetic stimulation of cholinergic/muscarinic receptors in the bladder wall causes detrusor contraction.

There is evidence that the smooth muscle of the bladder neck is more highly developed in the male than in the female. There is also evidence that interstitial cells interspersed throughout the smooth muscle of the bladder neck may function as "pacemakers" to promote contractility and maintain urethral closure during the filling cycle and that there is direct input from the pontine storage center (PSC) to the bladder neck promoting closure (Birder et al., 2017; Chai & Birder, 2015; Sadananda et al., 2011).

KEY POINT

The "internal sphincter" is comprised of smooth muscle fibers within the bladder neck, which are innervated by the autonomic nervous system and controlled by the pons.

Striated Muscle

The voluntary sphincter (also known as the external urethral sphincter [EUS] or rhabdosphincter) consisting of striated muscle is located just distal to the prostate gland in men (at the level of the membranous urethra) and at approximately midurethra in women. In men, the rhabdosphincter is one omega-shaped muscle; in women, it is more semicircular (horseshoe) in shape and consists of three separate but connected muscles (sphincter urethrae, compressor urethrae, and sphincter urethrovaginalis) that work together to support, compress, and elongate the urethra (**Fig. 2-6B**) (Hinata & Murakami, 2014; Jung et al., 2012). The EUS contains both fast-twitch (quick and strong contraction) and slow-twitch (sustained contraction) fibers. Ratio of fast-twitch to slow-twitch fibers in women is 13% to 87% and 35% to 65% in men, respectively (Chai & Birder, 2015). Fast-twitch fibers provide a rapid burst of contractile force when sudden increases of abdominal pressure, that is, cough, while the slow-twitch offers a sustained contraction that is slow to fatigue to maintain continence. The voluntary sphincter is innervated by branches of the pudendal nerve; voluntary contraction significantly increases urethral closure pressure and helps to prevent leakage during periods of increased intra-abdominal pressure.

KEY POINT

The "external" urethral sphincter is comprised of striated muscles located just distal to the prostate gland in men and at midurethra in women; it is under voluntary control and can be strengthened by pelvic muscle exercises.

PELVIS

The pelvis is a ring of bones composed of the sacrum and fusion of paired bones of the iliac, ischial, and pubic bones. The female pelvis accommodates both locomotion

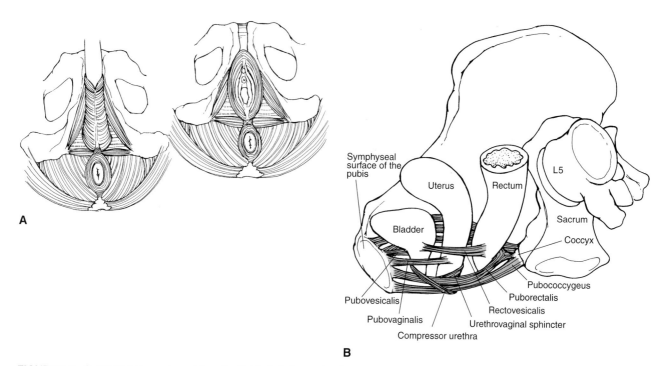

FIGURE 2-5. **A.** Pelvic floor, male and female. **B.** Medial view pelvic floor muscles. (From Oatis, C. A. (2004). *Kinesiology—The mechanics and pathomechanics of human movement.* Baltimore, MD: Lippincott Williams & Wilkins.)

and childbirth by being larger and broader than that of a male (tall, narrow, and compact) as well as having an ovoid-shaped inlet in contrast to the male heart-shaped inlet.

PELVIC FLOOR

The pelvic floor consists of several muscle groups, fascia, and ligaments that help support the pelvic viscera (urethra, bladder, vagina, uterus, prostate) and promote anal and urethral sphincter function (**Fig. 2-5A and B**); there are many descriptors given to these muscles by authors, which creates confusion even for the savviest continence specialist. Basically, the pelvic floor is made up of three primary layers beginning from the inferior to the most superior view of the pelvis: (1) superficial perineum (houses erectile tissues, external genitalia muscles, superficial perineal space, created by superficial facia interfacing with the perineal membrane); (2) urogenital diaphragm (deep perineum) contains the deep perineal space (superior aspect or roof of the perineal membrane), urethral and vaginal sphincter muscles; and (3) pelvic diaphragm that consist of the levator ani, coccygeus, and pelvic wall muscles (Bordoni et al., 2019). See **Figure 2-6A–C**.

 PELVIC FLOOR PART I & II

Key support structures within these three layers provide vital support to the pelvic soft organs (viscera) and the urethral continence mechanism: (1) levator ani muscle; (2) endopelvic fascia; and (3) perineal membrane, perineal body (PB) and external anal sphincter (Bordoni et al., 2019).

Levator Ani

Within the third layer (pelvic floor diaphragm) resides the principal source of support of the pelvic floor, the levator ani, which consists of the (1) pubococcygeous (includes pubourethralis, pubovaginalis), the central and major muscle, which extends from the symphysis pubis to the coccyx; (2) puborectalis, which forms a sling behind the anorectal junction; and (3) ileococcygeous, a smaller muscle that lies superior to the pubococcygeus (**Fig. 2-6C**). Although the levator ani is a group of muscles, they function as a single unit (Pradidarcheep et al., 2011; Sampselle & DeLancey, 1998). The principle function of the levator ani is to lift the anus, vagina, and urethra and to pull them forward; this anterior pull creates a compressive force against the lumen of these organs that promotes closure through increased intraurethral, intravaginal, and intra-anal pressures (Bordoni et al., 2019; Sampselle & DeLancey, 1998). The muscles are covered by endopelvic fascia, which condenses into ligaments that attach the pelvic organs to the bony pelvis (Siccardi & Valle, 2019).

Endopelvic Fascia

The pelvic floor layers and viscera must anchor to the bony structures of the pelvis in order to provide optimal support. The endopelvic fascia is complex internal system made of dense connective tissue composed of collagen, elastin, and smooth muscle. It provides suspensory support by encapsulating the pelvic viscera (urethra, vagina, bladder, uterus) as well as the levator ani and connecting them to the boney pelvis as well to each other. In general, endopelvic fascia serves to

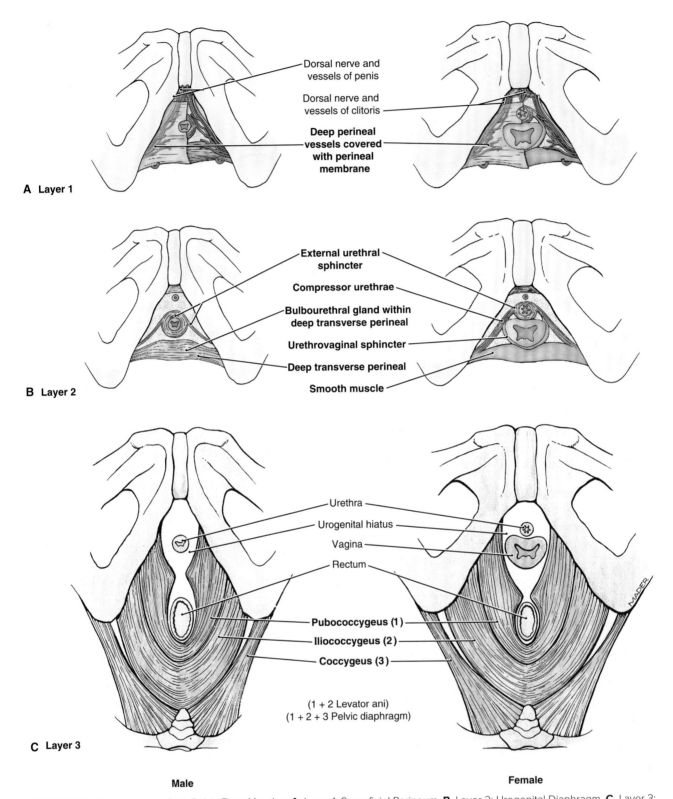

A Layer 1

Dorsal nerve and vessels of penis

Dorsal nerve and vessels of clitoris

Deep perineal vessels covered with perineal membrane

B Layer 2

External urethral sphincter

Compressor urethrae

Bulbourethral gland within deep transverse perineal

Urethrovaginal sphincter

Deep transverse perineal

Smooth muscle

C Layer 3

Urethra

Urogenital hiatus

Vagina

Rectum

Pubococcygeus (1)

Iliococcygeus (2)

Coccygeus (3)

(1 + 2 Levator ani)
(1 + 2 + 3 Pelvic diaphragm)

Male   **Female**

FIGURE 2-6. Three Layers of the Pelvic Floor Muscles. **A.** Layer 1: Superficial Perineum. **B.** Layer 2: Urogenital Diaphragm. **C.** Layer 3: Pelvic Diaphragm. (Used with permission from Moore, K. L., DAlley, A. F., & Agur, A. M. R. *Clinically oriented anatomy.* Philadelphia, PA: Wolters Kluwer.)

compartmentalize organs and muscles to maintain form and function, assists in sliding yet limits friction during motion, responds to stretch and distention and serves as a shock absorber (Siccardi & Valle, 2019).

Perineal Membrane and Perineal Body

The perineal membrane, PB, and anal sphincter comprise an inferior supportive layer of the pelvic floor (Siccardi & Bordoni, 2018) (**Fig. 2-6A,B;** and **Fig. 2-7**). The perineal membrane (urogenital diaphragm) is a triangular fibrous structure that spans the anterior pelvis, the vagina, and urethra pass through a central hole in this supportive membrane. The primary function of the perineal membrane is to limit descent of the pelvic organs by attaching the PB to the pubic bones. The perineal membrane provides secondary support by limiting descent of the PB and vagina when the levator ani is relaxed during the processes of defecation, urination, and birth (Sampselle & DeLancey, 1998).

The PB is a fibrous muscular structure that is centrally located between the urogenital and anal triangles. In women, it's between the anus and vagina and men, between the bulb of the penis and anus. It is often referred as the "central tendon" of the perineum because of the multiple attachments to the superficial and deep perineal muscles, urethral and anal sphincters, as well as a midline anchor for the perineal membrane and rectovaginal or recto prostatic facia (Siccardi & Bordoni, 2018). See **Figure 2-7**. Due to these attachments, the PB strengthens the pelvic floor. Some authors describe the PB as a knot made of many strings to simplify its image and visualization of function. For example, if tension is applied to one of the strings attached to the knot, the PB (knot) becomes imbalance or changes position (Nayak et al., 2008). Recently, the PB has received greater attention in the literature due to its crucial role in maintaining pelvic floor integrity especially in women (Larson et al., 2010; Siccardi & Bordoni, 2018). Injury often occurs during childbirth causing it to rupture from spontaneous tears, episiotomy or overstretching leading to nerve, muscle or fascial defects such as prolapse of the uterus, rectum, and occasionally the bladder leading to bowel and bladder dysfunction (Siccardi & Bordoni, 2018). Assessment of the PB is encouraged during the assessment of pelvic floor function (Chevalier et al., 2014). See Chapter 4 for further discussion. The role of the anal sphincter mechanism is outlined in Chapter 20.

Role in Continence

A healthy pelvic floor has sometimes been compared to a trampoline; when increased intra-abdominal pressure pushes pelvic organs caudally, the pelvic floor normally provides counterpressure and sufficient support to maintain the organs (vagina, bladder, and urethra) in their normal positions (Ashton-Miller et al., 2001). This is important because there is some evidence that loss of normal intrapelvic position compromises function of the striated sphincter; urethral "hypermobility" (distal displacement of the urethra in response to increased intra-abdominal pressure) is thought to be one factor contributing to stress incontinence in women (Aleksic & De, 2016; Bauer & Huebner, 2013). Pelvic floor support is enabled by the fact that there are connections between the pelvic floor and striated sphincter muscles, so contraction of the striated sphincter also causes contraction of the pelvic floor muscles. This means that pelvic muscle exercise programs strengthen both the striated sphincter and the

pelvic floor muscles, thus providing improved support for pelvic organs in addition to increasing sphincter muscle contractility and endurance (McLean et al., 2013; Dumoulin et al., 2017; Qaseem et al., 2014).

KEY POINT

A healthy pelvic floor has sometimes been compared to a trampoline; it serves to support the pelvic organs in normal anatomic position and to oppose downward displacement during activities that cause increased intra-abdominal pressure.

Fast-Twitch versus Slow-Twitch Muscle Fibers

The pelvic floor muscles are comprised of approximately 2/3 slow-twitch fibers and 1/3 fast-twitch fibers. Slow-twitch fibers provide sustained tonic contraction and improve baseline support for pelvic organs, while fast-twitch fibers provide rapid strong contractions that prevent leakage during periods of increased abdominal pressure (Marques et al., 2010). Pelvic muscle exercise programs are generally designed to strengthen both slow-twitch and fast-twitch fibers and thus to improve both continence at rest and continence during activities that increase stress on the continence mechanism (Dumoulin et al., 2017; Madill et al., 2013; Marques et al., 2010; Qaseem et al., 2014).

KEY POINT

Pelvic floor muscles contain both slow-twitch and fast-twitch fibers, which means they provide both baseline support for continence and increased contractility during periods of increased abdominal pressure.

GUARDING REFLEX

The guarding reflex helps to maintain continence by progressively increasing outlet resistance in response to bladder filling or sudden increase in bladder pressure, that is, cough (Birder et al., 2017; Vo & Kielb, 2018). There appears to be at least two pathways involved in the guarding reflex: (1) As the bladder distends with urine, stretch receptors in the bladder wall are activated, and these receptors send signals regarding bladder filling to the sacral cord; this activates the pudendal nerve (in addition to sending messages regarding bladder filling to the brain). The pudendal nerve then activates efferent (motor) pathways to the external sphincter that act on nicotinic receptors in the external sphincter muscle to increase outlet resistance. (2) In addition, afferent (sensory) signals from the distending bladder activate a pathway from the sacral cord to the thoracolumbar cord; this causes increased sympathetic stimulation of the bladder neck and bladder, which results in increased bladder neck tone and detrusor relaxation; (Chai & Birder, 2015;

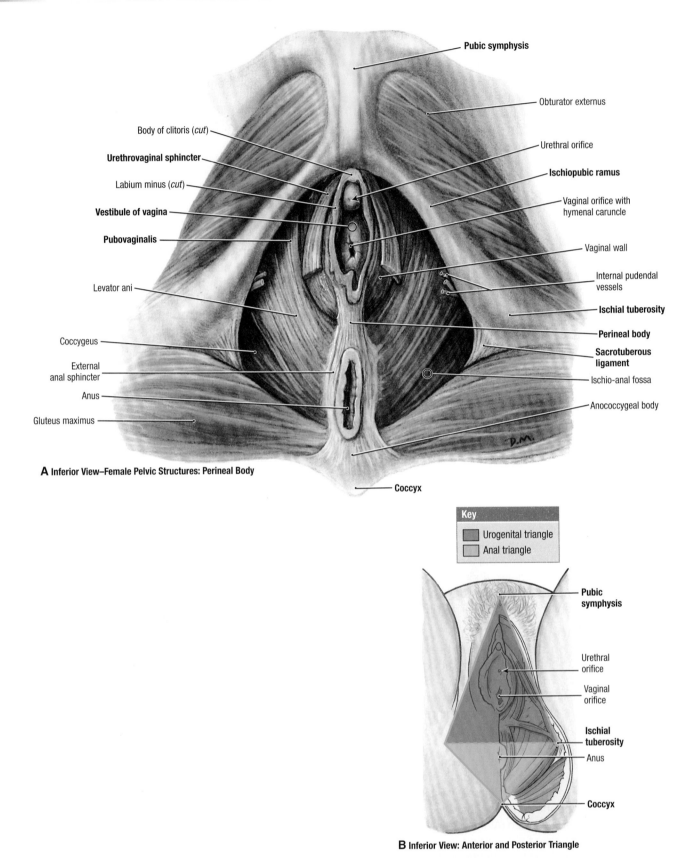

FIGURE 2-7. Perineal Body **(A)** and Anterior Posterior Triangle **(B)**. (Used with permission from Agur, A. M. R., & Dalley, A. F. *Grant's atlas of anatomy*. Philadelphia, PA: Wolters Kluwer.)

Vo & Kielb, 2018). Recently, there is a greater emphasis that sensory fibers within the urethra itself may in fact initiate the guarding reflex when urine is presented in the proximal urethra activating both pudendal motor pathways and sympathetic activation as described above (Birder et al., 2017).

KEY POINT

The guarding reflex helps to maintain continence by progressively increasing outlet resistance in response to bladder filling or an abrupt increase in bladder pressure.

Support for Voiding

In addition to maintaining closure during the filling cycle and thereby preventing incontinence, the normal urethra funnels and opens to provide unobstructed emptying during voiding. There is some evidence that afferent nerves in the urethra may contribute to effective bladder emptying by sensing flow rates and providing feedback that maintains the detrusor contraction as long as flow rates remain high (Deckmann et al., 2014; Girard et al., 2017).

NEURAL CONTROL OF MICTURITION

As noted, the bladder and its outlet constantly cycle between filling and periodic emptying, with synergistic activity during each phase (bladder relaxation and sphincter contraction during filling, followed by bladder contraction and sphincter relaxation during emptying). This coordinated and cyclical activity requires complex interaction among multiple signaling pathways and neurologic centers, in addition to an intact lower urinary tract (Birder et al., 2017; de Groat et al., 2015; Gill & Kim, 2018). The primary nervous systems involved include (1) CNS including the brain, brain stem, and spinal cord; (2) peripheral nervous system including the ANS providing sympathetic outflow tracts located in the thoracolumbar cord (T10–L2) and parasympathetic outflow tracts located in the sacral cord (S2–S4) and somatic nervous system controlling striated muscles through outflow tracts at Onuf nucleus also located in the sacral cord (S2–S4); and lastly (3) signaling neurons in the urothelium and detrusor (Birder et al., 2017; Chai & Birder, 2015; Gill & Kim, 2018; Girard et al., 2017; Griffiths, 2015) (see **Figs. 2-8 and 2-9**).

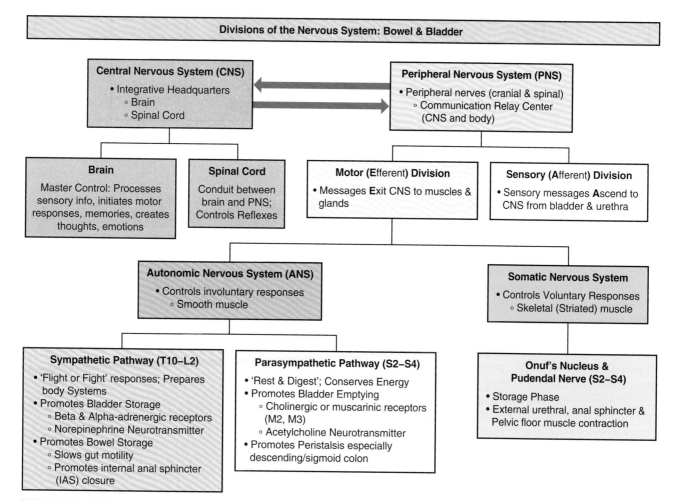

FIGURE 2-8. Divisions of the Nervous System. (Image created by JoAnn Ermer-Seltun.)

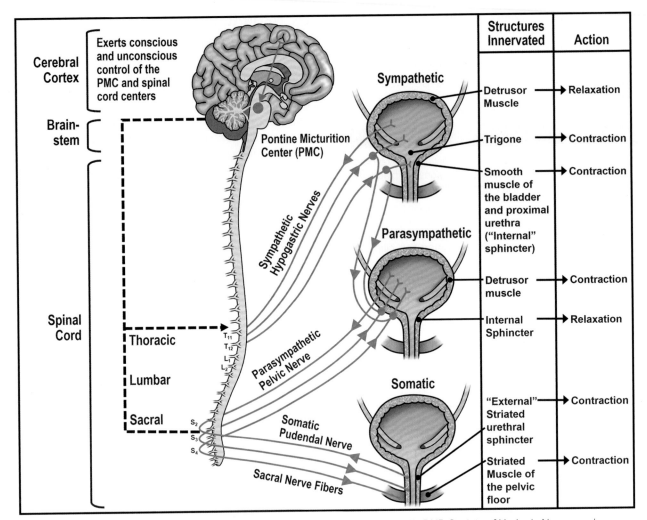

FIGURE 2-9. Neural Control of Voiding. (Reprinted with permission from Newman, D. K., DNP, Society of Urologic Nurses and Associates Core Curriculum.)

CENTRAL NERVOUS SYSTEM

Cerebral Cortex and Midbrain

The actual switch between bladder filling (storage) and bladder emptying (voiding) is controlled by midbrain structures (particularly the periaqueductal gray, or PAG) and the PMC; however, *decision-making* regarding voiding (social continence) is the responsibility of higher brain centers, specifically the prefrontal cortex (Yao et al., 2018). The decision regarding voiding is based on sensory input from mechanoreceptors within the bladder regarding bladder filling as well as environmental input and can involve delay of voiding despite a very full bladder (until an appropriate time and place can be found) or can involve volitional initiation of voiding in the absence of any urgency to void, such as the decision to void "prophylactically" before beginning a long car trip (Griffiths, 2015). The primary centers involved in processing signals regarding bladder filling include the periaqueductal gray, the insula, the locus coeruleus, the anterior cingulate gyrus, and the prefrontal cortex (Birder et al., 2017; Griffiths, 2015). This information is then relayed to the decision-making center (prefrontal cortex) to defer or initiate the micturition (voiding) reflex depending upon social acceptability. This reflex is usually under voluntary control by the higher brain center by age 3 to 5 but if any injuries or disease occur where the CNS cannot inhibit the micturition reflex when the bladder becomes full, involuntary voiding will result (reflex voiding) (Gill & Kim, 2018; Girard et al., 2017).

Functional neuroimaging suggests the following sequence of events: (1) The PAG processes sensory input regarding bladder filling and relays the information to the hypothalamus, insula, anterior cingulate gyrus, and lateral prefrontal cortex; (2) the information is then transmitted from these centers to the medial prefrontal cortex, which maintains inhibitory control of the PAG; (3) the medial prefrontal cortex makes a decision regarding whether or not to void; (4) if the decision is *not* to void, inhibition of the

PAG is maintained and voiding is delayed; and (5) when the decision is made to void, inhibitory control of the PAG is withdrawn and the PAG then activates the PMC (Barrington nucleus) to initiate coordinated voiding (de Groat et al., 2015; Girard et al., 2017; Griffiths, 2015; Yao et al., 2018). New insights regarding regulation of voiding validate the presence of other urination-related cortical neurons that may signal the PMC to permit or suppress voiding (Yao et al., 2018).

> **KEY POINT**
>
> The actual switch between bladder filling and bladder emptying is provided by the midbrain structures (e.g., periaqueductal gray and pons); however, *decision-making* regarding voluntary voiding is the responsibility of the prefrontal cortex.

PONS

The pons is located within the brainstem, which serves as specialized relay center between the brain and the bladder. The pons has two areas involved with continence and voiding: the pontine micturition center (PMC or Barrington nucleus) and the pontine storage center (PSC) (Birder et al., 2017). The PMC is responsible for assuring that both the bladder neck (internal sphincter) and rhabdosphincter (external sphincter) are relaxed before the bladder contracts, in order to provide unobstructed voiding. When activated by the PAG to initiate the micturition reflex, the PMC sends input to the cord that inhibits sympathetic stimulation of the bladder neck and innervation of the external sphincter via Onuf nucleus (thus causing both internal and external sphincter relaxation) and activates the parasympathetic pathways causing detrusor contraction (Birder et al., 2017; Gill & Kim, 2018; Griffiths, 2015). When the PSC is activated, there is direct stimulation of a somatic pathway to Onuf nucleus triggering continued contraction of the striated sphincter via pudendal nerve (Birder et al., 2017). Bladder filling (storage) begins again with sympathetic activation once the PAG inhibits the PMC (Birder et al., 2017; Gill & Kim, 2018; Vo & Kielb, 2018).

> **KEY POINT**
>
> The PMC is responsible for assuring that both the bladder neck (internal sphincter) and rhabdosphincter (external sphincter) are relaxed before the bladder contracts, in order to provide unobstructed voiding.

SPINAL CORD AND NERVE PATHWAYS

The spinal cord and its peripheral nerve pathways are essential to continence and to normal voiding, because these structures comprise the communication center of the controlled voiding system, transmitting messages from the bladder and sphincter to the brain and brain stem, and from the brain and brain stem to the bladder and sphincter. Thus, any disruption in the spinal cord causes loss of continence and disruption in effective coordinated voiding, a condition known as neurogenic bladder (Gill & Kim, 2018) (see also Chapter 9).

> **KEY POINT**
>
> Any disruption in the spinal cord causes loss of continence and disruption in effective coordinated voiding, a condition known as neurogenic bladder.

AUTONOMIC NERVOUS SYSTEM: SYMPATHETIC AND PARASYMPATHETIC PATHWAYS

Sympathetic Pathways

As explained earlier, sympathetic stimulation activates alpha-adrenergic receptors in the bladder neck (via neurotransmitters such as norepinephrine) to produce increased tone and resistance and also activates beta-adrenergic receptors in the bladder wall to cause detrusor relaxation. Thus, sympathetic pathways are active during the storage phase and quiescent during voiding. Sympathetic pathways exit the cord at the thoracolumbar level (T10–L2) via the hypogastric nerve (de Groat et al., 2015).

Parasympathetic Pathways

In contrast, parasympathetic stimulation causes bladder contraction and reflex relaxation of the bladder neck; the primary neurotransmitter is acetylcholine, which mediates contraction via muscarinic receptors (M2 and M3) in the bladder wall. In addition to its direct effects on detrusor contractility, acetylcholine is thought to affect sensory awareness of bladder filling (Sellers & Chess-Williams, 2012). Parasympathetic pathways are active during voiding and quiescent during filling. Parasympathetic pathways exit the cord at S2–S4 via the pelvic nerves (de Groat et al., 2015; Girard et al., 2017).

> **KEY POINT**
>
> Sympathetic pathways are active during the storage phase, causing bladder neck contraction and detrusor relaxation; parasympathetic pathways are active during voiding, causing reflex relaxation of the bladder neck and detrusor contraction.

SOMATIC NERVOUS SYSTEM

Pudendal Nerve (Onuf Nucleus)

The striated sphincter is under voluntary control, via a collection of cells in the sacral cord known as Onuf nucleus and the pudendal nerve. The cells of Onuf nucleus appear to receive direct input from the PSC; activation provides contraction of the striated sphincter via the pudendal nerve, which exits the cord at S2–S4 (de Groat et al., 2015). (As noted, inhibition of Onuf nucleus via the PMC causes striated sphincter relaxation.)

KEY POINT

The striated sphincter and pelvic floor are under voluntary control (pudendal nerve).

SIGNALING NEURONS IN THE DETRUSOR AND UROTHELIUM

As previously discussed, the urothelium and detrusor contain a number of receptors that respond to progressive bladder distention. The gradual increase in intravesical pressures that accompanies bladder filling activates thinly myelinated fibers that send increasingly strong signals of bladder filling along autonomic sensory nerve pathways to the cord; from the cord, they are transmitted to the brain, where there is a gradual increase in awareness that prompts decision-making regarding when and where to void (Birder et al., 2017; Chai & Birder, 2015). Studies of normal subjects revealed that bladder filling is perceived as "tingling" or "pressure" and that awareness proceeds along the following continuum: no sensation, weak awareness, stronger awareness, weak need to void, stronger need to void, and absolute need to void (Heeringa et al., 2011). Extreme distention may also activate C fibers, which transmit signals of severe discomfort and pain; C fibers are also activated by noxious substances in the urine or inflammation of the bladder wall (Birder et al., 2017; Girard et al., 2017; Gonzalez et al., 2014b).

INTACT COGNITION

Bladder control is dependent in part on normal cognitive function. The individual must be able to accurately interpret messages related to bladder filling, determine or locate a socially appropriate place to void, move to that location, and remove clothing in order to permit voiding (Griffiths, 2015; Yao et al., 2018). While the controlled voiding process is "automatic" for most individuals, it is in fact a complex process governed at each step by the CNS. This is reflected by the fact that incontinence is common among individuals with cognitive impairment, such as those who are sedated and those with advanced dementia. These individuals tend to void whenever the bladder reaches a certain point of filling, regardless of time and place (reflexive voiding) (de Groat et al., 2015; Gill & Kim, 2018). Incontinence due to cognitive impairment is labeled "functional incontinence" and is discussed in detail in Chapter 13.

KEY POINT

While the controlled voiding process is "automatic" for most individuals, it is in fact a complex process governed at each step by the central nervous system.

SUMMARY OF NORMAL LOWER URINARY TRACT FUNCTION

KEY POINT

The lower urinary tract cycles between "storage" and "emptying" via a complex sequence of events controlled by a myriad of signaling molecules and nerve pathways.

STORAGE PHASE

During storage, the sympathetic pathways are active, and the parasympathetic pathways are quiescent. Sympathetic stimulation of the alpha-adrenergic receptors in the bladder neck and proximal urethra maintains bladder neck closure, and sympathetic stimulation of the beta-adrenergic receptors in the bladder wall maintains bladder relaxation. The slow-twitch fibers in the pelvic floor muscles maintain resting tone, and direct input from the PSC to Onuf nucleus (in the sacral cord) maintains closure of the external sphincter via pudendal nerve innervation (Birder et al., 2017; Griffiths, 2015).

Progressive filling of the bladder activates stretch receptors in the bladder wall and release of signaling molecules by the urothelium that provide progressively stronger messages to the midbrain (via the cord) regarding bladder filling. Microcontractions of the detrusor muscle may also contribute to signaling regarding bladder filling. This progressive filling also activates the guarding reflex (i.e., activation of pathways that increase tone within the bladder neck and the voluntary sphincter via sympathetic stimulation and pudendal nerve stimulation, respectively). The guarding reflex assures that urethral resistance increases in proportion to the demands placed by a progressively distending bladder and increasing intravesical pressures (Birder et al., 2017; Griffiths, 2015).

Messages regarding bladder filling are integrated by the midbrain, primarily the PAG; these synthesized messages are forwarded to the medial prefrontal cortex, which maintains inhibitory control of the PAG and where decision-making regarding when and where to void takes place. If the decision is made to defer voiding, inhibitory control of the PAG is maintained, as is sympathetic input to the bladder and bladder neck and pudendal nerve input to the voluntary sphincter (Birder et al., 2017; Griffiths, 2015).

EMPTYING PHASE (MICTURITION)

If the decision is made to initiate voiding, inhibitory control of the PAG is released; the PAG then directs the PMC to mediate coordinated voiding (sphincter relaxation prior to detrusor contraction). The PMC inactivates sympathetic pathways and the pathways controlling Onuf nucleus, thus causing relaxation of the internal and external sphincters; the PMC also activates the parasympathetic pathways, thus causing detrusor contraction via acetylcholine stimulation of muscarinic receptors (Birder et al., 2017; Griffiths, 2015; Yao et al., 2018).

CHANGES ACROSS THE LIFESPAN

There are a number of changes that occur in lower urinary tract structure and function across the lifespan that impact on continence and the ability to empty the bladder effectively; these changes will be discussed briefly in this chapter and in more depth in Chapters 13 and 14.

INFANTS AND TODDLERS

Lower urinary tract development and urine production begin early in fetal life, at about 4 to 6 weeks gestation; by the 12th week of gestation, the three-layered structure of the bladder wall is evident, and by 16 weeks, the bladder exhibits limited reservoir capacity. During infancy, bladder function is characterized by lack of coordination between the bladder and sphincter and by interrupted voiding (two separate voids during a 5- to 10-minute period). For many years, it was thought that voiding in infants was a simple spinal reflex; however, recent studies suggest involvement of the CNS, based on evidence of varying degrees of arousal preceding voiding. When the child has matured to the level where she/he recognizes bladder filling and can control bladder emptying, toilet training is appropriate. Once the child has established voluntary control of voiding, the loss of coordination between bladder and sphincter disappears (sacral reflex voiding) and the filling emptying cycle characteristic of adult bladder function is established (de Groat et al., 2015). For most children, daytime continence is established first (attained by age 4 to 5), followed by nighttime control; girls typically achieve continence at an earlier age than boys (Bauer & Huebner, 2013; Milsom et al., 2017). Prevalence of daytime urinary incontinence (diurnal) at age 7 is 3.2% to 11.2% and nocturnal enuresis (bedwetting) at age 7 (11%), 11 to 12 (3.5%), and 16 (1.3%). In most cases, children who suffer diurnal incontinence or combination of day and nighttime incontinence are caused by overactive bladder (Milsom et al., 2017).

KEY POINT

Once the child has matured to the level where she/he recognizes bladder filling and can control emptying, toilet training is appropriate. For most children, daytime continence is established first, followed by nighttime continence; girls usually achieve continence at an earlier age than boys.

MIDDLE-AGED ADULTS

Urinary incontinence is especially prevalent in middle-age women (Burgio et al., 1991; Danforth et al., 2006; Hunskaar et al., 2000; Khoudary et al., 2019; Milsom et al., 2017). A longitudinal cohort study with an ethnically and racially diverse sample of women (age 42 to 52 years) from seven geographical sites across the United States named SWAN (Study of Women's Health at Midlife) reported 68% of the 3,302 participants suffered from at least one urinary incontinent episode per month (Khoudary et al., 2019). Danforth et al. (2006) reported in a cross-sectional analysis of 83,335 participants in the Nurses' Health Study II, 43% of women experienced at least one urinary incontinent episode per month. In addition, data identified primary risk factors: age, race/ethnicity, body mass index, parity, smoking, diabetes, and hysterectomy (Danforth et al., 2006). Prevalence data regarding UI in middle-age men are sparse (Milsom et al., 2017), but data indicate that lower urinary tract symptoms (LUTS) begin to manifest during the fourth decade of life in both sexes; among women, storage symptoms are more common, while voiding symptoms are more common among men. For both men and women, LUTS are associated with negative impact on quality of life, resulting in anxiety and depression. For women, symptoms associated with increased anxiety include nocturia, urgency, stress incontinence, leakage during sexual activity, weak stream, and split stream; symptoms associated with increased anxiety in men include nocturia, urgency, incomplete emptying, and bladder pain. Among women, stress incontinence, urgency, and weak stream are associated with depression; symptoms associated with depression in men include frequency and incomplete emptying (Bauer & Huebner, 2013).

KEY POINT

Urinary incontinence is especially prevalent in middle-age women compared to men. Women tend to suffer storage problems (stress incontinence) at midlife while men experience voiding problems.

ELDERLY

The elderly population has the highest prevalence rate of urinary incontinence (UI) compared to any other age group (Wagg et al., 2017). A novel study reported by Gorina et al. (2014) of national estimates for UI prevalence in the United States among people 65 years and older living in different care settings employed data from CDC (Centers for Disease Control), NCHS (Prevention's National Center for Health Statistics), and CMS (Centers for Medicare & Medicaid Services) based upon interviews with 2,625 noninstitutionalized individuals, 6,856 assisted living residents, 3,226 home care patients,

3,918 hospice discharges, and 2,416,705 nursing home residents. Prevalence rates of UI in men and women by place of residence includes (1) noninstitutionalized: women (54.8%), men (29.9%); (2) residential care facility: women (39.4%), men (32.7%); (3) long-term facility: women (73.5%), men (64.9%); (4) home care services; women (49.%), men (32.4%); and (5) hospice care: women (48.2%), men (39.9%). These data support previous reports of UI and voiding dysfunction as prevalent conditions among the elderly that increase with age (Wagg et al., 2017). The prevalence of UI and voiding dysfunction is due in part to changes in bladder and sphincter function and in part to increasing comorbid conditions and use of pharmacologic agents that can adversely affect bladder and sphincter function (Vahabi et al., 2017). Likewise, Inouye et al. (2007) classified multiple interacting risk factors in this age group as a "geriatric syndrome" that could greatly impact the elder's bladder health involving multiple comorbidities, polypharmacy, age-related physical and cognitive function (Wagg et al., 2017). Regrettably, studies have also confirmed a lack of knowledge by health care providers at all levels of licensure regarding the "symptom of incontinence" may in fact limit meaningful assessment and treatment and mistakenly promote the "normalization" of incontinence in the aged (Wagg et al., 2017). Conversely, it is important to realize that urinary incontinence and voiding dysfunction are not inevitable consequences of aging; it is also important to realize that most elderly men and women can be effectively treated.

KEY POINT

Elderly population have significant risk factors to develop urinary incontinence due to age-related changes to the lower urinary tract, comorbidities, and polypharmacy. Nevertheless, incontinence is not a normal part of the aging process but a symptom that deserves proper assessment and treatment.

Changes in Bladder Function

Aging is associated with increased collagen content in the bladder wall, which reduces elasticity and bladder capacity and also adversely affects contractility. There is also a reduction in M3 receptors and a loss of caveolae (specialized areas in the muscle cell that affect bladder smooth muscle contractility), which may further reduce contractility. Reduced contractility results in less effective emptying and higher postvoid residual volumes, and the combination of reduced bladder capacity and higher postvoid residuals can produce urinary frequency, a common complaint among older adults (Chai & Birder, 2015; Ranson & Saffrey, 2015; Wagg et al., 2017). In addition, older adults report less ability to inhibit bladder contractions, which may be due in part to failure of CNS centers or to increased presence of white matter hyperdensities (Wagg et al., 2017). Moreover, study findings posit that in

older adults, detrusor hyperactivity and underactivity can occur simultaneously due to an imbalance of purinergic and muscarinic signaling. Increased purinergic signaling in aging bladders leads to bladder overactivity but also suppresses muscarinic signaling, thereby reducing the ability to empty the bladder effectively as seen in detrusor hyperactivity with impaired contractility (DHIC) (Chai & Birder, 2015; Wagg et al., 2017). When one considers the fact that many elderly individuals have reduced mobility, changes in bladder function and CNS function that cause increased urinary frequency and urgency place them at significant risk for leakage.

KEY POINT

Aging is associated with reduced bladder capacity and contractility, which results in higher postvoid residuals and increased urinary frequency.

Changes in Sphincter Function

Changes in sphincter function and in bladder outlet resistance are due in part to hormonal changes resulting in benign prostatic enlargement in men (and increased risk of voiding dysfunction) and estrogen loss in women. Estrogen deficiency is known to adversely affect urethral coaptation and to increase the risk for storage symptoms such as urgency and frequency; in addition, estrogen affects the synthesis of collagen and muscle in the lower urinary tract and may influence neurologic control of voiding (Wagg et al., 2017).

Changes in Pelvic Floor Function

Currently, there are no studies that link ageing as a "direct" cause in the reduction of total collagen in pelvic muscles and fascia as well enhanced cross-linking and reduced elasticity (Wagg et al., 2017). The difficulty lies in the ability to differentiate the changes in pelvic floor structure from consequences of hormonal changes and number of vaginal deliveries (Wagg et al., 2017).

Comorbid Conditions and Impact of Pharmacologic Agents

Perhaps, the greatest impact of aging on bladder and sphincter function relates to the increasing number of comorbid conditions and the pharmacologic agents used for control of those conditions. Many commonly used pharmaceuticals can adversely affect bladder function, including diuretics, antihypertensives, alpha-adrenergic agonists and antagonists, angiotensin-converting enzyme (ACE) inhibitors, and drugs with anticholinergic effects (e.g., antipsychotics and antidepressants). Multiple comorbid conditions are linked in causing or promoting urinary incontinence in the frail elderly such as diabetes, congestive heart failure, sleep apnea, neurological disorders such as stroke, Parkinson disease, dementia, depression, functional impairments, as well as environmental factors such as inaccessible or unsafe toilet facilities or lack of toileting assistance or caregivers (Wagg et al., 2017). Thus, effective management of the older individual with urinary incontinence or voiding dysfunction must involve a holistic approach that includes a careful review of all medications being taken and management of comorbid conditions (Vahabi et al., 2017; Wagg et al., 2017).

KEY POINT

Factors contributing to bladder dysfunction in the elderly include hormonal changes and the increasing number of comorbid conditions and pharmacologic agents used to control those conditions.

 ## CONCLUSION

Urinary continence and effective emptying require an intact lower urinary tract (bladder, sphincter, and pelvic floor), normal neural innervation and control, and normal cognitive function. Neural control involves the cortex, midbrain, pons, and spinal cord pathways; the storage phase of the voiding cycle is primarily mediated by sympathetic inputs, while the voiding phase is primarily mediated by parasympathetic stimulation. Any neurologic lesion at any level can adversely affect bladder control and the ability to empty effectively. There are a number of changes in bladder and sphincter function associated with aging that can increase the risk of incontinence or impaired emptying; however, urinary incontinence and voiding dysfunction are never "normal" findings.

REFERENCES

Aleksic, I., & De, J. B. (2016). Surgical management of female voiding dysfunction. *Surgical Clinics of North America, 96*(3), 469–490.

Alperin, M., Burnett, L., Lukacz, E., et al. (2019). The mysteries of menopause and urogynecological health: clinical and scientific gaps. *Menopause, 26*(1), 103–111.

Andersson, K. E., & McCloskey, K. (2014). Lamina propria: The functional center of the bladder? *Neurourology and Urodynamics, 33*, 9–16.

Ashton-Miller, J. A., Howard, D., & DeLancey, J. O. (2001). The functional anatomy of the female pelvic floor and stress continence control system. *Scandinavian Journal of Urology and Nephrology. Supplementum*, (207), 1–125.

Bauer, R., & Huebner, W. (2013). Gender differences in bladder control: From babies to elderly. *World Journal of Urology, 31*, 1081–1085.

Birder, L., Blok, B., Burnstock, G., et al. (2017). Neural control. In P. Abrams, L. Cardozo, A. Wagg, et al., (Eds.), *Incontinence* (6th ed., pp. 259–363). Bristol, UK: International Continence Society.

Bolla, S. R., & Jetti, R. (2019). Histology, bladder [Updated September 20, 2019]. In *StatPearls [Internet]*. Treasure Island, FL: StatPearls Publishing. Retrieved from https://www.ncbi.nlm.nih.gov/books/NBK540963/

Bordoni, B., Sugumar, K., & Leslie, S. W. (2019). Anatomy, abdomen and pelvis, pelvic floor [Updated April 25, 2019]. In *StatPearls [Internet]*. Treasure Island, FL: StatPearls Publishing. Retrieved from: https://www.ncbi.nlm.nih.gov/books/NBK482200/

Burgio, K. L., Matthews, K. A., & Engel, B. T. (1991). Prevalence, incidence, and correlates of urinary incontinence in healthy, middle-aged women. *The Journal of Urology, 146*, 1255–1259.

Chai, T. C., & Birder, L. A. (2015). Physiology and pharmacology of the urinary bladder and urethra. In A. J. Wein, L. R. Kavoussi, A. C. Novick, et al., (Eds.), *Campbell-Walsh urology* (11th ed., pp. 1631–1684). St Louis, MO: Elsevier.

Chevalier, F., Fernandez-Lao, C., & Cuesta-Vargas, A. I. (2014). Normal reference values of strength in pelvic floor muscle of women: A descriptive and inferential study. *BMC Womens Health, 14*, 143.

Danforth, K. N., Townsend, M. K., Lifford, K., et al. (2006). Risk factors for urinary incontinence among middle-aged women. *American Journal of Obstetrics and Gynecology, 194*(2), 339–345.

de Groat, W. C., Griffiths, D., & Yoshimura, N. (2015). Neural control of the lower urinary tract. *Comprehensive Physiology, 5*, 327–396.

Deckmann, K., Filipski, K., Krasteva-Christ, G., et al. (2014). Bitter triggers acetylcholine release from polymodal urethral chemosensory cells and bladder reflexes. *Proceedings of the National academy of Sciences of the United States of America, 111*, 8287–8292.

Dumoulin, C., Adewuyi, T., Bradley, C., et al. (2017). Adult conservative management. In P. Abrams, L. Cardozo, A. Wagg, et al., (Eds.), *Incontinence* (6th ed., pp. 1443–1491). Bristol, UK: International Continence Society.

Eastham, J., & Gillespie, J. (2013). The concept of peripheral modulation of bladder sensation. *Organogenesis, 9*(3), 224–233.

Fry, C. H., & Vahabi, B. (2016). Role of the mucosa in normal and abnormal bladders. *Basic Clinical Pharmacology Toxicology, 119*(Suppl 3), 57–62.

Gill, B. C. (2019). Urinary incontinence relevant anatomy. Retrieved from https://emedicine.medscape.com/article/1988009-overview#a1

Gill, B. C., & Kim, E. D. (2018). Neurogenic bladder. Retrieved from https://emedicine.medscape.com/article/453539-overview#showall

Girard, B. M., Tooke, K., & Vizzard, M. A. (2017). PACAP/receptor system in urinary bladder dysfunction and pelvic pain following urinary bladder inflammation or stress. *Frontiers in Systems Neuroscience, 11*, 90. doi: 10.3389/fnsys.2017.00090.

Gonzalez, E. J., Arms, L., & Vizzard, M. A. (2014a). The role(s) of cytokines/chemokines in urinary bladder inflammation and dysfunction. *BioMed Research International, 2014*, 120525.

Gonzalez, E., Merrill, L., & Vizzard, M. (2014b). Bladder sensory physiology: Neuroactive compounds and receptors, sensory transducers, and target-derived growth factors as targets to improve function. *American Journal of Physiology—Regulatory, Integrative and Comparative Physiology, 306*, R869–R878.

Gorina, Y., Schappert, S., Bercovitz, A., et al. (2014). Prevalence of incontinence among older Americans. National Center for Health Statistics. *Vital and Health Statistics, 3*(36), 1–33.

Griffiths, D. (2015). Neural control of micturition in humans: A working model. *Nature Reviews Urology, 12*, 695–705. doi: 10.1038/nrurol.2015.266.

Heeringa, R., deWachter, S., van Kerrebroeck, P., et al. (2011). Normal bladder sensations in healthy volunteers: A focus group investigation. *Neurourology and Urodynamics, 30*(7), 1350–1355.

Hinata, H., & Murakami, G. (2014). The urethral rhabdosphincter, levator ani muscle, and perineal membrane: A review. *BioMed Research International, 2014*, 906921. doi: 10.1155/2014/906921.

Huether, S. E. (2019). Structure and function of the renal and urologic system. In S. E. Huether, & K. L. McCance (Eds.), *Understanding pathophysiology* (8th ed., pp. 1228–1243). St. Louis, MO: Elsevier.

Hunskaar, S., Arnold, E. P., Burgio, K., et al. (2000). Epidemiology and natural history of urinary incontinence. *International Urogynecology Journal and Pelvic Floor Dysfunction, 11*, 301–319.

Inouye, S. K., Studenski, S., Tinetti, M. E., et al. (2007). Geriatric syndromes: Clinical, research, and policy implications of a core geriatric concept. *Journal of the American Geriatric Society, 55*(5), 780–791.

Jung, J., Ahn, H., & Huh, Y. (2012). Clinical and functional anatomy of the urethral sphincters. *International Neurourology Journal, 16*(3), 102–106.

Khoudary, S. E., Greendale, G., Crawford, S. et al. (2019). The menopause transition and women's health at midlife: a progress report from the Study of Women's Health Across the Nation (SWAN). *Menopause, 26*(10), 1213–1227.

Kurz, D. A., & Guzzo, T. J. (2017). Genitourinary anatomy and physiology. In D. K. Newman, J. F. Wyman, & V. W. Welch (Eds.), *SUNA core curriculum for urologic nursing* (1st ed., pp. 375–443). Pitman, NJ: SUNA.

Larson, K. A., Yousuf, A., Lewicky-Gaupp, C., et al. (2010). Perineal body anatomy in living women: 3-dimensional analysis using thin-slice magnetic resonance imaging. *American Journal of Obstetrics and Gynecology, 203*(5), 494.e15–494.e21.

Lukacz, E. S., Sampselle, C., Gray, M., et al. (2011). A healthy bladder: a consensus statement. *International Journal of Clinical Practice, 65*, 1026–1036. doi: 10.1111/j.1742-1241.2011.02763.x.

Lukacz, E. S., Whitcomb, E. L., Lawerence, J. M., et al. (2009). Urinary frequency in community-dwelling women: What is normal? *American Journal of Obstetrics and Gynecology, 200*(5), 552.e1–552.e7.

Madill, S., Pontbriand-Drolet, S., Tang, A., et al. (2013). Effects of PFM rehabilitation on PFM function and morphology in older women. *Neurourology and Urodynamics, 32*(8), 1086–1095.

Marques, A., Stothers, L., & Macnab, A. (2010). The status of pelvic floor muscle training for women. *Canadian Urological Association Journal, 4*(6), 419–424.

McLean, L., Varette, K., Gentilcore-Saulnier, E., et al. (2013). Pelvic floor muscle training in women with stress urinary incontinence causes hypertrophy of the urethral sphincters and reduces bladder neck mobility during coughing. *Neurourology and Urodynamics, 32*(8), 1096–1102.

Milsom, I., Altman, D., Cartwright, R., et al. (2017). Epidemiology of urinary incontinence and other lower urinary tract symptoms, pelvic organ prolapse, and anal incontinence. In P. Abrams, L. Cardozo, A. Wagg, et al., (Eds.), *Incontinence* (6th ed., pp. 4–90). Bristol, UK: International Continence Society. ISBN: 978-0956960733.

Nayak, S. B., David, W., & Rodenbaugh, D. W. (2008). Modeling the anatomy and function of the pelvic diaphragm and perineal body using a string model. *Advances in Physiology Education, 32*, 169–170. doi: 10.1152/advan.00106.2007. Accessed on October 25, 2019.

Pradidarcheep, W., Wallner, C., Dabhoiwala, N. F., et al. (2011). Anatomy and histology of the lower urinary tract. In K. E. Andersson & M. C. Michel (Eds.), *Urinary tract, handbook of experimental pharmacology* (pp. 117–148). Berlin/Heidelberg, Germany: Springer-Verlag.

Qaseem, A., Dallas, P., Forciea, M. A., et al. (2014). Nonsurgical management of urinary incontinence in women: A clinical practice guideline from the American College of Physicians. *Annals of Internal Medicine, 161*(6), 429–440.

Ranson, R. N., & Saffrey, M. J. (2015). Neurogenic mechanisms in bladder and bowel ageing. *Biogerontology, 16*(2), 265–284.

Sadananda, P., Vahabi, B., & Drake, M. (2011). Bladder outlet physiology in the context of LUT dysfunction. *Neurourology and Urodynamics, 30*(5), 708–713.

Sampselle, C. A., & DeLancey, O. L. (1998). Anatomy of female continence. *Journal of Wound, Ostomy, and Continence Nursing, 25*(2), 63–74.

Sellers, D., & Chess-Williams, R. (2012). Muscarinic agonists and antagonists: Effects on the urinary bladder. *Handbook of Experimental Pharmacology, 208*, 375–400.

Shier, D., Butler, J., & Lewis, R. (2019). Urinary system. In D. Shier, J. Butler, & R. Lewis (Eds.), *Hole's human anatomy & physiology* (15th ed., pp. 767–802). New York, NY: McGraw-Hill.

Siccardi, M. A., & Bordoni, B. (2018). Anatomy, abdomen and pelvis, perineal body [Updated December 20, 2018]. In *StatPearls [Internet]*. Treasure Island, FL: StatPearls Publishing. Retrieved from https://www.ncbi.nlm.nih.gov/books/NBK537345/?report=classic

Siccardi, M. A., & Valle, C. (2019). Anatomy, bony pelvis and lower limb, pelvic fascia [Updated January 24, 2019]. In *StatPearls [Internet]*. Treasure Island, FL: StatPearls Publishing. Retrieved from https://www.ncbi.nlm.nih.gov/books/NBK518984/

Vahabi, B., Wagg, A. S., Rosier, P., et al. (2017). Can we define and characterize the aging lower urinary tract? ICI-RS 2015. *Neurourology and Urodynamics, 36*(4), 854–858. doi: 10.1002/nau.23035.

Vo, A., & Kielb, S. J. (2018). Female voiding dysfunction and urinary incontinence. *Medical Clinics of North America, 102*(2), 313–324. doi: 10.1016/j.mcna.2017.10.006.

Wagg, A., Chen, L. K., Johnson, T., et al. (2017). Incontinence in the frail older person. In P. Abrams, L. Cardozo, A. Wagg, et al., (Eds.), *Incontinence* (6th ed., pp. 1311–1442). Bristol, UK: International Continence Society.

Wyndaele, J., Gammie, A., Bruschini, H., et al. (2011). Bladder compliance: What does it represent, can it be measured, and is it clinically relevant? *Neurourology and Urodynamics, 30*, 714–722.

Yao, J., Zhang, Q., Liao, X., et al. (2018). A corticopontine circuit for initiation of urination. *Nature Neuroscience, 21*, 1541–1550.

Zderic, S., & Chacko, S. (2012). Alterations in the contractile phenotype of the bladder: Lessons for understanding physiological and pathological remodeling of smooth muscle. *Journal of Cellular and Molecular Medicine, 16*(2), 203–217.

QUESTIONS

1. The continence nurse is assessing bladder compliance in an older adult. Which of the following accurately describes this property of the urinary tract system?
  A. The ability to delay voiding until a socially acceptable time and place are found
  B. The ability of the bladder to distend with urine while maintaining low intravesical pressures
  C. The ability of the bladder to contract with enough force and duration to expel all or most of stored urine
  D. Detrusor relaxation in response to beta-adrenergic stimulation

2. Which layer of the bladder secretes signaling molecules that provide input to the brain regarding bladder filling and messaging to the bladder muscle that help to modulate relaxation and contractility?
  A. Urothelium
  B. Trigone
  C. Propria
  D. Detrusor

3. The lamina propria contributes to normal bladder distensibility by maintaining the balance between type III and type I collagen and

A. Secreting signaling molecules that provide input to the brain regarding bladder filling
B. Secreting signaling molecules that provide input to the brain regarding the need to void
C. Allowing smooth muscle cells to stretch slowly without inducing a contraction until emptying is initiated
D. Producing elastic fibers that allow the bladder to return to normal shape after voiding

4. Which of the following describes the main function of the urethra?
A. Serving as a conduit for elimination of urine from the bladder
B. Providing stretch receptors that signal bladder filling
C. Preventing leakage during periods of increased intra-abdominal pressure
D. Supporting the pelvic organs in normal anatomic position

5. Which anatomic feature of the male urethra predominately contributes to the maintenance of continence?
A. Rich suburethral vascular plexus
B. Coaptation of the urethral walls
C. Greater length and curvature
D. Prostatic hypertrophy

6. A continence nurse recommends pelvic muscle exercises for a female patient experiencing stress incontinence. What anatomical structure is strengthened by these exercises?
A. Internal sphincter
B. External sphincter
C. Detrusor muscle
D. Urethra

7. What mechanism is involved in the guarding reflex function that helps to maintain continence?
A. Increased detrusor contractility in response to increased abdominal pressure
B. Closing of the urethra during the storage phase
C. Support of the pelvic organs in normal anatomic position
D. Progressive increase in outlet resistance in response to bladder filling

8. Which structure controls the actual switch between bladder filling (storage) and bladder emptying (voiding)?
A. Midbrain
B. Prefrontal cortex
C. Spinal cord
D. Neuronal pathways

9. Which structure is responsible for assuring that both the bladder neck (internal sphincter) and rhabdosphincter (external sphincter) are relaxed before the bladder contracts, in order to provide unobstructed voiding?
A. Periaqueductal gray (PAG)
B. Onuf nucleus
C. Pontine micturition center (PMC)
D. Sympathetic pathways

10. A continence nurse assessing elderly patients in a nursing home takes into consideration age-related changes in the urinary system, such as
A. Lower postvoid residuals
B. Reduced bladder contractility
C. Increased bladder capacity
D. Decreased urinary frequency

ANSWERS AND RATIONALES

1. B. Rationale: The ability to distend with urine while maintaining low intravesical pressures is a property known as compliance and is important both to preservation of upper tract (renal) health and to normal voiding intervals and quality of life.

2. A. Rationale: Numerous receptors located in the urothelium detect mechanical, thermal, and chemical stimuli; in response to these stimuli, the urothelium secretes signaling molecules (such as ATP, ACh, and NO) that provide input to the brain regarding bladder filling and messaging to

the bladder muscle that help regulate bladder relaxation and contractility.

3. D. Rationale: The *lamina propria* is the layer lying between the urothelium and the detrusor and often referred as the "functional center" of the bladder by coordinating detrusor muscle and uroepithelium activities. It contributes to normal bladder distensibility (compliance) by maintaining a balance between type III and type I collagen (25% and 75%, respectively) and by production of the elastic fibers that allow the bladder to return to its normal shape following emptying.

4. A. Rationale: The urethra serves as a conduit for elimination of urine from the bladder (and for semen in men) and plays an important role in both effective bladder emptying and in maintenance of continence.

5. C. Rationale: The male urethra can be subdivided into three sections: the prostatic urethra (the section surrounded by the prostate gland), the membranous urethra (the section involving the voluntary sphincter mechanism), and the penile urethra. The greater urethral length and curvature in men provides increased urethral resistance to promote continence.

6. B. Rationale: The "external" sphincter is comprised of striated muscles located just distal to the prostate gland in men and at midurethra in women; it is under voluntary control and can be strengthened by pelvic muscle exercises.

7. D. Rationale: The guarding reflex helps to maintain continence by progressively increasing outlet resistance by sympathetic stimulation of the internal bladder sphincter resulting in enhance urethral tone and pudendal nerve stimulation of striated external sphincter to boost outlet closure in response to bladder filling or sudden increase in bladder pressure.

8. A. Rationale: The actual switch between bladder filling (storage) and bladder emptying (voiding) is controlled by midbrain structures (particularly the periaqueductal gray, or PAG) and the pontine micturition center (PMC); however, *decision-making* regarding voiding (social continence) is the responsibility of higher brain centers, specifically the prefrontal cortex.

9. C. Rationale: When activated by the PAG to initiate the micturition reflex, the PMC sends input to the cord that inhibits sympathetic stimulation of the bladder neck and innervation of the external sphincter via Onuf nucleus (thus causing both internal and external sphincter relaxation) and activates the parasympathetic pathways causing detrusor contraction.

10. B. Rationale: Aging is associated with increased collagen content in the bladder wall, which reduces elasticity and bladder capacity and adversely affects contractility.

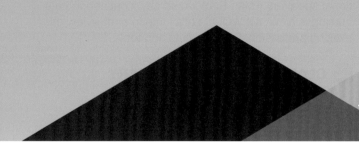

CHAPTER 3

CONTINENCE CARE NURSING: AN OVERVIEW

JoAnn M. Ermer-Seltun and Sandra Engberg

OBJECTIVES

1. Discuss the impact of incontinence and implications for WOC nurses and other health care providers.

2. Describe reversible factors contributing to incontinence and implications for assessment and management.

3. Define the term "lower urinary tract symptoms" (LUTS), and differentiate among storage symptoms, voiding symptoms, and postvoiding symptoms.

4. Synthesize assessment data to determine type of incontinence/voiding dysfunction and goals for management.

5. Discuss current thinking regarding the difference between "functional factors contributing to incontinence" and "functional incontinence" and implications for management.

TOPIC OUTLINE

INTRODUCTION OF THE WOCN® CORE CURRICULUM: CONTINENCE MANAGEMENT

This chapter provides a brief overview of the various types of urinary incontinence (UI) and voiding dysfunction; the pathology, presentation, assessment, and management of each type are discussed in greater depth in subsequent chapters. Bowel dysfunction and fecal incontinence are briefly highlighted as these conditions often impact bladder health. In addition, the coeditors would like to take this opportunity "call out" notable content featured in each of the chapters and highlight chapters new to the second edition of the WOCN® Core Curriculum: Continence Management.

PROFESSIONAL PRACTICE: YOU ARE A CONTINENCE CARE NURSE

Chapter 1 is a fresh addition in all three WOCN® Core Curriculum textbooks. It begins with the scope and role of the wound, ostomy, and continence (WOC) nurse and a historical perspective of WOC nursing. It outlines specific scopes of practice based upon licensure of the WOC nurse. It is the hope of the coeditors that the scope and role of the continence care nurse is specifically reflected in each chapter of this textbook. Many WOC nurses have unfortunately dropped their certification in "Continence." As a codirector of one of the WOCN® Nursing Education Programs, this coeditor has had the opportunity to witness numerous reasons why WOC nurses either drop their certification or choose not to embrace the continence care role. Much of the feedback provided by nurses encompass three basic themes: (1) lack of understanding of the scope and role of the continence care nurse; (2) feelings of already being overwhelm with their current role as a wound and or ostomy care nurse specialist therefore lacking the time and energy to address the topic of incontinence or voiding dysfunction; and (3) notions that the topic or pathophysiology of continence issues are "too difficult to understand and learn." The scope and role of the continence care nurse can be embraced at many different practice levels depending upon the nurse's licensure, care setting, interests, and patient population (WOCN, 2018). The WOC nurses' "roots" date back to ostomy care; however, the underpinnings of this profession are that WOC nurses are *experts in maintaining skin integrity* (see first-hand by reviewing Chapter 17 on incontinence-associated dermatitis better known as IAD)! Every WOC nurse, no matter how they choose to "walk out" their practice, will *always* encounter individuals with altered skin integrity due to continence issues especially in light of the expediential aging population. The coeditors hope the following chapters will ignite a *passion* to care for the patient with a bowel and bladder disorder at whatever comfort level, even if it is to

initiate lifestyle and behavioral management techniques, which as the reader will learn, can dramatically reduce, or even cure most types of incontinence. Remember, you ARE and CAN be a CONTINENCE CARE NURSE. The coeditors believe continence care nursing is a "**W**indow **O**f **O**pportunities" or as one of JoAnn's favorite motivational speakers (Brian Biro) would say, continence care nursing is a "WOO! WOO!" Let's jump in and review this exciting professional nursing field and topic.

CLASSIFICATION OF URINARY INCONTINENCE/VOIDING DYSFUNCTION

PREVALENCE OF THE PROBLEM

UI is a common problem, although prevalence rates vary by sex and age. The estimated prevalence of UI in community-dwelling women is 25% to 45% for occasional urinary leakage and 10% for UI at least weekly. Reported prevalence rates are lower in men, varying from 4.81% to 32.71% with rates increasing with age. The prevalence in both men and women increases with age and as individuals become more functionally impaired. UI is less common in children, with reported prevalence rates between 3.2% and 9% reported at age 7 years and 1.2% to 3% at age 15 to 17 years (Milsom et al., 2017).

UI is also costly; according to 2000 data, $19.5 billion is spent annually on management of UI, with 50% to 75% of the money being spent on management (absorptive products, etc.) and only 25% to 50% spent on diagnosis and correction of the underlying problem (Hu et al., 2004). This disproportionate expenditure on management products as opposed to diagnostic studies and corrective therapies may be due in part to the widely held perception that UI is a normal part of aging and that "nothing can be done." In addition to the fiscal costs, UI is costly to the individual, adversely affecting quality of life and causing significant psychological distress (e.g., anxiety and embarrassment); moreover, UI increases the risk of falls and skin breakdown (Gorina et al., 2014).

DEFINITION

UI is the complaint of any involuntary leakage of urine (Abrams et al., 2002). During the interview, the health care professional should ask about specific factors relating to the symptom of UI such as frequency; severity; precipitating factors; social impact; effect on hygiene; effect on quality of life; coping strategies such as pads, frequent toileting, or social isolation; preferences and goals for management/treatment; and previous investigations/treatments (Abrams et al., 2002). As explained in Chapter 2, the lower urinary tract is responsible for alternately storing and then emptying urine; normal function is characterized by the ability to store 300 to 500 mL of urine at low intravesical pressures and to delay voiding until a socially convenient time and place and by the ability to empty the bladder completely during voiding, with minimal postvoid urine volumes. Lower urinary tract symptoms (LUTS) are symptoms related to lower urinary tract structures and can result from alternations in bladder, urethral, prostate, or pelvic floor function. The symptoms include (1) storage symptoms such as urinary frequency and nocturia, bladder filling symptoms (e.g., urgency or reduced awareness of bladder filling), and incontinence symptoms (e.g., urge or stress incontinence); (2) voiding symptoms (e.g., hesitancy, slow and reduced stream strength and urinary retention); and (3) postvoiding symptoms (e.g., revoiding ["encore" or "double voiding"], postvoid incontinence (dribbling), and post-micturition urgency) (D'Ancona et al., 2019). Alterations in the ability to store urine effectively and to control the time and place for voiding result in *urinary incontinence* and altered ability to empty urine effectively results in *voiding dysfunction* and *urinary retention*. Both of these conditions negatively impact quality of life (QoL); some forms of voiding dysfunction and urinary retention are also associated with increased risk for upper tract (kidney) damage.

Several chapters in this edition discussion voiding dysfunction and UI in specific patient populations. Four chapters (10, 11, 13, 14) also featured in the first edition textbook discuss voiding dysfunction and UI in *specific* patient populations and how to effectively assess, evaluate, and manage it. Two new chapters appear in the textbook addressing voiding dysfunction in specific populations: (1) Chapter 12 draws attention to advance pelvic health disorders in women including the debilitating and difficult to treat chronic pelvic pain and pelvic organ prolapsed and (2) Chapter 15 explores obesity and its effect on bladder and bowel health.

UI may be classified as either *acute/transient* or *chronic*.

ACUTE/TRANSIENT UI

Transient UI is generally defined as newly occurring UI of relatively sudden onset; it typically lasts <6 months and is the result of reversible factors. By definition, transient UI is usually curable, and the focus of management is on correction of the etiologic factors. There are several mnemonics designed to help clinicians remember the potentially reversible causes of UI, including TOILETED, DRIP, and DIAPPERS (Dowling-Castronovo & Specht, 2009; Wound, Ostomy, and Continence Nurses Society, 2007). TOILETED is considered by many to be the preferred mnemonic due to the negative connotations of "diapers" and "drip" in relation to adults with urinary leakage.

> **KEY POINT**
>
> Transient UI is caused by reversible factors and is usually curable. A mnemonic commonly used to help clinicians remember to assess for and manage reversible factors is TOILETED (thin dry urethral epithelium; obstruction; infection; limited mobility; emotional/psychological issues; therapeutic medications; endocrine disorders; delirium).

T: Thin, Dry Urethral Epithelium

Genitourinary syndrome of menopause, previously known as atrophic vaginitis or vulvovaginal atrophy (Alperin et al., 2019; Faubion et al., 2017), is a relatively new term used to describe symptomatic vulvovaginal atrophy as well as LUTS related to a decrease in estrogen and other sex hormones. As explained in Chapter 2, continence in the female is at least partially dependent on normal coaptation of the urethral walls, which is affected by the softness and stickiness of the urethral tissue. Estrogen deficiency is associated with thinning and drying of the urethral tissues, which reduces coaptation and also contributes to the symptoms of urinary urgency and frequency; in addition, atrophic urethritis has been associated with increased incidence of recurrent urinary tract infections (UTIs) in menopausal women as well as elderly females in long-term care settings. Therefore, postmenopausal women presenting with symptoms of urinary leakage or with recurrent UTIs should be carefully evaluated for evidence of atrophic urethritis (manifest by inflamed hypertrophic urethral meatus) and should be considered for a trial of transvaginal estrogen therapy (ACOG, 2014; Anger et al., 2019; Bonkat et al., 2019).

O: Obstruction (Stool Impaction/Constipation)

The bladder and rectum share the limited space available in the bony pelvis; thus, chronic rectal distention can adversely affect bladder function. Specifically, chronic rectal distention can compromise bladder filling and can exacerbate symptoms of overactive bladder (OAB) (urgency, frequency, and low voided volumes). Severe rectal distention (as may occur with fecal impaction) can also cause bladder outlet obstruction and urinary retention. Assessment of bowel function and interventions to eliminate retained stool and to restore effective bowel elimination patterns are therefore important responsibilities for the continence nurse (Wound, Ostomy, and Continence Nurses Society, 2016). Other types of acute obstructions can occur and cause transient or acute UI. For instance, individual who suffer from abrupt onset of bladder outlet obstruction or poor bladder contractility due to a variety of causes such as benign prostatic hypertrophy (Chapter 10), pelvic organ prolapse (Chapter 12), non-neurogenic and neurogenic (Chapters 8 and 9) etiologies. Check out Chapter 20 (Physiology of Defecation), Chapter 21 (Motility Disorders), Chapter 22 (Fecal Incontinence), and Chapter 23 (Bowel Dysfunction in the

Pediatric Population) for all your *need to know* regarding defecation disorders leading to bowel dysfunction and fecal incontinence.

I: Infection

Urinary tract infection (UTI) causes inflammation of the bladder wall and urethra, which, in the continent individual, results in urinary urgency, frequency, and dysuria. For the individual with preexisting issues with urgency and frequency, and for the individual with mobility issues, UTI can overwhelm the continence system, resulting in urinary leakage. In addition, infectious processes such as UTI can cause acute alteration in mental status among elders with any degree of preexisting dementia; UTI in these individuals may manifest as sudden onset of incontinence accompanied by acute worsening of mental and functional status (Wound, Ostomy, and Continence Nurses Society, 2016). Another original chapter (Chapter 18) making its debut is on the topic of UTIs. It provides an excellent discussion regarding UTIs etiologies, risk factors, assessments, effective prevention, and management in the adult population without an indwelling urinary catheter (IUC). An overview of catheter-associated UTIs (CAUTIs) is provided in Chapter 19.

L: Limited Mobility (Restricted Mobility)

Continence depends on cognitive awareness of the need to void, normal function of the bladder and sphincters, and the ability to move to an appropriate place (and to manipulate clothing in preparation for voiding) in a timely manner. Any condition that reduces the individual's ability to get to a toilet or suitable alternative (e.g., dependency on ambulatory aids such as walkers) and/or to remove his or her clothing in preparation for voiding (e.g., arthritis) can contribute to incontinence. This is particularly problematic for elderly individuals, who may have less ability to control urgency and to delay voiding due to changes in the central nervous system (CNS). The combination of reduced ability to manage urgency and to delay voiding and increased time required to get to the toilet and prepare for voiding may combine to produce incontinence, even though the individual retains cognitive function and basic bladder control. Simple measures such as clothing alterations, use of bedside commodes and urinals, and scheduled voiding may be all that is needed to restore continence for these individuals (Wound, Ostomy, and Continence Nurses Society, 2016). Chapter 13 is an excellent resource featuring the overall continence care of the older and frail individual while Chapter 16 delivers key measures to provide dignity and "social continence" for all individuals with UI or FI (ability to go in public and engage in activities without the fear and embarrassment of leaking and being noticed) with body worn absorbent products (BWAPs), other external containment devices (ECDs), as well as adaptive aides to assist those with physical limitations in bladder management programs.

E: Emotional Issues (Psychological, Depression)

Many studies have reported an association between depression and UI although the cause and effect relationship is not clear (Wound, Ostomy, and Continence Nurses Society, 2016). In a large prospective study of women age >20 years ($n = 16,253$) followed for 10 years, anxiety or depression increased the likelihood of developing UI during follow-up. Conversely, women with UI at baseline were more likely to develop anxiety or depression during follow-up (Felde et al., 2017). Thus, the continence nurse must be alert to any indicators of depression and/or anxiety and must refer these individuals for treatment (Wound, Ostomy, and Continence Nurses Society, 2016).

T: Therapeutic Medications (Pharmacologic)

Medications are common contributing (exacerbating) factors for both storage disorders (incontinence) and emptying disorders (retention). For example, diuretics may cause sudden production of large volumes of urine, which may precipitate incontinence in the individual with OAB or mobility issues. Conversely, any medication with anticholinergic properties may compromise bladder contractility and precipitate or worsen urinary retention; medications with alpha-adrenergic properties can also cause or worsen retention, because they increase urethral resistance.

The impact of medications is of particular concern with older individuals and those with multiple comorbid conditions, because they may be taking multiple medications, any or all of which could affect the lower urinary tract. As a result, a careful medication history (to include prescription, over-the-counter, and herbal agents) is recommended for all individuals with urinary tract dysfunction; the pharmacist can frequently be of assistance in evaluating an individual's medications for potential adverse effects on bladder and sphincter function. The continence care nurse must then collaborate with the patient and the prescribing providers to determine whether any changes in prescribed medications are warranted (Wound, Ostomy, and Continence Nurses Society, 2016). Chapter 4 outlines the importance of reviewing all medications during the primary assessment and their effects on bowel and bladder health.

E: Excessive Urine Output

Endocrine disorders, such as diabetes mellitus with hyperglycemia, can compromise continence by causing production of excessive volumes of urine (polyuria) that can overwhelm the bladder and sphincter, producing sudden urgency and, in some cases, leakage. Diabetes insipidus is another endocrine disorder resulting in production of abnormally high volumes of dilute urine that can contribute to incontinence. Other possible causes of polyuria include diuretics, lithium, caffeine, alcohol, obstructive sleep apnea, and heart failure. If the polyuria is occurring during the night (nocturnal polyuria), obstructive sleep apnea should be considered as a possible cause. Other causes of nocturnal polyuria may include edema, excessive fluid intake at night, and taking a diuretic in the evening. Some individuals may take their diuretic in the evening rather in the morning because of concern about daytime urinary frequency particularly if they plan to be out. In older adults, age-related changes in vasopressin and atrial natriuretic hormone can result in nocturnal polyuria. The history for a person with incontinence must always include queries regarding other comorbid conditions, with specific focus on endocrine disorders, and management must include measures to normalize endocrine function and urinary output (Wound, Ostomy, and Continence Nurses Society, 2016).

D: Delirium

As noted in Chapter 2, intact cognition is essential to continence; the individual must be able to recognize bladder filling, make appropriate decisions regarding when and where to void, and then move to an appropriate location for voiding. Thus, any condition that adversely affects cognition places the individual at risk for incontinence. It is important for the continence nurse to differentiate between dementia, which is an irreversible decline in cognition, and delirium, which by definition is transient; the nurse must also be aware that delirium can be superimposed on dementia, causing a sudden but reversible worsening of cognitive impairment. Delirium may be caused by an infectious process (in the person with preexisting cognitive impairment), the adverse effects of medications, or electrolyte or chemical imbalance. Implications for the continence nurse include routine assessment of cognitive status and of any recent change in cognition and prompt attention to correction of factors causing cognitive impairment (Wound, Ostomy, and Continence Nurses Society, 2007).

If untreated, transient UI may become established (chronic) UI. In addition, reversible factors are frequently contributing factors to some types of chronic incontinence; thus, continence nurses should assess all incontinent individuals for transient conditions contributing to incontinence; when present, treatment of these factors is a critical "first step" in management of the incontinence.

The reader will want to dive into this novel chapter (Chapter 6) that delivers fundamental concepts to optimize bladder and bowel health in all populations. This engaging chapter is where the reader will find detailed content on lifestyle and behavioral modifications as well as the "How Tos"; plus, valuable education key concepts the continence care nurse will want to share with every patient. Moreover, this chapter features best practice tactics to assist those with cognitive changes to address functional limitations that impact continence status.

CHRONIC UI

UI that persists despite correction of reversible factors is known as *chronic incontinence*; the most common forms

of chronic incontinence are stress, urge, and mixed and functional incontinence. A brief description of each type is provided here, with in-depth discussion provided in subsequent chapters of this core curriculum.

> **KEY POINT**
>
> UI that does not resolve despite correction of reversible factors is defined as chronic UI; the most common forms of chronic UI are stress UI, urgency UI, and mixed UI.

Stress UI

Stress urinary incontinence (SUI) is defined as "the complaint of involuntary leakage on effort or exertion or on sneezing or coughing" (Drake, 2018, p. S14). Stress incontinence is also sometimes known as "activity-associated incontinence" because the leakage is associated with activities that increase intra-abdominal pressure (jumping, straining, lifting, coughing, sneezing, laughing, etc.). While the typical individual with SUI leaks small amounts of urine during activities that increase intra-abdominal pressure, if urethral sphincter function is severely impaired, leakage volumes can be larger and urine loss can occur with minimal physical activity. It is important to realize that stress incontinence occurs *in the absence of any urgency to void*; this is a significant finding because the lack of urgency means that the bladder is not contracting and is not contributing to the leakage.

Stress incontinence is much more common in women than in men, because the female urethra is short and straight and therefore provides less resistance than the male urethra, which is long and curved. In addition, the supporting pelvic floor muscles and ligaments are at risk for damage related to pregnancy and vaginal delivery. Chapter 11 provides in-depth evidence to the care of women suffering stress UI.

SUI is uncommon in men unless there is damage to the urethral sphincter mechanism. A common cause of SUI in men is a prostatectomy. This surgical procedure involves removal of the prostatic urethra with anastomosis of the distal urethra to the bladder neck. In addition to causing some reduction in urethral length and baseline resistance, radical prostatectomy can result in damage to the voluntary sphincter, which is located just distal to the prostate gland (Robinson et al., 2009) (see Chapter 10).

> **KEY POINT**
>
> Stress UI is associated with activities that increase intra-abdominal pressure and is most commonly caused by weakness of the pelvic floor and sphincter muscles; pelvic muscle rehabilitation is first-line therapy for most individuals.

Urge UI

Urge or urgency incontinence is involuntary urine leakage associated with a *strong* urge to void. It is caused by bladder (detrusor) overactivity and is often accompanied by urinary frequency and nocturia.

Urge urinary incontinence (UUI) is one of the common symptoms of OAB. The International Continence Society (ICS) defines OAB as, "urinary urgency, usually accompanied by frequency and nocturia with or without urgency urinary incontinence, in the absence of urinary tract infection or other obvious pathology" (Haylen et al., 2010, p. 7). When OAB occurs in the absence of UUI, it is sometimes called OAB dry, while OAB wet is sometimes used when OAB symptoms also include UUI. See Chapter 7 for a detailed discussion of UUI and OAB.

KEY POINT

Urge or urgency incontinence is involuntary urine leakage associated with a *strong* urge to void. It is caused by bladder (detrusor) overactivity and is often accompanied by urinary frequency and nocturia.

Mixed UI

Mixed incontinence is the complaint of involuntary leakage associated with urgency and also with exertion, effort, sneezing, or coughing. Patients with mixed UI have both sphincter dysfunction and bladder overactivity and therefore present with complaints of leakage associated with urgency as well as leakage associated with activity. Management strategies must address both etiologies and usually includes the lifestyle modification and behavioral therapies outlined in Chapters 6, 7, 10, and 11.

UI Due to Functional Impairment

"Functional incontinence" is caused by factors outside the urinary tract that compromise the individual's ability to respond appropriately to signals of bladder filling. The two most common types of functional impairments involve mobility and cognitive function. Patients with significant mobility impairments are frequently dependent on others for assistance with toileting and may require significantly greater time to reach the toilet and prepare for voiding; incontinence occurs when they do not get the assistance they need or are unable to reach the toilet in a timely manner. Patients with cognitive impairments frequently do not recognize the sensation of bladder filling or cannot remember the steps involved in toileting; in these individuals, voiding occurs in response to bladder filling as opposed to being a conscious and controlled act. Functional issues may be the *primary etiologic factor* for the incontinence (e.g., incontinence in the individual with advanced dementia); in this case, the incontinence is sometimes labeled "functional incontinence." Functional issues may also be a contributing factor to other types of incontinence, such as mobility issues contributing to

incontinence in the individual with OAB (Wound, Ostomy, and Continence Nurses Society, 2007). There are no objective tests for functional incontinence; diagnosis is based on patient history and physical exam and on simple tests such as the "get up and go" test for mobility and the Mini-Mental Status Exam or clock-drawing test for cognitive function.

Management of functional incontinence and functional issues is dependent on the specific functional impairment; for the patient with impaired mobility, management may involve use of a bedside commode, a raised toilet seat, physical therapy and occupational therapy consults for assistive devices, and/or modifications in clothing to facilitate toileting. For the patient with cognitive impairment, management begins with a toileting trial to determine responsiveness to a toileting program. Patients who are able to respond to toileting cues are placed on a scheduled toileting or prompted voiding program, augmented by appropriate absorptive products (see Chapter 16). Chapter 6 provides robust content to optimize bladder health especially in those with functional limitations.

KEY POINT

Functional factors such as cognitive impairment and mobility impairment may be either causative or contributing factors for UI; thus, all patients should be assessed for cognitive status and mobility.

Nocturnal Enuresis

Nocturnal enuresis, involuntary urine loss while asleep, is a common childhood issue, occurring in an estimated 10% of children at 7 years of age, 3.1% at ages 11 to 12 years, and 0.5% to 1.6% at age 16 to 17 years (Kuwertz-Broking & von Gontard, 2018). It can be very distressing for both children and parents. See Chapter 14 for more information on childhood enuresis.

In adults, the estimated prevalence is 2% to 3% overall with higher prevalence rates in women with voiding dysfunction and in nursing home residents. A number of normal physiologic mechanisms help to maintain nocturnal continence including normal bladder capacity (normally bladder volumes of 300 to 400 mL without needing to void), a closed bladder outlet, reduction to glomerular filtration rates by 30% and increased water reabsorption (via the action of arginine-vasopressin), and central mechanisms that awaken the individual before involuntary voiding occurs (Akhavizadegan et al., 2019). Disruptions in any of these normal physiologic mechanisms can result in enuresis.

Extraurethral Incontinence

Extraurethral incontinence is defined as urinary leakage through channels other than the urethra. This is most commonly due to a vesicovaginal fistula, which involves an abnormal opening between the bladder and the vagina that permits free flow of urine from the bladder into the vagina (and an almost constant flow of urine from the vagina). Vesicovaginal fistulas are common in the developing world, due to obstructed labor and obstetric trauma (Ayaz et al., 2012); in the United States, these fistulas are uncommon but occasionally occur as a result of radical gynecologic procedures and/or pelvic radiation therapy.

Diagnosis is suggested by the constant leakage of urine and the absence of any associated symptomatology, such as urgency; diagnosis is confirmed by radiologic studies, and management involves either surgical correction or use of absorptive products in conjunction with indwelling catheters to divert the urine. Chapter 12 addresses advance pelvic health considerations including vesicovaginal fistulas. In children, continuous urinary leakage is most commonly due to an ectopic ureter (ureter does not terminate at the bladder) that drains into the vagina or the urethra; management involves surgical reimplantation of the ureter (see Chapter 14).

Nocturia

The ICS defines nocturia as the number of times a person wakes up from their normal sleep period to void. Each episode must be followed by sleep or intention to sleep to be classified as nocturia (D'Ancona et al., 2019). Although the degree of bother reported by individuals with nocturia varies, most report moderate bother with two episodes per night and major bother with three or more. The prevalence of nocturia increases with age with 28.3% to 61.5% of women and 29% to 59.3% of men in their 70's and 80's reporting two or more episodes per night (Bliwise et al., 2019). Impaired bladder storage, nocturnal polyuria, and/or sleep disturbances can all contribute to nocturia. In older adults, these conditions often coexist making nocturia a multifactorial problem. Conditions associated with nocturia include those that cause detrusor hyperactivity such as OAB and benign prostatic hypertrophy; those associated with nocturnal polyuria such as heart failure, diuretic therapy, lower extremity edema, diabetes insipidus, obstructive sleep apnea, and poorly control diabetes; and those associated with sleep dysfunction such as restless leg syndrome and obstructive sleep apnea (Vaughan & Bliwise, 2018). Chapter 6 further reviews the ill effects of nocturia on sleep hygiene and provides practical solutions.

VOIDING DYSFUNCTION

The various forms of UI all relate to problems with storage of urine; in contrast, voiding dysfunction is the term used to denote problems with urine elimination.

Urinary retention, or incomplete bladder emptying, may be caused by two types of problems: (1) obstruction at the level of the bladder neck or urethra (e.g., incomplete emptying caused by prostate enlargement or urethral stricture) or (2) ineffective bladder contractions (e.g., neurologic conditions such as multiple sclerosis or long-standing diabetes). Retention can be classified as acute or chronic. Acute retention is of rapid onset and usually accompanied by painful suprapubic sensation (from a full bladder) due to inability to void despite persistent intensive effort to do so. Chronic urinary retention is characterized by complaints of repeated inability to empty the bladder, despite the ability to pass some urine. Individuals may report the frequent passage of small amounts of urine or UI and on abdominal examination, the bladder may be distended (D'Ancona et al., 2019).

"Acute retention is defined as a painful, palpable, or percussible bladder, when the patient is unable to pass any urine." Chronic retention, on the other hand, "is a non-painful bladder, which remains palpable or percussible after the patient has passed urine." Such patients may also experience urinary leakage (Abrams et al., 2002).

The patient with chronic retention typically reports a weak urinary stream and prolonged time required to void and may complain of a sensation of incomplete emptying. The patient may also report recurrent UTIs. Physical exam reveals bladder distention, which is confirmed by a postvoid residual test. Urodynamic studies are typically required to determine whether the problem is due to urethral obstruction or to ineffective bladder contractions; urodynamic studies allow the clinician to correlate the strength of the bladder contraction with the urinary flow rate (Abrams et al., 2002).

> **KEY POINT**
>
> Voiding dysfunction indicates impaired ability to empty the bladder effectively and may be caused by bladder outlet obstruction or by reduced contractility of the detrusor muscle; management depends on the underlying cause.

Management of urinary retention depends on the cause; obstruction can usually be eliminated through medical surgical intervention, while management of ineffective bladder contractions typically requires intermittent catheterization or insertion of an indwelling catheter.

Chapter 8 provides details on acute and chronic urinary retention and its management.

NEUROGENIC BLADDER

Neurogenic bladder dysfunction refers to lower urinary tract dysfunction caused by disturbance of the neurologic control mechanisms; it is thus only diagnosed in the presence of neurologic pathology, most commonly a lesion between the sacral cord and the brain. Common specific etiologic factors include spinal cord injury or multiple sclerosis (MS) lesions (Stöhrer et al., 1999). In 2017, the ICS recommended replacing the terms "neurogenic bladder" and "neurogenic bladder dysfunction" with neurogenic lower urinary tract dysfunction (NLUTD) clinically confirmed relevant neurologic disorder (Gajweski et al., 2017).

Patients with NLUTD typically lack sensory awareness of bladder filling, are unable to voluntarily initiate voiding, and have no control over the urinary sphincter, because there is a loss of communication between the cortex and brain stem and the bladder and sphincter. In the absence of voluntary control of voiding, the bladder empties by a reflex arc triggered by bladder filling. However, patients with neurogenic lower urinary tract dysfunction are at risk for a serious complication known as detrusor sphincter dyssynergia (DSD); this denotes failure of sphincter relaxation in response to detrusor contraction and is associated with significant risk of upper tract dysfunction.

KEY POINT

Neurogenic lower urinary tract dysfunction (NLUTD) refers to loss of normal neural control of bladder and sphincter function; it is usually caused by a spinal cord lesion and results in impaired sensory awareness of bladder filling, inability to consistently initiate voiding on a voluntary basis, loss of sphincter control, and possibly loss of "coordinated voiding."

Diagnosis of NLUTD is suggested by reports of urinary leakage or voiding dysfunction in a patient with a known neurologic diagnosis and is confirmed by urodynamic studies. Urodynamic studies are an essential element of workup for these patients since it is critical to determine the presence or absence of DSD. Chapter 5 provides a review of advance assessment through urodynamic testing.

Management most commonly involves intermittent catheterization to assure complete emptying and to prevent leakage; selected patients with minimal or no DSD may elect management with containment products (such as external catheter to bedside drainage bag). Indwelling catheters have been used in the past for management of these individuals but are associated with unacceptably high complication rates; therefore, their use is generally limited to short-term management or patients who cannot be effectively managed with other interventions. Chapter 9 provides a comprehensive overview of etiology and management of NLUTD.

The continence care nurse plays a vital role in educating individuals regarding the proper technique in intermittent self-catheterization (ISC), obtaining adaptive equipment aides if needed, supply procurement, encouraging consistent and adequate fluid intake, teaching signs and symptoms to monitor, and assuring close follow-up especially when starting an ISC program. Most individuals are fearful, reluctant, may have limited knowledge regarding their genital anatomy, may be embarrassed, and even resistance to engage in learning ISC. Adequate time is mandatory to dispelling myths or incorrect information and provides education in a respectful and calm manner at a level that the patient can understand. This patient-centered approach can make learning this procedure much less anxiety producing and increase the likelihood of success. Teaching points for ISC, positions, and adaptive aides especially for those with dexterity or mobility issues are featured in Chapter 16.

ASSESSMENT AND DIAGNOSIS: OVERVIEW

The evaluation of an individual with UI or voiding dysfunction begins with a thorough assessment of the presenting signs and symptoms. Signs are objective indicators that can be observed by the health care professional, for example, leaking when coughing, cystocele with straining, bladder distention, or high postvoid residual volumes. Symptoms are the individual's experience of a problem such as pain or the sensation of incomplete emptying; symptoms are subjective and qualitative in nature. Additional qualitative and quantitative data can be obtained via bladder diaries, pad tests, and quality of life questionnaires.

LOWER URINARY TRACT SYMPTOMS

LUTS can be categorized as

- Storage symptoms
- Voiding symptoms
- Postvoiding symptoms (Abrams et al., 2002)

Storage LUTS

These symptoms, as the name suggests, are indicators of problems related to the storage phase of the voiding cycle and are common among individuals with UI and irritative bladder disorders. Storage LUTS include frequency, urgency, dysuria (pain on voiding), nocturia, nocturnal polyuria, and urinary leakage associated with urgency or activity or both (symptoms of OAB with urge incontinence, stress incontinence, or mixed stress–urge incontinence).

Voiding LUTS

In contrast to storage LUTS, voiding LUTS suggest problems with bladder emptying and include hesitancy, poor and/or intermittent stream, straining to void, and terminal dribble. These symptoms are common among individuals with some degree of voiding dysfunction and urinary retention. Voiding symptoms in men are most likely to be caused by bladder outlet obstruction related to prostatism; in women, outlet obstruction and voiding symptoms may be caused by severe cystocele or pelvic organ prolapse. These symptoms may also be caused by a poorly contractile detrusor, which can occur in individuals with long-standing diabetes or other conditions affecting detrusor innervation.

Postvoiding LUTS

Individuals with voiding dysfunction and urinary retention may also report postvoiding LUTS, which include postvoid dribbling and the sensation of incomplete emptying.

DIAGNOSTIC WORKUP

Definitive determination of the type of incontinence or voiding dysfunction begins with a careful review of symptomatology, followed by a careful history, focused physical examination, and limited diagnostic studies (e.g., bladder diary, urinalysis, and postvoid residual urine measurement). Individuals with complex problems may require advanced assessment including urodynamic studies and possibly serum and radiologic studies. Chapter 4 provides in-depth review of the components of primary assessment of the individual with incontinence or voiding dysfunction, and Chapter 5 provides in-depth information on advanced assessment techniques such as urodynamics.

KEY POINT

Diagnostic workup for the individual with UI or voiding dysfunction begins with a careful exploration of presenting signs and symptoms, followed by an appropriately focused history and physical and limited diagnostics (bladder chart, urinalysis, postvoid residual if indicated); serum studies and urodynamics may be required for the individual with complex or nonresponsive conditions.

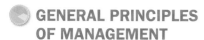 **GENERAL PRINCIPLES OF MANAGEMENT**

Management of UI or voiding dysfunction has two major goals: (1) prevention of any upper tract damage or deterioration and (2) enhanced quality of life for the individual and/or caregivers. If the individual presents with a condition that creates a threat to the kidneys (e.g., high-pressure chronic retention), the primary goal is to reduce the high intravesical pressures in order to restore normal urinary drainage from the kidneys to the bladder; this typically involves medical–surgical interventions to eliminate bladder outlet obstruction (see Chapter 8).

KEY POINT

Management for the patient with UI or voiding dysfunction is focused on prevention of upper tract distress and measures to optimize the patient's and/or caregiver's quality of life. Behavioral strategies are considered first-line therapy for most individuals; pharmacologic therapy and surgical intervention are usually reserved for patients with complex or refractory conditions.

However, for most individuals, the focus is on eliminating, minimizing, and/or effectively managing the problem with urinary leakage or voiding dysfunction in order to improve quality of life. In general, behavioral strategies are considered first-line interventions; pharmacologic and/or surgical interventions are typically recommended for individuals with inadequate response to behavioral therapies. However, the treatment plan must always be established based on the goals and priorities of the patient (and/or caregiver). For example, the patient who presents with signs and symptoms of OAB and urgency incontinence is typically managed initially with behavioral strategies (elimination of potential bladder irritants, instruction in urge suppression strategies, and bladder training); however, anticholinergic medications may be added to the initial management plan for the individual with severe urgency or the patient who requests medication. Similarly, pelvic floor rehabilitation is typically recommended as initial therapy for the individual with stress incontinence caused by weak sphincter and pelvic floor muscles; however, the individual who requests evaluation for surgical intervention should be referred appropriately *in addition to* receiving education about pelvic floor muscle exercises and their importance as adjunct therapy. The individual with functional incontinence due to significant cognitive impairment who is cared for by a family member may be managed with a toileting program and adjunct absorbent products or with absorbent products alone; the choice is up to the caregiver.

 CONCLUSION

UI and voiding dysfunction are common problems that typically have a profound impact on quality of life and may also place the individual at risk for physical complications. Workup begins with a thorough exploration of presenting signs and symptoms and with assessment for and correction of any reversible factors commonly associated with bladder dysfunction. This should be followed by an appropriately focused history and physical examination; individuals with complex conditions may also require advanced assessment including urodynamic studies. Management is directed toward two major goals: protection of the upper tracts (in selected situations where the voiding dysfunction creates upper tract distress) and enhancement of the individual's quality of life. Behavioral strategies are usually considered "first-line" therapy; pharmacologic and surgical interventions are usually reserved for individuals who fail to respond adequately to behavioral therapy. However, medical and surgical intervention may be first-line therapy in selected situations, due to the complexity or severity of the problem or the patient or caregiver's preferences. The content provided in each of these chapters provide elementary evidence-based concepts in evaluating and managing individuals with bowel and bladder disorders but also are an excellent resource for the experienced or expert continence care nurse as well as the advance practice continence nurse. The coeditors recommend the reader continues to visit these chapters to build a strong foundational knowledge base that will quickly grow into a passionate and thriving practice that provides meaningful, evidence-base quality care for those who suffer from these disorders. Remember, Continence Care Nursing is a Window of Opportunity!

REFERENCES

Abrams, P., Cardozo, L., Fall, M., et al.; Standardization Sub-committee of the International Continence Society. (2002). The standardization of terminology in lower urinary tract dysfunction: Report form the standardization sub-committee of the International Continence Society. *Neurourolology and Urodynamics, 21*(2), 162–178.

Akhavizadegan, H., Locke, J. A., Stothers, L., et al. (2019). A comprehensive review of adult enuresis. *Canadian Urological Association Journal, 13*(8), 282–287.

Alperin, M., Burnett, L., Lukacz, E., et al. (2019). The mysteries of menopause and urogynecologic health: Clinical and scientific gaps. *Menopause, 26*(1), 103–111.

American College of Obstetricians and Gynecologists (ACOG). (2014). Practice Bulletin No. 141: Management of menopausal symptoms. *Obstetrics & Gynecology, 123*(1), 202–216. doi: 10.1097/01. AOG.0000441353.20693.7.

Anger, J., Una, L., & Ackerman, L. A. (2019). Recurrent uncomplicated urinary tract infections in women: American Urological Association (AUA)/Canadian Urological Association (CUA)/Society of Urodynamics, Female Pelvic Medicine & Urogenital Reconstruction (SUFU) Guideline. American Urological Association Education and Research, Inc.

Ayaz, A., unNisa, R., Anwar, S., et al. (2012). Vesicovaginal and rectovaginal Fistulas: 12-year results of surgical treatment. *Journal of Ayub Medical College, Abbottabad, 24*(3–4), 25–27.

Bliwise, D. L., Wagg, A., Sand, P. K. (2019). Nocturia: A highly prevalent disorder with multifaceted consequences. *Urology, 133*, 3–13.

Bonkat, G., Bartoletti, R., Bruyere, T., et al. (2019). *European Association of Urology (EAU) guidelines on urological infections*. Arnhem, The Netherlands: EAU Guidelines Office. Retrieved from http://uroweb. org/guidelines/compilations-of-all-guidelines/

D'Ancona, C., Haylen, B., Oelke, M., et al. (2019). The International Continence Society (ICS) report on the terminology for adult male lower urinary tract and pelvic floor symptoms and dysfunction. *Neurourology and Urodynamics, 38*(2), 433–447.

Dowling-Castronovo, A., & Specht, J. K. (2009). Assessment of transient urinary incontinence in older adults. *American Journal of Nursing, 109*(2), 62–71.

Drake, M. J. (2018). Fundamentals of terminology in lower urinary tract function. *Neurourology and Urodynamics, 37*, S13–S19.

Faubion, S. S., Sood, R., & Kapoor, E. (2017). Genitourinary syndrome of menopauses: Management strategies for the clinician. *Mayo Clinic Proceedings, 92*(12), 1842–1849.

Felde, G., Ebbesen, M. H., & Hunskaar, S. (2017). Anxiety and depression associated with urinary incontinence. A 10-year follow-up study from the Norwegian HUNT study (EPINCONT). *Neurourology and Urodynamics, 36*, 322–328.

Gajweski, J. B., Schurch, B., Hamid, R., et al. (2017). An International Continence Society (ICS) report on the terminology for adult neurogenic lower urinary tract dysfunction (ANLUTD). *Neurourology and Urodynamics, 37*(3), 1–10. doi: 10.1002/nau.23397.

Gorina, Y., Schappert, S., Bercovitz, A., et al. (2014). *Prevalence of incontinence among older Americans*. Vital Health Statistics. Series 3, # 36. Washington, DC: National Center for Health Statistics, Department of Health and Human Services.

Haylen, B. T., de Ridder, D., Freeman, R. M., et al. (2010). An International Urogynecological Association (IUGA)/International Continence Society (ICS) joint report on the terminology for female pelvic floor dysfunction. *Neurourology and Urodynamics, 29*(1), 4–20.

Hu, T., Wagner, T., Bentkorn, J., et al. (2004). Costs of urinary incontinence and overactive bladder in the United States: A comparative study. *Urology, 63*(3), 461–465.

Kuwertz-Broking, E., & von Gontard, A. (2018). Clinical management of nocturnal enuresis. *Pediatric Nephrology, 33*, 1145–1154.

Milsom, I., Altman, D., Cartwright, R., et al. (2017) Epidemiology of urinary incontinence (UI) and other lower urinary tract symptoms (LUTS), pelvic organ prolapse (POP) and anal (AI) incontinence. In P. Abrams, L. Cardozo, A. Wagg, et al., (Eds.), *Incontinence* (6th ed., pp. 13–141). ICUD-EAU 2017.

Robinson, J., Weiss, R., Avi-Itshak, T., et al. (2009). Pilot testing of a theory-based pelvic floor training intervention for radical prostate patients. *Neurourology and Urodynamics, 28*(7), 682–683.

Stöhrer, M., Goepel, M., Kondo, A., et al. (1999). The standardization of terminology in neurogenic lower urinary tract dysfunction with suggestions for diagnostic procedures. *Neurourology and Urodynamics, 18*(2), 139–158.

Vaughan, C. P., & Bliwise, D. L. (2018). Sleep and nocturia in older adults. *Sleep Medicine Clinics, 13*, 107–116.

Wound, Ostomy, and Continence Nurses Society. (2007). *Reversible causes of urinary incontinence: A guide for clinicians*. Mt. Laurel, NJ: Author.

Wound, Ostomy and Continence Nurses Society. (2016). *Reversible causes of acute/transient urinary incontinence: Clinical resource guide*. Mt. Laurel, NJ: Author.

Wound, Ostomy and Continence Nurses Society. (2018). *Role of the wound, ostomy and continence nurse in continence care*. Mt. Laurel, NJ: Author.

QUESTIONS

1. The continence nurse is assessing an 80-year-old female patient who complains that she is unable to get to a bathroom in time when she feels the need to urinate. What is the term for this urinary alteration?

A. Urinary retention

B. Voiding dysfunction

C. Urinary incontinence

D. Postvoiding LUTS

2. What is the *main* characteristic of acute/transient urinary incontinence (UI) that distinguishes it from chronic UI?

A. It mainly occurs in the evening hours and overnight.

B. It is short term and usually curable.

C. It is caused by irreversible factors.

D. It comes and goes over a long period of time.

3. The continence nurse is using the mnemonic TOILETED to assess a patient for reversible factors causing urinary incontinence (UI). Which of the following describes one of these factors?
A. O= Obstruction
B. L = LUTS
C. T = Time frame
D. D = Diabetes

4. For which of the following conditions associated with urinary incontinence (UI) might the continence nurse recommend a trial of topical estrogen therapy?
A. Atrophic urethritis
B. Dementia
C. Urinary infection
D. Endocrine disorders

5. An elderly patient is prescribed an anticholinergic medication to treat depression. For what adverse side effect affecting urinary continence would the continence nurse monitor this patient?
A. Sudden production of large volumes of urine precipitating incontinence
B. Depression altering motivation to manage urinary symptoms
C. Increased urethral resistance worsening urinary retention
D. Compromise in bladder contractility worsening urinary retention

6. A 65-year-old female patient is diagnosed with urge incontinence. What is the usual cause of this urinary disorder?
A. Weak pelvic floor
B. Bladder (detrusor) overactivity

C. Weak sphincter muscles
D. Cognitive impairment

7. The continence nurse is assessing a patient with multiple sclerosis for urinary dysfunction. For which of the following voiding dysfunctions is this patient at risk?
A. Obstruction of the bladder neck
B. Obstruction of the urethra
C. Ineffective bladder contractions
D. Pelvic floor dysfunction

8. What therapeutic measure might the continence nurse recommend for a patient with chronic urinary retention related to ineffective bladder contractions?
A. Instruction in intermittent catheterization
B. Surgical intervention
C. Pharmacologic intervention
D. Interventions to improve pelvic muscle strength

9. Which of the following is a common cause of neurogenic bladder?
A. Spinal cord lesion
B. Dementia
C. Brain tumor
D. Diabetes

10. The continence nurse is assessing a patient diagnosed with storage lower urinary tract symptoms (LUTS). Which of the following is a common symptom of this urinary alteration?
A. Intermittent stream
B. Straining to void
C. Terminal dribble
D. Urinary frequency

ANSWERS AND RATIONALES

1. C. Rationale: The patient is describing urinary incontinence, the involuntary loss of urine.

2. B. Rationale: Incontinence of recent onset caused by a potentially reversible condition is characteristic of acute or transient UI.

3. A. Rationale: The O in TOILETED stands for obstruction, one of the reversible factors associated with UI. Obstruction can result from bowel distention due to severe constipation or

impaction, which can compromise bladder filling and can exacerbate symptoms of overactive bladder. Conditions such as prostatic hypertrophy can obstruct the bladder outlet and cause urinary retention.

4. A. Rationale: Estrogen deficiency after menopause can lead to atrophic changes in the urethra, which, in turn, can cause UI. Topic estrogen is often beneficial in women with atrophic urethritis.

5. D. Rationale: Anticholinergic medications can impair bladder contractility and cause urinary retention. Older adults who already often have age-related reductions in bladder contractility are at higher risk for this adverse effect.

6. B. Rationale: Urge incontinence is usually caused by detrusor overactivity. It is typically part of the syndrome called overactive bladder syndrome (OAB) and is accompanied by urgency and urinary frequency.

7. C. Rationale: Multiple sclerosis (MS) can have a number of effects on lower urinary tract function, one of which is impaired bladder contractility.

8. A. Rationale: When patients cannot empty their bladder secondary to ineffective bladder contractions, intermittent catheterization is often required to ensure adequate bladder emptying.

9. A. Rationale: Spinal cord lesions are a common cause of neurogenic bladder.

10. D. Rationale: Frequency is a common lower urinary tract symptom associated with bladder storage problems.

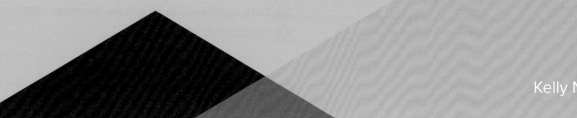

CHAPTER 4

PRIMARY ASSESSMENT OF PATIENTS WITH URINARY INCONTINENCE AND VOIDING DYSFUNCTION

Kelly Nelles

OBJECTIVES

1. Identify goals for the assessment of the individual with urinary incontinence.

2. Describe data to be gathered during the patient interview and the significance of these data to accurate diagnosis.

3. Describe key elements of a focused physical examination for the patient with urinary incontinence or voiding dysfunction to include interpretation of findings.

4. Describe data provided by a bladder chart and the importance of a completed bladder chart to

assessment and management of the patient with urinary incontinence.

5. Utilize data gathered during the interview and physical assessment to determine appropriate laboratory testing for the patient with urinary incontinence or voiding dysfunction.

6. Synthesize assessment data to determine type of incontinence/voiding dysfunction and goals for management.

TOPIC OUTLINE

A comprehensive and accurate assessment of the individual with urinary incontinence (UI) or voiding dysfunction is the foundation for effective management. This chapter addresses primary assessment strategies; advanced diagnostic tests such as urodynamic studies are addressed in Chapter 5.

ASSESSMENT GOALS

The goals of primary assessment are to

1. Screen for and identify conditions that mandate further evaluation and/or referral
2. Determine the type(s) of UI
3. Develop collaborative patient-centered goals for treatment

KEY POINT

The goals of primary (initial) assessment of the individual with urinary incontinence or voiding dysfunction are to identify conditions that require further evaluation or medical/surgical intervention, determine the specific type of incontinence or voiding dysfunction, and determine the individual's goals for treatment.

KEY PRINCIPLES UNDERLYING ACCURATE ASSESSMENT

Accurate diagnosis and management of urinary incontinence (UI) and voiding dysfunction is based on the data obtained through a tailored urologic assessment. The continence nurse uses basic and advanced health assessment skills to perform a focused health history and physical assessment and obtains appropriate laboratory and diagnostic studies as indicated.

As discussed in Chapter 2, *Voiding Physiology*, and Chapter 3, *Continence Care Nursing: An Overview*, continence and voiding dysfunction symptoms are usually caused by a disruption in anatomical, physiological, psychological, and/or neurologic function. Continence requires an intact lower urinary tract, the cognitive ability to recognize the urge to void, and the functional ability to get to the bathroom to use the toilet or commode. In addition, the patient must be motivated to maintain

continence and have an environment that supports the process (Thompson & Bradway, 2017). When performing a health history, it is important for the nurse to remember these concepts and to assess urologic function in relation to the person's medical and surgical history; social history and health habits; neurologic, cognitive, and psychological function; gastrointestinal and bowel function; and obstetric/gynecologic history in women and genitourinary/prostate history in men. In addition, when assessing an older individual, the continence nurse should be alert to changes associated with aging that can affect continence and voiding, for example, reduced bladder capacity, benign prostatic hypertrophy (BPH) in men, and loss of estrogen in postmenopausal women (Vahabi et al., 2017; Wagg et al., 2017).

KEY POINT

When assessing an older individual, the continence nurse should be alert to changes associated with aging that can affect continence and voiding, for example, reduced bladder capacity, BPH in men, and estrogen deficiency in women.

REVIEW OF ONSET AND DURATION OF THE PROBLEM

When obtaining the history of a person with UI or voiding dysfunction, it is important to ask specific questions regarding the onset and duration of the problem, in order to differentiate between transient and established problems. Transient UI or voiding dysfunction is considered acute and generally reversible, while established UI or voiding dysfunction is described as chronic or persistent (Newman & Wein, 2009). Established UI or voiding dysfunction may develop either suddenly or gradually, and initial onset may be associated with an acute illness, hospitalization, or a sudden change in environment or daily routine (Palmer, 1996). Types of established UI and voiding dysfunction include stress, urge, mixed, and functional incontinence, neurogenic lower urinary tract dysfunction (NLUTD), and urinary retention; the continence nurse should ask questions and conduct testing to determine the specific type of incontinence or voiding dysfunction affecting this individual.

Stress UI

Stress UI is characterized by an involuntary loss of urine associated with an increase in intra-abdominal pressure (e.g., position change, cough, sneezing). Urine loss usually occurs in small amounts and is observable on physical examination during a cough test. Stress UI is more common in women although it also occurs in some men postprostatectomy (see Chapters 10 and 11).

Urge UI

Urge incontinence is described as an involuntary loss of urine associated with a strong urge to void. Persons with urge UI (UUI) often report they are unable to hold their urine and leak on the way to the bathroom; they typically report frequency and nocturia as well as urgency. Individuals may also report symptoms of urgency, frequency, and nocturia without urine loss; this is a characteristic of the syndrome of overactive bladder or OAB. UUI and OAB become more prevalent with aging and put older adults at risk for sleep disruption and falls (Bolz et al., 2012) (see Chapter 7).

Mixed UI

Mixed incontinence is the term used to denote a combination of stress and urge UI; these individuals experience involuntary loss of urine associated with increased intra-abdominal pressure and also experience leakage associated with urgency and frequency (Jayasekara, 2009).

Functional UI

Functional incontinence is caused by conditions outside the urinary tract itself that cause leakage, such as cognitive impairment and/or mobility impairment; these individuals may be unaware of the leakage or may report leakage that occurs because they are unable to get out of the bed or chair and to the bathroom (see Chapter 13).

Neurogenic UI

NLUTD is caused by a neurologic lesion (such as a spinal cord injury or multiple sclerosis) that disrupts the neurologic pathways that provide voluntary control of voiding; these individuals typically are unable to sense bladder filling and unable to voluntarily initiate voiding. In addition, they are at risk for detrusor–sphincter dyssynergia, which means loss of coordination between the detrusor and the sphincter; failure of the sphincter to relax during a bladder contraction places the person at high risk for impaired emptying and ureteral reflux. These individuals require referral for advanced assessment including urodynamic studies (see Chapter 9).

Voiding Dysfunction

Voiding dysfunction (also known as retention) is characterized by difficulty emptying the bladder and may be either acute or chronic. Acute onset retention is usually characterized by total inability to void and severe pain and requires emergent intervention. In contrast, chronic retention is characterized by bladder distention and by symptoms of dribbling, urinary hesitancy, and an uncomfortable sensation of fullness or pressure in the lower abdomen; some individuals also experience leakage that may or may not be associated with urgency. Voiding dysfunction requires further workup to determine the underlying cause, which is usually either outlet obstruction (e.g., retention associated with BPH) or hypocontractility of the detrusor muscle (Jayasekara, 2009; Moore, 2006) (see Chapter 8).

KEY ELEMENTS OF CONTINENCE ASSESSMENT

Critical components of a comprehensive assessment include (1) focused health history; (2) focused physical examination; (3) appropriate selection of laboratory and diagnostic tests; and (4) a synthesis of the data collected to determine the type of UI and/or voiding dysfunction and to develop an individualized management plan.

HEALTH HISTORY/INTERVIEW GUIDELINES

The history is the most critical element of the comprehensive assessment; it includes an in-depth review of the chief complaint; discussion of the impact of the problem on the individual's quality of life and their goals and expectations for treatment; and a focused review of systems and medication profile.

CHIEF COMPLAINT

The interview begins with a discussion of the problem(s) prompting the individual to seek care, the impact of those symptoms on quality of life, and the individual's goals for treatment.

Symptoms

Individuals may present with a variety of incontinence or voiding dysfunction symptoms, including storage symptoms (involuntary loss of urine, urgency, frequency, nocturia, or enuresis), voiding symptoms (difficulty starting the stream, poor or intermittent stream, straining to void), or postvoiding symptoms (postvoid leaking or dribbling and/or a sensation of pressure or incomplete bladder emptying). Each symptom should be fully investigated, including the onset, duration, frequency with which the symptom occurs, precipitating factors, and symptom severity. Questions regarding current management of symptoms and previous treatments and effectiveness are also important; the answers provide insight into the individual's understanding of the problem, access to resources, and self-efficacy. Using the nursing acronym, "OLDCART" can help the nurse provide a systematic approach when interviewing the patient about the characteristics of their UI (see **Box 4-1**).

KEY POINT

Questions regarding current management of symptoms and previous treatments and effectiveness provide insight into the individual's understanding of the problem, access to resources, and self-efficacy. Using the nursing acronym, "OLDCART" can help the nurse provide a systematic approach when interviewing the patient about the characteristics of their UI.

Impact on Quality of Life

Validated tools can be beneficial in assessing health-related quality of life and symptom distress related to UI and voiding dysfunction, see **Table 4-1** (Dowling-Castronovo & Spiro, 2013). The Urinary Distress Inventory-6 (UDI-6) and the Incontinence Impact Questionnaire-7 (IIQ-7) are shortened versions of the original UDI and IIQ and are appropriate for assessing chronic UI. The UDI-6 describes a set of six UI symptoms and asks individuals to identify the degree of distress related to each symptom over the past 3 months. The IIQ-7 consists of seven questions specific to accidental urine loss and asks individuals to rate the effect on activities, relationships, and feelings using a rating scale from 0 to 3. While tested predominately in community-dwelling women, IIQ-7 has also been validated in men (Moore & Jensen, 2000), correlates strongly with the original long versions, and may be useful as part of the general assessment (Dowling-Castronovo & Spiro, 2013; Lemack & Zimmern, 1999; Shumaker et al., 1994; Uebersax et al., 1995; Van der Vaart et al., 2003). The Male Urogenital Distress Inventory (MUDI) and the Male Urinary Symptoms Impact

---

BOX 4-1   GUIDE TO SYSTEMATIC INTERVIEW ABOUT CHARACTERISTICS OF UI

Onset of UI symptoms: When did symptoms start? Was onset abrupt or gradual? Initiation or change in medications, diet/fluid intake, activity level, bowel pattern?

Location of Symptoms: Abdominal/suprapubic pressure, pain or distension; genital/urethral irritation, burning, itching, or discomfort?

Duration: How often do symptoms occur? How long do the symptoms last?

Character: Awareness of urge to void? Able to hold/delay void? Loss of urine with laughing/coughing/position change? Sense of urgency, frequency, or not emptying bladder completely? Nocturia? Straining to initiate voiding, weak or intermittent stream, dribbling?

Consistency: experiences symptoms with each void or at certain times of the day?

Aggravating Factors: Recent UTI? Increase or restriction of fluids? Dietary irritants including caffeine, NutraSweet, spicy foods? Smoking? Cough? Constipation? Medications? Weight gain? Recent abdominal or pelvic surgery? Relationship of UI symptoms to pregnancy or menopause for women? Relationship to prostate problems (e.g., BPH, prostatitis, etc.) for men?

Relieving Factors: What has the patient tried to relieve their UI symptoms? What was the response?

Timing/**T**ests Treatments: Frequency of voiding? Relationship between meals/fluid intake, medications, smoking, or constipation? Past diagnostics to evaluate bowel or bladder issues? Past treatments to address bowel or bladder symptoms? If so, outcomes?

Questionnaire (MUSIQ), variations of the UDI and IIQ specific to males, are also reliable in measuring health-related quality of life for men with UI or voiding dysfunction (Dowling-Castronovo & Spiro, 2013; Robinson & Shea, 2002) (**Table 4-1**).

Goals for Treatment

An initial step in the assessment is to establish the individual's goals and expectations for the visit and for management of the problem, while the nurse gathers objective data and considers appropriate strategies. It is critical to understand expectations and previous experiences as these can strongly influence care going forward. Patient-centered continence care involves partnering with the individual to discuss potential goals and outcomes and working together to develop an individualized plan of care. This process involves discussion of the individual's motivation and ability to self-manage as well as explaining possible treatment and management options and prioritizing continence-related concerns. While UI is not always reversible, appropriate management and support can always improve outcomes.

TABLE 4-1 VALIDATED ASSESSMENT TOOLS	
ASSESSMENT	INSTRUMENT
Symptoms and health-related quality of life	Urinary Distress Inventory-6 (UDI-6) and the Incontinence Impact Questionnaire-7 (IIQ-7). Access online at http://www.gericareonline.net/tools/eng/urinary/attachments/UI_Tool_2_IIQ7_SF.pdf and https://www.womenscare.com/wp-content/uploads/2013/04/inconques.pdf International Prostate Symptom Score (IPSS). Access online at https://www.baus.org.uk/_userfiles/pages/files/Patients/Leaflets/IPSS.pdf
Activities of daily living, function	Katz Index of Independence of Activities of Daily Living (ADL). Access online at https://www.alz.org/careplanning/downloads/katz-adl.pdf The Lawton Instrumental Activities of Daily Living (IADL) Scale. Access online at https://www.alz.org/careplanning/downloads/lawton-iadl.pdf
Cognitive assessment	Mental status assessment of older adults: The Mini-Cog. Access online at http://mini-cog.com/wp-content/uploads/2018/03/Standardized-English-Mini-Cog-1-19-16-EN_v1-low-1.pdf
Depression	The Geriatric Depression Scale (GDS). Access online at https://hign.org/sites/default/files/2020-06/Try_This_General_Assessment_4.pdf Patient Health Questionnaire (PHQ-9). Access online at https://www2.gov.bc.ca/assets/gov/health/practitioner-pro/bc-guidelines/depression_patient_health_questionnaire.pdf
Risk of falls	Fall Risk Assessment in Older Adults: The Hendrich II Fall Risk Model. Access online at http://www.wsha.org/wp-content/uploads/Hendrich-II-Fall-Risk.pdf Assessment of Fear of Falling in Older Adults: The Falls Efficacy Scale-International (FES-1). Access online at https://medicine.osu.edu/-/media/files/medicine/departments/orthopaedics/research/clinical-trials/ffp-fes-i.pdf?la=en&hash=17E635EACC101A11BB68537E5DD2A0B9CC014C98
Medication	AGS Beers Criteria for Potentially Inappropriate Medication Use in Older Adults. Access online at https://geriatricscareonline.org/ProductAbstract/beers-criteria-pocketcard-2019/PC007
Mobility	Timed Up and Go (TUG) Test. Access online at https://www.cdc.gov/steadi/pdf/TUG_Test-print.pdf

MEDICAL/SURGICAL HISTORY AND RELATED REVIEW OF SYSTEMS

Obtaining a pertinent medical and surgical history and accurate review of systems allows the continence nurse to identify health conditions that may directly impact continence status and/or contribute to voiding dysfunction.

KEY POINT

Obtaining a pertinent medical and surgical history and review of systems allows the continence nurse to identify health conditions that may impact on continence status and/or contribute to voiding dysfunction.

General Assessment/Review of Constitutional Symptoms

The nurse should begin by assessing for *general constitutional* symptoms that would affect ability and motivation to toilet, such as fatigue, weakness, depression, and confusion. Sensory impairments, specifically alterations in vision and hearing, may negatively affect the individual's ability to find the bathroom and to respond appropriately to caregiver instructions regarding toileting.

Cardiovascular System

Cardiovascular issues, especially hypotension, heart failure, and arrhythmias, place the individual at risk for dizziness, weakness, and falls. Peripheral dependent edema is an indicator of impaired perfusion and third spacing and is typically associated with increased nocturnal urine production, nocturia, and increased risk of falls. In addition, diuretics are commonly used to treat heart failure, and the marked increase in urine production is frequently associated with urinary urgency and frequency. In hypertensive patients with peripheral edema, symptoms of urinary urgency and transient UI can also result from diuresis (Gray & Moore, 2009; Krieg, 2017).

Respiratory System

It is also important to identify *respiratory* conditions resulting in acute or chronic coughing, which increases intra-abdominal pressure and can cause or contribute to episodes of stress UI. The nurse should ask about nicotine use. Smoking contributes to chronic cough, which increases the risk of UI, and nicotine has been shown to act as a bladder irritant in some individuals, which increases the risk of frequency and urgency (Moore et al., 2013). A well-known side effect of ACE inhibitors is chronic cough; thus, these medications increase the risk for UI. An acute upper respiratory infection can cause severe coughing that results in transient stress incontinence; the stress incontinence will resolve when the URI resolves. In contrast, coughing related to chronic obstructive pulmonary disease is an example of a chronic condition associated with increased risk of UI that is not spontaneously reversible. Effective management of this patient would involve measures to control cough. Assessing readiness to quit smoking and offering assistance to do so is an appropriate role for the continence nurse.

KEY POINT

Coughing related to the use of ACE inhibitors, acute URI, and smoking all contribute to an increased risk for UI. Presence of these factors should cue the continence nurse to assess and consider management strategies to effectively address.

Endocrine System

Metabolic conditions such as diabetes and obesity are risk factors for bladder dysfunction and incontinence. This is significant since these conditions are increasingly prevalent (Shamliyan et al., 2007; Subak et al., 2009). Poorly controlled DM results in hyperglycemia and polyuria, which increases the risk for urgency, frequency, and urge UI. In addition, longstanding DM can cause autonomic neuropathy (diabetic cystopathy) and chronic urinary retention (Gray & Moore, 2009; Krieg, 2017). Truncal obesity is associated with increased intra-abdominal pressure, which increases the risk for episodes of stress UI (Lamerton et al., 2018). Thus, education and support for weight reduction can be an important strategy for improving continence.

KEY POINT

Metabolic conditions such as diabetes and obesity are risk factors for bladder dysfunction and incontinence. Support for weight reduction can be an important strategy for improving continence.

Gastrointestinal System

Gastrointestinal problems are common contributing factors to UI and voiding dysfunction; thus, assessment of bowel history (to include surgical procedures) and current bowel function and control is a critical element of the assessment. Conditions such as acute or chronic diarrhea and diarrhea-predominant irritable bowel syndrome are risk factors for fecal urgency and fecal incontinence and will be addressed further in Chapter 21. Constipation is associated with increased urinary urgency and frequency, due to the effects of a full rectum and sigmoid on bladder filling and detrusor irritability. Severe constipation and fecal impaction can cause urethral compression and bladder outlet obstruction, which causes or exacerbates urinary retention. This is sometimes the cause of worsening retention in a male with mild retention due to BPH. Finally, fecal incontinence may be indicative of a neurologic lesion affecting the sacral nerve pathways; these individuals would also be at risk for UI and/or voiding dysfunction (Gray & Moore, 2009; Krieg, 2017).

KEY POINT

Constipation is associated with urgency and frequency, due to the effects of a full rectosigmoid on bladder filling and detrusor instability. Impaction can cause urethral obstruction and bladder outlet obstruction.

Genitourinary System

When assessing a male with UI or voiding dysfunction, the *genitourinary* (GU) history is of critical importance and should include questions regarding UI episodes, urinary tract infections (UTIs), BPH, prostatitis, any urologic surgical procedures, and history of bladder/kidney stones. A clear understanding of the person's GU history may provide insight into factors contributing to current symptoms and into appropriate management, that is, interventions to mitigate symptoms and to reduce the risk for recurrence. For example, finding that the person has been diagnosed with BPH and has had problems with retention in the past provides the foundation for education and counseling regarding current symptom management and measures to prevent recurrent episodes (such as assuring appropriate bowel management and avoidance of medications that could increase outlet resistance or reduce detrusor contractility).

Such measures will help to prevent episodes of acute retention, which increase the risk for UTIs, upper urinary tract damage, bladder and renal calculi, and eventual renal insufficiency (Gray & Moore, 2009; Krieg, 2017). Similarly, prostatitis is known to contribute to irritative voiding symptoms including urge UI, and treatment of prostate cancer with radical prostatectomy and radiation therapy increases the risk for UI and voiding problems (Gray & Moore, 2009; Krieg, 2017; Shamliyan et al., 2007). Symptoms can be assessed using the International Prostate Symptom Score (IPSS) (see **Table 4-1**). This validated tool consists of eight questions with the first seven designed to measure irritative and obstructive symptoms, while the eighth captures the degree to which symptoms are bothersome and negatively affect quality of life.

> **KEY POINT**
>
> A history of BPH and retention should prompt education regarding prevention of constipation and avoidance of medications that reduce bladder contractility or increase the risk of bladder outlet obstruction (e.g., anticholinergics and alpha-adrenergic agonists).

Obstetric/Gynecologic System

In women, the obstetric and gynecologic history should include information regarding pregnancies, deliveries, and menopausal status as well as any gynecologic or urologic surgical procedures. The number of pregnancies, type of delivery (vaginal vs. C-section), and use of episiotomy are factors known to affect UI risk (Shamliyan et al., 2007). Multiple deliveries, episiotomy, breech delivery, and traumatic deliveries involving perineal tears have all been shown in various studies to increase the risk of pelvic floor denervation and stress UI (Gray & Moore, 2009; Van Geelen et al., 2018).

In women who are still menstruating, it is helpful to obtain a menstrual history including use of contraception and the specific method(s) used. Recent data indicate that some progestin-only contraceptives (i.e., Depo-Provera) can contribute to estrogen depletion and can therefore increase the risk for UI (Schulling & Likis, 2013). For women who are no longer menstruating, determining the age and type of menopause (i.e., natural vs. medically or surgically induced) is useful as bladder problems often begin or become more noticeable around the time of menopause. Gathering information about current or previous hormone replacement therapy and any indicators of urogenital atrophy (e.g., dyspareunia, itching, irritation, vaginal dryness or pain, urinary urgency and frequency, and dysuria) is critical since atrophic changes are thought to contribute to both SUI and UUI and are generally reversible with topical estrogen therapy (Greenblum et al., 2008; Kinsberg et al., 2009; Lekan-Rutledge, 2004; North American Menopause Society, 2017; Schulling & Likis, 2013). Irritative bladder symptoms or urge UI may occur in women with endometriosis or vaginitis; thus, the nurse should ask about any history of endometriosis and any symptoms of vaginitis (i.e., vaginal discharge, odor, or itching) (Gray & Moore, 2009). The woman should be asked about pelvic pressure or pain, history of pelvic organ prolapse, prior pelvic procedures, and any sensation of a vaginal "bulge," because pelvic organ prolapse increases the risk of stress UI and UTI. In addition, severe prolapse can result in significant urinary retention (ACOG, 2019).

> **KEY POINT**
>
> Information about current or past hormone replacement therapy and indicators of urogenital atrophy is critical since atrophic changes are thought to contribute to both stress incontinence and urge incontinence and are generally reversible with topical estrogen therapy.

Skin

The patient with atypical alterations in perineal skin integrity should be asked about systemic dermatologic conditions such as dermatitis, eczema, and psoriasis, because these conditions can recur in the urogenital area with similar symptoms.

Musculoskeletal System

Some musculoskeletal problems can contribute to alterations in function and mobility that impact continence status (Offermans et al., 2009; Shamliyan et al., 2007). Arthritis (either osteo- or rheumatoid arthritis) and/or back problems including spinal stenosis should be identified as these conditions impact on dexterity and clothing management, sensory awareness of bladder filling, and overall mobility and ability to toilet safely. In many individuals, motivation to toilet is impacted by chronic pain and fatigue due to musculoskeletal disorders; this increases the risk for functional UI (Gray, 2006).

> **KEY POINT**
>
> In many individuals, motivation to toilet is impacted by chronic pain and fatigue due to musculoskeletal disorders.

Neurologic System

Neurologic conditions are an essential area of investigation. In addition to affecting overall function and mobility, neurologic conditions and lesions can adversely affect neural control of voiding. For example, CVA (stroke) and Parkinson disease are associated with increased risk of urge UI due to impaired ability to inhibit voiding (Gray & Moore, 2009; Shamliyan et al., 2007). Spinal cord disorders resulting in paralysis (e.g., spinal cord injury and progressive multiple sclerosis of the spinal cord) are associated with neurogenic bladder, increased risk of reflux and upper tract damage, and/or urinary retention (Gray & Moore, 2009). Clinicians should also ask about surgeries of the spine, since these procedures can result in denervation injuries that profoundly affect bladder function and continence. Both musculoskeletal and neurologic alterations can contribute to alterations in functional status, which should be fully assessed on physical examination.

Cognitive and Psychological Status

Cognitive and psychological alterations including dementia and depression have a significant impact on the ability and motivation to toilet and are risk factors for functional UI. Delirium is a reversible alteration in mental status that is associated with acute or transient UI, while dementia is a generally irreversible deterioration in cognitive function that contributes to progressively more severe functional incontinence. Psychiatric disorders may also increase the risk for UI or voiding dysfunction, due to impact on motivation to toilet and to the medications used for treatment. For example, the medications used to treat anxiety, schizophrenia, and other psychiatric conditions increase the risk for urinary retention due to their anticholinergic properties. Depression is common and underdiagnosed in the elderly and in individuals with cognitive impairment, and depression increases the risk for UI; thus, the nurse needs to be alert to indicators of depression in these individuals. In addition, many persons with UI are reluctant to seek health care due to embarrassment or fear of stigma; they often attempt to self-manage their symptoms by limiting or avoiding social activities, which increases their risk of social isolation and depression (Diokno et al., 2000; DuBeau et al., 2006). Therefore, accurate screening and assessing for both depression and cognitive impairment is an important part of the continence assessment.

The nurse may find validated tools beneficial in assessing for these conditions. The Mini-Cog is a brief assessment tool designed to identify dementia and cognitive changes. Easy to administer, this 3-minute tool assesses cognitive function, memory, language comprehension, visual–motor skills, and executive function. The Mini-Cog is appropriate for older adults and can be used in all health care settings to track cognitive changes over time (Doerflinger, 2013). The Geriatric Depression Scale is used in community, acute, and long-term care settings to screen for depression among the elderly, including those with mild to moderate cognitive impairment (Greenberg, 2012). The Patient Health Questionnaire-9 (PHQ-9) is another short and easily administered tool designed to screen and monitor depressive symptoms over time. It is most commonly used in adults, but there is also an adolescent version. **Table 4-1** lists several of the most commonly used assessment tools.

> **KEY POINT**
>
> Dementia and depression are risk factors for functional incontinence.

MEDICATION PROFILE

Medications are known to affect bladder function and continence; therefore, the interview must include queries regarding all over-the-counter, herbal, and prescription medications with current dosages, administration routes, and frequency of use. Each medication should be assessed for efficacy and side effects, with particular attention to the elderly and those persons using multiple medications. The *2019 American Geriatrics Society Updated Beers Criteria for Potentially Inappropriate Medication Use in Older Adults* (American Geriatrics Society, 2019) is an important medication reconciliation resource for the continence nurse who is working with older adults. This safety tool provides an in-depth review of all medication categories and the potential side effects and contraindications for use in older adults (Molony & Greenberg, 2013) (**Table 4-1**). The pharmacist can also provide invaluable assistance in evaluating the individual's medications for potential interactions and for potential adverse effects on bladder function and continence.

There are multiple medications that have the potential to impact continence status; some are more likely to contribute to UI and voiding dysfunction than others (**Box 4-2**). For example, diuretics increase urinary output and are associated with increased urinary frequency, urgency, and risk of urge UI; therefore, the clinician should be alert to initiation of a diuretic or an increase in dosing. α-Adrenergic blockers (alpha blockers) are associated with increased risk of stress incontinence (due to reduced urethral tone). The chronic cough associated with ACE inhibitors also increases the risk for stress incontinence. Many medications cause drowsiness or sedation, which can compromise sensory awareness of bladder filling and the ability to respond to toileting cues and can therefore result in functional and/or transient UI as well as risk of falls. Risk of urinary retention is increased with the use of calcium channel blockers, beta-3 adrenergic agonists, anticholinergic medications, antispasmodics, antidepressants, antipsychotics, sedative/hypnotics, and narcotic analgesics. Decongestants are sympathomimetic agents that increase urethral resistance and therefore increase the risk for retention in men with prostate enlargement; they are therefore considered contraindicated in this group (Bolz et al., 2012; Gray & Moore, 2009). All patients on sedating or anticholinergic medications should be monitored for side effects (e.g., confusion, cognitive changes, dry mouth, constipation) as these interfere with function and increase fall risk. The nurse should consult/refer for adjustment of medications when there are identified concerns regarding safety, efficacy, or duplicative medications.

> **KEY POINT**
>
> Multiple medications have the potential to impact on continence and voiding; the pharmacist can be invaluable in assessing an individual's medications for potential adverse effects on bladder and sphincter function.

BOX 4-2	**EXAMPLES OF MEDICATIONS THAT IMPACT CONTINENCE STATUS**

MEDICATION EXAMPLE	EFFECT ON CONTINENCE
Diuretics	Increased urinary output resulting in increased frequency, urgency, and risk of urge UI
α-Adrenergic antagonists (alpha blockers)	Reduced urethral tone associated with increased risk of stress UI
ACE inhibitors	Side effect of chronic cough increases risk of stress UI
Calcium channel blockers, beta-3 adrenergic agonists, anticholinergic medications, antispasmodics, antidepressants, antipsychotics, sedative/hypnotics, and narcotic analgesics	Increased risk of urinary retention
α-Adrenergic agonists (decongestants)	Sympathomimetic agents that increase urethral resistance and therefore increase the risk for retention in men with prostate enlargement; they are therefore considered contraindicated in this group

SOCIAL HISTORY

The social history provides the continence nurse an opportunity to examine additional contributing factors to UI, voiding dysfunction, and quality of life. Asking about *primary or significant relationship* status and the impact of the continence or bladder problem on the relationship is important. Issues surrounding sexuality, social isolation, and sleep disruption should be explored along with the willingness and ability of the significant other to provide emotional support and/or assistance when considering the management plan. Determining the person's *occupation* may provide insight into other contributing factors. For example, individuals with jobs that require heavy lifting are at increased risk for stress UI. Others may work in jobs that limit opportunities for toileting and may have to postpone voiding until a scheduled break (e.g., factory line worker, teacher); this may increase the risk for urge UI or for retention.

Asking about *exercise and activity* level provides insight into alterations in quality of life and/or activities associated with risk of UI. For example, high-impact physical activities are associated with an increased risk of leaking and stress UI. Female athletes and participants

in exercise classes and fitness training, when compared with the rest of the female population, have increased rates of UI (Angelini, 2017). Reduced mobility and a sedentary lifestyle may contribute to a loss of core strength that makes it difficult for the individual to get up from a chair or the toilet. In addition, these alterations may contribute to a loss of pelvic floor muscle tone, which increases the likelihood for pelvic floor relaxation and urine loss consistent with stress UI.

NUTRITIONAL ASSESSMENT

A brief nutritional assessment can be useful in determining special dietary considerations and the presence of any swallowing difficulties that could impact the management plan. A brief 24-hour dietary recall can provide a snapshot of usual food and fluid intake, including usual intake of dietary fiber and the pattern, types, and amounts of fluids ingested. The use and number of beverages consumed daily that contain caffeine, artificial sweeteners (e.g., NutraSweet, aspartame), or alcohol should be assessed, and the relationship between their use and an increase in bladder symptoms should be explored (Gray, 2006). Lifestyle changes that include reducing or eliminating these types of beverages can be beneficial in reducing symptoms of urgency and frequency in some individuals (Newman & Wein, 2009). Dietary review and bladder diary may reveal excessive fluid intake, and further assessment is indicated to determine the reasons for the high volume intake. Poorly controlled or undiagnosed diabetes mellitus and deliberate use of water intake to control appetite and reduce food intake are two common reasons that would require very different management approaches (Gray, 2006).

KEY POINT

The use and number of beverages consumed daily that contain caffeine, alcohol, or artificial sweeteners should be assessed.

While excessive fluid intake can be an issue for some individuals, voluntary restriction is more common as many persons with UI limit their fluid intake in an attempt to manage their incontinence. While understandable, it is important for the nurse to be able to emphasize the benefits of adequate fluid intake. Specifically, excessive fluid restriction results in highly concentrated urine that may increase irritative bladder symptoms (e.g., urgency and frequency), UTI risk, and constipation. For the elderly, dehydration can contribute to transient changes in cognitive status. A bladder record that includes fluid intake and voided amounts is helpful in gathering objective data to correlate fluid intake with voiding frequency, irritative symptoms, and UI. In providing patient and education, the nurse should be aware that most adults need about 1,500 mL of fluid per day (or 30 mL/kg).

ENVIRONMENTAL AND FUNCTIONAL ASSESSMENT

Environmental assessment should include toilet availability and safety issues, while functional assessment focuses on the ability of the individual to independently perform toileting and related activities of daily living (ADL).

Environmental Assessment

During the patient interview, the nurse should identify the setting where the person lives (e.g., home, assisted living, nursing home) and the support needed to toilet successfully. The nurse should ask specifically about toileting regimes, bathroom accessibility, and available assistive devices (e.g., urinal, raised toilet seat, grab bars, bedside commode or bedpan) and should be alert to safety issues, such as obstacles in the path to the toilet, poor lighting, ambulatory instability, and footwear with slick soles. Conducting the evaluation in the person's residence allows the nurse to assess the environment firsthand and to identify barriers to continence. Cleanliness and presence of urine odor should be assessed as well as accessibility of laundry facilities; this helps assure appropriate recommendations related to reusable versus disposable absorptive products.

Determining the sleeping situation (i.e., where they sleep and presence of a sleeping partner) is helpful, as some persons opt to sleep in a bed, while others choose other alternatives due to various health problems (e.g., a recliner). In either situation, the person's ability to get up to toilet and the potential benefit of assistive devices should be assessed. Protective bed coverings and use of absorptive products should be explored. Types of products used, frequency of use, hygiene, and appropriate disposal of used products should be reviewed. Availability and responsiveness of caregivers is also important as is the presence of community resources and family support, particularly for the elderly and those with disability (Gray, 2006).

Functional Assessment

The functional assessment should be conducted at the same time as the environmental assessment and should focus on the level of independence and assistance needed to carry out ADL (see Table 4-1). This is another area where the use of validated tools can be helpful. The Katz Index of Independence of ADL and the Lawton Instrumental Activities of Daily Living (IADL) Scale are two such tools. The Katz ADL assesses independence in six areas, with yes/no answers to questions about bathing, dressing, toileting, transferring, continence, and feeding. A score of 6 indicates fully independent function, 4 indicates moderate functional impairment, and 2 or less correlates with severe functional impairment. This tool can be used with adults in a variety of care settings and can capture baseline function as well as changes over time (Shelkey & Wallace, 2012).

The Lawton IADL assesses independent living skills that are considered more complex than those assessed with the Katz Index of ADLs. This tool may be used for both men and women and assesses ability to use the telephone, shop, prepare food, complete housekeeping chores and laundry, manage transportation, manage medications, and handle finances. It is useful for identifying current function and for reflecting functional changes over time. Persons are scored on a scale of 0 (lowest function) to 8 (highest function, independent) for activities in each category. The tool can be used in clinic, community, and hospital settings but is not applicable for institutionalized adults (Graf, 2013) (**Table 4-1**).

Assessing both environment and functional status as part of the focused health history not only provides an opportunity to identify barriers to continence but also identifies safety issues that include fall risk. Many older adults are at risk for falling on the way to the bathroom, and this risk increases in the presence of bladder symptoms (e.g., urgency, leaking of urine) and accompanying alterations in function and mobility (Brown et al., 2000; Morris & Wagg, 2007). The Hendrich II Fall Risk Model and the Falls Efficacy Scale-International (FES-I) are two validated tools for identifying fall risk in older adults (Greenberg, 2011; Hendrich, 2013). Originally tested in the acute care setting, the Hendrich II Fall Risk Model has demonstrated validity and has been adapted for use across a variety of settings. Advantages of this tool are that it is short, includes assessment of risk related to medications, and includes the "Get Up and Go" test. The "Get Up and Go" test is a short assessment designed to test an individual's ability to safely rise from a chair, an essential function for safe toileting, and fall prevention (Mathias et al., 1986). This tool also helps the nurse to identify specific areas of risk and to design and implement interventions that address those areas (Hendrich, 2013).

The FES-I is designed to assess fear of falling; while it does not specifically ask about continence or toileting, it does assess related areas of function and may provide additional insight regarding persons at risk for depression and social isolation. The short tool asks about fall concern related to social and daily activities and uses a Likert scale (1 = not at all, 4 = very concerned) to measure concern (Greenberg, 2011).

KEY POINT

Assessment of the individual's environment and functional status permits identification of barriers to continence as well as safety issues such as fall risk.

BLADDER DIARY

The bladder record or diary is an important tool in gathering objective data related to voiding patterns, fluid intake, and incontinence. When possible, this should be included as a routine part of the assessment. In persons with cognitive impairment who are not able to complete the diary, a caregiver may complete a "modified" diary if she/he is willing to do so. (A "modified" diary typically involves hourly documentation as to wet or dry status, which provides insight into voiding frequency and is helpful in developing an individualized toileting schedule. The caregiver may also elect to take the person to the bathroom every 2 hours and provide verbal cues to void; the caregiver should then record the individual's response. This also provides very helpful information as to whether or not the person is likely to benefit from a toileting program.)

Many variations on bladder diaries exist, ranging from very basic to quite detailed. Bladder diaries can also be tailored to a variety of settings. It can be helpful for the continence nurse to have several different types of bladder diaries available for use and to select the specific tool depending on care setting and the symptoms to be monitored.

All bladder diaries require the willingness of the individual or caregiver to complete them. In the simplest of bladder records, the person simply documents the time of each voluntary voiding episode and each episode of leakage. More involved diaries also capture fluid intake, activities or symptoms surrounding the loss of urine (e.g., lifting, urgency), and the amount of urine lost (e.g., minimal urine loss = several drops or wet spot on underwear, moderate urine loss = several teaspoons or tablespoons of urine, large urine loss = several ounces soaking clothing or saturating a large pad or absorbent brief) (Gray, 2006).

KEY POINT

Bladder diaries provide important objective data regarding voiding frequency, fluid intake, and incontinence.

Bladder diaries (see **Fig. 4-1**) can be completed for varying lengths of time with 1- to 14-day diaries shown to produce reliable results with or without intensive instruction (Gray, 2006). Since it is difficult for many persons or caregivers to collect data for an extended time, the nurse should realize that diaries maintained for 1 to 3 days produce valuable information (Gray, 2006). To increase the likelihood of completion, it is important for the nurse to explain the purpose of the bladder record, how the information collected will be used, and strategies for ensuring completion (e.g., place record near the toilet or at

the bedside, or download an electronic diary to one's phone).

All bladder diaries provide data regarding voiding frequency and frequency of leakage episodes and therefore help to quantify the severity of the leakage. More complex diaries provide insight as to type of incontinence and the potential role of fluid intake; for example, leakage that is always associated with activity is indicative of stress incontinence, and normal voided volumes associated with urgency in a person with daily fluid intake of 4 L suggest that the problem relates to volume of intake and not to bladder dysfunction.

KEY POINT

The caregiver can complete a modified bladder diary for the person with cognitive impairment; data to be gathered would include "wet/dry" status on an hourly basis, response to q2-hour toileting attempts, and fluid intake.

FOCUSED PHYSICAL EXAMINATION

During the interview, the continence nurse has the opportunity to observe the individual and begins to collect objective data that are part of the focused physical examination. For example, the nurse assesses general appearance, gait, dexterity, and mobility when meeting the individual and throughout the interview as well as general demeanor, cognition, and affect. As stated, validated tools can be used throughout the interview to provide quantifiable objective data regarding cognition, presence or absence of depression, and functional status.

The interview also provides time and opportunity for establishment of the nurse–patient relationship. This relationship enhances patient comfort during the physical examination and is further developed by a respectful and sensitive approach to the examination. Specifically, the nurse should ask permission to examine the person, explain the examination process, assist with positioning and draping, and convey consistent respect for the individual's privacy and the sensitive nature of the examination. As the nurse moves from one part of the examination to the next, the patient should be informed of the next steps in the examination and permission sought to continue.

GENERAL ASSESSMENT

In addition to the observations and interactions described in the previous paragraph, general assessment includes an overall impression of the client's state of health. This general assessment is documented, for example, healthy-appearing adult and frail-appearing older adult. Each patient should have height, weight,

Your Daily Bladder Diary

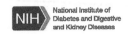

This diary will help you and your health care team figure out the causes of your bladder control trouble.
The "sample" line shows you how to use the diary.

Time	Drinks		Trips to the Bathroom		Accidental Leaks	Did you feel a strong urge to go?	What were you doing at the time?
	What kind?	How much? oz, mL, cups	How many times?	How much urine?	How much urine?		Sneezing, lifting, arriving home, sleeping, etc.
Sample	Juice	8 ounces	✓✓	⬤ sm ◯ med ◯ lg	⬤ sm ◯ med ◯ lg	(Yes) No	Running
6–7 a.m.				◯ ◯ ⬤	◯ ◯ ⬤	Yes No	
7–8 a.m.				◯ ◯ ⬤	◯ ◯ ⬤	Yes No	
8–9 a.m.				◯ ◯ ⬤	◯ ◯ ⬤	Yes No	
9–10 a.m.				◯ ◯ ⬤	◯ ◯ ⬤	Yes No	
10–11 a.m.				◯ ◯ ⬤	◯ ◯ ⬤	Yes No	
11–12 noon				◯ ◯ ⬤	◯ ◯ ⬤	Yes No	
12–1 p.m.				◯ ◯ ⬤	◯ ◯ ⬤	Yes No	
1–2 p.m.				◯ ◯ ⬤	◯ ◯ ⬤	Yes No	
2–3 p.m.				◯ ◯ ⬤	◯ ◯ ⬤	Yes No	
3–4 p.m.				◯ ◯ ⬤	◯ ◯ ⬤	Yes No	
4–5 p.m.				◯ ◯ ⬤	◯ ◯ ⬤	Yes No	
5–6 p.m.				◯ ◯ ⬤	◯ ◯ ⬤	Yes No	
6–7 p.m.				◯ ◯ ⬤	◯ ◯ ⬤	Yes No	
7–8 p.m.				◯ ◯ ⬤	◯ ◯ ⬤	Yes No	
8–9 p.m.				◯ ◯ ⬤	◯ ◯ ⬤	Yes No	
9–10 p.m.				◯ ◯ ⬤	◯ ◯ ⬤	Yes No	
10–11 p.m.				◯ ◯ ⬤	◯ ◯ ⬤	Yes No	
11–12 mid.				◯ ◯ ⬤	◯ ◯ ⬤	Yes No	
12–1 a.m.				◯ ◯ ⬤	◯ ◯ ⬤	Yes No	
1–2 a.m.				◯ ◯ ⬤	◯ ◯ ⬤	Yes No	
2–3 a.m.				◯ ◯ ⬤	◯ ◯ ⬤	Yes No	
3–4 a.m.				◯ ◯ ⬤	◯ ◯ ⬤	Yes No	
4–5 a.m.				◯ ◯ ⬤	◯ ◯ ⬤	Yes No	
5–6 a.m.				◯ ◯ ⬤	◯ ◯ ⬤	Yes No	

Use this sheet as a master for making copies that you can use as a bladder diary for as many days as you need.

I used _____ pads today. I used _____ diapers today (write number).

Questions to ask my health care team: _____

FIGURE 4-1. Example of a Bladder Diary. (Courtesy of NIDDK. Retrieved from https://www.niddk.nih.gov/media Files/Urologic-Diseases diary_508)

blood pressure, and pulse recorded (Vasavada & Kim, 2019).

MENTAL STATUS

The purpose of the mental status examination is to assess the individual's cognitive status and functional ability, including ability to respond appropriately to information and instruction. Physical appearance, appropriateness of dress, facial expression, and body posture are all indicators of mental function. Orientation to person, place, and time is an important indicator of memory and cognition. Emotional affect and alertness should also be assessed. As discussed previously, when there are any concerns as to cognitive status or depression, a validated tool should be used for objective assessment and documentation.

KEY POINT

When there are concerns regarding cognitive status or depression, a validated tool should be used for objective assessment and documentation.

MUSCULOSKELETAL EXAMINATION

Observation and assessment of dexterity, gait, and mobility are important components of the examination in relation to continence. Dexterity includes the ability of an individual to manage their own clothing and toileting hygiene. Gait and mobility include the individual's ability to walk to the bathroom with reasonable speed and to transfer to the toilet independently versus walking or moving slowly, needing assistance of one or two persons, or being totally dependent on caregivers for mobility. Observation for any visible abnormalities in the extremities and palpation for detection of edema are also important. Many continence clinicians measure the time required by an elderly patient with UI to get to the bathroom, manage clothing, and sit on the toilet (Gray, 2006). The continence nurse can often provide recommendations that facilitate clothing management (e.g., suspenders instead of belts, elastic waist pants rather than zippers) and safe toileting (e.g., urinal or bedside commode, grab bar, or elevated toilet seat).

NEUROLOGIC EXAMINATION

Although much information can be gained from simple conversation with the patient and observation of gait, any abnormalities should prompt more in-depth investigation. Strength, sensation, and deep tendon reflexes of the lower extremities should be tested along with assessment of mobility, dexterity, and cognition (Vasavada & Kim, 2019). The back, buttocks, and lower extremities may be assessed for signs of neurologic lesions such as spina bifida occulta. For example, if there are any concerns regarding neurologic function, the back should be inspected for indicators of spinal dysraphism (e.g., lipomatous area, hairy tuft, or skin tag near the lumbosacral spinal area) (Gray, 2006). When indicated, the buttocks should be inspected for asymmetry or signs of muscle atrophy, and the lower extremities and feet can be assessed for atrophy or other obvious signs of neurologic abnormality (Gray, 2006). If there is ambulatory instability, the clinician should assess for diminished or absent position sense, which is associated with increased fall risk. Additional components of the neurologic examination are included in the examination of the perineum, genitalia, and rectum when indicated.

SKIN ASSESSMENT

Skin temperature, turgor, and condition are the main components of this examination. Temperature and turgor reflect hydration, which is of great importance. In addition, general skin assessment includes inspection for significant bruising or lesions. Perineal skin assessment is the main focus; the nurse should assess for redness and denudement consistent with incontinence-associated dermatitis (IAD) and for a maculopapular rash with distinct satellite lesions, consistent with candidiasis. Both are common findings in persons with persistent urinary leakage and individuals managed with containment devices; individuals with combined urinary and fecal incontinence are at even higher risk for skin damage. Skin changes range in severity; mild IAD is characterized by erythema that may be more intense in skin folds, while advanced IAD is characterized by extensive erosion with or without candidiasis (Beeckman et al., 2018; Borchert et al., 2010; Doughty et al., 2012). Chapter 17 elaborates on visual assessment tools available to evaluate the severity of IAD that may be useful depending upon the continence nurses work setting.

ABDOMINAL EXAMINATION

Inspection of the abdomen begins with general observation for symmetry, obvious distension or masses, and skin abnormalities; any pathologic findings should prompt referral for further evaluation (e.g., evidence of hernia or mass, areas of intense erythema, and induration suggestive of abscess). *Auscultation* of bowel sounds should be performed if there are any concerns regarding obstruction or ileus but is not routinely indicated for the individual with UI. *Percussion* is utilized to detect fluid, gaseous distention, stool retention, and masses. The entire abdomen should be lightly percussed with tympany expected throughout most of the abdomen due to the presence of gas in the large and small bowel. Solid masses will produce a dull percussion note as will a distended bladder (Jarvis, 2011).

To assess for bladder distention, the nurse percusses from the xiphoid to the symphysis, noting any change in percussion note; a distended bladder is usually visible and percussible in a thin individual but may be difficult to appreciate in an obese person. In a relatively thin person, percussion can be used to define the outline of the distended bladder. Evidence of bladder distention mandates measurement of postvoid residual (PVR) urine volume, either by catheterization or by ultrasound. Percussion along the length of the colon is helpful in determining the presence or absence of retained stool (fecal loading). As stated, the percussion note along the colon is normally tympanic, due to presence of gas; however, the percussion note over areas of retained stool is dull. Evidence of fecal loading should prompt initiation of a bowel cleansing regimen and bowel management program. Light and deep *palpation* may be performed to assess for hypersensitivity, muscle spasticity, liver or spleen enlargement, and masses. The bladder is not normally palpable on examination unless it is distended with urine, in which case it is felt as a smooth, round, somewhat tense mass (Hull, 2017; Lajiness, 2017).

> **KEY POINT**
>
> The abdominal examination should include percussion to assess for bladder distention and/or fecal loading.

GENITOURINARY EXAMINATION IN MEN

A thorough inspection of the external genitalia and perineal skin should be respectfully performed assessing for skin integrity. *Examination of the penis* includes observation of the absence or presence of the foreskin (circumcised vs. uncircumcised). The foreskin when present should be easily retractable with the glans and urethra easily visualized. The condition of phimosis should be considered when the foreskin is not easily retractable or is difficult to return to normal position. The urethra should be midline on the glans and patent with intact skin integrity. Urethral discharge, redness, or irritation should be further investigated. The presence of urethral stricture or hypospadias requires further assessment to rule out voiding dysfunction and urinary retention (Lajiness, 2017). (Hypospadias is a congenital condition in which the opening of the urethra is located on the underside of the penis rather than on the glans.)

In older men, atrophic changes, including penile retraction, may be evident. The *scrotum* should be inspected for areas of diffuse or localized redness, excoriations, or ulcerations. It is appropriate for continence nurses to perform a *testicular examination* assessing for

symmetry, masses, swelling, or tenderness. Any positive findings should be referred for further evaluation. In individuals with a previous history of infections, the advanced practice registered nurse (APRN) may expand the examination by palpating the epididymis in each testicle. Previous infections may present as fibrosis or scarring and can be a contributing factor in individuals with long-standing detrusor–sphincter dyssynergia or prostatitis resulting in bladder outlet obstruction (Gray, 2006; Lajiness, 2017).

GENITOURINARY EXAMINATION IN WOMEN

The examination begins with inspection of the external genitalia. Hair pattern, skin condition of the perineum (e.g., presence of lesions, scars, rashes, erythema, discharge, or discoloration), and size and shape of the labia majora are observed. Diminished size of the clitoris and labia majora is consistent with aging and hypoestrogenic effects. Tissues that are pale, thin, dry, or fissured are indicative of significant atrophic changes due to estrogen deficiency. Palpation of the area includes separation of the labia majora to inspect and palpate the labia minora. Atrophic changes include diminution in size of the labia and, in some cases, fusion of the tissues. The urethral meatus should be inspected for relaxation or gaping, redness, or discharge. In some cases, urinary leakage may be readily observable when the woman bears down or changes position; this signifies major sphincter dysfunction. Atrophic changes may include a urethral caruncle, a cherry red protruding (prolapsed) urethral meatus. The introitus to the vagina should be assessed for narrowing, erythema, adhesions, and stenosis (Hull, 2017).

The woman should be asked to bear down, and the nurse should observe for an observable bulge or protrusion of tissue that extends to the introitus or beyond; this is indicative of pelvic organ prolapse (addressed in detail in Chapter 12). The vaginal and vulvar tissues may be tender or sensitive due to irritation or dryness caused by a decline in estrogen levels. Vaginal discharge is generally not present in postmenopausal women and should be investigated further if observed. A change in vaginal discharge, odor, and itching should be further investigated in all sexually active women regardless of age as vaginitis and/or sexually transmitted infections can contribute to irritative bladder symptoms (Hull, 2017; Robinson & Cardozo, 2011; Schulling & Likis, 2013).

> **KEY POINT**
>
> Pelvic examination in women should include assessment for atrophic changes (thinning and drying of the vaginal mucosa, urethral caruncle), pelvic organ prolapse, and pelvic muscle strength and endurance.

Digital vaginal examination is done to assess pelvic muscle tone and sensation; the advanced practice continence nurse also conducts a bimanual examination to evaluate pelvic organ structures. The nurse gently inserts one or two gloved fingers into the vagina and asks the woman if she is able to feel the presence of the finger in the vagina. The woman is then asked to contract the vaginal muscles around the examiner's finger as if trying to stop her urine stream or keep from passing gas. This allows the nurse to determine the individual's ability to identify, isolate, contract, and relax the pelvic floor muscles. In addition, the nurse can observe for use of accessory muscles (such as abdominal and buttocks muscles) and the presence of hypertonus or muscle spasm. Pelvic muscle tone, accessory muscle use, and muscle hypertonus/spasm can all be scored using the Oxford grading system, an internationally accepted muscle grading system (Laycock, 1994; Messelink, et al., 2005) (**Box 4-3**). This assessment of pelvic muscle strength provides an excellent opportunity for the nurse to teach and provide feedback regarding the performance of pelvic muscle exercises. The digital vaginal examination also presents an opportunity to further palpate for pelvic organ prolapse. With one to two fingers in the vagina, the nurse can ask the woman to bear down and can palpate for any descent of the bladder (cystocele), uterus (uterine prolapse), or rectum (rectocele) into the vaginal vault (Hull, 2017). When these structural changes are identified, the woman should be referred for further evaluation. All continence nurse specialists providing continence assessment should be able to provide inspection and palpation of the external genitalia and vagina including pelvic muscle tone (**Box 4-3**).

BOX 4-3   PELVIC FLOOR MUSCLE ASSESSMENT

Scale for Grading Digital Evaluation of Pelvic Muscle Strength

(Check one)_____Vaginal Examination_____Rectal Examination

SCALE	GRADE	DESCRIPTION
None	0	No discernable muscle contraction, pressure, and/or displacement of examiner's finger
Flicker	1/5	Trace but instant contraction <1 second, very slight compression of examiner's finger
Weak	2/5	Weak contraction or pressure with or without elevation/lifting of examiner's finger, held for >1 second but <3 seconds
Moderate	3/5	Moderate contraction or compression of examiner's finger with or without elevation/lifting of finger, held for at least 4–6 seconds, repeated 3 times
Firm	4/5	Firm contraction with good compression of examiner's finger with elevation/lifting of finger toward the pubic bone, held for at least 7–9 seconds, repeated 4–5 times
Strong	5/5	Unmistakable strong contraction and grip of examiner's finger with posterior elevation/lifting of finger, held at least 10 seconds, repeated 4–5 times

Use of Accessory Muscle Groups

Abdominal	_____Yes	_____No
Gluteal	_____Yes	_____No
Thigh/Abductor	_____Yes	_____No

Evaluation during Examination—Muscle Hypertonus/Spasm

0	No pressure or pain
1	Comfortable pressure
2	Uncomfortable pressure
3	Moderate pain that interferes with muscle contraction
4	Severe pain; patient unable to perform muscle contraction because of pain

Based on Oxford Grading System (Laycock, 1994; Messelink et al., 2005).

APRN GENITOURINARY EXAMINATION

The APRN has additional health assessment skills that include the vaginal speculum and pelvic examination. It is important for APRNs performing this part of the examination to be competent in pelvic examination in order to ensure accuracy and to reduce the risk of inadvertent pain with speculum insertion. The speculum examination is used to visualize the vaginal tissues and the cervix, and the size and type of speculum should be selected based on clinical presentation of the vagina. For example, in multiparous women or obese women, the larger Graves speculum will likely allow for better visualization, while the smaller and narrower Pederson or pediatric speculum may be required for nulliparous or postmenopausal women.

Following insertion of the speculum into the vagina, the vaginal tissue is assessed for rugae, color, moisture, and flexibility. An absence of vaginal rugae and the presence of tissue thinning and dryness are all consistent with vaginal atrophy due to estrogen deficiency. The cervix may or may not be present depending on surgical history; if present, paleness and retraction into the pelvic floor are also common findings consistent with atrophy and hypoestrogenism. The vaginal pH can be determined by touching litmus paper to the lower third of the vaginal wall; an alkaline pH in postmenopausal women is consistent with estrogen deficiency. If obtaining a vaginal culture, the swab is taken from the posterior vaginal vault. In order to assess for anterior vaginal compartment descent, gently place a closed speculum or using just the posterior blade, apply pressure to the posterior wall of the vagina and then ask the woman to bear down; bulging of the anterior wall may be an indicator of urethral hypermobility and/or cystocele. The diagnosis of stress UI is supported by an observable loss of urine during the maneuver. The APRN can then gently rotate the position of the speculum blade so that it is now stabilizing the anterior vaginal wall to assess the posterior compartment. The woman should again be asked to bear down while the nurse observes for bulging of the posterior vaginal wall consistent with rectocele.

Throughout both procedures, descent of the cervix into the vaginal vault may be observed and can be more specifically assessed by placing the speculum blades in the distal vaginal vault and asking the woman to bear down (Gray, 2006; Hull, 2017; Laycock, 1994; Messelink et al., 2005; Schulling & Likis, 2013). The Baden-Walker system is a five-point grading system for pelvic organ prolapse that is in widespread use and is summarized in **Table 4-2** (Newman & Wein, 2009).

Following removal of the speculum, the bimanual examination is performed to assess the internal pelvic organs. With the first two fingers of the dominant hand inserted into the vagina and the nondominant hand

TABLE 4-2 BADEN-WALKER FIVE-POINT SYSTEM FOR GRADING PELVIC ORGAN PROLAPSE

GRADE	AMOUNT OF PROLAPSE
0	No prolapse
1	Prolapse descends or bulges halfway down to the hymen/vaginal opening
2	Descent of the prolapse to the hymen/vaginal opening
3	Prolapse protrudes halfway from the hymen/vaginal opening
4	Maximal descent: the vagina with the vaginal vault and uterus protrudes completely outside the body without a Valsalva maneuver Procidentia: the most severe form of prolapse

Adapted from Newman, D. K. (2009). *Managing and treating urinary incontinence* (2nd ed.). Baltimore, MD: Health Professions Press.

positioned on the abdomen, the presence or absence of pelvic organs should be discerned. Uterine position, size, shape, and consistency should be assessed. The presence of uterine position in relation to the bladder should be determined as uterine enlargement or displacement can put pressure on the bladder, thus affecting voiding. The adnexa should be assessed for palpable masses, fullness, or tenderness with a rectal–vaginal examination completing the examination.

RECTAL EXAMINATION

The rectal examination is an essential component of the continence assessment for men as it is the only approach to evaluate pelvic muscle strength; it is also essential for women with coexisting fecal incontinence (Hull, 2017; Lajiness, 2017). For women with UI but no issues with fecal incontinence, it is not as critical but does provide the opportunity to more fully assess for anal sphincter/pelvic muscle strength, masses, and the presence of stool impaction (Gray, 2006; Hull, 2017). In addition, inspection of the perianal skin may reveal the presence of external hemorrhoids and anal fissures as well as anal irritation or skin changes. Determination of perineal sensation in relation to light touch as well as differentiation of sharp and dull stimuli can be included when there is concern regarding altered neurologic function. Inspection of the anus for prolapse, gaping, or incomplete closure is important in identifying issues related to bowel evacuation and is usually indicative of neurologic dysfunction (Hull, 2017; Lajiness, 2017). The presence of the bulbocavernosus reflex (BCR) and anal reflex (anal wink) indicates intact neurologic pathways between the motor neurons in the sacral spinal cord and the pelvic muscles (Kirshblum & Eren, 2020; Previnaire, 2018). The BCR can be assessed on digital rectal examination (DRE) or through anal observation. In both situations, the reflex is stimulated by gently tapping the clitoris in women or squeezing the glans of the penis in men. On DRE, contraction is felt, whereas on anal observation, the contraction or "wink" is visualized.

The BCR, while helpful, is a somewhat limited test in that it only tests gross neurologic function. The "anal wink" or anal reflex may be assessed to detect intact pudendal nerve pathways that innervate the pelvic floor muscles, external anal and urethral sphincters (Possover & Forman, 2012; Previnaire, 2018). This reflex may be assessed in both men and women by gently stroking next to the anus bilaterally (5 o'clock and 7 o'clock positions) with a cotton-tip swab. The anus should reflexively contact or "wink" if pudendal nerve pathways are intact. This reflex may be difficult to assess in obese individuals since the buttocks may be snuggly approximated, limiting visualization of anus and is often absent or diminished in the elderly (Lajiness, 2017). For persons with diminished or absent BCR and anal (wink) reflex, this finding may or may not be significant in relation to urinary problems (Hull, 2017). Gray (2006) recommends that further assessment of neurologic denervation be pursued when additional indicators of neurologic deficits are identified. For example, women with neurologic voiding dysfunction who also have chronic constipation or fecal incontinence and vaginal dryness or dyspareunia not explained by estrogen deficiency should be evaluated for perineal denervation. In men, voiding dysfunction, constipation or fecal incontinence, and erectile or ejaculatory dysfunction are representative of neurologic deficits. In both situations, referral for further neurologic consultation and multichannel urodynamics testing may be indicated (Gray, 2006).

KEY POINT

Rectal examination is an essential component of continence assessment for men as it permits evaluation of pelvic muscle function; it is essential for women who have any coexisting issues with fecal incontinence.

The DRE can be used to test pelvic floor muscle tone in men and in women who are unable to tolerate a vaginal examination (Hull, 2017; Lajiness, 2017). With a single gloved finger inserted into the rectum, the person is asked to contract their rectal muscles around the examiner's finger. The same Oxford grading system can be used to assess pelvic muscle tone on rectal examination (**Box 4-3**). For men, DRE also provides an opportunity to identify the presence and consistency of stool in the rectum and to assess the prostate for size, consistency, and symmetry (Lajiness, 2017). The presence of tenderness or pain on palpation of the prostate raises concerns about prostatitis. Symmetric enlargement of the prostate is consistent with BPH, while asymmetric enlargement is

characteristic of cancer (Lajiness, 2017). The consistency of the prostate is normally rubbery; therefore, a boggy, firm, or hardened prostate warrants further evaluation. Prostate examination is generally considered the purview of the APRN.

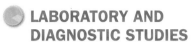

LABORATORY AND DIAGNOSTIC STUDIES

URINALYSIS

A urinalysis is an important component of continence evaluation in those individuals who are exhibiting symptoms of UI, voiding dysfunction, and UTI (Robertson & Hamlin, 2017). Urinalysis can be conducted using urine dipstick or microscopic analysis and is best obtained midstream or clean catch to decrease the likelihood of bacterial contamination. In those individuals who are unable to perform perineal hygiene or obtain a clean catch urine specimen, sterile straight catheterization is an alternative. For best results, the urine should be tested within 15 to 30 minutes or if refrigerated within 2 hours following its collection (Jarvis, 2011; Robertson & Hamlin, 2017).

Components of the UA include specific gravity, pH, glucose, nitrites and leukocytes, hemoglobin, and protein. Specific gravity provides an indicator of the kidneys' ability to concentrate urine. The test is reported as the ratio of the weight of the urine tested to the weight of water. Low specific gravity can be related to excessive fluid intake or to renal tubular dysfunction associated with some metabolic conditions (e.g., diabetes insipidus), while an elevated specific gravity may reflect inadequate fluid intake. The pH of freshly voided urine is normally acidic; alkaline urine is associated with some bacterial UTIs. The presence of glucose is not a normal finding; when glucose is present on UA, the individual should be evaluated for uncontrolled or undiagnosed diabetes mellitus. Nitrites and leukocytes in general should be absent; however, among older adults living in community or institutional settings (e.g., assisted living, nursing homes), there is an increased likelihood for these indicators to be present.

Positive nitrites and leukocytes without urinary symptoms are consistent with asymptomatic bacteriuria (ASB), which does not require treatment (Benton et al., 2006; Henderson et al., 2019; Nicolle et al., 2005). Microscopic analysis should be performed in those individuals in whom symptoms of UTI are present. Hemoglobin should also be negative; positive hemoglobin is consistent with hematuria and infection and should be further evaluated. Negative protein is a normal finding but may be positive when leukocytes are also present. Proteinuria that persists after treatment of infection may be indicative of renal disease, and the individual should be referred for further evaluation.

URINE CULTURE AND SENSITIVITY

This test is done when the UA findings are consistent with UTI, and the patient has symptoms of UTI (Robertson & Hamlin, 2017). Urine in the bladder is normally sterile; when bacteria are present, the urine can be cultured and monitored for bacterial growth. Little to no growth is considered a negative culture, while bacterial growth is microscopically and chemically analyzed to determine the amount and type(s) of bacteria as well as the organisms' sensitivity or resistance to antibiotics that could be used for treatment. Reassessment of UTI symptoms is important after completion of treatment to determine if treatment has been effective. Unresolved symptoms require further workup to determine whether they are caused by persistent UTI or by another type of pathology (see Chapter 14 regarding UTI symptoms in children and Chapter 18 in adults).

POSTVOID RESIDUAL VOLUME

PVR should be measured on anyone at risk for incomplete bladder emptying or urinary retention. Indicators for PVR measurement include the following: signs and symptoms of incomplete emptying (bladder distention on physical examination; sensation of incomplete emptying; urinary hesitancy; straining to void; intermittent or poor stream; postvoid dribbling); history of voiding dysfunction/urinary retention; recurrent UTIs; known or suspected BPH; evidence of pelvic organ prolapse; neurologic conditions; spinal or endocrine disorders; and stool impaction. Antidepressants, antipsychotics, sedatives and hypnotics, alpha-adrenergic agonists, anticholinergics, and calcium channel blockers also increase the risk of urinary retention, and patients taking one or more of these medications should be considered for PVR evaluation (Gray & Moore, 2009; Wooldridge, 2017).

KEY POINT

PVR should be measured on anyone at risk for urinary retention or incomplete bladder emptying.

PVR can be obtained by the use of ultrasound or catheterization and should be done as soon as possible after voiding. Catheterization done by an experienced clinician can be inexpensive and accurate; however, there is a slight risk of UTI associated with the procedure and some individuals experience varying degrees of discomfort (Bolz et al., 2012; Gray, 2006; Gray & Moore, 2009). Ultrasound is more expensive; however, it is less invasive and presents minimal risk of infection or discomfort. Both ultrasound and catheterization are considered accurate PVR methods. There is no clear consensus on a specific PVR volume that signifies urinary retention; however, comparison of the voided amount to the PVR is important in obtaining a clear picture regarding completeness of

bladder emptying. In general, PVRs of 50 to 100 mL are considered on the low end of abnormal (Wooldridge, 2017); typically, these individuals are managed with monitoring and conservative strategies to improve bladder emptying. PVRs that exceed 250 mL are considered significant, and those above 350 mL increase the risk for upper urinary tract dilatation and renal insufficiency (Gray, 2006; Kelly, 2004).

KEY POINT

PVR > 250 mL is considered significant; PVR > 350 mL increases the risk for upper tract dilatation and renal damage.

SERUM STUDIES

There are instances when serum studies are indicated as part of the continence assessment. These studies most commonly include BUN (blood, urea, nitrogen) and creatinine, electrolytes, complete blood count (CBC), fasting blood sugar (FBS), and hemoglobin A1c (Robertson & Hamlin, 2017). Often, the chemistry panel will include all of these measures including the estimated glomerular filtration rate (eGFR), see Table 4-1. Together, these studies provide a snapshot of overall renal and endocrine function. BUN and creatinine should be monitored for elevation caused by medications, metabolic disorders, or voiding dysfunction related to outlet obstruction (e.g., BPH). If upper urinary tract distress is suspected (e.g., recurring pyelonephritis, renal insufficiency), urology consultation is indicated (Gray, 2006). An electrolyte panel may be needed when low specific gravity is noted on UA, there are concerns related to dehydration, or a change in cognition is observed. The CBC provides an overall measurement of white and red blood cell activity. FBS and Hgb A1c are helpful in understanding the individual's blood sugar control at present and retrospectively over the past 3 months, which is essential since elevated and uncontrolled blood sugars play a significant role in voiding dysfunction as well as the development of neuropathy and urinary retention.

The eGFR is helpful in determining how well the kidneys are functioning and is estimated using the individual's creatinine level as well as gender, age, race, and weight. Medications, chronic illness, and upper urinary tract dysfunction can all contribute to an elevation in eGFR; thus, this value should be monitored in these patients. In addition, the eGFR is used to monitor the progression of chronic kidney disease over time and is used to guide decision-making surrounding treatment (National Kidney Foundation, Inc., 2014; **Table 4-3**).

● DATA SYNTHESIS: PULLING IT ALL TOGETHER

Once the key elements of the continence assessment have been completed, the next step is for the continence

TABLE 4-3 GLOMERULAR FILTRATION RATES AND KIDNEY DISEASE

STAGES OF CHRONIC KIDNEY DISEASE		GFR*	% OF KIDNEY FUNCTION
Stage 1	Kidney damage with **normal** kidney function	90 or higher	90–100%
Stage 2	Kidney damage with **mild loss** of kidney function	89–60	89–60%
Stag 3a	**Mild to moderate** loss of kidney function	59–45	59–45%
Stage 3b	**Moderate to severe** loss of kidney function	44–30	44–30%
Stag 4	**Severe** loss of kidney function	29–15	29–15%
Stag 5	Kidney **failure**	<15	Less than 15%

*Your GFR number tells you how much kidney function you have. As kidney disease gets worse, the GFR number goes down.
Stages of Chronic Kidney Disease, GFR and Percentage of Kidney Function National Kidney Foundation. 2018. https://www.kidney.org/atoz/content/gfr

nurse to determine the diagnosis using data collected from the focused history, physical, bladder diary, and laboratory tests. Type(s) of UI and related voiding dysfunction should be identified along with factors that could worsen symptoms or interfere with treatment and management. These findings should be reviewed with the individual and the goals of care prioritized in joint discussion. Based on input from the patient, an individualized, patient-centered plan of care should be developed that includes treatment and management options as well as the goals for care. Discussion of barriers in following the prescribed plan of care need to be explored, that is health literacy, cultural, educational, financial, physical, emotional or psychosocial disparities (Nix et al., 2016). Patient education should be provided along with support for any needed lifestyle and health behavior changes. Designing patient education materials that are one page, easy to read (font size 10 to 14), and at an eight-grade reading level should emphasize critical information the patient needs to know "now" rather than "nice to know" (Nix et al., 2016). In addition, offering educational materials in patient preferred formats may improve patient education, that is brochures, YouTube videos, DVDs, smartphone apps, demonstrations, or group classes. Studies show that patients forget 80% what the health care provider tells them at face to face encounters so lean on reliable health technology (Heath, 2017). Ensuring patients are knowledgeable regarding the type of incontinence or voiding dysfunction, treatment recommendations and their role in following the plan of care will enhance health literacy and adherence. With the patient's permission, it may be helpful to include family members and/or caregivers in this process as well. Strategies to improve patient and family engagement include (1) assess patient health literacy (ability to obtain, process, and understand basic health-related information through AHRQ [Agency for Healthcare Research and Quality] resources), (2) employ patient "teach-back" (patient repeats the instructions in their own words or demonstrates procedure), (3) develop educational resources that define key terms, ideas, and contains written instructions, (4) teach relevant information and the benefit, (5) provide time at end of each encounter for questions to reinforce and repeat information, and (6) timely follow-up (Heath, 2017; Rolstad, 2020). Recommendations for monitoring and follow-up should be determined, and referrals for further consultation should be made. Communication with the patient, the family, the primary provider, and other members of the health care team completes the assessment process. Mutually agreed-upon goals should be included in the overall plan of care to promote patient engagement and adherence.

CONCLUSION

Continence nurses are in prime positions to assess UI and voiding dysfunction and to develop patient-centered plans of care that treat and manage symptoms, reduce risk, and improve overall quality of life. Critical elements of assessment include a patient history and review of systems, focused physical examination, completion and assessment of a bladder diary, and selected diagnostic procedures (e.g., UA and PVR). A comprehensive assessment provides the data needed to determine the type of incontinence or voiding dysfunction and appropriate evidence-based treatment options or to identify the need for referrals for additional workup or for medical–surgical intervention.

REFERENCES

American College of Obstetrics & Gynecology (ACOG). (2019). Pelvic organ prolapse: ACOG practice Bulletin, Number 214. *Obstetrics & Gynecology, 134*(5), e126–e142.

American Geriatrics Society 2019 Beers Criteria Update Expert Panel. (2019). American Geriatrics Society 2019 updated AGS Beers Criteria for potentially inappropriate medication use in older adults. *Journal of the American Geriatric Society, 67*(4), 674–694.

Angelini, K. (2017). Effect of physical activity on urinary incontinence in women: Implications for providers. *Women's Healthcare, 5*(3), 36–40.

Beeckman, D., Van den Bussche, K., & Alves, P. (2018). Towards an international language for incontinence-associated dermatitis (IAD): Design and evaluation of psychometric properties of the Ghent Global IAD Categorization Tool (GLOBIAD) in 30 countries. *British Journal of Dermatology, 178*(6), 1331–1340.

Benton, T., Young, R., & Leeper, S. (2006). Asymptomatic bacteriuria in the nursing home. *Annals of Long-Term Care: Clinical Care and Aging, 14*(7), 17–22.

Bolz, M., Capezuti, E., Fulmer, T., et al. (2012). *Evidence-based geriatric nursing protocols for best practice* (4th ed.). New York, NY: Springer Publishing Co.

Borchert, K., Bliss, D. Z., Savik, K., et al. (2010). The incontinence-associated dermatitis and its severity instrument: Development and validation. *Journal of Wound, Ostomy, and Continence Nursing, 37*(5), 527–535.

Brown, J. S., Vittinghoff, E., Wyman, J. F., et al. (2000). Urinary incontinence: Does it increase risk for falls and fractures? *Journal of the American Geriatrics Society, 48*, 721–725.

Diokno, A., Burgio, E., Arnold, P., et al. (2000). Epidemiology and natural history of urinary incontinence. *International Urogynecology Journal, 11*, 301–319.

Doerflinger, D. (2013). Mental status assessment of older adults: The Mini-Cog. *Try this: Best practices in nursing care of older adults*. The Hartford Foundation. Retrieved from http://consultgerirn.org/uploads/File/trythis/try_this_3.pdf

Doughty, D., Junkin, J., Kurz, P., et al. (2012). Incontinence-associated dermatitis consensus statements, evidence-based guidelines for prevention and treatment, and current challenges. *Journal of Wound Ostomy & Continence Nursing, 39*(3), 303–315.

Dowling-Castronovo, A., & Spiro, E. (2013). *Urinary incontinence assessment in older adults: Part II—Established urinary incontinence. Best practices in geriatric nursing*. The Hartford Institute for Geriatric Nursing, 11, 2. Retrieved from http://consultgerirn.org/uploads/File/trythis/try_this_11_2.pdf

DuBeau, C., Kuchel, G., Johnson, T., et al. (2010). Incontinence in the frail elderly: Report from the 4th International Consultation on Incontinence. *Neurourology and Urodynamics, 29*(1), 165–178.

DuBeau, C., Simon, S., & Morris, J. N. (2006). The effect of urinary incontinence on quality of life in older nursing home residents. *Journal of the American Geriatrics Society, 54*(9), 1325–1333.

Graf, C. (2013). The Lawton Instrumental Activities of Daily Living (IADL) Scale. *Try this: Best practices in nursing care of older adults*. The

Hartford Foundation. Retrieved from http://consultgerirn.org/uploads/File/trythis/try_this_23.pdf

Gray, M. (2006). Assessment of the patient with urinary incontinence or voiding dysfunction. In D. Doughty (Ed.), *Urinary and fecal incontinence: Current management concepts* (3rd ed.). St. Louis, MO: Mosby Elsevier.

Gray, M., & Moore, K. N. (2009). Urinary incontinence. In M. Gray & K. N. Moore (Eds.), *Urologic disorders: Adult and pediatric care* (pp. 119–159). St. Louis, MO: Mosby Elsevier.

Greenberg, S. (2011). Assessment of fear of falling in older adults: The Falls Efficacy Scale-International (FES-1). *Try this: Best practices in nursing care of older adults.* The Hartford Foundation. Retrieved from http://consultgerirn.org/uploads/File/trythis/try_this_29.pdf

Greenberg, S. (2012). The Geriatric Depression Scale (GDS). *Try this: Best practices in nursing care of older adults.* The Hartford Foundation. Retrieved from http://consultgerirn.org/uploads/File/trythis/try_this_4.pdf

Greenblum, C., Greenblum, J., & Neff, D. (2008). Vaginal estrogen use in menopause: Is it safe? *American Journal for Nurse Practitioners, 13*(9), 26–34.

Heath, S. (2017). 4 patient education strategies that drive patient activation. Patient Data Access News, Patient Engagement HIT. Retrieved from https://patientengagementhit.com/news/4-patient-education-strategies-that-drive-patient-activation

Henderson, J. T., Webber, E. M., & Bean, S. (2019). Screening for asymptomatic bacteriuria in adults: Updated evidence report and systematic review for the U.S. Preventive Services Task Force. *JAMA, 322*(12), 1195–1205. doi: 10.1001/jama.2019.10060.

Hendrich, A. (2013). Fall risk assessment in older adults: The Hendrich II Fall Risk Model. *Try this: Best practices in nursing care of older adults.* The Hartford Foundation. Retrieved from http://consultgerirn.org/uploads/File/trythis/try_this_8.pdf

Hull, M. A. (2017). Assessment of women. In D. K. Newman, J. F. Wyman, & V. W. Welch (Eds.), *Core curriculum for urological nursing* (pp. 235–246). Pittman, NJ: SUNA.

Jarvis, C. (2011). *Physical examination and health assessment* (6th ed.). St. Louis, MO: Elsevier.

Jayasekara, R. (2009). Urinary incontinence: Evaluation. *JBI Database Evidence Summaries*, Publication ES-610.

Kelly, C. (2004). Evaluation of voiding dysfunction and measurement of bladder volume. *Reviews in Urology, 6*(Supp1), 532–537.

Kinsberg, S. A., Kellogg, S., & Krychman, M. (2009). Treating dyspareunia caused by vaginal atrophy: A review of treatment options using vaginal estrogen therapy. *International Journal of Women's Health, 1*, 105–111.

Kirshblum, S., & Eren, F. (2020). Anal reflex versus bulbocavernosus reflex in evaluation of patients with spinal cord injury. *Spinal Cord Series and Cases, 6*, 2. doi: 10.1038/s41394-019-0251-3.

Krieg, C. B. (2017). Urologic signs and symptoms. In D. K. Newman, J. F. Wyman, & V. W. Welch (Eds.), *Core Curriculum for Urological Nursing* (pp. 225–234). Pittman, NJ: SUNA.

Lajiness, M. J. (2017). Assessment of men. In D. K. Newman, J. F. Wyman, & V. W. Welch (Eds.), *Core curriculum for urological nursing* (pp. 247–255). Pittman, NJ: SUNA.

Lamerton, T. J., Torquati, L., & Brown, W. J. (2018). Overweight and obesity as major modifiable risk factors for urinary incontinence in young to mid-aged women: A systematic review and meta-analysis. *Obesity Reviews, 19*(12), 1735–1745. doi: 10.1111/obr.12756.

Laycock, J. (1994). Clinical evaluation of the pelvic floor. In B. Schussler, J. Laycock, P. Norton, et al. (Eds.), *Pelvic floor re-education: Principles and practice* (pp. 42–48). London, UK: Springer-Verlag.

Lekan-Rutledge, D. (2004). Urinary incontinence strategies for frail elderly women. *Urologic Nursing, 24*(4), 281–301.

Lemack, G., & Zimmern, P. (1999). Predictability of urodynamic findings based on the Urogenital Distress Inventory-6 questionnaire. *Urology, 54*(3), 461–466.

Mathias, S., Nayak, U. S. L., & Isaacs, B. (1986). Balance in elderly patients: The "get-up and go" test. *Archives of Physical Medicine and Rehabilitation, 67*, 387–389.

Messelink, B., Benson, T., Berghamans, B., et al. (2005). Standardization of terminology of pelvic floor muscle function and dysfunction: Report from the pelvic floor clinical assessment group of the International Continence Society. *Neurourology & Urodynamics, 24*, 374–380.

Molony, S., & Greenberg, S. (2013). The 2012 American Geriatrics Society updated Beers Criteria for potentially inappropriate medication use in older adult. *Try this: Best practices in nursing care of older adults.* The Hartford Foundation. Retrieved from http://consultgerirn.org/uploads/File/trythis/try_this_16.pdf

Moore, K. N. (2006). Urinary retention. In D. Doughty (Ed.), *Urinary and fecal incontinence: Current management concepts* (3rd ed.). St. Louis, MO: Mosby Elsevier.

Moore, K. N., Dumoulin, C., Bradley, C., et al. (2013). Adult conservative management. In P. H. Abrams, L. Cardoza, A. E. Khoury, et al. (Eds.), *5th International consultation on incontinence* (5th ed., pp. 1–200). London, UK: European Association of Urology. ISBN: 978-9953-493-21-3.

Moore, K. N., & Jensen, L. (2000). Testing of the Incontinence Impact Questionnaire (IIQ-7) with men after radical prostatectomy. *Journal of Wound Ostomy & Continence Nursing, 27*(6), 304–312.

Morris, V., & Wagg, A. (2007). Lower urinary tract symptoms, incontinence and falls in elderly people: Time for an intervention study. *International Journal of Clinical Practice, 61*, 320–323.

National Kidney Foundation, Inc. (2014). Frequently asked questions about GFR estimates. Retrieved from http://www.kidney.org/sites/default/files/docs/12-10-4004_abe_faqs_aboutgfrrey1b_singleb.pdf

Newman, D., & Wein, A. (2009). *Managing and treating incontinence* (2nd ed.). Baltimore, MD: Health Professionals Press.

Nicolle, L., Bradley, S., Colgan, R., et al. (2005). Infectious Disease Society of America guidelines for diagnosis and treatment of asymptomatic bacteriuria in adults. *Clinical Infectious Diseases, 40*(5), 643.

Nix, D. P., Peirce, B., & Haugen, V. (2016). Eliminating non-compliance. In R. A. Bryant & D. P. Nix (Eds.), *Acute and chronic wounds: Current management concepts* (5th ed., pp. 428–440). St. Louis, MO: Elsevier.

North American Menopause Society. (2017). The 2017 Hormone therapy position statement of The North American Menopause Society. *Menopause, 24*(7), 728–753. doi: 10.1097/GME.0000000000000921. Retrieved from https://www.menopause.org/docs/default-source/2017/nams-2017-hormone-therapy-position-statement.pdf

Offermans, M., du Moulin, M., Hamers, J., et al. (2009). Prevalence of urinary incontinence and associated risk factors in nursing home residents: A systematic review. *Neurourology and Urodynamics, 28*(4), 288–294.

Palmer, M. (1996). *Urinary incontinence assessment and promotion.* Gaithersburg, MD: Aspen.

Possover, M., & Forman, A. (2012). Voiding dysfunction associated with pudendal nerve entrapment. *Current Bladder Dysfunction Reports, 7*(4), 281–285. doi: 10.1007/s11884-012-0156-5.

Previnaire, J. G. (2018). The importance of the bulbocavernosus reflex. *Spinal Cord Series and Cases, 4*, 2. doi: 10.1038/s41394-017-0012-0.

Robertson, T. M., & Hamlin, A. S. (2017). Laboratory tests. In D. K. Newman, J. F. Wyman, & V. W. Welch (Eds.), *Core curriculum for urological nursing* (pp. 257–267). Pittman, NJ: SUNA.

Robinson, D., & Cardozo, L. (2011). Estrogens and the lower urinary tract. *Neurourology and Urodynamics, 30*, 754–757.

Robinson, J. P., & Shea, J. A. (2002). Development and testing of a measure of health-related quality of life for men with urinary incontinence. *Journal of the American Geriatrics Society, 50*(5), 935–945.

Rolstad, B. S. (2020). *Education and adaptation across the scopes.* WEB WOC® Nursing Education Program.

Schulling, K. D., & Likis, F. E. (2013). *Women's gynecologic health* (2nd ed.). Burlington, MA: Jones & Bartlett Learning.

Shamliyan, T., Wyman, J., Bliss, D., et al. (2007). Prevention of urinary and fecal incontinence in adults. *Evidence Report/Technology Assessment (Full Rep)*, (161), 1–379.

Shelkey, M., & Wallace, V. (2012). Katz index of independence of activities of daily living (ADL). *Try this: Best practice in nursing care of older adults*. The Hartford Foundation. Retrieved from http://consultgerirn.org/uploads/File/trythis/try_this_2.pdf

Shumaker, S. A., Wyman, J. F., Uebersax, J. S., et al. (1994). Health related quality of life measures for women with urinary incontinence: The Incontinence Impact Questionnaire and the Urogenital Distress Inventory. *Quality of Life Research, 3*, 291–306.

Subak, L., Richter, H., & Hunskaar, S. (2009). Obesity and urinary incontinence: Epidemiology and clinical research update. *The Journal of Urology, 182*(6 Suppl), S2–S7.

Thompson, D. L., & Bradway, C. K. (2017). The older urologic patient. In D. K. Newman, J. F. Wyman, & V. W. Welch (Eds.), *Core curriculum for urological nursing* (pp. 709–724). Pittman, NJ: SUNA.

Uebersax, J. S., Wyman, J. F., Shumaker, S. A., et al. (1995). Short forms to assess life quality and symptom distress for urinary incontinence in women: The Incontinence Impact Questionnaire and the Urogenital Distress Inventory. *Neurourology and Urodynamics, 14*, 131–139.

Vahabi, B., Wagg, A. S., Rosier, P., et al. (2017). Can we define and characterize the aging lower urinary tract? ICI-RS 2015. *Neurourology and Urodynamics, 36*(4), 854–858. doi: 10.1002/nau.23035.

Van der Vaart, C. H., De Leeuw, J. R. J., Roovers, J. P., et al. (2003). Measuring health-related quality of life in women with urogenital dysfunction: The Urogenital Distress Inventory and Incontinence Impact Questionnaire revisited. *Neurourology and Urodynamics, 22*, 97–104.

Van Geelen, H., Ostergard, D., & Sand, P. (2018). A review of the impact of pregnancy and childbirth on pelvic floor function as assessed by objective measurement techniques. *International Urogynecology Journal, 29*, 327–338. doi: 10.1007/s00192-017-3540-z.

Vasavada, S. P., & Kim, E. D. (September 23, 2019). Urinary incontinence. *eMedicine*. Retrieved December 11, 2019, from https://emedicine.medscapte.com/article/452289-overview

Wagg, A., Chen, L. K., Johnson, T., et al. (2017). Incontinence in the frail older person. In P. Abrams, L. Cardozo, A. Wagg, et al., (Eds.), *Incontinence* (6th ed., pp. 1311–1442). Bristol, UK: International Continence Society.

Wooldridge, L. S. (2017). Urinary incontinence. In D. K. Newman, J. F. Wyman, & V. W. Welch (Eds.), *Core curriculum for urological nursing* (pp. 467–486). Pittman, NJ: SUNA.

QUESTIONS

1. A continence nurse is assessing older adults in a long-term care facility for urinary incontinence. What age-related change places this population at greater risk for this condition?
A. Increased bladder capacity
B. Benign prostatic hypertrophy in men
C. Increased estrogen production in women
D. Decreased will to remain continent

2. Distinguishing characteristics of onset related to incontinence is an important part of the continence assessment. Which condition would the continence nurse document as transient urinary incontinence as opposed to established urinary incontinence?
A. Stress UI (leakage with activity)
B. Urge UI (leakage associated with urgency)
C. Mixed UI (leakage associated with both activity and urgency)
D. New-onset incontinence in a patient with UTI

3. A patient tells a continence nurse that he is unable to hold his urine and leaks on the way to the bathroom. What type of incontinence would the nurse suspect?
A. Urge UI
B. Stress UI
C. Neurogenic UI
D. Mixed UI

4. Which patient would the continence nurse consider at high risk for detrusor–sphincter dyssynergia?
A. A patient with stress UI
B. A patient with acute diarrhea
C. A patient with neurogenic UI
D. A patient with diabetes mellitus

5. In reviewing the medical history which medical condition would the continence nurse recognize as placing the patient at risk for urinary retention?
A. Fecal impaction
B. Newly diagnosed diabetes mellitus
C. Truncal obesity
D. Hypertension

6. The continence nurse is performing an abdominal examination of a patient with urinary incontinence. Which assessment technique would the nurse use to detect fluid, gaseous distention, stool retention, and masses?
A. Inspection
B. Auscultation
C. Palpation
D. Percussion

7. The continence nurse is performing a genitourinary examination of a 68-year-old female who is experiencing stress UI. Which finding is *NOT* an expected age-related condition?

A. Diminished size of the clitoris
B. Observable bulge extending to the introitus or beyond
C. Tissues that are pale, thin, and/or dry
D. Lack of vaginal moisture

8. A continence nurse examining a female patient for pelvic muscle strength documents the following findings: trace but instant contraction <1 second, very slight compression of examiner's finger. What grade would the nurse document?
A. 0
B. 1/5
C. 2/5
D. 4/5

9. When assessing quality of life, which validated tool would be appropriate for the continence nurse to select?
A. The Mini-cog
B. Get Up and Go Test
C. Urinary Distress Inventory (UDI-6)
D. Patient Health Questionnaire (PHQ-9)

10. Which test finding indicates to the continence nurse the possibility of inadequate fluid intake in a patient?
A. Elevated specific gravity
B. Bacteria present in the urine
C. Postvoid residual volume exceeding 250 mL
D. Nitrites and leukocytes present in the urine

ANSWERS AND RATIONALES

1. B. Rationale: The continence nurse should be alert to changes associated with aging that can affect continence and voiding: reduced bladder capacity, benign prostatic hypertrophy (BPH) in men, and loss of estrogen in postmenopausal women.

2. D. Rationale: Transient UI or voiding dysfunction is considered acute and generally reversible, while established or UI or voiding dysfunction is described as chronic or persistent.

3. A. Rationale: Persons with urge UI often report they are unable to hold their urine and leak on the way to the bathroom; they typically report frequency and nocturia as well as urgency.

4. C. Rationale: Neurogenic lower urinary tract dysfunction (NLUTD) is caused by a neurologic lesion (spinal cord injury or multiple sclerosis) that disrupts the neurologic pathways that provide voluntary control of voiding and are at risk for detrusor–sphincter dyssynergia, which means loss of coordination between the detrusor and the sphincter.

5. A. Rationale: Severe constipation and fecal impaction can cause urethral compression and bladder outlet obstruction leading to urgency, frequency, and even urinary retention.

6. D. Rationale: *Percussion* is utilized to detect fluid, gaseous distention, stool retention, and masses.

7. B. Rationale: An observable vaginal bulge at or beyond the introitus is NOT a normal age-related change. The rest of the answers are age-related changes that can affect continence and voiding in women.

8. B. Rationale: Based upon the Oxford Grading System, a flicker or trace of a pelvic muscle contraction <1 second is graded 1 out of 5 scale of strength.

9. C. Rationale: Urinary Distress Inventory (UDI-6) and Incontinence Impact Questionnaire-7 (IIQ-7) evaluate how incontinence is impacting the patient's quality of life issues. See Table 4-1.

10. A. Rationale: Specific gravity test is reported as the ratio of the weight of the urine tested to the weight of water. An elevated specific gravity may reflect recent inadequate fluid intake while a low specific gravity can be related to excessive fluid intake or some metabolic conditions (e.g., diabetes insipidus).

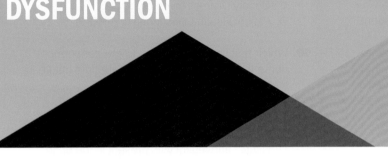

CHAPTER 5

ADVANCED ASSESSMENT OF THE PATIENT WITH URINARY INCONTINENCE AND VOIDING DYSFUNCTION

Tamara Dickinson

OBJECTIVES

1. Identify goals for advanced assessment of the patient with urinary incontinence and voiding dysfunction.
2. Describe indications for urodynamic testing.
3. Identify basic interpretation of urodynamic findings.
4. Name basic components of urodynamic testing.

TOPIC OUTLINE

Evaluation and management of lower urinary tract dysfunction requires a carefully obtained history and a thorough physical exam. Even with carefully doned patient interview and physical assessment skills, the clinical diagnosis may be unclear and more advanced assessment may be required. Advanced assessment may include laboratory studies, endoscopic procedures, radiologic evaluation, and/or urodynamic studies (Hanno et al., 2007; Winters et al., 2012). Urodynamic studies are of particular value in evaluation of lower urinary tract function and will be the focus of this chapter.

The goal of urodynamics is to reproduce the patient's symptoms in an effort to provide a clearer clinical diagnosis. Urodynamic testing evaluates the filling and voiding phases of the micturition cycle and provides information regarding the functionality of the lower urinary tract. Specifically it evaluates the bladder's ability to store urine at low pressures and to empty effectively, and evaluates the ability of the sphincter to maintain closure during filling and to open for voiding.

INDICATIONS

Urodynamic testing is invasive and relatively expensive in the United States, and the quality of the studies is largely dependent on the skill of the urodynamicist and requires clear clinical indications critical for its use (Rosier et al., 2016). This has remained a controversial topic in the field in the United States, so much so that the American Urologic Association (AUA) and the Society of Urodynamics, Female Pelvic Medicine and Urogenital Reconstruction (SUFU) reviewed the literature and developed guidelines to assist clinicians in determining which patients should undergo urodynamic testing (**Box 5-1**) (Rosier et al., 2016; Winters et al., 2012).

KEY POINT

The goal of urodynamics is to reproduce the patient's symptoms in an effort to provide a clearer clinical diagnosis.

 OVERVIEW AND DESCRIPTION

Urodynamics is a broad term that involves several components to evaluate the lower urinary tract and, combined, to create a picture of its functional status. Conventional urodynamic testing is performed in a clinical setting; the test involves filling the bladder in an artificial and retrograde manner and then having the patient void while bladder pressures and urinary flow are measured (Rosier et al., 2016). The specific components included in urodynamic testing are described in **Table 5-1**.

A patient who is to undergo urodynamic testing should be given written information about what will occur during the test. Specifically, the patient should know that a small catheter will be placed into the bladder and a small balloon-tipped tube will be placed into the rectum to measure pressures within the bladder and the abdomen and that the bladder will be slowly filled and then he/she will be asked to urinate into a special commode. (A sample patient fact sheet to explain urodynamic testing is available at https://suna.org/download/members/urodynamics.pdf) The patient should be assured that typically testing is not painful and should be instructed to arrive with a comfortably full bladder. Urodynamic testing should not be a traumatic event for the patient; the clinician should be skilled at providing a calming environment. This is critical not only because it minimizes stress for the patient but also because it impacts significantly on the accuracy of the test results. Postprocedure, patients may experience mild dysuria and possibly some mild hematuria and should be encouraged to increase fluid intake for approximately 24 hours postprocedure.

Testing should *not* be performed in the presence of a urinary tract infection, because the accuracy of the results can be compromised. Screening for infection should be done prior to the procedure. It is controversial whether or not periprocedural antibiotics should be used and there is a lack of evidence to support the use of periprocedural antibiotics (Hirakauva et al., 2017).

TABLE 5-1 URODYNAMIC TESTS	
URODYNAMICS COMPONENT	**DESCRIPTION**
Uroflowmetry	The noninvasive measurement of the flow of urine over time
Simple cystometrogram	The measurement of bladder pressure (Pves) in response to being filled
Complex cystometrogram	The measurement of bladder pressure (Pves) and estimated abdominal pressure (Pabd) to estimate detrusor pressure (Pdet)
Pressure flow study	The measurement of Pves, Pabd, and Pdet while voiding to assess pressure and flow relationships
Valsalva leak point pressure	The measurement of the amount of abdominal force needed to cause leakage across the urethral sphincter
Electromyography	Study of pelvic floor muscle activity during filling and voiding
Urethral pressure profile	Study measuring pressures and landmarks along the length of the urethra

BOX 5-1   AUA/SUFU GUIDELINE SUMMARY

- Stress urinary incontinence/prolapse: Assess urethral function, postvoid residual, and occult urinary incontinence in the presence of high-grade prolapse.
- Overactive bladder, urge urinary incontinence, mixed urinary incontinence: Assess for evidence of altered compliance and evidence of bladder outlet obstruction (BOO).
- Neurogenic bladder: Assess postvoid residual and perform multichannel urodynamics including pressure flow studies and electromyography as part of a baseline evaluation (with or without symptoms), when symptoms change and when there is concern of upper tract compromise.
- Lower urinary tract symptoms: Assess postvoid residual and uroflowmetry initially and during routine follow-up, and assess pressure flow studies for evidence of obstruction when invasive treatments are considered.

Data from Winters et al. (2012).

KEY POINT

Urodynamic testing should not be a traumatic event for the patient; the clinician should be skilled at providing a calming environment.

UROFLOWMETRY

Uroflowmetry involves measurement of the rate of urine flow over time and is measured in milliliters/second. It is noninvasive and is often used as an initial screening tool for lower urinary tract (voiding) dysfunction (Rosier et al., 2016). Patients are instructed to arrive with a comfortably full bladder as they are able. The patient urinates into a commode with a funnel that utilizes a weight and force sensing transducer or a rotating disk style sensor to measure the rate of urine flow. The patient should be given adequate privacy and instructions about the uroflow commode and should be asked to void as normally as possible. Once the patient voids into the uroflow commode, a bladder scanner can be used to obtain a noninvasive postvoid residual volume; the combination of uroflow and postvoid residual provides a complete screening assessment of the emptying phase of the micturition cycle. These tests can also be used to evaluate the response to treatment of urinary retention, either medical or surgical.

Normal uroflowmetry should be a bell-shaped curve. Abnormal uroflowmetry manifests as intermittent or uneven bursts of flow, or a low velocity flat flow rate; however, the clinician must remember that abnormal results can also be the result of low voided volumes. This is the reason for preparing patients for the test by instructing them to come to the clinic with a full bladder. **Figure 5-1A** depicts a normal voiding pattern, and **Figure 5-1B** indicates a uroflow from a patient with probable voiding dysfunction or bladder outlet obstruction (BOO). The area under each curve represents the volume of urine voided.

> ### KEY POINT
> Normal uroflowmetry should be a bell-shaped curve. Normal values vary depending upon sex and age. Women have minimal change with age while men's flow rates decline with age.

An abnormal uroflow such as that in **Figure 5-1B** suggests problems with bladder emptying, but it does not provide enough information to determine the clinical cause, that is, reduced bladder contractility versus BOO (Rosier et al., 2016). Consistently low voided volumes and low flow rates can be indicative of decreased detrusor contractility, increased outlet resistance, overactive detrusor, or a combination of these factors, and further urodynamic testing is indicated to confirm the diagnosis (Hanno et al., 2007; Hashim et al., 2019). Obstruction that is constrictive such as a urethral stricture typically creates a plateau pattern, whereas obstruction caused by prostatic hypertrophy usually creates a compressed pattern that tapers off at the end (Rosier et al., 2016) (**Figs. 5-2 and 5-3**). However, these patterns may also be produced by a weak detrusor contraction. Intermittent bursts of flow can be caused by detrusor sphincter dys-

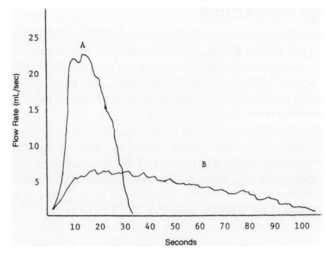

FIGURE 5-1. Urinary Flow Studies. **A.** Normal voiding. **B.** Obstructed voiding. The area under each curve represents the volume. (From Goroll, A. H., & Mulley, A. G. (2009). *Primary care medicine*. Philadelphia, PA: Lippincott Williams & Wilkins.)

synergia (as may be seen in the patient with a neurologic condition), pelvic floor dysfunction in the absence of a neurologic condition, or abdominal straining. **Box 5-2** lists the uroflowmetry data points.

> ### KEY POINT
> Abnormal uroflow may be the result of obstruction or poor detrusor contractility but may also be due to low voided volume. Patient preparation includes instruction on attending the appointment with a full bladder.

> ### KEY POINT
> Abnormal uroflow results indicate an emptying problem thus further evaluation is needed to determine the cause.

FILLING CYSTOMETRY

Filling cystometry evaluates the filling phase of the micturition cycle and begins when filling is initiated and lasts until the urodynamicist gives the patient permission to void (Rosier et al., 2016). Data gathered include bladder capacity, sensory awareness of bladder filling, bladder wall compliance (the ability to stretch and store at low volumes), and the presence or absence of overactive bladder contractions (Rosier et al., 2016).

> ### KEY POINT
> Cystometrogram (CMG) or filling cystometry evaluates the filling phase of the micturition cycle, a measurement of bladder pressure in response to being filled. CMG assesses bladder capacity, sensory awareness, bladder wall compliance, and detrusor instability (bladder spasms) if present.

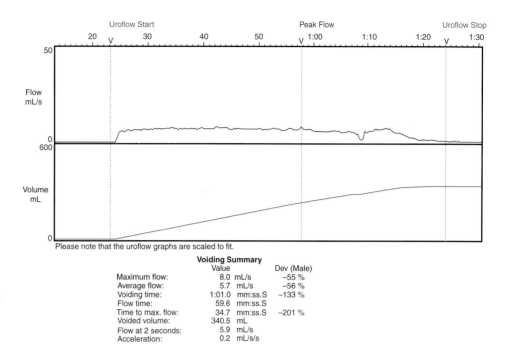

Voiding Summary

	Value		Dev (Male)
Maximum flow:	8.0	mL/s	−55 %
Average flow:	5.7	mL/s	−56 %
Voiding time:	1:01.0	mm:ss.S	−133 %
Flow time:	59.6	mm:ss.S	
Time to max. flow:	34.7	mm:ss.S	−201 %
Voided volume:	340.5	mL	
Flow at 2 seconds:	5.9	mL/s	
Acceleration:	0.2	mL/s/s	

FIGURE 5-2. Obstruction that is Constrictive, such as a Stricture, Typically Creates a Plateau Pattern.

SIMPLE VERSUS COMPLEX CYSTOMETRY

There are two types of filling cystometry, simple and complex. Simple cystometry was historically the initial method of evaluating bladder capacity and compliance. It was accomplished by placing a catheter in the bladder and performing a retrograde filling. Capacity was obtained by simple calculation and compliance by watching the meniscus of the column of water. It has been used as a screening tool to assess bladder sensation and to detect involuntary bladder contractions especially in the frail elderly in settings where urodynamic testing is not practical nor available (Fonda et al., 1993; Ouslander et al., 1998; Wall et al., 1994). When compared to traditional urodynamics, it was found to have an 88% sensitivity and 75% specificity in detecting bladder overactivity (Fonda et al., 1993). Ouslander et al. (1998) evaluated 164 geriatric incontinent

patients and noted comparable results with 75% sensitivity and 79% specificity and positive predictive of 85% in diagnosing detrusor instability. Wall et al., (1994) evaluated 77 incontinent women and reported simple CMG as a

---

BOX 5-2   UROFLOWMETRY DATA POINTS

Maximum Flow Rate (Qmax): Maximum measured flow rate 30–35 mL/s for women; 25 mL/s in men under 40, and 15 mL/s in men over 60 years of age

Average Flow Rate: Voided volume divided by flow time. Normal values vary depending on age and sex (Wein et al., 2012). In men, urine flow declines with age. Women have less change with age:

- Ages 4–7
  - The average flow rate for both males and females is 10 mL/s.
- Ages 8–13
  - The average flow rate for males is 12 mL/s.
  - The average flow rate for females is 15 mL/s.
- Ages 14–45
  - The average flow rate for males is 21 mL/s.
  - The average flow rate for females is 18 mL/s.
- Ages 46–65
  - The average flow rate for males is 12 mL/s.
  - The average flow rate for females is 18 mL/s.
- Ages 66–80
  - The average flow rate for males is 9 mL/s.
  - The average flow rate for females is 18 mL/s.

Time to Maximum Flow: Time from onset of measurable flow to the maximum flow rate

Flow Time: Time that measureable flow occurs

Voided Volume: Total volume voided

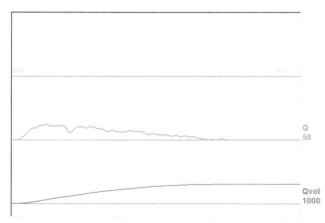

FIGURE 5-3. Obstruction Caused by Prostatic Hypertrophy Usually Creates a Compressed Pattern that Tapers off at the End of the Void.

reliable predictor of detrusor overactivity (DO) (64% sensitivity and 86.8% specificity) and stress urinary incontinence (sensitivity of 88.1% and a specificity of 77.1%). Simple CMG as a screening tool is advantageous due to its portability, testing ease, and convenience, especially where complex urodynamics may not be readily available in underserved communities. It may also assist in selecting patients who may need more of thorough evaluation. Disadvantages include the inability to differentiate between pressure changes caused by forces outside the bladder wall and those resulting from bladder contractions or bladder wall stiffness, and limitations in providing accurate diagnosis of voiding dysfunctions. Simple cystometry should be reserved as a screening tool especially in the geriatric population to guide treatment of incontinence to formulate an awareness of patient's ability to sense bladder filling, presence of sensory urgency, or unstable bladder, verification of postvoid residual, and presence of stress incontinence if patient is asked to perform provocative maneuvers with a full bladder following testing. It offers the continence nurse specialist a practical, safe, and low cost approach to evaluate select incontinent patients (Rayome, 1995). Since it may not determine specific voiding dysfunctions, it should not be used when traditional urodynamic evaluation is indicated (see **Box 5-1**) (Chapple et al., 2009; Rosier et al., 2017).

KEY POINT

Simple CMG is an easy, practical, and cost-effective approach to assist the continence nurse specialist in evaluating incontinent patients in settings where formal urodynamics are not available nor practical.

Complex filling cystometry involves measurement of both intravesical and intra-abdominal pressures; the pressure-sensitive catheter equipped with a transducer in the bladder measures bladder pressures (Pves), and a similar catheter placed into the rectum measures abdominal pressures (Pabd). A computer-based software then subtracts the abdominal pressures from the bladder pressures, and the subtracted pressure (Pdet) represents the pressures exerted by the detrusor muscle and bladder wall. Complex cystometry is currently considered the gold standard because it provides for differentiation between abdominal pressures and bladder wall pressures. **Figure 5-4** provides an illustration of how the urodynamic parameters are monitored.

KEY POINT

In contrast to simple cystometry, complex filling cystometry involves measurement of both intravesical and intra-abdominal pressures converted into numerical data by the computer-based software provides a more accurate representation of bladder filling and emptying thus considered to be the gold standard.

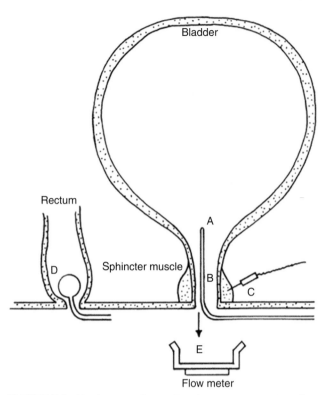

FIGURE 5-4. Urodynamics Setup. Simultaneous monitoring of various urodynamics parameters is shown. Intravesical pressure minus intra-abdominal pressure will produce the detrusor pressure (Pdet). **A.** Intravesical pressure, Pves. **B.** Urethral sphincter pressure, Pur. **C.** Urethral sphincter electromyography. **D.** Intra-abdominal pressure, Pabd. **E.** Urine flow rate. (From Frontera, W. R. (2010). *DeLisa's physical medicine and rehabilitation*. Philadelphia, PA: Lippincott Williams & Wilkins.)

CYSTOMETRY TECHNOLOGY

Many catheter and transducer technologies have entered the urodynamics marketplace over the years. Three primary types are widely available. These include water-filled manometry system catheters with an external pressure transducer (**Figs. 5-5 and 5-6**), electronic catheter-mounted transducers (microtip, **Fig. 5-7**), and the newest air-charged catheter technology (Digesu et al., 2014). Air-charged catheters have been marketed as easier to use, but many argue that the results are not comparable to those of water-filled manometry catheters, which are the gold standard according to the International Continence Society (ICS) (Gammie et al., 2014). Studies have demonstrated significant variation in pressure measurements obtained simultaneously by the different catheter systems (Digesu et al., 2014).

After the catheters are placed in the bladder and rectum, all pressures are zeroed or balanced to atmospheric pressure giving a picture of the baseline pressure of the patient not an absolute zero value (Gammie et al., 2014). The patient should be asked to cough to assure accurate transmission of intra-abdominal pressures, and baseline resting pressures should be obtained prior to the start of filling. The bladder is then filled with sterile water or saline, and the patient is asked to inform the urodynamicist of sensations throughout the filling cycle.

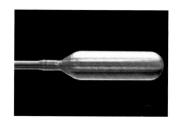

FIGURE 5-5. Examples of Water-Filled Manometry Catheters.

DATA PROVIDED BY FILLING CYSTOMETRY

As noted, filling cystometry provides data regarding bladder capacity, sensory awareness of bladder filling, detrusor stability, and bladder wall compliance.

Bladder Capacity

Cystometric bladder capacity differs from the patient's functional capacity (obtained from a voiding diary or frequency/volume chart). The cystometric capacity is the volume in the bladder at the end of filling cystometry (Dickinson, 2016). This includes any residual urine (unless removed prior to filling) as well as the filling solution. A normal adult bladder can be filled to approximately 500 mL before a strong desire to void is felt. The determination of normal bladder capacity in children is based on the following formula (Dickinson, 2016; Hanno et al., 2007).

Age (years) × 30 + 30 = bladder capacity in mL

Abnormally low capacity can be caused by chronic DO, irritative disorders such as interstitial cystitis, or long-term indwelling catheter use resulting in a small contracted bladder. Neurologic conditions causing loss of sensory awareness of bladder filling can lead to abnormally high capacity, as can chronic distention (e.g., the patient with diabetic cystopathy).

Sensory Awareness of Bladder Filling

Definitions related to sensory awareness of bladder filling are listed in **Table 5-2**. There are no data to support specific volumes at which the individual should report first sensation or first desire to void; strong desire to void normally occurs at about 500 mL, as noted (Dickinson, 2016). Increased bladder sensation occurs when, during filling, the patient experiences an early desire to void that is persistent, with or without urgency. This abnormally heightened awareness of bladder filling is typically seen in patients with overactive bladder, pelvic floor dysfunction, or interstitial cystitis. Reduced bladder sensation means that the desire to void is felt later in the filling phase than expected, but does occur, as opposed to absent bladder sensation, which indicates that the individual is completely unaware of bladder filling and does not experience the urge to void (Abrams et al., 2003). Diminished or absent awareness of bladder filling is usually seen in patients with chronic over distention, diabetes, or lower motor neuron lesions.

Bladder capacity and sensation are closely related. For example, the sensation of fullness reflects the volume of urine the individual is able to hold comfortably, and the volume associated with the sensation of being unable to delay voiding is considered maximum

KEY POINT

Chronic DO, interstitial cystitis or painful bladder disorders, long-term indwelling catheters, and upper motor neuron dysfunction (lesion above the sacral cord) may result in a low capacity bladder, in contrast lower motor neuron dysfunction (sacral cord lesion) and other neurologic conditions causing reduced sensory awareness of bladder filling may lead to a high bladder capacity.

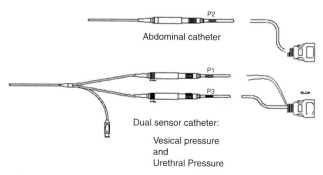

FIGURE 5-6. Examples of Electronic Urodynamic Catheters.

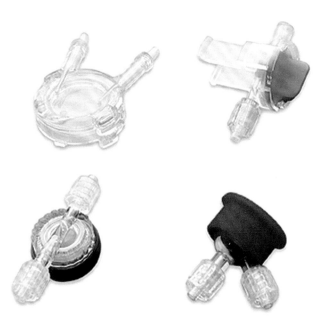

FIGURE 5-7. Examples of Transducers that are Used with Water-Filled Catheters. (Courtesy of LABORIE.)

TABLE 5-2 SENSATIONS OF BLADDER FILLING DURING URODYNAMIC TESTING

SENSATION	DEFINITION
First sensation	When he/she first becomes aware of filling
First desire	When he/she would urinate at the next appropriate time, but it can be delayed
Strong desire	Continuing desire to void but without a fear of leaking
Urgency	Sudden strong desire to void
Maximum cystometric capacity	When the patient feels they can no longer delay voiding

Data from Abrams et al. (2003).

cystometric bladder capacity. Pain during bladder filling is an abnormal sensation.

KEY POINT

Heightened awareness of bladder filling is typically seen in patients with overactive bladder, pelvic floor dysfunction, or interstitial cystitis. Reduced bladder sensation or absent awareness of bladder filling is usually seen in patients with chronic over distention, diabetes, or lower motor neuron lesions.

Detrusor Stability

Stability of the detrusor refers to the absence or presence of involuntary detrusor contractions. During filling, the bladder should remain relaxed and there should be no contractile activity even if the urodynamicist employs provocative maneuvers such as asking the patient to cough or putting the patient's hand in water that may initiate a primitive voiding reflex (Dickinson, 2016). Absence of contractile activity is normal and indicative of a stable detrusor muscle. Any involuntary contractions of the detrusor are considered abnormal and are termed DO (Dickinson, 2016). These involuntary contractions may be phasic (**Fig. 5-8**) or terminal (**Fig. 5-9**); phasic contractions occur during filling and may or may not result in urinary leakage, while terminal detrusor contractions typically result in complete loss of bladder volume and thereby terminate the study. When unstable bladder contractions cause urinary leakage, the condition is labeled detrusor overactivity incontinence (DOI), which may be neurogenic or idiopathic in origin (Dickinson, 2016).

KEY POINT

When unstable bladder contractions cause urinary leakage, the condition is labeled detrusor overactivity incontinence (DOI), which may be neurogenic or idiopathic in origin.

Figure 5-8 tracing shows phasic increases in Pves and Pdet. Since Pabd has no activity, the phasic contractions are the detrusor. The increase in electromyogram (EMG) activity is likely a guarding reflex. The slow rise in both Pves and Pdet reflect an increase in intra-abdominal pressure with a Valsalva maneuver to assess for urodynamic stress in continence (**Fig. 5-9**).

KEY POINT

When unstable bladder contractions cause urinary leakage, the condition is labeled detrusor overactivity incontinence (DOI), which may be neurogenic or idiopathic in origin.

Bladder Wall Compliance

Bladder wall compliance describes the bladder's ability to stretch and to maintain low pressures throughout the

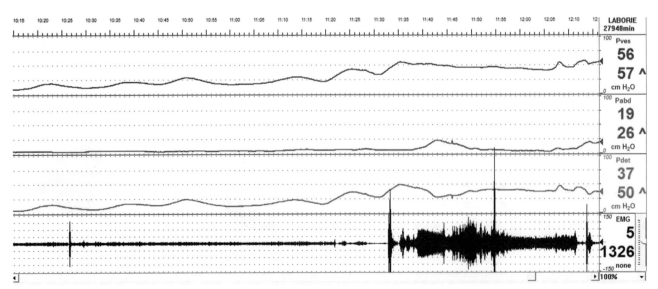

FIGURE 5-8. Phasic Contractions Occur During Filling. (Courtesy of LABORIE.)

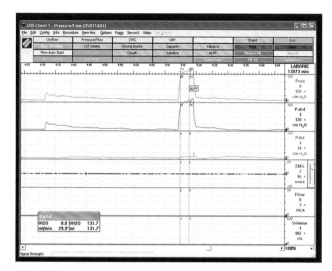

FIGURE 5-9. Increase in Intra-Abdominal Pressure with a Valsalva Maneuver to Assess for SUI.

filling cycle (Dickinson, 2007; Gajewski et al., 2018). The formula for determining bladder compliance is

$$\text{Compliance (mL/cm } H_2O) = \text{change in volume }(\Delta V)/\text{change in detrusor pressure }(\Delta Pdet)$$

The ICS recommends use of the following points for calculation of bladder compliance: the detrusor pressure at the point when filling begins and detrusor pressure at capacity or just before any detrusor contraction. Using the formula above, normal bladder compliance is >30 to 40 mL/cm H_2O; this means that the

pressures within the bladder wall rise only 1 cm H_2O for every 30 to 40 mL of urine. The urodynamic tracing of a poorly compliant bladder would show a steady steep rise in bladder pressure, often with small infused volumes. When leakage occurs in association with poor bladder compliance, the pressure when the leakage occurs is called the detrusor leak point pressure (LPP). Poor compliance can be caused by long-standing obstruction, which may result from pelvic organ prolapse, an enlarged prostate, or neurogenic bladder with detrusor–sphincteric dyssynergia. A poorly compliant bladder with high filling pressures (i.e., ≥40 cm H_2O change from baseline) creates resistance to the inflow of urine and places the individual at great risk for upper tract damage (Dickinson, 2007; Gajewski et al., 2018).

Figure 5-10 shows a slow, steady steep rise in Pves and Pdet pressures in response to filling. The elongated trabeculated bladder shape is typical of obstructive neurological disease, particularly lower motor neuron lesions. The compliance change is >40 cm H_2O, which is considered a *hostile bladder pressure* or low compliance and creates significant upper tract damage (Dickinson, 2007).

KEY POINT

Normal bladder compliance is >30 to 40 mL/cm H_2O; this means that the pressures within the bladder wall rise only 1 cm H_2O for every 30 to 40 mL of urine; hostile bladder pressures (>40 mL/cm H_2O) can result in upper tract damage.

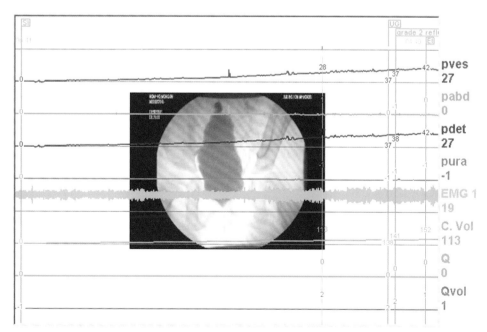

FIGURE 5-10. A Slow Steady Steep Rise in Pves and Pdet in Response to Filling. Bladder is elongated and trabeculated typical of obstructive neurologic disease. Compliance change is >40 cm H_2O, which is considered a hostile bladder. (Courtesy of LABORIE.)

PRESSURE FLOW STUDIES

When cystometric capacity is reached (i.e., when the patient states he/she can no longer delay voiding), permission to void is given. This begins the voiding phase of urodynamics, which is known as a pressure flow study. The patient voids into the uroflow commode with the pressure-sensitive catheter still in place in the bladder; thus, the pressure flow study allows for simultaneous measurement of urine flow and pressures generated by detrusor muscle contraction.

KEY POINT

The voiding phase of urodynamics is known as a pressure flow study.

URINE FLOW PATTERN

The urine flow is defined as either continuous or intermittent, and a continuous flow pattern is further defined as smooth or fluctuating (Dickinson, 2016). A pressure flow study is essential in assessing incomplete bladder emptying, because it provides the answer to the following question: Is the bladder contracting effectively and working hard to pass urine through a BOO, or is the detrusor contraction inadequate? (Hashim et al., 2019; Rosier et al., 2016).

KEY POINT

A pressure flow study identifies the *cause* of incomplete emptying or urinary retention, which may be due to BOO as seen in BPH or severe pelvic organ prolapse or a poorly contractile bladder from damage to the nerves controlling the bladder.

BOX 5-3	**PRESSURE MEASUREMENTS DURING URODYNAMIC TESTING**

- Opening pressure: Pressure immediately before the detrusor contraction
- Opening time: Time from the rise in detrusor pressure to the start of urine flow
- Maximum pressure: Maximum pressure measured during voiding
- Pressure at maximum flow: Pressure measured at Q_{max}
- Closing pressure: Pressure at the end of urine flow

Data from Abrams et al. (2003).

DETRUSOR CONTRACTION STRENGTH

The pressure flow study provides data regarding the strength of detrusor contraction in addition to data regarding urinary flow (**Box 5-3**). A normal bladder should empty fully with a maximum detrusor pressure of 25 to 50 cm H_2O.

Normal detrusor function involves a voluntary sustained contraction that results in continuous flow of urine and that empties the bladder over a normal time span. Detrusor underactivity is manifested by a poorly sustained contraction and a prolonged flow of urine, while BOO is characterized by high voiding pressures and low flow rates as seen in **Figure 5-11**. An acontractile detrusor typically has a pressure-flow pattern consistent with Valsalva voiding, as illustrated in **Figure 5-12**. An explosive flow pattern with high maximum flow rates and low pressures likely indicates very little outlet resistance and may be seen in patients with stress urinary incontinence or postprostatectomy incontinence.

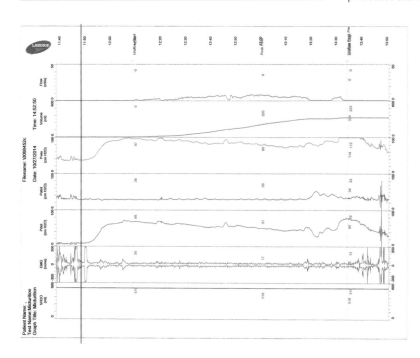

FIGURE 5-11. Example of BOO with Very Slow Flow and High-pressure Detrusor Contraction. (Courtesy of LABORIE.)

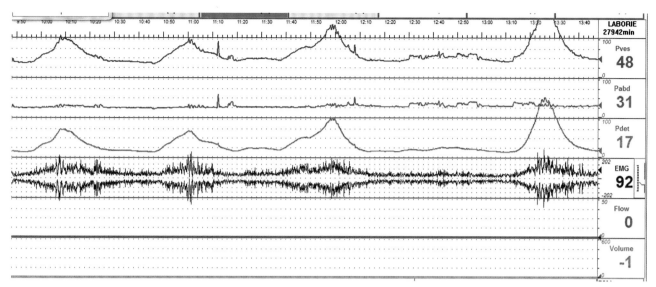

FIGURE 5-12. Phasic Detrusor Sphincter Dyssynergia; EMG Rises with Each Detrusor Contraction Causing Obstruction at the Urethral Sphincter and Impeding Bladder Emptying. Increase in Pves and Pdet mimics each other. EMG activity increases as Pdet rises in an attempt to empty the bladder. (Courtesy of LABORIE.)

In **Figure 5-11**, the patient is voluntarily voiding. Pves and Pdet pressures begin to rise, quite some time before flow is initiated. EMG remains quiet during voiding, signaling normal sphincter relaxation and a synergic voiding event. Flow is very slow and poor despite a very high-pressure contraction (so high that it bleeds into the next pressure channel on the tracing). This is consistent with BOO. This patient was an elderly male with an enlarged prostate, but the same pattern could be seen in a female with significant pelvic organ prolapse or following a surgical procedure for stress incontinence that resulted in excessive urethral resistance.

KEY POINT

The pressure flow study provides data regarding the strength of detrusor contraction in addition to data regarding urinary flow. A normal bladder should empty fully with a maximum detrusor pressure of 25 to 50 cm H$_2$O.

In **Figure 5-12**, there is no contraction of the detrusor. The Pves and Pabd pressures mimic each other, indicating that the increase in pressure is due to abdominal muscle contraction as opposed to bladder contraction (a Valsalva voiding event). The increase in EMG activity can also be consistent with Valsalva voiding. The flow pattern is intermittent, reflecting bursts of urine flow coinciding with Valsalva as seen in phasic detrusor sphincter dyssynergia.

ELECTROMYOGRAPHY

Historically performed using needle electrodes, most EMG studies are now done with surface electrodes, similar to those used for the standard electrocardiogram.

Surface electrodes record the total electrical output from the pelvic floor muscles (Gajewski et al., 2018). During the filling phase, it is normal to see a slight increase in EMG activity; this is known as the "guarding reflex." During voiding, the pelvic floor muscles should relax, producing little or no EMG activity. Increased EMG activity during voiding is abnormal. If it is continual, it may be due to dysfunctional voiding, detrusor sphincter dyssynergia, or Valsalva artifact (apparent increase in sphincter activity during Valsalva voiding caused by use of surface electrodes to measure pelvic floor activity, as opposed to use of needle electrodes that measure actual sphincteric activity).

Dysfunctional voiding or pelvic floor dysfunction is manifested by an intermittent flow pattern, intermittent detrusor contractions, and increased EMG activity during voiding in neurologically normal individuals. Dysfunctional voiding can be a learned behavior or can be due to pelvic floor muscle dysfunction. Pelvic floor dysfunction can be characterized by high tone or spasm of the pelvic floor musculature, which can result in various lower urinary tract symptoms. The same pattern in those with a neurologic diagnosis is called detrusor sphincter dyssynergia (Gajewski et al., 2018) (**Fig. 5-13**). This is commonly seen in patients with certain spinal cord injuries and in multiple sclerosis and occurs when the sphincter fails to relax during the emptying phase due to loss of normal neural control.

KEY POINT

During voiding, the pelvic floor muscles should relax, producing little or no EMG activity. Increased EMG activity during voiding is abnormal. If it is continual, it may be due to dysfunctional voiding, detrusor sphincter dyssynergia, or Valsalva artifact.

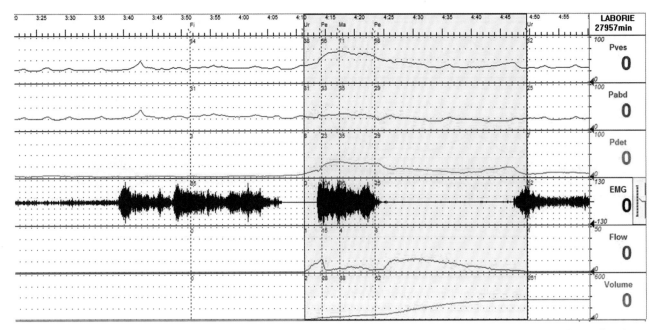

FIGURE 5-13. Pves and Pdet Pressures Rise and at the Same Time EMG Activity Increases (Rather than Relaxing as is Normal) and Results in Bladder Neck Obstruction and Obstructed Voiding. (Courtesy of LABORIE.)

In **Figure 5-13**, Pves and Pdet pressures rise during a voiding event, whether voiding is voluntary or involuntary. At the same time, the EMG activity increases significantly, thus resulting in BOO and obstructed voiding. This places the patient at risk for incomplete emptying, urinary tract infections, and vesicoureteral reflux.

 URETHRAL PRESSURE PROFILES

A urethral pressure profile (UPP) provides a graphic representation of the pressures along the entire length of the urethra (Dickinson, 2016). Urethral pressures can be measured at rest, during stress maneuvers (cough, strain), or during voiding. The UPP is obtained by utilizing a pulling apparatus or withdrawal unit to precisely and steadily withdraw a pressure-sensitive catheter through the urethra (**Fig. 5-14**). A resting UPP provides data regarding urethral resistance during the filling cycle; it is thought that a low maximum urethral closure pressure (**Fig. 5-15**) is associated with low outlet resistance and may help to confirm a diagnosis of stress urinary incontinence.

KEY POINT

Urethral pressure profile measures the pressures along the entire length of the urethra while at rest, during provocative (stress) maneuvers, and during voiding. Low maximum urethral resting pressures during the filling cycle are associated with stress urinary incontinence due to low outlet resistance although. This study is cumbersome and not easily reproducible thus led to the development of the abdominal leak point pressure study.

 ABDOMINAL LEAK POINT PRESSURE

In the early 1990s, clinicians and urodynamicists began to look for alternatives to UPP studies. New research and new options warranted a need to identify patients with intrinsic sphincter deficiency (ISD) who needed surgical procedures that would provide increased urethral resistance and who would not benefit from procedures

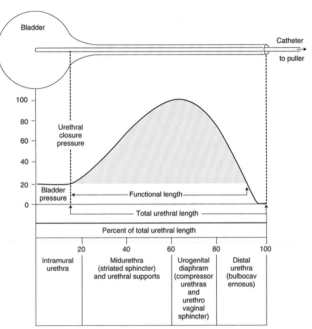

FIGURE 5-14. Correlation of Mid-Urethral Anatomy with Urodynamic Anatomy (EMG). (Adapted from DeLancey, J. O. (1986). Correlative study of paraurethral anatomy. *Obstetrics and Gynecology, 68*, 91–97, with permission.)

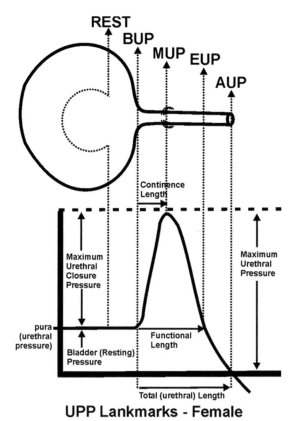

UPP Lankmarks - Female

FIGURE 5-15. Urethral Pressure Profile Data Points. REST, resting pressure; BUP, baseline urethral pressure; MUP, maximum urethral pressure; EUP, end urethral pressure; AUP, atmospheric urethral pressure.

designed simply to provide support or bulk at the bladder neck. It was thought that the UPP, although correlated with poor urethral function, was cumbersome and not easily reproducible (Dickinson, 2007). This led to the development of the abdominal LPP study, which measures the level of intra-abdominal pressure required to push urine across a (partially) closed sphincter.

The abdominal LPP (ALPP) is assessed during the course of the filling cystometry; the patient is placed in the upright position (seated or standing) and is asked to perform coughing and straining maneuvers at certain standardized bladder volumes (**Fig. 5-16**). The ALPP is easily reproducible and quantifies the ability of the urethra to resist increases in abdominal pressure. In **Figure 5-16**, the ALPP is 114 cm H_2O (the abdominal pressure at which the patient leaked urine). There is a lack of agreement regarding normal and ALPP pressures but general consensus notes pressures <60 cm H_2O reflect poor bladder outlet resistance or ISD, pressures between 60 and 90 cm H_2O is unclear or "gray area" although Centers for Medicare/Medicaid Services and third-party payers require ALPP <100 cm H_2O for a diagnosis of ISD to qualify for urethral bulking therapies (AUGS, 2018; Burden et al., 2015). According to Burden et al. (2015), ALPP has evidence to support or refute its use; it clearly assists the surgeon in understanding anatomical causes for the

stress UI, thereby clarifying all options available to the patient to make a better informed decision in selecting UI treatment modalities. However, ALLP does not measure SUI severity nor does it assist in predicting success of surgeries for SUI; it should never be used as a stand-alone diagnostic but as an integral part of urodynamic testing (Rosier et al., 2017). Certainly there is a need for randomized trials to further demonstrate the validity and utility of ALLP but at this time is an integral part of urodynamic studies and it is especially important to qualify for insurance coverage when considering urethral bulking therapies for SUI (AUGS, 2018; Burden et al., 2015).

KEY POINT

Compared with UPP, abdominal LPP may be a more accurate assessment of the ability of the urethral sphincter to resist increases in abdominal pressure such as cough or straining. However, the utility of these tests remains controversial.

VIDEO URODYNAMICS

Video urodynamic testing involves filling cystometry utilizing contrast medium and simultaneous use of fluoroscopic evaluation. The addition of radiology equipment is quite costly, and many centers do not have this capability. So when is video urodynamic testing recommended? Those with known or suspected neurologic disorders may benefit from the more complex video urodynamic investigation. Complex cases involving lower urinary tract symptoms not responding to medical therapy, suspected primary bladder neck obstruction, suspected or known pelvic floor dysfunction, and/or failure of previous operative procedures may also benefit from video urodynamics (Dickinson, 2016; Winters et al., 2012). Video urodynamics permit assessment of vesicoureteral reflux in an individual with neurologic disease and can also be used to identify the level of urethral obstruction.

KEY POINT

Video urodynamics is usually reserved for complex cases: those with known or suspected neurologic disorders; when lower urinary tract symptoms have not responded to medical therapy; if bladder neck obstruction is suspected; if pelvic floor dysfunction is known or suspected; and/or when previous operative procedures have failed.

FURTHER DIAGNOSTICS

In evaluation of lower urinary tract dysfunction, urinalysis for evaluation of hematuria, proteinuria, glucose, and infection is considered standard. Measurement of postvoid residual either by bladder scan or catheterization is indicated whenever there are concerns about the patient's ability to empty effectively. Renal ultrasound

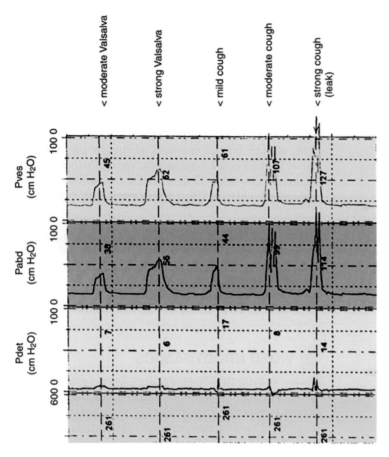

FIGURE 5-16. The Abdominal Leak Point Pressure (LPP) is 114 cm H_2O (the Abdominal Pressure at which the Patient Leaked Urine). (From Berek, J. S. (2011). *Berek and Novak's gynecology*. Philadelphia, PA: Lippincott Williams & Wilkins.)

can provide a noninvasive means of evaluating for hydronephrosis and stones (Hanno et al., 2007). Cystoscopy not only permits evaluation of the bladder mucosa for malignancy, stones, or foreign bodies but also provides visual confirmation of trabeculation (thickening of the bladder wall) caused by overwork of the detrusor, bladder neck abnormalities, and presence or absence of bladder diverticulum. Patients should be referred for these additional studies whenever there are concerns about renal function or bladder complications. Laboratory studies may also be needed to assess for renal damage.

 CONCLUSION

Urodynamic testing is considered an advanced assessment reserved for patients with complex histories or for those who have not responded to initial treatment. It provides a graphic picture of bladder and sphincter function and, combined with patient history and presenting symptoms, can be very helpful in identifying the cause of voiding or pelvic floor dysfunction.

REFERENCES

Abrams, P., Cardozo, L., Fall, M. et al. (2003). The standardization of terminology in lower urinary tract function: Report from the standardization sub-committee of the International Continence Society. *Urology, 61*, 37–49.

American Urogynecologic Society (AUGS) Coding and Reimbursement Committee. (2018). Coding for urethral bulking. Retrieved from https://www.augs.org/assets/1/6/Coding_Fact_Sheet_for_Urethral_bulking_2017_v2.pdf

Burden, H., Warren, K., & Abrams, P. (2015). Leak point pressures: How useful are they? *Current Opinion, 25*, 317–322. doi: 10.1097/MOU.0000000000000176.

Chapple, C.R., MacDiarmid, S. A., & Patel, A. (2009). *Urodynamics made easy* (3rd ed., pp. 117). Oxford, UK: Elsevier.

Dickinson, T. (2007). Demystifying leak point pressures: The valuable tool for functional assessment. *Urologic Nursing, 27*, 128-132.

Dickinson, T. (2016). Advanced assessment of the patient with urinary incontinence and voiding dysfunction. In D. B. Doughty & K. N. Moore (Eds.), *Wound ostomy and continence nurses society core curriculum: Continence Management* (pp. 42–53). Philadelphia PA: Wolters Kluwer.

Digesu, G. A., Depapas, A., Robshaw, P., et al. (2014). Are the measurements of water-filled and air-charged catheters the same in urodynamics? *International Urogynecology Journal, 25*, 123–130. doi: 10.1007/s00192-013-2182-z.

Fonda, D., Brimage, P. J., & D'Astoli, M. (1993). Simple screening for urinary incontinence in the elderly: Comparison of simple and multichannel cystometry. *Urology, 42*(5), 536–540.

Gajewski, J. B., Schurch, B., Hamid, R. T., et al. (2018). An international continence society (ICS) report on the terminology for adult neurogenic lower urinary tract dysfunction (ANLUTD). *Neurourology and Urodynamics, 37*, 1152–1161. doi: 10.1002/nau.23397.

Gammie, A., Clarkson, B., Constantinou, C., et al. (2014). International continence society guidelines on urodynamic equipment performance. *Neurourology and Urodynamics, 33*, 369. doi: 10.1002/nau.22546.

Hanno, P. M., Malkowicz, S. B., & Wein, A. J. (2007). *Penn clinical manual of urology*. Philadelphia, PA: Saunders Elsevier.

Hashim, H., Blanker, M. H., Drake, M. J., et al. (2019). International continence society (ICS) report on the terminology for nocturia and nocturnal lower urinary tract function. *Neurourology and Urodynamics, 38*, 499–508. doi: 10.1002/nau.23917.

Hirakauva, E. Y., Bianchi-Ferraro, A. H., Zucchi, E., et al. (2017). Incidence of bacteriuria after urodynamic study with or without antibiotic prophylaxis in women with urinary incontinence. *Revista Brasileira de Ginecologia e Obstetrícia, 39*, 534–540. doi: 10.1055/s-0037-1604006.

Ouslander, J., Leach, G., Abelson, S., et al. (1988). Simple versus multichannel cystometry in the evaluation of bladder function in an incontinent geriatric population. *The Journal of Urology, 140*(6), 1482–1486.

Rayome, R. (1995). Simple urodynamic techniques. *Journal of Wound, Ostomy and Incontinence, 22*(1), 17–26.

Rosier, P. F., Kuo, H. C., Agro, E. F., et al. (2017). Urodynamic testing. In P. Abrams, L. Cardozo, A. Wagg, et al., (Eds.), *Incontinence* (6th ed., pp. 599–670). ICI-ICS. Bristol, UK: International Continence Society.

Rosier, P. F., Schaefer, W., Lose, G., et al. (2016). International continence society good urodynamic practices and terms 2016: Urodynamics, uroflowmetry, cystometry and pressure-flow study. *Neurourology and Urodynamics, 36*, 1243–1260. doi: 10.1002/nau.23124.

Wall, L. L., Wiskind, A. K., & Taylor, P. A. (1994). Simple bladder filling with a cough stress test compared with subtracted cystometry for the diagnosis of urinary incontinence. *American Journal of Obstetrics and Gynecology, 171*(6), 1472–1479.

Wein, A. J., Kavoussi, L. R., Novick, A. C., et al. (2012). Urodynamic and video-urodynamic evaluation of the lower urinary tract. In A. J. Wein, L. R. Kavoussi, A. C. Novick, et al. (Eds.), *Campbell-Walsh Urology* (Chapter 62, pp.1847-1870). Philadelphia, PA: Elsevier/Saunders.

Winters, J. C., Dmochowski, R. R., Goldman, H. B., et al. (2012). Urodynamic studies in adults: AUA/SUFU guideline. *Journal of Urology, 188*, 2464–2472. doi: 10.1016/j.uro.2012.09.081.

QUESTIONS

1. A continence nurse orders urodynamic testing for a patient with urinary incontinence. Which statement accurately describes an aspect of this type of testing?
   A. Urodynamic testing evaluates the filling and voiding phases of the micturition cycle.
   B. Urodynamic testing provides information regarding the functionality of the upper urinary tract.
   C. Urodynamic testing is noninvasive and relatively inexpensive in the United States.
   D. Urodynamic testing can be used to detect the presence of a urinary tract infection or hematuria.

2. Which of the following describes normal uroflowmetry results?
   A. Low velocity flat flow rate
   B. Intermittent burst of flow
   C. Plateau pattern of flow
   D. Bell-shaped curve of flow

3. The continence nurse records test results for a patient experiencing incontinence and notes the following data: bladder capacity, sensory awareness of bladder filling, detrusor stability, and bladder wall compliance. Which test provides this information?
   A. Electromyogram
   B. Filling cystometry
   C. Pressure flow study
   D. Urethral pressure profile

4. What is the major advantage of using complex cystometry as opposed to simple cystometry?
   A. It provides for differentiation between abdominal pressures and bladder wall pressure.
   B. It is noninvasive and is often used as an initial screening tool for lower urinary tract (voiding) dysfunction.
   C. It determines if the bladder is contracting effectively or if the detrusor contraction is inadequate.
   D. It provides data regarding the strength of detrusor contraction in addition to data regarding urinary flow.

5. Which catheter used for performing filling cystometry is considered to be the gold standard according to the International Continence Society?
   A. Air-charged catheters
   B. Catheter-mounted transducers
   C. Water-filled manometry system catheters
   D. Suprapubic urinary catheter

6. Which patient would the continence nurse place at higher risk for reduced bladder sensation? A patient with
   A. Overactive bladder
   B. Pelvic floor dysfunction
   C. Interstitial cystitis
   D. Diabetes

7. Which condition occurring during filling is indicative of a normal, stable detrusor muscle?
   A. Absence of bladder sensation
   B. Absence of contractile activity
   C. Phasic contractions of the detrusor
   D. High filling pressures

8. The continence nurse records bladder compliance in a patient as 40 mL/cm H_2O. What does this information signify?
   A. High potential for upper tract damage
   B. High potential for lower tract damage
   C. Risk for pelvic floor dysfunction
   D. This is a normal bladder compliance result

9. A continence nurse is performing the pressure flow study involved in urodynamic testing. What condition does this test assess?
A. Sensory awareness of bladder filling
B. Bladder wall compliance
C. Bladder emptying
D. Bladder capacity

10. Which condition is indicative of normal voiding patterns tested by electromyogram?
A. Intermittent flow pattern
B. Tensing of the pelvic floor muscles increasing EMG activity during voiding
C. Dramatic increase in EMG activity during filling phase
D. Little or no EMG activity during voiding

ANSWERS AND RATIONALES

1. A. Rationale: Urodynamic testing evaluates the filling and voiding phases of the micturition cycle and provides information regarding the functionality of the lower urinary tract. Specifically it evaluates the bladder's ability to store urine at low pressures, to empty effectively, and to evaluate the ability of the sphincter to maintain closure during filling and to open for voiding. It is invasive and expensive testing and should be ordered with a clear question needing answered.

2. D. Rationale: Normal uroflowmetry should be a bell-shaped curve. Normal values vary depending upon sex and age. Low velocity or plateau patterns are indicative of obstruction. Intermittent bursts of flow show straining to void (due to obstruction), dysfunctional elimination, or potential detrusor sphincter dyssynergia (in the setting of a neurologic condition).

3. B. Rationale: Filling cystometry evaluates the filling phase of the micturition cycle, a measurement of bladder pressure in response to being filled. It assesses bladder capacity, sensory awareness, bladder wall compliance, and detrusor instability (bladder spasms) if present.

4. A. Rationale: Complex cystometry is able to differentiate between pressure changes caused by forces outside the bladder wall and those resulting from bladder contractions, assesses bladder wall stiffness (compliance), and helps in determining an accurate diagnosis in voiding dysfunctions.

5. C. Rationale: The water-filled manometry system is the technique on which the foundations of urodynamics have been tested. Suprapubic catheters should not be used for urodynamic testing unless there is no urethral access. Air-charged and catheter-mounted transducers are felt to be an easier set up and less margin for technical error but have not been as widely studied over a long period of time.

6. D. Rationale: It is known that diabetic patients often develop neuropathy over time. Diabetic patients also can develop diabetic cystopathy in which bladder sensation becomes diminished and is often accompanied by decreased detrusor contractility and elevated postvoid residual.

7. B. Rationale: During the filling phase, the detrusor should not contract. Contraction of the detrusor should occur during a voluntary voiding event.

8. A. Rationale: Bladder compliance ≥40 has been documented since the 1980s as a high-risk factor for upper tract damage. This is often seen in patients with neurologic conditions (such as spinal cord injury) or in response to long-standing obstruction. During filling, the detrusor should remain low and stable without any significant change in response to filling.

9. C. Rationale: The voiding phase of urodynamics is known as a pressure flow study. This study allows for simultaneous measurement of urine flow and pressures generated by detrusor muscle contraction.

10. D. Rationale: During normal voiding, the detrusor contracts and the sphincter and pelvic floor relax for effective emptying. Tension or increased activity during voiding can indicate Valsalva voiding, detrusor sphincter dyssynergia, or dysfunctional elimination (as in pelvic floor dysfunction).

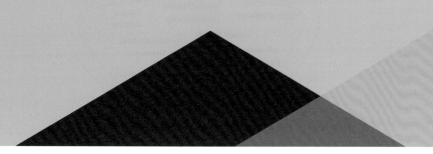

CHAPTER 6

MANAGEMENT FUNDAMENTALS FOR INCONTINENCE

Donna L. Thompson

1. Define the eight fundamental components of continence nursing that are key contributors to a healthy bladder.

2. Develop an exercise prescription for pelvic floor muscle exercises for the prevention or treatment of urinary and/or fecal incontinence.

3. Discuss fundamental nursing interventions to promote bowel health.

4. Integrate knowledge of the components of functional and cognitive impairment into the development of a plan of care for patients with incontinence.

5. Compare and contrast scheduled toileting programs in relationship to candidates, implementation, and expected outcomes.

6. Utilize first-line behavioral and lifestyle change interventions in the treatment of incontinence.

TOPIC OUTLINE

A fundamental component of continence nursing is promoting a healthy bladder lifestyle. Promotion of health and prevention of disease are important components of all nursing care and especially continence nursing. The Wound Ostomy Continence Nurses Society™ has identified in the *Scope and Standards of WOC Practice, 2nd Edition* (Lawrence et al., 2018) the role of the continence nurse as promoting a healthy bladder lifestyle though education about preventative strategies and providing counseling for lifestyle changes. Until recently, research and clinical practice have focused primarily on incontinence assessment and treatment with few randomized clinical trials addressing strategies to prevent urinary incontinence (UI) in men and women. Palmer et al. (2020) conducted a comprehensive literature review focused on the prevention of incontinence and identified little in the way of prevention research other than Grade B recommendations in pregnant and postpartum women. Fortunately, there has been a relatively recent movement, sponsored by the National Institute of Diabetes and Digestive and Kidney Diseases (NIDDK) to refocus research, clinical practice and health care policy on bladder health. In 2015, the Prevention of Lower Urinary Tract Symptoms (PLUS) Research Consortium was established using a transdisciplinary research network focusing on bladder health in girls and women (Harlow et al., 2017). The PLUS Research Consortium has developed a working definition of bladder health to focus research initiatives (**Box 6-1**).

Continence nursing finds at its core a focus on interventions that promote and restore bladder health as much as possible. Lukacz et al. (2011) developed a healthy bladder consensus statement that helps identify components of a healthy bladder lifestyle. The authors acknowledge a dependence on secondary prevention research given limited research in the area of primary prevention. Their framework has been adapted here in **Figure 6-1** to illustrate the fundamental components of continence nursing in terms of promoting a healthy bladder as well as restoring as much health as possible by implementing continence nursing interventions.

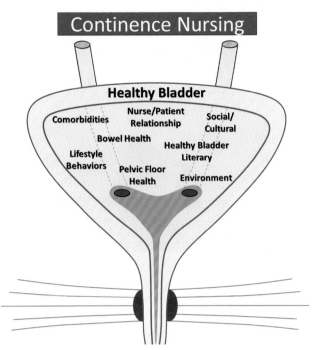

FIGURE 6-1. Eight Fundamental Components of Continence Nursing. (Created by Donna L. Thompson.)

FUNDAMENTAL COMPONENTS OF CONTINENCE NURSING

NURSE/PATIENT RELATIONSHIP

A core component of continence nursing is the unique relationship the nurse has with the patient, whether it be short interactions as part of a busy inpatient practice or the protracted relationships that form as part of the care of those with chronic illnesses and conditions. Nurses are in the unique position to form helping relationships founded on trust and respect, relationships that nurture hope and are based on sensitivity to the holistic needs of the patient. Continence nursing involves implementing evidence-based specialty nursing care as patient advocate, educator, researcher, and communicator.

HEALTHY BLADDER LITERACY

Promoting bladder health and treating incontinence starts with recommending lifestyle changes. Long-term adherence to a healthy bladder lifestyle may be enhanced if the patient understands the reasons behind the recommended changes. Increasing knowledge about the urinary tract and a bladder healthy lifestyle may contribute to overall bladder health (Lukacz et al., 2011; Newman et al., 2017). **Box 6-2** lists a sample outline for patient education.

BOX 6-1	**PLUS NETWORK DEFINITION OF BLADDER HEALTH**

A complete state of physical, mental, and social well-being related to bladder function and not merely the absence of LUTS. Healthy bladder function permits daily activities, adapts to short-term physical or environmental stressors, and allows optimal well-being (e.g., travel, exercise, social, occupational, or other activities).

From: Lukacz, E. S., Bavendam, T. G., Berry, A., et al. (2018). A Novel Research Definition of bladder health in women and girls: Implications for research and public health promotion. *Journal of Women's Health, 27*(8), 978.

KEY POINT

Increasing knowledge about the urinary tract and a bladder healthy lifestyle may contribute to overall bladder health.

| BOX 6-2 | SAMPLE PATIENT EDUCATION |

BOX 6-2   SAMPLE PATIENT EDUCATION

A. The normal urinary tract
   a. Kidney, ureters, bladder, urethra
   b. Urinary sphincters
   c. Pelvic floor muscles
   d. Normal micturition
B. Healthy bladder habits
C. Healthy pelvic floor
D. Healthy bowel habits

SOCIAL/CULTURAL

UI as well as related symptoms of urgency, frequency, and nocturia have a significant impact on quality of life (QoL) and have been reported to be associated with depression, anxiety, and sexual dysfunction (Chu et al., 2015; Coyne et al., 2011a, 2012; Tang et al., 2014). Inadequate control of the bladder and bowel are stigmatized in western societies resulting in efforts to conceal the problem due to fear of embarrassing leakage and odor (Southall et al., 2017). Social estrangement and isolation increase intrapersonal stress and impact interpersonal relationships as well as delay and even prevent access to treatment (Hagglund & Wadensten, 2007). Elstad et al. (2010) reported, based on findings from the Boston Area Community Health Survey, that stigma associated with urgency, frequency, and incontinence resulted in feelings of embarrassment and shame as well as fear of being discovered as being *different* or with a problem. Perceptions of incontinence included a fear of others' opinions as being unclean and lacking adequate hygiene. Hispanic men and woman coped with their bladder control problems with secrecy or silence creating an even greater barrier to adequate treatment (Elstad et al., 2010). In other social groups, such as older adults, incontinence is often viewed as an inevitable result of aging and thus not amenable for treatment. In nursing home populations, incontinence is inaccurately labeled as chronic and resistant to treatment with poor expectations for improvement when treatment is started. The continence nurse is in the unique position to approach patients in a nonjudgmental way and, through accurate assessment and case finding, educate patients and caregivers in all care settings that incontinence is a *treatable* problem.

KEY POINT

The continence nurse is in the unique position to approach patients in a nonjudgmental way and, through accurate assessment and case finding, educate patients and caregivers in all care settings that incontinence is a treatable problem.

ENVIRONMENT

Timely and acceptable access to toilet facilities can have a significant impact on healthy voiding. Unsanitary public toilets prompt many to avoid and/or delay bladder emptying. Some women, when using public restrooms, will assume a hovering position to empty the bladder, a position that can inhibit complete bladder emptying. Others will avoid public restrooms altogether, pre-emptively void prior to going out, and restrict fluids to avoid the need to void. All such behaviors have a potential to impact overall bladder health with the delay of voiding associated with the development of bothersome urinary urgency (Palmer et al., 2018).

An important factor to consider when addressing a healthy bladder lifestyle is the impact the work/school environment has on normal voiding. Pierce et al. (2019) looked at the relationship between the work environment, voiding habits, urinary symptoms, and work productivity. Female nurses and midwives were surveyed with one in five nurses reporting restricted toilet access and delay voiding while at work. One in four nurses self-limited fluids while at work to avoid the need to use the toilet. Half of the surveyed nurses reported urinary symptoms while at work with voiding postponement impacting mental concentration and fluid limitations impacting time management. Camenga et al. (2019) conducted a qualitative study that explored adolescent and adult women's experiences in accessing restrooms in schools, in work environments, and in public areas. One of the findings in the study was the significant role gatekeepers played in regulating adolescents' access to toilet facilities in the school, a finding that recurred when interviewing adolescents as well as women recalling experiences in their youth. Common responses to toilet restrictions included limiting fluid intake and delayed voiding, both of which can contribute to incontinence, dysfunctional voiding, and risk for urinary tract infections (UTIs) (von Gontard et al., 2017).

It has also been suggested that other work conditions may impact bladder function such as shift work and night work. Von Gontard et al. (2017) suggests that melatonin production may be suppressed by artificial light, which may be a mechanism that potentially affects bladder contractility. Further research is needed in this area.

The role of the continence nurse is evolving and may be realized in advocating for our patients through local and national avenues. A high priority goal for promoting bladder health is to advocate for adequate toilet access and removal of barriers to toilet facilities in the workplace and school. The continence nurse should actively support research to study behavioral, societal, and environmental determinants of bladder health.

COMORBIDITIES

There are several health conditions that are associated with incontinence and/or bothersome voiding symptoms. Encouraging and in some cases facilitating adequate disease management can promote bladder health and improve existing bladder symptoms and incontinence. **Table 6-1** summarizes some of the more common

TABLE 6-1 COMORBIDITIES AND INCONTINENCE RISK

PROBLEM	IMPACT OF BLADDER HEALTH	NURSING INTERVENTIONS
Urinary tract infections	Irritative voiding symptoms; can precipitate incontinence, urgency, and frequency	• Preventative strategies (see Chapter 18)
Pulmonary disease—chronic cough (Button et al., 2019; Hrisanfow & Hagglund, 2011)	Can impact the pelvic floor increasing risk for pelvic muscle weakness, stress incontinence, and pelvic organ prolapse	• Disease management to minimize cough • Pelvic floor muscle exercises • Stress incontinence prevention strategy "The Knack"
Cardiovascular disease/heart failure/hypertension (Daugirdas et al., 2020; Everaert et al., 2019; John, 2020)	Increased nighttime urine production (nocturnal polyuria) that can aggravate nocturia and nighttime incontinence	• Encourage compliance with disease treatment plan • Fluid modifications such as reducing evening fluid intake • Management of lower extremity edema • Adjust timing of diuretics • Timed voiding for diuretic-induced frequency and urgency • Pelvic floor muscle exercises • Urge suppression strategies
Obstructive sleep apnea (Everaert et al., 2019)	Nocturia, nocturnal polyuria	• Education related to the regular use of CPAP and impact on nocturia and improved sleep. • Fluid modifications such as reducing evening fluid intake
Acute and chronic pain	Functional impairment impacting timely toilet access	• Facilitate pain management plan • Modify barriers to toilet access
Stroke (Holroyd, 2019; Thomas et al., 2019)	Urinary urgency, frequency, urgency incontinence, to a lesser degree impaired bladder emptying, functional impairment impacting timely toilet access	• Modify barriers to toilet access • Lifestyle modification—fluid and diet modifications • Toileting programs • Bladder retraining with urge suppression strategies • Pelvic floor muscle exercises
Multiple sclerosis (Meduba-Polo et al., 2020; Zecca et al., 2016)	Urgency, frequency, nocturia, urgency incontinence, impaired bladder emptying, functional impairment impacting timely toilet access	• Referral to Urology for voiding symptoms to facilitate early diagnosis, treatment, and follow-up • Lifestyle modification—fluid and diet modifications • Bladder retraining with urge suppression strategies • Pelvic floor muscle exercises • Modification of barriers to toileting • Timed voiding—especially in the presence of impaired bladder sensation • Double voiding—to promote adequate emptying • Monitor for incomplete bladder emptying
Parkinson disease (PD) (Sakakibara et al., 2016)	Urgency urinary incontinence, urinary frequency, urgency, urinary hesitancy, weak urinary stream, double voiding, incomplete bladder emptying, functional impairment impacting timely toilet access	• Lifestyle modification—fluid and diet modifications • Bladder retraining with urge suppression strategies • Pelvic floor muscle exercises • Modification of barriers to toileting • In older men, referral for evaluation for BPH (benign prostatic enlargement) • Women: assess for stress incontinence, instruct in pelvic muscle exercises, stress incontinence prevention ("The Knack") • Watch for associated increase in PD symptoms and incontinence—refer for PD medication management • If treated with OAB medications—assess for incomplete emptying
Dementia	Functional impairment impacting timely toilet access	• Individualized plan of care that considers specific cognitive deficits • Lifestyle modification—fluid and diet modifications • Bladder retraining with urge suppression strategies • Pelvic floor muscle exercises • Modification of barriers to toileting • Toileting programs

TABLE 6-1 COMORBIDITIES AND INCONTINENCE RISK (*continued*)

PROBLEM	IMPACT OF BLADDER HEALTH	NURSING INTERVENTIONS
Diabetes (inadequate blood sugar control), metabolic syndrome (John, 2020)	Nocturia Osmotic diuresis induced by hyperglycemia Increases risk for UTI Increased risk for UUI due to microvascular damage Autonomic neuropathy causing impaired bladder sensation, underactive bladder, impaired bladder emptying	• Counseling on blood sugar control • Referral for disease management • Lifestyle modification—fluid and diet modifications • Bladder retraining with urge suppression strategies • Pelvic floor muscle exercises • Modification of barriers to toileting • Timed voiding—especially in the presence of impaired bladder sensation • Double voiding—to promote adequate emptying • Monitor for incomplete bladder emptying
Urogenital syndrome of menopause (Gandhi et al., 2016; Steele et al., 2016)	Urgency, frequency, nocturia, incontinence, dysuria, recurrent UTI	• Education related to the causal relationship between urinary symptoms and urogenital syndrome of menopause • Referral for vaginal estrogen therapy

health care problems that can impact bladder function and some nursing interventions to help guide patient care. Changes associated with aging (Chapter 13), obesity (Chapter 15), UTIs (Chapter 18), and neurogenic lower urinary tract diseases (Chapter 9) are addressed in much more detail in the listed chapters in this textbook.

LIFESTYLE AND BEHAVIORS

Fluids and Diet

Fluid intake and dietary preferences play a major role in normal bladder and bowel function. There is a commonly held belief that drinking large amounts of water is beneficial and healthy. In 2005 the *Institute of Medicine* (IOM, 2005) recommended that total water intake for adult men should be 3.7 L/day and adult women 2.7 L/day. The IOM recommendations incorporated that this fluid intake includes fluids with meals, extra water, as well as water contained in foods. The recommendations clearly state that there is a wide range of fluid intake outside their recommended volumes that constitute normal hydration (IOM, 2005). Lukacz et al. (2011) in their expert consensus statements on health bladder recommended adequate fluid intake to be 25 to 30 mL/kg body weight per day with the goal to void every 3 to 4 hours.

Fluid intake volume does impact bothersome voiding symptoms such as urgency, frequency, nocturia, and urgency incontinence. Callan et al. (2015) completed a systematic review that addressed the question if increasing or decreasing fluids impacted OAB (overactive bladder) symptoms. The results of that review found normal hydration was key to a healthy bladder (Callan et al., 2015). Another systematic review of the literature (Wood et al., 2018) concluded that the commonly held belief that drinking eight glasses of water a day carries no benefit other than in patients with nephrolithiasis. What is known is that excessive fluid intake does increase

urinary urgency and frequency and can exacerbate OAB symptoms including UI (Hashim and Abrams, 2008; IOM, 2005; Lightner et al., 2019). Drinking large volumes over a short time span can also contribute to urinary urgency and frequency. Fluid intake in the hours before sleep can precipitate bothersome nocturia.

Promoting bladder health and initial treatment for incontinence includes normalizing fluid intake. Fluid volume recommendations should include education related to what constitutes normal daily intake of fluids. Thirst is generally an excellent indicator of need for more water. Unfortunately, thirst is a poor indicator of hydration if a patient has dry mouth, which can occur in conditions such as mouth breathers, Sjogren syndrome, and taking medications with anticholinergic effects. In most people, adequate fluid intake will produce pale yellow urine, a concept that patients can easily understand. A common response to urinary urgency, frequency, and UI is to self-restrict fluids (Anger et al., 2011). Fluid restriction or inadequate fluid intake can precipitate increased urinary urgency and increase risk for incontinence (von Gontard et al., 2017). A consistent day-to-day pattern of fluid intake will produce a more consistent pattern of urine elimination, which is critical especially in conjunction with timed voiding strategies or a toileting program. **Box 6-3** summarizes strategies to normalize fluid intake.

The type of fluid intake also impacts bladder function and can aggravate OAB symptoms. Caffeine is one of the most common triggers for urinary urgency and frequency. Common sources of caffeine are coffee, teas, chocolate, soft drinks, and energy drinks, and it is found in some medications. **Box 6-4** contains a list of common bladder irritants based upon dietary triggers identified by patients with interstitial cystitis/painful bladder syndrome (Friedlander et al., 2012; Sutcliffe et al., 2018). The best approach to identifying fluids and foods that trigger

BOX 6-3	STRATEGIES TO NORMALIZE FLUID INTAKE

- Education: role of water for normal body functions, effects of overhydration and dehydration on the bladder
- Recommendations should
  - Specify the type and volume of fluid
  - Approximate timing of fluid intake
  - Space fluid intake throughout the day
- Consistent day-to-day fluid intake
- Avoid excessive fluid intake
- Avoid restricting fluid intake
- Avoid drinking large volumes in one sitting
- Avoid fluid intake within 4 hours of sleep
- Individualize the plan to address fluid preferences, lifestyle, and any concurrent medical conditions

symptoms is to systematically eliminate one item at a time to determine if elimination improves symptoms.

KEY POINT

Caffeine is one of the most common triggers for urinary urgency and frequency.

When counseling a patient on fluid modification, it is helpful to *negotiate* a plan that works best for the patient. Such a plan will promote patient involvement in the plan of care and ultimately will increase adherence. For example, a fluid management plan may involve a gradual weaning of the symptom-producing fluid. In the case of caffeinated beverages, a gradual decrease in caffeinated coffee may

BOX 6-4	COMMON BLADDER IRRITANTS

- Caffeine: coffee, tea, chocolate, iced tea
- Carbonated drinks (especially cola based)
- Dairy products: aged cheese, sour cream, yogurt
- Alcohol: beer, wine, champagne
- High acid fruits: grapefruit, lemon, orange, pineapple
- High-acid fruit juices: cranberry, grapefruit, orange, pineapple
- Tomato and tomato products
- Spicy Foods: hot peppers, chili, horseradish, highly spiced foods
- Artificial sweeteners: NutraSweet, Sweet' Low, Equal, Saccharin
- Vinegar and vinegar-based dressings and sauces
- Foods and beverages containing monosodium glutamate (MSG)

Adapted from: Friedlander, J. I., Shorter, B., & Moldwin, R. M. (2012). Diet and its role in interstitial cystitis/bladder pain syndrome (IC/BPS) and comorbid conditions. *BJU International, 109*, 1584–1591. Sutcliffe, S., Jemielta, T., Lai, H. H., et al. (2018). A case-crossover study of urologic chronic pelvic pain syndrome flare triggers in the Mapp research network. *Journal of Urology, 199*(5), 1245–1251.

start with suggesting ½ caffeinated coffee or decreasing daily morning coffee intake by one cup every week.

Nocturia

Nocturia is defined as waking up from sleep one or more times to void preceded and followed by sleep (van Kerrebroeck et al., 2002). It is a bothersome voiding symptom that is complex and multifaceted requiring careful evaluation to understand the underlying cause. OAB and benign prostatic hypertrophy (BPH) are common causes of frequent nighttime awakening for small-volume voiding. Nocturia can also be the result of increased urine production (nocturnal polyuria) caused by heart disease, obstructive sleep apnea, or chronic kidney disease (Lombardo et al., 2020). An initial assessment should always include a determination of the cause of nighttime voiding: awakening due to an urge to void (true nocturia) or awaking from some other cause, which then prompts the need to empty the bladder. Improving sleep hygiene (**Table 6-2**) promotes bladder health as well as enhances sleep quality, which in turn impacts bothersome nighttime voiding. For patients with true nocturia, first-line strategies include lifestyle modifications such as fluid intake modifications in addition to addressing underlying causes (**Box 6-5**).

KEY POINT

Improving sleep hygiene promotes bladder health as well as improves sleep quality thereby impacting bothersome nighttime voiding.

TABLE 6-2 PATIENT EDUCATION: SLEEP HYGIENE

Lifestyle modifications	• Regular exercise • Avoid exercise in the evening—exercise close to the hour of sleep can affect ability to get to sleep • Avoid caffeine (coffee, tea, chocolate, power drinks) after midday • Alcohol in the evening can cause sleepiness but can also cause interrupted sleep later in the sleep cycle • Avoid eating a heavy meal before bed • Avoid going to bed hungry • Avoid nicotine close to bedtime—also applies to secondhand smoke exposure
Sleeping environment	• Cool, dark, quiet, and comfortable • Light exposure can suppress melatonin making sleep difficult • Avoiding use of electronics before hour of sleep • Use the bedroom only for sleep • Reduce noise in the bedroom
Sleep/wake schedule	• Eliminate naps • Keep a consistent bedtime as well as your wake-up time.

Adapted from Ellis, J. G., & Allen, S. F. (2019). Sleep hygiene and the prevention of chronic insomnia. In M. A. Grandner (Ed.), *Sleep and health* (pp. 137–145). Cambridge, MA: Academic Press.

BOX 6-5	STRATEGIES FOR NOCTURIA MANAGEMENT

- Limiting fluids within 4 hours of sleep
- Avoid fluid intake when awakened from sleep
- Edema management: Elevation of lower extremities, compression therapy
- Avoid use of diuretics in evening

Weight Management

Evidence points toward increased body mass index (BMI) and obesity as risk factors for UI in both men and women (Khullar et al., 2014). The Symptoms of Lower Urinary Tract Dysfunction Research Network (LURN) observational study (*n* = 920) identified a positive association between obesity and urgency incontinence, urgency, and frequency in both men and women and stress incontinence and OAB symptoms in women (Lai et al., 2019). Research has shown that weight loss strategies such as diet and exercise decrease stress incontinence episodes in women (Yazdany et al., 2020) and positively impact QoL (Auwad et al., 2008). Given the association between obesity and incontinence, and the fact that obesity increases risk for other health care problems, the continence nurse should include interventions to promote sustained weight loss in individuals who are overweight and obese (Dumoulin et al., 2017). When addressing obesity-related risk for coronary heart disease, type 2 diabetes, cancer, and disability, the United States Preventative Services Task Force (USPSTF) recommends that practitioners in the primary care setting offer or refer patients with a BMI 30 or higher for behavior-based interventions (Curry et al., 2018). The USPSTF review of literature identified weight loss interventions as weight monitoring by the patient, exercise, and monitoring tools such as scales, pedometers, or videos (Curry et al., 2018). Referral for weight loss counseling may also be an effective strategy. For further discussion on the link between obesity and bladder dysfunction, see Chapter 15.

Physical Activity

Regular physical exercise is a lifestyle modification that positively impacts overall health (USHHS, 2018). There is some evidence to support that moderate levels of exercise may decrease risk of developing UI (Bo & Nygaard, 2020; Dumoulin et al., 2017; Moreno-Vecino et al., 2015). Regular physical exercise is proposed to strengthen the pelvic floor muscles (PFMs) given that there seems to be a co-contraction of the abdominal and hip muscles and the PFMs (Lasak et al., 2018; Luginbuehl et al., 2015). An analysis of data from the 2005 to 2006 *National Health and Nutrition Examination Survey* (NHANES) revealed an association between severity of urgency-related UI and increased duration of sedentary behavior in a sample of 459 women aged 60 and older with the clear implication

that decreasing time sitting may reduce urgency UI (Jerez-Roid et al., 2020). Further research is certainly needed but the continence nurse can safely recommend moderate exercise to promote bladder health, if not contraindicated by other health care conditions.

KEY POINT

Continence nurses can safely recommend moderate exercise to promote bladder health, if not contraindicated by comorbid conditions, but further research is necessary.

Smoking

Urinary tract health is significantly impacted by smoking. Tobacco use is a leading risk factor for urinary tract cancers such as bladder, prostate and upper track cancers with an associated upsurge in cancer mortality (NIH, 2019). Smoking also has been linked to nephrolithiasis, infertility, benign prostatic hyperplasia, and interstitial cystitis (Mobley & Baum, 2015). Chronic cough, a common consequence of smoking and related chronic lung disease, has been identified as a risk factor for incontinence in women (Button, et al., 2019; Hrisanfow & Hagglund, 2011). Chronic cough contributes to pelvic floor dysfunction and stress incontinence (Mobley & Baum, 2015). The impact of vaping on the urinary tract is yet to be determined. Patients who smoke should be counseled on cessation and referred to a smoking cessation provider.

Toileting Habits

There are behaviors related to the frequency of voiding and toileting habits that impact bladder health and may also indicate underlying bladder overactivity. Normal bladder emptying occurs every 3 to 4 hours depending on fluid volume intake (Lukacz et al., 2011). There are many factors that impact voiding frequency including the volume and type of fluid intake, sensation of bladder urgency, unavailability of socially acceptable toilet facilities resulting in voiding postponement, voiding more frequently without the sensation of urgency, preemptive voiding to prevent urgency and incontinence, infrequent voiding due to being too busy, and voiding frequently due to a fear of incontinence (Wu et al., 2019). Over time, increased voiding frequency is thought to lower bladder capacity and contribute to voiding dysfunction. Increased voiding frequency also may indicate possible underlying and nondiagnosed bladder overactivity (Peng et al., 2017). Voiding postponement is thought to cause bladder mucosa irritation increasing the risk for developing lower urinary tract symptoms (LUTS) such as urgency, frequency, and nocturia as well as increasing the risk for UTI (Palmer et al., 2018; Wan et al., 2017). Evidence suggests that women who routinely delay voiding or preemptively void without urge and strain to void are

BOX 6-6	HEALTHY VOIDING BEHAVIORS FOR WOMEN

- Void every 3 to 4 hours
- Relaxed position for voiding
- Feet flat on the floor
- Use of a small stool for voiding, especially if the feet are dangling
- Use of toilet seat covers when in public restrooms (are available in small travel packages)
- Allow adequate time for voiding
- Avoid Valsalva during voiding
- Avoid hovering position to void

more likely to have an OAB (Daily et al., 2019; Kowalik et al., 2019).

Toileting habits can also impact bladder emptying. Poor understanding of normal voiding has been associated with Valsalva's or straining during voiding and failure to relax the pelvic floor during voiding (Burgio et al., 2013). Women who hover over the toilet to avoid contact with perceived unclean toilet seats do not completely relax the pelvic floor and external urinary sphincter and therefore are at risk for incomplete bladder emptying, UTIs, and voiding dysfunction (Yang et al., 2010).

The continence nurse is a key source of information related to healthy toileting behaviors (**Box 6-6**). The continence nurse can be a source of *referral* for advanced evaluation and treatment for men and women who routinely exhibit toileting behaviors such as delaying voiding, preemptive voiding, and straining to void.

KEY POINT

The continence nurse can be a source of referral for advanced evaluation and treatment for men and women who routinely exhibit toileting behaviors such as delaying voiding, preemptive voiding, and straining to void.

PELVIC FLOOR HEALTH

A healthy pelvic floor supports the abdominopelvic organs that lie above it and is a critical component of overall bladder health and continence (Burgio et al., 2013). Inadequate support contributes to urgency and stress incontinence and fecal incontinence, as well as pelvic organ prolapse. Failure of the pelvic floor is complex and can be linked to muscle and endopelvic fascia injury such as during childbirth, muscle weakness due to aging, damage to connective tissue that contributes to overall support, or denervation of critical neural control such as damage to the pudendal nerve or S2-S4 nerve roots. See Chapters 2, 11 and 12 for more detail.

PFM exercises are recommended as first-line treatment for the prevention and treatment of stress and

urgency incontinence in men and women (Dumoulin et al., 2017; Lightner et al., 2019; Nambiar et al., 2018; Qaseem et al., 2014; Tse et al., 2016). In a 2014 systematic review, Dumoulin et al. (2018) concluded after a review of 38 trials that women with stress incontinence receiving treatment with PFMT (pelvic floor muscle training) were 5 times more likely to report cure of as well as to demonstrate decreased urine leakage. Chang et al. (2016a) in a systematic review and meta-analysis of 11 studies concluded that PFMT instruction prior to radical prostatectomy improves the early return of continence but did not necessarily impact long-term continence rates. There is growing evidence that PFM can positively impact the bothersome symptoms of pelvic organ prolapse (Hagen et al., 2017).

KEY POINT

Pelvic floor muscle exercises are recommended as first-line treatment for the prevention and treatment of stress and urgency incontinence in men and women.

Teaching Pelvic Floor Muscle Exercises

Promoting bladder health involves teaching the "why, where, and how" of performing PFM exercises. Patient education improves exercise adherence and is an essential component of the treatment plan (Dumoulin et al., 2015; Hay-Smith et al., 2015). Start education with a discussion on the role the pelvic floor plays in overall prevention and treatment of urinary and fecal incontinence and pelvic organ prolapse. Always be alert for any potential barriers to compliance such as long workdays, problems remembering to exercise, or lack of confidence to perform PFM exercises correctly. Offer suggestions to improve compliance such as an individualized exercise schedule, prompts to remember, and setting mutual and realistic goals. The use of pictures and/or pelvic models is helpful when reviewing pelvic anatomy (see **Figs. 6-2 and 6-3**). The continence nurse should keep the discussion simple and practical. **Tables 6-3 and 6-4** give a simple review of the pelvic floor anatomy with implications for patient teaching.

KEY POINT

When teaching patients, it is more important to stress correct technique in performing pelvic floor muscle exercises than in doing lots of repetitions improperly.

Motor learning, such as learning how to perform PFM exercises, is dependent on practice and feedback. Adequate learning is not only dependent on demonstration of the ability to correctly perform a muscle contraction but also involves being able *repeat* (learning retained) and *apply* learning to varied situations (generalizable learning). When teaching patients, it is

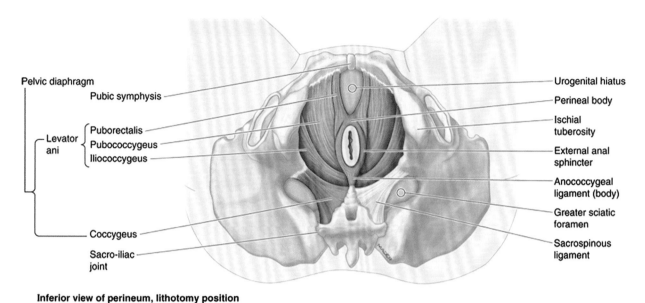

Inferior view of perineum, lithotomy position

FIGURE 6-2. Structures of the Pelvic Floor. (From Moore, K. L., Agur, A. M. R., & Dalley, A. F. (2013). *Clinically oriented anatomy.* Philadelphia, PA: Lippincott Williams & Wilkins.)

important to emphasize that doing a PFM exercise *correctly* is more important than doing multiple repetitions. **Box 6-7** lists the elements of teaching patients how to perform PFM exercises. Underscore the importance of the *rest period* after a muscle contraction; muscle strength is dependent upon adequate rest. Explain that muscle control is as important as muscle strength and daily exercise reinforces what has been learned. Giving feedback about contracting and relaxing the correct muscles is best achieved by digital palpation of the PFMs through the vagina (see **Fig. 6-4**) and in men by observing for the lifting of the scrotum or palpating the PFMs through the rectum. In addition to using the correct muscles, it is important to give feedback related to the ability to isolate the PFM and avoid contraction of the adnominal muscles, gluteals, or the hip abductors. An effective strategy is to observe for use of accessory muscles (abdomen, thighs, buttocks) during pelvic muscle contraction and watching to make

sure there is no breath holding or bearing down (Valsalva) during muscle contraction. If there is poor muscle isolation, ask the patient to place a hand over the abdomen or buttocks to be better aware of accessory muscle use. In some cases, asking the patient to decrease the strength or duration of the PFM contraction, especially if the muscle is weak, helps to improve muscle isolation. Patients who hold their breath during muscle contraction can be asked to count out loud, which effectively prevents breath holding. Valsalva during PFM contraction increases intra-abdominal pressure and pressure on the pelvic floor and should be stopped. Ask the patients to decrease the strength and duration of muscle contraction until they can perform the exercise correctly. PFM exercises should not be painful and pain may indicate a high-tone pelvic floor or PFM spasms. Some patients may be unable to isolate the PFM or elicit a muscle contraction. These patients should be referred to a continence provider such as a continence advanced practice registered nurse (APRN), urologist, or urogynecologist for further evaluation and advanced treatment modalities such as pelvic floor biofeedback, electrical stimulation, and/or pelvic physical therapy.

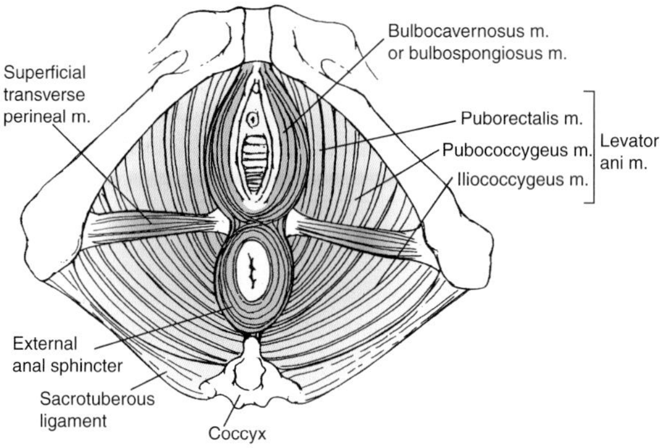

Once the patient has learned how to do a PFM exercise, an exercise prescription should be given. **Table 6-5** lists the components of a PFMT exercise prescription. Available evidence varies widely when describing the exact components of an optimal exercise prescription in terms of number of repeated muscle contractions per day and duration of muscle contraction (Dumoulin et al., 2011; Hay-Smith et al., 2012; Luginbuehl et al., 2015). This author advocates an exercise prescription that is a middle approach based upon available evidence and in my own practice has proven effective due to an "easy to remember" formula of contractions, and repetitions.

FIGURE 6-3. Puborectalis and Levator Ani. (From Pfeifer, S. M. (2011). *NMS obstetrics and gynecology.* Philadelphia, PA: Lippincott Williams & Wilkins.)

TABLE 6-3 PELVIC FLOOR LEVELS OF SUPPORT

PELVIC FLOOR LEVELS OF SUPPORT	STRUCTURES	IMPLICATIONS WITH PFM EXERCISES
Level I Endopelvic fascia	• Lining consisting of ligaments, nerves, blood vessels, connective tissue • Covers bladder, intestine, uterus, upper vagina • Ligaments connect to lumbar spine and symphysis pubis	Improving strength to the pelvic diaphragm (2nd layer) creates better support for the pelvic organs. If there has been damage to the endopelvic fascia, reduction of stress on ligaments by strengthening the pelvic diaphragm can improving symptoms such as lower back pain and reduce risk for pelvic organ prolapse.

Level II Pelvic diaphragm	• Consists of the skeletal muscle the levator ani
	• Hammock-like muscle that stretches from the public bone to the coccyx.
	• Consists of:
	  • Puborectalis muscle—with contraction pulls the rectum forward
	  • Pubococcygeus muscle—supports proximal urethra and bladder neck
	  • Iliococcygeus muscle—provides support especially during times of increased intra-abdominal pressure
		Levator ani muscle is the main support for the pelvic organs and maintains a higher resting tone than other skeletal muscles. It contracts to keep the urethra closed and relaxes to allow for voiding. Strengthening this muscle can improve continence and impact symptoms and progression of pelvic organ prolapse.

Level III Urogenital diaphragm	• Consists of several muscles that include the:
	  • Deep transverse perineal muscle
	  • Superficial transverse perineal muscle
	  • Bulbocavernosus muscle
	  • Anal sphincter muscle
	• These muscles do not support the pelvic organs but do contribute to continence as well as sexual function.
		The strengthening of the anal sphincter muscle in conjunction with the puborectalis muscle is a component in preventing and treating fecal incontinence.

"The 'Knack' Maneuver" to Prevent Stress Incontinence

Once a patient has learned how to do effective PFM exercises, there are other strategies that are extremely effective in preventing and treating UI. One strategy, commonly known as "the Knack" (Miller et al., 1989), the stress maneuver or "squeeze before you sneeze" is effective in preventing stress incontinence during times of increased intra-abdominal pressure, such as coughs, sneezes, moving from sitting to standing, or lifting a grandchild (see **Box 6-8**). Contraction of the striated muscles of the urethral sphincter as well as the pubococcygeus and puborectalis muscles increases pressure within the urethra additionally supporting the urethra by elevating the proximal urethra during times of increased intra-abdominal pressure preventing urine leakage (Miller et al., 2008). The "Knack" is effective in women with stress incontinence as well as men with postprostatectomy stress incontinence.

KEY POINT

One strategy, commonly known as "the Knack" stress maneuver or "squeeze before you sneeze" is effective in preventing stress incontinence during times of increased intra-abdominal pressure, such as coughs, sneezes, moving from sitting to standing, or lifting a grandchild.

TABLE 6-4 PELVIC FLOOR MUSCLE FIBERS

MUSCLE FIBER TYPE	IMPLICATIONS WHEN TEACHING PFM EXERCISES
Type I fiber—slow twitch fibers Approximately 70% of the PFM	• Maintains overall muscle tone • The "holding" muscles—helps with getting to the bathroom in time • Strengthened by teaching endurance "holding" muscle contractions • Used to help control bladder urgency, frequency, urgency incontinence as well as strengthening to prevent or treat fecal incontinence
Type II fibers—fast-twitch fibers Approximately 30% of the PFM	• Increases pressure in the urethra to prevent urine leakage during times of increased intra-abdominal pressure (cough, sneeze, running, jumping) • Quick to turn on and off muscles • Strengthened by teaching strong "quick" flick muscle contractions • Used to prevent and treat stress incontinence

| BOX 6-7 | PATIENT EDUCATION: PELVIC FLOOR MUSCLE TRAINING |

1. Ask the patient to empty the bladder.
2. Review the location of the PFM using picture/diagram/ pelvic model.
3. Position patient in a comfortable position—supine with knees bent, head on a pillow.
4. Teach about muscle isolation: "Squeeze like you are trying to control the passage of gas, keep your abdomen, thighs and buttocks relaxed."
5. Palpate the pelvic floor muscles/observe for use of accessory muscles (buttocks, abdomen, thighs, breath holding).
6. Ask patient to squeeze for a count of 10 (10 seconds) and relax for a count of 10 (10 seconds).
7. Repeat the squeeze and relax 10 times.
8. Assess for consistently in performance and for muscle fatigue
   a. poor control during muscle contraction
   b. decreasing ability to hold
   c. problems relaxing the muscle after contraction
9. Provide feedback about performance giving specific strategies to improve performance.
10. Develop an exercise prescription.

Urge Suppression and Bladder Retraining

Urinary urgency, frequency, and urgency UI are very bothersome symptoms associated with OAB (see Chapter 7). Psychological stress, anxiety, and depression often are associated with OAB symptoms (Lai et al., 2016; Vrijens et al., 2015). Helping patients with bothersome urgency requires attention to far more than just urinary symptoms. Acknowledging the patient's distress as a compo-

nent of their urinary symptoms is therapeutic and helps gain insight into behaviors that precede or occur with urgency. Counseling patients on relaxation strategies such a deep breathing and progressive relaxation can help in selected cases. Some clinicians refer patients to yoga as a strategy to manage the stress, depression, and anxiety associated with their incontinence. Unfortunately, there are limited data to support efficacy of yoga in the treatment of incontinence (Wieland et al., 2019). Referral to a mental health provider may also be helpful.

Urinary urgency is a strong and "not to be delayed" sensation of the need to empty the bladder immediately. "Lachkey" or "key in the lock" urgency and incontinence is a particularly bothersome symptom of OAB described as an overwhelming need to urinate when reaching home. O'Connell et al. (2014) used an online questionnaire to compare patients with and without self-reported symptoms of OAB experiencing urinary urgency associated with environmental cues (e.g., exposed to cold, drinking cold water, near a bathroom, running water, getting up in the morning after sleep). Their findings revealed that both groups reported urgency related to a bathroom trip or opening the front door after being out. Patients with OAB reported a higher occurrence of urinary urgency with environmental cues. Identification of a patient's unique urgency cues is the first step in managing them. In many cases the urgency cue is repeated behavior—such as "I drive down the street and pull into the driveway and then the urgency starts." Some patients will just pass the bathroom door, hear running water, or start cooking dinner and experience urgency. Changing the sequence of events such as driving a different way

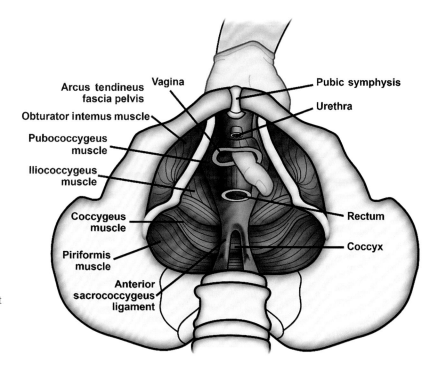

FIGURE 6-4. Providing Feedback on Correct Isolation of the PFM Exercise in Women. (Reprinted with permission from Newman, D. K., DNP. Pelvic Muscle Rehabilitation Clinical Manual.)

TABLE 6-5 THE PFM EXERCISE PRESCRIPTION

PRESCRIPTION	DEFINITION	EXAMPLE
Exercise type	Describes the contraction of the PFM and body position for exercise Doing exercises in different positions (supine vs. sitting vs. standing) changes the resistance, like adding weights to a leg lift type exercise. If the muscle is weak, the supine position may be the best position to start with progression to sitting and then standing when stronger.	PFM exercises in the lying position for 2 sets a day and sitting position for 1 set a day
Duration	The time period during which the muscle is contracted and is often called the hold time. The hold of the muscle contraction should be equal in strength for each repetition. The ability to hold the muscle contraction can be gradually increased as strength improves to a maximum duration of 10 seconds (count of 10).	Hold muscle contraction for a count of 5 (5 seconds).
Rest	Time period when the muscle is at rest and allows recovery after muscle contraction. Relaxation can be facilitated by taking deep breaths. The rest time should be at least equal to the hold time, and in the case of muscle weakness or inability to quickly relax may need to be greater than the hold time.	Relax the muscle for a count of 10 seconds.
Intensity	Describe the strength of muscle contraction for exercise. In the case of muscle weakness, it may be necessary to decrease the strength of the muscle contraction to a percentage of the strongest contraction and gradually increase intensity as the muscle strengthens.	Hold the muscle contraction at 50% strength.
Frequency	Lists the number of repetitions in each exercise session or "set" as well as how many times a day exercise should occur. Initially exercise sets should be 10 repetitions at least 3–4 times a day. Long term, one exercises set a day is sufficient.	Do 10 repetitions (1 set) 3 times a day.

home, relaxation strategies, and diverting thoughts away from the bothersome cue can impact symptoms.

Urge suppression utilizes both the pelvic floor and cognitive strategies to inhibit bladder contractions, reduce the sensation of urgency, delay voiding, and prevent urine leakage. With urinary urgency there is increased anxiety usually over the fear of an embarrassing leak. The first step in suppressing that urge is to promote relaxation with some deep breaths. With an increase in pelvic floor muscle tone (PFM contraction) there is a corresponding inhibiting response of the detrusor muscle. Performing quick and strong PFM contractions followed by mental distraction inhibits urgency (see **Box 6-9**). Working on urgency suppression is difficult, like climbing a mountain (see **Fig. 6-5**). Support and encouragement by the continence nurse is an important component of success. Bladder training (Wallace et al., 2004) is a behavioral program that gradually increases intervals between voiding to reduce urinary frequency through urge suppression techniques. A bladder diary is used as a tool to identify voiding intervals and to measure success with deferred voiding. Goals are mutually agreed upon with the patient on how long to suppress urge before using the toilet. In this way, the interval between voiding is gradually increased with the continence nurse there as coach and cheerleader.

BOX 6-8   PATIENT EDUCATION: PREVENTION OF STRESS INCONTINENCE

The "Knack Maneuver"
Quickly and strongly contract the PFM immediately before:
- Cough
- Sneeze
- Bending over
- Lifting heavy object
- Laughing
- Or other activities identified to cause a leak of urine

Created by Donna L. Thompson.
References
Miller, J., Ashton-Miller, J., & DeLancey, J. O. O. (1989). A pelvic muscle precontraction can reduce cough related urine loss in selected women with mild SUI. *Journal of the American Geriatric Society, 46*, 870–874.
Miller, J. M., Sampselle, C. M., Ashton-Miller, J. A., et al. (2008). Clarification and confirmation of the effect of volitional pelvic floor muscle contraction to preempt urine loss (The Knack Maneuver) in stress incontinent women. *International Urogynecology Journal Pelvic Floor Dysfunction, 19*(6), 773–782.

KEY POINT

Urge suppression utilizes both the pelvic floor and cognitive strategies to inhibit bladder contractions, reduce the sensation of urgency, delay voiding, and prevent urine leakage.

BOWEL HEALTH

The lower bowel and lower urinary tract have similarities in function and innervation as well as in proximity with each other (Grundy & Brierley, 2018). Thus, it makes sense that bladder and bowel dysfunction often occur together (Panicker et al., 2019). Constipation has long

BOX 6-9 PATIENT EDUCATION: URGE SUPPRESSION AND BLADDER RETRAINING

Patient Teaching: Steps to Control Urgency
- Stop the rush to the bathroom.
- Take some deep breaths.
- Contract the PFM quickly and strongly 6 times in a row.
- Take your mind off going to the bathroom: for example count backwards from 100, recite a favorite poem, name the state capitals, list your grandchildren in order of birth.
- When the urge has gone away, slowly walk to the bathroom.

Teaching talking points
- Start practicing at home.
- Inside your head repeat the phrase "I can do this; I am in control."
- Rushing to the toilet only makes the urge worse.
- If urgency returns while on the way to the toilet, repeat the process.
- A urine leak does not mean failure.

Bladder Training
- Using a bladder diary, identify the baseline voiding interval.
- Develop realistic goals with the patient.
- Using urge suppression, progressively lengthen intervals between voiding.
- Use a bladder diary to measure success.
- Provide encouragement and positive reinforcement.
- End Goal: 3- to 4-hour voiding interval

been identified as a risk factor for developing LUTS. Bowel management is a critical component in both promoting a healthy bladder as well as being a part of the treatment plan in the management of UI, OAB, urinary urgency, and frequency (Coyne et al., 2011b; Thurmon et al., 2013). Fecal incontinence, or accidental bowel leakage (ABL) (Brown et al., 2012) is a common problem that is underrecognized and undertreated (Whitehead et al., 2016). ABL varies from embarrassing flatus incontinence to full incontinence of bowel contents. First-line treatment for constipation and ABL includes healthy bowel habits and normalizing stool consistency. In-depth discussion of constipation and ABL resistant to simple first-line strategies is covered in Chapters 21 and 22.

Teaching patients about healthy bowel habits and dietary strategies to normalize stool consistency is a fundamental component of any treatment plan for a healthy bladder and bowel, and managing simple constipation and ABL. There are strategies that promote normal and regular bowel emptying such as responding to the urge or "call" to move the bowels rather than repeatedly inhibiting the urge, assuming a proper position for optimum defecation (see **Fig. 6-6**), normalizing stool consistency, and promoting bowel motility (**Box 6-10**).

KEY POINT

There are several strategies that promote normal and regular bowel emptying such as responding to the urge to move the bowels rather than repeatedly inhibiting urgency, assuming a proper position for optimal defecation, normalizing stool consistency, and promoting bowel motility.

Normalizing Stool Consistency

Normalizing stool consistency includes addressing both constipation as well as stools that have a more liquid texture. The Bristol Stool Scale (Chumpitazi et al., 2016; Heaton & Lewis, 1997) was adopted by the ROME III committee (Longstreth et al., 2006) as a tool to categorized stool types in irritable bowel syndrome (IBS) but is now commonly used in many settings to help assess a patient's stool consistency (see **Fig. 6-7**). The softness or water content in the stool affects the speed at which bowel contents travel through the large bowel and the ease of defecation (McRorie and McKeown, 2017). Stool types 5 and 6 are described as having a soft, mushy, loose, pasty, or sticky consistency. Overly soft stools

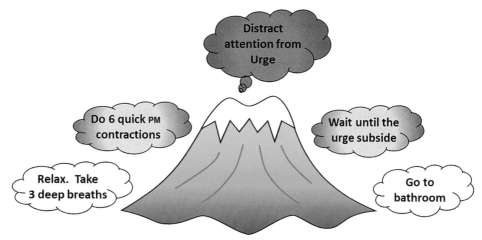

FIGURE 6-5. Urge Suppression Strategy.

Correct position for opening your bowels

Step one

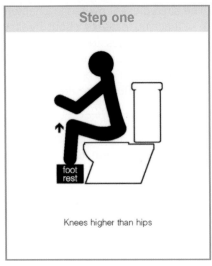

Knees higher than hips

Step two

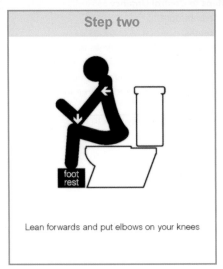

Lean forwards and put elbows on your knees

Step three

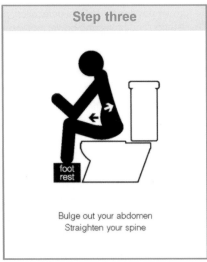

Bulge out your abdomen
Straighten your spine

Correct position

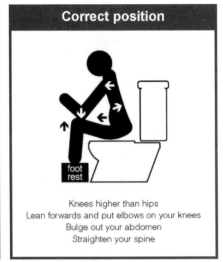

Knees higher than hips
Lean forwards and put elbows on your knees
Bulge out your abdomen
Straighten your spine

Reproduced by the kind permission of Ray Addison, Nurse Consultant in Bladder and Bowel Dysfunction.
Wendy Ness, Colorectal Nurse Specialist.

Produced as a service to the medical profession by Norgine Ltd.

MO/03/11 (6809792) November 2003

FIGURE 6-6. Correct Position for Opening the Bowels. (Reproduced by the kind permission of Ray Addison, Nurse Consultant in Bladder and Bowel Dysfunction. Wendy Ness, Colorectal Nurse Specialist. Produced as a service to the medical profession by Norgine Ltd.)

have a higher fluid content, which reduces transit time, increases the number of stools, and, in some cases such as women with rectocele, can impair complete rectal emptying resulting in difficult hygiene, fecal smearing, and fecal stress incontinence. Stools with a higher fluid content can increase fecal urgency and an inability to hold, especially if the external anal sphincter is weak. Hard and difficult to pass stools (Bristol Stool Scale types 2 and 1) have a lower water content, take longer to transit the large bowel, and can result in straining. It takes more time and effort to evacuate a small hard stool.

Stool retention in the rectum, if severe and obstructive, can cause fecal overflow incontinence. Hard stool in the lower bowel also negatively impacts OAB symptoms. The optimal stool size and consistency is reflected in the Bristol Stool Scale types 3 and 4.

There are food triggers that affect bowel motility resulting in a change in stool consistency and adequate elimination and in some cases increase risk for ABL. For example, a diet high in fat slows bowel motility increasing the risk for constipation. Caffeine is a bowel stimulant and can increase bowel motility with resultant increase in

BOX 6-10   HEALTHY BOWEL STRATEGIES

- Answer the "call to stool."
- Take your time.
- Avoid straining.
- Position for easing the passing of stool
  - Feet flat on the floor
  - Keep the back straight, lean forward, rest your forearms on your knees or
  - Use a modified "squat" position: Elevate the knees above the hips when on the toilet with a small stool so to promote straightening of the anorectal angle (see Fig. 4)
- Normalizing stool consistency to prevent constipation and incontinence
  - Fiber healthy diet
  - Fiber supplementation (e.g., psyllium)
  - Adequate hydration
- Regular Exercise—promotes bowel motility
- Pelvic floor muscle exercises
- Best time of day for a bowel movement is about ½ hour after the AM meal when the gastrocolic reflex is at work.
- Identify and eliminate foods that trigger unwanted changes in bowel motility (use a bowel diary).
  - Vegetables: Gas-producing vegetables, onions
  - Spicy foods
  - Caffeinated foods and beverages
  - Fatty/greasy foods
  - Sugar/candy
  - Popcorn, seeds
  - Cheese

Adapted from: Bliss, D. Z., Savik, K., Jung, H. J., et al. (2014). Dietary fiber supplementation for fecal incontinence: a randomized clinical trial. *Research in Nursing & Health, 37*(5), 367–378.

Bove, A., Bellini, M., Battaglia, E., et al. (2012). Consensus statement AIGO/SICCR diagnosis and treatment of chronic constipation and obstructed defecation (Part II: Treatment). *World Journal of Gastroenterology, 18*(36), 4994–5013.

Carter, D. (2016). Conservative and novel treatment options for fecal incontinence. *Journal of Gastrointestinal & Digestive System, 6,* 428. doi: 10.4172/2161-069X.1000428.

Chang, J., McLemore, E., & Tejirian, T. (2016). Anal health care basics. *Permanente Journal, 20*(4), 15–222.

Colavita, K., & Andy, U. U. (2016). Role of diet in fecal incontinence: A systematic review of the literature. *International Urogynecology Journal, 27,* 1805–1810.

Croswell, E., Bliss, D. Z., & Savik, K. (2010). Diet and eating pattern modifications used by community-living adults to manage their fecal incontinence. *Journal of Wound, Ostomy, and Continence Nursing, 37*(6), 677–682.

Hansen, J. L., Bliss, D. Z., & Peden-McAlpine, C. (2006). Diet strategies used by women to manage fecal incontinence. *Journal of Wound, Ostomy, and Continence Nursing, 33*(1), 52–61; discussion 61–62.

Paquette, I. M., Barma, M., Kaiser, A., et al. (2015). The American Society of Colon and Rectal Surgeons' clinical practice guideline for the treatment of fecal incontinence. *Diseases of the Colon and Rectum, 58,* 623–636.

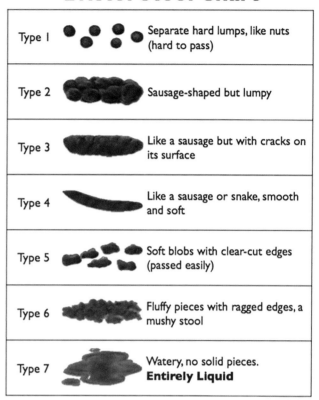

Bristol Stool Chart

Type 1		Separate hard lumps, like nuts (hard to pass)
Type 2		Sausage-shaped but lumpy
Type 3		Like a sausage but with cracks on its surface
Type 4		Like a sausage or snake, smooth and soft
Type 5		Soft blobs with clear-cut edges (passed easily)
Type 6		Fluffy pieces with ragged edges, a mushy stool
Type 7		Watery, no solid pieces. **Entirely Liquid**

FIGURE 6-7. Bristol Stool Scale. (From Lewis, S. J., & Heaton, K. W. (1997). Stool form scale as a useful guide to intestinal transit time. *Scandinavian Journal of Gastroenterology, 32*(9), 920–924.)

stool fluid content, which, in turn, can precipitate fecal incontinence. In some cases, a morning cup of coffee facilitates bowel motility and can be a helpful strategy for constipation. Personal experience with foods should guide dietary limitations (Colavita & Andy, 2016; Croswell et al., 2010; Hansen et al., 2006), which illustrates the importance of a diet/stool diary to identify bothersome foods (see **Fig. 6-8** for an example) and eliminate them from the diet. Advanced management of bowel motility disorders is addressed in Chapter 21.

KEY POINT

Adequate dietary fiber intake as well as hydration and physical activity are major components in bowel health.

Adding Fiber to the Diet

Adequate dietary fiber intake as well as hydration and physical activity are major components in bowel health. The 2015–2020 Dietary Guidelines for Americans (U.S. Department of Health and Human Services and U.S. Department of Agriculture, 2015) recommends a daily intake of 25 g/day for women and 38 g/day for men. The average daily fiber intake of Americans ranges from

Instructions:
Use the space provided on the following pages to document your eating habits and bowel movements for the next week. Each page represents a day of the week. Remember to record **every** meal, bowel movement, and accident.
See the example below for completed entry.

Date: Sunday, January 1, 2017

Time	Meal/Food Intake	BM?	Stool Score	Urgency Y=Yes, N=No	Accidental Bowel *Leakage* S=Small, M=Medium, L=Large	Comments	Bristol Stool Score
9 am	Oatmeal						
11 am		✔	7	Y		Ran to the bathroom	
12 pm	Almonds Apple						
2 pm	Brown rice Ground turkey Vegetables						
6 pm	Chicken Mashed potatoes Gravy						
7 pm		✔	6	Y	M		

Type 1
Type 2
Type 3
Type 4
Type 5
Type 6
Type 7

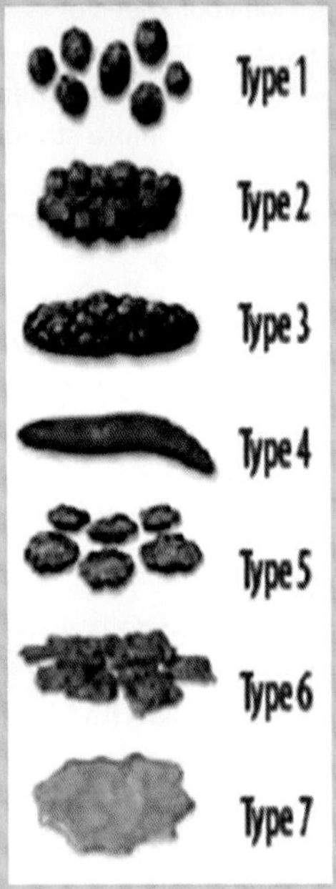

FIGURE 6-8. Diet/Stool Diary. (Used with permission from Andy, U. U., MD. Philadelphia, PA).

15 to 17 g/day with only 5% of the population meeting national recommended intake (Academy of Nutrition and Dietetics, 2015; McGill et al., 2015). The large prospective Nurses Health Study, n = 58,330 women, revealed that that higher long-term dietary fiber intake was associated with lower risk of developing fecal incontinence (Staller et al., 2018).

Increasing fiber in the diet can normalize the stool to a soft and formed stool (Bristol Scale type 4) that is completely evacuated thus minimizing constipation and, in some cases, decreasing ABL. To improve bowel elimination, fiber must increase stool bulk as well as soften the stool by increasing stool water content. Dietary fiber must also resist fermentation and remain intact in the stool the full length of the colon. Wheat bran consists of large insoluble fiber, resistant to fermentation, that stimulates secretion of water and mucus through an irritating effect on the mucosa of the colon thus producing higher water content in the stool and faster colonic transit. Psyllium is a soluble gel-forming fiber that increases colonic water content thus also increasing colonic transit

(McRorie & McKeown, 2017). Gel-forming fiber also has the benefit of modulating stool consistency that is too soft, improving ABL due to incomplete rectal emptying. Many high-fiber foods contain both soluble and insoluble fiber, both contributing to overall health as well as bowel health. **Table 6-6** lists high-fiber foods that can be slowly incorporated into the diet to promote bowel health and/or normalize stool consistency. Refer to Chapters 21 and 22 for a more detailed discussion in the use of fiber in patient with ABL and problems with bowel motility where careful attention to types of fiber is critical.

Pelvic Floor Muscle Exercises and Bowel Health

PFM exercises improve bowel health and are often incorporated in a plan to treat ABL. In addition, they improve external anal sphincter tone (Rao et al., 2015; Whitehead et al., 2015) and are proposed to strengthen the puborectalis muscle as it surrounds the anorectal junction thus creating a 90-degree angle between the rectum and anal canal that enhances anal continence. See **Figure 20-6** to appreciate the anorectal angle created by the puborectalis

TABLE 6-6 HIGH-FIBER FOODS		
FIBER SOURCE	PORTION SIZE	DIETARY FIBER (G)
CEREALS AND GRAINS		
Bran cereals	½–¾ cup	9.1–14.3
Wheat bran flakes cereal	¾ cup	5.0–5.5
Cooked bulgur	½ cup	4.1
Multigrain bread	1 slice	4.3
Cooked pearled barley	½ cup	3.0
BEANS		
Chickpeas	½ cup	8.1
Cooked lentils	½ cup	7.8
Cooked pinto beans	½ cup	7.7
Cooked black beans	½ cup	7.5
Cooked kidney beans	½ cup	5.7
Cooked quinoa	½ cup	2.6
FRUIT		
Pear	Medium	5.5
Avocado	½ cup	5.0
Apple with skin	Medium	4.4
Raspberries	½ cup	4.0
Blackberries	½ cup	3.8
Stewed prunes	½ cup	3.8
Dried figs	¼ cup	3.7
Orange	Medium	3.1
Banana	Medium	3.1
Guava	1 fruit	3.0
Dates	¼ cup	2.9
SEEDS AND NUTS		
Whole roasted pumpkin seeds	1 oz	5.2
Almonds	1 oz	3.5
Dry roasted sunflower seeds	1 oz	3.1
Dry roasted pistachios	1 oz	2.8
Peanuts	1 oz	2.7
VEGETABLES		
Frozen mixed vegetables	½ cup	4.0
Cooked collards	½ cup	3.8
Baked sweet potato	Medium	3.8
Green peas	½ cup	3.5–4.4
Baked potato with skin	Medium	3.6
Vegetable soup	1 cup	2.9
Cooked broccoli	½ cup	2.6
Baby spinach leaves	3 oz	2.1
Carrot	1 medium	1.7

Adapted from U.S Department of Agriculture. *Agricultural Research Service Food Data Central*. Retrieved from https://fdc.nal.usda.gov/. Accessed March 15, 2020.
U.S. Department of Health and Human Services and U.S. Department of Agriculture. (December, 2015). *2015–2020 dietary guidelines for Americans* (8th ed.). Retrieved from http://health.gov/dietaryguidelines/2015/guidelines/. Accessed March 15, 2020.

muscle. Use the techniques for teaching PFM exercises addressed previously (**Box 6-7**; **Table 6-5**).

Anal/Rectal Sensitivity

Anal/rectal sensitivity to the presence of stool is also an important component of fecal continence. ABL may be attributed to altered sensation of the need to move the bowels. Increased sensitivity to rectal distention is associated with bowel urgency and ABL. Impaired ability to recognize a sensation of rectal fullness or to distinguish rectal fullness with gas, liquid, or solid stool can precipitate ABL. **Table 6-7** addresses strategies that can be taught to patients so to help them increase sensitivity to rectal distention or inhibit fecal urgency (Lee et al., 2013; Rao et al., 2015). Patients with ABL may need referral for anorectal manometry and biofeedback. Biofeedback is used to help patients learn to recognize their unique signals of rectal distention by using an inflatable balloon in the rectum that is slowly inflated until a sensation of fullness is identified. The same technique can be used for patients with significant fecal urgency due to increased sensitively to rectal distention. The rectal balloon volume is progressively increased as the patient practices relaxation and urge resistance (see Chapter 22).

CONTINENCE NURSING: ADDRESSING FUNCTIONAL COMPONENTS OF INCONTINENCE

One of the fundamental components of the continence nurse role is to identify and modify as best as possible, barriers to timely toilet access. Frail older adults, adults with multisystem impairment or impaired fine or gross

TABLE 6-7 STRATEGIES FOR ALTERED RECTAL SENSATION ASSOCIATED WITH ABL	
ALTERED SENSATION	STRATEGY
Increase sensitivity to rectal distention	Teach "hypervigilance" to rectal distention • Identify subtle sensations to rectal fullness that could be pressure, fullness, sensation of gas, abdominal pressure • Attend to that sensation and use the toilet
Fecal urgency	Teach urge resistance training • Take deep breaths • Relax the abdomen • Perform anal sphincter squeezes • With the reduction of urgency, walk slowly to the toilet

Created by Donna L. Thompson.
References
Lee, H. J., Jung, K. W., & Myung, S. (2013). Technique of functional and motility test: How to perform biofeedback for constipation and fecal incontinence. *Journal of Neurogastroenterology and Motility, 19*(4), 532–537.
Rao, S. S. C., Benninga, M. A., Bharucha, A. E., et al. (2015). ANMS-ESNM position paper and consensus guidelines on biofeedback therapy for anorectal disorders. *Neurogastroenterology and Motility, 27*(5), 594–609.

motor function, and those who are developmentally disabled, have a greater risk for the development of incontinence due to motivational, physical, and/or cognitive impairments. Chapter 13 reviews in detail the unique needs of older adults with incontinence.

KEY POINT

Frail older adults, adults with multisystem impairment or impaired fine or gross motor function, and those who are developmentally disabled, have a greater risk for the development of incontinence due to motivational, physical, and/or cognitive impairments.

A continence plan of care should always include strategies to prevent, improve and/or maintain continence by overcoming barriers and increasing access to a toilet or toilet substitute (urinal, bedpan, bedside commode). In developing a plan of care, the continence nurse must remember that there are times when the incontinent patients and/or their caregivers choose not to initiate treatment because the burden of treatment far exceeds the burden of the incontinence. It is imperative in these situations (and in fact in all situations) that the ultimate plan reflect collaboration between the patient/caregiver and the continence nurse. In some cases, the most appropriate goal for treatment may be odor and wetness control through the use of an appropriate body-worn absorptive product (see Chapter 16). **Table 6-8** defines realistic continence outcomes for adults with incontinence and functional impairment (Fonda & Abrams, 2006; Palmer et al., 1997). Management strategies can be categorized into two major areas: modification of barriers and toileting

programs. **Tables 6-9 and 6-10** address barriers to toileting and nursing interventions to modify those barriers with the outcome to achieve as much continence as realistically possible (Fletcher, 2012; Grand et al., 2011; Thompson & Bradway, 2017; Walid, 2009).

TOILETING PROGRAMS

Toileting programs are an effective treatment strategy for incontinence due to impaired mobility and cognition. Inherent in the process of developing and implementing toileting programs is the assumption that other barriers to continence (**Tables 6-9 and 6-10**) have been addressed and appropriate interventions implemented. Scheduled toileting programs involve reminding and/or assisting the individual to use the toilet, urinal, or bedpan at prescheduled times. These programs can be implemented on a fixed schedule or can be individualized based on the patient's voiding patterns and ability to participate. All toileting programs involve caregiver support to maintain some degree of continence. There are three commonly used scheduled toileting programs that can be successfully implemented in home care and institutional settings: routine scheduled toileting (RST), habit training, and prompted voiding. See **Table 6-11** for a detailed review of scheduled toileting programs (Colling et al., 1992, 1994; Jirovec, 1991; Lyons and Pringle Specht, 2000; Newman, 2019). Chapter 13 addresses the unique challenges of implementing toileting programs in extended care facilities.

KEY POINT

All toileting programs involve caregiver support to maintain some degree of continence.

TABLE 6-8 REALISTIC CONTINENCE OUTCOMES IN ADULTS WITH FUNCTIONAL IMPAIRMENT

	NURSING INTERVENTIONS	EXPECTED OUTCOMES
Independent continence	• Patient is actively involved in the treatment plan • Healthy bladder strategies	• Continence • Improved continence • Decrease incontinence episodes
Partial continence	• Patient actively involved in the treatment plan • Healthy bladder strategies • Caregiver support needed	• Decrease incontinence episodes • Improve self-esteem • Increase participation in a toileting program • Prevent incontinence-associated skin damage
Dependent continence	• Continent solely through efforts of caregivers as part of a toileting program • Plan includes appropriate use of body-worn absorptive products.	• Decrease wetness • Improve self-esteem • Promote dignity • Prevent incontinence-associated skin damage
Social continence	• Dependent on caregivers • Not continent • Plan includes appropriate use of body-worn absorptive products.	• Maintain patient comfort and dignity • Keep dry and odor-free as possible • Prevent incontinence-associated skin damage

Adapted from: Fonda, D., & Abrams, P. (2006). Cure sometimes, help always—A "continence paradigm" for all ages and conditions. *Neurourology and Urodynamics, 25*(3), 290–292. Based upon: Palmer, M., Reid Czarapata, D., Wells, T., et al. (1997). Urinary outcomes in older adults: Research and clinical perspectives. *Urologic Nursing, 17*(3), 2–9.

TABLE 6-9 MODIFICATION OF BARRIERS TO TOILETING: MOBILITY IMPAIRMENT AND NURSING INTERVENTIONS FOR CONTINENCE

BARRIER TO CONTINENCE	INTERVENTIONS
Immobility	• Physical therapy consultation for transfer techniques, transfer aides, muscle strengthening, joint rehabilitation, gait training • Refer/treat foot and toe deformities (bunions, corns, hammer toes, Charcot foot, fractures) • Refer/treat lower extremity wounds that impact mobility/toilet access • Referral for compromised range of motion and strength of the shoulders and arms (fracture, rotator cuff tear, joint deformities, deconditioning) • Appropriate assistive devices such as canes, walkers, wheelchairs, grab bars, transfer boards • Shoes, supportive and well fitted with nonskid soles • Caregiver training: safe transfer techniques, use of transfer equipment such as transfer discs, transfer belts • Use of bedside commodes, urinals • Raised toilet seats • Provide access to bathroom or commode on same level as living area. • Ensure bed is at a height where when sitting on the side, feet are flat on the floor • Ensure chair cushions are firm, chairs have arms to assist with safe standing • Avoid recliners that are difficult to reposition for standing • Avoid cushions or pillows that restrict easy movement out of chairs and beds • Avoid restraints
Impaired manual dexterity	• Referral to physical and occupational therapy for assistive aides • Modify clothing: stretch waist bands, pants without buttons or zippers, loose-fitting clothing • Avoid clothing with buttons, zippers, hooks, and eyes; tight or ill-fitting clothing; multilayered clothing • Replace bathroom doorknobs with lever-type handles • Use pull-up-type containment products or inserts/pads that can be easily applied and removed • Use of perineal wipes for personal hygiene
Poor visual acuity	• Ensure adequate lighting in bathrooms and areas leading to bathrooms • Motion detection lighting in bathrooms • Night lights • Create clear access to the bathroom by moving trash, equipment, furniture, or any other items that could impede access
Pain	• Referral for adequate pain management
Poor motivation	• Referral for the management of depression • Referral for the management of fatigue, dyspnea, pain • Positive reinforcement of desired behaviors

TABLE 6-10 MODIFYING BARRIERS TO TOILETING: COGNITIVE IMPAIRMENT AND NURSING INTERVENTIONS FOR CONTINENCE

COGNITIVE IMPAIRMENT	CHARACTERISTICS	IMPACT ON BLADDER FUNCTION/CONTINENCE	NURSING INTERVENTIONS
Memory	• Problems with immediate, short-term, and/or long-term memory • Tends to mix up recent and distant memory events • Loses the link of the present to the past • Problems retaining new information	• Difficulty with articulating health history • May forget to take medications • Negative impact on toileting and hygiene behaviors, such as: • May forget to change wet/soiled clothing and/or containment products • Difficulty learning new treatments/therapies • May forget to eat or drink	• With permission, include caregivers in obtaining subjective health information. • Be specific when asking about common complaints such as frequency or dysuria. • Provide individualized suggestions for implementing a consistent daily routine for toileting and other ADLs. • Consider a toileting program that includes prompting for toileting and toileting behaviors, scheduled toileting, habit training, or prompted voiding. • Provide written and verbal instructions for new skills, for example, Kegel exercises, timed toileting, sequence for hygiene, flushing the toilet, dressing changes. • Consider using clocks, calendars, and check-off lists as reminders of daily tasks. • Supervision for medications as needed

(continued)

TABLE 6-10 MODIFYING BARRIERS TO TOILETING: COGNITIVE IMPAIRMENT AND NURSING INTERVENTIONS FOR CONTINENCE (*continued*)

COGNITIVE IMPAIRMENT	CHARACTERISTICS	IMPACT ON BLADDER FUNCTION/CONTINENCE	NURSING INTERVENTIONS
Language	• Expressive or receptive aphasia • Use of incoherent words	• Difficulty communicating needs • Offers of toileting assistance may not be understood • Instructions may not be understood thus increasing anxiety or creating behavioral disturbances	• Calm and reassuring approach essential • Avoid open-ended questions. • Do not rush the patient. • Break instructions into simple short phrases. • Anxiety or other behavioral changes may be an indication of discomfort, needs to void, or needing a change of clothing. • Toileting program may include scheduled toileting or habit training.
Orientation and attention	• Poor concentration • Easily distracted • Misidentification of persons, places, objects • May get lost more easily	• Instructions may be missed or misunderstood • May be unable to attend to long teaching or examination session • May have difficulty finding the bathroom or recognizing the toilet	• Patient education needs to be in short sessions. • Minimize background noise. • With permission, caregivers should be included in patient education. • Toileting program may include cueing for toileting, scheduled toileting, habit training, or prompted voiding. • Picture of toilet on bathroom door may help with recognition.
Thinking and Executive Function	• Poor reasoning and judgment • Difficulty with grasping abstract ideas or concepts or complete multitask steps • Difficulty with planning and organizing	• May have difficulty with toileting behaviors • Difficulty with medication regimens or completing treatment instructions • May have difficulty applying containment products • May not respond to the urge to void appropriately and use inappropriate other objects (e.g., flowerpot) for voiding	• Simple, easy to understand written instructions in addition to verbal instructions may be helpful. • Use one-step instructions if more complex directions are hard to follow. • Allow time to adjust to a new type of containment product. • Underwear-like containment briefs may be preferable to diaper-like product. • Toileting program may include cue and prompt for toileting and toileting behaviors, scheduled toileting, habit training, and prompted voiding.
Apraxis	• Difficulty directing or coordinating • Difficulty with accurately naming objects and their uses	• Difficulty writing or using objects such as toilet paper or lifting the lid of a toilet • Difficulty executing toileting behaviors • May not be able to apply or remove containment products • Difficulty communicating the need to use the toilet	• Consider underwear-like containment products. • Supervised toileting and hygiene • Label the bathroom with the word "Toilet" and a picture of a toilet. • Toileting program may include cue and prompt for toileting and toileting behaviors, scheduled toileting, and habit training
Agnosias	• Inability to recognize items in environment	• May void in inappropriate places • May have difficulty locating toilet • May have difficulty recognizing medications, particularly those taken in a nonoral (e.g., transdermal) fashion • May "play" with urinary catheters increasing risk for traumatic dislodgement	• Cue and prompt to use the bathroom. • Label bathroom with the word "Toilet" or use a photograph of a toilet on the bathroom door to assist with recognition. • Keep a light on in the bathroom. • "Camouflage" urinary catheters. • Toileting program may include cue and prompt for toileting and toileting behaviors, scheduled toileting, and habit training.

TABLE 6-10 MODIFYING BARRIERS TO TOILETING: COGNITIVE IMPAIRMENT AND NURSING INTERVENTIONS FOR CONTINENCE (continued)

COGNITIVE IMPAIRMENT	CHARACTERISTICS	IMPACT ON BLADDER FUNCTION/CONTINENCE	NURSING INTERVENTIONS
Cognitive impairment-linked conditions or behaviors that may influence continence: • Depression • Paranoid ideation • Delusions • Hallucinations • Aggression • Wandering	• Older adults with dementia, depression, and schizophrenia are at higher risk for urinary incontinence.	• Motivation for continence may be impaired • Increased use of antipsychotic and antidepressant medications increase risk for incontinence due to sedation, polyuric effects, and anticholinergic effects	• Request a medication review. • Assignment of consistent caregivers when in institutional settings • Recommend recreation therapy (music, art, pets) to help reduce anxiety and agitation. • Toileting program may include cue and prompt for toileting and toileting behaviors, scheduled toileting, and habit training.

From Fletcher, K. (2012). DEMENTIA Nursing Standard of Practice Protocol: Recognition and Management of Dementia. Retrieved from http://consultgerirn.org/topics/dementia. Accessed on March 28, 2020.
Grand, J. H. G., Caspar, S., & MacDonald, S. W. S. (2011). Clinical features and multidisciplinary approaches to dementia care. *Journal of Multidisciplinary Healthcare, 4*, 125–147.
Hoe, J., & Thompson, R. (2010). Promoting positive approaches to dementia care in nursing. *Nursing Standard, 25*(4), 47–56.
Thompson, D. L., & Bradway, C. K. (2017). The older urologic patient. In D. K. Newman, J. F. Wyman, & V. W. Welch (Eds.), *SUNA core curriculum for urologic nursing* (1st ed., pp. 709–724). Pittman, N.J.: Anthony J. Jannetti, Inc.
Walid, M. S. (2009). Prevalence of urinary incontinence in female residents of American nursing homes and association with neuropsychiatric disorders. *Journal of Clinical Medicine Research, 1*, 37–39.
Source: © 2017 Society of Urologic Nurses and Associates. Reprinted from the Core Curriculum for Urologic Nursing, 2017, p. 720. Used with permission of the publisher, the Society of Urologic Nurses and Associates, Inc.

TABLE 6-11 SCHEDULED TOILETING PROGRAMS

TYPE	DEFINITION	CANDIDATES	IMPLEMENTATION	EXPECTED OUTCOME
Routine scheduled toileting Also known as: Timed voiding, routine toileting, toilet training, scheduled toileting	Toileting program with a fixed schedule of assisted toileting where there is no attempt to individualize the schedule to conform to normal voiding patterns and there is no attempt made to motivate the individual to remain continent.	• Cognitive impairment • Cooperative with toileting • Able to use a toilet, bedpan, or urinal with the assistance of one • Unable to identify and/or communicate the need to void and/or defecate	• Patient toileted on a predetermined schedule such as every 2–4 hours or an institutionally defined schedule such as: Upon awakening, before and after meals, and before bed • Does not include awakening at night, but if awakened at night, can be toileted at that time	• May prompt the patient to delay voiding until toileting times • Reduced wetness • Reduced cost for laundry and BWAP • Improved quality of life • Preserve dignity • Reduced risk for incontinence-associated skin damage
Habit training PURT "patterned urge response training"	• Toileting program based upon the premise that the incontinent persons will improve their continence if they have timely access to a toileting facility when their bladder is full • Requires motivated caregivers that need extensive education concerning program	• Moderate cognitive impairment • Able to use a toilet, bedpan, or urinal with the assistance of one • Cooperative with toileting • Consistently voids when toileted or reminded to toilet per bladder diary • Inconsistently able or unable to identify or communicate the need to void and/or defecate	• Keep a bladder diary that records voiding/defecation times and continence for 3–5 days • Toileting schedule is designed with toileting scheduled just before the most common times the patient had voided/defecated per the diary • Maintain consistent fluid intake • Requires caregiver to implement the plan	• Continence or partial continence • Consistent compliance to the schedule is essential for success, which may not be realistic in many care environments • Reduced wetness • Reduced cost for laundry and BWAP • Improved quality of life • Preserve dignity • Reduced risk for incontinence-associated skin damage

(continued)

TABLE 6-11 SCHEDULED TOILETING PROGRAMS (*continued*)

TYPE	DEFINITION	CANDIDATES	IMPLEMENTATION	EXPECTED OUTCOME
Prompted voiding	• Toileting program designed to retrain the ability to recognize and to act upon the urge to void, increase self-initiated toileting	• Mild to moderate cognitive impairment (able to recognize their name and common elements in the environment, able to follow 1- to 2-step instructions) • Able to use a toilet, bedpan, or urinal with the assistance of one • Cooperative with toileting • Consistently voids (50% of the time) when toileted per bladder diary • Able to inhibit the urge to void • Requires motivated caregivers that need extensive education concerning the program	• At regular intervals, ask the patient if he or she is wet or dry. • Prompt the patient to void—ask the patient if he or she needs to void, and then assist the patient with toileting. • Encouragement and praise—each continent episode is positively reinforced • Consistent compliance to the schedule is essential for success, which may not be realistic in many care environments.	• Continence or partial continence • Increased self-initiated toileting • Reduced wetness • Reduced cost for laundry and BWAP • Improved quality of life • Preserved dignity • Reduced risk for incontinence-associated skin damage

From Colling, J., Ouslander, J., Hadley, B. J., et al. (1992). The effects of patterned urge-response toileting (PURT) on urinary incontinence among nursing home residents. *Journal of the American Geriatric Society, 40*, 135–141.
Colling, J. C., Owen, T. R., & McCreedy, M. R. (1994). Urine volumes and voiding's among incontinent nursing home residents. *Geriatric Nursing, 15*, 188–192.
Jirovec, M. M. (1991). Effect of individualized prompted toileting on incontinence in nursing home residents. *Applies Nursing Research, 4*, 188–191.
Lyons, S. S., & Pringle Specht, K. (2000). Prompted voiding protocol for individuals with urinary incontinence. *Journal of Gerontological Nursing, 26*(6), 5–12.
Newman, D. K. (2019). Evidenced-based practice guideline for prompted voiding for individuals with urinary incontinence. *Journal of Gerontological Nursing, 45*(2), 14–26.
Ostaszkiewicz, J., Johnson, L., & Roe, B. (2004). Habit retraining for the management of urinary incontinence in adults. *Cochrane Database of Systematic Reviews*, (4), CD002801.

Prompted voiding is the most studied scheduled toileting program with research showing that prompted voiding is a successful behavioral treatment modality for the moderately cognitively impaired in both institutional settings and in the home. Studies of nursing home residents placed on a prompted voiding protocol have shown significant decreases in frequency of incontinence (Eustice et al., 2000; Hu et al., 1989; Kaltreider et al., 1990; Lai & Wan, 2017; Ouslander et al., 2001). Prompted voiding has also been shown to be effective in homebound older adults (Adkins and Mathews, 1997). In a small study of cognitively impaired adults in the home, Engberg et al. (2002) found a mean 60% reduction in daytime incontinence for subjects in a prompted voiding protocol as compared to only a 37% reduction for those in the control group.

 CONCLUSION

The continence nurse brings a full portfolio of skills that promote and restore bladder health. The purpose of this chapter was to present the fundamental components of continence nursing emphasizing the role of the specialty continence nurse in prevention, practice based in evidence, patient educator, referral agent for further treatment, and the expert on first-line treatment of urinary and fecal incontinence.

CASE STUDY

A 90-year-old woman with incontinence has a long history of small volume urinary leakage with getting out of her chair, coughing, and sneezing that is managed with an absorbent pad. Over the past month, since returning home after hospitalization for surgical repair after a fall and hip fracture, the home care personal care aide has reported observing difficulty finding the way to the toilet and episodes of large-volume incontinence once or twice a day. The patient is very bothered by her increased incontinence. The home care continence nurse is called because the family is very concerned and fears she may need to be transferred to a skilled nursing facility. The continence nurse reviews the home care chart and notes that with the first complaint of large-volume incontinence, a urinalysis and urine culture were checked and were negative for infection. A review of medications shows no recent changes, and she is no longer on pain medication other than acetaminophen. A cognitive evaluation was completed prior to hospital discharge and showed mild cognitive impairment with impaired ability with activities of daily living involving toileting and dressing.

What barriers might there be for toilet access for this patient?

1. Immobility: This patient has had recent surgery after a fall and hip fracture with expected problems with independent mobility. The nurse should assess the patient's ability to get out of the chair and walk to the toilet in a timely manner. If assistive devices are in the home (walker, cane, raised toilet seat), is the patient using them and using them correctly? Has physical therapy or occupational therapy been consulted for this patient? When walking, is the patient using supportive shoes? Do the caregivers know how to properly assist her? Where is the bathroom and can she safely access it? Is the pathway from her chair/bed to the bathroom clear of clutter, dangerous throw rugs, and furniture?

2. Pain: Does pain with movement interfere with her ability to use the toilet in a timely manner? Is the current pain management plan with acetaminophen adequate to manage her pain?

3. Manual dexterity: Can the patient remove clothing easily when in the bathroom. If not, does she have available pull-on-type pants with an elastic waistband? Does she use a body-worn absorptive

product; if so, is it appropriate? Does that product interfere with timely toilet access? If she can self-toilet, how much help does she need, especially since the previous assessment shows problems with dressing? How long is the personal care aide in the home? In many cases, health aides are only there long enough for morning hygiene needs such as bathing and dressing.

4. Cognitive: This patient has been evaluated to have mild cognitive impairment. The caregiver in the home has noticed that the patient is having difficulty finding the bathroom. Does she have problems identifying common objects and places that may explain her problems finding the bathroom? If she has eyeglasses, is she wearing them? Does she need reminders to complete the steps in dressing herself and toilet hygiene?

The nurse addresses identified barriers to toilet use and determines that a toileting program would be an effective strategy to reduce incontinence. What type of toileting program should be recommended?

The nurse has the family and caregiver complete a bladder diary for 3 days. The diary shows that with toileting there were only 1 to 2 incontinence episodes a day, with all other voids continent. In this case, given the patient's mild cognitive impairment, >50% continent voids on bladder diary, ability to dress herself with cuing from the caregiver, ability to use the toilet with assistance, and caregivers available most of the day, she is a candidate for prompted voiding. A toileting schedule based upon voiding patterns identified in the bladder diary is developed. The family and caregivers are educated on the implementation of the program. The nurse teaches them that with each toileting the patient is asked about wetness or dryness as well as a need to void. If the patient is found dry with that toileting, praise and encouragement is given. With each toileting, the patient is told when the caregiver will return to check on them. The nurse also stresses how important it is to consistently implement the program. The nurse discusses with the caregivers the outcomes for the program and helps them develop a realistic goal. In this case, the most realistic goal would be partial continence given the dependence on caregivers. After the patient fully recovers from her surgery, works with physical therapy to regain as much toileting independence as possible, she may return to her previous continence level of occasional stress incontinence managed by a pad.

REFERENCES

Academy of Nutrition and Dietetics. (2015). Position of the Academy of Nutrition and Dietetics: Health implications of dietary fiber. *Journal of the Academy of Nutrition and Dietetics, 115*, 1861–1870.

Adkins, V. K., & Mathews, R. M. (1997). Prompted voiding to reduce incontinence in community-dwelling older adults. *Journal of Applied Behavioral Analysis, 30*, 153–156.

Anger, J. T., Nissim, H. A., Le, T. X., et al. (2011). Women's experience with severe overactive bladder symptoms and treatment: Insight revealed from patient focus groups. *Neurourology and Urodynamics, 30*, 1295–1299.

Auwad, W., Steggle, S. P., Bombieri, L., et al. (2008). Moderate weight loss in obese women with urinary incontinence: a prospective longitudinal study. *International Urogynecology Journal Pelvic Floor Dysfunction, 19*(9), 1251–1259.

Bliss, D. Z., Savik, K., Jung, H. J., et al. (2014). Dietary fiber supplementation for fecal incontinence: a randomized clinical trial. *Research in Nursing and Health, 37*(5), 367–378.

Bo, K., & Nygaard, I. E. (2020). Is physical activity good or bad for the female pelvic floor? A Narrative review. *Sports Medicine, 50*, 471–484. doi: 10.1007/s40279-019-01243-1.

Bove, A., Bellini, M., Battaglia, E., et al. (2012). Consensus statement AIGO/SICCR diagnosis and treatment of chronic constipation and obstructed defecation (Part II: Treatment). *World Journal of Gastroenterology, 18*(36), 4994–5013.

Brown, H. W., Wexner, S. E., Segall, M. M., et al. (2012). Accidental bowel leakage in the mature women's health study: prevalence and predictors. *International Journal of Clinical Practice, 66*, 1101–1108.

Burgio, K. L., Newman, D. K., Rosenberg, M. T., et al. (2013). Impact of behavior and lifestyle on bladder health. *International Journal of Clinical Practice, 67*(6), 495–504.

Button, B. M., Holland, A. E., Sherburn, M. S., et al. (2019). Prevalence, impact and specialized treatment of urinary incontinence in women with chronic lung disease. *Physiotherapy, 105*(1), 114–119.

Callan, L., Thompson, D. L., & Netsch, D. (2015). Does increasing or decreasing the daily intake of water/fluids by adults affect OAB symptoms. *Journal of Wound, Ostomy, and Continence Nursing, 42*(6), 614–620.

Carter, D. (2016). Conservative and novel treatment options for fecal incontinence. *Journal of Gastrointestinal and Digestive System, 6*, 428. doi: 10.4172/2161-069X.1000428.

Camenga, D. R., Brady, S. S., Hardacker, D. T., et al. (2019). U.S. Adolescent and adult women's experiences accessing and using toilets in schools, workplaces, and public spaces: A multi-site focus group study to inform future research in bladder health. *International Journal of Environmental Research & Public Health, 16*(18), 3338.

Chang, J. I., Lam, V., & Patel, M. I. (2016a). Preoperative pelvic floor muscle exercise and postprostatectomy incontinence: A systematic review and meta-analysis. *European Urology, 69*, 460–467.

Chang, J., McLemore, E., & Tejirian, T. (2016b). Anal health care basics. *Permanente Journal, 20*(4), 15–222.

Chu, C. M., Arya, L. A., & Andy, U. U. (2015). Impact of urinary incontinence on female sexual health in women during midlife. *Women's Midlife Health, 1*, 6. doi: 10.1186/s40695-015-0007-6.

Chumpitazi, B. P., Self, M. M., Czyzewski, D. I., et al. (2016). Bristol stool form scale reliability and agreement decreases with determining Rome III stool form designations. *Neurogastroenterology and Motility, 28*(3), 443–448.

Colling, J., Ouslander, J., Hadley, B. J., et al. (1992). The effects of patterned urge-response toileting (PURT) on urinary incontinence among nursing home residents. *Journal of the American Geriatric Society, 40*(2), 135–141.

Colling, J. C., Owen, T. R., & McCreedy, M. R. (1994). Urine volumes and voiding's among incontinent nursing home residents. *Geriatric Nursing, 15*(4), 188–192.

Colavita, K., & Andy, U. U. (2016). Role of diet in fecal incontinence: A systematic review of the literature. *International Urogynecology Journal, 27*, 1805–1810.

Coyne, K. S., Cash, B., Kopp, Z., et al. (2011a). The prevalence of chronic constipation and faecal incontinence among men and women with symptoms of overactive bladder. *BJU International, 107*, 254–261.

Coyne, K. S., Kvasz, M., Ireland, A. M., et al. (2012). Urinary incontinence and its relationship to mental health and health-related quality of life in men and women in Sweden, the United Kingdom, and the United States. *European Urology, 61*, 88–95.

Coyne, K. S., Sexton, C. C., Thompson, C., et al. (2011b). The impact of OAB on sexual health in men and women: results from EpiLUTS. *Journal of Sexual Medicine, 8*, 1603–1615.

Croswell, E., Bliss, D. Z., & Savik, K. (2010). Diet and eating pattern modifications used by community-living adults to manage their fecal incontinence. *Journal of Wound, Ostomy, and Continence Nursing, 37*(6), 677–682.

Curry, S. J., Krist, A. H., Owens, D. K., et al. (2018). Behavioral weight loss interventions to prevent obesity-related morbidity and mortality in adults: U.S. Preventive Services Task Force Recommendation Statement. *JAMA, 320*(11), 1163–1171.

Daily, A. M., Kowalik, C. G., Delpe, S. D., et al. (2019). Women with overactive bladder exhibit more unhealthy toileting behaviors: a cross-sectional study. *Urology, 134*, 97–102.

Daugirdas, S. P., Markossian, T., Mueller, E. R., et al. (2020). Urinary incontinence and chronic conditions in the US population age 50 years and older. *International Urogyecology Journal, 31*, 1013–1020. doi: 10.1007/s00192-019-04137-y.

Dumoulin, C., Adewuyi, T., & Booth, C., et al. (2017). Adult conservative management. In P. Abrams, L. Cardozo, A. Wagg, et al. (Eds.), *Incontinence* (6th ed., pp. 1443–1628). Bristol, UK: International Continence Society.

Dumoulin, C., Cacciari, L. P., & Hay-Smith, E. J. C. (2018). Pelvic floor muscle training versus no treatment, or inactive control treatments, for urinary incontinence in women. *Cochrane Database of Systematic Reviews*, (10), CD005654. doi: 10.1002/14651858.CD005654.pub4.

Dumoulin, C., Glazener, C., & Jenkinson, D. (2011). Determining the optimal pelvic floor muscle training regimen for women with stress urinary incontinence. *Neurourology and Urodynamics, 30*(5), 746–753.

Dumoulin, C., Hay-Smith, J., Frawley, H., et al. (2015). Consensus statement on Improving pelvic floor muscle training adherence: International Continence Society 2011 state of the science seminar. *Neurourology and Urodynamics, 34*, 600–605.

Ellis, J. G., & Allen, S. F. (2019). Sleep hygiene and the prevention of chronic insomnia. In M. A. Grandner (Ed.), *Sleep and health* (pp. 137–145). Cambridge, MA: Academic Press.

Elstad, E. A., Taubenberger, S. P., Botelho, E. M., et al. (2010). Beyond incontinence: The stigma of other urinary symptoms. *Journal of Advanced Nursing, 66*(11), 2460–2470.

Engberg, S. J., Sereika, S. M., McDowell, B. J., et al. (2002). Effectiveness of prompted voiding in treating urinary incontinence in cognitively impaired homebound older adults. *Journal of Wound, Ostomy, and Continence Nursing, 29*(5), 252–265.

Eustice, S., Roe, B., & Paterson, J. (2000). Prompted voiding for the management of urinary incontinence in adults. *Cochrane Database of Systematic Reviews*, (2), CD002113.

Everaert, K., Herve, F., Bosch, R., et al. (2019). International Continence Society consensus on the diagnosis and treatment of nocturia. *Neurourology and Urodynamics, 38*, 478–498.

Fletcher, K. (2012). *DEMENTIA nursing standard of practice protocol: Recognition and management of dementia*. Retrieved from http://consultgerirn.org/topics/dementia. Accessed on March 28, 2020.

Fonda, D., & Abrams, P. (2006). Cure sometimes, help always—A "continence paradigm" for all ages and conditions. *Neurourology and Urodynamics, 25*(3), 290–292.

Friedlander, J. I., Shorter, B., & Moldwin, R. M. (2012). Diet and its role in interstitial cystitis/bladder pain syndrome (IC/BPS) and comorbid conditions. *BJU International, 109*, 1584–1591.

Gandhi, J., Chen, A., Gautam Dagus, M. S., et al. (2016). Genitourinary syndrome of menopause: An overview of clinical manifestations, pathophysiology, etiology, evaluation, and management. *American Journal of Obstetrics & Gynecology, 215*(6), 704–711.

Grand, J. H. G., Caspar, S., & MacDonald, S. W. S. (2011). Clinical features and multidisciplinary approaches to dementia care. *Journal of Multidisciplinary Healthcare, 4*, 125–147.

Grundy, L., & Brierley, S. M. (2018). Cross-organ sensitization between the colon and bladder: to pee or not to pee? *American Journal of Physiology—Gastrointestinal and Liver Physiology, 314*, G301–G308.

Hagen, S., Glazner, C., McClurg, D., et al. (2017). Pelvic floor muscle training for secondary prevention of pelvic organ prolapse (PREVPROL): A multicenter randomized controlled trial. *Lancet, 389*, 393–402.

Hagglund, D., & Wadensten, B. (2007). Fear of humiliation inhibits women's care-seeking behavior for long-term urinary incontinence. *Scandinavian Journal of Caring Science, 21*(3), 305–312.

Hansen, J. L., Bliss, D. Z., & Peden-McAlpine, C. (2006). Diet strategies used by women to manage fecal incontinence. *Journal of Wound, Ostomy, and Continence Nursing, 33*(1), 52–61; discussion 61–62.

Harlow, B. L., Bavendam, T. G., Palmer, M. H., et al. (2017). The prevention of lower urinary tract symptoms (PLUS) research consortium: A transdisciplinary approach toward promoting bladder health and preventing lower urinary tract symptoms in women across the life course. *Journal of Women's Health, 27*(3), 283–289.

Hashim, H., & Abrams, P. (2008). How should patients with an overactive bladder manipulate their fluid intake? *BJU International, 102*, 62–66.

Hay-Smith, J., Dean, S., Burgio, K., et al. (2015). Pelvic–Floor-Muscle-Training Adherence "Modifiers": a review of primary qualitative studies 2011 ICS stat of the science seminar research paper III of IV. *Neurourology and Urodynamics, 34*(7), 622–631.

Hay-Smith, J., Herderschee, R., Dumoulin, C., et al. (2012). Comparisons of approaches to pelvic floor muscle training for urinary incontinence in women: An abridged Cochrane systematic review. *European Journal of Physical Rehabilitation Medicine, 48*, 689–705.

Heaton, K. W., & Lewis, S. J. (1997). Stool form scale as a useful guide to intestinal transit time. *Scandinavian Journal of Gastroenterology, 32*(9), 920–924.

Hoe, J., & Thompson, R. (2010). Promoting positive approaches to dementia care in nursing. *Nursing Standard, 25*(4), 47–56.

Holroyd, S. (2019). Urinary incontinence after stroke. *British Journal of Community Nursing, 24*(12), 590–594.

Hrisanfow, E., & Hagglund, D., (2011). The prevalence of urinary incontinence among women and men with chronic obstructive pulmonary disease in Sweden. *Journal of Clinical Nursing, 20*, 1895–1905.

Hu, T. W., Igou, J. F., Kaltreider, D. L., et al. (1989). A clinical trial of a behavioral therapy to reduce urinary incontinence in nursing homes: Outcome and implications. *JAMA, 261*(18), 2656–2662.

Institute of Medicine. (2005). *Dietary reference intakes for water, potassium, sodium, chloride, and sulfate*. Washington, DC: The National Academies Press.

Jerez-Roid, J., Booth, J., Skelton, D. A., et al. (2020). Is urinary incontinence associated with sedentary behavior in older women? Analysis of data from the National Health and Nutrition Examination Survey. *PLoS One, 15*(2), e0227195. doi: 10.1371/journal.pone.0227195.

Jirovec, M. M. (1991). Effect of individualized prompted toileting on incontinence in nursing home residents. *Applied Nursing Research, 4*(4), 188–191.

John, G. (2020). Urinary incontinence and cardiovascular disease: a narrative review. *International Urogynecology Journal, 31*, 857–863. doi: 10.1007/s00192-019-04058-w.

Kaltreider, D. L., Hu, T. W., Igou, J. F., et al. (1990). Can reminders curb incontinence? *Geriatric Nursing, 11*(1), 17–19.

Khullar, V., Sexton, C. C., Thompson, D. L., et al. (2014). The relationship between BMI and urinary incontinence subgroups: Results from EpiLUTS. *Neurourology and Urodynamics, 33*, 392–399.

Kowalik, C. G., Daily, A., Kaufman, R. R., et al. (2019). Toileting behaviors of women-What is healthy? *Journal of Urology, 201*(1), 129–134.

Lai, H. H., Helmuth, M. E., Smith, A. R., et al. (2019). Relationship between, central obesity, general obesity, overactive bladder syndrome and urinary incontinence among male and female patients seeking care for their lower urinary tract symptoms. *Urology, 123*, 34–43.

Lai, H. H., Rawal, A., Shen, B., et al. (2016). The relationship between anxiety and overactive bladder or urinary incontinence symptoms in the clinical population. *Urology, 98*, 50–57. doi: 10.1016/j.urology.2016.07.013.

Lai, C. K. Y., & Wan, X. (2017). Using prompted voiding to manage urinary incontinence in nursing homes: Can it be sustained? *Journal of the American Medical Directors Association, 18*(6), 509–514.

Lasak, A. M., Jean-Michel, J., Le, P. U., et al. (2018). The role of pelvic floor muscle training in the conservative and surgical management of female stress urinary incontinence: Does the strength of the pelvic floor muscles matter? *Physical Medicine and Rehabilitation, 10*(11), 1198–1210.

Lawrence, K. G., Bauer, C. A., Jacobson, T., et al. (2018). Wound, Ostomy, and Continence Nursing: Scope and standards of WOC practice, 2nd edition: An executive summary. *Journal of Wound Ostomy & Continence Nursing, 45*(4), 369–387.

Lee, H. J., Jung, K. W., & Myung, S. (2013). Technique of functional and motility test: How to perform biofeedback for constipation and fecal incontinence. *Journal of Neurogastroenterology and Motility, 19*(4), 532–537.

Lightner, D. J., Gomeisky, A., Souter, L., et al. (2019). Diagnosis and treatment of overactive bladder (Non-Nuerogenic) in adults: AUA/SUFU guideline amendment 2019. *Journal of Urology, 202*(3), 558–563.

Lombardo, R., Tubaro, A., & Burkhard, F. (2020). Nocturia: The complex role of the heart, kidneys, and bladder. *European Urology Focus, 6*, 534–536. doi: 10.1016/j.euf.2019.07.007.

Longstreth, G. F., Thompson, W. G., Chey, W. D., et al. (2006). Functional bowel disorders. *Gastroenterology, 130*, 1480–1491.

Lukacz, E. S., Bavendam, T. G., Berry, A., et al. (2018). A novel research definition of bladder health in women and girls: Implications for research and public health promotion. *Journal of Women's Health, 27*(8), 974–981.

Lukacz, E. S., Sampselle, C., Gray, M., et al. (2011). A healthy bladder: a consensus statement. *International Journal of Clinical Practice, 65*(10), 1026–1036.

Luginbuehl, H., Lehmann, C., Baeyens, J. P., et al. (2015). Pelvic floor muscle activation and strength components influencing female urinary continence and stress incontinence: A systematic review. *Neurourology and Urodynamics, 34*, 498–506.

Lyons, S. S., & Pringle Specht, K. (2000). Prompted voiding protocol for individuals with urinary incontinence. *Journal of Gerontological Nursing, 26*(6), 5–12.

McGill, C. R., Fulgoni, V. L., & Devareddy, L. (2015). Ten-year trends in fiber and whole grain intakes and food sources for the United States population: National Health and nutrition examination survey 2001–2010. *Forum Nutrition, 7*, 1119–1130.

McRorie, J. W., & McKeown, N. M. (2017). Understanding the physics of functional fibers in the gastrointestinal tract: An Evidence-Based approach to resolving enduring misconceptions about insoluble and soluble Fiber. *Journal of the Academy of Nutrition and Dietetics, 117*, 251–264.

Meduba-Polo, J., Adot, J. M., Allue, M., et al. (2020). Consensus document on the multidisciplinary management of neurogenic lower urinary tract dysfunction in patients with multiple sclerosis. *Neurourology and Urodynamics, 39*(2), 1–9.

Miller, J., Ashton-Miller, J., & DeLancey, J. O. O. (1989). A pelvic muscle pre-contraction can reduce cough related urine loss in selected women with mild SUI. *Journal of the American Geriatric Society, 46*, 870–874.

Miller, J. M., Sampselle, C. M., Ashton-Miller, J. A., et al. (2008). Clarification and confirmation of the effect of volitional pelvic floor muscle contraction to preempt urine loss (The Knack Maneuver) in stress incontinent women. *International Urogynecology Journal and Pelvic Floor Dysfunction, 19*(6), 773–782.

Mobley, D., & Baum, N. (2015). Smoking: its impact on urologic health. *Reviews in Urology, 17*(4), 220–225.

Moreno-Vecino, B., Arija-Blazquez, A., Pedrero-Chamizo, R., et al. (2015). Associations between, obesity, physical fitness, and urinary incontinence in non-institutionalized postmenopausal women: The elderly EXERNET multi-center study. *Maturitas, 82,* 208–214.

Nambiar, A. K., Bosch, R., Cruz, F., et al. (2018). EAU Guidelines on assessment and nonsurgical management of urinary incontinence. *European Urology, 73*(4), 596–609.

National Institutes of Health. (2019). *SEER cancer stat facts.* Retrieved from https://seer.cancer.gov/statfacts/. Accessed March 7, 2019.

Newman, D. K. (2019). Evidenced-based practice guideline for prompted voiding for individuals with urinary incontinence. *Journal of Gerontological Nursing, 45*(2), 14–26.

Newman, D. K., Cockerell, R., Griebling, T. L., et al. (2017). Primary prevention, continence promotion, models of care and education. In P. Abrams, L. Cardozo, A. Wagg, et al. (Eds.), *Incontinence* (6th ed., pp. 2429–2478). Bristol, UK: International Continence Society.

O'Connell, K., Torstrick, A., & Victor, E. (2014). Dues to urinary urgency and urge incontinence: How those diagnosed with overactive bladder differ from undiagnosed persons. *Journal of Wound, Ostomy, and Continence Nursing, 41*(3), 259–267.

Ostaszkiewicz, J., Johnson, L., & Roe, B. (2004). Habit retraining for the management of urinary incontinence in adults (Cochrane review). *Cochrane Database of Systematic Reviews*, (4), CD002801.

Ouslander, J. G., Al-Samarrai, N., & Schnelle, J. F. (2001). Prompted voiding for nighttime incontinence in nursing homes: Is it effective? *Journal of the American Geriatric Society, 49*(6), 706–709.

Palmer, M. H., Cockerell, R., Greibling, T. L., et al. (2020). Review of the 6th International Consultation on Incontinence: Primary prevention of urinary incontinence. *Neurourology and Urodynamics, 39,* 66–72.

Palmer, M., Reid Czarapata, D., Wells, T., et al. (1997). Urinary outcomes in older adults: Research and clinical perspectives. *Urologic Nursing, 17*(3), 2–9.

Palmer, M. H., Willis-Gray, M. G., Zhou, F., et al. (2018). Self-reported toileting behaviors in employed women: Are they associated with lower urinary tract symptoms? *Neurourology and Urodynamics, 37*(2), 735–743.

Panicker, J. N., Marcelissen, T., von Gontard, A., et al. (2019). Bladder-bowel interactions: Do we understand pelvic organ cross-sensitization? International Consultation on Incontinence Research Society (ICI-RS) 2019. *Neurourology and Urodynamics, 38,* S25–S34.

Paquette, I. M., Barma, M., Kaiser, A., et al. (2015). The American Society of Colon and Rectal Surgeons' clinical practice guideline for the treatment of fecal incontinence. *Diseases of the Colon and Rectum, 58,* 623–636.

Peng, C. H., Chen, S. F., & Kuo, H. C. (2017). Videourodynamic analysis of the urethral sphincter overactivity and the poor relaxing pelvic floor muscles in women with voiding dysfunction. *Neurourology and Urodynamics, 36*(8), 2169–2175.

Pierce, H. M., Perry, L., Gallagher, R., et al. (2019). Delaying voiding, limiting fluids, urinary symptoms, and work productivity: A survey of female nurses and midwives. *Journal of Advanced Nursing, 75,* 2579–2590.

Qaseem, A., Dallas, P., Forciea, M. A., et al. (2014). Nonsurgical management of urinary incontinence in women: A clinical practice guideline from the American College of Physicians. *Annals of Internal Medicine, 161,* 429–444.

Rao, S. S. C., Benninga, M. A., Bharucha, A. E., et al. (2015). ANMS-ESNM position paper and consensus guidelines on biofeedback therapy for anorectal disorders. *Neurogastroenterolgy and Motility, 27*(5), 594–609.

Sakakibara, R., Panicker, J., Finazzi-Agro, E., et al. (2016). A guideline for the management of bladder dysfunction in Parkinson's Disease and other gait disorders. *Neurourology and Urodynamics, 35,* 551–563.

Southall, K., Tuazonk J. R., Djokhdem, A. H., et al. (2017). Assessing the stigma content of urinary incontinence intervention outcome measures. *Journal of Rehabilitation and Assistive Technologies Engineering, 4,* 1–13.

Staller, K., Song, M., Grodstein, F., et al. (2018). Increased long-term dietary fiber intake is associated with a decreased risk of fecal incontinence in older women. *Gastroenterology, 155,* 661–667.

Steele, N. M., Ledbetter, C. A., & Bernier, F. (2016). Genitourinary Syndrome of Menopause and Vaginal Estrogen Use. *Urologic Nursing, 36*(2), 59–65.

Sutcliffe, S., Jemielta, T., Lai, H. H., et al. (2018). A case-crossover study of urologic chronic pelvic pain syndrome flare triggers in the Mapp research network. *Journal of Urology, 199*(5), 1245–1251.

Tang, D. H., Colayco, D. C., Kkhalaf, K. M., et al. (2014). Impact of urinary incontinence on healthcare resource utilization, health-related quality of life and productivity in patients with overactive bladder. *BJU International, 113*(3), 484–491.

Thomas, L. H., Coupe, J., Cross, L. D., et al. (2019). Interventions for treating urinary incontinence after stroke in adults. *Cochrane Database of Systematic Reviews*, (2), CD004462. doi: 10.1002/14651858. CD004462.pub4.

Thompson, D. L., & Bradway, C. K. (2017). The older urologic patient. In D. K. Newman, J. F. Wyman, & V. W. Welch (Eds.), *Core curriculum for urologic nursing* (1st ed., pp. 709–724). Pittman, N.J.: Anthony J. Jannetti, Inc.

Thurmon, K. L., Breyer, B. N., & Erickson, B. A., (2013). Association of bowel habits with lower urinary tract symptoms in men: Findings from the 2005-2006 and 2007-2008 National Health and Nutrition Examination Survey. *Journal of Urology, 189,* 1409–1414.

Tse, F., King, J., Dowling, C., et al. (2016). Conjoint Urological Society of Australia and New Zealand (USANZ) and Urogynaecological Society of Australasia (UGSA) guidelines on the management of adult non-neurogenic overactive bladder. *BJU International, 117*(1), 34–47.

U. S. Department of Agriculture, Agricultural Research Service. *FoodData Central*, 2019. fdc.nal.usda.gov.

U.S. Department of Health and Human Services (USDHHS) and U.S. Department of Agriculture (USDA). (December 2015). *2015–2020 dietary guidelines for Americans* (8th ed.). Retrieved from http://health. gov/dietaryguidelines/2015/guidelines/. Accessed March 15, 2020.

U.S. Department of Health and Human Services (USDHHS), Physical Activity Guidelines Advisory Committee I. (2018). *Physical Activity Guidelines Advisory Committee scientific report.* Retrieved from https://health.gov/sites/default/files/2019-09/paguide.pdf. Accessed February 28, 2020.

van Kerrebroeck, P., Abrams, P., Chaikin, D., et al. (2002). The standardisation of terminology in nocturia: Report from the Standardisation Sub-committee of the International Continence Society. *Neurourology and Urodynamics, 21*(2), 179–183.

von Gontard, A., de Jong, T. P., Badawi, J. K., et al. (2017). Psychological and physical environmental factors in the development of incontinence in adults and children: A comprehensive review. *Journal of Wound, Ostomy, and Continence Nursing, 44*(2), 181–187.

Vrijens, D., Drossaerts, J., van Koeveringe, G., et al. (2015). Affective symptoms and the overactive bladder—A systematic review. *Journal of Psychosomatic Research, 78,* 95–108.

Wallace, S. A., Roe, B., Williams, K., et al. (2004). Bladder training for urinary incontinence in adults. *Cochrane Database of Systematic Reviews*, (1), CD001308. doi: 10.1002/14651858.CD001308.pub2.

Walid, M. S. (2009). Prevalence of urinary incontinence in female residents of American nursing homes and association with neuropsychiatric disorders. *Journal of Clinical Medicine and Research, 1*(1), 37–39.

Wan, X., Wu, C., Xu, D., et al. (2017). Toileting behaviors and lower urinary tract symptoms among female nurses: A cross-sectional questionnaire survey. *International Journal of Nursing Studies, 65,* 1–7.

Whitehead, W. E., Palsson, O. S., & Simren, M. (2016). Treating fecal incontinence: an unmet need in primary care medicine. *North Carolina Medical Journal, 77*(3), 211–215.

Whitehead, W. E., Rao, S. C., Lowry, A., et al. (2015). Treatment of Fecal Incontinence: State of the science summary for the national institute of diabetes and digestive and kidney disease workshop. *American Journal of Gastroenterology, 110*, 138–146.

Wieland, L. S., Shrestha, N., Lassi, Z. S., et al. (2019). Yoga for treating urinary incontinence in women. *Cochrane Database of Systematic Reviews*, (2), CD012668. doi: 10.1002/14651858.CD012668.pub2.

Wood, L. N., Markowitz, M. A., Parameshwar, P. S., et al. (2018). Is it safe to reduce water intake in the overactive bladder population? A systematic review. *Journal of Urology, 200*, 375–381.

Wu, C., Zue, K., & Palmer, M. H. (2019). Toileting behaviors related to urination in women: A scoping review. *International Journal of Envi-ronmental Research and Public Health, 16*, 4000. doi: 10.3390/ijerph16204000.

Yang, K. N., Chen, S. C., Chen, S. Y., et al. (2010). Female voiding postures and their effects on micturition. *International Urogynecology Journal, 21*, 1371–1376.

Yazdany, T., Jakus-Waldman, S., Jeppsonk, P. C., et al. (2020). American Urogynecologic Society systematic review: The impact of weight loss intervention on lower urinary tract symptoms and urinary incontinence in overweight and obese women. *Female Pelvic Medicine and Reconstructive Surgery, 26*, 16–29.

Zecca, C., Riccitelli, G. C., Disanto, G., et al. (2016). Urinary incontinence in multiple sclerosis: prevalence, severity and impact on patients' quality of life. *European Journal of Neurology, 23*, 1228–1234.

QUESTIONS

1. What is the *first* step when teaching a patient to suppress strong urinary urge?
   A. Distract attention away from the urge by counting backwards.
   B. Wait a few minutes and then walk to the bathroom.
   C. Squeeze and hold the pelvic floor muscles for 10 seconds.
   D. Quickly squeeze and relax the pelvic floor muscles 6 times.

2. When counseling a patient on healthy bowel habits, what time of day should be recommended as optimal for normal bowel movements?
   A. After a meal
   B. Before bed
   C. Only when there is a strong urge
   D. Prior to walking or exercise

3. A mother of two small children reports small volume urine leakage associated with a strong cough and when picking up her baby. The continence nurse expects to educate this woman about which of the following?
   A. Regular daily exercise
   B. Increasing fiber in the diet
   C. Identification and contraction of pelvic floor muscles
   D. Avoiding caffeinated beverages

4. A 66-year-old woman returns to the continence clinic 2 weeks after starting a pelvic floor muscle (PFM) exercise program stating she has trouble holding a muscle contraction. What strategy should the continence nurse add to her current treatment plan?
   A. Do pelvic muscle contractions in rapid succession.
   B. Add abdominal and buttock muscle contractions with each PFM contraction.
   C. Ensure that with each muscle contraction she takes a deep breath and holds it.
   D. Do her exercises supine until she can hold the contraction for 5 seconds.

5. What nursing intervention should be included in the INITIAL plan to improve continence in a frail older woman with severe arthritis that experiences occasional incontinence episodes when on the way to the toilet at night?
   A. Recommend a disposable undergarment for use at night.
   B. Counseling about decreasing intake of fluids 6 to 8 hours prior to bed.
   C. Obtain a commode to be placed near the bed.
   D. Referral for physical therapy and pain management.

6. The home care continence nurse is evaluating a cognitively impaired man with incontinence for a toileting program. What finding BEST establishes him as a candidate for a prompted voiding program?
   A. Three-day bladder diary shows 1 to 2 continent voids per day.
   B. The primary caregiver works outside the home.
   C. Requires 1 to 2 people to transfer to the toilet.
   D. Can dress himself if cued to put on each clothing item.

7. What is an important component of a healthy bowel program in a patient with constipation?
   A. Encourage fluids and restrict bran and beans in the diet.
   B. Educate about engaging in daily walks.
   C. Encourage vigorous pushing throughout toilet time.
   D. Use a raised toilet seat so that hips are higher than knees.

8. What fluid intake pattern is a likely trigger for urinary urgency and frequency?
   A. 8 oz Milk with cereal in the morning, 1 cup of coffee
   B. 8 oz Water with morning medications, 1 cup of tea
   C. Iced tea with dinner, 2 glasses of wine after dinner
   D. Two 8-oz water glasses and 4 oz of soup with dinner

9. A patient is observed to have difficulty isolating the pelvic floor muscles when performing a pelvic floor muscle contraction. What strategy should be part of this patient's exercise prescription?
   A. Do the exercises in the standing position.
   B. Squeeze the muscle as hard as possible.
   C. Increase the number of repetitions.
   D. Decrease the duration of the squeeze.

10. What should the continence nurse include in a talk about healthy bladder to a women's group?
    A. To shorten toilet time, strain to start the urinary stream.
    B. Avoid public toilet use; restrict fluid intake.
    C. Ensure feet are flat on the floor and avoid toilet hovering.
    D. Practice pelvic muscle exercises when using the toilet.

ANSWERS AND RATIONALES

1. **D. Rationale:** With an increase in pelvic floor muscle tone such as with a PFM contraction, there is a corresponding inhibiting response of the detrusor muscle. Performing quick and strong PFM contractions followed by mental distraction inhibits urgency.

2. **A. Rationale:** Colonic motor activity is most active after a meal.

3. **C. Rationale:** The patient in this case exhibits classic symptoms of stress incontinence of which PFM exercises are first-line treatment to improve strength and tone of the pelvic floor muscles to prevent incontinence.

4. **D. Rationale:** Difficulty with holding a PFM contraction is characteristic of muscle weakness. The exercise prescription should be modified to decrease resistance (occurs in sitting or standing positions) by recommending exercise in the supine position.

5. **C. Rationale:** In frail older adults with severe arthritis, getting out of bed at night is painful and prolonged creating a barrier to timely toilet access. Providing a bedside commode would be the best initial intervention.

6. **D. Rationale:** The best candidate for a prompted voiding program should show 50% or better continent voids on a bladder diary, have a consistent caregiver in the home, be able to safely use a toilet with minimal assistance of one person, and be able to follow 1- to 2-step instructions.

7. **B. Rationale:** A component of a healthy bowel program includes regular exercises, which contribute to normal bowel motility.

8. **C. Rationale:** Fluids that function as bladder irritant such as the caffeine in iced tea and fluids that exert a diuretic effect such as alcohol are common triggers for urine urgency and frequency.

9. **D. Rationale:** Difficulty isolating the correct muscle during a PFM contraction is characteristic of muscle weakness. The exercise prescription should be modified by decreasing the duration of the squeeze so to help the patient better contract the correct muscle. As the muscle gets stronger, the duration of muscle contraction can be gradually increased.

10. **C. Rationale:** Toilet hovering and feet dangling when on the toilet can contribute to inadequate bladder emptying.

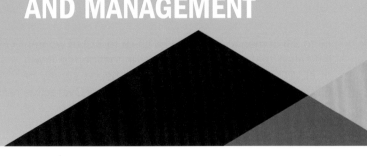

CHAPTER 7

OVERACTIVE BLADDER/URGENCY UI: PATHOLOGY, PRESENTATION, DIAGNOSIS, AND MANAGEMENT

Leslie Sazsteinlt Wooldridge

OBJECTIVES

1. Explain how bladder and sphincter functions change with aging and how these changes affect voiding patterns and continence.

2. Describe current theories regarding the etiology and pathology of overactive bladder (OAB) with/without urgency incontinence.

3. Outline indications and guidelines according to AUA/SUFU and ICS for treatment and evaluation of

behavioral interventions, medication management, third-line therapy including percutaneous tibial nerve stimulation (PTNS), sacral neuromodulation (SNS), and onabotulinumtoxinA and surgical options/catheter options for refractory OAB patients.

TOPIC OUTLINE

INTRODUCTION

Overactive bladder (OAB) is a clinically defined symptom complex that consists of urinary urgency, with or without urgency incontinence, usually with increased daytime frequency and nocturia in the absence of urinary tract infection (UTI) or other obvious pathology (Abrams et al., 2009; Drake, 2018). The single defining symptom, said to drive the others, is urinary *urgency*, a sudden, overwhelming desire to pass urine that is difficult to defer (Haylen et al., 2010) and is often accompanied by fear of leakage. This is different from the normal *urge* to void, the physiological sensation that can be deferred until it is convenient to do so.

KEY POINT

OAB is a symptom complex involving urgency (with or without urgency incontinence), frequency, and nocturia in the absence of UTI or other obvious pathology.

OAB is a clinical diagnosis, made on the basis of a detailed history, and is not generally reliant on invasive tests such as multichannel cystometry. OAB with urgency urinary incontinence (UUI) denotes the symptoms of OAB associated with urinary leakage; the leakage is the result of involuntary bladder (detrusor) contractions. Not all individuals with OAB have objectively documented involuntary detrusor contractions; indeed, only approximately 60% of people with clinical OAB will have demonstrable detrusor overactivity (DO), the observation of involuntary detrusor contractions during filling cystometry (see Chapter 5). Furthermore, 36% of people with DO on filling cystometry *do not* have symptomatic OAB (Hashim & Abrams, 2006). Lower urinary tract symptoms (LUTS), of which urinary frequency, nocturia, and urinary urgency are the most prevalent, are common in the general population.

PREVALENCE AND INCIDENCE

In the EPIC (European Prospective Investigation into Cancer and Nutrition) study of adults over 40, based upon a structured telephone interview of over 19,000 people from four European countries and Canada, 19.1% (95% CI 17.5 to 20.7) of community dwelling men and 18.3% (95% CI 16.9 to 19.6) of women over the age of 60 years indicated that they had urinary urgency, and 2.5% (95% CI 1.9 to 3.1) of men and 2.5% (95% CI 1.9 to 3.0) of women indicated that they had urgency incontinence (Irwin et al., 2006). Similarly, a population-based survey of 5,204 adults in the United States, the National Overactive Bladder Evaluation (NOBLE) study, found a prevalence of OAB of 16% in men and 16.9% in women; prevalence increased with age (Stewart et al., 2003). Overall, in multiple studies, prevalence of OAB in both men and women has been estimated to be as low as 2% and up to 53% (Milsom et al., 2017, Table 18). However, the bothersome of symptoms was not measured in the majority of these studies (Milsom et al., 2017).

Thus, it is clear that OAB symptoms are prevalent in both men (Malmsten et al., 2010) and women, especially in those in the older age range. **Figure 7-1** shows the proportion of urgency and stress urinary incontinence in women. **Figure 7-2** reflects the spectrum of OAB and illustrates that it often coexists with stress urinary incontinence (SUI), the condition termed *mixed urinary incontinence*. Note that OAB is defined by the symptom of *urgency* with (OAB wet) or without urinary incontinence (OAB dry) and usually with frequency and nocturia.

The cost of OAB wet is forecasting to be a staggering $82.6 billion dollars by 2021 including absorbent products, treatment, services, and indirect costs such as loss of productivity due to disability (Coyne et al., 2014).

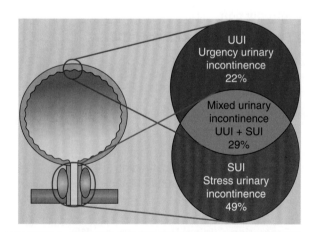

FIGURE 7-1. Definition and Classification of UI. UUI occurs with a strong sudden and uncontrollable desire to urinate as a result of involuntary detrusor contractions; overactive bladder is defined by the symptom of urgency with or without urgency incontinence; SUI is involuntary leakage on effort or exertion or on sneezing or coughing, as a result of insufficient urethral closure pressure. (Reproduced with permission from 3rd ICI 2005.)

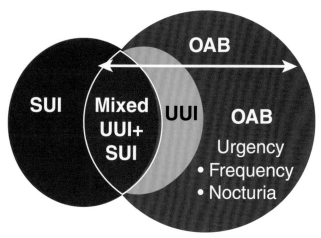

FIGURE 7-2. Spectrum of OAB. (Reproduced with permission from 3rd ICI 2005.)

KEY POINT

OAB wet or dry is quite prevalent in both men and women, increases with age and associated with staggering costs in the United States.

 PATHOLOGY

Following the development of urinary continence in the 2nd or 3rd year of life, micturition should only occur at a time and in a place of one's own choosing, when it is convenient and socially acceptable to do so. The bladder has only two modes—storage and voiding. The switch between the two is under conscious control. The brain receives sensory information generated by both the urothelium and detrusor muscle via the pudendal, hypogastric, and pelvic nerves. Afferent (sensory) signals from the bladder may arise from the urothelium, the detrusor muscle, or both (**Fig. 7-3**).

UROTHELIAL HYPOTHESIS

The urothelium is not, as previously thought, merely a passive barrier separating urine from person. It is a highly active organ, responding to stretch and to substances in the urine by expressing numerous signaling molecules including acetylcholine (ACh), nitric oxide, prostaglandins, and adenosine triphosphate (ATP). The multiple receptors in the urothelium include alpha A_1 and β_3 adrenoreceptors, muscarinic (principally M_2) (Bschleipfer

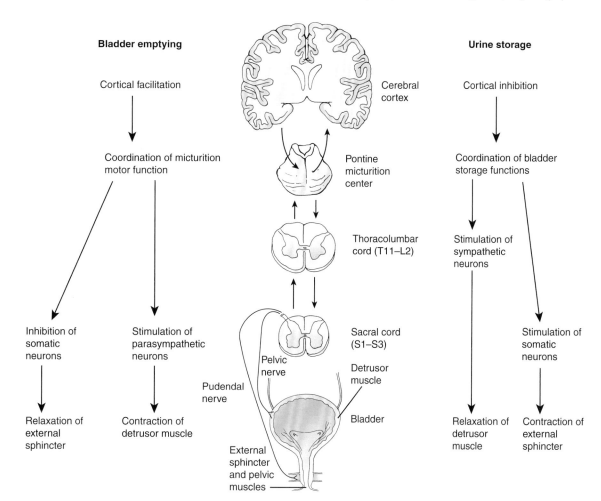

FIGURE 7-3. Pathways and Central Nervous System Centers Involved in the Control of Bladder Emptying (*left*) and Storage (*right*) Functions. Efferent pathways for micturition (*left*) and urine storage (*right*) also are shown. (From Porth, C. (2010). *Essentials of pathophysiology*. Philadelphia, PA: Lippincott Williams & Wilkins.)

et al., 2007) and nicotinic (Beckel & Birder, 2012) receptors, and purinergic (Rapp et al., 2005), cannabinoid (Tyagi et al., 2009), and vallinoid receptors (Birder & Andersson, 2013).

The urothelium is innervated by afferent (sensory) and autonomic efferent (motor) nerves, and as such the urothelium can be thought of as a "first responder" to mechanical and noxious stimulation associated with bladder filling. In addition, there is a suburothelial layer of myofibroblasts that may respond to ATP produced by the urothelium, and the detrusor muscle itself has stretch receptors. Thus, the urothelium, suburothelial layer, and detrusor act as a sensory organ that provides information to the brain on the fullness of the bladder and communicates the need to void. In OAB, there is evidence that this system is dysfunctional. For example, in vitro urothelium samples from OABs released three times the amount of ATP released by normal urothelium when exposed to capsaicin (Birder et al., 2013).

normally limited to isolated parts of the bladder, which could be interpreted as an urgent desire to void.

These two models of OAB are termed the urothelial and myogenic hypotheses, respectively. The reality is likely to be that they are both important in the generation of urgency.

The sensation of needing to void is processed by numerous areas of the brain, including the pons (Barrington nucleus) also called pontine micturition center (PMC), periaqueductal gray matter (PAG), hypothalamus, and the medial frontal cortex (Fowler et al., 2008) (see Chapter 2). These areas allow an individual to assess the need to void and the convenience and social acceptability of voiding. In children with primary nocturnal enuresis, there is evidence of underdevelopment of continence-related areas, in particular the thalamus, the frontal lobe, the anterior cingulate cortex, and the insula (Lei et al., 2012); in older adults, age-related changes to the brain are associated with OAB symptoms (Tadic et al., 2010).

KEY POINT

The exact pathology leading to OAB and urgency incontinence is not clearly defined; theories include abnormal sensory input regarding bladder filling and/or abnormalities in detrusor muscle function.

KEY POINT

OAB may arise from an increase in sensory signals from the bladder to the brain, from a failure of the brain to correctly handle these signals and control the bladder, or from both.

MYOGENIC HYPOTHESIS

There is also evidence that the detrusor muscle itself is abnormal in OAB. In several species, including humans, the detrusor muscle produces spontaneous microcontractions, the amplitude of which increases with increasing bladder volume (Coolsaet, 1985). The physiological role, if any, of these contractions is unknown, and they are not detectable by standard urodynamic measurement (Chacko et al., 2014). There is evidence that these contractions are exaggerated in DO; isolated strips of detrusor taken from patients with urodynamically proven DO demonstrate higher levels of intracellular calcium, greater oscillations in the levels of calcium, and more spontaneously active cells than the normal bladder (Sui et al., 2009).

Alterations in regulation of contractile protein function have also—been implicated in the pathogenesis of DO. In the presence of bladder outlet obstruction, proteins within the detrusor muscle undergo chemical changes that increase contractile strength (Su et al., 2003); it is conceivable that similar processes are involved in idiopathic DO. Denervation is frequently observed in detrusor muscle biopsies from OABs, and it has been proposed that partial denervation of detrusor myocytes leads to increased coupling between cells and therefore increased excitability (Mills et al., 2000). This may lead to the spread throughout the detrusor of contractions

OAB RISK FACTORS

Risk factors that have been identified in several studies include

- Increasing age
- Obesity
- Lifestyle
- Diet
- Urinary outflow obstruction
- Childhood continence issues
- Pregnancy
- Ethnicity
- Medications
- Chronic disease

AGE

Age is a key risk factor as the prevalence of all LUTS rises with age (Irwin et al., 2006), and numerous studies, both cross-sectional (Hannestad et al., 2000; Irwin et al., 2006) and longitudinal (Irwin et al., 2010), support this statement. Numerous changes occur in the bladder in association with aging. These include increased collagen content, changes to gap junctions, increased space between myocytes, and changes in the sensitivity of sensory afferents (Siroky, 2004). ATP-dependent detrusor contractions rise with age, whereas cholinergic-dependent contractions decline (Yoshida et al., 2004). There is also a reduction in the number of detrusor M_3 receptors (Mansfield et al., 2005). Additionally, the aging brain is less able to suppress the sensation of urgency (Griffiths et al., 2009). The presence of white matter hyperintensities in the brain is associated with LUTS in older adults (Kuchel et al., 2009), and there is a correlation between vascular risk factors such as hypertension and hypercholesterolemia and incontinence (Ponholzer et al., 2006). OAB, particularly in the elderly, may be considered as a neurological as much as a urological disease. These physiologic features relate to symptoms of decreased bladder capacity, increased tendency for bladder to contract in response to filling and to "triggers" such as running water or cold, decreased awareness of bladder filling, decreased pressure flow from reduced strength of bladder contractions, and delay in the desire to void. Most older adults adapt to these "normal" changes. However, in the presence of OAB, it is very difficult.

KEY POINT

Age is a key risk factor for OAB/UUI as the prevalence of all LUTS rises with age. Age-related changes include reduced bladder capacity, increase in detrusor contractions in response to "triggers," decreased awareness of bladder filling, reduced bladder contractility strength, and the desire to void is delayed.

OBESITY

Obesity is a strong risk factor for UI (Wyman et al., 2009), although the effect is greater for SUI than OAB (Subak et al., 2009). In a most recent study (Hagovska et al., 2020) of subjects with a BMI indicating obesity, it was noted that after 12 weeks of an intense exercise program to lose weight, there was a significant decrease in OAB symptoms with a 5% or greater weight loss. Continence appears to be definitely improved with weight management in those with OAB/UUI (Parker & Griebling, 2015).

LIFESTYLE FACTORS AND DIET

High caffeine intake (over 400 mg/day) has been shown to be associated with DO (Arya et al., 2000), and a relationship between the consumption of "diet" soft drinks and OAB has been demonstrated (Cartwright et al., 2007). Wyman et al. (2009) also state that overindulging in bladder irritants can exacerbate symptoms by "causing detrusor excitability and increased detrusor pressure." There is also a reported but inconsistent association with smoking (Dallosso et al., 2003; Maserejian et al., 2012; Tahtinen et al., 2011) as well as other diet and lifestyle factors and OAB. In a model tracking incidence of OAB over a period of 3 years, low physical exercise levels and a high-carbohydrate diet, in conjunction with obesity and diabetes, were associated with doubling of the risk for developing OAB (McGrother et al., 2012).

URINARY OUTFLOW OBSTRUCTION

There also appears to be a relationship between bladder outflow obstruction (BOO) and DO (see also Chapter 8, Urinary Retention). Spontaneous detrusor contractions are associated with BOO in animal models (Su et al., 2003), and BOO causes detrusor hypertrophy and hyperactivity (Zhang et al., 2004). In humans, there is a reported association between BOO and DO; the relief of BOO with prostatectomy has been shown to reduce DO. The histological detrusor denervation associated with BOO appears to improve after prostatectomy. DO can be induced by surgical treatment for SUI if the procedure results in some degree of bladder outlet obstruction (Brading & Turner, 1994).

CHILDHOOD CONTINENCE ISSUES

Childhood continence problems, including urgency and enuresis, are also strong risk factors for the development of OAB in adult life; children who wet the bed are more than twice as likely to have OAB as adults than those who do not (Fitzgerald et al., 2006).

PREGNANCY

Symptoms of urinary urgency are also common during pregnancy, with increasing prevalence as pregnancy progresses (Liang et al., 2012).

ETHNICITY

There is mixed evidence for the influence of ethnicity. The multinational EpiLUTS study suggested a higher prevalence in Hispanic and African American men but no differences in women (Coyne et al., 2009), and studies in hospital populations have found no differences in prevalence between different ethnic groups (Finkelstein et al., 2008). A Swedish twin study suggested genetic influences on UI, frequency, and nocturia but not for the development of OAB (Wennberg et al., 2011).

KEY POINT

Risk factors for OAB include age, obesity, BOO, childhood continence issues, pregnancy, and most likely "high" caffeine intake and "diet" sodas.

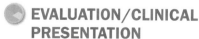 ## EVALUATION/CLINICAL PRESENTATION

Up to half of people with significant LUTS will never present to health care professionals (Irwin et al., 2008; Shaw et al., 2001). LUTS, particularly incontinence, are associated with high levels of embarrassment, not just because of wetness and odor but also of embarrassment related to going to the toilet frequently, fear of being seen to be "unclean" or being mocked, and, in men, a fear of being thought to be impotent (Elstad et al., 2010). Patients also fail to seek help because they believe that incontinence is a normal part of aging, an unavoidable consequence of childbirth, or that UI and LUTS are untreatable (Shaw et al., 2001). As such, it is imperative that health care professionals specifically ask people at risk of LUTS/UI if they have any bladder problems; this includes older people; women post-childbirth; and those with neurological disease such as multiple sclerosis, Parkinson disease, stroke, or diabetes.

CLINICAL SYMPTOMS

The classic triad of symptoms associated with OAB are urgency, frequency, and nocturia.

Urgency

The hallmark symptom of OAB is *urinary urgency*. Patients report a sudden sensation of needing to empty their bladder, which they struggle to suppress; they are unable to delay voiding until a socially convenient time. This sensation is often accompanied by the fear of leaking urine or by actual incontinence (UUI). Individuals often report increased daytime frequency; some of these findings reflect adaptive behaviors, such as "going frequently, just in case" in an attempt to avoid symptoms and unplanned toilet visits. The volume of urine passed is usually relatively small, often as little as 50 to 75 mL because of the frequency of voiding, but typically results in complete bladder emptying.

KEY POINT

The hallmark symptom of OAB is *urgency*, the inability to delay voiding until a socially acceptable time. Frequency and nocturia often accompany urgency creating a triad of symptoms associated with OAB.

Frequency

It is generally accepted that urinary *frequency* becomes bothersome if it occurs more than 13 times per day, although this has not been formally evaluated in research trials, which use a diurnal frequency of *eight* as a defining criterion. Moreover, frequency of voiding is subjective, and for some people, every 2 hours is interpreted as "frequency." In all cases, bladder diaries are invaluable as a baseline assessment tool. Note that 3 days of diaries have been shown to be most reliable (Bright et al., 2012). There can be compliance issues related to completing bladder diaries due to the amount of information requested, not understanding how to complete them, and forgetfulness. It is important to use a diary that is going to be useful to both the patient and the provider. Explaining to the patient why the bladder diary is important can be helpful in it being completed. Patients frequently feel completing the diary changes the way they view their symptoms and also gives them insight into the severity of their problem, which in turn helps understand their treatment and importance of possibly changing behaviors (see Chapter 4, Fig. 4-1).

Nocturia

The complaint of waking at night one or more times to void is a particularly bothersome symptom. It is important to differentiate true nocturia, where the desire to void causes the person to wake, from waking for another reason and deciding to visit the toilet. Most people will accept nocturia once per night but waking twice or more is associated with increasing levels of bother (Bing et al., 2006). The symptom associated with most bother has been reported variably as UI during sexual intercourse (Coyne et al., 2009), urgency incontinence (Liberman et al., 2001), or urinary urgency (Coyne et al., 2004), depending on the study and the framing of the question. Unfortunately, women rarely voice the worsening of sexual function, especially those who already have OAB. Despite OAB having a potentially debilitating effect on sexual function, its effect is rarely reported by women (Levy & Lowenstein, 2020). Treating OAB can positively impact sexual functioning and can thus improve quality of life.

KEY POINT

The most bothersome symptom associated with OAB varies and includes urinary incontinence during intercourse, urgency incontinence, and urinary urgency.

Other Symptoms

In addition to urgency, frequency, and nocturia, patients with OAB often report symptoms such as toilet mapping, where they will make a conscious effort to know the locations of facilities when out in public, and latch-key, or key in the door syndrome (or garage door) incontinence, which is the sensation of a sudden onset of urgency at the point of putting the key in the door or opening the garage when arriving home. Other anecdotal exacerbating factors to explore are cold weather, running water, and psychological stress and anxiety.

Validated questionnaires such as the OAB-q determine what is most bothersome to the patient in regard to their bladder issues. The short form, OABq SF, has been validated and is just as useful (Coyne et al., 2015). This questionnaire also helps the patient realize how OAB is actually affecting quality of life and how treatment is improving it.

HISTORY

As already mentioned, the diagnosis of OAB is a clinical one and is not reliant on any diagnostic tests. The National Institute of Clinical Excellence (NICE) issued guidelines in 2013, which state "history taking is regarded as the cornerstone of assessment of UI" (NICE, 2013). Guideline, Statement 1 (Gormley et al., 2019) states that in addition to a careful history, physical exam, and urinalysis, other disorders that could be contributing to the patient's symptoms should be ruled out. Chapter 4 provides a detailed overview of primary assessment of UI and voiding dysfunction in adults. At the end of the initial assessment, a diagnosis of the type and cause of UI and its impact on the patient can generally be made without needing further investigation. However, if diagnosis is unclear or conflicting, urodynamics may be necessary (see Chapter 5, Box 5-1).

The history should cover the following specifically in relation to evaluating OAB triad of symptoms:

- General health, presence of functional or cognitive impairments
- Fluid intake amounts and types, particularly carbonated, caffeinated drinks and other potential bladder irritants such as citrus
- Diet
- Smoking and alcohol habits
- A detailed obstetric history: number and mode of delivery or deliveries, menstrual patterns, or menopause symptoms
- Genitourinary history: report of recurrent UTIs, genitourinary symptoms of menopause (GSM), prostate issues such as BPH, prostatitis, kidney or bladder stones, episodes of hematuria
- Sexuality history: dyspareunia, leakage with intercourse and/or orgasm, erectile dysfunction, sexually transmitted diseases
- Bowel regularity, consistency of stool, and constipation, which can exacerbate OAB symptoms and irritable bowel symptoms. UI and fecal incontinence (FI) frequently coexist
- Family history: first-line relatives with history of colon, bladder, kidney, prostate, uterine, and ovarian cancer
- All prescribed and over-the-counter medications taken
- Medical conditions that predispose to incontinence (**Table 7-1**), which should be treated, if possible, to ameliorate the impact on continence status
- The individual's beliefs about the cause of the problem, impact on quality of life, and his or her goals for treatment

The impact of UI on a person's quality of life is extremely variable. There is little correlation between severity and impact (Barentsen et al., 2012), but there is evidence that urgency incontinence leads to greater detriment including depression and social isolation than stress incontinence, perhaps due to its unpredictability (Shaw, 2001). Therefore, the assessment should include the impact of an individual's symptoms on their quality of life, to allow the formulation of realistic and acceptable goals of treatment. This may include use of the Quality of Life Short-Form (OAB-q SF), a questionnaire that is condition specific that assesses symptom bother and health-related quality of life impact of OAB (Coyne et al., 2015). This objective questionnaire is useful in helping the patient see symptom bother has changed at each point in treatment and allow the continence nurse to focus on those that have little change.

KEY POINT

There is evidence that urgency incontinence leads to greater detriment in QoL including depression and social isolation than stress incontinence, perhaps due to its unpredictability. Therefore, an assessment should be made of the impact of an individual's symptoms on their quality of life, to allow the formulation of realistic and acceptable goals of treatment.

Continence-specific aspects that need to be covered in detail include

- Daytime and nighttime frequency and intensity of symptoms (see Chapter 4, Fig. 4-1 bladder diary)
- Urgency
- The length of time they can "hold on," and any symptoms of stress incontinence, reported or noted on the bladder diary
- Coping strategies

Inquiry should be made about strategies used to cope with urine loss as well as over-the-counter products for UI, many of which are perceived as expensive. A study on willingness to pay for a treatment for UI in Sweden found that people would be prepared to pay up to an eighth of their net income to reduce UI episodes by half, when given a hypothetical model (Johannesson et al., 1997). Having UI is costly, with direct and indirect annual costs per person of around $900 in a 2006 US study (Subak et al., 2006). In the United Kingdom, the total annual National Health Service (NHS) cost of UI in community-dwelling adults was £536 (2,000 prices), with total costs borne by individuals of an additional £207. Women spent much more than men (Turner et al., 2004). A European study in 2005 found the average annual out-of-pocket expenses to be between €359 and €655 (approximately US $480 to $900) (Papanicolaou et al., 2005). Many patients with UI improvise, using things such as sanitary towels, wadded toilet tissue, or towels cut in pieces to absorb urine. See Chapter 16 for details on the many continence products available. Be aware that the cost of urge urinary incontinence is increasing throughout the world, and in the United States alone is predicted to reach $82.6 billion dollars by 2021 (Coyne et al., 2014).

Consideration should also be given to the fact that successful toileting relies not just on the ability to con-

TABLE 7-1 ASSOCIATED CONDITIONS AFFECTING CONTINENCE STATUS

CONDITION	IMPACT	MITIGATING FACTORS
Diabetes mellitus	Poor control can cause polyuria and precipitate or exacerbate incontinence; also associated with increased likelihood of urgency incontinence and diabetic neuropathic bladder	Better control of diabetes can reduce osmotic diuresis and associated polyuria and improve incontinence
Degenerative joint disease	Can impair mobility and precipitate UUI	Optimal pharmacologic and nonpharmacologic pain management can improve mobility and toileting ability
Chronic pulmonary disease	Associated cough can cause SUI	Cough suppression can reduce stress incontinence and cough-induced UUI
Congestive heart failure Lower extremity venous insufficiency	Redistribution of edema when lying flat increases nighttime urine production and can contribute to nocturia and UI	Optimizing pharmacologic management of congestive heart failure, sodium restriction, support stockings, leg elevation, and a late-afternoon dose of a rapid-acting diuretic may reduce nocturnal polyuria and associated nocturia and nighttime UI
Sleep apnea	May increase nighttime urine production by increasing production of atrial natriuretic peptide	Diagnosis and treatment of sleep apnea, usually with continuous positive airway pressure devices, may improve the condition and reduce nocturnal polyuria and associated nocturia and UI
Stroke	Can precipitate urgency and less often retention; also impairs mobility	UI after an acute stroke often resolves with rehabilitation; persistent UI should be further evaluated Regular toileting assistance essential for those with persistent mobility impairment
Parkinson disease	Associated with UUI; also causes impaired mobility and cognition in late stages	Optimizing management may improve mobility and improve UI. Regular toileting assistance is essential for those with mobility and cognitive impairment in late-stage disease
Normal pressure hydrocephalus	Presents with UI, along with gait and cognitive impairments	Patients presenting with all three symptoms should be considered for brain imaging to rule out this condition, as it may improve with a ventricular–peritoneal shunt
Dementia (Alzheimer, multi-infarct, others)	Associated with UUI; impaired cognition and apraxia interfere with toileting and hygiene	Regular prompt voiding and toileting assistance essential for those with mobility and cognitive impairment in all stages of dementia, but most important in later stages
Depression	May impair motivation to be continent; may also be a consequence of incontinence	Optimizing pharmacologic and nonpharmacologic management of depression may improve UI

Adapted from Wagg, A., Gibson, W., Johnson, T., III., et al. (2014b). Urinary incontinence in frail elderly persons: Report from the 5th International Consultation on Incontinence. *Neurourology and Urodynamics, 34*(5), 398–406.

trol urgency but also on being able to locate and get to the toilet, undress and redress. Therefore, when relevant, the clinician should assess mobility, cognition, visual impairment, and functional impairment, with the goal of intervening to address modifiable associated factors.

PHYSICAL EXAMINATION

- General assessment including any functional limitations
- Cognitive status
- Abdominal exam (checking for scars, distended bladder, fecal loading)
- Perineal examination (perigenital skin status, health of vaginal mucosa, evidence of prolapse)
- Evaluation of pelvic floor muscle strength and the ability to perform a pelvic floor contraction

- Rectal examination if constipation or poor rectal tone is suspected and prostate health in men
- Bladder diary as previously discussed
- Pad test to improve objectivity of the volume of urine lost described in Chapter 11

In people who experience urgency incontinence, a quantification of the frequency, circumstance, and volume of urine lost should be made. Quantification may be obtained using a bladder diary documenting the frequency of urine loss, the presence of urgency, and voiding frequency. A pad test is useful in providing a more objective quantification of the volume of urine loss (see Chapter 11). Certainly the clinician should ask about situations and factors that aggravate OAB symptoms, such as caffeine intake, stressful situations, being cold, or hearing running water during history intake.

BASELINE TESTS

- Standard urinalysis with urine dipstick if there is a history or symptoms of UTI, diabetes, or hematuria
- Postvoid residual (PVR) urine if incomplete emptying suspected or in the presence of vaginal prolapse

URODYNAMICS

Urodynamic testing is seldom necessary in the initial assessment of OAB and is usually reserved for individuals with neurologic conditions, those with a complex history such as prior surgery, those where the diagnosis is unclear, or those who have not responded to treatment. (See Chapter 5, Advanced Assessment [Urodynamics].)

KEY POINT

Urodynamic testing is not usually indicated for individuals with OAB, unless there is an associated neurologic condition, prior surgery for UI, unclear diagnosis, or failure to respond to treatment.

 ## MANAGEMENT OPTIONS

Many national and international guidelines for the management of UI have been published, including those by the American Urological Association (Gormley et al., 2019), the European Association of Urology (Thuroff et al., 2011), the National Institute of Clinical and Healthcare Excellence in the United Kingdom (NICE, 2010, 2013), and the Canadian Urological Association (Bettez et al., 2012).

CONSERVATIVE TREATMENT

Conservative treatment of OAB includes lifestyle interventions such as weight loss, reduction in caffeine intake, reduction/cessation of smoking, treatment of constipation, and fluid management. While these are all healthy lifestyle choices, there is very little research to support these recommendations as being of particular benefit in the treatment of OAB (Moore et al., 2013). However, using a treatment algorithm that includes conservative interventions can improve symptoms and patient satisfaction especially in primary care (Bartley et al., 2013). AUA Guidelines for OAB also recommend conservative treatment as first-line therapy (Gormley et al., 2019). Chapter 6 provides an excellent review of conservative treatment options as well as educational tips for continence nurses.

For cases of pelvic floor weakness or mixed UI, pelvic floor muscle therapy (PFMT) may be helpful, especially in combination with bladder training. Contraction of the pelvic floor has been known to prevent urinary leakage occurring with increased abdominal pressure. However, contraction can cause reflexive relaxation of detrusor contractions, thereby decreasing leakage (Lamin et al., 2016). Older studies (Burgio et al., 1998) have also

reported that PFMT is more effective than treatment with anticholinergics. More recently 65 elderly women were evaluated after utilizing biofeedback followed by verbal coaching over 8 to 12 weeks. Forty-six percent of participants experienced a 50% or greater improvement in the frequency of urgency episodes and 15% were dry at the completion of the study (Griffiths et al., 2015). A barrier to the use of PFMT might be availability of experienced clinicians, cost, length of treatment, and provider fear of losing their patients to follow-up visits. The 2019 AUA/SUFU guidelines for the diagnosis and treatment of non-neurogenic OAB recommend behavioral therapies including PFMT as first-line treatments (Gormley et al., 2019).

KEY POINT

Lifestyle interventions such as weight loss, reduction in caffeine intake, smoking cessation, and constipation management are commonly recommended, although there is little robust research to prove effectiveness. Other noninvasive approaches include bladder training techniques and lifestyle changes.

General Measures

Once a diagnosis of OAB is made, the first step is to consider and treat any coexisting medical conditions, functional impairments, or reversible causes (see Chapter 3) that may be contributing to the overall symptom load. Bowel function should be normalized to avoid constipation and if present, fecal incontinence should be treated (see Chapters 21 and 22).

Weight Loss

For individuals who are overweight or obese, weight loss should be tactfully encouraged. The continence nurse should share with patients the overall benefits of weight loss as well as the evidence that weight loss has been shown to improve incontinence (Parker & Griebling, 2015). Exploring the patients' current dietary and physical activity habits to identify opportunities to improve both diet and physical activity opens dialogue to developing a patient-centered weight loss strategy.

Smoking Cessation

Those who smoke should be strongly encouraged to stop, although, again, there are no intervention trials to support this practice in the treatment of OAB. Despite the lack of research examining the effect of smoking cessation on OAB, the adverse health effects of smoking on health are well known including the risk for chronic obstructive pulmonary disease (COPD) (chronic COPD-related coughing can exacerbation SUI), lung cancer, and cardiovascular disease, as well as smoking being a strong risk factor for bladder cancer (Parker & Griebling, 2015).

Caffeine Reduction

Caffeine is a known stimulant and diuretic that has direct effects on voiding through multiple pathways. Studies have shown increased risk for UUI with high caffeine intake and there is some research evidence showing that reducing caffeine intake is associated with a decrease in incontinence episodes (Parker & Griebling, 2015). It is common practice to advise a reduction in the intake of caffeinated drinks in patients who experience urgency. There has been one randomized controlled trial of caffeine reduction, which compared bladder training with caffeine reduction to bladder training alone in men; these investigators found that a reduction of caffeine intake to below 100 mg/day was associated with statistically significant reductions in episodes of urgency and urgency incontinence (Bryant et al., 2002). Gleason et al. (2013) examined the association between caffeine intake and UI in women and reported that caffeine intake of 204 mg or greater per day was associated with an increased risk of UI. Another small trial ($n = 11$) in which participants were randomized to decaffeinated versus caffeinated coffee also found a significant improvement in urgency and frequency and improved scores on the ICI-Q OAB questionnaire (Wells et al., 2014). Based on current evidence, the continence nurse should encourage patients, particularly those with high caffeine intake to reduce their caffeine intake and to monitor its effect on OAB symptoms. If it does not change symptoms, the individual may reintroduce caffeine into their diet.

Fluid Intake

It is generally held that fluid intake should be around 2 L/day. There is a widespread belief that concentrated urine is irritating to the urothelium and worsens OAB symptoms, although there is no supporting evidence for this. Overhydration predictably leads to polyuria and therefore increased urinary frequency. However, analysis of the Nurses' Health Study cohort found no link between fluid intake and the development of incontinence (Townsend et al., 2011). In a study of older adults in hospital, older people with DO were found to drink less than those without DO, possibly as a result of voluntary fluid restriction. In this study, there was also a strong correlation between increased fluid intake and increased frequency of micturition (Griffiths et al., 1993).

There is a paucity of high-quality evidence to support fluid intake changes as treatment for UUI. A small trial (Dowd et al., 1996) suggested that increasing fluid intake reduced episodes of UUI, but adherence to the study protocol was poor. A trial of medication alone versus medication and lifestyle interventions (including general advice on fluid intake and specific advice to reduce fluid intake for those who habitually drank more than 2.1 L/day) found no additional benefit of lifestyle intervention and little impact of specific advice on drinking habits (Zimmern et al., 2010). A systematic review published in 2018 (Wood et al., 2018) examined which health conditions require increased fluid intake and whether patients with high fluid intake can safely be advised to decrease their fluid intake. They included studies (study designs were variable and included systematic reviews, meta-analysis, clinical trials, and case series) examining water intake in relation to risk of the primary onset or recurrence of a variety of medical conditions in adults. The authors concluded that, "Although sources continue to lead the population to believe that it is necessary to drink 8 glasses of water daily, there is a lack of evidence supporting this belief and it can exacerbate OAB symptoms. Other than for the prevention of urolithiasis, physicians should reconsider routinely recommending increased fluid intake in the majority of patients" (p. 379).

Constipation

The effect of regulating bowel function on UI has not been well studied, the data that exist are old, and to date, there are no intervention trials that address the effect of resolving constipation on UI (Moore et al., 2013). In a small observational study, 30% of women with SUI and 61% of women with uterovaginal prolapse reported straining at stool as a young adult, compared to 4% of women without urogynecological symptoms (Spence-Jones et al., 1994). In a large population-based study of 1,154 women over age 60 years, those with UI were slightly more likely to report constipation than those who were continent of urine (31.6% vs. 24.7%) (Diokno et al., 1990). After adjusting for demographic and obstetric confounders, women who reported straining at stool were more likely to report SUI and urgency (Alling-Møller et al., 2000). It has been suggested that straining and pudendal nerve function may be related, but more research is required to explore this relationship. It should be stressed that, although "lifestyle" interventions are common practice in the initial treatment of OAB, there is very little high-quality evidence to support their use. However, as they are low cost and low risk and are general recommendations for healthy living, there is little to be lost through their adoption. Simple diet adjustments, fluid, fiber management, and exercise can all safely and effectively affect constipation status (see Chapter 6, Box 6-10 regarding healthy bowel strategies).

Urgency Suppression/Bladder Training

Patients can be taught techniques to override the sensation of urgency, allowing them to delay voiding until convenient. Several methods have been described, including rapid pelvic floor contraction at the onset of urgency, sitting on a hard surface, and distraction techniques. Bladder drill, also known as bladder training or bladder retraining, is a self-guided method of increasing the time between onset of urge to void and the actual time of voiding. Although it requires significant patient engagement, bladder training has been shown to be effective in reducing urgency and urge incontinence episodes (Roe et al., 2007). Chapter 6 provides a detailed discussion and "how to do" regarding urgency suppression and bladder training. **Figure 7-4** provides an example of a patient teaching brochure that can be used for bladder training.

KEY POINT

Urgency suppression and bladder training (bladder drill) have been proven to be effective in management of OAB and/or urgency incontinence.

Introduction

Forty-two million people in the United States experience symptoms of over active bladder (OAB) syndrome including urgency, frequency and urge urinary incontinence. OAB affects both men and women of any age group.

Despite being so common, bladder difficulties are often hidden. As a result, many people do not get the help they need and they suffer in silence.

This pamphlet contains useful and practical advice about bladder training, a simple technique that can help people who have an urgent need to go to the washroom.

Bladder urgency is also called **over-active bladder**.

Overactive bladder

Many bladder problems are caused by an overactive bladder:

- A sudden urge to go to the washroom (**urgency**)
- Unable to hold the urgency and reach the toilet in time (**urgency incontinence**)
- Needing to go very often - (**frequency**)
- Getting up during the night (**nocturia**)
- Wetting the bed at night (**nocturnal enuresis**)

These problems are caused when the bladder is very sensitive, or the bladder muscle squeezes when it shouldn't—even when you want to hold on.

How the bladder works

The bladder is made of muscle. It is positioned in the lower part of the tummy just behind the pubic bone.

In between visits to the bathroom the bladder relaxes and fills up. When you go to the bathroom, it is important to relax whether you sit (generally female) or stand (male). The brain then tells the bladder to contract or "squeeze" and the bladder empties through a tube called the urethra.

The pelvic floor is made of layers of muscle, which support the bladder and bowel. The pelvic floor also helps to stop leaks from the bladder and bowel.

The urethral sphincter is a circular muscle that goes around the urethra. The sphincter muscle normally squeezes as the bladder is filling up—it creates a seal so urine can't leak out. When you go to the toilet, the sphincter muscle relaxes and lets the urine flow.

Bladder training

Many people with urgency will get into the habit of going to the toilet too often—trying to make sure they are never "caught short" or to the bathroom "just because". This can result in confusing your bladder.

Bladder training is a method that helps the bladder hold more urine and allows you to hold on for longer.

Keep a record of when you pass urine and how much you drink for at least three days. You can ask for one of our bladder diaries to help you.

Gradually increase the time between visits to the bathroom. This can be done by practicing "Urge reduction techniques" when you get the urge to urinate or "pass water".
This includes:
- Stop what you are doing
- RELAX!
- Take a deep breath
- Do a few Kegel exercises 3-5
- Distract yourself
- Repeat if necessary

This should stop the urge. When the urge subsides, slowly walk to the toilet to empty your bladder. Try to extend the time between toileting using this technique. It will take time and determination on your part but it will eventually be successful if you keep at it.

Note that normal voiding is 6-8 times per day. This should be your goal. Fluid management is also very important in reaching your goals

Resources:

There are a number of online patient information sites. Here are a few:
National Association for Continence: www.nafc.org
Simon Foundation: www.simonfoundation.org
Patient Pictures: www.PatientPictures.com

Please ask your provider for any other information or clarification.

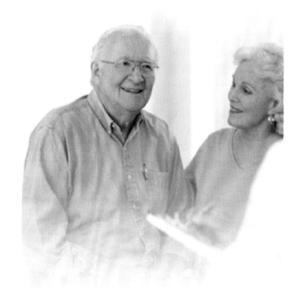

FIGURE 7-4. Example of a Bladder Training Brochure.

Interventions for Individuals with Impaired Cognitive and/or Mobility Function

For individuals with OAB who have mobility or cognitive impairment, the ability to get to the toilet in a timely manner when there is an urge to urinate is often a contributing factor to incontinence. For these individuals, toileting programs and/or functional training may improve their incontinence.

Toileting Programs

Behavioral interventions have been especially designed for frail older people with cognitive and physical impairments or younger individuals with functional and cognitive impairments. Because they have no side effects, they have been the mainstay of UI treatment in frail older people (Roe et al., 2007). Toileting programs require caregiver involvement to assist in the acquisition of continence. Three commonly used scheduled toileting programs that can be successfully implemented in long-term care facilities and at home include routine scheduled toileting (RST), habit training, and prompted voiding. These are discussed in detail in Chapter 6, Table 6-11.

Functional Intervention Training

Functional training incorporates musculoskeletal strengthening exercises into toileting routines by nursing home care aides or nursing assistants (Schnelle et al., 1995). There is increasing evidence for the effectiveness of physical exercise as an intervention for UI in populations in diverse settings. In a Veterans nursing home population in the United States, the combination of individualized prompted voiding and functionally oriented endurance and strength-training exercises (offered four times per day, 5 days per week, for 8 weeks) delivered by trained research staff was effective in significantly reducing UI (Ouslander et al., 2005). An intervention that provided exercise and incontinence care every 2 hours from 8:00 AM to 4:30 PM (total of 4 daily care episodes) for 5 days a week over 32 weeks in a nursing home population was also found to be effective in significantly reducing incontinence (Bates-Jensen et al., 2003). Similarly, a study of walking exercise for 30 minutes per day in a small group of cognitively impaired residents over 4 weeks resulted in a significant reduction in daytime incontinence episodes and an increase in gait speed and stamina (Jirovec, 1991). In community-dwelling older people, a 30-minute evening walk proved effective in reducing nocturia, while also improving daytime urinary frequency, blood pressure, body weight, body fat ratio, triglycerides, total cholesterol, and sleep quality (Sugaya et al., 2007).

Cognitive and functional impairment, common in frail elderly people, may preclude the use of some of these interventions. Additionally, the context in which care is provided needs to be considered (Booth et al., 2009; Dingwall, 2008; Wright et al., 2007). Many of these interventions are time consuming and need staff engagement for effective delivery (Vinsnes et al., 2007). Although pelvic floor muscle rehabilitation has not been studied extensively in frail older people, age and frailty alone should not preclude their use in appropriate patients with sufficient cognition to participate. The research supporting the above interventions is older, and little recent examination of these strategies has occurred. With an ever-increasing aging population and increasing prevalence of OAB, there is a major need for research in this area. Refer to Chapter 6 for further techniques to engage frail elderly people and their carers to optimize bladder health.

KEY POINT

There is increasing evidence that physical exercise programs can be beneficial in the treatment of UI in diverse care settings.

PHARMACOLOGIC TREATMENT

Should conservative management fail, then a pharmacological approach should be considered.

Antimuscarinics (See Table 7-2, Medications for OAB or UUI)

For many years, the mainstay of drug therapy for OAB has been the bladder antimuscarinics, including darifenacin, fesoterodine, imidafenacin (Japan), oxybutynin, propiverine (non-US), solifenacin, tolterodine, and trospium chloride. These agents block activation of the muscarinic receptors in the urothelium and detrusor, thereby reducing the sensation of urgency and increasing bladder storage capacity. Although initially effective, long-term adherence to treatment is poor, with discontinuation rates of up to 80% after 12 months' treatment (Wagg et al., 2012) due in part to lack of compliance, cost, side effects, and perceived lack of efficacy (Yeaw et al., 2009). Treatment failure has been found to be high regardless of anticholinergic therapy choice, and adherence is suboptimal (Chancellor et al., 2013). Despite new evidence confirming that there are small differences among the drugs in efficacy, side effects still lead to discontinuance; therefore, the continence care nurse needs to assess side effect profile and provide guidance in how to reduce or ameliorate the symptoms or trial another type of medication (Hsu et al., 2019). Common side effects include xerostomia (dry mouth) and constipation. Some of the bladder antimuscarinics, particularly oxybutynin, have been shown to cause cognitive impairment in older people, and its use in the elderly is therefore not recommended (Gibson et al., 2014).

In contrast to oxybutynin, darifenacin, trospium, solifenacin, and tolterodine have much lower central nervous system (CNS) concentrations, as they do not cross the blood–brain barrier (BBB) well, and some (5-hydroxymethyl tolterodine, the active metabolite of both tolterodine and fesoterodine, darifenacin, and trospium) are actively removed from the CNS by the permeability glycoprotein (P-GP) system, further lowering CNS levels and the potential for related adverse effects. The BBB becomes more permeable with increasing age and in association with some other diseases, and perhaps because of this, older people are more prone to CNS side effects of many drugs (Popescu et al., 2009). Thus, one advantage of the newer antimuscarinics is the absence of deleterious effects on cognition, at least in the short term, in cognitively intact older persons (Wagg, 2012); however, the newer agents do have similar rates of other adverse effects (such as xerostomia) as the older drugs (Buser et al., 2012).

Mirabegron

Mirabegron, a β_3 agonist, introduced in 2012 (Sacco et al., 2014) and has shown to be an effective option for OAB in both young and older people. The side effect profile avoids typical antimuscarinic side effects most commonly dry mouth and constipation but includes a concern about either new-onset or worsening hypertension (Wagg et al., 2014a).

Combination Therapy

Refractory OAB can be a very difficult, challenging and a long-term treatment regimen that can utilize many different options. In all studies reviewed by Andersson et al. (2017), patients all showed improvement by adding another medication when the first OAB drug was not as efficacious as hoped. There is some suggestion that adding mirabegron to a current treatment with antimuscarinic, especially solifenacin, may improve outcomes (Hsu, et al., 2019). Combining mirabegron with an antimuscarinic agent may allow a lower dose of the antimuscarinic to be administered with fewer bothersome antimuscarinic side effects (Allison & Gibson, 2018). Adding an antimuscarinic to another antimuscarinic has been shown to be effective in reducing refractory OAB symptoms, but the increase in anticholinergic load or side effects often leads to termination.

Topical Estrogens

Topical estrogens, in the form of cream, a ring, or vaginal suppository, is commonly used in the treatment of OAB in postmenopausal women. It is known that estrogen has a major role in the function of the female urogenital tract and well recognized that urogenital atrophy can lead to dysuria. According to the Cochrane group in 2012 (Cody, 2012) in multiple trials (34) including 19676 incontinent women of whom 9,599 received estrogen therapy (1,464 received topical estrogens), it was found that oral estrogens resulted in worse incontinence than placebo. However, there was some evidence that topical estrogens used locally as vaginal creams or pessary (rings) improved continence. Overall, there was less urgency and frequency in women using local estrogen (Robinson et al., 2014) (see **Table 7-2** for medication types, dosing and nursing considerations). Chapter 18 provides greater in-depth discussion regarding the benefits of transvaginal estrogen in postmenopausal women.

KEY POINT

Pharmacologic therapy should be considered for any patient for whom conservative therapy provides insufficient improvement; the major types of medications include antimuscarinics, mirabegron, combination therapy, vaginal estrogen, and Botox. Choice of medication should be determined by medication action, patient's medical status, age, complicating factors, side effect profile, and cost.

OnabotulinumtoxinA

OnabotulinumtoxinA (Botox®), one of the subtypes of the neurotoxin produced by the bacterium *Clostridium botulinum*, is a potent inhibitor of acetylcholine release from the motor axon (Proft, 2009). It has been shown to be of value in the treatment of refractory OAB, leading to increased bladder capacity, decreased intravesical pressure, and reduced incontinence episodes (Kuo & Kuo, 2013). Treatment involves injection of botulinum toxin into the suburothelium via a cystoscope and can be performed as an outpatient procedure under local anesthesia. It has been shown to be safe in older people, although there is an increased risk of large PVR and treatment failure compared to younger patients (Liao & Kuo, 2013). Postprocedure clean intermittent catheterization (CIC) may be needed if postvoid residual volumes (PVRs) are too high, with elevated PVRs generally lasting 2 to 12 weeks. Abnormal PVRs were reported at about 5.4% of study participants (Nitti et al., 2017). The patient is generally taught preprocedure how to perform CIC. Infection (UTI) can also be a potential side effect. Re-injection rate of Botox® is generally required in about 24 weeks (Chapple et al., 2013; Nitti et al., 2017). When evaluating patients for this treatment option, the individual's willingness and ability to perform CIC needs to be part of the assessment; this criterion eliminates numerous eligible candidates who otherwise might benefit from Botox®. **Figure 7-5** shows Botox® injection patterns.

NEUROMODULATION

Neuromodulation is a therapeutic modality that uses electrical signals to alter the involuntary reflexes of the lower urinary tract, thus inhibiting the voiding reflex, reducing involuntary detrusor contractions, and assisting patients to regain voluntary control of micturition. The

TABLE 7-2 MEDICATIONS USED FOR OAB OR UUI

MEDICATION	DOSAGE	ADVERSE EVENTS (>4%)	COMMENTS
Anticholinergic or Antimuscarinic			
Darifenacin (Enable®)	Enablex 7.5 mg QD Enablex 15 mg QD	Constipation 21% Dry mouth 19% Headache 7%	• All oral medications in these two classes cannot be crushed • Drug/drug interactions noted with digoxin, ketoconazole, clarithromycin • Best used with patients who have concurrent fecal incontinence
Fesoterodine (Toviaz®)	Toviaz 4 mg QD Toviaz 8 mg QD	Dry mouth 19% Constipation 5%	• Hot environment caution • Better choice than trospium for patients with >2–3 episodes UI daily

Oxybutynin (Ditropan®, Ditropan XL®, Oxytrol®, Gelnique®)	Ditropan IR, 5–15 mg, 1–3/day
	Ditropan XL 5–30 mg QD
	Gelnique sachet (10%), topical, QD
	Oxytrol patch 3.9 mg q3-4 days
		Dry mouth 29%
		Constipation
		Headache 6%
			• Likely to cross blood brain barrier (Kay et al., 2005)
			• Not recommended for elderly (AGS, 2019)
			• Monitor cognitive effects
			• Consider Oxytrol and Gelnique for patients with swallowing difficulties
			• Oxytrol patch a more convenient form of delivery with fewer side effects and is available over the counter
			  • Change patch q3-4 days on the same 2 days every week
			  • Apply to a different area with each change
			  • Less GI side effects
			• Studies unavailable to drug/drug interactions
			• Topical gel considerations
			  • Can be applied anywhere o shoulders, upper arms, stomach, or thighs; a different site should be used every day
			  • Do not apply to skin that has recently been shaved, has open sores, rashes, or tattoos
			  • Do not take a bath, swim shower, exercise, or get the application site wet for 1 hour after application
			  • Gel is flammable and patients should be instructed to avoid open flames and smoking until gel has dried
			  • Gel can cause redness, rash, itching, or irritation where applied

Solifenacin (Vesicare®)	Vesicare 5 mg QD Vesicare 10 mg QD	Dry mouth 10.2% Constipation 5% Blurred vision 4.1%	• Head to head study with Detrol LA • No known drug/drug interactions • Favorable tolerability profile • Better choice for patients with 2–3 UI episodes daily • No central nervous system effects
Tolterodine (Detrol®, Detrol LA®)	Detrol 2 mg QD or BID Detrol LA 4 mg QD	Dry mouth 23% Headache 6% Constipation 6%	• No known drug/drug interactions
Trospium (Sanctura®, Sanctura XR®)	Sanctura 20 mg BID Sanctura XR 60 mg QD	Dry mouth 19% Constipation 5%	• Needs to be taken on an empty stomach, 1 hour prior to meals • Avoid alcohol 1–2 hours prior to taking dose • No known drug/drug interactions

TABLE 7-2 MEDICATIONS USED FOR OAB OR UUI (Continued)

MEDICATION	DOSAGE	ADVERSE EVENTS (>4%)	COMMENTS
β₃-Adrenergic Agonist			
Mirabegron (Myrbetriq®)	• Myrbetriq 25 mg and 50 mg QD • Effectiveness within 8 weeks (25 mg), 4 weeks with 50 mg	Hypertension 9% Nasopharyngitis 4% UTI 4%	• May be taken in combination with anticholinergics • Better taken at bedtime • No food effects • A moderated CYP inhibitor. Caution with metoprolol and desipramine • Monitor blood pressure and possible drug interactions • Administer with caution to patients with chronic disease. Use only 25 mg with caution and monitor kidney function
Hormone Therapy			
Topical Estrogen (Premarin®, Estrace®, estradiol, estriol, Estring®, Femring®)	• Application of all creams in the presence of atrophic vaginitis should be nightly for 1–2 weeks then 2–3 times per week at bedtime • Premarin and Estrace, 0.5 g • Estradiol (0.1 mg/g) or Estriol (0.5 mg/g) compounded • Estring (estradiol) vaginal ring 2 mg q3mo • Femring (estradiol) vaginal ring 0.5 or 0.1 mg/day q3mo • Estradiol vaginal tablets, 10 mcg; insert one tablet nightly for 2 weeks then twice weekly	• Few adverse effects • Caution in patients with breast cancer	• Application can be with applicator or finger • NOT appropriate treatment for stress incontinence • Also helpful with urethritis (pea size application to urethra 3 per week) • Seek permission from oncologist with history of breast cancer • In higher, long-term usage, consider opposing progesterone in women with intact uterus especially with Femring • Women find rings more convenient and less messy as well as tablets • They are good alternative to cream but may take longer initially to improve atrophic vaginitis and its effect on urinary urgency

NOTE: DO NOT administer these oral medications to adults with uncontrolled narrow angled glaucoma, significant bladder outflow obstruction, gastrointestinal obstructive disorders, or renal or hepatic dysfunction.

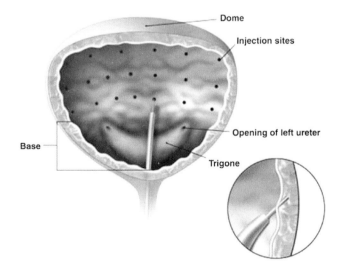

FIGURE 7-5. Example of an Injection Template for Botulinum, with 20 Injections and Sparing of the Trigone and Dome. (From Nitti, V. W. (2006). Botulinum toxin for the treatment of idiopathic and neurogenic overactive bladder: State of the art. *Reviews in Urology, 8*(4), 198–208.)

exact mode of action is still unclear (Leng & Chancellor, 2005). There are two commonly used approaches to neuromodulation that are used when conservative and pharmacological therapies have failed to improve OAB or UUI symptoms.

Percutaneous Tibial Nerve Stimulation

Percutaneous tibial nerve stimulation (PTNS) is a minimally invasive therapy that is delivered in the office setting for 30 minutes. There is a series of 12 treatments, typically once a week. Adverse events are relatively uncommon. It is used in patients for whom behavioral therapy and medication are not helpful or not meeting the patient's goals. PTNS is contraindicated in pregnancy and in patients with a pacemaker or internal defibrillator. Objective improvement is best monitored by having the patient complete a bladder diary prior to treatment, after the 6th treatment and at the conclusion of the 12th treatment. The OAB-q SF is also very helpful. Pharmacotherapy may be used concomitantly with PTNS. The nonimplanted stimulator system includes a

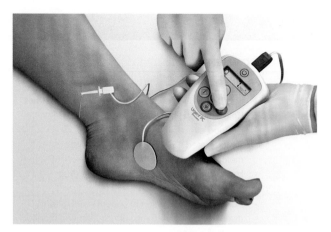

FIGURE 7-6. Percutaneous Tibial Nerve Stimulation (PTNS). (Used with permission from Laborie Medical Technologies. ©Laborie Medical Technologies All rights reserved.)

stimulator and lead set (see **Figure 7-6**). The needle is 34 g, inserted two finger breadths (5 cm) cephalad (toward the individuals head) from the medial malleolus and just posterior to the margin of the tibia at a 60 degrees angle. The grounding electrode pad is placed on the medial surface of the calcaneus. The stimulator is activated until there is a neuro response indicator (i.e., toe flexion or report of tingling sensation) of proper placement. Timer is set for 30 minutes. If PTNS therapy is found therapeutic following the 12-week treatment, ongoing maintenance treatments for continued attainment is individualized but generally monthly to every few months (Yates, 2019).

A blinded trial of PTNS versus sham treatment found that 55% of those treated had moderate or marked improvements in their OAB symptoms, compared to 20% in the sham group (Peters et al., 2010). Peters et al. (2009) compare objective measures of improvement

(UUI, urinary frequency, urge severity, and nocturia) episodes in adults with OAB randomly assigned to PTNS or tolterodine and improvements were similar in both groups. Peters et al. (2013) followed 29 patients completing a 12-week randomized controlled trial comparing PTNS to a shame treatment for OAB. After completing the 12-week trial, participants completed a fixed schedule gradual tapering 3-month protocol and then were assessed and individual treatment plans were implemented based on patient-reported symptoms with the goal of sustaining symptom improvement. Participants were followed for 36 months and most sustained improvement in their OAB symptoms with a median of 1.1 treatments per month.

Sacral Nerve Stimulation

Sacral neuromodulation (SNS) uses an implantable electrode placed in a sacral foramen, commonly S3 (Fig. 7-7). Although effective, with reported success rates of 70% and cure rates of 20% for incontinence and 33% cure for urinary urgency, around 40% of patients will require reintervention, most commonly for lead migration or infection (Peters et al., 2014). Pain at the site can also be an issue and could result in removal of device. It is normal practice to first use a temporary system and, should a bladder diary show benefit (>50% symptom resolution) during a trial period of 4 days to 2 weeks, a permanent device is implanted, usually under the skin of the buttock. The patient is given a programmable external device that can be used to turn the stimulator on or off or change programs. Obviously, the right patient for SNS must be cognitively intact and have the ability to learn how to use the device. Placement of the device is under local anesthesia and with fluoroscopic guidance. MRI is contraindicated with the device in place.

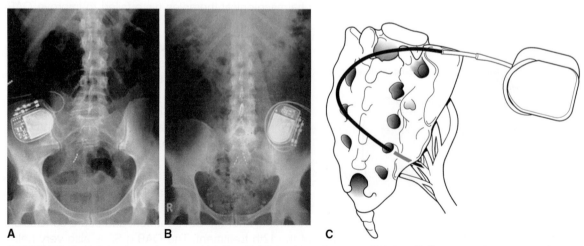

A   B   C

FIGURE 7-7. A. Unilateral sacral neuromodulation. **B.** Bilateral sacral neuromodulation. **C.** Illustration showing sacral neuromodulation. (From Schrier, R. W. (2006). *Diseases of the kidney and urinary tract*. Philadelphia, PA: Lippincott Williams & Wilkins; Keighley, M. R. B., & Williams, N. S. (2008). *Surgery of the anus, rectum, and colon* (3rd ed.). Philadelphia, PA: W.B. Saunders, with permission.)

SURGERY: AUGMENTATION CYSTOPLASTY

When all else has failed, augmentation cystoplasty can be considered (Fig. 7-8). This is a surgical procedure, performed either open or laparoscopically, that uses a length of small intestine to enlarge the bladder and increase bladder capacity. Although effective in reducing OAB symptoms, the procedure carries not only the operative risks but also postprocedure risks of UTI, with rates between 4% and 46% depending on definition and study method. Perforation of the augmented bladder is reported, occurring in between 6% and 9% of cases, and can be fatal (Reyblat & Ginsberg, 2010). Reliance on intermittent self-catheterization is extremely common, with between 26% and 100% of patients needing to self-catheterize; however, reliance on self-catheterization is much less common in patients undergoing augmentation cystoplasty for idiopathic OAB as compared to those with neurogenic bladder or postradiotherapy cystitis (Veeratterapillay et al., 2013). An inability to self-catheterize is a contraindication to cystoplasty.

CONCLUSION

OAB is a common and potentially debilitating condition, which is underreported and undertreated. It can usually be diagnosed on the basis of a detailed history and examination, without the need for invasive testing. Behavioral and lifestyle interventions are the most appropriate first-line therapy for many patients with OAB. For patients who are not candidates for behavioral interventions or who do not have an acceptable reduction in OAB symptoms, pharmacotherapy should be considered. The recent development of newer pharmaceutical treatments has improved the options for patients. Pharmacotherapy is not appropriate for some patients with OAB, some patients will either find side effects too bothersome to continue treatment, and some who tolerate the medications will not achieve an acceptable reduction in their OAB symptoms. For these patients, there are other treatment options including onabotulinumtoxinA and neuromodulation. The continence nurse needs to

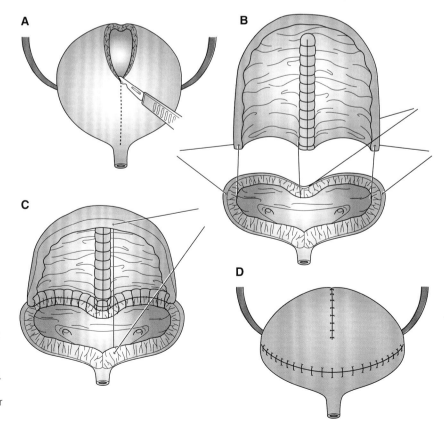

FIGURE 7-8. Bladder Augmentation with an Intestinal Segment. **A.** The bladder is opened as a "clam shell." **B.** The intestinal segment is detubularized by longitudinal incision along the antimesenteric border. A cup-patch is fashioned by suturing one edge of the resultant rectangle to itself. **C.** The cup-patch is sutured to the remnant bladder plate. **D.** Final appearance. (From Sheldon, C. A., & Bukowski, T. (1995). Bladder function. In M. I. Rowe, J. A. O'Neal, J. L. Grosfeld, et al. (Eds.), *Essentials of pediatric surgery*. St. Louis, MO: Mosby-Year Book, with permission.)

BOX 7-1   RESOURCES

Patient:
   National Association for Continence: www.nafc.org
   National Kidney and Urologic Diseases Information Clear-inghouse: http://kidneuy.niddk.nih.gov
   Simon Foundation: www.simonfoundation.org
   Patient Pictures: www.PatientPictures.com
   Voices for Pelvic Floor Disorders: www.voicesforpfd.org
Professional:
   Agency for Healthcare Research and Quality: www.effec-tivehealthcare.ahrq.gov
   American Urogynecologic Association: www.augs.org
   American Urological Association: www.auanet.org
   International Continence Society: www.ics.org
   OAB-q short form symptom bother ©Pfizer: www.pfizerpcoa.com/sites/default/files/oabqsf_us_enreview_only.pdf
   Society of Urologic Nurses and Associates: www.SUNA.org

be mindful that OAB is a chronic disease and should be treated as such requires continuous follow-up for treatment success (Yates, 2019).

OPPORTUNITIES FOR CLINICAL PRACTICE

Continence nurse specialists are on the front lines to address this debilitating, embarrassing, life-altering disorder. Lifestyle modifications and effective behavioral interventions provide first-line measures to reduce OAB and UUI that can help individuals regain control and impact their quality of life. Advance practice registered nurse (APRN) continence specialists provide additional skills to assess, evaluate, and manage the patient with OAB including the ability to prescribe pharmacologic and PTNS modalities in individuals unresponsive to first-line interventions. Referrals should be made for any individuals who fail to improve with therapeutic treatment; this act reflects standards of collaboration and enhanced coordination of care that will ultimately improve patient outcomes and QoL. Additional patient and professional resources are listed in **Box 7-1**.

REFERENCES

Abrams, P., Artibani, W., Cardozo, L., et al. (2009). Reviewing the ICS 2002 terminology report: The ongoing debate. *Neurourology and Urodynamics, 28*, 287.

Alling-Møller, L., Lose, G., & Jørgensen, T. (2000). Risk factors for urinary tract symptoms in women 40 to 60 years of age. *Obstetrics and Gynecology, 96*(3), 446–451.

Allison, S. J., & Gibson, W. (2018). Mirabegron alone and in combination in the treatment of overactive bladder: Real-world evidence and experience. *Therapeutic Advances Urology, 10*(12), 411–419. doi: 10.1177/1756287218801282.

American Geriatrics Society 2019 Beers Criteria Update Expert Panel. (2019). American Geriatrics Society 2019 Updated AGS Beers Cri-teria for potentially inappropriate medication use in older adults. *Journal of American Geriatric Society, 67*(4), 674–694.

Andersson, K-E., Cardozo, L., Cruz, F., et al. (2017). Pharmacological treatment of urinary incontinence. In P. Abrams, L. Cardozo, A. Wagg, et al. (Eds.), *Incontinence* (6th ed, pp. 805-857) ICUS-EAU 2017. ISBN: 978-0-9569607-3-3.

Arya, L. A., Myers, D. L., & Jackson, N. D. (2000). Dietary caffeine intake and the risk for detrusor instability: A case–control study. *Obstetrics and Gynecology, 96*, 85–89.

Barentsen, J. A., Visser, E., Hofstetter, H., et al. (2012). Severity, not type, is the main predictor of decreased quality of life in elderly women with urinary incontinence: A population-based study as part of a randomized controlled trial in primary care. *Health Quality Life Out-comes, 10*, 153. doi: 10.1186/1477-7525-10-153.

Bartley, J. M., Blum, E. S., Sirls, L. T., et al. (2013). Understanding clinic options for overactive bladder. *Current Urology Report, 14*(6), 541–548. doi: 10.1007/s11934-013-0353-6.

Bates-Jensen, B. M., Alessi, C. A., Al-Samarrai, N. R., et al. (2003). The effects of an exercise and incontinence intervention on skin health outcomes in nursing home residents. *Journal of the American Geri-atric Society, 51*, 348–355.

Beckel, J. M., & Birder, L. A. (2012). Differential expression and function of nicotinic acetylcholine receptors in the urinary bladder epithe-lium of the rat. *Journal of Physiology, 590*, 1465–1480.

Bettez, M., Tu, L. M., Carlson, K., et al. (2012). 2012 update: Guidelines for adult urinary incontinence collaborative consensus document for the Canadian Urological Association. *Canadian Urological Association Journal, 6*, 354–363.

Bing, M. H., Møller, L. A., Jennum, P., et al. (2006). Prevalence and bother of nocturia and causes of sleep interruption in a Danish pop-ulation of men and women aged 60–80 years. *BJU International, 98*, 599–604.

Birder, L., & Andersson, K. E. (2013). Urothelial signaling. *Physiological Reviews, 93*, 653–680.

Birder, L. A., Wolf-Johnston, A. S., Sun, Y., et al. (2013). Alteration in TRPV1 and Muscarinic (M3) receptor expression and function in idiopathic overactive bladder urothelial cells. *Acta Physiologica (Oxford, England), 207*, 123–129.

Booth, J., Kumlien, S., & Zang, Y. (2009). Promoting urinary continence with older people: Key issues for nurses. *International Journal of Older People Nursing, 4*, 63–69.

Brading, A. F., & Turner, W. H. (1994). The unstable bladder: Towards a common mechanism. *British Journal of Urology, 73*, 3–8.

Bright, E., Cotterill, N., Drake, M., et al. (2012). Developing a validated urinary diary phase 1. *Neurourology and Urodynamics, 31*(5), 625–633.

Bryant, C. M., Dowell, C. J., & Fairbrother, G. (2002). Caffeine reduction education to improve urinary symptoms. *British Journal of Nursing, 11*, 560–565.

Bschleipfer, T., Schukowski, K., Weidner, W., et al. (2007). Expression and distribution of cholinergic receptors in the human urothelium. *Life Sciences, 80*, 2303–2307.

Burgio, K. L., Locher, J. L., Goode, P. S., et al. (1998). Behavioral vs drug treatment for urge urinary incontinence in older women: A randomized controlled trial. *JAMA, 280*(23), 1995–2000. doi: 10.1001/jama.280.23.1995.

Buser, N., Ivic, S., Kessler, T. M., et al. (2012). Efficacy and adverse events of antimuscarinics for treating overactive bladder: Network meta-analyses. *European Urology, 62*, 1040–1060.

Cartwright, R., Srikrishna, S., Cardozo, L., et al. (2007). Does Diet Coke cause overactive bladder? A 4-way crossover trial, investigating the effect of carbonated soft drinks on overactive bladder symptoms in normal volunteers. Annual Meeting of the International Continence Society (Abstract 19), Rotterdam. Retrieved from http://www.ics.org/Abstracts/Publish/45/000019.pdf

Chacko, S., Cortes, E., Drake, M. J., et al. (2014). Does altered myogenic activity contribute to OAB symptoms from detrusor overactivity? ICI-RS 2013. *Neurourology and Urodynamics, 33*, 577–580.

Chancellor, M., Migliaccio-Walle, K., Bramley, T., et al. (2013). Long-term patterns of use and treatment failure with anticholinergic agents for overactive bladder. *Clinical Therapeutics, 35*(11), 1744–1751.

Chapple, C., Sievert, K. D., MacDiarmid, S., et al. (2013). Onabotulinum-toxinA 100 U significantly improves all idiopathic overactive bladder and urinary incontinence: A randomized, double-blind, placebo-controlled trial. *European Urology, 64*(2), 249–256.

Cody, J. D. (2012). Oestrogen therapy for urinary incontinence in post-menopausal women. *The Cochrane Database of Systematic Review, 4*, CD001405. doi: 10.1002/14651858.CD001405.pub3.

Coolsaet, B. (1985). Bladder compliance and detrusor activity during the collection phase. *Neurourology and Urodynamics, 4*, 263–273.

Coyne, K. S., Payne, C., Bhattacharyya, S. K., et al. (2004). The impact of urinary urgency and frequency on health-related quality of life in overactive bladder: Results from a national community survey. *Value in Health, 7*, 455–463.

Coyne, K. S., Sexton, C. C., Thompson, C. L., et al. (2009). The prevalence of lower urinary tract symptoms (LUTS) in the USA, the UK and Sweden: Results from the Epidemiology of LUTS (EpiLUTS) study. *BJU International, 104*, 352–360.

Coyne, K. S., Thompson, C. L., Lai, J. S., et al. (2015). An overactive bladder symptom and health-related quality of life short-form: Validation of the OAB-q SF. *Neurourology and Urodynamics, 34*, 255–263.

Coyne, K., Wein, A., Nicholson, S., et al. (2014). Economic burden of urgency urinary incontinence in the United States: A systematic review. *Journal of Managed Care Pharmacy, 20*(2), 130–140.

Dallosso, H. M., McGrother, C. W., Matthews, R. J., et al.; Leicestershire MRC Incontinence Study Group. (2003). The association of diet and other lifestyle factors with overactive bladder and stress incontinence: A longitudinal study in women. *BJU International, 92*, 69–77.

Dingwall, L. (2008). Promoting effective continence care for older people: A literature review. *British Journal of Nursing, 17*, 166–172.

Diokno, A. C., Brock, B. M., Herzog, A. R., et al. (1990). Medical correlates of urinary incontinence in the elderly. *Urology, 36*(2), 129–138.

Dowd, T. T., Campbell, J. M., & Jones, J. A. (1996). Fluid intake and urinary incontinence in older community-dwelling women. *Journal of Community Health Nursing, 13*, 179–186.

Drake, M. J. (2018). Fundamentals of terminology in lower urinary tract function. *Neurourology and Urodynamics, 37*, S13–S19. doi: 10.1002/nau.23768.

Elstad, E. A., Taubenberger, S. P., Botelho, E. M., et al. (2010). Beyond incontinence: The stigma of other urinary symptoms. *Journal of Advanced Nursing, 66*, 2460–2470.

Finkelstein, K., Glosner, S., Sanchez, R. J., et al. (2008). Prevalence of probable overactive bladder in a private obstetrics and gynecology group practice. *Current Medical Research and Opinion, 24*, 1083–1090.

Fitzgerald, M. P., Thom, D. H., Wassel-Fyr, C., et al.; Reproductive Risks for Incontinence Study At Kaiser Research, Group. (2006). Childhood urinary symptoms predict adult overactive bladder symptoms. *Journal of Urology, 175*, 989–993.

Fowler, C. J., Griffiths, D., & de Groat, W. C. (2008). The neural control of micturition. *Nature Reviews Neuroscience, 9*, 453–466.

Gibson, W., Athanasopoulos, A., Goldman, H. B., et al. (2014). Are we short-changing the elderly when it comes to the pharmacological treatment of urgency urinary incontinence? *International Journal of Clinical Practice, 68*(9), 1165–1173. doi: 10.1111/ijcp.12447.

Gleason, J. L., Richter, H. E., Redden, D. T., et al. (2013). Caffeine and urinary incontinence in US women. *International Urogynecology Journal, 13*(24), 295–302.

Gormley, E. A., Lightner, D. J., Burgio, K. L., et al. (2019). *Diagnosis and treatment of non-neurogenic overactive bladder (OAB) in adults: An AUA/SUFU guideline*. Amended 2014, 2019 Endorsed by the American Urogynecologic Society (AUGS). Retrieved from https://www.auanet.org/guidelines/overactive-bladder-(oab)-guideline

Griffiths, D., Clarkson, B., Tadic, S., et al. (2015). Brain mechanisms underlying urge incontinence and its response to pelvic floor muscle training. *Journal of Urology, 194*(3), 708–715.

Griffiths, D. J., McCracken, P. N., Harrison, G. M., et al. (1993). Relationship of fluid intake to voluntary micturition and urinary incontinence in geriatric patients. *Neurourology and Urodynamics, 12*, 1–7.

Griffiths, D. J., Tadic, S. D., Schaefer, W., et al. (2009). Cerebral control of the lower urinary tract: How age-related changes might predispose to urge incontinence. *Neurology Image, 47*, 981–986.

Hagovska, M., Svihra, J., Bukova, A., et al. (2020). Effect of an exercise program for reducing abdominal fat on overactive bladder symptoms in young overweight women. *International Urogynecology Journal, 31*, 895–902. doi: 1007/s00192-019-04157-8.

Hannestad, Y. S., Rortveit, G., Sandvik, H., et al. (2000). A community-based epidemiological survey of female urinary incontinence: The Norwegian EPINCONT study. Epidemiology of Incontinence in the County of Nord-Trondelag. *Journal of Clinical Epidemiology, 53*, 1150–1157.

Hashim, H., & Abrams, P. (2006). Is the bladder a reliable witness for predicting detrusor overactivity? *Journal of Urology, 175*, 191–194; discussion 194–195.

Haylen, B. T., De Ridder, D., Freeman, R. M., et al.; International Continence Society. (2010). An International Urogynecological Association (IUGA)/International Continence Society (ICS) joint report on the terminology for female pelvic floor dysfunction. *Neurourology and Urodynamics, 29*, 4–20.

Hsu, F. C., Weeks, C. E., Selph, S. S., et al. (2019). Updating the evidence on drugs to treat overactive bladder: A systematic review. *International Urogynecology Journal*, (10), 1603–1617. doi: 10.1007/s00192-019-04022-8.

Irwin, D. E., Milsom, I., Chancellor, M. B., et al. (2010). Dynamic progression of overactive bladder and urinary incontinence symptoms: A systematic review. *European Urology, 58*, 532–543.

Irwin, D. E., Milsom, I., Hunskaar, S., et al. (2006). Population-based survey of urinary incontinence, overactive bladder, and other lower urinary tract symptoms in five countries: Results of the EPIC study. *European Urology, 50*, 1306–1314; discussion 1314–1315.

Irwin, D. E., Milsom, I., Kopp, Z., et al. (2008). Symptom bother and health care-seeking behavior among individuals with overactive bladder. *European Urology, 53*, 1029–1037.

Jirovec, M. M. (1991). The impact of daily exercise on the mobility, balance, and urine control of cognitively impaired nursing home residents. *International Journal of Nursing Studies, 28*, 145–151.

Johannesson, M., O'Conor, R. M., Kobelt-Nguyen, G., et al. (1997). Willingness to pay for reduced incontinence symptoms. British Journal of Urology, *80*, 557–562.

Kay, G. G., Abou-Donia, M. B., Messer, W. S., Jr, et al. (2005). Antimuscarinic drugs for overactive bladder and their potential effects on cognitive function in older patients. *Journal of the American Geriatrics Society, 53*(12), 2195–2201.

Kuchel, G. A., Moscufo, N., Guttmann, C. R., et al. (2009). Localization of brain white matter hyperintensities and urinary incontinence in community-dwelling older adults. *The Journals of Gerontology Series A: Biological Sciences and Medical Sciences, 64*, 902–909.

Kuo, Y. C., & Kuo, H. C. (2013). Botulinum toxin injection for lower urinary tract dysfunction. *International Journal of Urology, 20*, 40–55.

Lamin, E., Parrillo, L. M., Newman, D. K., et al. (2016). Pelvic floor muscle training: Underutilization in the USA. *Current Urology Reports, 17*(2), 10. doi: 10.1007/s11934-015-0572-0.

Lei, D., Ma, J., Shen, X., et al. (2012). Changes in the brain microstructure of children with primary monosymptomatic nocturnal enuresis: A diffusion tensor imaging study. *PLoS One, 7*, e31023. doi: 10.1371/journal.pone.0031023.

Leng, W. W., & Chancellor, M. B. (2005). How sacral nerve stimulation neuromodulation works. *Urologic Clinics of North America, 32*, 11–18.

Levy, G., & Lowenstein, L. (2020). Overactive bladder syndrome treatments and their effect on female sexual function: A review. *Sexual Medicine, 8*(1), 1–7. doi: 10.1016/j.esxm.2019.08.013.

Liang, C. C., Chang, S. D., Lin, S. J., et al. (2012). Lower urinary tract symptoms in primiparous women before and during pregnancy. *Archives of Gynecology and Obstetrics, 285*, 1205–1210.

Liao, C. H., & Kuo, H. C. (2013). Increased risk of large post-void residual urine and decreased long-term success rate after intravesical onabotulinumtoxinA injection for refractory idiopathic detrusor overactivity. *Journal of Urology, 189*, 1804–1810.

Liberman, J. N., Hunt, T. L., Stewart, W. F., et al. (2001). Health-related quality of life among adults with symptoms of overactive bladder: Results from a U.S. community-based survey. *Urology, 57*, 1044–1050.

Malmsten, U. G., Molander, U., Peeker, R., et al. (2010). Urinary incontinence, overactive bladder, and other lower urinary tract symptoms: A longitudinal population-based survey in men aged 45–103 years. *European Urology, 58(1)*, 149–156.

Mansfield, K. J., Liu, L., Mitchelson, F. J., et al. (2005). Muscarinic receptor subtypes in human bladder detrusor and mucosa, studied by radioligand binding and quantitative competitive RT-PCR: Changes in ageing. *British Journal of Pharmacology, 144*, 1089–1099.

Maserejian, N. N., Kupelian, V., Miyasato, G., et al. (2012). Are physical activity, smoking and alcohol consumption associated with lower urinary tract symptoms in men or women? Results from a population based observational study. *Journal of Urology, 188*, 490–495.

McGrother, C. W., Donaldson, M. M., Thompson, J., et al. (2012). Etiology of overactive bladder: A diet and lifestyle model for diabetes and obesity in older women. *Neurourology and Urodynamics, 31*, 487–495.

Mills, I. W., Greenland, J. E., Mcmurray, G., et al. (2000). Studies of the pathophysiology of idiopathic detrusor instability: The physiological properties of the detrusor smooth muscle and its pattern of innervation. *Journal of Urology, 163*, 646–651.

Milsom, I., Altman, D., Cartwright, R., et al. (2017). Epidemiology of urinary incontinence (UI) and other lower urinary tract symptoms (LUTS), pelvic organ prolapse (POP) and anal (AI) incontinence. In P. Abrams, L. Cardozo, A. Wagg, et al. (Eds.), *Incontinence* (6th ed.). Volumes 1 & 2. ICS/ICUD. ISBN: 978-0-9569607-3-3.

Moore, K. N., Dumoulin, C., Bradley, C., et al. (2013). Adult conservative management. In P. Abrams, L. Cardozo, S. Khoury, et al. (Eds.), *Incontinence* (5th ed., pp. 1101–1227). Arnhem, The Netherlands: European Association of Urology.

National Institute for Health and Care Excellence (NICE). (2010). *CG97 Lower urinary tract symptoms: The management of lower urinary tract symptoms in men* [Online]. Retrieved from www.nice.org.uk/guidance/cg97/chapter/introduction

National Institute for Health and Care Excellence (NICE). (2013). *CG171 Urinary incontinence in women* [Online]. Retrieved from http://guidance.nice.org.uk/CG171/NICEGuidance/pdf/English

Nitti, V. W., Dmochowski, R., Herschorn, S., et al. (2017). EMBARK Study Group. OnabotulinumtoxinA for the treatment of patients with overactive bladder and urinary incontinence: Results of a phase 3, randomized, placebo-controlled trial. *Journal of Urology, 197*, S216–S223. doi: 10.1016/j.juro.2016.10.109.

Ouslander, J. G., Griffiths, P., McConnell, E., et al. (2005). Functional Incidental Training: Applicability and feasibility in the Veterans Affairs nursing home patient population. *Journal of the American Medical Directors Association, 6*, 121–127.

Papanicolaou, S., Pons, M. E., Hampel, C., et al. (2005). Medical resource utilization and cost of care for women seeking treatment for urinary incontinence in an outpatient setting. Examples from three countries participating in the PURE study. *Maturitas, 52*(Suppl 2), S35–S47.

Parker, W. P., & Griebling, T. L. (2015). Nonsurgical treatment of urinary incontinence in elderly women. *Clinical Geriatric Medicine, 31*(4), 471–485.

Peters, K. M., Carrico, D. J., Perez-Marrero, R. A., et al. (2010). Randomized trial of percutaneous tibial nerve stimulation versus sham efficacy in the treatment of overactive bladder syndrome: Results from the SUmiT trial. *Journal of Urology, 183*, 1438–1443.

Peters, K. M., Carrico, D. J., Wooldridge, L. S., et al. (2013). Percutaneous tibial nerve stimulation for the long-term treatment of overactive bladder: Three-year results of the STEP study. *Journal of Urology, 189*, 2194–2201.

Peters, K. M., Macdiarmid, S. A., Wooldridge, L. S., et al. (2009). Randomized trial of percutaneous tibial nerve stimulation versus extended-release tolterodine: Results from the overactive bladder innovative therapy trial. *Journal of Urology, 182*(3), 1055–1061.

Peters, K., Sahai, A., De Ridder, D., et al. (2014). Long-term follow-up of sacral neuromodulation for lower urinary tract dysfunction. *BJU International, 113*, 789–794.

Ponholzer, A., Temml, C., Wehrberger, C., et al. (2006). The association between vascular risk factors and lower urinary tract symptoms in both sexes. *European Urology, 50*, 581–586.

Popescu, B. O., Toescu, E. C., Popescu, L. M., et al. (2009). Blood–brain barrier alterations in ageing and dementia. *Journal of the Neurological Sciences, 283*, 99–106.

Proft, T. (2009). *Microbial toxins: Current research and future trends.* Norfolk, UK: Caister Academic Press.

Rapp, D. E., Lyon, M. B., Bales, G. T., et al. (2005). A role for the P2X receptor in urinary tract physiology and in the pathophysiology of urinary dysfunction. *European Urology, 48*, 303–308.

Reyblat, P., & Ginsberg, D. A. (2010). Augmentation enterocystoplasty in overactive bladder: Is there still a role? *Current Urology Reports, 11*, 432–439.

Robinson, D., Cardozo, L., Milsom, I., et al. (2014). Oestrogens and overactive bladder. *Neurourology and Urodynamics, 33*(7), 1086–1091. doi: 10.1002/nau.22464.

Roe, B., Ostaszkiewicz, J., Milne, J., et al. (2007). Systematic reviews of bladder training and voiding programmes in adults: A synopsis of findings from data analysis and outcomes using metastudy techniques. *Journal of Advanced Nursing, 57*, 15–31.

Sacco, E., Bientinesi, R., Tienforti, D., et al. (2014). Discovery history and clinical development of mirabegron for the treatment of overactive bladder and urinary incontinence. *Expert Opinion on Drug Discovery, 9,* 433–448.

Schnelle, J. F., Macrae, P. G., Ouslander, J. G., et al. (1995). Functional Incidental Training, mobility performance, and incontinence care with nursing home residents. *Journal of the American Geriatric Society, 43*, 1356–1362.

Shaw, C. (2001). A review of the psychosocial predictors of help-seeking behaviour and impact on quality of life in people with urinary incontinence. *Journal of Clinical Nursing, 10*, 15–24.

Shaw, C., Tansey, R., Jackson, C., et al. (2001). Barriers to help seeking in people with urinary symptoms. *Family Practice, 18*, 48–52.

Siroky, M. B. (2004). The aging bladder. *Reviews in Urology, 6*(Suppl 1), S3–S7.

Spence-Jones C., Kamm M. A., Henry M. M., et al. (1994). Bowel dysfunction: A pathogenic factor in ureterovaginal prolapse and urinary stress incontinence. *British Journal of Obstetrics and Gynecology, 101*(2), 147–152.

Stewart, W. F., Van Rooyen, J. B., Cundiff, G. W., et al. (2003). Prevalence and burden of overactive bladder in the United States. *World Journal of Urology, 20*, 327–336.

Su, X., Stein, R., Stanton, M. C., et al. (2003). Effect of partial outlet obstruction on rabbit urinary bladder smooth muscle function. *American Journal of Physiology. Renal Physiology, 284*, F644–F652.

Subak, L. L., Brown, J. S., Kraus, S. R., et al.; Diagnostic Aspects of Incontinence Study Group. (2006). The "costs" of urinary incontinence for women. *Obstetrics and Gynecology, 107*, 908–916.

Subak, L. L., Wing, R., West, D. S., et al. (2009). Weight loss to treat urinary incontinence in overweight an obese women. *New England Journal of Medicine, 360*, 481–490.

Sugaya, K., Nishijima, S., Owan, T., et al. (2007). Effects of walking exercise on nocturia in the elderly. *Biomedical Research, 28*, 101–105.

Sui, G., Fry, C. H., Malone-Lee, J., et al. (2009). Aberrant Ca^{2+} oscillations in smooth muscle cells from overactive human bladders. *Cell Calcium, 45*, 456–464.

Tadic, S., Griffiths, D., Murrin, A., et al. (2010). Structural damage of brain's white matter affects brain-bladder control in older women with urgency incontinence. Joint Annual Meeting of the International Continence Society, ICS and International Urogynecological Association, IUGA Toronto, ON Canada, 29, 1109–1110. Retrieved from http://www.ics.org/Abstracts/Publish/105/000211.pdf

Tahtinen, R. M., Auvinen, A., Cartwright, R., et al. (2011). Smoking and bladder symptoms in women. *Obstetrics and Gynecology, 118,* 643–648.

Thuroff, J. W., Abrams, P., Andersson, K. E., et al. (2011). EAU guidelines on urinary incontinence. *European Urology, 59,* 387–400.

Townsend, M. K., Jura, Y. H., Curhan, G. C., et al. (2011). Fluid intake and risk of stress, urgency, and mixed urinary incontinence. *American Journal of Obstetrics and Gynecology, 205*(73), e1–e6.

Turner, D. A., Shaw, C., McGrother, C. W., et al. (2004). The cost of clinically significant urinary storage symptoms for community dwelling adults in the UK. *BJU International, 93,* 1246–1252.

Tyagi, V., Philips, B. J., Su, R., et al. (2009). Differential expression of functional cannabinoid receptors in human bladder detrusor and urothelium. *Journal of Urology, 181,* 1932–1938.

Veerattterapillay, R., Thorpe, A. C., & Harding, C. (2013). Augmentation cystoplasty: Contemporary indications, techniques and complications. *Indian Journal of Urology, 29,* 322–327.

Vinsnes, A. G., Harkless, G. E., & Nyronning, S. (2007). Unit-based intervention to improve urinary incontinence in frail elderly. *Nordic Journal of Nursing Research & Clinical Studies, 27,* 53.

Wagg, A. (2012). The cognitive burden of anticholinergics in the elderly—implications for the treatment of overactive bladder. *European Urological Reviews, 7*(1), 42–49.

Wagg, A., Cardozo, L., Nitti, V. W., et al. (2014a). The efficacy and tolerability of the beta3-adrenoceptor agonist mirabegron for the treatment of symptoms of overactive bladder in older patients. *Age and Ageing, 43*(5), 666–675. doi: 10.1093/ageing/afu017.

Wagg, A., Compion, G., Fahey, A., et al. (2012). Persistence with prescribed antimuscarinic therapy for overactive bladder: A UK experience. *BJU International, 110,* 1767–1774.

Wagg, A., Gibson, W., Johnson, T, III., et al. (2014b). Urinary incontinence in frail elderly persons: Report from the 5th International Consultation on Incontinence. *Neurourology and Urodynamics, 34*(5), 398–406.

Wells, M. J., Jamieson, K., Markham, T. C. W., et al. (2014). The effect of caffeinated versus decaffeinated drinks on overactive bladder: A double-blind, randomized, crossover study. *Journal of Wound, Ostomy, and Continence Nursing, 41*(4), 371–378. doi: 10.1097/WON.0000000000000040.

Wennberg, A. L., Altman, D., Lundholm, C., et al. (2011). Genetic influences are important for most but not all lower urinary tract symptoms: A population-based survey in a cohort of adult Swedish twins. *European Urology, 59,* 1032–1038.

Wright, J., Mccormack, B., Coffey, A., et al. (2007). Evaluating the context within which continence care is provided in rehabilitation units for older people. *International Journal of Older People Nursing, 2,* 9–19.

Wyman, J. F., Burgio, K. L., & Newman, D. K. (2009). Practical aspects of lifestyle modifications and behavioral interventions in the treatment of overactive bladder and urgency urinary incontinence. *International Journal of Clinical Practice, 63*(8), 1177–1191. doi: 10.1111/j.1742-1241.2009.02078x.

Yates, N. L. (2019). Moving evidence into practice for an overactive bladder program: A literature review. *Urologic Nursing, 39*(4), 163–183. doi: 10.7257/1053-816X.2019.39.4.163.

Yeaw, J., Benner, J. S., Walt, J. G., et al. (2009). Comparing adherence and persistence across 6 chronic medication classes. *Journal of Managed Care Pharmacy, 15*(9), 728–740.

Yoshida, M., Miyamae, K., Iwashita, H., et al. (2004). Management of detrusor dysfunction in the elderly: Changes in acetylcholine and adenosine triphosphate release during aging. *Urology, 63,* 17–23.

Zhang, E. Y., Stein, R., Chang, S., et al. (2004). Smooth muscle hypertrophy following partial bladder outlet obstruction is associated with overexpression of non-muscle caldesmon. *American Journal of Pathology, 164,* 601–612.

Zimmern, P., Litman, H. J., Mueller, E., et al. (2010). Effect of fluid management on fluid intake and urge incontinence in a trial for overactive bladder in women. *BJU International, 105,* 1680–1685.

QUESTIONS

1. When determining a plan of care for the patient with OAB, what sequence of interventions is most appropriate?
   A. Drugs, pelvic floor therapy, PTNS
   B. Pelvic floor therapy, drugs, BOTOX®
   C. Fluid management, SNS, drugs
   D. PTNS, behavioral management, medications

2. The continence nurse is planning on starting the patient on anticholinergic medication due to residual symptoms following conservative measures were implemented. Which of the following should be taken into consideration first?
   A. Constipation
   B. Presence of diabetes
   C. Diagnosis of narrow angled glaucoma
   D. High blood pressure

3. Combination drug therapy should be considered if
   A. The patient failed behavioral interventions
   B. After pelvic floor therapy, the patient is voiding six times per day and up once at night
   C. The patient has no complaints of constipation
   D. The patient is voiding ten times per day despite fluid management, a toileting program and solifenacin

4. The continence nurse is teaching a patient about proven risk factors that may double the risk for developing overactive bladder. One of these factors is:
   A. High caffeine intake
   B. High physical activity level
   C. Diet high in protein/low in carbohydrates
   D. Obesity or diabetes

5. For which patient with urinary urgency would the continence nurse include a recommendation for urodynamic testing to be performed to diagnose overactive bladder?
A. A patient with a history of childhood enuresis
B. A patient who is a poor historian and cannot verbalize her symptoms, but leaks "a lot"
C. A patient who has frequency and nocturia in addition to urgency
D. A patient who is a smoker

6. When you get a strong urge to void, what is the *first* thing you should do when practicing urge suppression techniques
A. Quick Kegels
B. Find a hard surface
C. Rush to the bathroom
D. Stop what you are doing

7. The continence nurse is caring for frail older people who have urinary incontinence. Which behavioral intervention is a mainstay of UI treatment in this population?
A. Prompted voiding
B. Pelvic floor rehabilitation
C. Double voiding
D. Use of absorptive products

8. The continence nurse is explaining the technique of functional intervention training to a nursing home resident who is experiencing urinary incontinence. Which element combined with toileting routines comprises this method?
A. Pharmacological treatment
B. Restricted fluid intake
C. Pelvic floor muscle rehabilitation
D. Musculoskeletal strengthening exercises

9. For which patient would a continence nurse recommend the use of a topical estrogen for overactive bladder?
A. A 78-year-old male with prostate cancer
B. A 38-year-old pregnant woman
C. A postmenopausal woman
D. A 45-year-old female with diabetes

10. Which of the following has been shown to provide positive outcomes for many patients with OAB who "fail" pharmacologic therapy?
A. Surgical denervation of the bladder
B. Indwelling catheter
C. Neuromodulation
D. Urodynamics

ANSWERS AND RATIONALES

1. B. Rationale: Conservative treatment (lifestyle modification, behavioral therapies) is considered to be first-line, pharmacological therapies as an adjunct to conservative therapy, thus are considered second-line interventions; Botox, neuromodulation, and bladder augmentation are modalities reserved for patients who failed to respond to first and second-line interventions.

2. C. Rationale: The use of anticholinergic is contraindicated in narrow angle glaucoma because it will increase pressures in the eye.

3. D. Rationale: Some individuals who have refractory OAB (failed conservative measures and single drug treatment), benefit from dual medications that reduces cholinergic activation (induces relaxation of bladder) and stimulates β-adrenergic receptors to relax the bladder such as seen with combination use of solifenacin (anticholinergic) and mirabegron (β$_3$-adrenergic agonist).

4. D. Rationale: In a study tracking incidence of OAB over a period of 3 years, low physical exercise levels and a high-carbohydrate diet, in conjunction with obesity and diabetes, were associated with doubling of the risk for developing OAB.

5. B. Rationale: Urodynamic testing is not usually indicated for individuals with OAB, unless there is an associated neurologic condition, history of prior surgery for UI, unclear diagnosis, or failure to respond to treatment.

6. D. Rationale: Proper sequence in performing urgency suppression is 1. Stop, stay still, sit down if possible, 2. Squeezed PFM quickly 3-5 times, 3. Relax, take a deep breath, 4. Distract yourself to get your mind off the urge, 5. Wait till urge subsides, then walk slowly to BR; if the urge resurges, repeat the sequence.

7. A. Rationale: Toileting programs have been designed for frail older people with cognitive and physical impairments. Prompted voiding has the most evidence for its use. Individuals are prompted to use the toilet and encouraged with social reward when successfully toileted. This technique increases patient requests for toileting and self-initiated toileting and decreases the number of UI episodes.

8. D. Rationale: Functional intervention training incorporates musculoskeletal strengthening exercises into toileting routines by nursing home care aides or nursing assistants.

9. C. Rationale: The application of topical estrogens, in the form of cream, a ring, or vaginal suppository, is commonly used in the treatment of OAB in postmenopausal women to reduce urgency, frequency, and dysuria.

10. C. Rationale: Neuromodulation has been shown to be effective in management of OAB refractory to other therapies; options include "percutaneous tibial nerve stimulation" and "sacral nerve stimulation."

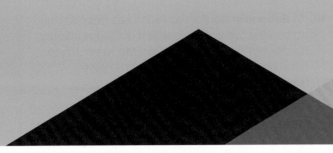

CHAPTER 8

RETENTION OF URINE

Phyllis Sheldon and Margaret Mary Santos

OBJECTIVES

1. Discuss the pathophysiology and classification of urinary retention (UR) and potential impact on upper urinary tract function.

2. Explain distinguishing factors between retention caused by impaired detrusor contractility and retention caused by outlet obstruction and the implications for treatment.

3. Evaluate the patient with suspected UR.

4. Describe common treatments available for specific presentations of UR.

5. Understand the continence nurse's role in patient education for each of the following: alpha-adrenergic antagonists; double voiding/scheduled voiding; clean intermittent catheterization; and indwelling catheter.

TOPIC OUTLINE

INTRODUCTION

An overview of voiding dysfunction was discussed in Chapter 3. The term voiding dysfunction is a broad term that denotes problems emptying the bladder effectively. There are different manifestations of voiding dysfunction and difficulty with emptying frequently results in acute or chronic urinary retention (CUR). This chapter will focus on the prevalence, incidence, pathophysiology, presentation, and management of urinary retention.

Retention of urine implies the inability to empty the bladder to completion (Kaplan et al., 2008). It is often stressful for patients and may have significant implications for their health. In many cases, retention merits immediate catheterization of the bladder to alleviate the patient's distress. Prompt recognition and effective management are essential, as inadequate management may lead to further morbidity and even mortality.

DEFINITION

Acute urinary retention (AUR) is defined by the International Continence Society (ICS) as a painful, palpable, or percussable bladder, when the patient is unable to pass any urine (Abrams et al., 2003). The retained volume of urine is usually significantly greater than normal bladder capacity. While this is the classic presentation, the clinician should be aware that bladder pain is not always a presenting complaint and that the bladder is not always palpable or percussable. For example, pain may not be a presenting feature in retention following regional anesthesia such as an epidural anesthetic or during the immediate postoperative period following abdominal surgery, the bladder may not be painful, palpable, or percussable, due to anterior abdominal wall pain or dressings in the lower abdomen.

CUR is characterized by a nonpainful bladder that remains palpable or percussable after the patient has passed urine. Such patients may also be incontinent of urine. The ICS no longer recommends the term "overflow incontinence" although this is still commonly used in clinical practice. The recommended term, retention with overflow is found in the ICS glossary 2019. CUR is defined as non-neurogenic urinary retention with a post-void residual (PVR) of more than 300 mL that is persistent for more than 6 months and has been documented on two separate occasions (American Urological Association [AUA], 2016).

Acute-on-chronic retention implies that an individual with a background of CUR presents with an episode of AUR.

KEY POINT

Retention is the inability to empty the bladder to completion; it can be classified as acute, chronic, or acute on chronic.

The International Continence Society (ICS) (2016) defines subcategories of urinary retention based on

- The ability of a patient to release any urine (complete or partial)
- The duration (acute or chronic)
- The symptoms (painful or silent)
- The mechanism (obstructive or nonobstructive)

KEY POINT

Acute urinary retention is the total inability to pass urine, requires immediate intervention, and is usually painful. Chronic retention is inability to empty the bladder completely and develops slowly over time thus minimal discomfort.

 ## EPIDEMIOLOGY AND ETIOLOGY OF URINARY RETENTION

The likelihood of urinary retention (UR) increases in both men and women with age. However, retention is much more common in men than in women. The ratio of UR in men to women is 13:1 (Oelke et al., 2015). The most common cause of UR in men over 60 is progression of benign prostatic hypertrophy (BPH), prostatic enlargement. Other causes of UR in men are urethral strictures, foreign body in the bladder, pelvic trauma, neurologic conditions, medications, and blood clots in the bladder. The most common causes of urinary retention in women are pelvic masses or pelvic prolapse causing urethral compression or following pelvic surgery. A frequent cause of transient retention in both sexes is infection.

ACUTE URINARY RETENTION

AUR refers to the sudden inability to pass any urine. It causes a "painful, palpable, or percussable bladder" (ICS). AUR may be further classified into precipitated or spontaneous retention (Emberton & Fitzpatrick, 2008; Fitzpatrick & Kirby, 2006; Kaplan et al., 2008).

Precipitated AUR

In precipitated AUR, there is typically a definable *triggering event*, such as a surgical or urologic procedure with anesthesia. Triggers also include urinary tract infection (UTI), medications, or neurologic disorder. See **Box 8-1** for triggering events for precipitated AUR. Postoperative UR (POUR) is a common cause of precipitated UR. Medications that are given intraoperatively, pain medication and sedation given postoperatively as well as relative immobility due to type of surgery, vascular access with intravenous therapy or other vascular devices, or even simply the fact that a patient is expected to urinate in a position that is not a natural position for them all can contribute to a patient's inability to void (Simsek & Sureyya, 2016). Patients can and should be assessed preoperatively for known risk factors that may increase the likelihood of POUR. The preoperative assessment information, in collaboration with other team members, may allow for interventions to minimize development of POUR or at the least, recognize the development of POUR more quickly, to minimize the discomfort and distress to the patient (Simsek & Sureyya, 2016). The nurse may be able to employ simple interventions such as providing privacy, running tap water (provides relaxation and masks sound of urination), assisting the patient to a sitting on the side of the bed or commode, or standing (if indicated) to allow the patient a more usual voiding position, may facilitate voiding in some patients (Simsek & Sureyya, 2016).

Spontaneous AUR

When no triggering event is identified, AUR is considered spontaneous. Spontaneous AUR is most commonly associated with prostatic enlargement due to BPH and is indeed considered as a sign of BPH progression (Emberton & Fitzpatrick, 2008; Fitzpatrick & Kirby, 2006; Kaplan et al., 2008). The difference between precipitated and spontaneous retention has treatment implications because BPH-related surgery is less commonly required in cases of precipitated AUR (Emberton & Fitzpatrick, 2008; Kaplan et al., 2008).

KEY POINT

Acute urinary retention can occur spontaneously (usually as a result of BPH) or can be precipitated by anesthesia, medications, UTI, or a neurologic process such as stroke.

Role of Benign Prostatic Hypertrophy

BPH is the most common benign neoplasm in men and a major etiological factor in the occurrence of AUR. Its prevalence increases with age, with approximately 50% of men in their 50s and 90% of men in their 80s showing evidence of the disease (Berry et al., 1984; National Institute of Diabetes and Digestive and Kidney Diseases [NIDDK], Prostate Enlargement, 2014). BPH may be evident clinically as benign prostatic enlargement (BPE). The enlargement in the periurethral and transitional zones of the prostate can lead to compression of the urethra and bladder outflow obstruction (BOO) (see **Fig. 8-1**). This may result in the clinical manifestations of the disease such as lower urinary tract symptoms (LUTS) and AUR. LUTS include frequency, urgency, hesitancy, slowed urinary stream, and postvoid dribble. Nurse practitioners and advanced practice nurses (APN) will undertake a

---

BOX 8-1	**TRIGGERING EVENTS FOR PRECIPITATED ACUTE URINARY RETENTION**

Triggering Events:
- Postoperative state
- Urological procedures (e.g., prostate biopsy)
- General/spinal/epidural/local anesthesia
- UTI
- Immobility
- Constipation
- Neurological disorder (multiple sclerosis, diabetes, stroke, spinal injury)
- Pelvic surgery (injury to bladder innervations)
- Alcohol
- Drugs (amphetamines, antihistamines, anticholinergics, muscle relaxants, NSAIDs, pseudoephedrine, some antipsychotics, some older antidepressants, and some opioid pain medications)

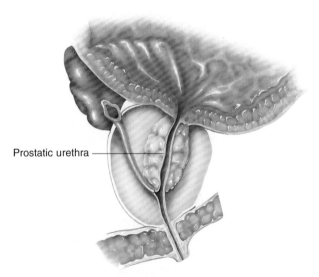

Prostatic urethra

FIGURE 8-1. Early Prostatic Hyperplasia Showing Area of Urethral Obstruction.

CASE STUDY #1 POUR

Mary, the 7 PM medical–surgical nurse, has taken report and makes rounds to check on her patients.

Her patient, Mr. James, is a 78-year-old male, postopen inguinal hernia repair under general anesthesia this morning. He was transferred to the unit at 1 PM and was initially stable. Mental status awake, alert, and cooperative. Saline lock intact in left forearm. Vital signs were stable upon transfer, ice packs were applied to surgical area to minimize swelling and decrease pain. Appetite was good for lunch and is tolerating oral fluids well.

Pain medication, hydromorphone (Dilaudid) was administered at 3:30 PM for complaint of pain level 6/10 in abdomen near surgical site.

Pain reevaluation at 4 PM showed vital signs: BP 130/70, P 84 bpm, R 16, SaO$_2$ 99%, T 98.8 oral. Pain reported 3/10 at surgical site. Dressing dry and intact. Patient noted to have dark purple discoloration of groin, penis, scrotum, and upper thigh and edema of his scrotum. The nurse elevated the scrotum on a rolled washcloth. Ice packs were continued.

When Mary made her rounds, she noted the patient to be restless, agitated, and diaphoretic. His 7:30 PM BP was 170/100, P 100 bpm, R 22, SaO$_2$ 99% on room air, T 99.2 oral.

Patient complains of severe abdominal pain, 10/10. When questioned further, he pointed to the suprapubic area. Suprapubic area noted to be distended, firm, and tender to touch. Surgical dressings were dry and intact.

Mary checks the transfer notes and determines the patient had an indwelling catheter in the recovery room that was discontinued just prior to transfer. Mr. James has no recorded urine output since transfer. Portable ultrasonic bladder scan shows 750 mL urine in the bladder.

Provider notified and an order was obtained for indwelling catheter to be left in place for 24 hours to allow for the swelling to subside. The bladder drained 800 mL urine with relief of pain, and the patient immediately appeared relaxed and was able to rest. Vital signs returned to baseline when rechecked after the bladder was emptied.

Reflection: Mary made the correct assessment of Mr. James in having Mr. James point to the area of pain, then palpating for distention and taking a bladder scan to determine urine volume. Her prompt actions provided relief for the patient.

What could have been done differently?

Patients should be assessed for risks of POUR prior to surgery. Depending on the patient's medical history and home medications, the type of surgery and anesthesia to be administered needs to be considered for potential risk factors. The patient had an "open" procedure as opposed to the laparoscopic procedure so there was more trauma to the area.

The patient had an indwelling catheter in the recovery room that was removed prior to being transferred to inpatient unit.

Postoperatively, postcatheter removal, opportunity to void should be offered to patients on a regular basis (every 2 hours) as well as recording any voids is an important tool to assess voiding status.

---

digital rectal examination (DRE). **Figure 8-2** shows DRE. A lubricated, gloved index finger is inserted to palpate prostate size, shape, sensitivity, and consistency as well as perianal skin integrity, sensation or pain, anal sphincter tone, presence of stool (and consistency), and hemorrhoids or fissures. Any abnormalities are referred to a urologist (see Chapter 4 regarding prostatic examination details).

Data from the placebo arm of the Prostate Long-Term Efficacy and Safety Study (PLESS) demonstrated that the higher the serum PSA levels, larger prostate volume and the more severe symptoms, there is a greater likelihood of AUR (Roehrborn et al., 2001). **Box 8-2** lists risk factors for AUR in men with prostatic obstruction.

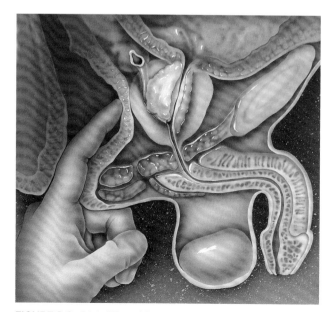

FIGURE 8-2. Digital Rectal Examination for Abnormalities in the Anus, Rectum, and Prostate. (Anatomical Chart Company. Philadelphia, PA: Lippincott Williams & Wilkins, 2000.)

KEY POINT

For the patient with BPH, prostate size/volume, PSA levels, and symptom severity are all predictors for development of AUR.

BPH-RELATED RISK FACTORS ASSOCIATED WITH SPONTANEOUS ACUTE URINARY RETENTION

Prostate volume (>30 to 40 mL)
PSA (>1.4 ng/mL)
Previous episode of AUR
Worsening LUTS (increasing IPPS by ≥4 points)
Lack of response to medical treatment (α-blocker ± 5-ARI)

An individual's response to treatment has recently been identified as a predictor of the risk for BPH disease progression and AUR (Armitage & Emberton, 2005). Response is frequently measured by the International Prostate Symptom Score (IPSS), a validated tool used widely to assess effect of treatment that asks questions regarding LUTS that indicate dysfunction and factors that may affect the patient's quality of life (QOL) (see **Fig. 8-3**). Increased severity of an individual LUTS or the overall LUTS score was associated with increased risk of AUR, independent of baseline severity (Meigs et al., 1999). This observation was supported by data from the Alf-One study, in which a prior episode of AUR was the most important predictor of AUR (Emberton & Fitzpatrick, 2008).

Transient Cause of UR: Infection & Inflammation
UTIs, sexually transmitted infections (STIs) cause swelling of the urethra, which causes inability to pass urine.

	Not at all 0	Less than 1 time in 5 1	Less than half the time 2	About half the time 3	More than half the time 4	Almost always 5
1. INCOMPLETE EMPTYING Over the last month or so, how often have you had a sensation of not emptying your bladder completely after you finished urinating?	0	1	2	3	4	5
2. FREQUENCY During the last month or so, how often have you had to urinate again <2 hours after you finished urinating?	0	1	2	3	4	5
3. INTERMITTENCY During the last month or so, how often have you stopped and started again several times when you urinated?	0	1	2	3	4	5
4. URGENCY During the last month or so, how often have you found it difficult to postpone urination?	0	1	2	3	4	5
5. WEAK STREAM During the last month or so, how often have you had a weak urinary stream?	0	1	2	3	4	5
6. STRAINING During the last month or so, how often have you had to push or strain to begin urination?	0	1	2	3	4	5
7. SLEEPING During the last month, how many times did you most typically get up to urinate from the time you went to bed at night until the time you got up in the morning?	0	1	2 (times at night)	3	4	5

SCORE: (0-35)_____

The International Prostate Symptom Score (IPSS) uses the same 7 questions as the AUA Symptom Index, but adds a "Disease Specific Quality of Life Question" (sometimes referred to as the "bother score") and scored from 0 to 6 points ("delighted" to "terrible").

If you were to spend the rest of your life with your urinary condition just the way it is now, how would you feel about that?

Delighted 0	Pleased 1	Mostly satisfied 2	Mixed 3	Mostly disappointed 4	Unhappy 5	Terrible 6

FIGURE 8-3. International Prostate Symptom Score Is Also Known as the American Urological Association Assessment Tool. It is a validated tool for assessing voiding dysfunction and the effect on quality of life. (Based on American Urological Association. (2003). *Guideline on the management of benign prostatic hyperplasia (BPH)*. Linthicum, MD: American Urological Association Education and Research, Inc., with permission.)

This blockage will resolve as the infection is treated and cleared.

Pathophysiology of AUR

Several mechanisms have been proposed to explain why AUR occurs, although it is still not very clear. Possible mechanisms include sudden increased resistance to flow of urine due to mechanical obstruction (urethral stricture, clot retention), dynamic obstruction (increased α-adrenergic activity, prostatic inflammation), bladder overdistension (immobility, constipation, drugs inhibiting bladder contractility), and/or neuropathic or metabolic conditions causing impaired bladder contractility (e.g., diabetic cystopathy) (Choong & Emberton, 2000; Emberton & Fitzpatrick, 2008; Fitzpatrick & Kirby, 2006; Kaplan et al., 2008).

CHRONIC URINARY RETENTION

CUR is defined as non-neurogenic urinary retention with a PVR of more than 300 mL that is persistent for more than 6 months and has been documented on two separate occasions (AUA, 2016). CUR is more complex and can be classified as either high-pressure chronic retention (HPCR) or low-pressure chronic retention (LPCR); the two are distinguished by the detrusor pressure at the end of micturition (i.e., at the start of the next filling phase) (Abrams et al., 1978; George et al., 1983).

High-Pressure Chronic Retention

BOO is the usual cause for HPCR, so flow rate is generally poor even though detrusor pressure is high. The continually elevated bladder pressure in HPCR, during both the storage and voiding phases of micturition, often results in bilateral hydronephrosis. **Figure 8-4** shows hydronephrosis as a result of chronic prostatic obstruction of the lower urinary tract.

Low-Pressure Chronic Retention

Other patients may have large-volume retention caused by a poorly contractile but very compliant (the bladder has the ability to stretch to accommodate large volumes) bladder that keeps the pressure low. These patients are said to have LPCR and typically exhibit no hydronephrosis or renal failure. Urodynamic studies in these patients show low detrusor pressures, low flow rates, and very large PVR volumes. LUTS can be of mild severity in CUR, at least in the early stages. LPCR can sometimes be discovered during the course of an examination for another complaint, as many patients with the condition have few bothersome symptoms. However, some patients may complain of frequency because their bladder never completely empties. Patients may also suffer from recurrent UTIs owing to stasis of urine in the bladder. Nocturnal enuresis may also be symptomatic presentation and may result from a slight reduction in urethral pressure when asleep.

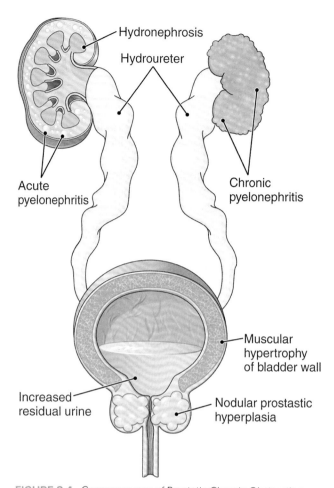

FIGURE 8-4. Consequences of Prostatic Chronic Obstruction of the Lower Urinary Tract. Incomplete emptying of the bladder causes nocturia, urgency, frequency, and loss of control. Ureteral reflux may cause infection and chronic kidney disease. (From McConnell, T. H. (2013). *Nature of disease*. Philadelphia, PA: Lippincott Williams & Wilkins.)

KEY POINT

Chronic urinary retention can be classified as HPCR (high-pressure chronic retention) and LPCR (low-pressure chronic retention); HPCR creates resistance to delivery of urine from the kidneys and can cause eventual hydronephrosis.

LESS COMMON CAUSES OF URINARY RETENTION

There are a number of other processes that can cause urinary retention, though they are relatively uncommon including cancer, pelvic masses or prolapse, bladder neck dyssynergia, detrusor underactivity, and paruresis.

Cancer

Malignancies of the urinary tract can cause urinary obstruction, but the process is more gradual and generally indicates a more advanced stage of malignancy. Cancer of the ureters, bladder, prostate, penis, or urethra can gradually obstruct urine output. Cancers often present with hematuria, weight loss, and lower back and/or groin pain.

Retention in Women

Urinary retention in women is much less common but may be caused by pelvic masses (e.g., uterine, ovarian) or pelvic prolapse (cystocele, rectocele, uterine) causing urethral compression or following pelvic surgery such as surgery to treat stress urinary incontinence, urethral stenosis, or urethral diverticulum. Transient retention may occur as a result of infection or inflammation occurring postpartum or secondary to herpes simplex infection, Bartholin abscess, acute urethritis, or vulvovaginitis. Fowler syndrome can also cause retention; this is a condition involving impaired relaxation of the external sphincter that occurs in premenopausal women, often in association with polycystic ovaries.

Bladder Neck Dyssynergia

Bladder neck obstruction/dyssynergia is another functional cause of BOO (rather than a mechanical cause) that is more commonly seen, absent of neurological abnormality, in relatively younger men it is due to failure of the bladder neck muscle fibers (internal sphincter) to relax during voiding. Detrusor sphincter dyssynergia (DSD) is often seen in motor neuron disease such as multiple sclerosis as well as spinal cord injury (SCI). DSD can also be behavioral.

Detrusor Underactivity

Nonobstructive causes of retention include detrusor underactivity (hypotonia, atonia) and can occur in both sexes. Specific etiologic factors include underlying neurological disorders (e.g., stroke, multiple sclerosis) or idiopathic detrusor underactivity, which is usually an age-related phenomenon seen in the elderly. Neurological disease can cause obstruction or retention by impairment of bladder contractility, nonrelaxation of the outlet, or failure of coordination between bladder contraction and sphincter/pelvic floor relaxation, depending on the precise level of the neurological deficit(s). Chapter 9 provides information regarding neurogenic lower urinary tract dysfunction (NLUTD) and how it impacts continence and bladder health.

Retention in Children

AUR is rare in children and is usually associated with infection or occurs postoperatively (e.g., circumcision).

Paruresis

Paruresis is the inability to urinate in the presence of others, such as in public toilets; this is also called "shy bladder syndrome," which, in extreme cases, can result in urinary retention.

Medications

Medications with anticholinergic properties can cause retention due to reduced contraction strength of the detrusor. In an individual at risk for AUR, taking medications with anticholinergic or alpha-adrenergic agonist properties (such as some decongestants or medications used to treat hypotension or bradycardia) may precipitate AUR. Psychoactive substances can cause retention due to enhanced outlet resistance; drugs in this category include stimulants such as MDMA (ecstasy) and other amphetamines.

Common causes of urinary retention in both men and women are listed in **Table 8-1**.

TABLE 8-1 CAUSES OF URINARY RETENTION BASED ON THE LEVEL OF THE URINARY TRACT INVOLVED		
	MALE	**FEMALE**
Urethra	Congenital urethral valves	Pelvic prolapse compressing the urethra
	Phimosis and/or pinhole meatus	Urethral stenosis
	Circumcision	Urethral diverticulum
	Obstruction in the urethra caused by stricture, calculus, or tumor	Postsurgery for stress urinary incontinence
	STD lesions (gonorrhea commonly causes multiple strictures, leading to a "rosary bead" appearance, whereas chlamydia usually causes a single stricture)	Postpartum infection/inflammation
		Genital herpes
		Bartholin abscess
		Acute urethritis/vulvovaginitis
Prostate/bladder neck	Benign prostatic hyperplasia (BPH)	Fowler syndrome
	Prostate cancer and other pelvic malignancies invading the prostate	Pelvic mass compressing/invading bladder neck
	Acute prostatitis	Bladder neck obstruction (dyssynergia, stenosis—scarring due to indwelling catheters, bladder neck surgery)
	Bladder neck obstruction (dyssynergia, stenosis—iatrogenic scarring following prostate surgery, indwelling catheters)	
Bladder	Detrusor sphincter dyssynergia	
	Neurogenic bladder (commonly pelvic splanchnic nerve damage, cauda equina syndrome, descending cortical fibers lesion, pontine micturition or storage center lesions, demyelinating diseases, or Parkinson disease)	

CASE STUDY #2 PRECIPITATED AUR

CAST STUDY DRUG-INDUCED AUR

A 38-year-old male factory worker who presents to the emergency department after leaving his job at noon. He in severe abdominal pain is diaphoretic and restless. VS T 99.8°F oral, P 106 radial, R 20 BP 144/90, O$_2$sat 100%.

On interview the patient reveals that he has not voided since before he went to bed the night before and only voided "a few drops" before he left home for work at 6 AM. Over the past 2 days, he noticed that when he urinates, he must strain and when finished there is a feeling that "he has to do more." This morning "only a few drops came out" and nothing since. Over the course of the morning, the pain became so severe prompting him to leave work early to seek medical attention.

The patient has no significant medical issues and is not on regular medications. He occasionally takes Tylenol for headache. The patient reports that he had been suffering with severe allergies for the past 3 days. His symptoms are nasal congestion, watery eyes, and sneezing. He has been self-treating with Claritin D (loratadine and pseudoephedrine).

Targeted physical examination reveals distended painful suprapubic area. Portable ultrasonic bladder scan showed 700 mL urine in bladder. The provider orders straight catheterization to relieve bladder distention.

The bladder is drained of 750 mL slightly cloudy, dark amber urine. Urine specimen sent for urinalysis and culture to rule out infection. The patient's discomfort is relieved, and the patient is observed to be more relaxed. Vital signs repeated 15 minutes after catheterization revealed T 99.2, P 92, R18 BP 130/80, O$_2$sat 100%.

Patient is prepared for discharge with instructions to discontinue use of products with pseudoephedrine and return ER if symptoms of urinary dysfunction return.

The information about allergies and the medication taken containing the decongestant pseudoephedrine is essential to the patient's condition and formulation of a diagnosis. Sometimes further investigation into over the counter, nonprescription medications is required, as patients do not report them because they do not think there are adverse effects of taking them.

In this case, the patient reported dysuria over the previous days prior to complete inability to void. Pseudoephedrine is known to potentially cause urinary retention as it acts to promote contraction of the bladder neck, urethra, and prostate causing increased outlet resistance. While this is a particular problem for older males with enlarged prostates, voiding dysfunction has been reported in all ages (Shao et al., 2016).

Fortunately for this patient, due to his age and no prior history of voiding dysfunction, he should do well after discontinuation of medications containing pseudoephedrine with resolution of his retention.

COMPLICATIONS OF URINARY RETENTION

Urinary retention should be treated as soon as possible in order to prevent long-term complications. It is important to note that UR in neurologic patients may trigger a potentially life-threatening condition, autonomic dysreflexia (AD). AD is an abnormal, overreaction of the autonomic (sympathetic) nervous system to stimulation by external or bodily stimuli that occurs below the level of the SCI. The most common causes include bladder or bowel overdistension, disimpaction procedures, blocked urinary catheters, or UTIs. It can also be precipitated by procedures such as cystoscopy or debridement of a pressure injury. AD occurs most often in individuals with SCI with lesions at or above the level of T6 but may appear in other neurologic conditions such as multiple sclerosis (MS) as well. AD is characterized by uncontrolled hypertension and bradycardia, often the patient will initially complain of headache and appear flushed and diaphoretic (above the level of injury). If unrecognized or untreated, severe hypertension may result in seizure or cerebral vascular accident (CVA), even death. Continence nurses are instrumental in being alert to and recognizing symptoms of AD. Initial treatment involves sitting the patient upright in a semi-Fowler position, removing any constrictive clothing (including abdominal binders and support stockings), checking the blood pressure, and then investigating and quickly removing the trigger. This may require urinary catheterization, searching for an indwelling catheter blockage, aborting digital manual removal of impacted stool, or other procedures. If systolic blood pressure remains elevated after initial steps, fast-acting short-duration antihypertensives (e.g., transdermal nitroglycerin) are considered while other potential triggering causes are investigated and resolved (Cowan, 2015).

Long-term complications associated with obstruction of the urinary tract and urinary retention include bladder and renal calculi (stones), atrophy or hypertrophy of the detrusor muscle, hydronephrosis, renal failure, diverticula (pouching) in the bladder wall, and UTI.

KEY POINT

Autonomic dysreflexia or AD is a dangerous syndrome caused from overstimulation of the sympathetic nervous system in patients with SCI at or above T6. It is characterized by uncontrolled hypertension and bradycardia, pounding headache, and the individual appears flushed and diaphoretic. If unrecognized or untreated, severe hypertension may result in seizure or cerebral vascular accident (CVA), even death.

 ## OBSTRUCTIVE UROPATHY

PROSTATISM AND OBSTRUCTIVE UROPATHY

The most common cause of blockage of the urethra in men is enlargement of the prostate. The prostate gland surrounds the urethra; thus, as it enlarges, the hypertrophy may lead to urethral compression and UR. Prostatic cancer can lead to the same sequela. In addition, AUR may be caused by prostatitis, an inflammation or infection of the prostate causing prostatic swelling. Prostatism is a disorder of the prostate associated with BOO at the bladder neck. If the obstruction continues over time, it can lead to bladder hypertrophy and trabeculation of the bladder wall (cord-like thickening into the bladder lumen), diverticulum formation (pouch or hernia of the bladder mucosa through a weakness in the smooth muscle layer), and ultimately hydronephrosis due to urine refluxing toward the kidneys from high pressures created from the inability to empty the bladder due to the obstruction (George et al., 1983). This viscous cycle then causes changes to the bladder wall compliance potentially to the point of detrusor failure (George et al., 1983). Bladder wall compliance is discussed in the next section.

LOSS OF BLADDER WALL COMPLIANCE

It appears likely that secondary structural changes in the bladder wall as a result of the pressure caused by the obstruction alter the filling-phase properties of the bladder. Of these, the most important is probably the property of "compliance," which is the ability of the normal bladder to stretch to accommodate changes in volume with almost no change in pressure. Compliance reflects normal detrusor muscle function and altered structure of the bladder wall will affect it, especially if there is connective tissue infiltration. If the bladder doesn't stretch to accommodate the increasing volume, this crucial property is lost, pressure rises with bladder filling and hampers the drainage of the ureters. That is to say, urine has difficulty flowing from the ureters into the bladder. The urine continues to flow from the kidney into the ureters and the accumulation of the urine causes the "swelling" of the ureters and eventually the kidney. This is particularly important if the bladder fails to empty completely with voiding, as the consequence will be high bladder pressures almost continuously. Another structural influence

causing elevated bladder pressure is the thickening of the bladder wall, which may compress or distort the vesicoureteric (bladder/ureter) junction, impairing the effective drainage of the ureter. It is not clear to what extent either process contributes, but the consequence is potentially the onset of progressive upper tract dilation (George et al., 1983).

KEY POINT

Loss of compliance (the inability of the bladder to stretch) causes high intravesical pressures throughout most of the filling/voiding cycle and is a major risk factor for upper tract damage.

In a normally compliant bladder, the rise in intravesical pressure associated with filling from empty to physiological bladder capacity (typically around 500 mL) is <5 cm H_2O. Uncomplicated BOO does not affect bladder compliance, so upper tract dilation (hydroureter/hydronephrosis) does not result. Only if there is a poorly compliant bladder is there risk of structural damage to the upper urinary tract and impaired renal function.

 ## CLINICAL PRESENTATION AND ASSESSMENT OF PATIENTS WITH URINARY RETENTION

ACUTE URINARY RETENTION

AUR is a medical emergency and requires prompt treatment. Lower abdominal pain can be severe when urine cannot be expelled. The individual in AUR can develop severe sweating, chest pain, anxiety, and high blood pressure, and there is a risk of precipitating angina or myocardial infarction. Patients with AUR may or may not have a history of previous LUTS. Some of these patients will not report prior LUTS, either because they did not recognize the significance of their symptoms or because they have learned to live with them. In AUR, there is a palpable mass that arises from the pelvis (i.e., the lower border of the mass is not palpable), which is dull on percussion.

The continence nursing assessment should include a history of present illness, medical, surgical and medication history, vital signs, pain assessment, and targeted physical examination (abdomen and bladder) as well as a bladder scan. A sample patient evaluation is demonstrated in **Box 8-3** with further elaboration in Chapter 4. This information obtained on assessment if promptly reported will lead the provider to the diagnosis of UR and the relieving of the retention (via catheterization). The volume of urine obtained is important to note and will be helpful in determining the type of retention (acute or chronic).

Symptoms such as lower abdominal pain, urinary incontinence, inability or difficulty voiding or incomplete

BOX 8-3   SAMPLE COMPREHENSIVE ASSESSMENT FOR URINARY RETENTION

History of present illness: What brings you in today?

Duration and onset: How long has this been going on? Why is today different?

Were there any precipitating factors? Recent surgery/procedure with general anesthesia?

Continence: leakage, postvoid dribble. Is the patient aware of need to void or urine leaked?

Hematuria: Do you notice blood in the urine?

Postvoiding symptoms: weak stream, pain on urination, feeling of incomplete emptying

Medical history: hypertension, diabetes, neurologic disorder, diagnosis of urinary tract or renal disorder

Medication history: Does the patient report use of amphetamines, antihistamines, heart medications such as beta-blockers or calcium channel blockers, medication to treat Parkinson disease, anticholinergics for urinary incontinence, muscle relaxants, nonsteroidal anti-inflammatory drugs (NSAIDs), pseudoephedrine, antipsychotics, tricyclic antidepressants, opioid pain medications.

Physical examination:

General observation: Patients with acute retention are usually in severe pains and restless, while those with chronic retention are calm.

Facial puffiness, pedal edema, anemia, acidotic breath, and elevated blood pressure may be found in patients with impaired renal function.

Focused abdominal examination:

Check for suprapubic swelling and tenderness, a full bladder will be dull to percussion.

In low-pressure chronic retention, bladder outline may or may not be palpable. The abdomen should be examined for suprapubic swelling and tenderness.

Genital examination: quick check for urethral discharge (or bleeding) obvious swelling or deformities

If neurologic illness or injury is suspected, lower limb motor and sensory evaluation including deep tendon and plantar reflexes

Advanced practice: additional examination

Prostate examination DRE for enlargement

Vaginal examination for prolapse

Neurologic disorders: check perianal and perineal sensations, anal sphincteric tone, and bulbocaerrnosal reflex (checks sensory and motor pathways of the pudendal nerves)

---

bladder emptying, and agitation and/or distress in cognitively impaired patients all raise suspicion for AUR. Medical conditions of note such as BPH, neurogenic disease or injury, and diabetes as well as medications that may contribute to AUR are discussed in more detail in other sections.

Due to the emergent nature of UR and the severe discomfort of the patient, it will be easier for the patient and will be more informative for the clinician if the rectal or vaginal examination is carried out after the patient has been catheterized and the retention has been relieved. Although AUR is primarily a clinical diagnosis, a bladder scan will further confirm the diagnosis before catheterization. The volume of urine drained in AUR is usually <1 L. If the volume drained is >1 L, it suggests the possibility of an acute-on-chronic retention, particularly if the level of discomfort is moderate rather than severe (Kalejaiye & Speakman, 2009).

Once the bladder has been emptied, advanced practice nurses or physicians can perform more invasive examinations such as DRE in men and pelvic examinations in women. DRE should include assessment of the size and consistency of the prostate, anal sphincter tone, and presence or absence of retained stool (see **Fig. 8-2**, DRE). The pelvic examination should include assessment for prolapse or other mass (using a speculum), any tenderness or mass in the vaginal fornices, and bimanual palpation of organs and any pelvic mass. See Chapter 4 for more information about the pelvic examination.

CHRONIC URINARY RETENTION

CUR occurs when a patient retains a substantial volume of urine in the bladder after each void (Kaplan et al., 2008). The threshold volume for CUR has not been standardized. The finding of persistent residual volumes of >300 mL, although some authors suggest >500 mL, after voiding is often used as evidence of CUR. Patients may be asymptomatic, they may void little and often, or they may have difficulty with initiating and completing micturition. Other features of CUR include nocturnal enuresis and a painless palpable bladder; at its extreme, there may be symptoms attributable to chronic renal failure (malaise, loss of appetite, anorexia, fatigue) (Ghalayini et al., 2005; Kaplan et al., 2008). In general, previous LUTS are uncommon in patients with CUR (Abrams et al., 1978; George et al., 1983).

DIAGNOSTIC STUDIES

In both types of retention, urinalysis should always be performed and a catheter specimen of urine (CSU) should be sent if there are signs of infection so that a urine culture can be performed. Urinary infection should be treated with appropriate antibiotics. Blood urea, serum creatinine, electrolytes, and estimated glomerular filtration rate (eGFR) should be checked; this is especially important in HPCR. Renal ultrasound is indicated in patients with high-volume retention and in patients with abnormal renal function. Any abnormalities require referral to the appropriate specialist, usually a urologist. PSA testing is best avoided during the acute episode, since any instrumentation of the prostate leads to a spurious false rise in PSA (Pruthi, 2000). Interpreting the PSA after the acute episode is settled requires recognition that PSA is a nonspecific test that can be elevated in prostate cancer, BPH, and prostatitis. A TRUS (transrectal ultrasound)-guided biopsy of the prostate can distinguish between these prostate conditions.

> **KEY POINT**
>
> Assessment of the patient with retention should include a urinalysis to assess for infection and BUN, creatinine, and eGFR to rule out renal damage.

When AUR is associated with neurologic symptoms, specific evaluation is required, which may be urgent, since irreversible change can result in some circumstances. New-onset pain in the lumbar spine, numbness in the perianal area, paresthesia, diminished anal sphincter tone, or altered deep tendon reflexes may be indicative. In these circumstances, an urgent neurological referral may be required. An MRI of the lumbar spine should be considered to further assess for possible spinal cord compression or cauda equina syndrome.

Differentiating AUR from other possible diagnoses is not usually difficult. However, other potentially more serious conditions such as diverticulitis, perforated or ischemic bowel, and abdominal aortic aneurysm can inappropriately be referred into hospital as AUR. Urinary retention may occur secondary to many medical conditions; accordingly, the patient should be reexamined soon after catheterization to confirm that the symptoms and signs have resolved. Additionally, any patient with a lower abdominal mass should be considered for catheterization to exclude a distended bladder prior to further examination or investigation (Kalejaiye & Speakman, 2009). Occasionally, an obese patient with anuria or oliguria due to renal failure may mistakenly be thought to be in AUR. A bladder ultrasound scan can be helpful in this situation. Urodynamics is not a first-line assessment method for etiology of urinary retention but is useful when conservative treatment has failed (see Chapter 5 for more information regarding urodynamics).

 TREATMENT OF URINARY RETENTION

ACUTE URINARY RETENTION

Treatment of AUR requires urgent catheterization. Whether patients are catheterized in the community or primary care by a general practitioner, in accident and emergency departments, or in surgical or urology wards depends mainly on local circumstances, as does the decision to admit or send home after catheterization (Bates et al., 2003; Emberton & Fitzpatrick, 2008;

Fitzpatrick & Kirby, 2006). Keeping patients in hospital awaiting definitive treatment results in a longer total hospital stay. The urine volume drained in the first 10 to 15 minutes following catheterization must be accurately recorded in the patient's notes to enable a distinction between acute and acute-on-chronic retention. This has important clinical implications because it will help the continence nurse determine who most likely will be successful in voiding completely after an AUR (successful voiding trial without catheter) versus those who continue to have high PVRs as seen in CUR potentially leading to another AUR crisis. The results of the Alfuzosin in Acute Urinary Retention (ALFAUR) study demonstrated a significantly increased risk of failure for trial without catheterization (TWOC) in the elderly (>65 years) and in patients with a drained volume >1 L (Emberton & Fitzpatrick, 2008). In the second part of the study, patients with initially successful TWOC were more likely to have recurrent AUR if their post-TWOC residual volume was high. It has been proposed that these patients should be offered elective transurethral resection of prostate (TURP) at an earlier stage.

> **KEY POINT**
>
> Treatment of acute urinary retention requires urgent catheterization; the volume drained during the first 10 to 15 minutes should be accurately recorded to help differentiate acute from acute-on-chronic retention. Catheterization volumes >1 L raise concern about a pattern of acute-on-chronic retention and increase the likelihood that the patient will fail a TWOC.

CHRONIC RETENTION

Management of CUR is more complex. Catheterization is less urgent in CUR because the condition is generally less painful or painless. If a patient has no symptoms and a kidney ultrasound scan and renal function tests are normal, there is no need to do anything except monitor the situation closely. But if the patient complains of frequency or nocturia, or is having recurrent urinary infections, intermittent self-catheterization (ISC) is an option. Early catheterization is indicated if renal dysfunction or hydronephrosis is present. Following relief of the obstruction, the majority of individuals have complete recovery of kidney function. However, a few will have marked polyuria (>4 to 5 L/day) after bladder drainage, which effectively restores the ability of each kidney to drain fully. This is termed "postobstructive diuresis." There are several physiological and pathologic factors that lead to the development of this condition.

Postobstructive Diuresis

Following catheter placement, the volume of urine output can be considerably greater than the PVR volume. This can result from correction of excess sodium and water retention in patients with HPCR and improved renal function, along with an osmotic diuresis that is caused by the accumulation of urea and other nonreabsorbable solutes (Sparks, 2010). Postobstructive diuresis is usually self-limiting and resolves over several days to a week, once surplus waste products (e.g., urea) are eliminated. It is critical, however, to monitor urine output closely. If the postobstructive diuresis condition becomes pathologic, it can cause serious consequences such as dehydration, electrolyte abnormalities (potassium especially), hypotension, hypovolemic shock, and even result in death. Persistent polyuria beyond a week is often due to overzealous volume replacement (Sparks, 2010).

Potassium levels, which are often high prior to catheterization, should be monitored and will usually (but not always) fall with the diuresis. Replacement should be guided by electrolyte levels, the patient's oral intake, and presence of comorbid conditions (such as heart disease). Most of the early improvement in the glomerular filtration rate (GFR) is related to tubular recovery, although a late glomerular recovery phase occurs as well (Jones et al., 1989).

Catheterization for CUR is often followed by hematuria; this is caused by the small vessels in the bladder bleeding as the pressure on the bladder wall is released. Bleeding may also be due to trauma by the catheter itself. If blood clots are present, it is important to check that the catheter is draining and is not blocked. The hematuria usually resolves after 48 to 72 hours. The past practice of slow decompression of the bladder is unnecessary as there is no evidence to support this practice.

KEY POINT

Catheterization for CUR is often followed by hematuria; this is caused by the small vessels in the bladder bleeding as the pressure on the bladder wall is released. The practice of slow decompression of the bladder is not evidence based; it does not reduce the episodes of hematuria postcatheterization.

Continence Care Nurse Considerations

Depending upon licensure, the continence care nurse may oversee care or encourage staff to carefully measure intake (both oral and intravenous) and output; monitor and report any signs and symptoms of dehydration, electrolyte abnormalities, hypotension, and hypovolemic shock to the health care provider; initiate and oversee catheter-associate UTI (CAUTI) prevention bundle; promote only competency-based staff placing catheters; and initiate interventions postcatheter removal.

Definitive Management of an Obstructive Condition

Even if renal failure resolves with catheterization, the patient should not undergo a TWOC (trial without catheterization) until the patient has been evaluated for a definitive procedure such as TURP. Patients with LPCR tend to do poorly after TURP, frequently failing to void completely after surgery, even after prolonged periods of catheterization; this is probably due to detrusor changes over time (Bates et al., 2003; Ghalayini et al., 2005). Patients with LPCR should be warned of this possibility prior to consenting them for a TURP. In these patients, ISC should be considered as an option prior to and potentially after a TURP (Ghalayini et al., 2005).

KEY POINT

Patients with low-pressure chronic retention may not do well following TURP and should be informed of this prior to surgery; they may require self-catheterization to empty the bladder.

CATHETERIZATION FOR URINARY RETENTION

Catheterization for management of urinary retention may be done via the urethral route or via suprapubic placement. Guidelines for urethral catheter selection for ISC or IUC including catheter and balloon size, tip, and construction as well as CAUTI prevention are featured in Chapter 19. Brief overview of ISC is highlighted; Chapter 16 provides practical tips on teaching ISC and explores adaptive aides for individuals who have physical limitations that may affect their ability to manage their bladder emptying effectively. In addition to ISC and IUC, suprapubic catheters are another option for bladder management especially for individuals with longstanding CUR. Indications, contraindications, potential complications, and principle advantages will be discussed here as well as the role of the continence care nurse in teaching patients bladder emptying through catheterization.

Intermittent Self-Catheterization

ISC is an alternative to an indwelling catheter. It is a safe, simple, and well-accepted technique that may result in fewer UTIs than indwelling catheterization. There are no external devices, and maintenance of sexual activity is possible. It may also increase the rate of successful spontaneous voiding. ISC can be used instead of an indwelling catheter after an episode of AUR or CUR, or it can be used in patients who fail to void following a prostatectomy. A period of ISC prior to TURP may be useful in patients with low pressure CR, as it may allow recovery of bladder contractility. For those with spinal cord lesions and neurogenic bladder dysfunction, IC is a standard method for bladder emptying. Patients' QOL may also be enhanced (Choong & Emberton, 2000; Ghalayini et al., 2005).

Suprapubic Catheterization

When placement of a urethral catheter is contraindicated or unsuccessful, percutaneous suprapubic urinary bladder catheterization can be performed to relieve urinary retention. Suprapubic catheterization (SPC) is another form of indwelling catheter that enters the bladder directly through the abdominal wall. Some of the most common reasons for SPC are urethral injuries, urethral obstruction, bladder neck masses and BPH, and prostate cancer. It is also used for long-term management of SCI patients who are unable or unwilling to use intermittent catheterization to empty the bladder.

SPC placement is contraindicated in the absence of an easily palpable or distended urinary bladder visualized by ultrasound (Ramos-Fernandez et al., 2013). Relative contraindications to SPC placement include coagulopathy (until the abnormality is corrected) and previous lower abdominal or pelvic surgery (due to potential bowel adherence to the bladder or anterior abdominal wall). In the latter situation, it is safer for the urologist to perform an open cystostomy. SPC is also relatively contraindicated in pelvic cancer, with or without pelvic radiation, owing to increased risk of adhesions (Harrison et al., 2011).

Figure 8-5 shows SPC in a male.

SPC is essentially a surgical procedure as it requires an entry through the abdominal wall into the bladder and is a painful procedure, even with proper local anesthesia. Patients may require parenteral analgesia, with or without sedation. As a result, this procedure is usually done in the procedure/surgical area of the facility by a urologist. SPC procedure requires the usual preoperative nursing and medical assessments and consents. The distended bladder is palpated, and the site of insertion is marked in the midline. During the procedure, a sterile suprapubic catheter kit is used that has a device that will help guide the catheter into the bladder. A catheter is placed through the skin just above the pubic bone into the bladder, often with the assistance of ultrasound imaging. Access to the bladder will result in immediate return of urine from the bladder through the cannula. Before the bladder empties of urine, a size 12 to 16 Fr

indwelling catheter is quickly placed into the bladder through the cannula and the catheter balloon is inflated (usually with 10 mL of sterile water). Sometimes the catheter is held in place with an anchoring suture. Initially, the catheter remains in place for up to a month while the tissue around it scars and forms a tract (sinus) between the bladder and the outside of the body. After the formation of scar tissue is complete, the catheter is replaced periodically in order to help prevent infection.

The nurse does not usually change the SPC until the tract is formed. The first change is usually performed by the urologist. When changing an SPC via an established track, it is important that the new catheter should be inserted immediately following removal of the old catheter; an SPC should not be removed unless the nurse or provider is ready to insert the replacement catheter.

Potential complications of SPCs include hematuria (typically transient), cellulitis and abscess formation, catheter blockage, UTIs, dermatitis at the stoma site from urine leak, urethral leakage in females with stress incontinence, and urinary calculi (late complication).

Urethral Versus Suprapubic Catheterization

The principal advantages of SPC are reduced urethral irritation and stricture formation, ability to have sexual intercourse in the absence of a urethral catheter, and the ability to provide a trial without catheter by simply clamping the catheter (as opposed to removing the catheter). This is often referred to as "trial of voiding (TOV)"; the SPC is clamped and the patient is allowed to void urine naturally, following which the SPC can be unclamped and the residual volume measured (Horgan et al., 1992). Although it has been suggested that UTI is lower with SPC, in long-term use, there appears to be no difference in UTI rates (Hunter et al., 2013).

A significant number of patients with retention will fail TWOC and will require repeat catheterization, with all the resulting discomfort (Emberton & Fitzpatrick, 2008). The benefits of SPC in AUR have been shown in many studies, and SPC may be regarded as the preferred route of catheterization. Additionally, studies have shown that there are similar complication rates for both types of catheters and there was no difference in asymptomatic bacteriuria, UTI, or urosepsis between indwelling and SPC. In classic papers on the use of SPCs, it is noted that patients frequently expressed a preference for SPC, specifically indicating increased comfort and ease of sexual intercourse with an SPC (Abrams et al., 1978; Ahluwalia et al., 2006; Horgan et al., 1992; Ichsan & Hunt, 1987). The latter is often overlooked when deciding on the type of catheter to provide patients but should be routinely considered; the ability to maintain active sexual function is particularly important to some patients. Despite this, the Reten-World survey reported that most urologists perform urethral catheterization (>80%), with SPCs inserted only for urethral catheter failures (Emberton & Fitzpatrick, 2008).

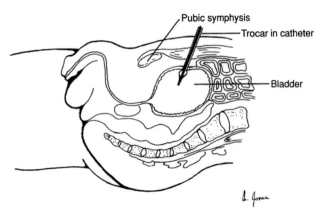

FIGURE 8-5. Technique of Suprapubic Catheterization by Using a Trocar with a Catheter. (From Simon, R. R., Ross, C., Bowman, S. H., et al. (2011). *Cook county manual of emergency procedures.* Philadelphia, PA: Lippincott Williams & Wilkins.)

Trial without Catheterization

TWOC involves catheter removal (typically after 1 to 3 days) and patients are allowed to void spontaneously and are monitored for recurrent retention. TWOC is considered for most patients. The patients who are able to effectively empty the bladder are able to return home without the potential risks associated with an indwelling catheter. TWOC also allows surgery to be delayed to an elective setting or may eliminate the need for surgery (Emberton & Fitzpatrick, 2008; Fitzpatrick & Kirby, 2006).

Factors leading to a better chance of success with TWOC include

- Younger age (<65 years)
- UTI with no previous voiding LUTS
- Identified precipitating cause (e.g., gross constipation)
- Recent initiation of anticholinergic or sympathomimetic drugs (which should be discontinued for TWOC)
- Drained volume/PVR <1,000 mL

Conversely, factors leading to a high probability of unsuccessful TWOC include

- Patient age >75 years
- Drained volume >1 L
- Previous LUTS
- Voiding detrusor contraction (on urodynamics) of <35 cm H_2O (Abrams et al., 1978; Emberton & Fitzpatrick, 2008; Fitzpatrick & Kirby, 2006)

The clinician should be aware that initial success with TWOC does not necessarily mean the patient will continue to be successful voiding. Half of those for whom initial TWOC is successful will experience recurrent AUR over the next year and 35% undergo surgery within the following 6 months (Emberton & Fitzpatrick, 2008; Fitzpatrick & Kirby, 2006). Patients with PVR > 500 mL, no precipitating factor for AUR, and maximum flow rate <5 mL/s were at increased risk of further retention (Shergill et al., 2008). This emphasizes the importance of follow-up for patients with risk factors for recurrent AUR, even if they are initially successful with TWOC.

Continence Care Nurse Considerations: Patient Education

Regardless of the type of catheter used, the patient needs information regarding the procedure itself; explaining why catheterization is necessary and how the procedure will be accomplished. Many patients are upset and overwhelmed by the idea of having to perform ISC. The nurse can help patients and families by supporting them and teaching them so that they can regain independence. The nurse assesses the patient both physically and mentally for their ability to perform self-catheterization. The catheterization technique is demonstrated and explained and then the patient is supervised performing self-catheterization prior to discharge. Instruction is given on hand hygiene and infection prevention. The patient who is performing CIC will be taught to handle the equipment, suggesting a schedule for catheterization (every 4 to 6 hours), how to minimize potential of infection, recognizing signs and symptoms of UTI and other complications, and when to call the provider or seek emergency care. Contact information of the hospital or clinic is provided for the patient to address any questions or concerns until the follow-up appointment.

ALPHA-ADRENERGIC ANTAGONISTS (ALPHA-BLOCKERS) AND TRIAL WITHOUT CATHETER

AUR due to BPH may be associated with an increase in α-adrenergic activity (Fitzpatrick & Kirby, 2006; McNeill et al., 1999). Inhibition of these receptors by α1-blockers (alpha-adrenergic antagonists) may decrease bladder outlet resistance, thereby facilitating normal voiding (Fitzpatrick & Kirby, 2006; McNeill et al., 1999; Zeif & Subramonian, 2009). There is some evidence that men catheterized for AUR can void more successfully after catheter removal if treated with medications such as tamsulosin or alfuzosin (α-blockers). The likelihood of a successful TWOC increases, even in patients who are elderly (>65 years) with PVR more than 1,000 mL (Emberton & Fitzpatrick, 2008; Fitzpatrick & Kirby, 2006; McNeill et al., 1999). Patients at risk for recurrent AUR after successful TWOC included those with a high PSA and PVR (Emberton & Fitzpatrick, 2008; Fitzpatrick & Kirby, 2006). The Reten-World survey revealed that 82% of patients received an α1-blocker before catheter removal; TWOC success was greater in those receiving α1-blockers, regardless of age (Emberton & Fitzpatrick, 2008). Use of alpha-blockers almost doubles the likelihood of successful trial without catheter.

HOSPITALIZATION FOR URINARY RETENTION

The decision regarding whether to admit patients or to send them home is dependent on local resources and preference

(Emberton & Fitzpatrick, 2008; Fitzpatrick & Kirby, 2006; McNeill et al., 2004). Admission is more common in patients with impaired renal function or another comorbidity.

KEY POINT

Alpha-adrenergic antagonists or α1-blockers such as tamsulosin of alfuzosin relax the alpha receptor of the bladder neck to help reduce bladder outlet resistance, thereby facilitating normal voiding. Individuals undergoing a TWOC were almost twice as likely to be successful when prescribed alpha blockers.

SURGICAL TREATMENT

Previously, AUR was considered an absolute indication for TURP (Choong & Emberton, 2000; Emberton & Fitzpatrick, 2008; Fitzpatrick & Kirby, 2006), but now most men with BPH can be managed well with medications to reduce BOO. At present, AUR is the indication for prostatectomy in 25% of patients in the United States and in 50% of patients in the United Kingdom. In men with large prostates (>100 g), an open prostatectomy may be required, which may be performed through a retropubic, transvesical, or perineal approach (Bouchier-Hayes et al., 2006; Choong & Emberton, 2000). Complications

---

CASE STUDY #3 AUR ON CUR

A 71-year-old male presents with "trouble voiding" for 2 days, fever, chills, diaphoresis, nausea, and vomiting

Current vitals are temp. 101.8°F, HR 134, RR 26, SpO_2 92 on room air

PMH: BPH for 4 years, DM for 20 years, hypertension, arthritis

PSH: Lumbar surgery 10 years ago, TURP 3 years ago

Medications: Glyburide, metoprolol, tamsulosin, diclofenac sodium

On examination, the bladder is palpated above the symphysis pubis

Patient denies CVA tenderness, chest pain, or shortness of breath. Denies pain with examination

Bladder scan results >1,000 mL

Lab results: WBC 14.2 k/μL, H/H 14/41, platelets 243 chemistry BUN 78, creatine 3.2, all other chemistries are WNL

What is the suspected diagnosis and cause? Sepsis related to urinary tract infection

UTI likely caused by incomplete emptying allowing for urine stasis that promotes bacterial growth.

AUR likely related to BPH causing the narrowing of the prostatic urethra. In addition, the patient has a long-standing history of diabetes affecting the detrusors muscle, impairing sensation, bladder contraction, and emptying.

Why didn't the patient feel pain with the distended bladder? Complications of diabetes can cause a triad of symptoms, sometimes called diabetic cystopathy. These symptoms are impaired sensation, decreased detrusor contractility, and increased bladder capacity. Because of the patient having

impaired sensation, he likely does not feel his bladder is full until volume is greater than normal. The decreased bladder contractility causes inability to empty the contents of the bladder and causes increased bladder volume due to urine being continually produced adding to the residual from incomplete emptying (Brown, 2009; Choong & Emberton, 2000; Emberton & Fitzpatrick, 2008; Fitzpatrick & Kirby, 2006; Kaplan et al., 2008).

What are the next steps for this patient?

Urinary catheterization to obtain a urinalysis, urine culture, and sensitivity and to empty the patient's bladder. Renal ultrasound will be performed to evaluate upper tract (kidney and ureters) involvement. Broad-spectrum antibiotics will be started, pending results of the culture.

The patient will be observed for possible void and postvoid residual will be monitored. If larger residuals persist (>300 mL), or if the patient does not void, he will continue to perform intermittent catheterization when discharged. If the patient has larger than usual urinary output, an indwelling catheter may be indicated for the initial period to monitor for postobstructive diuresis.

The patient will be referred to his urologist.

Later management of this patient will include urodynamic testing to determine the cause of his bladder dysfunction (BOO or impaired bladder contractility). Bladder medications will be evaluated and may be added or adjusted. If the cause is BOO with good bladder contractility, a procedure may be recommended.

The continence nurse is essential in the instruction of the patient and caregiver in the catheterization procedure and ensures that the patient has the necessary supplies and support to successfully manage his bladder.

of prostatectomy are infection, perioperative bleeding, and need for transfusion. Additionally, a higher percentage of men undergoing TURP for AUR fail to void following surgery, as compared with men undergoing surgery for symptoms but no retention (Choong & Emberton, 2000). Complications of TURP also include retrograde ejaculation, erectile dysfunction, urinary incontinence, TUR syndrome (dilutional hyponatremia due to systemic absorption of the irrigation fluid), urethral stricture, and bladder neck stenosis. Nonetheless, advances in surgical techniques have made TURP a much safer procedure. Commonly used, newer, procedures are Green Light Laser photovaporization of the prostate (GLL-PVP) and holmium laser enucleation of the prostate (HoLEP). All of these procedures require general or spinal anesthesia, so the patient's overall health status needs to be considered. Equivalent improvements to TURP may be seen in urinary flow rates and symptoms, with reduced length of stay, length of catheterization, and adverse events for the GLL-PVP group (Bouchier-Hayes et al., 2006; Choong & Emberton, 2000). Certainly, advances in surgical and laser techniques have made TURP a much safer procedure but long-term outcomes need to be evaluated. Further details regarding LUTS in men are discussed in Chapter 10.

 PREVENTION OF URINARY RETENTION

POSTOPERATIVE URINARY RETENTION

Patients should be assessed preoperatively for known risk factors that may increase the likelihood of POUR (see **Table 8-2**). Patients who are at high risk for POUR should be counselled preoperatively about the condition. The preoperative assessment information, in collaboration with other team members, may allow for interventions to minimize development of POUR or at the least, recognize the development of POUR more quickly, to minimize the discomfort and distress to the patient (Simsek & Sureyya, 2016). Intraoperative preventive strategies primarily involve judicious fluid management and reduction of blood loss. Bailey and Ferguson (1976) evaluated 500 patients after anorectal procedures and reported that patients who received <250-mL fluid perioperatively had significantly lower incidence of POUR.

Management of postoperative pain also plays an important role in preventing POUR. Sympathetic stimulation secondary to pain results in decreased detrusor contraction and increased outflow resistance (closed sphincter) leading to difficulty in voiding (see **Table 8-2**). Various pharmacological methods have also been attempted for prevention of POUR. As previously mentioned, alpha-adrenergic antagonists such as tamsulosin can aid voiding by decreasing outflow resistance and thus reduce the incidence of POUR.

PREVENTION OF NON-POUR URINARY RETENTION

Randomized studies have identified predictive risk factors for AUR (Emberton & Fitzpatrick, 2008), which include age >70 years with LUTS, an IPSS > 7 (i.e., moderate or severe LUTS), a flow rate of <12 mL/s, and/or a prostate volume of >40 g or a PSA > 1.4 ng/mL (**Box 8-2**). Studies have suggested that hesitancy may also predict a greater risk of subsequent AUR.

Further research found and confirmed that combination therapy with an alpha1-blocker (tamsulosin, doxazosin) and 5-alpha reductase inhibitor (dutasteride, finasteride) reduced the risk of clinical progression of BPH (McConnell et al., 2003; Roehrborn et al., 2010). Thus, identifying patients who are high risk for retention of urine and treating them with alpha1-blockers and 5-alpha reductase inhibitor may help prevent urinary retention. It is also essential to ensure patient follow-up, avoid the use of medications that could precipitate AUR, and prevent constipation.

CONCLUSION

Urinary retention remains a significant burden for both the patient and the health care system. The continence care nurse is instrumental in the management of this condition as the patient requires monitoring and support. In addition, education must be provided for patients and their significant others regarding UR symptom recognition and self-care pre- and postsurgery. Management of UR should include modification of risk factors for developing AUR, possible use an alpha-adrenergic antagonists and

TABLE 8-2 PREDICTORS OF POUR		
PATIENT HISTORY	**SURGICAL FACTORS**	**COMMONLY USED MEDICATIONS ASSOCIATED WITH POUR**
Age, sex	Length of surgery	
PMH—BPH, cardiac arrhythmias, diabetes, Parkinson disease or other neurological disorder Psychiatric disorders—Anxiety, depression Previous episode of UR	Location of surgical issue: Pelvic, inguinal, lower abdominal area	Anticholinergics Antihistamines Opioids General or spinal anesthesia Antiarrhythmics Anti-Parkinson's Beta-blockers
	General or spinal anesthesia	

5-alpha reductase inhibitor, as well as TWOC and potential future surgical interventions. Once retention occurs, the timing of surgery must be based on the risk of perioperative morbidity and mortality. The patient may need to perform ISC or have an indwelling catheter to manage UR. If this is the case, the patient must be instructed in catheter care. Finally, the evidence base for use of SPC for long term in retention patients may support SPC as a first-line approach as opposed to urethral catheterization.

REFERENCES

Abrams, P., Cardozo, L., Fall, M., et al. (2003). Standardisation Sub-Committee of the International Continence Society. The standardisation of terminology in lower urinary tract function: Report from the standardisation sub-committee of the International Continence Society. *Urology, 61*(1), 37–49.

Abrams, P. H., Dunn, M., & George, N. (1978). Urodynamic findings in chronic retention of urine and their relevance to results of surgery. *British Medical Journal, 2*(6147), 1258–1260.

Ahluwalia, R. S., Johal, N., Kouriefs, C., et al. (2006). The surgical risk of suprapubic catheter insertion and long-term sequelae. *Annals of the Royal College of Surgeons of England, 88*(2), 210–213. doi: 10.1308/003588406X95101.

Armitage, J., & Emberton, M. (2005). Is it time to reconsider the role of prostatic inflammation in the pathogenesis of lower urinary tract symptoms? *BJU International, 96*(6), 745–746. doi: 10.1111/j.1464-410X.2005.05761.x.

AUA White Paper. (2016). *Non-neurogenic chronic urinary retention: Consensus definition, management strategies, and future opportunities.* Retrieved September 23, 2019, from https://www.auanet.org/guidelines/chronic-urinary-retention

Bailey, H. R., & Fergurson, J. A. (1976). Prevention of urinary retention by fluid restriction following anorectal operations. *Diseases of the Colon and Rectum, 19*(3), 250–252.

Bates, T. S., Sugiono, M., James, E. D., et al. (2003). Is the conservative management of chronic retention in men ever justified? *British Journal International, 92*(6), 581–583.

Berry, S. J., Coffey, D. S., Walsh, P.C., et al. (1984). The development of human benign prostatic hyerplasia with age. *Journal of Urology, 132*(3), 474–479.

Bouchier-Hayes, D. M., Anderson, P., Van Appledorn, S., et al. (2006). KTP laser versus transurethral resection: Early results of a randomized trial. *Journal of Endourology/Endourological Society, 20*(8), 580–585. doi: 10.1089/end.2006.20.580.

Brasure M, Fink HA, Risk M, et al. Chronic urinary retention: Comparative effectiveness and harms of treatments *[Internet]* (2014). Rockville, MD: Agency for Healthcare Research and Quality (US). (Comparative Effectiveness Reviews, No. 140). Available from: https://www.ncbi.nlm.nih.gov/books/NBK246864/

Brown, J. (2009). Diabetic cystopathy—What does it mean? *Journal of Urology, 181*(1), 13–14.

Choong, S., & Emberton, M. (2000). Acute urinary retention. *BJU International, 85*(2), 186–201.

Cowan, H. (2015). Autonomic dysreflexia in spinal cord injury. *Nursing Times, 111*(44), 22–24.

Emberton, M., & Fitzpatrick, J. M. (2008). The Reten-World survey of the management of acute urinary retention: Preliminary results. *BJU International, 101*(Suppl 3), 27–32. doi: 10.1111/j.1464-410X.2008.07491.x.

Fitzpatrick, J. M., & Kirby, R. S. (2006). Management of acute urinary retention. *BJU International, 97*(Suppl 2), 16–20; discussion 21–22. doi: 10.1111/j.1464-410X.2006.06100.x.

George, N. J., O'Reilly, P. H., Barnard, R. J., et al. (1983). High pressure chronic retention. *British Medical Journal (Clinical Research Ed.), 286*(6380), 1780–1783.

Ghalayini, I. F., Al-Ghazo, M. A., & Pickard, R. S. (2005). A prospective randomized trial comparing transurethral prostatic resection and clean intermittent self-catheterization in men with chronic urinary retention. *BJU International, 96*(1), 93–97. doi: 10.1111/j.1464-410X.2005.05574.x.

Harrison, S. C. W., Lawrence, W. T., Morley, R., et al. (2011). British Association of Urological surgeons' suprapubic catheter practice guidelines. *BJU International, 107*(1), 77–85.

Hedlund, H., Hjelmas, K., Jonsson, O., et al. (2001). Hydrophilic versus non-coated catheters for intermittent catheterization. *Scandinavian Journal of Urology and Nephrology, 35*(1), 49–53.

Horgan, A. F., Prasad, B., Waldron, D. J., et al. (1992). Acute urinary retention. Comparison of suprapubic and urethral catheterisation. *British Journal of Urology, 70*(2), 149–151.

Hunter, K. F., Bharmal, A., & Moore, K. N. (2013). Long-term suprapubic versus urethral catheterization: A scoping review. *Neurourology and Urodynamics, 32*(7), 944–951. doi: 10.1002/nau.22356.

Ichsan, J., & Hunt, D. R. (1987). Suprapubic catheters: A comparison of suprapubic versus urethral catheters in the treatment of acute urinary retention. *Australian & New Zealand Journal of Surgery, 57*(1), 33–36.

International Continence Society. (2016). *Urinary retention.* Retrieved from https://www.ics.org/committees/standardisation/terminology-discussions/urinaryretention

Jones, D. A., Atherton, J. C., O'Reilly, P. H., et al. (1989). Assessment of the nephron segments involved in post-obstructive diuresis in man, using lithium clearance. *British Journal of Urology, 64*(6), 559–563.

Kalejaiye, O., & Speakman, M. J. (2009). Management of acute and chronic retention in men. *European Urology Supplements, 8*(6), 523–529.

Kaplan, S. A., Wein, A. J., Staskin, D. R., et al. (2008). Urinary retention and post-void residual urine in men: Separating truth from tradition. *Journal of Urology, 180*(1), 47–54.

McConnell, J. D., Roehrborn, C. G., Bautista, O. M., et al.; Medical Therapy of Prostatic Symptoms Research Group. (2003). The long-term effect of doxazosin, finasteride, and combination therapy on the clinical progression of benign prostatic hyperplasia. *New England Journal of Medicine, 349*(25), 2387–2398.

McNeill, S. A., Daruwala, P. D., Mitchell, I. D., et al. (1999). Sustained-release alfuzosin and trial without catheter after acute urinary retention: A prospective, placebo-controlled. *BJU International, 84*(6), 622–627.

McNeill, A. S., Rizvi, S., & Byrne, D. J. (2004). Prostate size influences the outcome after presenting with acute urinary retention. *BJU International, 94*(4), 559–562. doi: 10.1111/j.1464-410X.2004.05000.x.

Meigs, J. B., Barry, M. J., Giovannucci, E., et al. (1999). Incidence rates and risk factors for acute urinary retention: The health professionals follow-up study. *Journal of Urology, 162*(2), 376–382.

National Institute of Diabetes and Digestive and Kidney Diseases. (September 2014). *Prostate enlargement (Benign Prostatic Hyperplasia).* Retrieved from www.niddk.nih.gov/health-information/urologic-diseases/prostate-problems/prostate-benign-prostatic-hyperplasia

Oelke, M., Speakman, M. J., Desgrandchamps, F., et al. (2015). Acute urinary retention rates in the general male population and in adult men with LUTS participating in pharmacotherapy trials: A literature review. *Urology, 86*, 654–665.

Pruthi, R. S. (2000). The dynamics of prostate-specific antigen in benign and malignant diseases of the prostate. *BJU International, 86*(6), 652–658.

Ramos-Fernandez, M. R., Medero-Colon, R., & Mendez-Carreno, L. (2013). Critical urologic skills and procedures in the emergency department. *Emergency Medicine Clinics of North America, 31*(1), 237–260.

Roehrborn, C. G. (2008). BPH progression: Concept and key learning from MTOPS, ALTESS, COMBAT, and ALF-ONE. *BJU International, 101*(Suppl 3), 17–21.

Roehrborn, C. G., Malice, M., Cook, T. J., et al. (2001). Clinical predictors of spontaneous acute urinary retention in men with LUTS and clinical BPH: A comprehensive analysis of the pooled placebo groups of several large clinical trials. *Urology, 58*(2), 210–216.

Roehrborn, C. G., Siami, P., Barkin, J., et al.; CombAT Study Group. (2010). The effects of combination therapy with dutasteride and tamsulosin on clinical outcomes in men with symptomatic benign prostatic hyperplasia: 4-year results from the CombAT study. *European Urology, 57*(1), 123–131. doi: 10.1016/j.eururo.2009.09.035.

Shao, I. H., Wu, C. C., Tseng, H. J., et al. (2016). Voiding dysfunction in patients with nasal congestion treated with pseudoephedrine: A prospective study. *Drug Design Development Therapy, 10*, 2333–2339. doi: 10:2147/DDDT.S108819.

Shergill, I. S., Shaikh, T., Arya, M., et al. (2008). A training model for suprapubic catheter insertion: The UroEmerge suprapubic catheter model. *Urology, 72*(1), 196–197. doi: 10.1016/j.urology.2008.03.021.

Simsek, Y. Z., & Sureyya, K. (2016). Postoperative urinary retention and nursing approaches. *International Journal of Caring Sciences, 9*(2), 1154–1161.

Sparks, M. (2010). *Post-obstructive diuresis*. Retrieved from http://renalfellow.blogspot.ca/2010/09/post-obstructive-diuresis.html

Zeif, H. J., & Subramonian, K. (2009). Alpha blockers prior to removal of a catheter for acute urinary retention in adult men. *The Cochrane Database of Systematic Reviews*, (4), CD006744.

QUESTIONS

1. Following an assessment of urinary functioning, which patient would the continence nurse suspect as having chronic urinary retention (CUR)?
   A. A postpartum female who cannot pass urine
   B. A patient who is unable to pass urine and has a painful, palpable bladder
   C. A patient with a nonpainful palpable bladder and 300-mL residual urine
   D. A male patient with CUR who presents with an episode of AUR

2. A 69-year-old male patient is diagnosed with spontaneous acute urinary retention (AUR). What is a common cause of this condition?
   A. Benign prostatic hyperplasia
   B. Urologic intervention
   C. Anesthesia
   D. Urinary tract infection

3. Drugs with _____ effects may cause urinary retention.
   A. Cholinergic
   B. Anticholinergic
   C. Diuretics
   D. Urinary analgesics

4. Which condition is NOT a potential complication of urinary retention?
   A. Vesical calculi (bladder stones)
   B. Benign prostatic hypertrophy (BPH)
   C. Hydronephrosis
   D. Urinary tract infection

5. What property of the bladder is one of the most important factors to consider as an etiology when assessing a patient for urinary retention?
   A. Reflux
   B. Compliance
   C. Ability to concentrate urine
   D. Spasticity

6. The provider orders a bladder scan for a patient who is manifesting signs and symptoms of urinary retention with moderate discomfort. The continence care nurse notes that the findings show the volume of urine drained is a little over 1 L. What condition would the nurse suspect?
   A. Acute-on-chronic retention
   B. Acute retention
   C. Chronic urinary retention
   D. Partial urinary retention

7. Which of the following is *false* about acute urinary retention?
   A. Benign prostatic hyperplasia is a common cause in males.
   B. AUR is frequently the initial presentation in men with prostate cancer.
   C. Tricyclic antidepressants can lead to AUR.
   D. Urinary retention can occur after inguinal hernia surgery.

8. For what complication would the continence nurse monitor a patient who develops postobstructive diuresis?
   A. Hyperkalemia
   B. Hypercalcemia
   C. Hypokalemia
   D. Hypophosphatemia

9. Which of the following scenarios is not suggestive of urinary retention?
   A. Straining to void with no urine output
   B. Postvoid residual urine of >500 mL
   C. Urine output of 100 mL on catheterization
   D. Lower abdominal discomfort with marked suprapubic distention

10. A trial without catheter (TWOC) is considered for most patients with urinary retention. Which patient would the continence care nurse consider at highest risk for TWOC being unsuccessful?

    A. A patient with a drained volume >1 L

    B. A patient with UTI with no previous voiding LUTS

    C. A patient with gross constipation as a precipitating cause

    D. A patient with drained volume/postvoid residual (PVR) <1,000 mL

ANSWERS AND RATIONALES

1. C. Rationale: Hallmark symptoms of CUR are nonpainful, palpable bladder, and urinary residuals >300 mL.

2. A. Rationale: As a man ages, his prostate grows. It is very common for a 69-year-old man to have some degree of BPH, and it is possible that his prostate has grown to where it is obstructing the prostatic urethra causing AUR.

3. B. Rationale: Anticholinergic medications cause the smooth muscle of the bladder to relax and may impair the bladder's ability to contract to empty, causing retention.

4. B. Rationale: BPH is a cause of urinary retention, not a complication.

5. B. Rationale: Compliance is the bladder's ability to "stretch" to expand for volumes of urine. Without the ability to stretch, the pressure increases in the bladder along with increased volumes. The increased pressure can cause upper tract damage, that is, hydronephrosis and if untreated, permanent kidney damage.

6. A. Rationale: Since the patient has only moderate abdominal discomfort with a urinary output of >1,000 mL, likely he normally has incomplete emptying, leaving a large residual, but now the patient is unable to void at all. There is now AUR on CUR.

7. B. Rationale: Early symptoms of prostate cancer are similar to early BPH: frequent urination, weak or interrupted urine flow, or the need to straining, frequency, and nocturia. Retention is later, after the obstruction of the urethra.

8. C. Rationale: Expelling large volumes of urine and/or diarrhea causes depletion of potassium (hypokalemia).

9. C. Rationale: This is likely not retention as the bladder holds >100 mL urine and would not normally have to empty at that volume.

10. A. Rationale: The patient who drained >1 L has chronic retention and does not effectively empty his bladder. If he is in complete retention, he likely will not be successful in a TWOC. Either he has lost bladder contractility, or his prostate is so big it is causing complete obstruction.

CHAPTER 9

NEUROGENIC BLADDER: ASSESSMENT AND MANAGEMENT

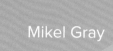

Mikel Gray

INTRODUCTION

The term "neurogenic" is defined as originating in or caused by the nerves (Oxford English Dictionary, 2014). Traditionally, the term neurogenic bladder was defined as lower urinary tract dysfunction arising from a nervous system origin (disease, disorder, or trauma of the nervous system). More recently, a working committee of the International Continence Society (ICS) has recommended renaming neurogenic bladder as neurogenic lower urinary tract dysfunction (NLUTD) (Gajewski et al., 2018). The rationale for this change is recognition of involvement of the entire lower urinary tract (bladder, urethra, urethral sphincter mechanism, and pelvic floor muscles) in what was historically described as neurogenic bladder dysfunction. For purposes of this chapter, these terms will be used interchangeably. NLUTD is caused by a variety of diseases or disorders affecting the central nervous system such as stroke, brain tumors, traumatic brain injury, parkinsonism, multiple sclerosis (MS), spinal cord injury (SCI), vertebral disk disease, transverse myelitis, polio, postpolio syndrome, Guillain-Barré syndrome, and spinal stenosis (Danforth & Ginsberg, 2014). It is also seen in infants, children, and adults with a number of congenital defects affecting central nervous system function and development, including spina bifida (especially myelomeningocele with or without hydrocephalus), anorectal malformations such as imperforate anus, and cerebral palsy. Finally, NLUTD is associated with metabolic or infectious diseases that indirectly influence central nervous system function such as diabetes mellitus or herpetic infections affecting the lumbosacral dermatomes (Powell, 2014).

Interest in the neurologic function of the bladder and the clinical challenges associated with neurogenic bladder dysfunction can be traced back to the 16th century, when Vicary described the urinary bladder as influenced by nerves that store and let go of urine (Hald & Bradley, 1982). Around the time of the American Civil War, Budge was the first to identify the bladder muscle (detrusor) as innervated by the parasympathetic nervous system (Budge, 1864). Despite these early pioneering works, care of persons with neurogenic bladder dysfunction remained rudimentary. During World War I, for example, management of NLUTD in patients with traumatic spinal cord injuries was primarily limited to indwelling catheterization or containment of urinary incontinence (Silver, 2011), although at least one surgeon described intermittent catheterization for management of neurogenic bladder dysfunction in five men with spinal cord injuries as early as 1889 (Thorburn, 1889).

Despite these early efforts, 60% of individuals suffering from spinal cord trauma died of complications within 3 years of their injury; urinary tract infection (UTI) in the era before antibiotic medications was a leading cause of these deaths (Bodner, 2009). Advances in health care, along with a sharp increase in the number of men who suffered from traumatic SCI, occurred during World War II and the Korean War. As a result, a number of hospital-based units were created across the globe dedicated to caring for persons with spinal cord injuries, including the Veteran's Administration Hospital in Long Beach, CA (Donovan, 2007). The unit in California was led by a urologist and a neurologist (E. Bors and A. Comarr, respectively), who focused on management of neurogenic bladder dysfunction in particular. Their research, combined with advances in antimicrobial therapy to manage UTI (Bors & Comarr, 1971), recent work in intermittent catheterization in 1966 by Guttman (Guttman & Frankel, 1966), and the popularization of clean intermittent catheterization (CIC) by Lapides (Lapides et al., 1972) in the early 1970s, provide the cornerstones of NLUTD that we continue to use in the 21st century.

CLASSIFICATION SYSTEMS FOR NEUROGENIC BLADDER DYSFUNCTION

Various classification systems for neurogenic bladder dysfunction have been proposed (Bors & Comarr, 1971; Lapides et al., 1972). While all of these systems provide clinically relevant insights, none enjoys widespread use owing to their inability to incorporate all of the factors that influence persons with NLUTD, including the variable effects of the underlying disease, the effects of bladder outlet obstruction on lower urinary tract dysfunction, and changes occurring over time, especially when NLUTD begins as an infant or child. Despite their lack of widespread use, two systems have led to the incorporation of concepts that remain widely used for NLUTD management today.

UPPER VERSUS LOWER MOTOR NEURON DYSFUNCTION

Bors and Comarr (1971) pioneered the concept of upper versus lower motor neuron NLUTD based on their clinical experiences with patients with spinal cord injuries. An upper motor neuron neurogenic bladder is characterized by detrusor overactivity (detrusor contraction without voluntary control), while the lower motor neuron neurogenic bladder is characterized by a noncontracting (underactive, acontractile, or areflexic) detrusor. They further described neurogenic bladders as balanced or imbalanced. A balanced bladder can be roughly defined as one that empties completely and is not associated with recurring UTI or upper urinary tract distress, while an imbalanced bladder does not empty completely and is associated with recurring UTI and/or upper urinary tract distress. Although continence clinicians do not use these concepts to describe NLUTD, they are sometimes used by neurosurgeons or rehabilitation clinicians in order to broadly categorize neurogenic bladder dysfunction.

LAPIDES CLASSIFICATION SYSTEM

Lapides (1970) also developed a taxonomy for classifying neurogenic bladder dysfunction. He included a description for reflex neurogenic bladder, which was characterized by detrusor overactivity and incoordination between the detrusor muscle and the striated sphincter mechanism, also referred to as detrusor sphincter dyssynergia. The term "reflex incontinence" remains widely used in many medical specialties, and it is a nursing diagnosis recognized by the North American Nursing Diagnosis Association and incorporated into the NIC and NOC nursing care schema (Gray, 2008).

URINARY CONTINENCE: A NEUROLOGIC PERSPECTIVE

Normal lower urinary tract function can be divided into two stages: storage and evacuation (de Groat et al., 2015; Gray, 2007). During bladder storage, the detrusor muscle remains in a relaxed state, allowing the upper urinary tracts to slowly fill the bladder with urine, while the urethral sphincter mechanism remains in a tonic (closed) state, preventing urinary leakage with physical activity. During the evacuation (voiding) phase, the detrusor muscle contracts and the urethral sphincter mechanism relaxes under neurological control, allowing urine to be expelled from the bladder via the urethra without excessive resistance. Urinary continence and effective bladder evacuation are based on three factors: anatomic integrity of the urinary system, neurological control of the detrusor muscles, and an intact urethral sphincter mechanism. For the purposes of this chapter focusing on NLUTD, a brief discussion of the physiology of the continent person will be limited to neurological control of the detrusor muscle and urethral sphincter mechanism.

HISTOLOGY OF DETRUSOR MUSCLE

The detrusor is a smooth muscle, but it has several properties that distinguish it from other smooth muscle found in the gastrointestinal tract or ureters. Specifically, the detrusor is characterized as single unit rather than multiunit smooth muscle (Yoshimura & Chancellor, 2012). Multiunit smooth muscle cells, such as those found in the ureter or intestinal tract, are linked electrically so that contraction in one smooth muscle cell (typically occurring in response to stretch) leads to a peristaltic contraction occurring independently of input from the neurological system (Weiss, 2012). These contractions are partly attributable to gap junctions; cytoplasmic bridges create communication that is independent of nervous system input. This coupling is so efficient that a ureter transplanted along with a donor kidney will continue to transport urine from the renal pelvis through the ureter and into the bladder despite being housed in a new host body. Such an arrangement would be disastrous to continence; a multiunit detrusor muscle would contract as it is filled with urine, resulting in involuntary voiding. Instead, the detrusor muscle has a single-unit arrangement, with a nearly 1:1 ratio of smooth muscle cells to nerve endings (neuromuscular junctions), which provides the neurological governance necessary for the voluntary control of detrusor muscle contractions essential to urinary continence.

NEUROTRANSMITTERS

The nervous system regulates relaxation and contraction of the urinary bladder using chemical messengers called neurotransmitters (Gray, 2007; Yoshimura & Chancellor, 2012). These neurotransmitters act at specific receptor sites on the smooth muscle; they carry two basic messages: contract or relax. The neurotransmitter acetylcholine acts at muscarinic receptor sites (mainly M2 and M3 receptor subtypes) on the detrusor muscle cell, signaling the bladder to contract (Andersson, 2011; de Groat et al., 2015; Frazier et al., 2008; Gray, 2007; Yoshimura & Chancellor, 2012). The neurotransmitter norepinephrine (also referred to as noradrenaline) acts on beta-3 adrenergic receptor sites on the detrusor smooth muscle cell, signaling the bladder to relax (de Groat et al., 2015; Ursino et al., 2009). Muscarinic and beta-adrenergic receptors are not only essential to neurological control of the detrusor muscle, they are also important pharmacologic targets for management of NLUTD.

URETHRAL SPHINCTER MECHANISM

The urethral sphincter mechanism is best conceptualized as containing two components: elements of compression and muscular elements that promote active urethral closure in response to physical exertion (Gray et al., 1995b). Smooth muscle cells within the bladder base, bladder neck, and proximal urethra are present in women and men. They are particularly abundant in the bladder neck and prostatic urethra in men (Yamata & Ito, 2011). Alpha-1 adrenergic receptors located on these urethral smooth cells cause muscle contraction and urethral closure in response to the neurotransmitter norepinephrine (Kojima et al., 2009). The urethral sphincter mechanism also contains periurethral striated muscle and a rhabdosphincter (also referred to as the external sphincter, sphincter urethrae, or urogenital diaphragm). These muscle cells have nicotinic receptors that react to the neurotransmitter acetylcholine, resulting in contraction of the periurethral and rhabdosphincter muscles and closure of the sphincter mechanism. No drug has been developed that is able to safely change the behavior of the striated muscles of the sphincter mechanism, but the alpha-1 adrenergic blocking drugs are used to reduce urethral resistance to urinary outflow in selected patients with neurogenic bladder.

BLADDER–SPHINCTER COORDINATION

The central nervous system is ultimately responsible for coordinating lower urinary tract function so that the bladder fills at low pressures with low tone within the detrusor coupled with closure of the urethral sphincter mechanism via contraction of smooth and striated muscles in the bladder sphincter mechanism (de Groat et al., 2015; de Groat & Wickens, 2013; Gray, 2007; Griffiths & Fowler, 2013; Yoshimura & Chancellor, 2012). Likewise, the act of voiding relies on input from the central nervous system, resulting in relaxation of smooth and striated muscle within the urethral sphincter mechanism and contraction of the detrusor muscle.

> ### KEY POINT
>
> Effective bladder emptying is dependent on both sphincter relaxation and detrusor muscle contraction.

VOLUNTARY CONTROL AND THE CENTRAL NERVOUS SYSTEM

Prior to toilet training, bladder filling and micturition follow a regular cycle of filling and evacuation without voluntary control. Lower urinary tract function is coordinated by neurons in the brain stem; collectively referred to as the pontine micturition center (PMC) and the periaqueductal gray (PAG) matter (de Groat & Wickens, 2013; Zare et al., 2019). Similar to the other areas in the brain, the PAG is functionally divided into groups (columns) of neurons that are connected to neurons in other areas of the brainstem that regulate lower urinary tract function (PMC and M region), the spine and peripheral nerves, and higher brain areas (thalamus, hypothalamus, cingulate gyrus, sulcus, prefrontal area of cerebral cortex). The PAG acts as a bridge between the central nervous system, brain, and peripheral nerves regulating bladder function, the PMC that coordinates contraction and relaxation of the detrusor and urethral sphincter mechanism, and the M center that promotes bladder storage (pontine storage center or PSC). As the bladder fills and stores urine, its walls are gradually stretched, provoking afferent (sensory) signals that enter the central nervous system in the sacral spinal cord (segments S2–S4) decussate (cross over) and travel the PAG, alerting the maturing brain to the presence of urine in the lower urinary tract. Storage of urine in the bladder is coordinated by the PAG and M region (PSC) via connections to the sympathetic nervous system; these nerves exit the spinal cord at thoracolumbar segments T10–L2 via the hypogastric nerve and terminate in the bladder wall (detrusor muscle). Other nerves exit the spine at sacral spinal segments S1–S3 enervating the smooth and striated muscles of the urethral sphincter mechanism and periurethral muscles with the pelvic floor, ensuring closure of the urethral sphincter mechanism during bladder storage/filling. Approximately once an hour (pending fluid intake and hydration), the bladder is sufficiently stretched and afferent signals sufficiently strong that micturition is provoked without voluntary control. Micturition occurs under the control of neurons in the PAG and PMC via connections to the parasympathetic nervous system; these nerves exit sacral spinal segments (S2–S4), traveling to the bladder via the pelvic nerve and resulting in contraction of the detrusor muscle along with relaxation of the urethral sphincter mechanism.

Successful toilet training is characterized by voluntary control over the lower urinary tract that persists throughout adulthood. Advances in functional brain imaging have vastly increased our understanding of how the brain influences both urine filling and storage and micturition in the continent child or adult (Griffiths & Fowler, 2013). While control of bladder filling and the micturition reflex are centered in the PAG, neurons in the frontal cortex, cingulate gyrus, and basal ganglia influence bladder filling/storage and voiding in the toilet trained child and continent adult. Multiple areas in the brain interact to control urine storage and evacuation in the adult; they can be roughly divided into three pathways (Arya & Weissbart, 2017).

The first pathway or circuit is active during normal lower urinary tract function (i.e., absence of UTI, neurologic disease, or trauma) (Arya & Weissbart, 2017; Griffiths, 2015). Afferent signals from the bladder respond to stretch and the chemical composition of urine; these signals travel to the PAG and are transmitted to the thalamus and insula to the prefrontal cortex and multiple other areas in the brain. The cerebral cortex (detrusor motor area in the medial prefrontal cortex) is part of the brain's executive decision-making center that employs a complex algorithm of psychosocial, cultural, and physiologic considerations that contribute to the decision to urinate. These factors include access to the proper room for voiding, arrangement of clothing to allow toileting, privacy during the act of micturition, and strength of the desire to urinate. If voiding is deemed appropriate, efferent nervous signals are sent to the PAG activating detrusor contraction and coordinate relaxation of the urethral sphincter mechanism. While our understanding of the precise pathways and mechanisms that modulate lower urinary tract function in the continent adult are not complete, current research indicates that the brain is essential for postponement of urination until micturition is deemed important *and* activation of effective voiding including a well-sustained detrusor contraction necessary for complete bladder emptying. Dysfunction of the brain seen in various dementias including Alzheimer disease is characterized by *both* neurogenic detrusor overactivity (loss of control over timing of micturition) and underactive bladder function (loss of a strong signal from the brain to bladder prompting a well-sustained detrusor contraction) required for effective bladder emptying with voluntary voiding. If micturition is deemed not appropriate (no access to a toilet, clothing not ready, timing not appropriate), inhibitory signals from the detrusor motor are in the prefrontal cortex signal the PAG, resulting in inhibition of detrusor contraction and sphincter relaxation via the PMC.

A second circuit or pathway is activated when the individual perceives a strong or imminent desire to urinate (Arya & Weissbart, 2017; Griffiths, 2015). In this case, afferent signals reach the dorsal anterior cingulate gyrus that, in turn, activates a different area of the cerebral cortex (supplementary motor area) that provokes increased sympathetic nervous system activity, and contraction of the smooth and striated muscle of the urethral sphincter mechanism. This system is activated when a patient is taught to forcefully and repeatedly contract the pelvic floor muscles as part of urge inhibition.

A third circuit or pathway activates neurons in the hippocampus, amygdala, and hypothalamus (Arya & Weissbart, 2017; Griffiths, 2015). Our understanding of this pathway is especially incomplete; it is hypothesized to act as a safety mechanism when conscious sensations of bladder filling are lost. For example, this circuit may become active following a stroke or traumatic brain injury resulting in micturition without voluntary control. This pathway is also postulated to be active in persons with overactive bladder dysfunction and bladder pain syndrome (interstitial cystitis).

KEY POINT

The ability to voluntarily initiate voiding and to delay voiding until a socially appropriate time and place requires modulation of multiple areas of the brain including the prefrontal cortex and intact pathways between the brain, brainstem, spine, and peripheral nerves in the lower urinary tract.

ETIOLOGY AND PATHOPHYSIOLOGY OF NEUROGENIC BLADDER DYSFUNCTION

Trauma or disease affecting the brain, spinal cord, or the rich supply of peripheral nerves required for healthy lower urinary tract function causes NLUTD. The nature of this dysfunction is dictated by the location and nature of the underlying neurological disorder and lower urinary tract function at the time of the neurological disorder (**Fig. 9-1**).

While classification schemas for neurogenic bladder dysfunction have failed to gain widespread use, the urodynamic-based system for neurogenic and non-NLUTD proposed by Wein (1981) will be incorporated in this chapter because of its ability to classify the various pathophysiologic mechanisms that characterize neurogenic bladder dysfunction (**Table 9-1**). The Wein classification system is based on urodynamic findings, a diagnostic test frequently used to evaluate neurogenic bladder dysfunction; it is particularly useful for characterizing the various dysfunctions that lead to urinary incontinence or retention seen with neurogenic bladder dysfunction. This discussion will be followed by an overview of the link between neurogenic bladder and upper urinary tract distress and its management.

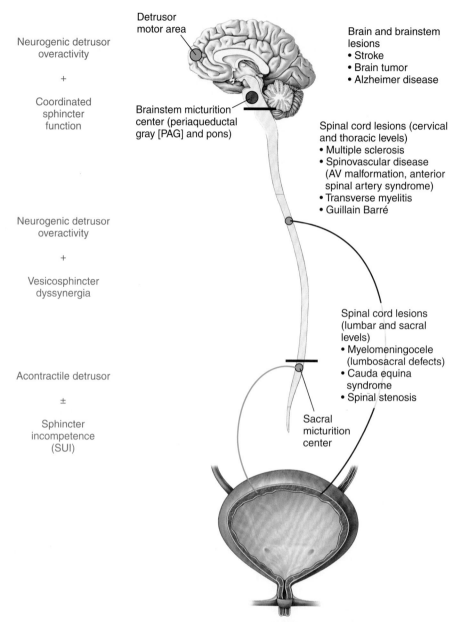

Neurogenic detrusor
overactivity

+

Coordinated
sphincter
function

Detrusor
motor area

Brainstem micturition
center (periaqueductal
gray [PAG] and pons)

Brain and brainstem
lesions
• Stroke
• Brain tumor
• Alzheimer disease

Spinal cord lesions (cervical
and thoracic levels)
• Multiple sclerosis
• Spinovascular disease
  (AV malformation, anterior
  spinal artery syndrome)
• Transverse myelitis
• Guillain Barré

Neurogenic detrusor
overactivity

+

Vesicosphincter
dyssynergia

Acontractile detrusor

±

Sphincter
incompetence
(SUI)

Spinal cord lesions
(lumbar and sacral
levels)
• Myelomeningocele
  (lumbosacral defects)
• Cauda equina
  syndrome
• Spinal stenosis

Sacral
micturition
center

FIGURE 9-1. Neurological Disorders Associated with Neurogenic Detrusor Overactivity and Urgency and/or Urge Urinary Incontinence. (Modified from McConnell, T. H., & Hull, K. L. (2010). *Human form, human function: Essentials of anatomy & physiology*. Philadelphia, PA: Lippincott Williams & Wilkins.)

KEY POINT

The Wein classification system is based on urodynamic findings and classifies lower urinary tract dysfunction as one of the following: failure to store because of the bladder; failure to store because of the sphincter; failure to empty because of the bladder; and failure to empty because of the sphincter.

FAILURE TO STORE URINE BECAUSE OF THE BLADDER

Failure to store urine because of the bladder is caused by a condition called detrusor overactivity (Abrams et al.,

2002; Wein, 1981). Detrusor overactivity is defined as an involuntary detrusor contraction of sufficient magnitude to cause urgency and/or urinary leakage. Neurogenic detrusor overactivity is defined as an overactive detrusor contraction associated with NLUTD. It is one of the most common dysfunctions among patients with neurogenic bladder. For example, it has been found in 50.9% of patients with MS, 52.3% of patients with SCI, 33.1% of persons with parkinsonism, and 23.6% of all patients who experience a stroke (Ruffion et al., 2013).

Among patients with preserved sensations of the lower urinary tract, detrusor overactivity is typically associated with daytime voiding frequency (more than eight

TABLE 9-1 WEIN'S URODYNAMICS-BASED CLASSIFICATION SYSTEM FOR NEUROGENIC VOIDING DYSFUNCTION

FAILURE TO STORE URINE	FAILURE TO EMPTY URINE
Because of the bladder (Neurogenic detrusor overactivity, low bladder wall compliance) [Urge urinary incontinence, urgency] [Reflex urinary incontinence]	Because of the bladder (Detrusor underactivity*) [Urinary retention†]
Because of the outlet (Urethral sphincter mechanism incompetence) [Stress urinary incontinence]	Because of the outlet (Bladder outlet obstruction) [Urinary retention†]

() = urodynamic abnormality.
[] = primary lower urinary tract symptom.
*Detrusor underactivity is defined as incomplete bladder emptying due to poor detrusor contraction strength or acontractile or hypocontractile detrusor.
†Urinary retention defined as inability to expel any urine from the bladder or chronic residual urine volumes despite the ability to partially evacuate urine from the bladder via micturition.
Data from Wein, A. J. (1981). Classification of neurogenic voiding dysfunction. *Journal of Urology, 125*(5), 605–609.

voids in a 24-hour period or voiding more often than every 2 hours while awake), nocturia (three or more episodes per night), and urgency (a sudden and compelling desire to urinate that cannot be deferred), with or without urge incontinence (urinary leakage associated with urgency). This cluster of lower urinary tract symptoms (LUTS) has been labeled overactive bladder (Abrams et al., 2002). (Refer to Chapter 7 for a more detailed discussion of the assessment and management of this prevalent form of incontinence.) **Figure 9-1** lists neurological disorders associated with neurogenic detrusor overactivity and urgency and/or urge urinary incontinence.

KEY POINT

Neurogenic detrusor overactivity is defined as bladder overactivity associated with neurogenic impairment; it can cause urgency, frequency, nocturia, and urge incontinence in the patient with intact sensation or incontinence without sensory awareness in those with diminished or absent sensation.

Depending on the underlying neurological disorder, persons with neurogenic bladder dysfunction also may experience neurogenic detrusor overactivity with absent or markedly decreased sensations of bladder filling. In contrast to urge incontinence, these individuals experience urinary incontinence without sensory awareness, although clinical experience reveals that some patients with SCI report atypical sensations associated with detrusor overactivity such as tingling of the jaw or side of the face. Rather than nocturia, these individuals often experience nocturnal enuresis. Neurogenic detrusor

overactivity with sensory impairment frequently occurs in patients with paralyzing spinal disorders such as SCI or transverse myelitis (**Fig. 9-1**) (Martens et al., 2010).

FAILURE TO STORE URINE BECAUSE OF THE OUTLET

Failure to store because of the outlet is caused by incompetence of the urethral sphincter mechanism, which results in stress urinary incontinence (Wein, 1981). Stress urinary incontinence presents as a LUTS or sign on physical assessment or as a urodynamic finding (Abrams et al., 2002). The symptom of stress incontinence is defined as the report of urine loss with coughing, sneezing, or physical activity. The sign of stress urinary incontinence occurs when a clinician observes urinary leakage from the urethra when the patient is asked to raise abdominal pressures by coughing or performing a Valsalva maneuver. Two urodynamic techniques, abdominal leak point pressure testing (Gray, 2011a) and urethral pressure profile (Gray, 2011b), are used to evaluate urodynamic stress urinary incontinence. Urodynamic stress incontinence is defined as urine loss in response to a rise in abdominal pressure or as part of a negative pressure transmission ratio on urethral pressure profilometry.

Stress urinary incontinence is especially prevalent in adult women (see Chapter 11 for a detailed discussion of the assessment and management of stress UI in women). Among patients with neurogenic bladder dysfunction, urethral sphincter incompetence occurs when disease or trauma damages lumbosacral spinal segments (including Onuf nucleus), leading to denervation of the striated sphincter muscle (Groen et al., 2012; Kulwin et al., 2013). The resulting stress urinary incontinence varies from mild leakage to nearly continuous urine loss when sphincter function is severely compromised. Neurological conditions associated with denervation of Onuf nucleus and stress urinary incontinence are shown in **Figure 9-1**.

KEY POINT

Stress incontinence (leakage with increased intra-abdominal pressure) is common among individuals with neurogenic bladder, due to loss of voluntary sphincter control caused by denervation of the striated sphincter mechanism.

In addition to denervation of the striated muscle component of the sphincter mechanism, the choice of bladder management program may result in erosion of the urethra and sphincter. Long-term indwelling catheterization has been linked to urethral erosion in both women and men; it often leads to a condition called catheter "bypassing," defined as leakage around an indwelling catheter associated with local damage or erosion of the urethral sphincter mechanism (Moore & Rayome, 1995).

In severe cases, the entire urethra is involved, leading to a condition called "stove-pipe" urethra where the urethra is unable to exert any closure pressure, resulting in continuous urinary leakage (Chapple et al., 2009).

FAILURE TO EMPTY BECAUSE OF THE BLADDER

Contraction of the detrusor muscle is an essential component of normal micturition. Failure to empty because of the bladder is caused by an underactive detrusor (Wein, 1981). Detrusor underactivity is defined as a contraction that has inadequate strength and/or duration to empty the bladder of urine in a reasonable period of time (Abrams et al., 2002; Aizawa & Igawa, 2017). Assessment of the strength of a detrusor contraction is challenging; LUTS commonly associated with detrusor underactivity include weak urinary stream, terminal dribble, postvoid dribbling, difficulty urinating, and feelings of incomplete bladder emptying. An elevated urinary residual volume is a common sign of detrusor underactivity, but the presence of an elevated residual volume is not exclusively caused by an underactive detrusor; incomplete bladder emptying is also caused by bladder outlet obstruction or a combination of detrusor underactivity and obstruction (Gray, 2010, 2012a,b).

Uroflowmetry is often used to evaluate incomplete bladder emptying, but it cannot differentiate an abnormal flow rate or elevated postvoid residual volume caused by detrusor underactivity from one caused by bladder outlet obstruction (Gray, 2010). The voiding pressure flow study provides a more definitive evaluation of detrusor underactivity; this test is used to measure the amplitude (maximal strength) and duration of a detrusor contraction during micturition (Gray, 2012a,b). Unfortunately, normal values for these parameters vary based on age and gender and have not been firmly established. In addition, the performance of the detrusor contraction, similar to all other smooth or striated muscles of the body, varies widely as evidenced by the widely variable residual volumes measured over multiple voiding episodes (Griffiths et al., 1996; Saaby & Lose, 2012).

> ### KEY POINT
>
> Detrusor underactivity refers to detrusor contractions that lack the strength and duration to effectively empty the bladder in a reasonable period of time.

Detrusor underactivity is prevalent in patients with neurogenic bladder dysfunction; conditions commonly associated with detrusor underactivity include MS, dementia/Alzheimer disease, Parkinson disease, and disorders affecting lower spinal segments such as spinal stenosis or tethered spinal cord (Aizawa & Igawa, 2017; Drake et al., 2014; van Koeveringe et al., 2011). Additional factors leading to detrusor underactivity in patients with neurogenic bladder dysfunction include constipation, use of drugs with anticholinergic activity, including the antimuscarinics, which are commonly used in the management of neurogenic detrusor overactivity.

FAILURE TO EMPTY BECAUSE OF THE OUTLET

Failure to empty because of the outlet occurs when urethral resistance is great enough to interfere with complete and efficient micturition (Wein, 1981). Similar to detrusor underactivity, there are no specific LUTS or physical signs that can reliably diagnose bladder outlet obstruction. Instead, the LUTS most closely associated with bladder outlet obstruction are not distinguishable as those linked with detrusor underactivity. Presence of an elevated residual urine volume is unreliable since it does not differentiate incomplete bladder emptying because of the outlet from incomplete emptying due to detrusor underactivity. Uroflowmetry detects abnormal flow rates, but it does not identify the cause of the abnormal flow (Gray, 2012b). Therefore, diagnosis of the presence and magnitude of bladder outlet obstruction relies on the voiding pressure flow study, preferably aided by a more quantitative analysis using a voiding pressure nomogram (Gray, 2012a,b).

A variety of factors can obstruct the bladder outlet, but the condition most closely associated with neurogenic bladder dysfunction is detrusor external sphincter dyssynergia, that is, loss of coordination between the detrusor muscle and external (striated) sphincter. Detrusor sphincter dyssynergia (also called vesicosphincter dyssynergia or detrusor-striated sphincter dyssynergia) occurs when the detrusor and striated sphincter contract simultaneously during micturition. Simultaneous contraction creates a functional obstruction of the bladder outlet that interferes with bladder emptying and increases the risk for UTI (Ahmed et al., 2006; Bacsu et al., 2012). It is caused by trauma or disease affecting spinal segments above S2 (suprasacral lesions) and below spinal segment C2.

In the continent individual, the PMC coordinates reflex activity of the detrusor and urethral sphincter mechanisms so that the urethral sphincter mechanism is closed (contracted) during bladder filling/storage and open (relaxed) during micturition. During voiding, the detrusor muscle contracts and the urethral sphincter mechanism opens (relaxes), enabling unobstructed outflow of urine. Spinal lesions below the brain stem and above the sacral micturition center (S2–S4) interfere with the pons' ability to coordinate detrusor and sphincter responses, resulting in incoordination (dyssynergia) between these elements of the lower urinary tract. Multiple neurological conditions cause neurogenic bladder dysfunction with detrusor sphincter dyssynergia. Approximately 75% to

87% of patients with spinal cord injuries above spinal segment S2, 35% of patients with MS, and 25% of patients with spina bifida have detrusor sphincter dyssynergia (Ahmed et al., 2006; De Seze et al., 2007; Weld et al., 2000).

> ## KEY POINT
>
> In the patient with neurogenic bladder dysfunction, failure to empty due to the sphincter is most commonly the result of detrusor external sphincter dyssynergia (persistent contraction of the sphincter during detrusor contraction), resulting from a lesion between the sacral cord and the pons.

Bladder neck dyssynergia (also called detrusor bladder neck dyssynergia) is defined as failure of the smooth muscle of the urethra to relax during a detrusor contraction (Stohrer et al., 1999). Similar to dyssynergia between the detrusor muscle and the striated sphincter, detrusor bladder neck dyssynergia increases resistance within the urethral sphincter mechanism, obstructing the bladder outlet and interfering with bladder emptying. It is uncommon in men without neurogenic bladder dysfunction and extremely rare in neurologically normal women (Coblentz & Gray, 2001; Yamanishi et al., 1997). Detrusor bladder neck dyssynergia is seen in patients with SCI; it is associated with complete spinal injuries occurring above spinal segment S2 and incomplete spinal injuries (usually T9 or lower) (Al-Ali & Haddad, 1996; Schurch et al., 1994).

Benign prostate hypertrophy (BPH) is defined as enlargement of the prostate and increased tone in the prostatic urethra, which may result in obstruction of the bladder outlet and a variety of LUTS. This condition is discussed in detail in Chapters 8 and 10. Nevertheless, it is included in this discussion because of its prevalence in aging men with parkinsonism, stroke, and dementia resulting in neurogenic bladder dysfunction. In addition, there is a growing body of evidence suggesting that BPH causes changes in the detrusor muscle that alter not only the local response of smooth muscle cells to the various neurotransmitters but also the spinal reflexes that regulate bladder filling/storage and micturition (Chai et al., 1998; Mirone et al., 2007).

NEUROGENIC BLADDER DYSFUNCTION AS A CAUSE OF UPPER URINARY TRACT DISTRESS

Upper urinary tract distress is defined as impaired function of the upper urinary tracts (the paired kidneys, renal pelves, and ureters), associated with neurogenic bladder dysfunction (Gray, 2011a; Killorin et al., 1992; Sung et al., 2018). Clinical manifestations include febrile UTI (recurring or chronic pyelonephritis), vesicoureteral reflux, ureterohydronephrosis, and impaired renal function. Two components of neurogenic bladder dysfunction, low

bladder wall compliance and increased urethral resistance (bladder outlet obstruction), increase the likelihood of upper urinary tract distress in patients with neurogenic bladder dysfunction (Ghoniem et al., 1989; McGuire et al., 1981; Nseyo & Santiago-Lastra, 2017; Perez et al., 1993).

Bladder wall compliance is defined as the relationship between bladder volume and intravesical pressure during bladder filling/storage (Gray, 2011a; Hosker et al., 2009). In the clinical setting, it is measured during urodynamic testing (Chapter 5). In the healthy bladder, intravesical pressures remain low despite filling to as much as 600 mL or more. Low bladder wall compliance occurs when intravesical pressures rise in proportion with bladder filling; whole bladder compliance ≤10 mL/cm H_2O or a detrusor pressure >40 cm H_2O is associated with increased risk for upper urinary tract distress (Gray, 2011a). Two characteristics of the bladder wall affect bladder compliance: detrusor smooth muscle tone and the viscoelastic properties of the vesical wall. In a person with normal bladder wall compliance, the detrusor muscle remains in a relaxed state until its owner makes a voluntary decision to urinate, and the viscoelastic components of the bladder wall (primarily collagen and elastin proteins) promote passive filling at low intravesical pressures.

> ## KEY POINT
>
> Neurogenic bladder dysfunction is a risk factor for upper tract distress, defined as impaired renal function and an increased risk for febrile urinary tract infection.

Urethral resistance is defined as the detrusor pressure required to overcome the urethral sphincter mechanism and create urinary flow (Gray, 2011b; Hosker et al., 2009; Schafer, 1995). In the person with normal lower urinary tract function, urethral resistance is defined as the magnitude of detrusor pressure required to open the urethra and initiate urine flow (voiding); it is measured during urodynamic testing as the urethral opening pressure (Gray, 2011b, 2012a,b). Bladder outlet obstruction is defined as increased resistance to urethral opening and urinary outflow (failure to empty because of the outlet). As noted previously, common causes of bladder outlet obstruction in the patient with neurogenic bladder dysfunction include detrusor sphincter dyssynergia and prostatic hyperplasia in aging men. However, the magnitude of urethral resistance is also clinically relevant in patients with neurogenic bladder and underactive detrusor function (failure to empty because of the bladder), along with low bladder wall compliance. Among these patients, urethral resistance is measured via the detrusor leak point pressure, defined as the sustained detrusor pressure required to open the urethra and create overflow incontinence (Ghoniem et al., 1989; Gray, 2011b McGuire et al., 1981).

Bladder outlet obstruction with an elevated urethral opening pressure or low bladder wall compliance with an elevated detrusor leak point pressure is sometimes described as an indicator of *hostile bladder function*, indicating a bladder that is likely to produce upper urinary tract distress unless a bladder management program is implemented to reduce urethral opening and/or detrusor leak point pressures while enhancing bladder wall compliance in order to prevent or alleviate upper urinary tract distress (Morrisroe et al., 2005; Perez et al., 1993).

KEY POINT

Bladder outlet obstruction resulting in elevated detrusor pressures and/or low bladder wall compliance are examples of *hostile bladder conditions* that are common among individuals with neurogenic bladder dysfunction. (Hostile bladder conditions are those that increase the risk of upper tract distress.)

ASSESSMENT OF THE PATIENT WITH NEUROGENIC BLADDER: GENERAL PRINCIPLES

Chapter 4 provides a detailed discussion of the assessment of the patient with urinary incontinence, and the principles and approaches described in that chapter apply to all patients with neurogenic bladder dysfunction. The brief discussion in this chapter will focus on components of the overall assessment unique to patients with neurogenic bladder dysfunction.

FOCUSED HISTORY: BLADDER MANAGEMENT PROGRAM

The focused history for patients with urinary incontinence must include assessment of LUTS (Abrams et al., 2002). Pertinent LUTS are subdivided into storage symptoms (daytime voiding frequency, nocturia, urgency, along with stress, urge, or mixed incontinence and incontinence without sensory awareness), voiding LUTS (weak or intermittent urinary stream, hesitancy, and terminal dribbling), and postvoid LUTS (feelings of incomplete bladder emptying and postvoid dribbling). However, many patients with neurogenic bladder dysfunction do not experience the typical cycle of bladder function: filling/storage, followed by micturition, followed by another cycle beginning with bladder filling/storage. Instead, they rely on a specific program to manage their bladder such as intermittent catheterization, involuntary voiding into an external collection device or body worn absorbent product (BWAP), indwelling catheterization, or some combination of these management strategies.

Therefore, it is important to first determine if the patient with neurogenic bladder dysfunction manages her or his bladder via spontaneous voiding. If this is not the case, questions about LUTS should be tailored to account for presence of a bladder management program. For example, patients who perform CIC should be queried about the frequency of catheterization, the size, length, and type of catheter used, and whether they use a new catheter each time they catheterize or clean and reuse catheters. Persons who rely on CIC should also be asked if they void or experience urinary incontinence between catheterizations or whether they rely on CIC exclusively for bladder emptying. The person who empties his or her bladder using CIC should be asked about nighttime urinary incontinence. While most are able to sleep through the night without catheterizing, some will report the need to catheterize once or more per night, and others (especially children with spina bifida) may be drained with an indwelling catheter that remains in place overnight, followed by resumption of CIC during waking hours.

KEY POINT

When conducting the interview for an individual with neurogenic bladder dysfunction, the nurse should ask about the patient's bladder management program (spontaneous voiding, clean intermittent catheterization, involuntary voiding into a collection device, etc.) as well as any problems or concerns associated with the current management program.

Patients who void into an external collection device or BWAP should be asked about the type of external collective device that they use (condom catheter or nonsheath external collection device), how often they change their external collection device, and whether they experience leakage due to an incomplete seal between device and penis (Gray et al., 2016). Those who involuntarily void into BWAP should be asked about the type of product they use, the average number used daily, and perceptions of wetness when the product is changed. The patient and care provider should be asked about skin problems associated with use of an external collection device or absorptive brief. They should also be asked if they perform CIC in addition to voiding into an external collection device.

Persons with neurogenic bladder dysfunction who use a long-term indwelling catheter should be asked about his or her catheterization site (urethral or suprapubic), the cumulative length of time that they have worn an indwelling catheter, the reason they use this bladder management strategy, and problems associated with catheter use. The average frequency of catheter changes should be explored, as well as experiences with catheter blockage resulting in the need to change the catheter urgently. They should be asked about possible problems associated with long-term catheterization including bypassing (leaking around the catheter), bladder spasms with leakage or pain, and episodes of hematuria. Patients using long-term indwelling catheters should be asked about his or her usual drainage system, including use of leg bags, overnight drainage bags, or belly bags. Problems associated with the urinary drainage system should be discussed, including leaks because of problems with their drainage system and skin problems related to leg bag straps (Fowler et al., 2014; Ostaszkiewicz & Paterson, 2012). Nighttime urinary drainage habits should be queried, along with strategies for repeated use of urinary drainage bags and how they are cleaned and prepared for reuse. Patients should be asked about catheter care (how the individual and/or care provider cleanses the perineal skin and exposed portion of the catheter) and how they manage the catheter during general bathing.

PHYSICAL ASSESSMENT: COGNITION, DEXTERITY, AND MOBILITY, AND NATURAL HISTORY OF UNDERLYING DISEASE

Functional and cognitive assessments are routine components of the physical assessment for all patients with urinary incontinence, and they are especially important for the patient with neurogenic bladder dysfunction. Because many patients with neurogenic bladder dysfunction experience incontinence without sensory awareness, a combination of urinary incontinence and incomplete bladder emptying, or hostile neurogenic bladder dysfunction with an increased risk of upper urinary tract distress, CIC is more widely used for bladder management in this population than in able-bodied, community-dwelling persons. Therefore, physical assessment of the person with neurogenic bladder dysfunction often includes evaluation of suitability for CIC or the need for long-term indwelling catheter use. This assessment should include consideration of body habitus, the physical ability of the patient to perform CIC, motivation to perform CIC, and the availability of a caregiver (partner, family member, paid care provider) to perform CIC if the patient is transiently unable to perform catheterization or able to perform the procedure only with some level of assistance.

The natural history of the underlying neurologic disorder should also be evaluated when considering CIC versus indwelling catheter use in selected patients with neurogenic bladder. For example, the person with a stable neurologic lesion such as a SCI resulting in paraplegia or relapsing–remitting MS may be expected to retain the ability to perform CIC over an extended period of time (Castel-Lacanal et al., 2013; Gray et al., 1995a). In contrast, the person with rapid physical deterioration due to progressive MS or recently diagnosed Guillain-Barré disease may only be able to perform CIC for a comparatively brief period of time before upper extremity function becomes so compromised that CIC is no longer possible. In this case, indwelling catheter use may be considered, provided all other options for bladder management have been explored and found not feasible.

KEY POINT

When conducting the physical assessment of an individual with neurogenic bladder, it is particularly important to assess functional status (mobility and dexterity), specifically the ability to access the urethra and perform intermittent catheterization.

Urinalysis Screening

Queries regarding recurrent UTI and screening urinalysis are routine components of evaluation in the community-dwelling adult with urinary incontinence (Gormley et al., 2014; Lucas et al., 2013). UTI is a frequent complication of neurogenic bladder dysfunction, and it is the most prevalent urologic complication among patients who use indwelling catheters (Gormley, 2010; Vasudeva & Madersbacher, 2014). Nevertheless, the purpose of the urinalysis and the use of data obtained from the urinalysis differ in patients with neurogenic bladder dysfunction who manage their bladder with CIC or indwelling urinary catheters. For example, while presence of leukocytes and nitrites on urinalysis indicates the need for additional evaluation in the patient with nonneurogenic stress, urge, or mixed urinary incontinence, these findings are highly prevalent in patients using CIC or an indwelling catheter and should *not* prompt further investigation unless a symptomatic UTI is suspected.

Urodynamic Testing

According to the American Urological Association/Society for Urodynamics, urodynamic testing is not indicated for the routine evaluation of persons with nonneurogenic urge, stress, or mixed urinary incontinence; rather, it is indicated in selected cases when surgical intervention that may permanently alter lower urinary tract function is anticipated (Winters et al., 2012). However, the guidelines do support consideration of urodynamic testing and the measurement of postvoid residual volume for evaluation of persons with NLUTD. The guidelines also support consideration of voiding pressure flow studies, pelvic floor muscle electromyography, and videourodynamic testing in patients with neurogenic bladder dysfunction and incomplete bladder emptying or other urologic symptoms, including suspicion of upper urinary tract distress.

KEY POINT

Urodynamic testing is commonly indicated for patients with neurogenic bladder dysfunction, to determine detrusor contractility, bladder wall compliance, and the presence and severity of any detrusor external sphincter dyssynergia.

MANAGEMENT OF THE PATIENT WITH NEUROGENIC BLADDER DYSFUNCTION: GENERAL PRINCIPLES

Multiple chapters in this book discuss management of patients with various types of nonneurogenic urinary incontinence and retention. The brief discussion in this chapter will focus on management options especially appropriate for patients with neurogenic bladder dysfunction. Management options will be divided into several categories: behavioral interventions, catheterization techniques, pharmacologic interventions, and surgical options.

KEY POINT

Management of the patient with neurogenic bladder must be individualized based on patient assessment and specific problems and issues; strategies include behavioral strategies, pharmacologic therapy, and surgical interventions.

BEHAVIORAL INTERVENTIONS

Behavioral interventions such as fluid and dietary modifications or changes in toileting behaviors (scheduled toileting, prompted voiding) have been shown to alleviate LUTS in patients with overactive bladder dysfunction and stress, urge, and mixed incontinence (Bradley et al., 2017; Gormley et al., 2014; Lucas et al., 2013). They may also be considered in the management of patients with neurogenic bladders, but the precise nature of these interventions varies according to the nature of the lower urinary tract dysfunction and the bladder management program. Patients with neurogenic detrusor overactivity and urge incontinence should be counseled similarly to those with nonneurogenic overactive bladder syndrome. Counseling focuses on maintenance of adequate fluid intake based on recommended daily allowances from the Institute of Medicine (Institute of Medicine, Food and Science Board, 2004) and avoidance or reduction of caffeine intake in persons with neurogenic overactive bladder dysfunction because of its role as a bladder irritant (Wells et al., 2014). Nevertheless, there is insufficient evidence to conclude that these behavioral interventions are clinically beneficial for patients with neurogenic detrusor overactivity and decreased or absent sensations of bladder filling, especially when combined with detrusor sphincter dyssynergia. Similarly, advice about fluid and caffeine intake must be individualized for the patient managed by CIC or indwelling catheterization. Prevention of constipation is recommended for maintenance of healthy bladder habits (Lukacz et al., 2011), but this advice must be individualized for those with neurogenic bladder dysfunction who may also utilize a structured bowel program for neurogenic bowel management. Chapter 6 provides detailed overview of lifestyle and behavioral modifications to promote healthy bowel and bladder habits.

CATHETERIZATION

Two forms of catheterization are used in the management of neurogenic bladder dysfunction: CIC and long-term indwelling catheterization.

Clean Intermittent Catheterization

CIC is indicated for patients with urinary retention, with or without urinary incontinence. Self-catheterization is taught whenever possible, and a care provider in the person's home is taught to catheterize as well. Teaching begins with an assessment of the patient's physical ability to manipulate and insert the catheter. This is particularly important for patients whose underlying neurological disorder may compromise upper arm movement, such as MS or cervical spinal cord injuries. This challenge was illustrated in a study of 44 community-dwelling persons practicing CIC for a variety of reasons; 21% of those with neurogenic bladder and MS cited poor dexterity as a problem when engaging in CIC (Bolinger & Engberg, 2013).

The continence nurse should be intimately involved in teaching principles of CIC and counseling patients about self-management of potential complications including symptomatic UTI, difficulty inserting a catheter, and urethral trauma or bleeding (Engberg et al., 2020; Gray et al., 2019; Newman & Willson, 2011; Wyndaele, 2002). For patients with urinary retention with or without urinary incontinence, patients are taught to catheterize every 4 to 6 hours or four times daily while awake. The nurse teaches CIC technique, including hand hygiene prior to catheterization, location of the urethral meatus (especially in women), gentle insertion of the catheter until urine returns, and maneuvers to encourage complete evacuation of the urine from the bladder. Teaching for those living at home should include the patient and at least one care provider (Gray et al., 2019). Chapter 16 provides examples of adaptive equipment, positioning, and environmental changes to support individuals who may have physical challenges in performing CIC.

KEY POINT

Clean intermittent catheterization is indicated for patients with urinary retention with or without incontinence; a common challenge is the physical mobility and dexterity required to perform the procedure.

Catheter selection is an important component of CIC teaching; adults are typically instructed to use a 14- to 16-French catheter, and families of infants and children are taught to use catheters ranging in size from 6 to 10 French. Patients should be educated about the various types of intermittent catheters, including red rubber, polyvinyl chloride (clear) catheters, prelubricated hydrophilic intermittent catheters, and enclosed catheter systems. Females and younger males should be counseled about the possibility of using intermittent catheters of shorter length, and males may be taught to use a coudé-tipped catheter if catheterization with a straight-tipped tube proves difficult. Children should be taught to self-catheterize as soon as feasible based on physical ability, cognitive function, maturation, and motivation (Faleiros et al., 2016).

Traditionally, patients managing their bladders with CIC were taught to clean and reuse catheters, but the U.S. Centers for Medicare and Medicaid Services has altered its policies and now covers 200 single catheters per month (WOCN White Paper, 2009). Prevention of complications associated with CIC must be taught, including UTI prevention. Strategies to reduce the risk for recurring UTI include consistent hand hygiene prior to catheter insertion, adherence to prescribed regimens for catheterization, and strategies to enhance complete evacuation of urine, such as catheterizing in an upright position whenever possible and slow removal of the catheter to enhance drainage. Prelubricated hydrophilic catheters and closed intermittent catheterization systems may reduce the potential for bacteriuria and/or UTI, and their use should be considered for patients who experience recurrent symptomatic UTI (Chartier, Kastler & Denys, 2011; Day et al., 2002; Engberg et al., 2020). Overwhelming clinical experience and limited evidence suggests that selected use of coudé-tipped catheters and prelubricated hydrophilic catheters also reduces the risk of urethral trauma (Engberg et al., 2020; Parker et al., 2009). Whenever any change is made to the bowel or bladder management program (such as a change to a closed system or prelubricated catheter), the continence nurse should track symptom improvement and antibiotic use.

KEY POINT

Strategies to reduce the risk of UTI among individuals managing with CIC include consistent hand hygiene, adherence to the prescribed schedule for catheterization, and measures to assure complete emptying.

Indwelling Catheterization

Short-term indwelling catheterization (see also Chapter 8) is often used to manage urinary drainage after an acute neurologic event such as a SCI or a stroke. These catheters typically remain in place for 30 days or less and should be managed using accepted principles for short-term catheters, including measures for prevention of catheter-associated UTI (Parker et al., 2009). Cyclical clamping and unclamping prior to removal of a short-term indwelling urinary catheter has been attempted in an effort to improve lower urinary tract function following removal of the catheter, but limited evidence demonstrates that this practice provides *no* benefit when compared to removal without clamping (Moon et al., 2012).

Transient indwelling catheterization also may be used in select females with NLUTD caused by SCI during pregnancy (Andretta et al., 2019).

Long-term use of indwelling catheters is associated with multiple adverse consequences including catheter-associated urinary tract infection (CAUTI), urethral erosion and catheter bypassing (leakage from around the catheter), medical devices related pressure injury of the urethra (also referred as catheter erosion), encrustation and catheter blockage, upper urinary tract distress, and impaired renal function (Lane et al., 2017; Linsenmeyer, 2018). As a result, it is typically reserved for patients with NLUTD and urinary retention (with or without urinary incontinence) that is not amenable to CIC or other bladder management techniques (Wisconsin Department of Health Services, 2001). It is also used in highly selected patients with neurogenic bladder and urinary incontinence who cannot be managed with CIC owing to specific social or economic circumstances. For example, a long-term indwelling catheter may be used for a quadriplegic female who cannot be managed with CIC because of lack of a full-time care provider in her home setting.

The continence nurse plays a primary role in management of the patient with a neurogenic bladder and long-term indwelling catheter. The decision to insert a long-term urinary catheter is typically made by an interdisciplinary team (including a nurse), with the order written by a physician. The team should counsel the patient and family regarding placement of a urethral versus suprapubic catheter. Evidence regarding the benefits and disadvantages of suprapubic versus urethral catheters remains sparse; several studies of patients with neurogenic bladder (due to spinal cord injuries, stroke, MS, and parkinsonism) found no difference in catheter-associated UTI occurrences, catheter bypassing (from the urethra or suprapubic site, respectively), or serum creatinine (Ahluwalia et al., 2006; Katsumi et al., 2010). Nevertheless, evidence suggests that some patients prefer suprapubic catheters, while others prefer urethral catheters (Ahluwalia et al., 2006; Fowler et al., 2014). Therefore, the selection between suprapubic versus urethral catheter should be based on a discussion of the advantages and disadvantages of urethral and suprapubic catheters from the perspective of the patient and family.

KEY POINT

Evidence regarding advantages of urethral versus suprapubic catheters is sparse; thus, the decision should be made based on a discussion with the patient and family to determine their preference.

Selection of catheter size, substrate (material of construction), and urinary drainage system is typically a nursing decision. A 14- to 16-French catheter is preferred for a long-term indwelling urethral catheter. Several substrates are available, including latex with a polytetrafluoroethylene coating, latex with a hydrogel coating, latex with a silicone coating, and all-silicone catheters (Curtis & Klykken, 2008). While all catheter substrates are susceptible to biofilm formation and encrustation, hydrogel-coated, silicone-coated, and all-silicone catheters are preferred to polytetrafluoroethylene catheters because they appear to produce less urethral inflammation and discomfort when left in place for a prolonged period of time (Parker et al., 2009). Evidence suggests that catheters impregnated with a silver alloy or antibiotic-coated catheters provide short-term protection against bacteriuria or CAUTI; they are not recommended for patients requiring long-term catheterization.

KEY POINT

Hydrogel-coated, silicone-coated, and all-silicone catheters are preferred for long-term use because they produce less urethral inflammation when left in place for prolonged periods of time.

Selection of a urinary drainage system is individualized based on patient preference, typical physical activity, and dexterity/ability to drain the system (Gray et al., 2008). While maintenance of a closed drainage system is feasible and desirable for the patient with a short-term indwelling catheter, it is not feasible for persons with long-term indwelling catheters. Daytime urinary drainage may be accomplished using a leg bag or a drainage bag attached to the lower abdominal area.

The optimal drainage bag should be comfortably attached to the patient, remain discreet under clothing, and create minimal noise when partially filled with urine during activity (Curtis & Klykken, 2008; Fowler et al., 2014). Leg straps should remain in place without irritating the underlying skin; in one study of nonneurogenic patients using leg bags, cloth leg straps with secure snaps were preferred over latex straps (Pinar et al., 2009). Patients who experience trouble with leg straps may be counseled regarding use of a cloth pouch device. Consideration should also be given to the backing of the leg bag (cloth is preferred to latex) and the connecting tubing; adjustable length and flexibility underneath clothing have been identified as important features by leg bag users (Fowler et al., 2014; Pinar et al., 2009). Evaluation of an optimal daytime drainage system should also take into account the dexterity required to open the spout, drain the leg bag, return the spout to a closed position, and distinguish between these positions. Overnight drainage usually relies on a bedside urinary drainage bag with sufficient volume to allow drainage without the need for emptying. Patients may be advised to place the bag in a bucket as added protection in the event of leakage (Fowler et al., 2014).

PHARMACOTHERAPY

A number of drugs are used in the management of neurogenic bladder. Drugs may be used to diminish or enhance urethral sphincter resistance, alleviate neurogenic detrusor overactivity, or improve bladder compliance by reducing detrusor muscle tone during bladder filling/storage (Cameron, 2010). **Table 9-2** summarizes pharmacologic options for management of neurogenic bladder dysfunction.

Medications used for neurogenic bladder management primarily include those designed to reduce or eliminate detrusor contractions (antimuscarinics, beta-3 agonists, and onabotulinum toxin A) and those designed to reduce urethral resistance (alpha-adrenergic antagonists, skeletal muscle relaxants, and onabotulinum toxin A).

Antimuscarinics

Pharmacotherapy is a cornerstone of therapy for neurogenic detrusor overactivity (failure to store because of the bladder). Antimuscarinics, also referred to as anticholinergics, block the neurotransmitter acetylcholine from binding to muscarinic receptors in the detrusor smooth muscle. Multiple pharmacologic options are available, including immediate- and extended-release oral agents, transdermal patches, and transdermal gels. In patients with preserved sensations of bladder filling, neurogenic detrusor overactivity is usually associated with urinary urgency, frequent urination while awake, nocturia or nocturnal enuresis, and urge incontinence. The typical goal of therapy in these patients is alleviation of urge incontinence and related LUTS (nocturia, daytime voiding frequency, and urgency) while preserving spontaneous voiding. Evidence strongly suggests that the clinical benefits of antimuscarinic drugs are enhanced when pharmacotherapy is combined with the behavioral interventions described earlier (Trocio et al., 2010). Refer to Chapter 7 for a more detailed discussion of the use of antimuscarinic drugs in persons with overactive bladder, including long-term use in older patients.

In contrast, patients with paralyzing spinal disorders such as SCI, transverse myelitis, and MS typically have significantly reduced or absent sensations of bladder filling; these individuals are usually unable to manage their bladders with spontaneous voiding owing to the combination of neurogenic detrusor overactivity and greatly reduced or absent sensory awareness of impending micturition. In addition, these individuals often experience detrusor sphincter dyssynergia, which results in incomplete emptying as well as leakage (a combination of failure to empty and failure to store). In this case, the goal of therapy is to abolish detrusor overactivity so that the bladder stores urine at low intravesical pressures and the individual remains free of incontinence between catheterizations (Amend et al., 2008; Kenelly et al., 2009; Mahfouz & Corcos, 2011; Nardulli et al., 2012). Because the goal is to eliminate detrusor overactivity, these

TABLE 9-2 PHARMACOLOGIC OPTIONS FOR MANAGEMENT OF NEUROGENIC BLADDER DYSFUNCTION

NEUROGENIC BLADDER DYSFUNCTION	DRUG CLASS: EXAMPLES	PHARMACOLOGIC ACTION	ADVERSE EFFECTS
Failure to store urine: because of the bladder (neurogenic detrusor overactivity, low bladder wall compliance)	**Antimuscarinics** (anticholinergics): Oxybutynin IR* Oxybutynin ER Oxybutynin TD patch Oxybutynin TD gel Tolterodine ER Fesoterodine Trospium ER Solifenacin Darifenacin	Binds with muscarinic receptors in bladder wall to block acetylcholine and abolish or reduce neurogenic detrusor overactivity	Dry mouth Blurred vision Constipation Flushing of skin Urinary retention
	Beta-3 adrenergic agonists Mirabegron	Adrenergic agonist, activates beta-3 receptors causing detrusor muscle relaxation and promoting bladder filling	Hypertension Stuffy nose Urinary tract infection Headache Constipation
	Injectable neurotoxin Onabotulinum toxin A	Cleaves SNAP-25 proteins preventing release of the neurotransmitter acetylcholine, abolishing or reducing neurogenic detrusor overactivity	Transient hematuria following injection Urinary tract infection Urinary retention Fatigue Constipation
Failure to store urine: because of the outlet (urethral sphincter incompetence)	**No drugs approved for this indication by U.S. FDA*** Alpha-adrenergic agonist pseudoephedrine and the tricyclic antidepressant imipramine have been used off label in the management of neurogenic bladder; imipramine also exerts anticholinergic effects used to alleviate or abolish neurogenic detrusor overactivity	Alpha-adrenergic agonists promote urethral sphincter closure by increasing smooth muscle tone in the bladder neck and proximal urethra	Hypertension Nervousness, restlessness Rapid pulse, palpitations Headache Imipramine also exerts anticholinergic side effects similar to antimuscarinic drugs
Failure to empty urine: because of the bladder (underactive detrusor function)	**Cholinergic agonists** Bethanechol chloride, no longer used for underactive detrusor function due to lack of effectiveness in clinical practice	Synthetic analog of acetylcholine, acts at muscarinic receptors in the detrusor muscle to stimulate and sustained detrusor muscle contraction	Abdominal cramps Nausea Diarrhea Sweating Bronchial constriction
Failure to empty urine: because of the outlet (bladder outlet obstruction, detrusor-striated sphincter dyssynergia, or detrusor bladder neck dyssynergia)	**Alpha-1 adrenergic blockers** Terazosin Doxazosin Tamsulosin Alfuzosin Silodosin	Binds with alpha-1 adrenergic receptors in smooth muscle of urethral sphincter mechanism to reduce urethral resistance to urinary outflow	Postural hypotension Dizziness Nasal congestion Headache Reflex tachycardia
	Skeletal muscle relaxants Baclofen (intrathecal)	Reduces skeletal muscle tone in the rhabdosphincter and periurethral skeletal muscles by inhibiting monosynaptic and polysynaptic reflexes at the spinal level	Drowsiness Dizziness Weakness Fatigue **Adverse side effects for intrathecal delivery** Sedation Respiratory and cardiovascular suppression Meningitis

(Continued)

TABLE 9-2 PHARMACOLOGIC OPTIONS FOR MANAGEMENT OF NEUROGENIC BLADDER DYSFUNCTION (*Continued*)

NEUROGENIC BLADDER DYSFUNCTION	DRUG CLASS: EXAMPLES	PHARMACOLOGIC ACTION	ADVERSE EFFECTS
	Injectable neurotoxin Onabotulinum toxin A (not approved for this indication by the U.S. FDA*)	Cleaves SNAP-25 proteins preventing release of the neurotransmitter acetylcholine, abolishing or reducing neurogenic detrusor overactivity	Generalized muscle weakness Transient urethral bleeding Transient autonomic dysreflexia

*U.S. Food and Drug Administration.
Data from Amend et al. (2008); Barrett (1981); Cameron (2010); Cruz (2014); Finkbeiner (1985); Kenelly et al. (2009); Lapeyre et al. (2010); Mahfouz and Corcos (2011); Marberger (2013); McIntyre et al. (2014); Mehta et al. (2012); Mertens et al. (1995); Nadulli et al. (2012); Nitti et al. (2014); Rapidi et al. (2007); Soljanik (2013); Trocio et al. (2010).

patients often require CIC and higher dosages of a single antimuscarinic agent, more than one oral antimuscarinic drug, an oral antimuscarinic drug combined with a transdermal formulation, an antimuscarinic combined with a beta-3 agonist (Nardulli et al., 2012). Evidence concerning the influence of long-term use of antimuscarinic drugs on cognitive function (taken over a period of 3 years or more) is mixed (Andre et al., 2019; Carriere et al., 2009; Richardson et al., 2018; Welsh et al., 2018), and the 2019 Beers criteria for potentially inappropriate use of medications in elder adults recommends against use of drugs with strong anticholinergic actions in adults aged ≥65 years (2019 American Geriatrics Society Beers Criteria° Update Expert Panel, 2019). Nevertheless, antimuscarinic drugs used to treat urinary incontinence are mentioned as an exception. A single study was located that examined cognitive function in patients with SCI (Krebs et al., 2018); no cognitive effects of ongoing administration of antimuscarinic drugs were identified, but the period of observation was short at 12 weeks and further research is needed to determine the long-term effects seen in community dwelling adults. Lacking more definitive evidence, caution is advised when administering antimuscarinic drugs to patients with NLUTD over a period of 3 years or more, and the continence nurse should carefully monitor all patients taking antimuscarinic drugs or multidrug therapy for adverse side effects.

KEY POINT

Individuals with detrusor overactivity and diminished or absent sensory awareness are frequently best managed with higher dosage or combination antimuscarinic agents (to eliminate detrusor contractions) in combination with CIC (to empty the bladder).

Beta-3 Agonists

Pharmacotherapy for patients with neurogenic detrusor overactivity has expanded to include a new drug class, the beta-3 agonists. Research is ongoing on several potential molecules, and one drug (mirabegron) has been approved for clinical use by the U.S. FDA (Nitti et al., 2014). Beta-3 agonists act differently than the antimuscarinics. Rather than blocking muscarinic receptors, they enhance the activity of the neurotransmitter epinephrine as it binds to beta-3 receptors in the bladder wall. Mirabegron may be administered for first-line management of neurogenic detrusor overactivity, or it may be used in combination with an antimuscarinic agent. Although additional research is needed, bladder management using both classes appears attractive for patients who prove refractory to a single agent because of the different sites of pharmacologic activity and different potential side effects.

Onabotulinum Toxin A

Onabotulinum toxin A is an attractive pharmacologic agent for patients with neurogenic detrusor overactivity because of its efficacy and comparatively long duration of action, even when injected repeatedly over a period of years (Ni et al., 2018). This neurotoxin is injected directly into the detrusor wall during a cystoscopic procedure (Soljanik, 2013). It cleaves SNAP-25 proteins in the nerve cell, which blocks the release of acetylcholine and thereby prevents contraction of the detrusor muscle (Cruz, 2014). Onabotulinum toxin A is injected approximately every 6 to 9 months. Many patients are able to reduce or discontinue oral or transdermal drugs for neurogenic detrusor overactivity after injection. Onabotulinum toxin A requires up to 36 injection sites; transient hematuria following injection occurs frequently, and prolonged hematuria was noted in 4.9% of a pooled sample of 2,301 patients with neurogenic detrusor overactivity. Urinary retention and UTIs are common side effects, affecting 23.7% and 16.7%, respectively. Given the high rate of urinary retention, patients with neurogenic bladder dysfunction who manage with spontaneous voiding must be counseled about the possible need to perform CIC following injection of onabotulinum toxin A.

Onabotulinum toxin A may also be injected directly into the striated muscles of the urethral sphincter mechanism in patients with detrusor-striated sphincter dyssynergia. Similar to its actions on the smooth muscle of the detrusor, it blocks contraction of the rhabdosphincter and periurethral striated muscles by cleaving SNAP-25 proteins in the nerve cells of the motor unit (Marberger, 2013). Although onabotulinum toxin A is not officially indicated or approved for treatment of detrusor-striated sphincter dyssynergia, a systematic review identified 2 randomized clinical trials and 6 nonrandomized trials involving 129 subjects with neurogenic bladder associated with SCI (Mehta et al., 2012). Pooled analysis of evidence from these trials found that treatment reduced postvoid residual volumes and the magnitude of obstruction caused by dyssynergia 30 days after injection. Findings from four studies showed reduction in CIC and results of three studies indicated a 50% reduction in UTI occurrence.

Baclofen

The pharmacologic management of patients with increased urethral resistance caused by detrusor–sphincter dyssynergia (failure to empty because of the outlet) is challenging. This problem is most commonly encountered in patients with neurogenic bladder and paralyzing spinal disorders such as spinal cord injuries, transverse myelitis, or MS. Baclofen administered by intrathecal pump has proved effective for skeletal muscle spasticity in patients with paralyzing spinal disorders (Lapeyre et al., 2010; McIntyre et al., 2014), and limited evidence suggests it may be effective for management of neurogenic detrusor overactivity with detrusor-striated sphincter dyssynergia (Mertens et al., 1995; Rapidi et al., 2007).

Alpha-Adrenergic Antagonists

The alpha-1 adrenergic antagonists reduce urethral sphincter mechanism resistance by blocking adrenergic receptors on the smooth muscle of the bladder neck and proximal urethra. They may be used to reduce urethral resistance in patients with detrusor-striated sphincter dyssynergia or detrusor–bladder neck dyssynergia (Ahmed et al., 2006; Yamanishi et al., 1997). They are also used in older men with neurogenic bladder dysfunction complicated by bladder outlet obstruction associated with benign prostatic enlargement (Mehta et al., 2012).

Cholinergic Agonists

Cholinergic agonists have been used in the past in an attempt to treat underactive detrusor function (failure to empty because of the bladder). A single agent, bethanechol chloride, is currently available. However, cholinergic agonists have been shown to be ineffective for improving bladder emptying in multiple studies, and they are *no longer recommended* for use in the management of neurogenic bladder dysfunction (Barrett, 1981; Finkbeiner, 1985).

Antidiuretic Hormone/Vasopressin Analogs

Several formulations of desmopressin have been approved for management of nocturia in adults (Cohn et al., 2017; Suman et al., 2019). The active molecule in both is desmopressin, a synthetic analog of the antidiuretic hormone. One drug is delivered as a sublingual tablet taken 1 hour before bedtime and the other as an intranasal spray administered 30 minutes before bedtime. Both are effective for adults with nocturia twice or

more nightly in patients with nocturnal polyuria. The ICS defines nocturnal polyuria as nocturnal output >20% of the daily total in younger adults and >33% of the daily total in older adults (van Doorn et al., 2013). Hyponatremia is a possible adverse side effect for both agents, and it may be severe or life threatening in some cases. Contraindications include patients at increased risk of severe hyponatremia, such as individual found to have high fluid intake on a bladder diary, disease associated with fluid or electrolyte imbalances, and those using loop diuretics or inhaled glucocorticoids. A diagnosis of nocturnal polyuria should be established via a bladder diary supported with voided volumes both day and night. The patient's serum sodium should be measured before initiating treatment, followed by careful instruction concerning dosage and administration of these agents. Serum sodium and advice concerning restriction of fluid 30 to 60 minutes prior to bedtime also may alleviate the risk of hyponatremia.

NEUROMODULATION

The International Neuromodulation Society defines neuromodulation alteration of neural activity via targeted delivery of a stimulus, such as electrical stimulation (International Neuromodulation Society). Neuromodulation for lower urinary tract dysfunction relies on electrical stimulation; it was originally developed for treatment of urge incontinence, now classified as a common component of overactive bladder syndrome. It can be delivered via a variety of approaches including transvaginal or transrectal sacral nerve stimulation, transcutaneous tibial nerve stimulation, percutaneous tibial nerve stimulation, or surgically implanted sacral nerve stimulation devices (Jaqua & Powell, 2017). Advanced practice continence nurses frequently provide percutaneous posterior tibial nerve stimulation, and they may provide transvaginal or transrectal electrical stimulation as an adjunct to pelvic floor muscle training.

Evidence concerning the efficacy of transvaginal or transrectal sacral nerve stimulation is sparse (Barroso et al., 2004), and it is not widely used in current practice. In contrast, percutaneous posterior tibial nerve stimulation for overactive bladder with urge incontinence is supported by robust evidence and was approved as third-line treatment for overactive bladder dysfunction with urge incontinence in 2006 (Burton et al., 2012; Jaqua & Powell, 2017). Posterior transcutaneous nerve stimulation is initially delivered as 12 weekly treatments; an acupuncture needle is placed in the ankle area near the posterior tibial nerve. Electrical stimulation is applied until the patient perceives a strong sensation (often described as tingling or throbbing) that is just below the pain threshold and a motor response (curling) of one or more toes is observed. The stimulation is continued for 30 minutes. Treatment may be repeated for patients who respond to initial therapy after 6 months, and monthly maintenance treatments have also been advocated. In addition to delivering treatments, continence nurses find these sessions valuable because they allow time to reinforce behavioral interventions such as fluid and dietary intake. Reported initial response rates to percutaneous posterior tibial nerve stimulation vary from 37% to 82%; an extension of the STEP trial found that 77% of initial responders had a durable and positive effect at 36 months (Jaqua & Powell, 2017; Peters, Carrico, et al., 2013).). Though the majority of research evaluating the efficacy of percutaneous tibial nerve stimulation was completed in patients with idiopathic overactive bladder dysfunction, limited evidence supports its effectiveness for patients with neurogenic detrusor overactivity (Canbaz-Kabay et al., 2017; Kabay et al., 2016); refer to Chapter 7, Overactive Bladder/Urgency UI: Pathology, Presentation, Diagnosis, and Management for a more detailed discussion of percutaneous tibial nerve stimulation for management of overactive bladder.

Limited evidence also suggests that *transcutaneous* posterior nerve stimulation may be used for treatment of patients with neurogenic detrusor overactivity (Booth et al., 2018; Chen et al., 2015; Perissinotto et al., 2015). Transcutaneous delivery of electrical stimulation is especially attractive in children and others who may not tolerate the multiple insertions of an acupuncture needle required for percutaneous therapy.

A surgically implanted device is also used to deliver neuromodulation in patients with idiopathic and neurogenic detrusor overactivity and incontinence; this device provides continuous stimulation when active (Graham et al., 2007). A study comparing 340 patients with and without neurogenic bladder dysfunction (including persons with stroke, MS, incomplete spinal cord injuries, and parkinsonism) demonstrated similar outcomes (Peters, Kandagatla et al., 2013). Persons contemplating implantation of a neuromodulation device should be counseled about the need for ongoing monitoring of his or her device including adjustment of the electrical signals used to stimulate the lower urinary tract and the potential need for additional surgery to ensure maximum function.

KEY POINT

Neuromodulation is effective for treatment of nonneurogenic bladder dysfunction; a growing body of evidence indicates that this therapy may also be of benefit to individuals with neurogenic overactive bladder dysfunction.

MINIMALLY INVASIVE AND SURGICAL MANAGEMENT

A comprehensive review of surgical options for treatment of neurogenic bladder dysfunction is beyond the scope of this chapter focusing on nursing management. **Table 9-3** provides an overview of surgical options for managing the neurogenic bladder (Graham et al., 2007).

TABLE 9-3 SURGICAL MANAGEMENT OPTIONS FOR NEUROGENIC BLADDER DYSFUNCTION

NEUROGENIC BLADDER DYSFUNCTION	SURGICAL PROCEDURE	DESCRIPTION
Failure to store urine: because of the bladder (neurogenic detrusor overactivity, low bladder wall compliance)	Augmentation enterocystoplasty Implantation of a sacral neuromodulation device	A segment of the bowel is isolated from the gastrointestinal tract, detubularized, and attached to the urinary bladder. A sacral neuromodulation device is implanted into the pelvis and leads are placed at the sacral roots that communicate with a remote control device. Activation of the device inhibits detrusor muscle contraction.
Failure to store urine: because of the outlet (urethral sphincter incompetence)	Injection of suburethral bulking agents (glutaraldehyde cross-linked collagen, calcium hydroxylapatite, pyrolytic carbon-coated beads, polydimethylsiloxane, ethylene vinyl alcohol copolymer) Suburethral sling procedures Artificial urinary sphincter	Biocompatible bulking agents are injected into the urethral submucosa just distal to the rhabdosphincter (membranous urethra in males, midurethra in females) under endoscopic guidance. Suburethral sling procedures using synthetic mesh or bolsters may be used to increase urethral resistance to urine outflow in both women and men. Artificial urinary sphincters may be implanted in both men and women to increase urethral resistance to urine outflow; the device is maintained in a closed position; activation of the sphincter shunts fluid from a urethral cuff to an abdominal reservoir, which transiently opens the cuff to enable spontaneous voiding or intermittent catheterization.
Failure to empty urine: because of the outlet (bladder outlet obstruction, detrusor-striated muscle dyssynergia, or detrusor bladder neck dyssynergia)	Transurethral sphincterotomy Multiple procedures may be used to relieve bladder outlet obstruction; common examples include transurethral or minimally invasive prostatectomy	Uses an endoscopic approach to incise the striated urethral sphincter in men in order to reduce urethral sphincter resistance to urine outflow. Uses an endoscopic approach to visualize the prostatic urethra; excess prostatic tissue is resected using a variety of instruments. Minimally invasive prostatectomy procedures use one of several forms of energy to destroy prostatic tissue such as microwave energy, direct contact laser energy, or high-intensity ultrasound.

Data from Atala (2014); Atala et al. (2006); Beirs et al. (2011); Boone (2009); Graham et al. (2007); Joseph et al. (2014); Kari et al. (2013); Liard et al. (2001); Nerli et al. (2013); Perkash (1996, 2009); Peters, Kandagatla et al., 2013; Revicky and Tincello (2014); Zuckerman et al. (2014).

Augmentation Enterocystoplasty

Augmentation enterocystoplasty is a reconstructive surgical procedure that enlarges bladder capacity, improves bladder wall compliance, and alleviates or abolishes neurogenic detrusor overactivity (Beirs et al., 2011). A bowel segment (usually the ileum) is isolated from the fecal stream and detubularized to interrupt peristaltic contractions. This segment is attached to the bladder, which is bivalved to create a spherical vesicle for maximum capacity. Patients who have undergone augmentation enterocystoplasty almost always use CIC to manage their bladder postoperatively, and they should be taught techniques to manage mucus production from the bowel segment, including adequate fluid intake and routine irrigation if mucus is significant. Patients must also be counseled about the long-term risk for carcinoma of the augmented bladder and the importance of routine follow-up with his or her physician.

Autologous Bladder Replacement

Tissue-engineered autologous bladders have been developed and successfully implanted into human hosts (Atala et al., 2006). These bladders are created from autologous cell cultures that are expanded using techniques originally developed and tested in animal models. A neobladder is formed using a scaffold constructed from homologous decellularized bladder submucosa, collagen, and/or a synthetic material used for hernia repair; the construction process requires approximately 7 to 8 weeks prior to surgical implantation. At the time of surgery, the engineered neobladder is attached onto the base of the native bladder and omentum is used to increase the vascularity of the reconstructed neobladder.

The engineered neobladder differs from augmentation enterocystoplasty in several important ways: (1) it replaces rather than augments the existing bladder body; (2) it is constructed from homologous bladder tissue rather than intestinal tissue; (3) surgery does not require loss of bowel from the gastrointestinal tract; and (4) it does not create mucus or reabsorb urinary constituents as does reconstructed bowel. Nevertheless, it must be remembered that CIC is needed for these bladders just as it is for bladders augmented by detubularized bowel. Short-term results in children with neurogenic bladder dysfunction associated with myelomeningocele were promising, but longer-term results have been disappointing (Atala, 2014; Joseph et al., 2014). Specifically, the engineered neobladders did not provide improved functional capacity or improved bladder wall compliance when compared to the patient's autologous bladder. As a result of this experience, this procedure remains experimental and additional research and refinement of techniques needed to create and implant-engineered neobladders are ongoing (Adamowicz et al., 2017).

Continent Catheterizable Stoma Construction

Several reconstructive procedures have been designed for persons who experience difficulty with CIC owing to urethral obstruction or prior urethral surgery, discomfort associated with catheterization, or the lack of mobility and dexterity required for urethral catheterization. Two procedures, creation of an appendicovesicostomy (attributed to Mitrofanoff) or an ileovesicostomy (attributed to Yang-Monti), allow children and adults with neurogenic bladder dysfunction to perform CIC who might not otherwise be able to perform these procedures (Liard et al., 2001; Nerli et al., 2013). The appendicovesicostomy involves attaching the appendix to the bladder and bringing the appendix to the umbilicus or abdominal wall to create a catheterizable stoma. The ileovesicostomy uses a small segment of reconstructed bowel to create a continent, catheterizable stoma. Research is limited but current evidence suggests that catheterizable abdominal or umbilical stomas remain continent over a 10-year period or longer, enhance adherence to CIC regimens, and reduce the psychosocial burden associated with urethral catheterization in selected children (Kari et al., 2013; Liard et al., 2001; Nerli et al., 2013).

Suburethral Slings

Multiple surgical procedures have been developed for the treatment of urethral sphincter incompetence in women; the most common procedure involves placement of a synthetic mesh creating a suburethral sling (Revicky & Tincello, 2014). Refer to Chapter 11 for a more detailed description of the management of stress incontinence. Suburethral sling procedures have also been adapted for male patients; short-term continence rates are impressive, but longer-term results (>1 year) show less robust dry rates (40%) (Zuckerman et al., 2014).

Artificial Urinary Sphincter

Artificial urinary sphincters (AUS) remain an attractive surgical option for some patients with neurogenic bladder and urethral sphincter incompetence (Graham et al., 2007; Marziale et al., 2018). The sling comprises three components: an abdominal reservoir, a baffling system with a pump implanted in the scrotum in men or underneath the labia majora in women, and a cuff that encircles the urethra distal to the rhabdosphincter. Similar to other surgical options, implantation of an AUS requires ongoing monitoring and repeated evaluation of its impact on neurogenic bladder dysfunction.

Transurethral Sphincterotomy

Multiple surgical procedures have been developed to manage bladder outlet obstruction associated with benign prostatic enlargement or urethral stricture disease. Refer to Chapters 8 and 10 for a more detailed discussion of these procedures. In contrast, transurethral sphincterotomy and associated procedures such as implantation of a urethral stent are used specifically for treatment of male patients with neurogenic bladder dysfunction and detrusor-striated sphincter dyssynergia (Perkash, 1996, 2009). Once considered a mainstay of the management of detrusor sphincter dyssynergia in men with neurogenic bladder and detrusor-striated sphincter dyssynergia caused by SCI, performance of this procedure has declined dramatically due to less than optimal long-term outcomes.

NEUROGENIC BLADDER MANAGEMENT: SPECIFIC EXAMPLES

As noted earlier in this chapter, taxonomies for classifying and managing neurogenic bladder dysfunction have not gained widespread use owing to limitations in their application to clinical practice. These limitations include failure to account for the natural history of the underlying neurologic condition and its impact on options for a bladder management program, the long-term impact of obstruction on lower urinary tract function, the risk for hostile neurogenic bladder dysfunction and upper urinary tract distress, and patient/family preference. The following examples of neurogenic bladder dysfunction associated with prevalent neurologic conditions illustrate the need to consider all of these factors when providing nursing care for these individuals.

SPINAL CORD INJURY

SCI is defined as trauma or damage to the spinal cord resulting in loss of motor and/or sensory function (Kirshblum et al., 2014). Approximately 270,000 Americans have an SCI, and 12,000 to 20,000 experience an SCI each year (Ma et al., 2014).

Classification

Spinal cord injuries are classified according to the International Standards for Neurological Classification of SCI (Kirshblum et al., 2014). This classification schema requires identification of sensory and motor impairments and matching of these deficits with the appropriate dermatome. The result is a spinal injury level that aids clinicians in determining physical rehabilitation needs and options for managing neurogenic bladder and bowel.

The American Spinal Injury Association (ASIA) has developed a complementary system to classify the severity of the impairment associated with SCI. An ASIA A SCI is defined as a "complete injury" with no sensory or motor function below the level of the SCI, and an ASIA B SCI is defined as "sensory incomplete" with preservation of sensory but no motor function below the level of the injury (van Middendorp et al., 2009). An ASIA C SCI is described as "motor complete" with preservation of less than half of the key muscle functions below the level of injury, while an ASIA D SCI indicates a "motor incomplete injury," with preservation of function of 50% or more of the key muscle groups below the level of injury. An ASIA E injury, sometimes referred to as an injury with no neurological deficit, is defined as absence of sensory or motor deficits despite a documented spinal trauma. Neurogenic bladder dysfunction is anticipated in all patients with ASIA A and B SCI and a high proportion of those with ASIA C and D injuries.

KEY POINT

Management of neurogenic bladder dysfunction is based on two main goals: preservation of upper urinary tract (renal) health and restoration of the greatest degree of continence possible.

Spinal Shock

Following SCI, the individual experiences a period of spinal shock characterized by four phases: (1) absent motor reflexes with flaccid paralysis of skeletal muscles, which lasts approximately 1 day postinjury; (2) denervation supersensitivity, which occurs approximately 1 to 3 days postinjury and involves initial return of affected skeletal muscle reflexes; (3) onset of hyperreflexia of the affected muscles, which occurs about 1 to 4 weeks after injury; and (4) onset of a chronic state of striated muscle hyperreflexia, which begins as soon as 1 month postinjury but can be delayed for as long as 12 months postinjury (Ditunno et al., 2004). The bulbocavernosus reflex is a contraction of the bulbospongiosus muscle (one of the pelvic floor muscles) that occurs in response to tapping of the dorsum of the penis, gentle compression of the glans penis, or tapping of the clitoris during physical assessment. This polysynaptic response is mediated by sacral spinal segments 2 to 4, and it is a common component of a physical examination in the person with urinary incontinence. It was historically used to determine the end of spinal shock, but it typically recovers during the first 24 hours following SCI, long before other signs of recovery from spinal shock in most patients. Despite flaccid paralysis of muscles below the level of injury, the *urethral sphincter* remains *closed* and the *detrusor* remains *acontractile* during spinal shock, resulting in urinary retention (failure to empty urine: because of the bladder) (Awad et al., 1977; Rossier & Ott, 1976).

An indwelling catheter is inserted immediately following SCI that is likely to remain in place during the early phases of spinal shock. This catheter is managed as a short-term indwelling catheter, and emphasis is placed on prevention of catheter-associated UTI. It serves two purposes, ongoing drainage of urine from the bladder and measurement of urine output. An acute SCI alters urine production, antidiuretic hormone production, and urinary output, predisposing the person to brisk urine production during the night and reduced production during waking hours when sitting upright (Denys et al., 2017; Viaene et al., 2019;). Intermittent catheterization is begun as soon as nighttime urine volumes diminish to a point that an intermittent catheterization schedule is reasonable; this usually occurs within a period of days to weeks after an acute SCI. Nevertheless, changes in urine production associated with SCI may create the need for an around the clock catheterization schedule until nighttime urine production subsides.

Selection of Bladder Management Program

Selection of an ongoing bladder management program is an important process based on careful consideration of multiple factors including characteristics of the specific individual's bladder dysfunction, level and severity of the SCI and its impact on mobility and dexterity, resources within the patient's home, patient preference, and long-term impact of the management program selected (Engkasan et al., 2014; Lane et al., 2017). Patients with an SCI that damages the sacral micturition center (sacral segments 2 to 4) are likely to experience chronic paralysis of the detrusor (underactive detrusor function), requiring ongoing CIC or continuous drainage using an indwelling urinary catheter. From a clinical perspective, these patients typically present as having ASIA A, B, or C SCI affecting vertebral levels T10–L2 (van Middendorp et al., 2009; Wyndaele, 1997).

Depending on the level of injury and whether spinal trauma has affected Onuf nucleus, these patients also may experience urethral sphincter incompetence (failure to store because of the outlet), with stress urinary incontinence noted during transfers in and out of the wheelchair or during coughing, sneezing, or straining. Depending on its severity, urethral sphincter incompetence may be managed by suburethral injection of a bulking agent, suburethral sling surgery, or implantation of an AUS (Bennett et al., 1995; Chartier Kastler et al., 2011; Davis et al., 2013; Groen et al., 2012).

The majority of patients with ASIA A, B, or C spinal injuries will have suprasacral level lesions, corresponding with injuries of vertebral levels of T10 to as high as C2 (van Middendorp et al., 2009; Wyndaele, 1997). As spinal shock subsides, the bladder exhibits neurogenic detrusor overactivity (failure to store because of the bladder), usually associated with detrusor-striated sphincter dyssynergia (failure to empty because of the outlet). A minority of patients with less severe SCI (ASIA C or D lesions), preserved sensations of bladder filling, and the ability to move to the toilet and prepare his or her clothing for urination may be able to maintain spontaneous voiding. These individuals may be managed by scheduled toileting, maintenance of a recommended daily intake of fluids, and avoidance of caffeine or other bladder irritants. Those with adequate detrusor contraction strength may benefit from an antimuscarinic or beta-3 agonist to reduce detrusor overactivity, possibly in combination with an alpha-1 adrenergic blocker to reduce sphincter resistance during micturition. These persons are at low risk for upper urinary tract distress, but they are at increased risk for UTI and should be monitored regularly (at least annually) to ensure optimal urinary tract function and maintenance of maximal social continence (Anson & Gray, 1993; Killorin et al., 1992).

Persons with neurogenic detrusor overactivity, reduced or absent sensations of bladder filling, and detrusor-striated sphincter dyssynergia are not able to void voluntarily and are typically managed by CIC, involuntary voiding into an external collection device, or long-term indwelling urinary catheterization (Anson & Gray, 1993; Killorin et al., 1992). CIC is preferred in these individuals, because of its ability to prevent upper urinary tract distress, in combination with its ability to maintain continence between catheterizations in most individuals (Gray et al., 1995a; Weld et al., 2000). Intermittent catheterization is typically combined with an antimuscarinic agent, beta-3 agonist, or onabotulinum toxin A injections. In this case, the goal of therapy is to ablate all overactive detrusor contractions between catheterizations, ensuring continence and preventing upper urinary tract distress. **Figure 9-2** and Case 1 describe management of a woman with an ASIA A SCI and NLUTD with detrusor neurogenic overactivity and detrusor-striated sphincter dyssynergia.

CASE STUDY #1

NEUROGENIC BLADDER IN A 34-YEAR-OLD FEMALE FOLLOWING T6 SPINAL CORD INJURY

Figure 9-2 illustrates the case of TA, a 34-year-old female who suffered a T6 (ASIA A, complete) spinal cord injury following a motor vehicle accident 3 years prior to attending our continence promotion center. She attended her initial evaluation with her partner; they have been together for 7 years. TA reported managing her bladder using adult containment briefs because of urinary incontinence without awareness. She states that she performs CIC twice daily. She stated that she originally catheterized every 4 hours and regularly took oxybutynin 5 mg twice daily but stopped the medication and CIC due to frequent episodes of urinary incontinence and occasional UTIs that she attributed to CIC. She began containing urinary leakage with adult absorptive briefs only. However, she restarted catheterizations twice daily when she began experiencing episodes of autonomic dysreflexia and a febrile UTI that required hospitalization and management with parenteral antibiotics. She initially approached her primary care WOC nurse requesting placement of an indwelling catheter. Her primary care provider declined and referred her for further evaluation of her NLUTD. Initial evaluation revealed a thin, alert, motivated Caucasian female with paraplegia and significant spasticity of her lower extremities. Her upper extremity strength was excellent and she reported no difficulty performing CIC. Her medications included nitrofurantoin 50 mg once daily for UTI suppression and baclofen 20 mg three times daily. Inspection of the perineal area revealed inflamed skin with some erosion of the skin surrounding the labia and inner thighs consistent with incontinence-associated dermatitis. Urinalysis revealed positive nitrites and small leukocytes with no red blood cells, glucose, or protein in her urine. Her serum creatinine was 0.6 mg/dL.

Urodynamic testing revealed small cystometric capacity (220 mL) with neurogenic detrusor overactivity causing urinary incontinence without awareness; detrusor-striated sphincter dyssynergia was noted on EMG causing functional obstruction of urinary outflow. Her postvoid residual volume was 150 mL. Testing did not provoke autonomic dysreflexia.

Based on these findings, TA was asked about her willingness to restart a regular CIC program. She expressed her willingness to restart pharmacotherapy and CIC but states she was concerned about the adverse side effects of dry mouth and significant flushing and fatigue when outdoors on warm, humid days.

She was initially started on CIC every 4 hours while awake and solifenacin 10 mg daily. On 6-week follow-up, she stated that she was encouraged that her new medication appeared to be more effective than her previous regimen but reported that she still experienced leakage episodes almost daily. After lengthy discussion, she underwent intradetrusor injection of onabotulinum toxin A. Following injection, she enjoyed complete dryness on her CIC program without any additional pharmacotherapy. She began experiencing UI episodes after a period of 8 months but regained continence after a second injection. She is currently scheduled to receive a third injection after 8 months.

This case illustrates the need for ongoing management in a young adult woman with paraplegia and NLUTD dysfunction following T6 SCI. Her original bladder management program, CIC with an antimuscarinic therapy, was appropriate for her bladder dysfunction, but her initial drug dosage proved insufficient to prevent neurogenic detrusor overactivity and incontinence between catheterizations. As a result, she abandoned her initial bladder management program but returned to care after experiencing autonomic dysreflexia and a febrile UTI. While a second antimuscarinic agent improved continence between catheterizations, it did not completely ablate leakage episodes. Second-line treatment, injection of onabotulinum toxin A, proved effective in preventing incontinence between catheterizations for a period of just over 8 months. The proposal of indwelling catheterization was not pursued because of its association with an increased risk for urologic complications with long-term use.

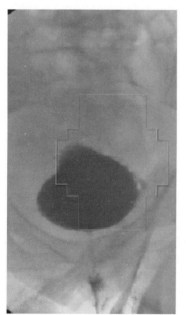
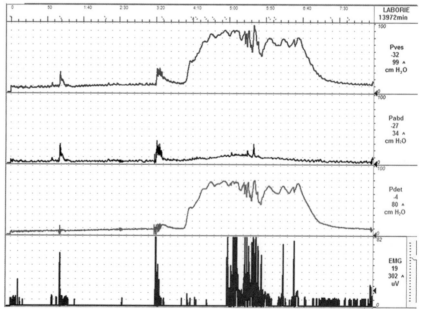

FIGURE 9-2. Management of a Female Patient with an ASIA A SCI and Neurogenic Bladder with Detrusor Neurogenic Overactivity and Detrusor-Striated Sphincter Dyssynergia. Refer to Case 1.

Quadriplegic males who are unable to perform CIC owing to motor deficits of their upper extremities or paraplegic males unwilling or unable to perform CIC may be managed by involuntary voiding into an external collection device (this program is sometimes referred to as a reflex, kickoff, or trigger voiding program) (Anson & Gray, 1993; Killorin et al., 1992). Involuntary voiding into an external collection device is dependent on the ability of the detrusor muscle to overcome any bladder outlet obstruction created by detrusor-striated sphincter dyssynergia. If there is sufficient outlet resistance to impede emptying, these men are at risk for recurring UTI and upper urinary tract distress. The risk for recurring UTI or upper urinary tract distress may be reduced by administration of alpha-1 adrenergic blockers to reduce urethral sphincter resistance, injection of onabotulinum toxin A into the rhabdosphincter, or a surgical sphincterotomy. The effectiveness of the program in preventing incontinence is determined by the ability of the external collection device and urinary drainage system to retain urine and prevent urine loss onto the clothing or skin.

KEY POINT

Males with SCI may elect to manage with condom drainage so long as the bladder is able to overcome any sphincter dyssynergia in order to provide complete emptying.

Because of challenges associated with normal female anatomy, no reliable external collection device has been developed for women. Therefore, quadriplegic women, or paraplegic women unwilling or unable to perform CIC, may require long-term use of an indwelling urinary catheter for bladder management. There are multiple potential complications associated with long-term use of indwelling catheters; therefore, meticulous management and routine follow-up is essential (see Chapter 19).

Ongoing Monitoring

Regardless of the bladder management program selected, ongoing monitoring and care are important for all patients with SCI. While the neurological impact of a traumatic SCI remains unchanged after spinal shock has subsided, the potential impact on lower urinary tract function is progressive and is affected by the presence and severity of bladder outlet obstruction, the variable impact of the bladder management program, and possibly the cumulative effects of recurring UTI or upper urinary tract distress. Monitoring of patients with SCI and NLUTD is recommended on an annual basis or more frequently when indicated. In a study of 96 patients with SCI and neurogenic bladder who were followed with annual visits for at least 2 years, 47.9% required adjustments in their bladder management programs either to enhance

continence or to manage recurring UTI or upper urinary tract distress (Linsenmeyer & Linsenmeyer, 2013).

The risk for upper urinary tract distress among persons with SCI and NLUTD dysfunction is significant (Anson & Gray, 1993; Killorin et al., 1992; Weld et al., 2000), due in part to the underlying bladder dysfunction and in part to the selected bladder management program. Spontaneous voiding and CIC are associated with lower complication rates than involuntary voiding into an external collecting device; thus, these approaches are encouraged and implemented whenever feasible (Anson & Gray, 1993; Killorin et al., 1992). In contrast, the greatest risk for upper urinary tract distress is associated with long-term indwelling catheterization (Anson & Gray, 1993; Killorin et al., 1992; Weld et al., 2000). Therefore, this program is reserved for patients who cannot manage NLUTD using an alternative program.

KEY POINT

Among individuals with NLUTD dysfunction due to SCI, the lowest incidence of upper tract distress is associated with spontaneous voiding and CIC, and the highest incidence of upper tract distress is associated with long-term use of indwelling catheters.

Surgical management is required in some persons with SCI and upper urinary tract distress. Augmentation enterocystoplasty may be indicated for patients with neurogenic detrusor overactivity or low bladder wall compliance who are able to perform CIC. An incontinent urinary diversion (ileal conduit) is performed in highly selected patients with SCI and NLUTD dysfunction that cannot be managed by any other means; individuals managed with diversion tend to be older with more physical limitations than those undergoing augmentation enterocystoplasty (Peterson et al., 2012).

MULTIPLE SCLEROSIS

MS is a chronic, immune-mediated inflammatory disease that affects multiple sites within the central nervous system (Milo & Miller, 2014). Several types of MS have been identified, including relapsing–remitting and primary progressive. Relapsing–remitting is the most common type of MS, accounting for 80% to 85% of all cases, followed by primary progressive, which comprises 10% to 15% of all cases. Additional categories based on the highly variable disease progression of MS have also been identified. Clinically isolated syndrome is defined as the first occurrence of clinical symptoms suggestive of MS. Secondary progressive MS is defined as an initial pattern of relapsing–remitting disease followed by slower progression with occasional remissions or plateaus; about half of patients who initially present with relapsing–remitting MS develop this pattern within 5 years, and 90% develop this pattern within 25 years.

Clinical Presentation

Approximately 400,000 persons living in the United States have some form of MS; the incidence is approximately 3.6 cases per 100,000 person-years in women and 2.0 per 100,000 person-years in men (Ma et al., 2014). The average time from disease onset to difficulty with ambulation is 8 years, and the mean time to complete reliance on assistive walking devices or a wheelchair is 15 to 30 years. NLUTD is prevalent in patients with MS; it is estimated to occur in 80% to 100% over the course of the disease (de Seze et al., 2007; Tubaro et al., 2012). Approximately 60% to 80% of persons with MS will have neurogenic detrusor overactivity with urgency, frequency, nocturia, nocturnal enuresis, and/or urge incontinence. Detrusor-striated sphincter dyssynergia occurs in as many as 25% of persons with MS, and underactive detrusor function is seen in about 20%.

KEY POINT

Neurogenic bladder dysfunction occurs in 80% to 100% of patients with MS, and sphincter dyssynergia occurs in 25% of these individuals.

Because of the variability in progression of neurological deficits caused by MS, and its ability to impair more than one area of the CNS, it is difficult to identify a predominant or typical type of NLUTD (de Seze et al., 2007; Tubaro et al., 2012). Instead, individualized assessment is required based on LUTS or signs of urological dysfunction present at the time of assessment. Most individuals with MS report urinary incontinence as the most bothersome urinary symptom, though others present because of recurring UTI or weak urinary stream with elevated residual volumes. Evaluation and selection of a bladder management program is based on a careful examination of lower urinary tract function, including routine measurement of residual urine volume and possibly urodynamic testing.

Management Options

Similar to the patient with an SCI, spontaneous voiding is maintained whenever feasible. Many persons with MS will present with LUTS consistent with neurogenic overactive bladder dysfunction (urgency, daytime voiding frequency, nocturia greater than three episodes per night with or without urge incontinence) and neurogenic detrusor overactivity seen on urodynamic testing. These LUTS may be managed using behavioral interventions for detrusor overactivity as described earlier, often combined with pharmacologic therapy. This approach also may be employed for persons with neurogenic detrusor overactivity and detrusor-striated sphincter dyssynergia provided their residual volumes are comparatively low (usually ≤200 mL) and they are not experiencing upper urinary tract distress. Alpha-1 adrenergic blocking agents may be considered in selected patients to further reduce residual urine volumes. Patients with MS and neurogenic overactive bladder dysfunction may be managed with neuromodulation (including percutaneous tibial nerve stimulation) and intradetrusor injection of onabotulinum toxin A as discussed earlier.

CIC with pharmacologic therapy designed to prevent all detrusor contractions may be used for patients with MS and markedly reduced or absent sensations of bladder filling. This program is also preferred in patients with neurogenic detrusor overactivity, detrusor-striated sphincter dyssynergia, and higher residual volumes. Although CIC plus pharmacotherapy for neurogenic detrusor overactivity is attractive from a urological perspective, it should be prescribed only after careful evaluation of the patient, who may experience impaired dexterity and difficulty with CIC (Bolinger & Engberg, 2013). Nevertheless, a study of 9,702 persons with MS revealed that 81% reported use of CIC at some point during the course of their disease (Mahajan et al., 2013).

Persons with MS and underactive detrusor function are also managed with CIC whenever possible (de Seze et al., 2007). However, indwelling urinary catheterization is occasionally necessary. Persons with MS who are managed with an indwelling catheter tend to have had the disease for a longer period of time resulting in greater impairment of both dexterity and mobility. Males are also more likely to be managed with an indwelling catheter. Despite the limited situations in which indwelling catheter use is recommended, 43% of a cohort of 9,702 persons with MS reported using an indwelling catheter at some point during the course of his or her disease (Mahajan et al., 2013).

KEY POINT

Studies indicate that 81% of individuals with MS use CIC at some point during their illness, and 43% report use of an indwelling catheter at some point.

Ongoing Monitoring

Because of the variable progression of neurologic impairment caused by MS, ongoing urologic monitoring and care is essential (de Seze et al., 2007). It is difficult to determine a routine time frame for follow-up assessments; timing should be based on the success of current bladder management strategies, changes in LUTS, occurrence of urologic complications such as UTI, or progression of MS resulting in a change in dexterity or mobility that affects the person's ability to continue a particular bladder management program.

MS is associated with an increased likelihood of upper urinary tract distress, but the magnitude of this risk is less than that associated with SCI. In one study, upper urinary tract distress was identified in 12.4% of 89 subjects with MS followed over a period of approximately 12 months (Fletcher et al., 2013). Risk factors associated with upper urinary tract distress include age ≥50 years, low bladder wall compliance, and duration of disease (de Seze et al., 2007; Fletcher et al., 2013). **Figure 9-3** and Case 2 describe a 34-year-old male with MS, urinary retention, and underactive detrusor function.

CASE STUDY #2

NEUROGENIC BLADDER IN A 34-YEAR-OLD MALE WITH MULTIPLE SCLEROSIS, URINARY RETENTION, AND UNDERACTIVE DETRUSOR FUNCTION

Figure 9-3 illustrates the case of a 34-year-old male with multiple sclerosis, urinary retention, and underactive detrusor function. AD is a 34-year-old male who was diagnosed with relapsing–remitting multiple sclerosis 8 years prior to evaluation at our continence service. He presented to our service based on self-referral, complaining of weak urinary stream and increasing difficulty urinating. Questioning about lower urinary tract symptoms revealed daytime voiding frequency, urgency with occasional episodes of urge incontinence, two to three episodes of nocturia per night, weak urinary stream, and postvoid dribbling. He reported difficulty initiating urination at times and feelings of incomplete bladder emptying. He denied any prior UTI, dysuria, or hematuria. A review of systems identified increasing weakness of his lower extremities with preservation of upper extremity strength and dexterity. He also reported frequent constipation and erectile dysfunction. Medications included fingolimod 5 mg daily (to prevent exacerbations of MS), baclofen 20 mg twice daily, and vitamin D 5,000 IU daily. He also reported taking the alpha-1 adrenergic blocker tamsulosin 0.4 mg daily but reported it has not improved his urgency as anticipated. Urinalysis was negative; his serum creatinine was 0.9 mg/dL. A 3-day bladder diary revealed voiding every 2 to 3 hours, three episodes of nocturia nightly, and two episodes of urge incontinence.

Urodynamic testing was performed to further evaluate his NLUTD. Testing revealed a large cystometric capacity (800 mL), normal bladder wall compliance, and increased sensations of bladder filling. He experienced neurogenic detrusor overactivity with urgency and dribbling UI at 773 mL of filling. Voiding pressure flow study revealed underactive detrusor function (poor detrusor contraction strength); no detrusor sphincter dyssynergia was noted. His voided volume was 373 mL and his residual volume was 400 mL.

Initially, he was informed of the purpose of tamsulosin (reduction of urethral sphincter resistance in an attempt to improve bladder emptying with micturition) rather than suppression of urgency or urge incontinence episodes. Because of the magnitude of his residual volumes in combination with underactive detrusor function, AD was counseled about the need to add CIC to his bladder management strategy. Two options were discussed in detail, CIC with maintenance of spontaneous voiding or CIC with pharmacotherapy to ablate all detrusor contractions and prevent leakage between catheterizations. He reported reluctance to perform CIC or stop spontaneous voiding. He initially agreed to perform CIC once daily before sleep to reduce frequency of nocturia and improve sleep, and he was encourage to add a morning catheterization if he desired. On follow-up 4 weeks later, he reported adding a second catheterization in the morning and expressed an interest in adding a drug to prevent all leakage with catheterization every 4 to 6 hours. Fesoterodine 4 mg was added to his regimen, with dosage titrated to 8 mg after a 2-week trial. On 6-week follow-up appointment, he reported catheterizing four to five times daily with no incontinence episodes over the past month.

This case illustrates a technique for introducing CIC to patient who was initially reluctant to give up spontaneous voiding. In these cases, teaching the patient to catheterize once daily is recommended because it greatly reduces or (as in AD's case) ablates nocturia entirely. Given the success of that strategy, the patient added a second catheterization episode and he ultimately elected a regular CIC program.

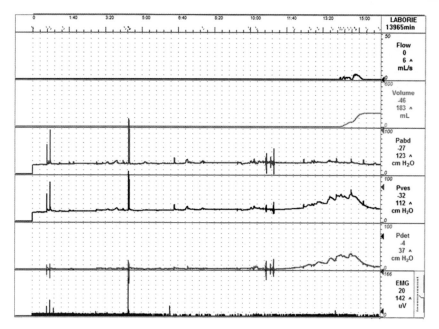

FIGURE 9-3. Neurogenic Bladder in a 34-Year-Old Male with Multiple Sclerosis, Urinary Retention, and Underactive Detrusor Function. Refer to Case 2.

PARKINSON DISEASE

Parkinson disease (PD) is a neurodegenerative disease characterized by a combination of motor deficits including bradykinesia and one or more of the following signs: tremor while at rest, rigidity, and/or postural instability (Bhidayasiri & Reichmann, 2013; Mahlknecht & Poewe, 2013). Various classification schemas have been proposed, but none has gained prominence and the diagnosis of parkinsonism is based on physical assessment and clinical evaluation rather than findings from a definitive diagnostic marker. Approximately 630,000 Americans suffer from PD; its incidence is approximately 13.4 per 100,000 persons making it the second leading form of neurodegenerative disease behind Alzheimer dementia (Kowal et al., 2013; van den Eeden et al., 2003). While dementia is not a characteristic feature of PD, slightly more than 10% also develop Lewy bodies (abnormal protein aggregates found in nerve cells) resulting in dementia, which further increases the likelihood of developing NLUTD dysfunction (Ransmayr et al., 2008; Savica et al., 2013).

Neurogenic Bladder in Parkinson Disease

The mechanisms that produce NLUTD in PD are not entirely understood. Some researchers suggest that the dopaminergic degeneration characteristic of PD causes NLUTD, while others state bladder dysfunction is an incidental finding more related to aging or comorbid conditions (Winge & Fowler, 2006). Clinical experience suggests that PD does cause identifiable NLUTD that is far more prevalent than can be explained by age or comorbid conditions alone. The reported prevalence of LUTS in persons with PD varies significantly; in a meta-analysis of 28 studies, prevalence rates ranged from as low as 7.7% to as high as 97% (Ruffion et al., 2013).

In a study of 271 males with PD in which the prevalence of LUTS was determined based on a validated instrument, slightly more than 40% of respondents reported at least one bothersome LUTS. The most prevalent was urge incontinence, followed by nocturia and voiding frequency (Robinson et al., 2013). Another study of 74 female and male patients found that nocturia was most prevalent, followed by voiding frequency and incontinence (Campos-Sousa et al., 2003). Clinical experience indicates that a minority of patients with PD experience urinary retention, though the cause of the retention is not well understood. A study of 23 men with PD who underwent transurethral resection of the prostate for benign prostatic enlargement found that 36% had persistent urinary retention postoperatively, indicating that retention in these men was at least partially attributable to underactive detrusor function (failure to empty because of the bladder) (Roth et al., 2009). Another study of 41 women and men correlated urodynamic findings and outcomes of PET scanning. Findings in this study suggest that urinary retention in these individuals was due to detrusor underactivity rather than outlet obstruction (Terayama et al., 2012).

While the pathology is not clear, LUTS are common among individuals with PD, ranging from 7.7% to 97%; the most common and problematic symptoms are urge incontinence, nocturia, and frequency. A minority of patients experience retention.

Management Options

Similar to care for patients with other neurological diseases, bladder management is based on the specific lower urinary tract dysfunctions, the physical and cognitive deficits produced by PD, resources in the home, and the patient and family's preferences. Most patients with PD have detrusor overactivity resulting in urge incontinence, frequent urination, and nocturia, as noted above.

Because these patients have intact sensations and they do not experience striated sphincter dyssynergia, they are able to void spontaneously. Behavioral interventions comprise first-line interventions, including fluid and dietary counseling along with scheduled toileting. These interventions are usually combined with pharmacotherapy for detrusor overactivity, as described earlier.

Particular attention should be paid to the symptoms of nocturia and nighttime urgency. Persons with PD have been shown to have a higher incidence of falls and hip fractures than age-matched controls, and nocturia and nighttime urgency have been shown to act as independent risk factors for these events (Asplund, 2006; Brown et al., 2000; Temml et al., 2009). In the case of patients with PD, nocturia is primarily attributable to two factors: nighttime urine production and detrusor overactivity. Options for managing nocturia include fluid restriction for 2 hours prior to sleep and elevation of the lower extremities prior to sleep for persons with dependent edema. Patients taking a diuretic may be advised to move the dose from morning to late afternoon or evening to reduce urine production at night. Pharmacotherapy using the sublingual or intranasal desmopressin also may be used (Cohn et al., 2017; Suman et al., 2019).

KEY POINT

Falls and hip fractures are more common among individuals with PD than age-matched controls, and nocturia and nighttime urgency are major risk factors for these events.

Patients with urinary retention and PD are managed with CIC whenever feasible or indwelling catheterization when CIC is not possible. Indwelling catheterization is more often necessary when retention occurs in a patient whose PD is associated with significant deficits in dexterity and mobility or complicated by Lewy bodies and dementia. Men with PD and evidence of prostatic enlargement and obstruction may be managed pharmacologically or with transurethral or minimally invasive prostatectomy procedures to alleviate obstruction. However, they should be counseled first about possible adverse outcomes of these procedures, including persistent urinary retention or urge incontinence due to detrusor overactivity (Roth et al., 2009).

Comorbid Conditions

Because persons with PD tend to be older when the disease is first diagnosed, they are also more likely to have comorbid conditions impacting lower urinary tract function. For example, a study of 271 male patients found that major depression, constipation, and dementia were present in more than half of men with PD and LUTS (Robinson et al., 2013). BPH, a known cause of LUTS, is also prevalent in older men. The impact of these comorbid conditions has not been extensively studied, but the likelihood that these conditions will influence lower urinary tract function is significant and should be accounted for when managing these challenging patients. **Figure 9-4** and Case 3 describe a 78-year-old male with PD and NLUTD complicated by benign prostatic enlargement.

CASE STUDY #3

NEUROGENIC BLADDER IN A 78-YEAR-OLD MALE WITH BENIGN PROSTATIC ENLARGEMENT

Figure 9-4 illustrates the case of PA, a 78-year-old male diagnosed with PD 2 years prior to evaluation for NLUTD. He is accompanied by his wife, who suffered a stroke approximately 1 year ago. He is able to walk for short distances with the aid of a walker; he requires a wheelchair for longer distances. His speech appears somewhat slowed, but he is alert and able to answer questions without assistance. Lower urinary tract symptoms include nocturia up to six episodes per night, daytime voiding frequency, urgency, and urge incontinence episodes. PA stated that he found paradoxical urgency to urinate, but difficulty initiating micturition when reaching the toilet, to be the most bothersome of all his lower urinary tract symptoms. He also described using an absorptive brief to manage urinary incontinence whenever traveling

away from home. Approximately 2 years prior to being diagnosed with PD, PA was evaluated for LUTS associated with benign prostatic enlargement. Notes from that examination revealed nocturia three episodes per night, weak urinary stream, and urgency but no urinary incontinence. Several postvoid residual volumes were measured, which varied from 60 to 90 mL. A minimally invasive prostatectomy was advised but PA declined surgery. He was advised about watchful waiting versus pharmacotherapy for LUTS but elected to pursue no further therapy at the time. Current medications include amantadine 100 mg twice daily, carbidopa–levodopa 25 to 100 mg three times daily, olmesartan–amlodipine 5/20, and furosemide 40 mg daily. Urinalysis was normal; his serum creatinine was 1.3 mg/dL.

Videourodynamic testing revealed small cystometric capacity (275 mL) with neurogenic detrusor overactivity resulting in urgency and involuntary urination.

No detrusor sphincter dyssynergia was noted, but voiding urethrography revealed narrowing and elongation of his proximal (prostatic) urethra; the voiding pressure flow study indicated moderately severe bladder outlet obstruction; his residual volume was 70 mL.

PA was counseled that his bladder dysfunction was attributable to his prostatic enlargement and his PD. He was counseled about fluid and dietary interventions for management of neurogenic detrusor overactivity. He was started on tamsulosin 0.4 mg daily and finasteride 5 mg daily for treatment of his prostatic enlargement. He was also counseled about management of his nocturia. He was provided a urinal to avoid the need to move from bed to his regular toilet, and he was advised about restriction of fluids within 2 hours of bedtime. He was also advised to move his furosemide dosage from breakfast to dinner in order to reduce nighttime urine production. Follow-up appointment 4 weeks later revealed that his nocturia had declined from six episodes per night to three. He reported that he was able to urinate with less hesitancy, but he also noted that he now had less warning before the onset of urge incontinence. Bladder ultrasound revealed a postvoid residual volume of 90 mL. In order to better manage his neurogenic detrusor overactivity, he began taking darifenacin 7.5 mg daily. After 4 weeks, PA reported that his nocturia had been reduced to two episodes per night, and

he was experiencing less than one urge incontinent episode per day. Bladder ultrasound revealed a post-void residual volume of 75 mL.

This case illustrates the multiple factors that may contribute to LUTS in an older man with NLUTD associated with PD. Initial treatment focused on addressing benign prostatic enlargement. Despite moderately severe bladder outlet obstruction, pharmacotherapy was favored over transurethral resection of the prostate because of concerns that surgery might worsen his underlying neurogenic detrusor overactivity and urge incontinence if urethral resistance were markedly reduced using a surgical approach. Rather, a pharmacological approach was adopted using one drug (finasteride) that acted to reduce prostate size and a second drug (tamsulosin) that acted to reduce smooth muscle tone within the urethra (**Table 9-2**).

Nocturia was addressed by altering the patient's environment (providing a urinal) and by reducing nighttime urine production. Two strategies were used to reduce nighttime urine production, restriction of fluids 2 hours prior to sleep and moving administration of his diuretic medication from the morning to dinner time. A final mediation, darifenacin, was added to reduce the LUTS urgency and urge incontinence. While this addition did not completely eradicate his urge incontinence episodes, it reduced these symptoms to an acceptable level without elevating his postvoid residual volumes.

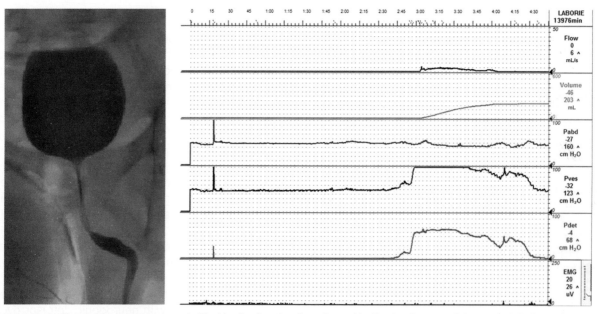

FIGURE 9-4. An Elderly Man with Neurogenic Bladder Dysfunction Complicated by Benign Prostatic Enlargement. Refer to Case 3.

STROKE

The term *stroke* (sometimes referred to as cerebrovascular accident or brain attack) is defined as an acute, focal injury of the central nervous system owing to a vascular cause such as cerebral infarction, intracerebral hemorrhage, or subarachnoid hemorrhage (Sacco et al., 2013). Strokes associated with cerebral infarction may be classified as ischemic or hemorrhagic. Approximately 6.8 million Americans have experienced a stroke in their lifetime, accounting for nearly 3% of the population (Ma et al., 2014). The physical consequences of a stroke vary significantly, but they tend to be more severe among older persons. Approximately 26% of older individuals who suffered a stroke remain dependent for one or more activities of daily living 6 months after the event, and 30% remain unable to walk without assistance. A systematic review and meta-analysis of 61 studies involving stroke patients reported that 64.7% of persons experiencing a stroke also experience NLUTD (Ruffion et al., 2013).

Stroke and Urologic Symptoms

Stroke produces a more homogenous group of LUTS than SCI or MS. A neurologic lesion that affects the brain alone tends to produce neurogenic detrusor overactivity with intact sensory function; thus, urgency, frequency, nocturia, and urge incontinence are the most commonly reported LUTS (McKenzie & Badlani, 2012). Several urodynamic studies have found evidence of underactive detrusor function in 33% to 40% of patients following cerebrovascular accident, but the magnitude of detrusor underactivity and its clinical relevance have not yet been established. While MS and PD are characterized by progression of neurologic deficits over time, functional impairments associated with a stroke may improve following the original insult (Hayward et al., 2014). For example, a longitudinal study of 340 patients with LUTS and a stroke found that 35% of the patients who reported new onset of urge urinary incontinence immediately following a stroke experienced resolution of urinary leakage at 12 months (Williams et al., 2012). Risk factors for persistent incontinence in this group included urinary leakage prior to the stroke and female gender.

KEY POINT

A total of 64.7% of individuals who sustain a stroke experience NLUTD (neurogenic overactive bladder), but 35% of these individuals experience spontaneous resolution within 12 months.

Management Options

Similar to the prior specific examples of NLUTD, assessment and care of the patient who has experienced a stroke must take into consideration the physical and cognitive disabilities created by the stroke, characteristics of the associated bladder dysfunction, resources in the home, and patient and family preference. Because most patients have intact sensation and do not experience striated sphincter dyssynergia, the vast majority are able to manage their bladder with spontaneous voiding.

Behavioral interventions, including fluid and dietary advice and scheduled toileting, are usual first-line interventions. Ultimately, many individuals will also require pharmacologic management for neurogenic detrusor overactivity. The efficacy of pharmacotherapy is enhanced when combined with behavioral interventions. In addition, because many persons with a stroke recover physical function over time, it is reasonable to consider pharmacotherapy over a 6- to 12-month period, followed by a drug holiday, and to discontinue drug therapy whenever possible. Because of the risk of detrusor underactivity, patients managed pharmacologically should be counseled about the risk of urinary retention and should be monitored with postvoid residual urine measurements as indicated.

The prevalence of stroke is highest among older adults, and management of the male patient should incorporate consideration of the potential for BPH and its impact on neurogenic dysfunction (McKenzie & Badlani, 2012). Because of the risk of obstruction and urinary retention associated with BPH, older men with bladder dysfunction following a stroke should undergo postvoid residual measurement as part of a continence evaluation, and many will benefit from multichannel urodynamic testing.

Neurogenic bladder dysfunction in patients with stroke is not associated with low bladder compliance or outlet obstruction caused by detrusor-striated sphincter dyssynergia; thus, the risk of hostile bladder dysfunction and upper urinary tract distress is low (McKenzie & Badlani, 2012). Patients who experience febrile UTI, vesicoureteral reflux, or deterioration of renal function should undergo evaluation for other potential causes of upper urinary tract distress. **Figure 9-5** and Case 4 describe a 75-year-old female with NLUTD and new-onset urge urinary incontinence following a stroke affecting the middle cerebral artery.

CASE STUDY #4

NEUROGENIC BLADDER IN A 75-YEAR-OLD FEMALE FOLLOWING A STROKE

Figure 9-5 illustrates the case of MK, a 75-year-old female who experienced an ischemic stroke involving the middle cerebral artery 16 weeks prior to evaluation. Prior to her stroke, she reported mild stress urinary incontinence that did not require regular use of pads. Upon presentation to our clinic, she reported voiding frequency of every hour and frequent incontinence episodes with complete loss of the ability to postpone urination. She tearfully reported the need for absorptive briefs at all times to prevent urinary leakage. She also reported four to five episodes of nocturia per night that usually resulted in incontinence before she was able to reach the toilet. Physical assessment revealed mild left hemiparesis; her speech was clear and she was alert and oriented throughout her evaluation. She was able to ambulate without assistance although she reported her gait as somewhat slowed. Current medications included lisinopril 5 mg daily and clopidogrel 75 mg daily. Urinalysis was normal and her serum creatinine was 0.9 mg/dL.

Urodynamic testing revealed small cystometric capacity (60 to 90 mL) with neurogenic detrusor overactivity and urge incontinence. Voiding pressure flow study demonstrated good detrusor contraction strength and no detrusor-striated sphincter dyssynergia. Residual volumes were 0 mL on sequential examinations.

Because of the severity of her voiding frequency and incontinence episodes, she was initially provided education about behavioral management of neurogenic detrusor overactivity (including dietary and fluid advice along with urge suppression techniques) and begun on a medication to alleviate her neurogenic detrusor overactivity (trospium extended release 60 mg daily). She was also advised that LUTS improve in some patients just as their physical function can improve over time. On follow-up, 3 weeks later, she reported significant improvement in her voiding frequency to every 1.5 hours and reduction of her nocturia to two episodes per night. Bladder ultrasound revealed a residual urine volume of 20 mL. Alternative medications were discussed, but she elected to continue with her current bladder management strategy. Telephone follow-up at 3 months revealed further reductions in daytime frequency to every 2 hours or more and reduction of nocturia to two episodes per night. During a scheduled follow-up visit at 6 months, the possibility of a medication holiday was discussed (stopping her daily antimuscarinic drug). MK expressed some anxiety but agreed to stop her medication. Telephone follow-up revealed that she remained off her medication and had not experienced the return of frequent urination and incontinence she had feared.

This case illustrates management of a sudden onset of urge incontinence caused by neurogenic detrusor overactivity following a stroke. It also emphasizes the importance of considering the natural history of the underlying neurological disorder when managing NLUTD. In this case, research has shown that many patients will experience a sudden onset of urge incontinence that may subside over the first 12 months following a stroke as the brain recovers and adapts. By providing a drug holiday, MK was able to determine that she was able to retain continence without ongoing drug therapy.

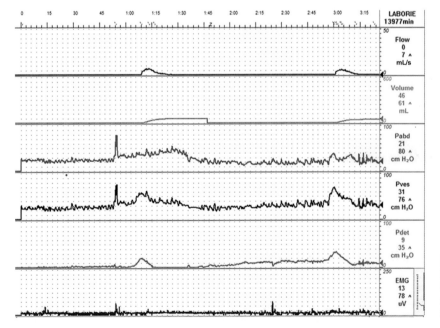

FIGURE 9-5. A 75-Year-Old Female with Neurogenic Bladder and New-Onset Urge Urinary Incontinence Following a Stroke Affecting the Middle Cerebral Artery. Refer to Case 4.

CONCLUSIONS

NLUTD is associated with a variety of underlying disorders resulting in a wide variety of negative consequences to lower urinary tract function. Assessment and treatment of patients with NLUTD relies on evaluation of bladder, urethral, and pelvic floor muscle dysfunction, combined with knowledge of the patient's physical and cognitive status, social situation, and knowledge of the natural history of the underlying neurological disorder.

REFERENCES

2019 American Geriatrics Society Beers Criteria® Update Expert Panel. (2019). American Geriatrics Society 2019 Updated AGS Beers Criteria® for Potentially Inappropriate Medication Use in Older Adults. *Journal of the American Geriatrics Society, 67*(4), 674–694.

Abrams, P., Cardozo, L., Fall, M., et al. (2002). The standardization of nomenclature for lower urinary tract function. *Neurourology and Urodynamics, 21,* 167–178.

Adamowicz, J., Pokrywczynska, M., Van Breda, S. V., et al. (2017). Concise review: Tissue engineering of urinary bladder; we still have a long way to go? *Nature Review in Urology, 6*(11), 2033–2043.

Ahluwalia, R. S., Johal, N., Kouriefs, C., et al. (2006). The surgical risk of suprapubic catheter insertion and long-term sequelae. *Annals of the Royal College of Surgeons England, 88,* 201–203.

Ahmed, H. U., Sherfill, I. S., Arya, M., et al. (2006). Management of detrusor-external sphincter dyssynergia. *Nature Clinical Practice Urology, 3*(7), 368–380.

Aizawa, N., & Igawa, Y. (2017). Pathophysiology of the underactive bladder. *Investigative and Clinical Urology, 58*(Suppl 2), S82–S89.

Al-Ali, M., & Haddad, L. (1996). A 10 year review of the endoscopic treatment of 125 spinal cord injured patients with vesical outlet obstruction: Does bladder neck dyssynergia exist? *Paraplegia, 34,* 34–38.

Amend, B., Hennenlotter, J., Schafer, T., et al. (2008). Effective treatment of neurogenic detrusor dysfunction by combined high dose antimuscarinics without increased side effects. *European Urology, 53*(5), 1021–1028.

Andersson, K. E. (2011). Muscarinic acetylcholine receptors in the urinary tract. *Handbook of Experimental Pharmacology, 202,* 319–344.

Andre, L., Gallini, A., Montastruc, F., et al. (2019). Anticholinergic exposure and cognitive decline in older adults: Effect of anticholinergic exposure definitions in a 3-year analysis of the multidomain Alzheimer preventive trial (MAPT) study. *British Journal of Clinical Pharmacology, 85*(1), 71–99.

Andretta, E., Landi, L. M., Cianfrocca, M., et al. (2019). Bladder management during pregnancy in women with spinal-cord injury: An observational, multicenter study. *International Urogynecology Journal, 30*(2), 293–300.

Anson, C., & Gray, M. (1993). Secondary complications after spinal cord injury. *Urologic Nursing, 13*(4), 107–112.

Arya, N. A., & Weissbart, S. J. (2017). Central control of micturition in women: Brain-bladder pathways in continence and urgency urinary incontinence. *Clinical Anatomy, 30,* 373–384.

Asplund, R. (2006). Hip fractures, nocturia and nocturnal polyuria in the elderly. *Archives of Gerontology and Geriatrics, 43*(3), 319–326.

Atala, A. (2014). Regenerative bladder augmentation using autologous tissue—When will we get there? *Journal of Urology, 191,* 1204–1205.

Atala, A., Bauer, S. B., Soker, S., et al. (2006). Tissue-engineered autologous bladders for patients needing cystoplasty. *Lancet, 367,* 1241–1246.

Awad, S. A., Bryniak, S. R., Downie, J. W., et al. (1977). Urethral pressure profile during the spinal shock stage in man: A preliminary report. *Journal of Urology, 117*(1), 91–93.

Bacsu, C., Chan, L., & Tse, V. (2012). Diagnosing detrusor sphincter dyssynergia in the neurological patient. *BJU International, 109*(Suppl 3), 31–34.

Barrett, D. M. (1981). The effect of bethanechol chloride on voiding in female patients with excessive residual urine: A randomized double-blind study. *Journal of Urology, 126,* 640–642.

Barroso, J. C. V., Ramos, J. G. L., Martins-Costa, S., et al. (2004). Transvaginal electrical stimulation in the treatment of urinary incontinence. *BJU International, 93,* 319–323.

Beirs, S. M., Venn, S. N., & Greenwell, T. J. (2011). The past, present and future of augmentation cystoplasty. *BJU International, 109,* 1280–1293.

Bennett, J. K., Green, B. G., Foote, J. E., et al. (1995). Collagen injections for intrinsic sphincter deficiency in the neuropathic urethra. *Paraplegia, 33*(12), 697–700.

Bhidayasiri, R., & Reichmann, H. (2013). Different diagnostic criteria for Parkinson disease: What are the pitfalls? *Journal of Neural Transmission, 120,* 619–625.

Bodner, D. R. (2009). Comarr memorial reward for distinguished clinical service: The legacy of A. Estin Comarr, MD. *Journal of Spinal Cord Medicine, 32*(3), 213–214.

Bolinger, R., & Engberg, S. (2013). Barriers, complications, adherence and self-reported quality of life for people using clean intermittent catheterization. *Journal of Wound, Ostomy, and Continence Nursing, 40*(1), 83–89.

Boone, T. B. (2009). External urethral sphincter stent for dyssynergia. *Journal of Urology, 181,* 1538–1539.

Booth, J., Connelly, L., Dickinson, F., et al. (2018). The effectiveness of transcutaneous tibial nerve stimulation (TTNS) for adults with overactive bladder syndrome: A systematic review. *Neurourology and Urodynamics, 37,* 528–541.

Bors, E., & Comarr, A. E. (1971). *Neurological urology.* Baltimore, MD: University Park Press.

Bradley, C. S., Erickson, B. A., Messersmith, E. E., et al. (2017). Evidence of the impact of diet, fluid intake, caffeine, alcohol and tobacco on lower urinary tract symptoms: A systematic review. *Journal of Urology, 198*(5), 1010–1020.

Brown, J. S., Vitinghoff, E., Wyman, J. F., et al. (2000). Urinary incontinence: Does it increase risk for falls and fractures? *Journal of the American Geriatrics Society, 48*(7), 721–725.

Budge, J. (1864). Uber den Einfluss des Nervebsystems auf die Bewegung der Blasé. Zietschr. F. *Rationelle Medizin, 21,* 1.

Burton, C., Sajja, A., & Latthe, P. M. (2012). Effectiveness of percutaneous posterior tibial nerve stimulation for overactive bladder: A systematic review and meta-analysis. *Neurourology and Urodynamics, 31*(8), 1206–1216.

Cameron, A. (2010). Pharmacologic therapy for the neurogenic bladder. *Urologic Clinics of North America, 37,* 495–506.

Campos-Sousa, R. N., Quagliato, E., de Silva, B. B., et al. (2003). Urinary symptoms in Parkinson's disease: Prevalence and associated factors. *Arquivos de Neuro-Psiquiatria, 61*(2B), 359–363.

Canbaz-Kabay, S., Kabay, S., Mestan, E., et al. (2017). Long term sustained therapeutic effects of percutaneous posterior tibial nerve stimulation treatment of neurogenic overactive bladder in multiple sclerosis patients: 12-months results. *Neurourology and Urodynamics, 36*(1), 104–110.

Carriere, I., Fourrier-Reglat, A., Dartigues, J. F., et al. (2009). Drugs with anticholinergic properties, cognitive decline, and dementia in an elderly general population: The 3-city study. *Archives of Internal Medicine, 169*(14), 1317–1324.

Castel-Lacanal, E., Game, X., De Boissezon, X., et al. (2013). Impact of intermittent catheterization on the quality of life in patients with multiple sclerosis. *World Journal of Urology, 31*(6), 1445–1450.

Chai, T. C., Gray, M. L., & Steers, W. D. (1998). The incidence of a positive ice water test on bladder outlet obstructed patients: Evidence for altered innervation. *Journal of Urology, 160,* 34–38.

Chapple, C. R., MacDiarmid, S. A., & Patel, A. (2009). *Urodynamics made easy* (3rd ed., p. 117). Oxford, UK: Elsevier.

Chartier Kastler, E., & Denys, P. (2011). Intermittent catheterization with hydrophilic catheters as a treatment of chronic neurogenic urinary retention. *Neurourology and Urodynamics, 30,* 21–31.

Chartier Kastler, E., Genevois, S., Game, X., et al. (2011). Treatment of neurogenic male urinary incontinence related to intrinsic sphincter insufficiency with an artificial urinary sphincter: A French retrospective multicenter study. *BJU International, 107*(3), 426–432.

Chen, G., Liao, L., & Li, Y. (2015). The possible role of percutaneous tibial nerve stimulation using adhesive skin surface electrodes in patients with neurogenic detrusor overactivity secondary to spinal cord injury. *International Urology and Nephrology, 47*(3), 451–455.

Coblentz, T., & Gray, M. (2001). Bladder neck obstruction in the female: A case study. *Urologic Nursing, 21*, 265–272.

Cohn, J. A., Kowalik, C. G., Reynolds, W. S., et al. (2017). Desmopressin acetate nasal spray for adults with nocturia. *Expert Review of Clinical Pharmacology, 10*(12), 1281–1293.

Cruz, F. (2014). Targets for botulinum toxin the lower urinary tract. *Neurourology and Urodynamics, 33*, 31–38.

Curtis, J., & Klykken, P. (2008). *A comparative assessment of three common catheter materials.* Retrieved from http://www.dowcorning.com/content/publishedlit/52-1116.pdf

Danforth, T. L., & Ginsberg, D. A. (2014). Neurogenic lower urinary tract dysfunction: How when and with which patients do we use urodynamics. *Urologic Clinics of North America, 41*, 445–452.

Davis, N. F., Kheradmand, F., & Creagh, T. (2013). Injectable biomaterials for the treatment of stress urinary incontinence: Their potential and pitfalls as urethral bulking agents. *International Urogynecology Journal, 24*(6), 913–919.

Day, R. A., Moore, K. N., & Albers, M. K. (2002). A study comparing 2 methods of intermittent catheterization: Limitations and challenges. *Urologic Nursing, 23*(2), 143–147.

de Groat, W. C., Griffiths, D., & Yoshimura, N. (2015). Neural control of the lower urinary tract. *Comprehensive Physiology, 5*, 327–396.

de Groat, W. C., & Wickens, C. (2013). Organization of the neural switching circuitry underlying reflex micturition. *Acta Physiologica (Oxford), 207*, 66–84.

De Seze, M., Ruffion, A., Denys, P., et al. (2007). GENULF study group. The neurogenic bladder in multiple sclerosis: Review of the literature and proposal of management guidelines. *Multiple Sclerosis, 13*, 915–928.

Denys, M. A., Viaene, A., Goessaert, A. S., et al. (2017). Circadian rhythms in water and solute handling in adults with a spinal cord injury. *Journal of Urology, 197*(2), 445–451.

Ditunno, J. F., Little, J. W., Tessler, A., et al. (2004). Spinal shock revisited: A four-phase model. *Spinal Cord, 42*, 383–395.

Donovan, W. H. (2007). Donald munro lecture: Spinal Cord Injury—Past, present and future. *Journal of Spinal Cord Medicine, 30*, 85–100.

Drake, M. J., Williams, J., & Bijos, D. A. (2014). Voiding dysfunction due to detrusor underactivity: An overview. *Nature Reviews in Urology, 11*, 454–464.

Engberg, S., Clapper, J., McNichol, L., et al. (2020). Current evidence related to intermittent catheterization: A scoping review. *Journal of Wound Ostomy & Continence Nursing, 47*(2), 140–165.

Engkasan, J. P., Ng, C. J., & Low, W. Y. (2014). Factors influencing bladder management in male patients with spinal cord injury: A qualitative study. *Spinal Cord, 52*(2), 157–162.

Faleiros, F., Käppler, C., Costa, J. N., et al. (2016). Predictive factors for intermittent self-catheterization in German and Brazilian individuals with spina bifida and neurogenic bladder dysfunction. *Journal of Wound Ostomy & Continence Nursing, 43*(6), 636–640.

Finkbeiner, A. E. (1985). Is bethanechol chloride clinically effective in promoting bladder emptying? A literature review. *Journal of Urology, 134*, 443–449.

Fletcher, S. G., Dillon, B. E., Gilchrist, A. S., et al. (2013). Renal deterioration in multiple sclerosis patients with neurovesical dysfunction. *Multiple Sclerosis, 19*, 1169–1174.

Fowler, S., Godfrey, H., Fader, M., et al. (2014). Living with a long-term indwelling urinary catheter: Catheter user's experiences. *Journal of Wound, Ostomy, and Continence Nursing, 41*(6), 597–603.

Frazier, E. P., Peters, S. L., Braverman, A. S., et al. (2008). Signal conduction underlying the control of urinary bladder smooth muscle tone by muscarinic receptors and beta-adrenoreceptors. *Naunyn-Schmiedebergs Archives of Pharmacology, 377*(4–6), 449–462.

Gajewski, J. B., Schurch, B., Hamid, R., et al. (2018). An International Continence Society (ICS) report on the terminology for adult neurogenic lower urinary tract dysfunction (ANLUTD). *Neurourology and Urodynamics, 37*, 1152–1161.

Ghoniem, G. M., Bloom, D. A., McGuire, E. J., et al. (1989). Bladder compliance in myelomeningocele children. *The Journal of Urology, 141*(6), 1404–1406.

Gormley, E. A. (2010). Urologic complications of the neurogenic bladder. *Urologic Clinics of North America, 37*(4), 601–607.

Gormley, E. A., Lightner, D. J., Burgio, K. L., et al. (2014). *Diagnosis and treatment of overactive bladder (non-neurogenic) in adults: AUA/SUFU Guideline.* Retrieved from http://www.auanet.org/common/pdf/education/clinical-guidance/Overactive-Bladder.pdf

Graham, S. D., Keane, T. E., & Glenn, J. F. (Eds.). (2007). *Glenn's urologic surgery* (7th ed.). Philadelphia, PA: Wolters Kluwer Health.

Gray, M. (2007). An update on the physiology of urinary continence. *Continence UK, 1*(2), 28–36.

Gray, M. (2008). Reflex urinary incontinence. In B. K. Ackely & G. B. Ladwig (Eds.), *Nursing diagnosis handbook* (8th ed., pp. 458–461). Philadelphia, PA: Elsevier.

Gray, M. (2010). Traces: Making sense of urodynamics testing—Part 2: Uroflowmetry. *Urologic Nursing, 30*(6), 321–326.

Gray, M. (2011a). Traces: Making sense of urodynamic testing—Part 6: Evaluation of bladder filling/storage: Bladder wall compliance and the detrusor leak point pressure. *Urologic Nursing, 31*(4), 215–221.

Gray, M. (2011b). Traces: Making sense of urodynamics testing-Part 7: Evaluation of bladder filling/storage: Evaluation of urethral sphincter incompetence and stress urinary incontinence. *Urologic Nursing, 31*(5), 267–277, 289.

Gray, M. (2012a). Traces: Making sense of urodynamics testing—Part 10: Evaluation of micturition via the voiding pressure-flow study. *Urologic Nursing, 32*(2), 71–78.

Gray, M. (2012b). Traces: Making sense of urodynamics testing—Part 11: Quantitative analysis of micturition via the voiding pressure-flow study. *Urologic Nursing, 32*(3), 159–165.

Gray, M., Joseph, A. C., Mercer, D. M., et al. (2008). Consensus and controversies in urinary drainage systems: Indications for improving patient's safety. *Safe Practice in Patient Care, 4*(1), 1–7.

Gray, M., Rayome, R., & Anson, C. (1995a). Incontinence and clean intermittent catheterization following spinal cord injury. *Clinical Nursing Research, 4*(1), 6–21.

Gray, M., Rayome, R., & Moore, K. N. (1995b). The urethral sphincter: An update. *Urologic Nursing, 15*(2), 40–55.

Gray, M., Skinner, C., & Kaller, W. (2016). External collection devices as an alternative to the indwelling urinary catheter: Evidence-based review and expert clinical panel deliberations. *Journal of Wound Ostomy & Continence Nursing, 43*(3), 301–307.

Gray, M., Wasner, M., & Nichols, T. (2019). Nursing practice related to intermittent catheterization: A cross-sectional survey. *Journal of Wound Ostomy & Continence Nursing, 46*(5), 418–423.

Griffiths, D. (2015). Neural control of micturition in humans: A working model. *Nature Reviews Urology, 12*(12), 695–705.

Griffiths, D. J., & Fowler, C. J. (2013). The micturition reflex and its forebrain influences. *Acta Physiologica (Oxford), 207*, 93–109.

Griffiths, D. H., Harrison, G., Moore, K., et al. (1996). Variability of post-void residual urine volume in the elderly. *Urological Research, 24*(1), 23–26.

Groen, L. A., Spinoit, A. F., Hoebeke, P., et al. (2012). The advance male sling as a minimally invasive treatment for intrinsic sphincter deficiency in men with neurogenic bladder sphincter dysfunction: A pilot study. *Neurourology and Urodynamics, 31*(8), 1284–1287.

Guttman, L., & Frankel, H. (1966). The value of intermittent catheterization in the management of traumatic paraplegia and tetraplegia. *Paraplegia, 4*, 63–84.

Hald, T., & Bradley, W. E. (1982). *The urinary bladder: Neurology and dynamics* (pp. 1–4). Baltimore, MD: Lippincott Williams & Wilkins.

Hayward, K. S., Barker, R. N., Carson, R. G., et al. (2014). The effect of altering a single component of a rehabilitation programme on the functional recovery of stroke patients: A systematic review and meta-analysis. *Clinical Rehabilitation, 28*(2), 107–117.

Hosker, G., Rosier, P., Gajewski, J., et al. (2009). Dynamic testing. In P. Abrams, L. Cardozo, S. Khoury, et al. (Eds.), *Incontinence* (4th ed., pp. 413–522). London, UK: Health Publication Ltd.

Institute of Medicine, Food and Science Board. (2004). Retrieved from http://www.iom.edu/Global/News%20Announcements/~/media/442A08B899F44DF9AAD083D86164C75B.ashx

International Neuromodulation Society. *About neuromodulation.* Retrieved November 9, 2020, from https://www.neuromodulation.com/about-neuromodulation

Jaqua, K., & Powell, C. R. (2017). Where are we headed with neuromodulation for overactive bladder? *Current Urology Reports, 18*(8), 59.

Joseph, D. B., Borer, J. G., DeFillipo, R. E., et al. (2014). Autologous seeded biodegradable scaffold for augmentation cystoplasty: Phase II study in children and adolescents with spina bifida. *Journal of Urology, 191,* 1389–1395.

Kabay, S., Canbaz-Kabay, S., Cetiner, M., et al. (2016). The clinical and urodynamic results of percutaneous posterior tibial nerve stimulation on neurogenic detrusor overactivity in patients with Parkinson's disease. *Urology, 87,* 76–81.

Kari, J., Al-Deek, B., Elkhatib, L., et al. (2013). Is Mitrofanoff a more socially acceptable CIC route for children and their families? *European Journal of Surgery, 23,* 405–410.

Katsumi, H. K., Kalisvaart, J. F., Ronningen, L. D., et al. (2010). Urethral versus suprapubic catheter: Choosing the best bladder management for male spinal cord injury patients with indwelling catheters. *Spinal Cord, 48,* 325–329.

Kenelly, M. J., Lemack, G. E., Foote, J. E., et al. (2009). Efficacy and safety of transdermal oxybutynin system in spinal cord injury patients with neurogenic detrusor overactivity and incontinence: An open label, dose titration study. *Urology, 74*(4), 741–745.

Killorin, W., Gray, M., Bennett, J. K., et al. (1992). The value of urodynamics and bladder management in predicting upper urinary tract distress in male spinal cord injury patients. *Paraplegia, 30,* 437–441.

Kirshblum, S. C., Biering-Sorenson, F., Betz, R., et al. (2014). International standards for neurological classification of spinal cord injury: Cases with classification challenges. *Journal of Spinal Cord Medicine, 37*(2), 120–128.

Kojima, Y., Kubota, Y., Sasaki, S., et al. (2009). Translational pharmacology in aging men with benign prostatic hyperplasia: Molecular and clinical approaches to alpha-1 adrenoreceptors. *Current Aging Science, 2*(3), 223–229.

Kowal, S. L., Dall, T. M., Chakrabarti, R., et al. (2013). Current and projected economic burden of Parkinson's disease in the United States. *Movement Disorders, 28*(3), 311–318.

Krebs, J., Scheel-Sailer, A., Oertli, R., et al., (2018). The effects of antimuscarinic treatment on the cognition of spinal cord injured individuals with neurogenic lower urinary tract dysfunction: a prospective controlled before-and-after study, *Spinal Cord, 56*(1), 22–27.

Kulwin, C. G., Patel, N. B., Ackerman, L. L., et al. (2013). Radiographic and clinical outcome of syringomyelia in patients treated for tethered spinal cord without other significant imaging abnormalities. *Journal of Neurosurgery Pediatrics, 11*(3), 307–312.

Lane, G. I., Driscoll, A., Tawfik, K., et al. (2017). A cross-sectional study of the catheter management of neurogenic bladder after traumatic spinal cord injury. *Neurourology and Urodynamics, 37*(1), 360–367.

Lapeyre, E., Kuks, J. B., & Meijler, W. J. (2010). Revisiting the role and the individual value of several pharmacological treatments. *Neurorehabilitation, 27*(2), 193–200.

Lapides, J. (1970). Neuromuscular, vesicle and ureteral dysfunction. In M. F. Campbell & J. H. Harrison (Eds.), *Campbell's urology* (3rd ed., pp. 1343–1379). Philadelphia, PA: Saunders.

Lapides, J., Diokno, A. C., & Silber, S. J. (1972). Clean intermittent catheterization in the treatment of urinary tract disease. *Journal of Urology, 107*(3), 458–461.

Liard, A., Seguier-Lipszyc, E., Mathiot, A., et al. (2001). The Mitrofanoff procedure: 20 years later. *Journal of Urology, 165*(6 Pt 2), 2394–2398.

Linsenmeyer, T. A. (2018). Catheter-associated urinary tract infections in persons with neurogenic bladders. *Journal of Spinal Cord Medicine, 41*(2), 132–141.

Linsenmeyer, T. A., & Linsenmeyer, M. A. (2013). Impact of annual urodynamic evaluations on guiding bladder management in individuals with spinal cord injuries. *Journal of Spinal Cord Medicine, 36*(5), 420–426.

Lucas, M. G., Bedretdinova, D., Bosch, J. L., et al. (2013). *Guidelines on urinary incontinence.* European Association of Urology. Retrieved from http://www.uroweb.org/gls/pdf/19_Urinary_Incontinence_LR.pdf

Lukacz, E. S., Sampselle, C., Gray, M., et al. (2011). A healthy bladder: A consensus statement. *International Journal of Clinical Practice, 65*(10), 1026–1036.

Ma, V. Y., Chan, L., & Carruthers, K. J. (2014). Incidence, prevalence, costs, and impact on disability of common conditions requiring rehabilitation in the United States: Stroke, spinal cord injury, traumatic brain injury, multiple sclerosis, osteoarthritis, rheumatoid arthritis, limb loss, and back pain. *Archives of Physical Medicine and Rehabilitation, 95,* 986–995.

Mahajan, S. T., Frasure, H. E., & Marrie, R. A. (2013). The prevalence of urinary catheterization in women and men with multiple sclerosis. *Journal of Spinal Cord Medicine, 36*(6), 632–637.

Mahfouz, W., & Corcos, J. (2011). Management of detrusor external sphincter dyssynergia in neurogenic bladder. *European Journal of Physical and Rehabilitation Medicine, 47*(4), 639–650.

Mahlknecht, P., & Poewe, W. (2013). Is there a need to redefine Parkinson's disease? *Journal of Neural Transmission, 120*(Suppl 1), S9–S17.

Marberger, M. (2013). Medical management of lower urinary tract symptoms in men with benign prostatic enlargement. *Advances in Therapy, 30*(4), 309–319.

Martens, F. M., van Kuppevelt, H. J., Beekman, J. A., et al. (2010). Limited value of bladder sensation as a trigger for conditional neurostimulation in spinal cord injury patients. *Neurourology and Urodynamics, 29*(3), 395–400.

Marziale, L., Lucarini, G., Mazzocchi, T., et al. (2018). Artificial sphincters to manage urinary incontinence: A review. *Artificial Organs, 42*(9), E215–E233.

McGuire, E. J., Woodside, J. R., Borden, T. A., et al. (1981). Prognostic value of urodynamic testing in myelodysplastic children. *Journal of Urology, 126*(2), 205–209.

McIntyre, A., Mary, R., Mehta, S., et al. (2014). Examining the effectiveness of intrathecal baclofen on spasticity in individuals with chronic spinal cord injury: A systematic review. *Journal of Spinal Cord Medicine, 37*(1), 11–18.

McKenzie, P., & Badlani, G. H. (2012). The incidence and etiology of overactive bladder in patients after cerebrovascular accident. *Current Urological Reports, 13,* 402–406.

Mehta, A., Hill, D., Foley, N., et al. (2012). A meta-analysis of botulinum toxin sphincteric injections in the treatment of incomplete voiding after spinal cord injury. *Archives in Physical Medicine and Rehabilitation, 93,* 597–603.

Mertens, P., Parise, M., Garcia-Larrea, L., et al. (1995). Long-term clinical electrophysiological and urodynamic effects of chronic intrathecal baclofen infusion for treatment of spinal spasticity. *Acat Neurochirurgica, 64*(Suppl), 17–25.

Milo, R., & Miller, A. (2014). Revised diagnostic criteria of multiple sclerosis. *Autoimmunity Reviews, 13,* 518–524.

Mirone, V., Imbimbo, C., Longo, N., et al. (2007). The detrusor muscle: An innocent victim of bladder outlet obstruction. *European Urology, 51*(1), 57–66.

Moon, H. J., Chun, M. H., Lee, S. J., et al. (2012). The usefulness of bladder reconditioning before indwelling urethral catheter removal from stroke patients. *American Journal of Physical Medicine & Rehabilitation, 91,* 681–688.

Moore, K. N., & Rayome, R. G. (1995). Problem solving and troubleshooting: The indwelling urinary catheter. *Journal of Wound, Ostomy, and Continence Nursing, 22*(5), 242–247.

Morrisroe, S. N., O'Connor, R. C., Nanigian, D. K., et al. (2005). Vesicostomy revisited: The best treatment for the hostile bladder is myelodysplastic child? *BJU International, 96*(3), 397–400.

Nardulli, R., Lasavio, E., Ranieri, M., et al. (2012). Combined antimuscarinics for treatment of neurogenic overactive bladder. *International Journal of Immunopathology and Pharmacology, 25*(1 Suppl), 35S–41S.

Nerli, R. B., Patil, S. M., Hiremath, M. B., et al. (2013). Yang-Monti's catheterizable stoma in children. *Nephro-urology Monthly, 5*(3), 801–805.

Newman, D. K., & Willson, M. M. (2011). Review of intermittent catheterization and current best practices. *Urologic Nursing, 31*(1), 12–28.

Ni, J., Wang, X., Cao, N., et al. (2018). Is repeat Botulinum Toxin A injection valuable for neurogenic detrusor overactivity-A systematic review and meta-analysis. *Neurourology and Urodynamics, 37*(2), 542–553.

Nitti, V. W., Chapple, C. R., Walters, C., et al. (2014). Safety and tolerability of the beta3-receptor agonist mirabegron for the treatment of overactive bladder: Results of a prospective analysis of three 12 week randomized Phase III trials and of a 1 year Phase III randomized trial. *International Journal of Clinical Practice, 68*(8), 972–985.

Nseyo, U., & Santiago-Lastra, Y. (2017). Long-term complications of the neurogenic bladder. *Urologic Clinics of North America, 44*(3), 355–366.

Ostaszkiewicz, J., & Paterson, J. (2012). Nurses advice concerning clean or sterile urinary drainage bags for persons with long-term indwelling catheters. *Journal of Wound, Ostomy, and Continence Nursing, 39*(1), 77–83.

Oxford English Dictionary. (2014). Retrieved October 1, 2014, from http://www.oed.com/view/Entry/126392?redirectedFrom=neurogenic#eid.

Parker, D., Callan, L., Harwood, J., et al. (2009). Nursing interventions to reduce risk of catheter-associated urinary tract infection. Part 1: Catheter selection. *Journal of Wound, Ostomy, and Continence Nursing, 36*(1), 23–34.

Perez, L. M., Barnes, N., MacDiramid, S. A., et al. (1993). Urological dysfunction in patients with diastematomyelia. *Journal of Urology, 149*(6), 1503–1505.

Perkash, I. (1996). Contact laser sphincterotomy: Further experience and longer follow-up. *Spinal Cord, 34*, 227–233.

Perkash, I. (2009). Transurethral sphincterotomy. *Journal of Urology, 181*, 1539–1540.

Perissinotto, M. C., D'Ancona, C. A. L., Lucio, A., et al. (2015). Transcutaneous tibial nerve stimulation in the treatment of lower urinary tract symptoms and its impact on health-related quality of life in patients with Parkinson disease: A randomized controlled trial. *Journal of Wound Ostomy & Continence Nursing, 42*(1), 94–99.

Peters, K. M., Carrico, D. J., Wooldridge, L. S., et al. (2013a). Percutaneous tibial nerve stimulation for the long-term treatment of overactive bladder: 3-year results of the STEP study. *Journal of Urology, 189*(6), 2194–2201.

Peters, K. M., Kandagatla, P., Killinger, K. A., et al. (2013b). Clinical outcomes of sacral neuromodulation in patients with neurologic conditions. *Urology, 81*, 738–744.

Peterson, A. C., Curtis, L. H., Shea, A. M., et al. (2012). Urinary diversions in patients with spinal cord injury in the United States. *Urology, 80*, 1247–1251.

Pinar, K., Moore, K. N., Smits, E., et al. (2009). Leg bag comparison. *Journal of Wound, Ostomy, and Continence Nursing, 36*(3), 319–326.

Powell, C. R. (2014). Is the diabetic bladder a neurogenic bladder? Evidence from the literature. *Current Bladder Dysfunction Reports, 9*(4), 261–267.

Ransmayr, G. N., Hilliger, S., Scheletterer, K., et al. (2008). Lower urinary tract symptoms in Lewy bodies, Parkinson disease, and Alzheimer disease. *Neurology, 70*(4), 299–303.

Rapidi, C. A., Panourias, I. G., Petropoulou, K., et al. (2007). Management and rehabilitation of neuropathic bladder in patients with spinal cord lesions. *Acta Neurochirurgia Supplement, 97*(Pt 1), 307–314.

Revicky, V., & Tincello, D. G. (2014). New surgical approaches for urinary incontinence in women. *Maturatis, 77*(3), 238–242.

Richardson, K., Fox, C., Maidment, I., et al. (2018). Anticholinergic drugs and risk of dementia: Case-control study. *BMJ Open, 361*, k1315. doi: 10.1136/bmj.k1315.

Robinson, J. P., Bradway, C. W., Bunting-Perry, L., et al. (2013). Lower urinary tract symptoms in men with Parkinson's disease. *Journal of Neuroscience Nursing, 45*(6), 381–392.

Rossier, A. B., & Ott, R. (1976). Bladder and urethral recordings in acute and chronic spinal cord injury patients. *Urologia Internationalis, 31*(1–2), 49–59.

Roth, B., Studer, U. E., Fowler, C. J., et al. (2009). Benign prostatic obstruction and Parkinson's disease—Should transurethral resection be avoided? *Journal of Urology, 181*, 2209–2213.

Ruffion, A., Castro-Diaz, D., Patel, H., et al. (2013). Systematic review of urinary incontinence and detrusor overactivity among patients with neurogenic overactive bladder. *Neuroepidemiology, 41*, 146–155.

Saaby, M. L., & Lose, G. (2012). Repeatability of post void urinary residual >100 ml in urogynecology patients. *International Urogynecology Journal, 23*(2), 207–209.

Sacco, R., Kasner, S. E., Broderick, J. P., et al. (2013). An updated definition of stroke for the 21st century: A statement for healthcare professionals from the American Heart Association/American Stroke Association. *Stroke, 44*, 2064–2089.

Savica, R., Grossardt, B. R., Bower, J. H., et al. (2013). Incidence of dementia with Lewy bodies and Parkinson disease dementia. *JAMA Neurology, 70*(11), 1396–1402.

Schafer, W. (1995). Analysis of bladder outlet function with the linearized passive urethral resistance relation, linPURR, a disease specific approach for grading obstruction: From complex to simple. *World Journal of Urology, 13*(1), 47–58.

Schurch, B., Yasuda, K., & Rossier, A. B. (1994). Detrusor bladder neck dyssynergia revisited. *Journal of Urology, 152*(6, Pt 1), 2066–2070.

Silver, J. R. (2011). Management of the bladder in traumatic injuries of the spinal cord during the First World War and its implications for current practice of urology. *BJU International, 108*, 493–500.

Soljanik, I. (2013). Efficacy and safety of botulinum toxin A intradetrusor injections in adults with neurogenic detrusor overactivity/ neurogenic overactive bladder: A systematic review. *Drugs, 73*, 1055–1066.

Stohrer, M., Goepel, M., Kondo, A., et al. (1999). The standardization of terminology in neurogenic lower urinary tract dysfunction. *Neurourology and Urodynamics, 18*, 139–158.

Suman, S., Robinson, D., Bhal, N., et al. (2019). Management of nocturia: Overcoming the challenges of nocturnal polyuria. *British Journal of Hospital Medicine 80*(9), 517–524.

Sung, B. M., Oh, D. J., Choi, M. H., et al. (2018). Chronic kidney disease in neurogenic bladder. *Nephrology, 23*(3), 231–236.

Temml, C., Ponholzer, A., Gutjahr, G., et al. (2009). Nocturia is an age-independent risk factor for hip fracture in men. *Neurourology and Urodynamics, 28*(8), 949–952.

Terayama, K., Sakakibara, R., Ogawa, A., et al. (2012). Weak detrusor contractility correlates with motor disorders in Parkinson's disease. *Movement Disorders, 27*(14), 1775–1780.

Thorburn, W. (1889). *A contribution to the surgery of the spinal cord.* London, UK: Griffin.

Trocio, J. N., Brubaker, L., Schavert, V. F., et al. (2010). Effects of combined behavioral and tolterodine on patient-reported outcomes. *Canadian Journal of Urology, 17*(4), 5283–5290.

Tubaro, A., Puccini, F., De Nunzio, C., et al. (2012). The treatment or lower urinary tract symptoms in patients with multiple sclerosis: A systematic review. *Current Urologic Reports, 13*, 335–342.

Ursino, M. G., Vasina, V., Raschi, E., et al. (2009). The beta-3 adrenoceptor as a therapeutic target: Current perspectives. *Pharmacological Research, 59*(4), 221–234.

van Doorn, B., Blanker, M. H., Kok E. T., et al. (2013). Prevalence, incidence, and resolution of nocturnal polyuria in a longitudinal community-based study in older men: The Krimpen study. *European Urology, 63*(3), 542–547.

Van den Eeden, S. K., Tanner, C. M., Bernstein, A. L., et al. (2003). Incidence of Parkinson's disease: Variation by age, gender and race/ethnicity. *American Journal of Epidemiology, 157*(11), 1015–1022.

Van Koeveringe, G. A., Vahabi, B., Andersson, K. E., et al. (2011). Detrusor underactivity: A plea for new approaches to a common bladder dysfunction. *Neurourology and Urodynamics, 30*, 723–728.

Van Middendorp, J. J., Hosman, A. J., Pouw, M. H., et al.; Em-SCI Study Group. (2009). ASIA impairment scale conversions in traumatic SCI: It is related with the ability to walk? *Spinal Cord, 47*, 555–560.

Vasudeva, P., & Madersbacher, H. (2014). Factors implicated in pathogenesis of urinary tract infections in neurogenic bladders: Some revered, few forgotten, others ignored. *Neurourology and Urodynamics, 33*, 95–100.

Viaene, A., Denys, M. A., Goessaert, A. S., et al. (2019). Evaluation of the occurrence and diagnose definitions for nocturnal polyuria in spinal cord injured patients during rehabilitation. *European Journal of Physical and Rehabilitation Medicine, 55*(1), 40–46.

Wein, A. J. (1981). Classification of neurogenic voiding dysfunction. *Journal of Urology, 125*(5), 605–609.

Weiss, R. M. (2012). Physiology and pharmacology of the renal pelvic and ureter. In A. J. Wein, L. R. Kavoussi, A. C. Novick, et al. (Eds.), *Campbell-Walsh urology* (10th ed., pp. 1755–1785). St. Louis, MO: Elsevier.

Weld, K. J., Graney, M. J., & Dmochowski, R. R. (2000). Clinical significance of detrusor dyssynergia type in patients with post-traumatic spinal cord injury. *Urology, 56*(4), 565–568.

Wells, M. J., Jamieson, K., Markham, T. C., et al. (2014). The effects of caffeinated versus decaffeinated drinks on overactive bladder: A double-blind, randomized cross-over study. *Journal of Wound, Ostomy, and Continence Nursing, 41*(4), 371–378.

Welsh, T.J., van der Wardt, V., Ojo, G., et al. (2018). Anticholinergic drug burden tools/scales and adverse outcomes in different clinical settings: A systematic review of reviews. *Drugs & Aging, 35*(6), 523–538.

Williams, M. P., Srikanth, V., Bird, M., et al. (2012). Urinary symptoms and natural history of urinary continence after first-ever stroke—A longitudinal population-based study. *Age and Ageing, 41*, 371–376.

Winge, K., & Fowler, C. J. (2006). Bladder dysfunction in Parkinsonism: Mechanisms, prevalence, symptoms and management. *Movement Disorders, 21*(6), 737–745.

Winters, J. C., Dmochowski, R. R., Goldman, H. B., et al. (2012). *Adult urodynamics: AUA/SUFU Guideline.* Retrieved January 2, 2020, from file:///C:/Users/Owner/Downloads/Adult-Urodynamics.pdf.

Wisconsin Department of Health Services. (2001). *Use of a catheter (F315) standard or practice resource.* Retrieved from http://www.dhs.wisconsin.gov/publications/p0/p00285.pdf

WOCN White Paper. (2009). *Clinical issues in clean intermittent catheterization.* Retrieved from http://c.ymcdn.com/sites/www.wocn.org/resource/resmgr/Publications/Clinical_Issues_in_Clean_Int.pdf

Wyndaele, J. J. (1997). Correlation between clinical neurological data and urodynamic function in spinal cord injured patients. *Spinal Cord, 35*, 213–216.

Wyndaele, J. J. (2002). Intermittent catheterization: Which is the optimal technique? *Spinal Cord, 40*, 432–437.

Yamanishi, T., Yasuda, K., Sakakibara, R., et al. (1997). The nature of detrusor bladder neck dyssynergia in non-neurogenic bladder dysfunction. *Neurourology and Urodynamics, 66*(3), 163–168.

Yamata, S., & Ito, Y. (2011). Alpha-1 adrenoreceptors in the urinary tract. *Handbook of Experimental Pharmacology, 202*, 283–306.

Yoshimura, N., & Chancellor, M. B. (2012). Physiology and pharmacology of the urinary bladder and urethra. In A. J. Wein, L. R. Kavoussi, A. C. Novick, et al. (Eds.), *Campbell-Walsh urology* (10th ed., pp. 1786–1853). St. Louis, MO: Elsevier.

Zare, A., Jahanshahi, A., Rahnama M. S., et al. (2019). The role of the periaqueductal gray matter in lower urinary tract function. *Molecular Neurobiology, 56*, 920–934.

Zuckerman, J. M., Edwards, B., Henderson, K., et al. (2014). Extended outcomes in the treatment of male stress urinary incontinence with a transobturator sling. *Urology, 83*(4), 939–945.

QUESTIONS

1. According to Wein's urodynamics-based classification system for neurogenic voiding dysfunction, which of the following is a urodynamic abnormality related to failure to store urine because of the outlet?
   A. Neurogenic detrusor overactivity
   B. Urethral sphincter mechanism incompetence
   C. Bladder outlet obstruction
   D. Detrusor underactivity

2. A continence nurse documents the condition "stove-pipe" urethra. What is the common cause of this alteration?
   A. Short-term indwelling catheterization
   B. Intermittent catheterization
   C. Long-term indwelling catheterization
   D. Surgical intervention

3. A patient is diagnosed with failure to empty urine due to the sphincter. What is the most common cause of this disorder among individuals with a neurogenic condition?
   A. Bladder outlet obstruction
   B. Detrusor external sphincter dyssynergia
   C. Weak pelvic floor
   D. Detrusor underactivity

4. Which of the following is an example of a "hostile bladder condition?"
   A. Low bladder wall compliance
   B. Decreased detrusor pressures
   C. Urgency
   D. Reflex urinary incontinence

5. The continence nurse is instructing patients with urinary retention related to neurogenic bladder and how to perform clean intermittent catheterization (CIC). Which teaching point would the nurse include in the plan?

A. Adult patients should use a 6- to 10-French catheter for the procedure.
B. Patients should remove the catheter quickly to prevent drainage.
C. Patients should clean and reuse catheters.
D. Catheterization should be performed in an upright position if possible.

6. The continence nurse recommends a silicone-coated catheter for long-term catheterization. What is the advantage of this type of catheter?
A. Protection against bacteriuria
B. Reduced urethral inflammation
C. Ease of insertion
D. Reduced risk of urinary leakage

7. A patient is diagnosed with detrusor-striated sphincter dyssynergia related to neurogenic bladder. What category of drugs is recommended for this condition?
A. Alpha-adrenergic antagonists
B. Beta-3 adrenergic agonists
C. Cholinergic agonists
D. Injectable neurotoxin

8. A female patient is diagnosed with urethral sphincter incompetence. What surgical intervention might be recommended for this patient?
A. Suburethral sling procedure
B. Augmentation enterocystoplasty
C. Implantation of a sacral neuromodulation device
D. Transurethral sphincterotomy

9. Which intervention is typically initiated immediately following spinal cord injury (SCI) for management of neurogenic bladder?
A. Intermittent catheterization
B. Insertion of an indwelling catheter
C. Prophylactic antibiotic therapy
D. Surgical intervention to create a urinary diversion

10. Which of the following is the typical first-line management strategy for patients experiencing neurogenic bladder related to stroke?
A. Surgical interventions
B. Pharmacotherapy
C. Behavioral interventions
D. Use of indwelling catheterization to prevent urinary retention

ANSWERS AND RATIONALES

1. B. Rationale: According to Wein's urodynamics-based classification system for neurogenic voiding dysfunction (**Table 9-1**), an incompetent urethral sphincter mechanism (an outlet) leads to stress UI, reflecting a storage problem at the outlet.

2. C. Rationale: Long-term use of an indwelling catheter causes a "stove pipe" urethra due to denervation and local damage to the urethra and urethral sphincter mechanism, resulting in an inability to exert any urethral closure pressure, which leads to continuous urinary leakage or bypassing of urine.

3. B. Rationale: In patients with neurogenic bladder dysfunction, detrusor external sphincter dyssynergia (persistent contraction of the sphincter during detrusor contraction) is the most common cause of failure to empty due to the sphincter.

4. A. Rationale: In the presence of inadequate bladder emptying, decreased bladder compliance can increase detrusor pressure and the risk of upper urinary tract distress.

5. D. Rationale: Performing catheterization in an upright position facilitates complete emptying of the bladder.

6. B. Rationale: Silicone-coated catheters are preferred for long-term use because they produce less urethral inflammation and discomfort when left in place for prolonged periods of time.

7. A. Rationale: Alpha-adrenergic antagonists (blockers) bind with alpha-1 adrenergic receptors in smooth muscle of urethral sphincter mechanism to reduce urethral resistance to urinary outflow.

8. A. Rationale: A suburethral sling procedure can help to decrease urine loss due to urethral sphincter incompetence by increasing urethral resistance to urine outflow.

9. B. Rationale: In the acute phase following spinal cord injury, there is a period of spinal shock during which the urethral sphincter remains closed and the detrusor remains acontractile, resulting in urinary retention, as well alterations in urine production, antidiuretic hormone production, and urinary output, predisposing the person to brisk urine production during the night and reduced production during waking hours when sitting upright. An indwelling catheter is typically used during this time period to provide ongoing drainage of urine from the bladder and measurement of urine output. Once nighttime urine output normalizes the catheter should be removed and intermittent catheterization initiated.

10. C. Rationale: When LUTS occurs secondary to a stroke they have to be characterized by neurogenic detrusor overactivity with intact sensory function; thus, urgency, frequency, nocturia, and urge incontinence are the most commonly reported LUTS. Behavioral interventions are generally considered the first-line therapy for these bladder symptoms.

CHAPTER 10

LOWER URINARY TRACT SYMPTOMS IN MEN

Joanne P. Robinson, Nicole L. Dugan, and Dorothea Frederick

OBJECTIVES

1. Describe the patterns, prevalence, impact, and pathophysiology of common lower urinary tract symptoms (LUTS) in men.

2. Identify key features of assessment for men who present with lower urinary tract symptoms.

3. Discuss behavioral and pharmacologic strategies for preventing and managing lower urinary tract symptoms in men.

TOPIC OUTLINE

LOWER URINARY TRACT SYMPTOMS IN MEN

Clinicians who provide care for men with lower urinary tract symptoms (LUTS) must have sufficient knowledge and expertise to support the development of a trusting collaborative relationship and therapeutic plan. This chapter provides an overview of common LUTS in men, including their patterns, prevalence, impact, and pathophysiology. Key features of assessment and conservative approaches for preventing and treating LUTS in men will also be addressed. Current terminology, definitions, and classifications of male LUTS endorsed by the International Continence Society are used (D'Ancona et al., 2018).

DEFINITION

LUTS is a general term that refers to subjective indicators of conditions and diseases related to the lower urinary tract, which consists of the bladder, urethra, and prostate gland. LUTS can be nonspecific in presentation and multifactorial in origin (Diaz et al., 2017a). For example, LUTS may originate from the bladder, prostate, urethra, and/or adjacent pelvic floor or pelvic organs, or at times referred from similarly innervated anatomy (e.g., a lower ureter) (D'Ancona et al., 2018). Three categories of male LUTS are commonly recognized: storage, voiding, and postvoiding symptoms. Mixed storage and voiding symptoms can also occur.

SYMPTOM PATTERNS

LUTS in men can be classified as storage symptoms, voiding symptoms, postvoiding symptoms, and mixed storage and voiding symptoms.

STORAGE SYMPTOMS

Storage symptoms affect the ability to hold urine in the bladder and are classified into four groups: general (e.g., urinary frequency, nocturia, polyuria), sensory (e.g., urgency, altered bladder filling sensation), urinary incontinence (UI) or involuntary urine loss (e.g., stress UI, urgency UI, mixed UI, overflow UI, enuresis, disability-associated UI, insensible UI, sexual arousal incontinence, climacturia), and storage symptom syndrome (i.e., overactive bladder). Storage symptoms arise from dysfunctions in detrusor (bladder muscle) sensation, activity, and elasticity, as well as from diminished strength of muscles in the bladder neck and/or urethral sphincter. Bladder oversensitivity, detrusor overactivity, reduced bladder compliance, and insufficiency/incompetence of the bladder outlet or urethral sphincter are common causes of LUTS that reduce the capacity to store urine (D'Ancona et al., 2018).

VOIDING SYMPTOMS

Voiding symptoms affect the ability to eliminate urine from the bladder and are generally observable as abnormally slow urine flow and/or abnormally high postvoid residual volume. Sixteen discrete voiding symptoms may be seen in men: hesitancy, paruresis ("bashful" or "shy" bladder), episodic inability to void, straining to void, slow stream, intermittency ("stopping and starting"), terminal dribbling, spraying (splitting) of urinary stream, position-dependent voiding, dysuria, stranguria ("drop by drop"), hematuria, pneumaturia (with air/gas), fecaluria (with feces), chyluria (pale or white, milky cloudy urine), and urinary retention (acute, chronic). Detrusor underactivity or acontractility, bladder outlet obstruction (BOO), retention of urine, and retention with overflow are common causes of LUTS that reduce the capacity to eliminate urine (D'Ancona et al., 2018).

POSTVOIDING SYMPTOMS

Postvoiding symptoms are experienced after the cessation of voiding and are classified as urinary, pain, or infection. Postvoiding urinary symptoms include incomplete emptying, revoiding ("encore" or "double voiding"), incontinence (dribbling), and postmicturition urgency. Postvoiding pain is considered to be discomfort that is general, bladder, urethral, scrotal, perineal, pelvic, ejaculatory, anorectal, coccygeal, or pudendal and also includes chronic pelvic pain syndrome (prostatitis). The postvoiding infection category includes urinary tract infection (UTI) (acute, recurrent) and urethral discharge (D'Ancona et al., 2018). While postvoiding urinary symptoms typically arise from dysfunctions of the bladder, postvoiding pain and infection symptoms often originate from dysfunctions or disorders external to the lower urinary tract.

MIXED STORAGE AND VOIDING SYMPTOMS

Storage and voiding symptoms are not mutually exclusive in men. A mixture of both can arise from the following combined dysfunctions: BOO and detrusor underactivity, detrusor overactivity and BOO, and detrusor overactivity with detrusor underactivity (D'Ancona et al., 2018).

KEY POINT

LUTS is a general term that refers to subjective indicators of conditions and diseases related to the lower urinary tract, which consists of the bladder, urethra, and prostate gland. Three categories of male LUTS are commonly recognized: storage, voiding, and postvoiding symptoms. Mixed storage and voiding symptoms can also occur.

PREVALENCE

The worldwide prevalence of LUTS is estimated at 2.3 billion, roughly 46% of the world's population (Zhang & Xu, 2018). Men constitute almost half of those affected, and prevalence rates in men rise steadily with age (Alawamlh et al., 2018; Zhang & Xu, 2018). In fact, the incidence of LUTS is estimated at 3.5% for middle-aged men, compared to an incidence of 30% for men over age 85 (Diaz et al., 2017a).

IMPACT

Men with LUTS suffer significant burden from symptoms such as nocturia, urgency, and incontinence. In addition, adverse psychological consequences can be substantial (Zhang & Xu, 2018). Evidence suggests that LUTS often diminishes quality of life in men as well as in their care-givers and partners. Anxiety and depression are common for many, and sexual function and satisfaction are impaired for some. LUTS can also place those affected at risk of potentially life-threatening injuries from falls (Diaz et al., 2017a). Economic burdens for patients and society also arise from LUTS, including costs associated with increased doctor and emergency room visits, hospital-izations, and loss of work productivity (Zhang & Xu, 2018).

KEY POINT

LUTS is a prevalent condition especially in men and rises steadily with age. Men with LUTS suffer significant burden from symptoms such as nocturia, urgency, and incontinence, and adverse psychological consequences can be substantial.

PATHOPHYSIOLOGY

The act of voiding requires the coordination of several structures, including bladder (detrusor) musculature and internal and external urethral sphincters. Notwithstand-ing contributions from an aging and/or dysfunctional

bladder (Diaz et al., 2017a), LUTS in men are commonly due to a complex interaction of structural and/or mechan-ical challenges to voiding that arise from benign and/or malignant diseases of the prostate and their treatment (Salvatore et al., 2017).

The Prostate Gland

The prostate is a walnut-sized gland that surrounds the proximal urethra. It sits just below the base of the bladder and just distal to the internal urinary sphincter. Seminal ducts pass through the prostate gland and empty into the urethra proximal to the external urethral sphincter, or rhabdosphincter. The bulbourethral glands or Cowper glands (not shown) are located on either side of the ure-thra just distal to the prostate.

The prostate gland along with the seminal vesicles and the bulbourethral glands serve primarily to enhance male sexual functioning and fertility. A normal prostate is important in the production of semen and plays a crucial role in orgasm and ejaculation. The prostate produces a slightly alkaline fluid that constitutes the majority of the volume of semen. The alkalinity of this fluid neutralizes the acidity of the vaginal tract and pro-longs the lifespan of sperm. The seminal vesicles store semen, and the bulbourethral glands secrete an alka-line fluid prior to ejaculation that neutralizes the acidity of urine to protect sperm. During orgasm, the nerve plexus surrounding the prostate stimulates rhythmic contractions of the prostate, urethral walls, seminal vesicles, and the bulbourethral glands. The normal anatomy of the prostate and surrounding structures is depicted in **Figure 10-1**.

KEY POINT

The prostate is a walnut-sized gland that surrounds the proxi-mal urethra. A normal prostate is important in the production of semen and plays a crucial role in orgasm and ejaculation.

Benign Prostatic Hyperplasia

Benign prostatic hyperplasia (BPH) refers to nonmalig-nant enlargement of the prostate gland. BPH affects half of all men by age 50 and up to 90% of men after age 80. Although not well understood, likely causes of BPH include the rising ratio of estrogen: testosterone that normally occurs as men age, as well as the continued production of dihydrotestosterone (DHT). Both estrogen and DHT are known to promote prostate cell growth (National Institute of Diabetes and Digestive and Kidney Diseases [NIDDK], Prostate Enlargement, 2014).

The proliferation of prostate connective tissue, smooth muscle, and glandular epithelium, accompa-nied by the increased smooth muscle tone and resis-tance that develops within the enlarged gland, leads to the voiding symptoms of LUTS (Foster et al., 2019).

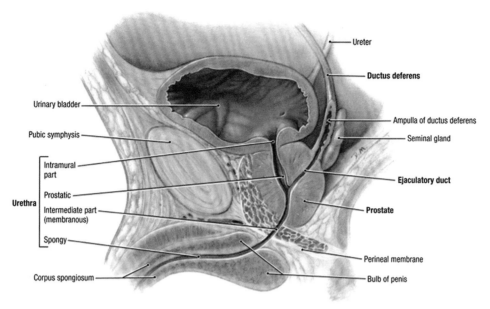

FIGURE 10-1. Normal Anatomy of the Prostate and Surrounding Tissues.

In addition, if the enlarged prostate begins to push up on the bladder as noted in **Figure 10-2**, changes in the mechanics and sensation of bladder filling can occur. The detrusor muscle may become overactive, resulting in problems with the storage of urine and symptoms of urgency and frequency.

> **KEY POINT**
>
> Benign prostatic hyperplasia (BPH) refers to nonmalignant enlargement of the prostate gland. BPH affects half of all men by age 50 and up to 90% of men after age 80.
> It frequently leads to storage and voiding symptoms in the lower urinary tract.

Prostatitis

Prostatitis refers to inflammation of the prostate gland that can be chronic, bacterial (acute or chronic), or asymptomatic (NIDDK, Prostatitis, 2014). Chronic prostatitis, also known as chronic pelvic pain syndrome, is thought to originate from factors such as a nonbacterial microorganism, chemicals in the urine, an immune system response to a previous UTI, or pelvic nerve damage; psychological stress enhances vulnerability in each scenario. Bacteria that travel from the urethra to the prostate are responsible for bacterial prostatitis. Asymptomatic prostatitis refers to prostate inflammation of unknown origin that presents without symptoms or complications. Whatever the cause, an inflamed prostate can trigger a host of storage, voiding, postvoiding, and systemic symptoms. Complete inability to void, dysuria and/or urgency with fever and chills, hematuria, or severe pelvic/lower urinary tract pain signal the need for immediate attention.

> **KEY POINT**
>
> Prostatitis refers to inflammation of the prostate gland that can be chronic, bacterial (acute or chronic), or asymptomatic and can trigger a host of storage, voiding, postvoiding, and systemic symptoms.

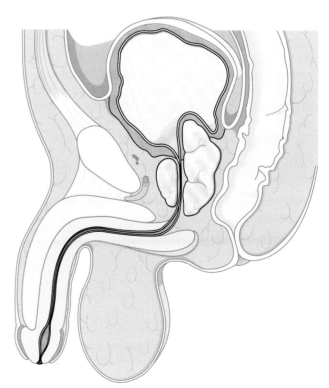

FIGURE 10-2. Anatomic Abnormalities of BPH and Bladder Dysfunction.

Prostate Cancer

Like BPH, an obstructive mass from locally invasive prostate cancer can precipitate voiding and/or storage symptoms (Alawamlh et al., 2018). Fortunately, approximately 90% of prostate cancers today are discovered at local or regional stages, prior to the appearance of any symptoms (American Cancer Society, n.d.). Although the 5-year survival rate for localized prostate cancer approaches 100%, important if, when, and what decisions regarding treatment options are complicated by concerns about inevitable LUTS side effects.

INCONTINENCE AFTER PROSTATE TREATMENT

Incontinence after prostate treatment (IPT) is an inclusive term that refers to involuntary urine loss and other LUTS that occur after undergoing radical prostatectomy (RP), radiation treatment (RT), or treatment for BPH (Sandhu et al., 2019). Evidence suggests that IPT is responsible for a significant degree of emotional and financial distress, delayed postoperative reentry into society, and inhibited relationships, as well as economic burden for patients and families are reported.

Radical Prostatectomy

In the context of RP, the primary cause of IPT is trauma to the external urethral sphincter (rhabdosphincter). With surgical removal of the prostatic urethra and its smooth muscle fibers that contract automatically as the bladder fills, a greater portion of the burden for bladder control falls on the rhabdosphincter and its specialized striated muscle fibers that contract on command to control urination. RP can traumatize the rhabdosphincter to the extent that it is unable to contract with sufficient strength or endurance to prevent urine leakage. Incompetence of the rhabdosphincter is typically temporary and often situational. In the case of stress UI, the rhabdosphincter lacks the capacity to remain sealed in situations when it is stressed by a sudden increase in intra-abdominal pressure.

Damage to the bladder may also account for some degree of IPT following RP. Although it is unclear how RP affects detrusor function, possible explanations include the presence of chronic obstructive pathology prior to surgery as well as bladder mobilization and/or denervation during surgery (Goldman et al., 2017; Salvatore et al., 2017).

Older RP patients with a larger prostate size, shorter membranous urethra, and deconditioned pelvic floor muscles are at greatest risk for IPT, as are RP patients who are obese or have undergone prior radiation therapy. Sexual arousal incontinence and climacturia (orgasm-associated UI) are relatively common forms of IPT, with an overall incidence rate of approximately 30%. Storage symptoms, including stress UI, urgency, and urge UI, are common in the short-term following RP but generally return to baseline by postoperative month 12 (Goldman et al., 2017; Sandhu et al., 2019).

Radiation Treatment

In the context of RT, IPT can be a direct effect of radiation or related to the treatment of other sequelae such as urinary retention. RT initially causes edema, small vessel obliteration, and endarteritis, which trigger a cascade of ischemic tissue changes including fibrosis, disorganization of musculature, and necrosis. While RT is primarily delivered to the prostate, portions of the bladder, distal urinary sphincter, and pelvic floor muscles may also be affected and damaged (Salvatore et al., 2017; Sandhu et al., 2019).

The risk of IPT after RT is variable. Older age and greater RT doses are risk factors for IPT in the salvage setting, while IPT in the adjuvant setting is worse among younger and/or hypertensive patients (Goldman et al., 2017). Following RT, IPT presents mostly as storage symptoms; however, urinary retention and other voiding symptoms are also common (Salvatore et al., 2017).

Benign Prostatic Hyperplasia

In the context of BPH, IPT after minimally invasive procedures and surgery includes storage, voiding, and post-voiding LUTS; complications of pharmacologic treatment are systemic and do not involve LUTS (NIDDK, Prostate Enlargement, 2014).

IPT after BPH surgery may be related to persistent or new-onset bladder dysfunction and/or injury to the sphincter. Possible causes of bladder dysfunction include denervation, super sensitivity of the detrusor, alterations in collagen composition over time in the chronically obstructed bladder, emergence of altered and increased sensory reflexes mediating the micturition reflex, physical changes in detrusor myocytes affecting neurological transmission, and inadvertent surgical resection of the bladder. Possible causes of sphincter dysfunction include inadvertent surgical, electrocautery, or thermal injury (Salvatore et al., 2017).

The incidence of IPT following open prostatectomy, transurethral removal of the prostate (TURP), transurethral incision of the prostate (TUIP), and laser therapies is low and does not differ appreciably among the various techniques. In fact, the rate of persistent stress UI in patients undergoing open, laparoscopic, or endoscopic surgical management of BPH ranges from 0% to 8.4%. Some evidence suggests that IPT following BPH surgery may be higher in older patients, mostly due to bladder dysfunction rather than sphincter insufficiency (Goldman et al., 2017). IPT for TURP following RT is high, with reported rates of up to 70%. Although there are no published rates of IPT for TURP following other local therapies (e.g., high-intensity focused ultrasound, cryotherapy), experts suggest that a history of these procedures also places TURP patients at high risk for IPT (Sandhu et al., 2019).

KEY POINT

Incontinence after prostate treatment (IPT) is an inclusive term that refers to involuntary urine loss and other LUTS that occur after undergoing radical prostatectomy (RP), radiation treatment (RT), or treatment for benign prostatic hyperplasia (BPH).

EVALUATION OF MEN WITH LUTS

Comprehensive history, physical assessment, and standardized assessment tools are used routinely to evaluate men with LUTS. Urodynamic studies are typically reserved for patients with a complex presentation of LUTS or LUTS that are refractory to conservative approaches to treatment.

INITIAL ASSESSMENT

Initial assessment of the patient with LUTS begins with a careful history and thorough focused physical examination. This includes a cognitive and functional assessment since many patients have cognitive and functional limitations that impact the management of symptoms. Serious conditions such as infection, prostate cancer, bladder cancer, and chronic kidney disease should be ruled out. The history should include the nature and frequency of symptoms, symptom progression, family history, and presence of comorbidities, particularly diabetes or other chronic conditions that cause peripheral or central nervous system dysfunction (Gormley et al., 2019). Continence specialists should also assess for daytime sleepiness and fatigue since nocturia can significantly interfere with the quality of sleep. That said, it is important to distinguish the nature of the primary problem causing the sleep disturbance (Zhou et al., 2020). For example, men who have insomnia and early awakening due to depression may void simply because they are awake rather than because of an overactive bladder. Chapter 4 provides primary assessment guidelines for the adult with incontinence and voiding dysfunction.

Guidelines from the International Continence Society recommend a comprehensive physical examination for men with LUTS to seek and rule in or out all potential influences on symptoms (D'Ancona et al., 2018) (see Chapter 4). Components of the comprehensive examination are described below.

- **General observations of overall function:** Observe general mobility, condition of the skin, and nutritional status with attention to extremes such as cachexia or obesity. Note skin irritations and edema of the genitalia and/or lower extremities that might be indicative of a circulatory or lymphatic condition.
- **Abdominal examination focusing on the suprapubic region:** Percuss and/or palpate the bladder for fullness/retention. Examine the abdomen, suprapubic region, and renal area noting any masses, scar tissue, interrupted skin integrity, or tenderness.
- **Lower urinary tract/genital examination:** Observe the skin condition around the genitals for excoriation, pigmentation, ulcerations, or evidence of sexually transmitted infections. Examine the penis for the presence of masses, mobility of tissue on the foreskin, position of the urethral meatus, and condition of the penile glans and shaft, noting in particular the presence of plaque, lichen sclerosus, redness, ulcers, warts, or discharge. Examine the scrotum for tenderness or signs of inflammation around the epididymis, and observe the perineum for dermatitis and fissures. Perform a digital rectal examination (DRE) to palpate the rectum and prostate, noting evidence of prostate enlargement, masses, reproduction of pain or LUTS, altered tone of the sphincter muscle, as well as the absence or presence of stool (see **Fig. 10-3**).
- **Focused neurological examination:** Observe for any global signs of abnormal sensory or motor function and assess for sensory deficits about the penis, scrotum, or perianal tissue. Evaluate the bulbospongiosus and cremasteric reflexes, which assess perineal innervation of S2–S4 and L1–L2 levels, respectively. The bulbospongiosus reflex (also called the bulbocavernosus reflex [BCR]) is elicited by tapping the dorsal penis or glans; this creates a contraction or pulling in of the bulbospongiosus muscle, which lies at the base of the penis, just anterior to the anus. The cremasteric reflex is elicited by stroking the inner thigh (3 inches below the groin fold) causing the cremaster muscle to contract leading to an elevation of the ipsilateral (same side) testicle toward the inguinal canal. This reflex is assessed in episodes of acute scrotal pain; absence of the reflex is potentially diagnostic for testicular torsion (Mellick & Al-Dhahir, 2020).

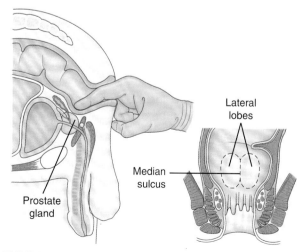

FIGURE 10-3. Digital Rectal Exam (DRE) and Assessment of the Prostate Gland.

- **UI signs:** Observe for signs of involuntary urine loss with physical exertion, cough, strong urge, or extraurethral leakage through a fistula. Complete this assessment with the patient's bladder comfortably full.
- **Pelvic floor muscle appearance and function:** Inspect the perineum for slight descent with a cough or bear down and for inward/cephalad lift with a voluntary active contraction, which is a normal finding. In males, the urethral rhabdosphincter itself is inaccessible for palpation, but pelvic floor muscles can be palpated during the DRE and assessed for increased or decreased resting tone, symmetry, and presence of myalgia. Palpation during a voluntary contraction allows for evaluation of muscle strength, endurance, repeatability, the presence of cocontractions or substitutions, response to abdominal contraction (e.g., with a sit up or cough), and finally the ability to return back to baseline position at rest. Based on this assessment, pelvic floor muscles can be classified as normal, overactive, underactive, or nonfunctioning. Any of these pelvic floor muscles presentations can accompany LUTS (see Chapter 4, Box 4-3 scale for grading digital evaluation of pelvic muscle strength).
- **Bladder diary or frequency–volume chart (FVC):** Objective measurement of input and output habits and the timing of LUTS can be obtained through the use of a bladder diary or FVC. These self-reported measures track indicators and triggers of bladder activity over a period 24 to 72 hours and are strongly correlated with cystometric test results (Diaz et al., 2017a). Voided volume (both daytime and nighttime), fluid intake, episodes of incontinence and associated activities, and number of pads used over the selected time period are recorded by the patient. Maximum and average volume voided is determined (see Chapter 4, Fig. 4-1).
- **Pad test:** The pad test is an objective measure of the volume of UI over a selected period of time. The record of pad use in an FVC or bladder diary may not accurately represent UI volume since some patients use pads as a safety net "just in case" and tolerance of leakage volume on pads varies among patients. The pad test involves measuring the weight of pads worn for a designated time interval (typically 2 hours) before and after use over a designated period of time. Compared to baseline weight of the dry pad, each 1 g of extra weight of the used pad is equivalent to 1 mL of urine loss. Urine leakage of ≥250 g over 24 hours represents more troublesome or severe leakage (Diaz et al., 2017a). The 24-hour pad test is most common since testing for longer durations reduces adherence to the protocol.
- **Urinalysis:** Urinalysis should be performed with a follow-up urine culture only if the urine dipstick suggests UTI. Any infection in a man is a *complicated UTI* until proven otherwise. Men with UTIs often have an infection beyond the bladder as seen in prostatitis therefore fall under a more complicated antibiotic regime to penetrate the prostate gland. Chapter 18 describes the assessment, evaluation, and treatment of UTIs in men. If RBCs are found in the urine without infection, the American Urological Association (AUA) guideline suggests any patient with gross or benign microscopic hematuria should be referred to urology for further workup to rule out bladder or kidney cancer or other pathologies of genitourinary system (Davis et al., 2016).
- **Postvoid residual:** Postvoid residual (PVR) volume is also usually quantified to assess bladder emptying relative to the normal PVR range of 10 to 30 mL for men without LUTS and up to 50 mL after double void for men with LUTS (D'Ancona et al., 2018).

In performing the comprehensive workup, the continence specialist can rule out causative factors of LUTS such as UTI, cystitis, decreased physical activity, neurologic disorders, and chronic diseases such as diabetes mellitus. The clinician can then decide whether LUTS are likely due to storage, voiding, postvoiding, or a mixture of dysfunctions such as an obstruction that restricts outflow, an overactive bladder, an incompetent sphincter, or prostate treatment. Treatment of LUTS should target the presenting problem(s).

> **KEY POINT**
>
> Initial assessment of the patient with LUTS begins with a careful history and thorough focused physical examination including cognitive and functional assessment since those types of limitations impact the management of symptoms.

> **KEY POINT**
>
> It is important to rule out serious pathology in the man with LUTS (e.g., infection, suspicion of prostate or bladder cancer, chronic kidney disease, uncontrolled diabetes, neurological disorders). In addition, any patient with gross or occult hematuria should be referred to a urologist.

STANDARDIZED ASSESSMENT TOOLS

Standardized assessment tools are integral to the evaluation of men with LUTS, yielding important information about symptom severity and perceived "bother" that informs treatment and its effectiveness from both clinical and patient perspectives (Diaz et al., 2017b). Data from standardized tools that are psychometrically robust can be used to guide initial treatment decisions as well as to monitor the efficacy of ongoing treatment. The International Prostate Symptom Score (IPSS) and the International Consultation on Incontinence Questionnaire—Male Lower Urinary Tract Symptoms (ICIQ-MLUTS or ICSmale-SF) both have high levels of validity and reliability and are used most often.

International Prostate Symptom Score

The IPSS assesses frequency of LUTS in seven domains, including sensation of incomplete emptying, urinary frequency, intermittency (starting and stopping of flow), weak stream, need to strain during urination, and need to get up at night to urinate. Each domain is scored on a scale that ranges from 0 to 5 ("not at all" to "almost always"). In addition, the patient is asked, "If you were to spend the rest of your life with your urinary symptoms just the way they are now, how would you feel about that?" This "degree of bother" item is rated on a scale that ranges from 0 to 6 ("delighted" to "terrible").

Treatment decisions are based on the total IPSS (sum of all domain scores) as well as the "degree of bother" item. Categories of symptom burden include mild (0 to 7), moderate (8 to 19), and severe (20 to 35). A cutoff score of 8 or greater is commonly used as an indicator of the need to start or advance treatment, as long as the patient is bothered by the symptoms. Watchful waiting (i.e., no medical treatment) may be indicated when the total IPSS is 7 or less or if the patient is not significantly bothered by the symptoms.

International Consultation on Incontinence Questionnaire—Male Lower Urinary Tract Symptoms

The IPPS tool neglects the symptoms of urgency and urge incontinence, which are associated with significant bother in many male patients with LUTS. In 1998, the International Consultation on Incontinence developed a series of modules to assess pelvic problems and, in 2004, finalized the format for a standard patient-reported outcome tool, the ICIQ (Bristol Urological Institute, n.d.). The ICIQ modular questionnaire was subsequently developed to meet the need for selected population and provide context-specific versions of the ICIQ that could be used in clinical practice and research (Diaz et al., 2017b). The ICIQ-MLUTS, formerly known as the International Continence Society's Male Questionnaire Short Form (ICSmaleSF), is a modular version of the ICIQ containing 13 items that assess the occurrence and perceived bother of a wide range of LUTS in men. The ICIQ-MLUTS contains two symptom subscales: voiding and incontinence. The frequency of each symptom is rated on a scale ranging from "never" to "all the time" (0 to 4), while bother associated with each symptom is rated on a scale ranging from "not at all" to "a great deal" (0 to 10). Both symptom and bother scores are used to determine symptom impact. Validated versions of the ICIQ-MLUTS are available in 24 languages (Bristol Urological Institute, n.d.).

> **KEY POINT**
>
> Standardized assessment tools are integral to the evaluation of men with LUTS, yielding important information about symptom severity and perceived "bother" that informs treatment and its effectiveness from both clinical and patient perspectives.

ADVANCED STUDIES

Beyond comprehensive physical assessment and the use of a standardized assessment tool, physiologic parameters related to LUTS can be obtained by uroflowmetry to assess the rate and volume of urine flow. Standardized flow rates have been established for men up to the age of 60. Cystometric testing can be performed to measure pressure–volume relationships of the bladder during filling. Cystometric testing is accomplished via artificial retrograde filling of the bladder. Correspondence between fluid volume and pressure rates in the bladder and abdomen is noted, as are sphincter and detrusor muscle activity with the initial sensation of bladder filling and subsequently with the first, normal, and strong desire to void. Bladder sensations and pain associated with filling are also noted. Urethral function is explored, observing for the closure mechanism, leak point pressures, and ability for the urethral rhabdosphincter to relax during voiding. This test allows the clinician to distinguish between BOO and dyssynergia of the detrusor and rhabdosphincter (D'Ancona et al., 2018). Refer to Chapter 5 for an advance discussion of urodynamic testing.

Imaging of the lower urinary tract and pelvic floor involves ultrasound measurement of bladder volume, urethral abnormality, prostate size, and pelvic floor muscle displacement to complement qualitative palpation that occurred during comprehensive physical assessment. Ultrasound can be conducted via transrectal, transabdominal, perineal, or scrotal access points. Currently, the AUA does not recommend advance diagnostics on initial evaluation of patients with uncomplicated LUTS but reserved for those who have failed treatment or have complicated symptoms, that is, BOO, urinary retention, neurologic abnormalities (Gormley et al., 2019).

> **KEY POINT**
>
> Advance diagnostics are rarely indicated as part of the initial workup of a male with uncomplicated LUTS.

> **KEY POINT**
>
> Analyzing the data from the history, physical examination, and standardized assessment tools, the continence nurse must determine whether LUTS are likely due to storage, voiding, postvoiding, or a mixture of dysfunctions such as an obstruction that restricts outflow, an overactive bladder, an incompetent sphincter, or prostate treatment. Treatment of LUTS should then target the presenting problem(s).

CONSERVATIVE MANAGEMENT STRATEGIES FOR MEN WITH LUTS

LUTS in men are known to increase with age but at a rate that is 50% greater than the rate in women. Additionally, men have a higher remission rate for LUTS than women, whether they have had treatment (Milsom et al., 2017). Although very few high-quality studies have yielded effective approaches for the prevention of LUTS (Dumoulin et al., 2017; Newman et al., 2017), continence education, self-management using a risk reduction tool, and a combination of these show promise. These behavioral approaches represent first-line strategies for both the prevention and conservative management of LUTS.

Conservative management of LUTS should target symptom relief as well as elimination or mitigation of the underlying cause(s). Perceived bother plays a major role in the patient's desire to pursue, initiate, and advance treatment. Although UI in men is less severe and occurs less frequently than in women, men tend to seek help sooner and more frequently due to fear of prostate cancer and/or an expectation that UI can be treated (Newman et al., 2017). While abnormalities of the prostate gland are a large contributor to LUTS, there are other noteworthy risk factors. Nocturnal polyuria, nocturia, obesity, snoring, sleep apnea, diabetes, and hypertension are all associated with LUTS (Milsom et al., 2017). Men with obstructive sleep apnea have a high incidence of nocturia (Zhou et al., 2020), while men with hypertension plus obstructive sleep apnea are 1.3 times more likely to have LUTS (Destors et al., 2015). Behavioral approaches to eliminate or mitigate these risk factors include nighttime fluid management, weight loss, exercise, and continuous positive airway pressure (CPAP) to address sleep apnea. Prevention of LUTS outside the context of prostate cancer has received little scientific attention. The primary conservative approach for prevention and treatment of LUTS in the RP population is pelvic floor muscle training (PFMT) (Dumoulin et al., 2017).

GENERAL HEALTH AND LIFESTYLE CONSIDERATIONS

Developing a treatment plan for LUTS begins by considering the patient's general health, lifestyle, and socioeconomic factors. For example, patients with diminished cognitive capacity may not be able to engage in behavioral interventions. Physical limitations that impede timely access to toilets will also limit the effectiveness of behavioral interventions. An overall lack of physical conditioning and activity is not only associated with higher symptom scores in men with LUTS but also coincides with diminished motivation for behavioral interventions. Finally, weight loss is dependent on access to affordable and healthy food options, which may be challenging for men with limited income, transportation, or food preparation capabilities.

There is a positive correlation between LUTS and body mass index. Evidence suggests that weight loss through lifestyle changes will reduce UI in overweight and obese men, particularly those with type 2 diabetes (Dumoulin et al., 2017). Education about food and medications that are bladder irritants is also recommended, particularly for men with storage symptoms.

EDUCATION

Published research on the efficacy of continence education is scant (Newman et al., 2017), but conservative management of LUTS logically begins with providing information about the basic anatomy and physiology of the bladder. The patient should also be informed about nuances of the neural and vascular supply that is shared by the bladder, prostate, and penis. The interaction between bladder functioning and erectile dysfunction, both at baseline and as a result of possible interventions, should be covered. **Figure 10-4** illustrates the important neural signaling pathways that are associated with bladder function. Understanding the anatomy and physiology of the lower urinary tract is fundamental to appreciating the rationale for behavioral interventions and has the potential to increase the patient's self-efficacy and adherence to lifestyle modifications. Of course, it is important to deliver continence education in a format that is compatible with the patient's level of education, literacy, and language skills.

The general public has little knowledge about UI and LUTS, and many older adults believe that UI is a normal part of aging. Older men would be well served by instruction about lifestyle changes that can prevent, eliminate, or reduce UI and LUTS (see Chapter 6 for further discussion on education and lifestyle modification to promote bladder health).

KEY POINT

Education regarding lifestyle modifications and behavioral approaches represents first-line strategies for both the prevention and conservative management of LUTS.

The bladder diary is not only a tool for evaluation but also a conservative approach to LUTS treatment that is especially important for patients with storage symptoms. Use of the bladder diary improves the patient's awareness of LUTS and engages him in the treatment plan. The diary should include the time interval between voids, the number of voids per day, and the volume voided. Recording the volume voided may particularly help to distinguish LUTS from other comorbid conditions associated with polyuria. In addition to recording output, the bladder diary improves awareness of fluid intake, in particular the time and volume of fluid consumption. In fact,

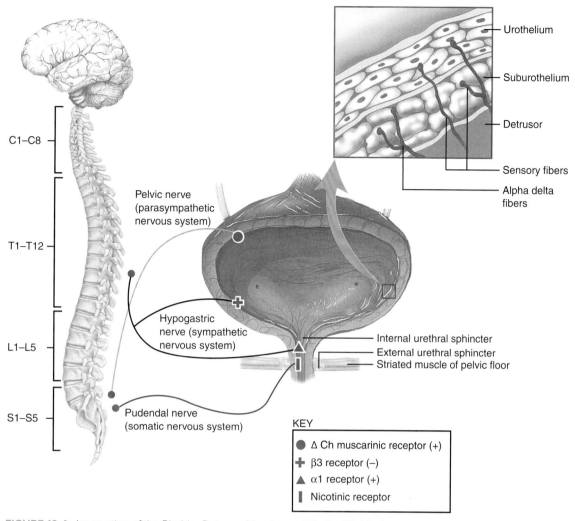

FIGURE 10-4. Innervation of the Bladder Detrusor Muscles and Urethral Sphincters.

combining the bladder diary with lifestyle education about fluid management may be enough to eliminate LUTS in some cases.

KEY POINT

The bladder diary is not only a tool for evaluation but also a conservative approach to LUTS treatment especially for patients with storage symptoms by improving the patient's awareness of LUTS and engages him in the treatment plan.

ABSORBENT PRODUCTS

Most men wear a body worn absorbent product (BWAP), which is advisable, at least in public, until they are confident about bladder control. As there is a wide range of products, men usually benefit from professional guidance regarding product selection. A general rule of thumb for patients is to wear the smallest possible amount of product and to advance gradually to "product-free" living, starting with low-stake circumstances

(e.g., around the house), as bladder control begins to return. A variety of BWAPs designed to fit the male genitourinary and pelvic anatomy are now on the market, but all are not alike. An excellent overview of absorbent products is available online from the National Association for Continence™ (NAFC, n.d.a). In addition, the Wound, Ostomy, and Continence Nurses Society™ (WOCN) appointed a BWAP Task Force to develop evidence-based recommendations for assessment, selection, use, and evaluation of BWAPs. The BWAP Task Force along with a panel of continence nurse specialists across the United States convened and developed validated consensus statements to generate consensus statements that were utilized to create an electronic algorithm to aid the clinician in decision-making for appropriate BWAP no matter the care setting. This evidence- and consensus-based WOCN® BWAP Guide can be accessed from any smart phone or computer at https://bwap.wocn.org to guide the clinician in optimal selection and use of incontinence products. Chapter 16 furthers the discussion regarding proper use of containment products.

There is no single best product design that suits all situations. Men should be encouraged to experiment with different product types and brands to maximize their satisfaction in terms of cost, comfort, absorbency, availability, and environmental impact. To maintain the highest quality of life, a range of products should be considered based upon time of use (i.e., day or night) and place of use (i.e., at home or away). Until bladder control is recovered, men should follow evidence-based best practice recommendations to prevent incontinence-associated dermatitis (IAD). Optimal skin care of incontinent patients, particularly for the dependent and nonambulatory, essentially involves gentle cleansing, moisturizing, and protecting the skin. It is recommended to clean the perigenital skin twice daily using either a no-rinse skin cleanser or warm water, followed by application of an emollient barrier to promote skin integrity in those suffering incontinence (Wound, Ostomy, and Continence Nursing Society™—Wound Guidelines Taskforce, 2017). Chapter 17 elaborates on a structured skin care program to prevent or treat IAD.

KEY POINT

There is no single best product design that suits all situations. Men should be encouraged to experiment with different product types and brands to maximize their satisfaction in terms of cost, comfort, absorbency, availability, and environmental impact.

WATCHFUL WAITING

Depending on results of a comprehensive assessment and evaluation, watchful waiting is a sound option for the initial treatment of BPH and accompanying LUTS. Decision-making about BPH treatment requires time and collaboration between the patient and his provider to balance the patient's expectations with the risk:benefit ratio of each treatment option. That said, conservative management of associated LUTS via education, behavioral therapy(s), PFMT, and appropriate absorbent products can be initiated immediately to improve quality of life. Modifiable risk factors for UI following surgery for BPH include obesity, physical inactivity, diminished well-being, presurgical bladder dysfunction, and presurgical presence of stress UI (Goldman et al., 2017). Thus, if surgery is a possible future treatment option, behavioral strategies to prevent or mitigate postprostatectomy UI, particularly stress UI, should be employed during the watchful waiting period.

CONSERVATIVE APPROACHES FOR TREATMENT OF STORAGE SYMPTOMS

PFMT and bladder training are the main conservative approaches used to treat LUTS that interfere with the ability to store urine.

Pelvic Floor Muscle Training

The rhabdosphincter does not connect directly to a skeletal structure but instead is surrounded by the levator ani, the skeletal muscle located deep within the pelvic floor. Composed of pubococcygeus, iliococcygeus, and puborectalis segments (Salvatore et al., 2017), the levator ani muscle and the urethral rhabdosphincter consist of both type I (slow twitch, nonfatiguing) and type II (fast twitch, fatiguing and nonfatiguing) fibers. Type I fibers maintain continence at rest, and the type II fibers are employed with sudden increases of intra-abdominal pressure such as laughing, sneezing, coughing, or orgasm. The pudendal nerve and the nerve to the levator ani provide innervation to both the levator ani and rhabdosphincter (**Fig. 10-5**).

The levator ani complex can be employed to maintain continence even if the sphincter is paralyzed (Salvatore et al., 2017). The contractile properties of the striated levator ani muscle and bulbospongiosus, a superficial perineal muscle covering the bulb of the penis, are also positively influenced by exposure to androgen hormones. The prevalence of LUTS in older men coincides with the reduction of muscle mass and decrease in androgen hormones that accompany aging. The striated muscles of the urethral rhabdosphincter and levator ani, which control urinary continence, are not spared from this effect (Fry et al., 2017). A decrease in urethral

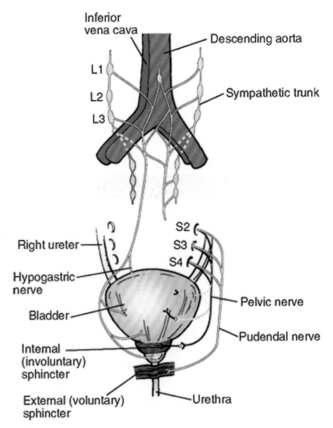

FIGURE 10-5. Innervation for the Internal and External Urethral Sphincters.

rhabdosphincter volume is also associated with stress urinary incontinence (SUI) and overall diminished pelvic floor function.

The prevalence of LUTS in older men coincides with the reduction of muscle mass and decrease in androgen hormones that accompany aging. The striated muscles of the urethral rhabdosphincter and levator ani, which control urinary continence, are not spared from this effect thereby increasing the risk for SUI.

General effects of exercise include muscle hypertrophy and improved endurance, which applies to pelvic floor muscles as well. Exercise of pelvic floor muscles continues to be the mainstay of behavioral interventions for UI. PFMT essentially involves building awareness, strength, and endurance of the levator ani muscle. PFMT begins by teaching the patient to identify and perform isolated contractions of the correct muscle group. There are a variety of published exercise protocols for development of muscle strength, including performance of sustained contractions of 6 to 12 seconds followed by a relaxation period of equal time, plus a series of quick contractions. PFMT for prevention of stress UI includes neuromuscular reeducation to achieve habitual contraction of pelvic floor muscles prior to activities that increase intra-abdominal pressure, such as coughing, climbing stairs, or lifting a heavy object. Chapter 6 provides an in-depth PFMT guide.

Comprehensive pelvic muscle rehabilitation includes training both slow- and fast-twitch muscle fibers since type II fast-twitch fibers are more predominant in the rhabdosphincter. In addition, comprehensive pelvic muscle rehabilitation includes behavioral strategies to avoid or reduce activities associated with a downward gravitational thrust onto the pelvic floor muscles. These strategies include reducing transabdominal fat, minimizing Valsalva maneuvers during lifting and bearing down, controlling breath during forceful exhale or speaking at loud volumes, and reducing forces during impact activities. The greatest benefit of PFMT for RP patients occurs with early postoperative implementation, which is associated with return of continence between postoperative months 3 to 6 (Dumoulin et al., 2017). Adjuncts to pelvic floor muscle rehabilitation, including biofeedback, electrical stimulation, and passive electromagnetic stimulation, are sometimes employed; however, evidence is equivocal concerning their beneficial effects (Dumoulin et al., 2017). The greatest limitations to implementation of these modalities are cost, access, and lack of clarity about optimal training protocols.

Information for men about pelvic floor muscle rehabilitation, including specific instructions for performing pelvic floor muscle exercise, is available online from the National Association for Continence (NAFC, What are Kegel exercises, n.d.b). Of note, in this document is that improved bladder control is often seen within 6 weeks but may take as long as 6 months.

The greatest benefit of PFMT for radical prostatectomy patients occurs with early postoperative implementation, which is associated with return of continence between postoperative months 3 to 6. Common adjuncts to pelvic floor muscle rehabilitation includes biofeedback and electrical stimulation.

Bladder Training

Bladder training is a behavioral strategy for urgency and urge UI that involves the use of purposeful relaxation, distraction, and self-assertion about the ability to delay voiding while tightening pelvic floor muscles. Relaxation and distraction techniques include focused breathing, progressive muscle relaxation, and guided imagery. Since the bladder is a smooth muscle, patients may also be taught urge deference (or urge suppression) techniques to gradually prolong the intervals between voiding so that bladder capacity increases over time. Urge suppression techniques include performance of a series of three to five quick pelvic floor muscle contractions and relaxations in the presence of an urge to void, which modifies signals from the central nervous system to the bladder to reduce bladder activity and tension; avoidance of preemptive ("just in case") voiding; and learning to "hold on" instead of rushing to the bathroom in the presence of urgency. For a compound benefit, lifestyle modifications such as fluid management, reduction in caffeine and alcohol (depending on intake as per the bladder diary), and weight loss are typically recommended along with bladder training (see Chapter 6).

In addition to lifestyle modification, pelvic floor muscle training and bladder training are the main conservative approaches used to treat LUTS that interfere with the ability to store urine.

CONSERVATIVE APPROACHES FOR TREATMENT OF VOIDING AND POSTVOIDING SYMPTOMS

Older men can have a number of voiding and postvoiding symptoms related to an enlarged prostate. Initial treatment should include behavioral approaches to enhance bladder emptying. Bladder emptying results from the combined effects of detrusor contraction, increased intra-abdominal pressure, sometimes with use of Valsalva maneuvers, and relaxation of urethral sphincters.

Goel and colleagues (2017) found that the most effective bladder emptying position for men over 50 years old was sitting rather than standing. Although flow rates were similar, postvoid residual volume was lower in the sitting position. Other studies report no differences; however, factors such as increased comfort, time to relax, less fatigue, and improved balance make the sitting position worthy of exploration as a recommended voiding practice in older men. In the standing position, it is also common practice to only partially lower the undergarments. Due to the superficial position of the urethra on the dorsal side of the penis, mild compression can occur, which will impede urine flow (see **Fig. 10-2**). Thus, men should be advised to fully lower their undergarments to avoid the risk of elastic banding compression of the urethra.

Historically, Crede maneuver, the application of external pressure to the suprapubic region to empty the bladder, has been used in patients with spinal cord injury. Although this method was thought to assist with voiding, a seminal study in neurologically intact subjects demonstrated that the procedure actually prompted contraction of the external urethral sphincter to maintain closure of the bladder neck (Barbalias et al., 1983).

Postmicturition dribbling can be managed by urethral and/or bulbar milking as well as by performing a series of pelvic floor muscle contractions. Where the path of the urethra takes a turn from vertical to horizontal, there is a small reservoir called the urethral bulb. In older age, when the urine stream is weaker and slower, there is a potential for urine to be trapped in the urethral bulb. Bulbar milking involves massaging the perineum behind the testicles in a forward direction and is often accompanied by urethral milking, which involves massaging along the length of the penis. Both are often recommended by primary care providers and urologists to compensate for the weaker, slower stream in men (Blanker et al., 2019). Additional advice for postvoid dribbling includes performing quick pelvic floor muscle contractions to help force urine out of the bladder. There is little evidence to support the efficacy of performing a strong pelvic floor muscle contraction immediately after voiding (Dumoulin et al., 2017).

KEY POINT

In older age, when the urine stream is weaker and slower, there is a potential for urine to be trapped in the urethral bulb. Bulbar milking involves massaging the perineum behind the testicles in a forward direction and is often accompanied by urethral milking, which involves massaging along the length of the penis to evacuate retained urine.

 ## PHARMACOLOGIC MANAGEMENT STRATEGIES FOR MEN WITH LUTS

Research has shown that contraction and relaxation of smooth muscle within the prostate gland contribute,

respectively, to the effective storage and evacuation of urine. During the last decade, the development of oral agents for LUTS in men has focused on maximizing or inhibiting these biological mechanisms (Uckert et al., 2020).

PHARMACOLOGIC AGENTS FOR TREATMENT OF STORAGE SYMPTOMS

Pharmacologic treatment of storage symptoms is recommended as an addition to behavioral therapy(s) that fails to produce the desired effect. Oral antimuscarinics and oral beta3-adrenoceptor agonists are the drugs of choice for storage symptoms. The goal of pharmacologic treatment of storage symptoms is to relax an overactive detrusor muscle.

Antimuscarinics

Detrusor contraction is triggered by acetylcholine. Antimuscarinic agents are one of two types of anticholinergic drugs that work by targeting the muscarinic class of acetylcholine receptors to counteract stimulation of the detrusor muscle by acetylcholine. Common side effects of antimuscarinic drugs include dry mouth, constipation, dry or itchy eyes, blurred vision, dyspepsia, UTI, urinary retention, and impaired cognitive function. Life-threatening arrhythmias have been reported as a rare side effect (Gormley et al., 2019).

Antimuscarinic drugs have been used for decades to mitigate storage symptoms. Examples include darifenacin, solifenacin, fesoterodine, tolterodine, oxybutynin, propiverine, and trospium chloride (Uckert et al., 2020). Of these, darifenacin and solifenacin primarily target muscarinic receptors in the bladder, which may decrease their peripheral side effects. Trospium chloride has limited ability to cross the blood–brain barrier and so may have less impact on cognitive function (Gormley et al., 2019) (see Chapter 7, Table 7-2).

Despite multiple available antimuscarinic agents, the most commonly prescribed drug is oxybutynin, possibly due to lower cost, better coverage by insurance, and prior provider experience (Anger et al., 2018). Extended-release (ER) formulation of antimuscarinics should preferentially be prescribed over immediate-release (IR) formulation due to lower rates of dry mouth. Transdermal oxybutynin (patch or gel) may be used if better tolerated than oral therapies. If one antimuscarinic medication offers inadequate symptom control and/or unacceptable adverse side effects, then a different antimuscarinic or a beta3-adrenoceptor agonist may be tried or combination therapy may be initiated (Gormley et al., 2019).

Antimuscarinics should not be used with narrow-angle glaucoma (unless approved by an ophthalmologist), and extreme caution should be used in prescribing for patients with impaired gastric emptying or a history of urinary retention. Extreme caution is also warranted in prescribing antimuscarinics for patients already taking medications with anticholinergic properties (such as tricyclic antidepressants, antiparkinsonian agents, and some antiemetics), as well as in prescribing antimuscarinics for frail patients (those with mobility deficits, weight loss, weakness, and cognitive deficits). Clinicians should manage associated constipation and dry mouth with bowel management, fluid management, dose modification, or alternative antimuscarinics before abandoning effective antimuscarinic therapy (Gormley et al., 2019).

Beta3-Adrenoceptor Agonists
Beta3-adrenoceptors are found in the bladder and are thought to have a direct role in relaxation of the detrusor muscle and prevention of urination. Beta3-adrenoceptor agonists are agents that bind to beta3-adrenoreceptors in the bladder, causing smooth muscle relaxation. Mirabegron, a beta3-adrenoceptor agonist, has been shown to perform similarly to tolterodine, an antimuscarinic, in terms of alleviating storage symptoms, but with lower rates of dry mouth and constipation (Gormley et al., 2019). Beta3-adrenoceptor agonists are recommended for patients who have bothersome symptoms related to the use of antimuscarinic agents.

KEY POINT

Oral antimuscarinics and oral beta3-adrenergic agonists are the drugs of choice for storage symptoms in addition to lifestyle modification and behavioral therapies. The goal of pharmacologic treatment of storage symptoms is to relax an overactive detrusor muscle.

Other Agents
Tadalafil, a phosphodiesterase type 5 (PDE5) inhibitor commonly used to treat erectile dysfunction, has also been shown to significantly improve storage and voiding symptoms, although the mechanism of action is not yet clear (Uckert et al., 2020).

Intradetrusor onabotulinumtoxinA (100 units, Botox®) is recommended for patients who are refractory to behavioral therapy and standard oral pharmacologic agents for treatment of storage symptoms. Patients treated with intradetrusor onabotulinumtoxinA must be able and willing to be evaluated frequently for postvoid residual volume and able to perform self-catheterization if necessary (Gormley et al., 2019) (see Chapter 7).

KEY POINT

Clinicians should manage associated constipation and dry mouth with bowel management, fluid management, dose modification, or alternative antimuscarinics before abandoning effective antimuscarinic therapy. Extreme caution is also warranted in prescribing antimuscarinics for patients already taking medications with anticholinergic properties as well as in the frail elderly.

PHARMACOLOGIC AGENTS FOR TREATMENT OF VOIDING AND POSTVOIDING SYMPTOMS
Like storage symptoms, pharmacologic treatment of voiding and postvoiding symptoms is recommended as an addition to behavioral therapy(s) that fails to produce the desired effect. Alpha-adrenergic antagonists and 5-alpha reductase inhibitors are the drugs of choice for voiding and postvoiding symptoms. The goal of pharmacologic treatment for voiding and postvoiding symptoms is to enhance bladder emptying.

Alpha1-Adrenergic Antagonists
Adrenergic receptors are located all over the body and are targets for catecholamines like norepinephrine and epinephrine. The binding of a catecholamine to an adrenergic receptor stimulates the sympathetic nervous system. Adrenergic receptors are generally classified as either alpha or beta. When stimulated, alpha receptors produce vasoconstriction and smooth muscle contraction, while beta receptors produce increased cardiac output and bronchodilation. Alpha1-adrenergic antagonists target alpha receptors (type 1) in the bladder neck, prostate, and urethra to produce smooth muscle relaxation and reduced resistance. Alpha1-adrenergic antagonists that are used to treat voiding and postvoiding symptoms include alfuzosin, doxazosin, silodosin, tamsulosin, and terazosin. The efficacy of these medications must be balanced against their side effects, including headache, orthostatic hypotension, and sexual dysfunction. Alfuzosin and silodosin have enhanced side effect profiles that minimize hypotension (Uckert et al., 2020). Terazosin and doxazosin should be initiated at bedtime to reduce postural light-headedness, and the dose may be titrated up over several weeks.

5-Alpha Reductase Inhibitors
5-Alpha reductases are enzymes involved in the metabolism of steroids, including the conversion of testosterone to DHT. 5-Alpha reductase inhibitors (5-ARI) block the production of DHT, a stimulant of prostate cell growth. 5-ARIs, including finasteride and dutasteride, act by reducing the size of the prostate gland with the potential for long-term reduction in prostate volume and need for prostate surgery. Combination treatment with a 5-ARI and an alpha1-adrenergic antagonist is recommended in patients with severe voiding or postvoiding symptoms, increased risk of disease progression, a prostate volume of >40 mL, and high postvoid residual. Treatment with 5-ARIs requires 6 to 12 months before symptom improvement, while alpha1-adrenergic antagonists provide immediate therapeutic benefits. Combination therapy results in greater improvement in LUTS and has been shown to be more effective in preventing disease progression and minimizing the risk of acute urinary retention (Uckert et al., 2020). The major side effects of 5-ARIs are decreased libido, ejaculatory/erectile dysfunction,

TABLE 10-1 EFFECTS AND ADVERSE EFFECTS OF MEDICATIONS USED FOR SYMPTOM MANAGEMENT OF BPH		
	ALPHA1-ADRENERGIC ANTAGONISTS	5-ALPHA REDUCTASE INHIBITORS
Decrease in prostate size	No	Yes
Peak onset	2–4 wk	6–12 mo
Sexual dysfunction	+	++
Hypotensive effects	++	—
Commonly used drugs	Tamsulosin, alfuzosin	Finasteride, dutasteride

and depression. These drugs should be avoided in couples trying to conceive. **Table 10-1** reviews the common effects of medications used for symptom management of BPH.

KEY POINT

For men with bothersome voiding LUTS unresponsive to lifestyle modifications, medications are recommended as the second-line intervention that is alpha-adrenergic antagonists to relax the bladder neck and 5-alpha reductase inhibitors to reduce the size of the prostate gland over time.

PHYTOTHERAPY

No guidelines published by urological professional organizations endorse the use of popular phytodrugs such as *Serenoa repens*, *Pygeum africanum*, *Urtica dioica*, *Cucurbita pepo*, or *Secale cereale*. These preparations are generally well tolerated and may ease LUTS secondary to BPH; however, plant extract preparations contain unknown quantities of chemicals, and positive effects are not consistently demonstrated in clinical studies (Uckert et al., 2020).

 ADVANCE MODALITIES FOR LUTS

NEUROMODULATION

Neuromodulation for an overactive bladder should be considered for patients with symptoms that are refractory to behavioral and pharmacologic therapy(s). Neuromodulation is thought to diminish abnormal reflex arcs associated with an overactive bladder by modulating afferent signals from the bladder to the spinal cord (also see Chapter 7).

Tibial nerve stimulation is a form of peripheral neuromodulation that may be considered in selected patients, especially those with overactive bladder and urge UI (Dumoulin et al., 2017). Percutaneous tibial nerve stimulation (PTNS) involves placement of a fine needle electrode

near the tibial nerve in the area of the medial malleolus of the ankle, with a grounding pad placed near the heel. Transcutaneous tibial nerve stimulation (TTNS) involves external electrodes that are placed near the ankle where the tibial nerve is located and has been shown to be as effective for overactive bladder symptoms as PTNS (Ramírez-García et al., 2019). An electrical impulse is generated that travels up the tibial nerve to the sacral region. The procedure requires weekly 30-minute treatments for a duration of up to 12 weeks, as determined by the patient's symptoms. In individuals sufficiently motivated to complete treatment, favorable short- and long-term improvement has been reported that is comparable to or slightly better than medications; however, no studies have yet compared PTNS to other forms of active treatment (Dumoulin et al., 2017). PTNS is recommended for men with overactive bladder and/or urge UI symptoms who do not achieve satisfactory results from lifestyle modification, behavioral interventions, and pharmacologic therapy (Dumoulin et al., 2017).

Sacral neuromodulation involves stimulation of the sacral nerves involved in the spinal reflex arc that controls bladder function. Sacral neuromodulation has been studied as an approach for urgency, frequency, urge UI, and other symptoms of overactive bladder and detrusor instability. Patients initially have a temporary surface electrode placed to gauge response. If successful, they may elect to have a pulse generator implanted, usually in the upper outer buttock or abdomen. Mean success rate, primarily in women, varies from 26% to 38% with 5-year revision rates of 39% to 42% (Goldman et al., 2017). Currently, support is mixed concerning the use of sacral neuromodulation for urgency, overactive bladder, and nonneurogenic LUTS in men (Goldman et al., 2017).

KEY POINT

Neuromodulation may be considered for patients who have failed conservative and pharmacological treatments. It is thought to diminish abnormal reflex arcs associated with an overactive bladder by modulating afferent signals from the bladder to the spinal cord thus reducing urgency, frequency, and urge incontinence.

SURGICAL INTERVENTION

Men who continue to have significant difficulty with bladder emptying despite the use of medications may be offered a variety of third-line invasive therapies to remove or ablate prostate tissue in the interest of improved urine flow. The selection of an intervention is influenced by age, prostate size, degree of symptom burden, and potential complications. These third-line therapies are listed and described in **Table 10-2**. In addition, surgical interventions resulting from postoperative complications

TABLE 10-2 CURRENT SURGICAL PROCEDURES TO REDUCE SYMPTOMS OF BPH/LUTS

TECHNIQUE	BRIEF DESCRIPTION	EFFICACY	SIDE EFFECT PROFILE
Invasive Surgery			
Simple prostatectomy	Surgical removal of the prostate through an abdominal or perineal approach Major surgery generally performed only if very large prostate or suspicion of coexisting prostate cancer; robotic-assisted prostatectomy with less complications and hospitalization but depends upon expertise of the urologist	Significant improvement in IPSS and quality-of-life scores; moderate recommendation; Grade C level of evidence	Significant blood loss with transfusion rates about 10% in some studies Long hospital stays (average 5 d) Long duration of indwelling catheter (average 5 d) Long-term complications include incontinence, bladder neck contracture
Transurethral resection of the prostate (TURP)	Typically, an endoscopic introduction of an electrocautery device into the prostatic urethra with layered removal of perurethral prostate tissue	High degree of long-term efficacy; moderate recommendation; Grade B evidence level	Requires spinal or general anesthesia Significant risks: Blood loss Hematuria TUR syndrome Long-term possible complications from urethral stricture or bladder neck abnormality Retrograde ejaculation
Transurethral incision of the prostate (TUIP)	Selective small incisions limited to the bladder neck using endoscopic guidance through the urethra; candidate has <30-g prostate	Indicated for men with smaller prostates and moderate symptoms who are at higher risk for more invasive procedures; moderate recommendation; Grade B evidence level	Fewer complications compared with TURP
Laser Therapy			
Holmium laser enucleation (HoLEP)	The laser is used to cut and remove the excess tissue that is blocking the urethra. Another instrument, called a morcellator, is then used to chop the prostate tissue into small pieces that are easily removed	Limited data that suggest acceptable efficacy; moderate recommendation; Grade B evidence level	Minimal complications and short procedure; consider for those with ↑ risk for bleeding
Holmium laser ablation of the prostate (HoLAP)	Holmium laser is used to melt away (vaporize) the excess prostate tissue	Limited data suggest acceptable efficacy	Minimal short- and long-term complications
Photoselective vaporization of the prostate (PVP)	A laser is used to melt away (vaporize) excess prostate tissue to enlarge the urinary channel	One study with sustained improvement in symptoms and significant reduction in prostate size; moderate recommendation; Grade B evidence level	Minimal short- and long-term complications; consider for those with ↑ risk for bleeding
Transurethral vaporization of prostate (TUVP)	An electrovaporization a prostate; closely resembles TURP	Conditional recommendation; Grade B evidence level	Less bleeding than standard TURP
Thulium laser enucleation (ThuLEP)	Uses a thulium laser to remove prostate tissue completely	Moderate recommendations; Grade B evidence level	Consider in patients with ↑ risk for bleeding
Minimally Invasive Therapies			
Transurethral radiofrequency needle ablation (TUNA)	Endoscopic transurethral placement of needles across lumen into surrounding prostate with radiofrequency energy used to cause prostate tissue necrosis and subsequent reduction in prostate volume	Expert opinion: NOT recommended for treatment for BPH Short-term outcomes similar to TURP. Long-term outcomes may not be quite as good	Does not require surgery Less sexual dysfunction including retrograde ejaculation

(Continued)

TABLE 10-2 CURRENT SURGICAL PROCEDURES TO REDUCE SYMPTOMS OF BPH/LUTS (Continued)

TECHNIQUE	BRIEF DESCRIPTION	EFFICACY	SIDE EFFECT PROFILE
Transurethral microwave therapy	Transurethral approach that uses devices to heat the prostate tissue while cooling the urethra allowing for maximal prostate tissue ablation while minimizing urethral damage	Conditional recommendation; Grade C evidence level; probably similar to TUNA, but data are limited due to evolving nature of the technology as well as lack of uniformity in study design to measure efficacy and adverse effects. Concerns about long-term efficacy	Does not require surgery Less sexual dysfunction
Prostatic urethral lift	Transurethral placement of small implants to reposition the prostate lobes to optimize urethral patency; prostate must be <80 g	Moderate recommendation; Grade C evidence level; limited data suggest adequate efficacy	Performed under local anesthesia Minimal to no ejaculatory or sexual dysfunction
Aquablation	Prostate should be >30/<80 g; Uses high-pressure saline to remove prostate without heat; minimally invasive	Conditional recommendation; Grade C evidence level; limited long-term evidence of efficacy	No sexual dysfunction reported; minimal bleeding
Water vapor thermal therapy	Candidate with >80 g prostate; uses radiofrequency energy and steamed water to eliminate prostate tissue; minimally invasive	Recommendation is conditional; Grade C evidence level; limited studies, some consider investigational	Can be done in urologist office; preserves sexual function
Prostate artery embolization (PAE)	Newer treatment; done by interventional radiologist; inserts catheter in wrist or groin and injects particles that ↓ prostrates blood supply; prostate shrinks	Expert opinion only; unproven efficacy; not recommended until more studies	Post PAE syndrome: N/V, pelvic pain, fever, bladder spasms, hematuria

*Ablation, the laser melts away excess tissue; enucleation, the laser cuts away excess prostate tissue. In all laser procedures, the laser is introduced into the urethra through a scope.

Adapted from Foster, H. E., Barry, M. J., Dahm, P., et al. (2019). *Surgical management of lower urinary tract symptoms attributed to benign prostatic hyperplasia: AUA Guideline.* American Urological Association. Retrieved from https://www.auanet.org/guidelines/benign-prostatic-hyperplasia-(bph)-guideline#x8189

for BOO or prostate cancer that leads to storage issues are discussed below.

Transurethral Resection of the Prostate

Transurethral resection of the prostate (TURP) is the gold standard third-line intervention with an 80% to 90% efficacy rate as measured by symptom improvement. Several complications are associated with its use; however, complication rates have decreased with newer techniques such as microprocessor-controlled electrocautery units. The most significant complications are bleeding leading to transfusion, urethral stricture, contracture of the bladder neck, SUI, sexual dysfunction including erectile dysfunction and retrograde ejaculation all leading to a reduced QOL (Foster et al., 2019). Newer protocols allow for a 1-day hospital stay, reduced risk of complications, and discharge without a catheter (Shum et al., 2014). Men who have failed pharmacological therapy to manage LUTS due to BPH and those who suffer comorbid conditions related to BPH including renal insufficiency, unmanaged urinary retention, and recurrent UTIs, bladder stones, or hematuria (Foster et al., 2019). **Figure 10-6** illustrates the most common approaches to a TURP.

KEY POINT

Surgical reduction of the prostate for treatment of voiding LUTS is recommended only for those whose bothersome symptoms not responsive to lifestyle modifications and pharmacologic therapy or those who suffer comorbid conditions secondary to BPH.

Simple Prostatectomy

Simple (total) prostatectomy is indicated only in cases in which the prostate is unusually large or prostate cancer is suspected. The literature on complications associated with simple prostatectomy is confusing due to wide variability in reporting types of complications and estimating complication rates (Hakimi et al., 2012). The greatest concerns are rates of postoperative UI and sexual dysfunction. These complications are more of an issue for younger men and men with higher baseline functioning (Brajtbord et al., 2014). Lifestyle modification, behavioral, and medical management of these problems should begin early in the recovery period. Limited evidence suggests that systematic exercise and training of pelvic

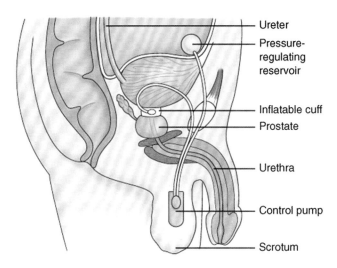

Ureter

Pressure-
regulating
reservoir

Inflatable cuff

Prostate

Urethra

Control pump

Scrotum

FIGURE 10-7. Artificial Urethral Sphincter Implant.

floor musculature can expedite recovery of bladder control following RP (Robinson et al., 2009). Any other surgical intervention to address SUI should be delayed for 6 to 12 months following surgery since spontaneous recovery can continue for several months postoperatively (Goldman et al., 2017).

KEY POINT

The most common complications following radical prostatectomy are urinary incontinence and erectile dysfunction.

Surgical Interventions for Storage Symptoms

Injection of a bulking agent, such as collagen, into the submucosa adjacent to the bladder neck may be helpful to many men suffering from SUI usually after a RP; however, the need for repeated injections due to migration and/or disintegration of the bulking agent is a drawback (ICS, 2013; Schaeffer et al., 2012). Due to the low success

rate, bulking agents should only be used if other alternatives are contraindicated (Goldman et al., 2017). Although required by few RP patients (Catalona & Han, 2012), two surgical interventions are considered definitive therapy for stress UI: implantation of a synthetic sling to restore urethral support and implantation of an artificial urinary sphincter (**Fig. 10-7**). Synthetic slings are associated with few complications and have shown efficacy and safety for men suffering from mild to moderate UI postprostatectomy (Goldman et al., 2017). While effective in eliminating stress UI, implantation of an artificial urinary sphincter is typically the option of *last resort* and can require surgical revision due to infection, erosion, or atrophy (Goldman et al., 2017; Gray & Moore, 2009a; Silva et al., 2011). It does, however, have the longest track record and remains the most predictably successful surgery for treating severe SUI following radical prostate surgery (Goldman et al., 2017).

CONCLUSION

LUTS are highly prevalent in older men, especially those past 50 years of age. Four categories of LUTS are recognized by the International Continence Society: storage, voiding, postvoiding, and mixed storage and voiding symptoms. LUTS in men primarily originate from benign and/or malignant diseases of the prostate and their treatment. Every man with LUTS deserves a comprehensive physical assessment, evaluation of LUTS severity and perceived bother with a standardized assessment tool, and further evaluation with advanced studies if necessary. Prevention and conservative management of LUTS should target symptom relief as well as elimination or mitigation of the underlying cause(s). Behavioral approaches are considered first-line therapy and include general health and lifestyle counseling, continence education, absorbent products, watchful waiting, and specific strategies to treat storage, voiding, and postvoiding symptoms. Pharmacologic agents are recommended as an addition

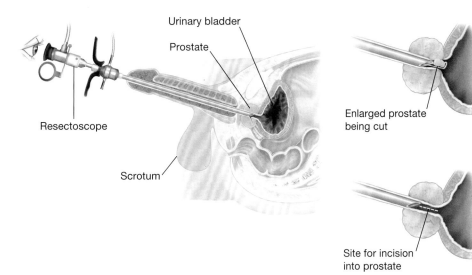

Urinary bladder

Prostate

Resectoscope

Scrotum

Enlarged prostate
being cut

Site for incision
into prostate

FIGURE 10-6. Transurethral Resection of the Prostate.

to behavioral therapy(s) that fails to produce the desired effect, while neuromodulation and surgical interventions may be a choice for those with refractory LUTS that have failed both conservative and pharmacological therapies.

The certified WOC nurse or continence specialist is well positioned to identify and evaluate LUTS in men and to assist with access to evidence-based continence care from a qualified continence care provider.

CASE STUDY

BACKGROUND

Mr. Damien is a 58-year-old African American man who presents to his primary care provider (PCP) with bothersome lower urinary tract symptoms (LUTS). He reports that he is getting up approximately three times a night to urinate, with small to moderate amounts of urine voided each time. He also reports having a weak urinary stream and feeling unable to empty his bladder completely. On further questioning, he admits to sudden urges to void on occasion and one to two episodes of urinary incontinence per week.

Mr. Damien drinks one to two cups of coffee per day and three to four beers per week. He does not smoke or drink diet beverages. His BMI is 23. His past medical history is significant for hypertension and hyperlipidemia but negative for diabetes and cardiovascular disease. His medications include hydrochlorothiazide, amlodipine, and simvastatin.

On physical examination, Mr. Damien has an enlarged symmetrical prostate with normal texture and no nodules. The prostate is not boggy or tender. Rectum is absent of stool or masses. Patient was able to contract and relax external anal sphincter on command. A dipstick urinalysis is negative for leukocytes, blood, protein, and glucose. He has no suprapubic tenderness. When Mr. Damien is asked what he thinks of his urinary symptoms, he says, "I have been bothered by them but felt that they were just normal for my age; however, if you can do something to help, it would be great."

DISCUSSION

Mr. Damien has mixed storage and voiding symptoms. His storage symptoms include nocturia, urgency, and urge incontinence. His voiding symptoms include a weak urinary stream and a sensation of incomplete bladder emptying. There is no evidence of a urinary tract infection. His prostate examination is normal with the exception of symmetrical enlargement. If the prostate was boggy or tender on examination, the clinical suspicion for prostate infection (prostatitis) would be increased. Also, if there was any asymmetry or nodules appreciated on examination, Mr. Damien would be referred for a worked up for prostate cancer.

Mr. Damien is diagnosed with LUTS secondary to benign prostatic hyperplasia (BPH), the nonmalignant enlargement of the prostate gland. BPH affects half of all men by age 50. The proliferation of prostate connective tissue, smooth muscle, and glandular epithelium, accompanied by the increased smooth muscle tone and resistance that develops within the enlarged gland, is the likely cause of the voiding symptoms that Mr. Damien is experiencing. The constant pressure of Mr. Damien's enlarged prostate on his bladder has likely led to overactivity of the detrusor muscle, resulting in problems with the storage of urine and symptoms of nocturia, urgency, and urge incontinence. Additional testing recommended for Mr. Damien includes determination of postvoid residual volume to assess bladder emptying, prostate-specific antigen (PSA) testing to screen for prostate cancer, completion of the International Consultation on Incontinence Questionnaire—Male Lower Urinary Tract Symptoms (ICIQ-MLUTS) to obtain a baseline measure of LUTS impact, and completion of a 3-day voiding diary to obtain information about patterns of voiding frequency and volume, fluid intake, episodes of incontinence and associated activities, and pad use.

Phase I of Mr. Damien's treatment plan begins with conservative management strategies introduced by the continence nurse toward the goal of relieving or eliminating storage symptoms. Education about the anatomy and physiology of the lower urinary tract is the first order of business so that Mr. Damien appreciates the rationale for behavioral interventions and feels competent and confident about his capacity to adhere to treatment. Adequate hydration and nighttime fluid management are emphasized, as well as either avoidance or strategic intake of bladder irritants (i.e., drinking coffee, beer, or other alcoholic beverages only in the presence of an accessible toilet). Use of absorbent products is discussed in the context of wearing the smallest possible amount of product and advancing to "product-free" living gradually, starting with low stakes circumstances as urgency and urge incontinence episodes begin to diminish. The continence nurse also assists Mr. Damien with the process of selecting a "best fit" absorbent product using the electronic WOCN° Body Worn Absorbent Guide on her smartphone found at https://bwap.

wocn.org. To prevent incontinence-associated dermatitis, Mr. Damien is taught to clean his perineum following an incontinent episode using either a no-rinse skin cleaner or warm water, followed by application of a barrier cream with dimethicone.

Phase II of Mr. Damien's treatment plan involves pelvic floor muscle training (PFMT) that is provided to Mr. Damien by either a trained continence nurse or specialized or physiotherapist. Urge suppression techniques are emphasized, followed by the introduction of bladder training to develop his ability to delay voiding. To mitigate the effects of BPH on Mr. Damien's voiding symptoms, he is taught to void in a sitting position with fully lowered undergarments and to perform bulbar and urethral milking to enhance urine flow. Following a collaborative discussion with Mr. Damien's PCP, he is prescribed an alpha-adrenergic antagonist or blocker (tamsulosin) to relax the bladder neck to optimize bladder emptying. In addition, he is instructed to take the first dose prior to bed and arise in the morning slowly to reduce the risk of dizziness from postural hypotension then take the remaining dosages at dinner time. He is informed of other possible side effects in addition to the dizziness including runny nose, headache, and abnormal ejaculation and encouraged to report any intolerances. Following completion of both phases of the treatment plan, Mr. Damien is scheduled for a follow-up visit with his PCP for medication recheck and in 3 months with the continence nurse to evaluate his progress.

REFERENCES

Alawamlh, O. A. H., Goueli, R., & Lee, R. K. (2018). Lower urinary tract symptoms, benign prostatic hyperplasia, and urinary retention. *Medical Clinics of North America, 102*(2), 301–311. doi: 10.1016/j.mcna.2017.10.005.

American Cancer Society. (n.d.). *Cancer facts and figures 2020*. Retrieved from https://www.cancer.org/content/dam/cancer-org/research/cancer-facts-and-statistics/annual-cancer-facts-and-figures/2020/cancer-facts-and-figures-2020.pdf

Anger, J. T., Goldman, H. B., Luo, X., et al. (2018). Patterns of medical management of overactive bladder (OAB) and benign prostatic hyperplasia (BPH) in the United States. *Neurourology and Urodynamics, 37*, 213–222.

Barbalias, G. A., Klauber, G. T., & Blaivas, J. G. (1983). Critical evaluation of the Credé maneuver: A urodynamic study of 207 patients. *Journal of Urology, 130*(4), 720–723.

Blanker, M. H., Brandenbarg, P., Slijkhuis, B. G. C., et al. (2019). Development of an online personalized self-management intervention for men with uncomplicated LUTS. *Neurourology and Urodynamics*, 38(6), 1685–1691.

Brajtbord, J. S., Punnen, S., Cowan, J. E., et al. (2014). Age and baseline quality of life at radical prostatectomy—who has the most to lose? *Journal of Urology*, 192(2), 396–401. doi: 10.1016/j.juro.2014.02.045.

Bristol Urological Institute. (n.d.). *The International Consultation on Incontinence Questionnaire*. Retrieved from http://www.iciq.net

Catalona, W. J., & Han, M. (2012). Definitive therapy for localized prostate cancer: An overview. In A. J. Wein, L. R. Kavoussi, A. C. Novick, et al. (Eds.), *Campbell-Walsh urology* (10th ed., pp. 2771–2788.e6). Philadelphia, PA: Elsevier.

D'Ancona, C., Haylen, B., Oelke, M., et al. (2018). The International Continence Society (ICS) report on the terminology for adult male lower urinary tract and pelvic floor symptoms and dysfunction. *Neurourology and Urodynamics, 38*(2), 433–477.

Davis, R., Jones, J. S., Barocas, A. D., et al. (updated, 2016). *Diagnosis, evaluation, and follow-up of asymptomatic microhematuria in adults*. American Urological Association Clinical Guidelines. Linthicum, MD: American Urological Association.

Destors, M., Tamisier, R., Sapene, M., et al. (May, 2015). Nocturia is an independent predictive factor of prevalent hypertension in obstructive sleep apnea patients. *Sleep Medicine, 16*(5), 652–658.

Diaz, D. C., Robinson, D., Bosch, R., et al. (2017a). Initial assessment of urinary incontinence in adult male and female patients. In P. Abrams, L. Cardozo, A. Wagg, et al. (Eds.), *Incontinence* (6th ed., pp. 521–540). Tokyo: International Consultation on Incontinence.

Diaz, D. C., Robinson, D., Bosch, R., et al. (2017b). Patient reported outcome assessment. In P. Abrams, L. Cardozo, A. Wagg, et al. (Eds.), *Incontinence* (6th ed., pp. 541–598). Tokyo: International Consultation on Incontinence.

Dumoulin, C., Adewuyi, T., Booth, J., et al. (2017). Adult conservative management. In P. Abrams, L. Cardozo, A. Wagg, et al. (Eds.), *Incontinence* (6th ed., pp. 1443–1631). Tokyo: International Consultation on Incontinence.

Foster, H. E., Barry, M. J., Dahm, P., et al. (2019). *Surgical management of lower urinary tract symptoms attributed to benign prostatic hyperplasia: AUA guideline*. American Urological Association. Retrieved from https://www.auanet.org/guidelines/benign-prostatic-hyperplasia-(bph)-guideline#x8189

Fry, C., Chess-Williams, R., Hashitani, H., et al. (2017). Cell biology. In P. Abrams, L. Cardozo, A. Wagg, et al. (Eds.), *Incontinence* (6th ed., pp. 143–258). Tokyo: International Consultation on Incontinence.

Goel, A., Kanodia, G., Sokhal, A. K., et al. (2017). Evaluation of the impact of voiding posture on uroflowmetry parameters in men. *World Journal of Men's Health, 35*(2), 100–106. doi: 10.5534/wjmh.2017.35.2.100.

Goldman, H. B., Averbeck, M. A., Bruschini, H., et al. (2017). Surgical treatment of urinary incontinence in men. In P. Abrams, L. Cardozo, A. Wagg, et al. (Eds.), *Incontinence* (6th ed., pp. 1629–1740). Tokyo: International Consultation on Incontinence.

Gormley, E. A., Lightner, D. J., Burgio, K. L., et al. (2019). *Diagnosis and treatment of non-neurogenic overactive bladder (OAB) in adults: An AUA/SUFU guideline*. American Urological Association (AUA)/Society of Urodynamics, Female Pelvic Medicine & Urogenital Reconstruction (SUFU). Retrieved from https://www.auanet.org/guidelines/overactive-bladder-(oab)-guideline

Gray, M., & Moore, K. N. (2009). Urinary incontinence. In M. Gray & K. N. Moore (Eds.), *Urologic disorders: Adult and pediatric care* (Chapter 6, pp. 119–159). St. Louis, MO: Elsevier.

Hakimi, A. A., Faleck, D. M., Sobey, S., et al. (2012). Assessment of complication and functional outcome reporting in the minimally invasive prostatectomy literature from 2006 to the present. *BJU International, 109*(1), 26–30; discussion 30. doi:10.1111/j.1464-410X.2011.10591.x.

International Continence Society. (2013). *ICS Factsheets (2013 Edition): Stress Urinary Incontinence*. http://www.ics.org/Documents/Documents.aspx?DocumentID=2172

Mellick, L. B., & Al-Dhahir, M. A. Cremasteric reflex [Updated February 17, 2020]. In *StatPearls* [Internet]. Treasure Island, FL: StatPearls Publishing. Retrieved from https://www.ncbi.nlm.nih.gov/books/NBK513348/

Milsom, I., Altman, D., Cartwright, R., et al. (2017). Epidemiology of urinary incontinence (UI) and other lower urinary tract symptoms

(LUTS), pelvic organ prolapse (POP) and anal incontinence (AI). In P. Abrams, L. Cardozo, A. Wagg, et al. (Eds.), *Incontinence* (6th ed., pp. 1443–1631). Tokyo: International Consultation on Incontinence.

National Association for Continence. (n.d.a). *Products*. Retrieved February 2, 2020, from https://www.nafc.org

National Association for Continence. (n.d.b). *What are Kegel exercises?* Retrieved February 3, 2020, from https://www.nafc.org

National Institute of Diabetes and Digestive and Kidney Diseases. (September, 2014a). *Prostate enlargement (Benign Prostatic Hyperplasia)*. Retrieved from www.niddk.nih.gov/health-information/urologic-diseases/prostate-problems/prostate-benign-prostatic-hyperplasia

National Institute of Diabetes and Digestive and Kidney Diseases. (July, 2014b). *Prostatitis: Inflammation of the prostate*. Retrieved from www.niddk.nih.gov/health-information/urologic-diseases/prostate-problems/prostatitis-inflammation-prostate

Newman, D. K., Cockrell, R., Griebling, T. L., et al. (2017). Primary prevention, continence promotion, models of care and education. In P. Abrams, L. Cardozo, A. Wagg, et al. (Eds.), *Incontinence* (6th ed., pp. 2427–2478). Tokyo: International Consultation on Incontinence.

Ramírez-García, I., Blanco-Ratto, L., Kauffmann, S., et al. (2019). Efficacy of transcutaneous stimulation of the posterior tibial nerve compared to percutaneous stimulation in idiopathic overactive bladder syndrome: A randomized controlled trial. *Neurourology and Urodynamics, 38*(1), 261–268. doi: 10.1002/nau.23843.

Robinson, J. P., Weiss, R., Avi-Itzhak, T., et al. (2009). Pilot-testing of a theory-based pelvic floor training intervention for radical prostatectomy patients [abstract]. *Neurourology and Urodynamics, 28*(7), 682–683.

Salvatore, S., Delancey, J., Igawa, Y., et al. (2017). Pathophysiology of urinary incontinence, faecal incontinence and pelvic organ prolapse. In P. Abrams, L. Cardozo, A. Wagg, et al. (Eds.), *Incontinence* (6th ed., pp. 431–440). Tokyo: International Consultation on Incontinence.

Sandhu, J. S., Breyer, B., Comiter, C., et al. (2019). *Incontinence after prostate treatment: AUA/SUFU guideline*. American Urological Association (AUA)/Society of Urodynamics, Female Pelvic Medicine & Urogenital Reconstruction (SUFU). Retrieved from https://www.auanet.org/guidelines/incontinence-after-prostate-treatment

Schaeffer, E. M., Partin, A. W., Lepor, H., et al. (2012). Radical retropubic and perineal prostatectomy. In A. J. Wein, L. R. Kavoussi, A. C. Novick, et al. (Eds.), *Campbell-Walsh urology* (10th ed., pp. 2801–2829.e4). Philadelphia, PA: Elsevier.

Shum, C. F., Mukherjee, A., & Teo, C. P. (2014). Catheter-free discharge on first postoperative day after bipolar transurethral resection of prostate: Clinical outcomes of 100 cases. *International Journal of Urology, 21*(3), 313–318. doi: 10.1111/iju.12246.

Silva, L. A., Andriolo, R. B., Atallah, A. N., et al. (2011). Surgery for stress incontinence due to presumed sphincter deficiency after prostate surgery (Review). *Cochrane Database of Systematic Reviews*, (4). Article No.: CD008306. doi: 10.1002/14651858. CD008306.pub2.

Uckert, S., Kedia, G. T., Tsikas, D., et al. (2020). Emerging drugs to target lower urinary tract symptomatology (LUTS)/benign prostatic hyperplasia (BPH): Focus on the prostate. *World Journal of Urology, 38*, 1423–1435. doi: 10.1007/s00345-019-02933-1.

Wound, Ostomy, and Continence Nurses Society—Wound Guidelines Taskforce. (2017). 2016 guideline for prevention and management of pressure injuries (ulcers): An executive summary. *Journal of Wound, Ostomy, and Continence Nursing, 44*(2), 241–246.

Zhang, A. Y., & Xu, X. (2018). Prevalence, burden, and treatment of lower urinary tract symptoms in men aged 50 and older: A systematic review of the literature. *SAGE Open Nursing, 4*, 1–24. doi: 10.1177/2377960818811773.

Zhou, J., Xia, S., Li, T., et al. (2020). Association between obstructive sleep apnea syndrome and nocturia: A meta-analysis. *Sleep and Breathing*. https://doi.org/10.1007/s11325-019-01981-6

QUESTIONS

1. A 50-year-old male patient tells the WOC nurse, "I have to get up twice a night and never feel like I'm emptying my bladder completely." He also reports urgency with occasional leakage. What category of LUTS would the nurse suspect?
A. Storage symptoms
B. Voiding symptoms
C. Postvoiding symptoms
D. Mixed storage and voiding symptoms

2. What is the main function of the prostate gland?
A. Controls the stream of urine
B. Prevents infection of the urinary tract
C. Prevents urine from mixing with semen
D. Produces seminal fluid

3. In addition to the aging process and bladder dysfunctions, which of the following represents the most common cause of LUTS in men?
A. Diseases of the prostate and their treatment
B. Urinary tract infections
C. Sexually transmitted infections
D. Neurological conditions and their treatment

4. Which of the following represents the method used to assess a male patient for observable signs of urinary incontinence?
A. Analysis of a frequency–volume chart/bladder diary.
B. Inspection of the perineum for slight descent with a cough or bear down and for inward/cephalad lift with a voluntary active contraction.
C. Observe for signs of involuntary urine loss with physical exertion or strong urge when the bladder is full.
D. Percussion and/or palpation of the bladder for fullness/retention.

5. Which standardized assessment tool best captures the symptoms of urgency and urge incontinence in male patients with LUTS?
A. International Prostate Symptom Score (IPSS)
B. International Consultation on Incontinence Questionnaire—Male Lower Urinary Tract Symptoms questionnaire (ICIQ-MLUTS)
C. Pad test
D. Uroflowmetry

6. Which statement represents the best advice from a WOC nurse for guiding male patients regarding selection and use of absorbent products for LUTS?
   A. Avoid the use of absorbent products as they are associated with incontinence-associated dermatitis.
   B. Wear the smallest amount of product and advance gradually to "product-free" living, starting with low stakes circumstances as bladder control begins to return.
   C. Wear the largest amount of product for as long as LUTS persist in the interest of protecting your skin and emotional well-being.
   D. All absorbent products, including feminine hygiene products, are generally equivalent in terms of cost, absorbency, comfort, availability, and environmental impact.

7. Which of the following conservative approaches should be initiated first by the WOC nurse to treat a gentleman who complains of urinary leakage in the presence of a cough, sneeze, or laugh?
   A. Pelvic floor muscle training (PFMT)
   B. Neuromodulation
   C. Bladder training
   D. Crede maneuver

8. Which of the following conservative approaches should be initiated by the WOC nurse to treat a gentleman who complains of postmicturition dribbling?
   A. Crede maneuver
   B. Bladder training
   C. Pelvic floor muscle training (PFMT)
   D. Urethral and/or bulbar milking

9. Pharmacologic treatment of LUTS in men should be considered by the WOC nurse under which of the following circumstances?
   A. When behavioral therapy(s) begins
   B. When behavioral therapy(s) fails to produce the desired effect
   C. When the patient is cognitively impaired
   D. When the patient has a busy life and demanding schedule

10. Which of the following statements reflects the goal of using antimuscarinic agents to treat men with LUTS?
    A. Reduction of voiding and postvoiding symptoms by relaxing an overactive detrusor muscle
    B. Reduction of voiding and postvoiding symptoms by enhancing bladder emptying
    C. Reduction of storage symptoms by relaxing an overactive detrusor muscle
    D. Reduction of storage symptoms by enhancing bladder emptying

ANSWERS AND RATIONALES

1. **D. Rationale:** Both storage and voiding symptoms are reported. Nocturia, urgency and leakage are storage symptoms; incomplete bladder emptying is a voiding symptom.

2. **D. Rationale:** The prostate gland is important in the production of semen and plays a crucial role in orgasm and ejaculation. The prostate gland does not control the stream of urine, prevent urinary tract infection, or prevent urine from mixing with semen.

3. **A. Rationale:** Compared to diseases of the prostate and their treatment, urinary tract infections, sexually transmitted infections, and neurological conditions and their treatment play a lesser role in the pathophysiology of LUTS in the majority of men.

4. **C. Rationale:** Signs of urinary incontinence are assessed by observing for leakage from a comfortably full bladder in the presence of an activity(s) that increases intraabdominal pressure. Analysis of a frequency–volume chart/bladder diary does not permit direct observation of UI. Inspection of the perineum for slight descent with a cough or bear down, and for inward/cephalad lift with a voluntary contraction is a method of assessing pelvic floor muscle function and may not produce UI. Percussion and/or palpation of the bladder for fullness/retention will not necessarily produce UI.

5. **B. Rationale:** The ICIQ-MLUTS has high levels of validity and reliability and captures the symptoms of urgency and urge incontinence in men. The IPSS is a similar instrument with high levels of

validity and reliability, however it neglects the symptoms of urgency and urge incontinence. The pad test and uroflowmetry are not standardized assessment instruments.

6. B. Rationale: Absorbent products are a necessary management strategy for LUTS until bladder control returns. Wearing the smallest amount of product and advancing gradually to "product fee" living is the established rule of thumb for guiding patients in their use of absorbent products. Wearing a large amount of product increases friction and heat, which can precipitate incontinence-associated dermatitis. A variety of absorbent products designed to fit the male pelvic floor are now on the market, but all are not alike.

7. A. Rationale: PFMT is the mainstay of behavioral therapies for stress UI. Neuromodulation and bladder training are appropriate for urgency and urge UI. Historically, Crede maneuver was used to promote bladder emptying in patients with spinal cord injury until it was found to prompt contraction of the external urethral sphincter to maintain closure of the bladder neck.

8. D. Rationale: Post micturition dribbling is a postvoiding symptom that can be alleviated by performing urethral and/or bulbar milking after each void. Historically, Crede maneuver was used to treat voiding symptoms, however its efficacy is no longer supported. Bladder training and PFMT are both conservative approaches for storage symptoms.

9. B. Rationale: Pharmacologic treatment of LUTS is considered a second-line therapy for LUTS. Several pharmacologic agents for LUTS require caution in the presence of cognitive impairment. A busy life and demanding schedule should not preclude the use of behavioral therapies for LUTS. In fact, pharmacologic agents are typically introduced in combination with behavioral therapy(s) when behavioral therapy(s) alone fails to produce the desired effect.

10. C. Rationale: Antimuscarinic agents are used to treat storage symptoms rather than voiding and postvoiding symptoms. Antimuscarinic agents work by relaxing an overactive detrusor muscle. Storage symptoms would be aggravated by an agent that enhanced bladder emptying.

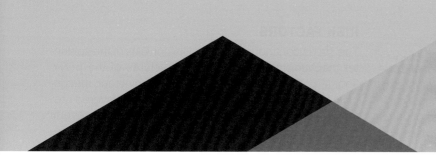

Sandra Engberg

OBJECTIVES

1. Describe data to be gathered during the patient interview and the significance of these data to accurate diagnosis.

2. Describe key elements of a focused physical exam for the patient with urinary incontinence, to include interpretation of findings.

3. Synthesize assessment data to determine type of incontinence/voiding dysfunction and goals for management.

4. Relate the basic pathology of stress urinary incontinence to risk factors, clinical presentation/ assessment findings, and treatment options.

5. Differentiate between stress incontinence caused by urethral hypermobility and stress incontinence caused by intrinsic sphincter deficiency in terms of pathology, presentation, and management.

6. Describe indications and guidelines for each of the following: pelvic muscle rehabilitation programs, pessaries, electrical stimulation, and surgical procedures.

TOPIC OUTLINE

STRESS URINARY INCONTINENCE

Stress urinary incontinence (SUI) is the involuntary loss of urine during sudden increases in intra-abdominal pressure. Incontinence occurs when intravesical (bladder) pressure exceeds urethral closure pressure.

DEFINITIONS

In their most recent update of the terminology describing female pelvic floor dysfunction, the International Urogynecological Association (IUGA) and the International Continence Society (ICS) defined SUI as a symptom, sign, and urodynamic diagnosis (Haylen et al., 2010). SUI, the symptom, is defined as a "complaint of involuntary loss of urine on effort or physical exertion (e.g., sporting activities), or on sneezing or coughing" (p. 5). SUI is also defined as a sign (objective finding): the "observation of involuntary leakage from the urethra synchronous with effort or physical exertion or on sneezing or coughing" (p. 7). Urodynamic SUI is defined as "the involuntary leakage of urine during filling cystometry, associated with increased intra-abdominal pressure, in the absence of a detrusor contraction" (p. 14). Stress incontinence is not related to psychological stress and to avoid confusion, some think that the term, "activity-related incontinence" might be better than "stress incontinence." However, because stress incontinence is still the widely used terminology for this type of incontinence and still advocated by the ICS, it is the terminology that will be used throughout this chapter.

> **KEY POINT**
>
> Stress incontinence is caused by sphincter dysfunction and involves leakage during activities that cause an increase in intra-abdominal pressure.

PREVALENCE AND INCIDENCE

SUI is primarily a women's health issue. Based on data from 17,850 adults (age 20+ years) participating in the National Health and Nutrition Examination Survey (2001 to 2008), the age-adjusted prevalence of SUI was 51% in women (95% CI 49.4% to 52.4%) as compared to 13.9% in men (95% CI 12.9% to 15.0%). The data also indicated that SUI was the most common subtype of UI among women (24.8% [95% CI 23.4% to 26.3%]) (Markland et al., 2011) (see Box 11-1 for an explanation of 95% CI). While SUI is the most common type of UI in women, the relative prevalence of SUI does vary across the lifespan. A number of studies report the following: SUI is typically first reported during pregnancy or the postpartum period; the prevalence of SUI increases with age, peaking about the fourth or fifth decade; and the prevalence of SUI then decreases, while the prevalence of urge UI (UUI) and mixed SUI and UUI increase (Buckley & Lapitan, 2010; Diokno, 2003; Minassian et al., 2008; Nygaard & Heit, 2004).

> **KEY POINT**
>
> SUI is typically first reported during pregnancy or the postpartum period; the prevalence of SUI increases with age, peaking about the fourth or fifth decade and then decreases, while the prevalence of urge UI (UUI) and mixed SUI and UUI increase.

RISK FACTORS

The stress continence mechanism consists of the sphincter mechanism and supporting structures of the pelvic floor (**Fig. 11-1**) (Delancey, 2010). The sphincteric mechanism includes the bladder neck and the multilayered urethra, which includes the vascular submucosa and several layers of muscle. As it traverses the bladder wall, the urethral lumen is surrounded by the smooth muscle of the trigonal ring. Below this point, the lumen is surrounded by an outer layer of striated muscle (the rhabdosphincter), a middle layer of smooth muscle, and an inner layer of longitudinal (smooth) muscle (Delancey, 2010).

The urethral support mechanism consists of the anterior vaginal wall, the surrounding muscles (levator ani), and the fascia; specifically, the connections between the vaginal walls and the muscles and fascia influence the position of the urethra, and inadequate urethral support has been thought to play a significant role in SUI. However, in a recent study, Delancey (2010) compared urethral closure pressure, urethral support, levator ani muscle function, and intravesical pressure in 103 women with daily documented SUI and 108 women without SUI; the women were matched in terms of race, age, parity, and hysterectomy status. In this study, urethral closure pressure was a more important factor in SUI than urethral support; maximal urethral closure pressure (MUCP)

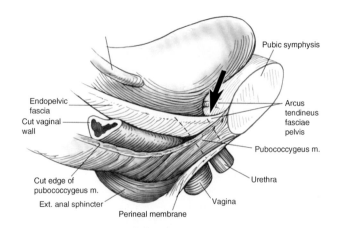

FIGURE 11-1. Stress Continence Mechanism. The urethra is compressed against the underlying supportive tissues by the downward force (*arrow*) generated by a cough or sneeze. (Delancey, J. (1994). Structural support of the urethra as it relates to stress urinary incontinence: the hammock hypothesis. *American Journal of Obstetrics and Gynecology, 170*, 1718, with permission.)

alone correctly classified 50% of the women with SUI. It should be noted that the level of urethrovaginal support and the cough strength (indicator of force exerted against continence mechanism) also contributed to accurate identification of women with SUI, suggesting that the level of support may be one factor affecting MUCP. Age may be another contributing factor; while there is individual variability in MUCP across all age groups, studies have shown a gradual decline with age. Delancey and colleagues have also found an age-related decrease in both the striated and smooth muscle of the urethra, which may explain the changes seen in MUCP. Although our understanding of the pathophysiology of SUI is increasing, these findings also indicate that our current understanding remains incomplete.

In addition to age, a number of other risk factors for SUI have been identified; these include pregnancy, menopause, hysterectomy, obesity, caffeine, smoking, and genetics. Pregnancy is associated with a number of changes in the continence support mechanisms including descent of the bladder neck, increased mobility of the bladder neck, decreased urethral resistance, and reduced pelvic floor contractility (Van Geelen et al., 2018). These changes may explain why many women experience SUI during pregnancy. Prevalence of SUI increases during pregnancy with rates varying from 18.6% (n = 10,098 in China) (Zhu et al., 2012) to 60% (n = 121 in the United States) (Thomason et al., 2007), with most studies reporting prevalence rates between 30% and 50% (Sangsawang & Sangsawang, 2013). Damage to the pelvic floor (stretching of connective tissues beyond their physiologic limits, injury to the levator ani muscles, and/or neurologic damage) occurs in most vaginal deliveries. In many women, subsequent reinnervation, wound healing, and muscle hypertrophy compensate for the delivery-related denervation and muscle injury (Van Geelen et al., 2018). In a meta-analysis examining the impact of method of delivery on the risk of having postpartum SUI, women who had a C-section were a little less than half as likely to have postpartum SUI compared to women delivered vaginally (OR = 0.48, 95% CI 0.39, 0.58) (see Box 11-1 for an explanation of OR and 95% CI). There was, however, no significant difference in the likelihood of developing severe SUI. Findings were similar in the studies that followed women for more than 1 year after delivery (Press et al., 2007). Later studies also support findings that women who have vaginal deliveries are at higher risk for developing SUI than those who undergo C-section (Altman et al., 2007a; Chang et al., 2014; Gyhagen et al., 2013; Leijonhufvud et al., 2011; Yang & Sun, 2019).

The EPINCONT study, a large population-based study conducted in Norway, examined the association between other delivery-related characteristics and SUI in a sample of 11,397 women between the ages of 20 and 64 years who had vaginal deliveries. The likelihood

of having SUI were 1.6 times greater in women who had a breech delivery (OR = 1.6, 95% CI 1.1, 2.2) and 1.4 time greater in those who had an epidural (OR = 1.4, 95% CI 1.1, 1.8) and 30% lower in those who had a vacuum delivery (OR = 0.7, 95% CI 0.4, 1.0) compared to women without these characteristics. There was no significant association between SUI and gestational age, head circumference, delivery-related injuries, prolonged labor or other functional delivery disorders, or forceps delivery (Rortveit et al., 2003). In a study that following women for 10 years following their first vaginal delivery, the prevalence of SUI increased over the 10-year follow-up period. None of the obstetric risk factors examined (age at index delivery, parity, maternal weight or fetal weight at index delivery, perineal lacerations during delivery, or instrumental delivery) were significant risk factors for SUI at 10-year follow-up. However, women who had SUI at 9 months postdelivery had a 12 times greater risk of having SUI at 10 years postdelivery compared to women who were continent at 9 months (RR = 12.3, 95% CI 3.9 to 33.1). Similarly, women who had SUI 5 years after their delivery had a 14 times greater risk of having SUI at 10 years compared to those who were continent at 5 years (RR = 14.1, 95% CI 2.5, 18.8) (Altman et al., 2006) (see Box 11-1 for an explanation of RR). In summary, the current evidence indicates that relative to C-section, vaginal delivery increases the risk for developing SUI. It is less clear, however, what obstetric and personal characteristics increase the risk for SUI following vaginal delivery.

KEY POINT

Damage to the pelvic floor (stretching of connective tissues beyond their physiologic limits, injury to the levator ani muscles, and/or neurologic damage) occurs in most vaginal deliveries. In many women, subsequent reinnervation, wound healing, and muscle hypertrophy compensates for the delivery-related denervation and muscle injury.

Other risk factors examined in relation to SUI include obesity, hysterectomy, caffeine intake, smoking, and genetics. Obesity has been identified as a risk factor for UI in numerous studies, and in most studies, the association was stronger for SUI than for urge urinary incontinence (Lamerton et al., 2018). In most studies, there was also a clear dose–response effect between weight and SUI. In a systematic review and meta-analysis of eight studies examining the effect of weight gain of the risk for SUI, each 5 kg/m^2 increase in BMI increased the risk for SUI 1.3 times (RR = 1.33, 95% CI 1.14 to 1.49) (Aune et al., 2019). The impact of obesity on SUI risk is further supported by studies showing a reduced prevalence of SUI among women who lost weight following surgical or behavioral interventions (Subak et al., 2009). The data regarding the effects of hysterectomy on risk of SUI are mixed; one issue that may contribute to this is the varying

BOX 11-1   STATISTICS MADE EASY: *p*-VALUE, OR, RR, CI

- *p-values* tell us whether the results of a study are statistically significant, that is, have a low likelihood of being due to chance. Typically *p*-values <0.05 are considered statistically significant because the probability of the findings being due to chance is <5%. Ideally, authors report the exact *p*-value, for example, $p = 0.001$. The smaller the p-value the less likely the probability that the study finding are due to chance. In many studies, however, you will see the p-value reported as <0.05 (statistically significant) or >0.05 (not statistically significant).

- *OR* stands for *odds ratio* and compares the likelihood (odds) of an outcome in individuals with a characteristic (risk factor) of interest (e.g., a breech delivery) to the likelihood in the group without the risk factor (those who did not have a breech delivery). One of the studies cited examining characteristics (risk factors) associated with SUI and reported that the OR for breech delivery 1.6. The simplest way to interpret this is that women in this study who had a breech delivery were 1.6 times more likely to have SUI than those who did not have a breech delivery. In a study like this that is comparing the likelihood of an outcome in individuals with and without a risk factor (delivery characteristics in this study), when the OR is >1 the outcome (SUI) is more likely in those with the risk factor and if it is <1 the outcome is less likely (the characteristic is often thought of as protective) than for women without the risk factor. An OR of 1 means that the outcome is equally likely in those with and without the characteristic being examined.

- *RR* stands for *relative risk* and compares the risk of an outcome in those with a risk factor (characteristic) and those without it. RR is interpreted the same way as the odds ratio; RR of 1 means there is no difference in the risk of the outcome, RR > 1 means the risk of the outcome is higher in individuals with the risk factor, and a RR < 1 means the risk is lower compared to individuals without the risk factor. RR is often reported

instead of OR in prospective studies where data collection starts with the presence of absence of the risk factors and individuals are followed over time to see who does and does not develop the outcome. In one of the cited studies, data collection started at the time of delivery and women were followed over time to determine who did and did not develop SUI. RR compared the risk of developing the outcome at the follow-up time point (in this study having SUI 10 years after delivery) in women with and without each of the risk factors measured at baseline (delivery characteristics) or 9 months or 5 years postdelivery (having SUI was the risk factor at these time points). The authors reported that the RR of being incontinent 10 years postdelivery was 12.3 in women who had SUI 9 months after delivery. This means that women in this study who had SUI 9 months postdelivery were 12.3 times more likely to have SUI 10 years later than women who were continent 9 months postdelivery.

- *CI* stands for confidence interval and studies typically report the 95% CI associated with an OR or RR. The 95% CI is typically reported with either a comma between the lower and upper limit or a dash between them (e.g., 95% CI 1.6, 10.2 or 95% CI 1.6–10.2). If the authors did not also report the *p*-value associated with the OR or RR, we can use the 95% CI to determine if it was significantly different (i.e., not likely to be due to chance) than 1 (remember 1 = no difference in likelihood or risk). If 1 is not between the lower and upper limit of the CI, the OR or RR is significantly different than 1 (e.g., 95% CI 0.2, 0.8 or 95% CI 1.3, 4.6). If 1 falls between the lower and upper value, the OR or RR is not significantly different than 1 (e.g., 95% CI 0.92, 3.2). The 95% CI are also sometimes reported with estimates such as prevalence rates where it provide an estimate of the upper and lower bound of the rate in the target population (e.g., all women in the United States with SUI).

definitions used to diagnose SUI. In two studies examining the risk of SUI following hysterectomy, the risk was significantly higher in women who had undergone hysterectomy than those who had not (Altman et al., 2007b; Forsgren et al., 2012). However, in other studies, no significant relationship was demonstrated between having a hysterectomy and self-reported SUI (De Tayrac et al., 2007; Gustafsson et al., 2006; Miller et al., 2008; van der Vaart et al., 2002). In a systematic review examining the relationship between hysterectomy and UI, Brown et al. (2000) reported that the odds of UI were increased in women age 60 and older (OR = 1.6, 95% CI 1.4, 1.8) but not for women <60 years of age. The association was not examined by subtype of UI.

KEY POINT

The impact of obesity on SUI risk is further supported by studies showing a reduced prevalence of SUI among women who lost weight following surgical or behavioral interventions.

Another proposed risk factor for UI is caffeine intake; however, the evidence supporting this in relation to SUI is limited, and findings are inconsistent. Two of the studies that examined the relationship between caffeine intake and SUI did not find a significant relationship (Gleason et al., 2013; Jura et al., 2011). In contrast, in the EPINCONT study, coffee had a weak but positive effect on SUI, with an odds ratio of 1.2 (95% CI 1.1, 1.5) for three or more cups per day relative to no coffee intake (Hannestad et al., 2003). Swithinbank et al. (2005) examined the impact of replacing caffeinated beverages with decaffeinated fluids on SUI and found no improvement in SUI symptoms. Smoking is another suggested risk factor for SUI; however, there is limited research examining the association between smoking and SUI, and in the three studies identified there was no significant association between smoking and SUI (Hannestad et al., 2003; Madhu et al., 2015; Tahtinen et al., 2011).

Finally, genetics has been suggested as a risk factor, and epidemiological studies do suggest that family history may be a risk factor for SUI. In a large twin study designed to examine genetic and environmental influences on SUI, Altman et al. (2008) found that genetic factors accounted for 43% of the variability in SUI after adjusting for age and parity. They also found, however, that nonshared environmental factors accounted for 40% of the variability. Based on these findings, they cautioned that the influence of genetics on SUI should not be overestimated. In a systematic review of meta-analysis of two studies, Cartwright et al. (2015) reported a significant association between variation in COL1A1 with SUI. Increased COL1AI expression is thought to be associated with reduced type 1 collagen content, a major structural component of the endopelvic fascia. McKenzie et al. (2010) also reviewed genetic influences on SUI and concluded that, while there is evidence to support the role of genetics, particularly genes encoding extracellular matrix (ECM) proteins, additional research is needed to understand genetic factors in SUI.

KEY POINT

Risk factors with the most research support in relation to SUI are pregnancy, vaginal delivery, and obesity. Current evidence, although limited, also suggests that genetics play a role in the risk for SUI.

PATHOLOGY AND CLINICAL PRESENTATION

Women with SUI typically present with involuntary urine loss that occurs during activities associated with sudden increases in intra-abdominal pressure such as coughing, sneezing, laughing, lifting, or exercise and that is not associated with a sense of urgency to void (**Fig. 11-2**). Frail older women with SUI who have difficulty getting up (e.g., from a sitting position) may also report involuntary urine loss when getting up from a chair. Women with SUI typically report leaking small amounts of urine during

the activities that precipitate their stress accidents. However, some women with SUI have "low-pressure urethras," which means the urethral sphincter mechanism has limited ability to withstand even minor increases in intra-abdominal pressure (Wilson et al., 2003); as a result, these women report severe SUI and leakage with minimal activity or "always being wet."

KEY POINT

Women with SUI typically present with involuntary urine loss that occurs during activities associated with sudden increases in intra-abdominal pressure such as coughing, sneezing, laughing, lifting, or exercise and that is not associated with a sense of urgency to void.

Historically, severe SUI has variously been labeled "grade 3 SUI" or "intrinsic sphincter deficiency (ISD)" (McGuire, 1981), a classification system based in part on the belief that the pathology of severe SUI was significantly different than the pathology of mild to moderate SUI. However, as knowledge regarding the pathophysiology of SUI evolves, there is increased recognition that the mechanisms underlying ISD and typical SUI (sometimes referred to as bladder neck hypermobility SUI) are not as distinctly different as once believed (Koelb et al., 2013). In addition, while a variety of diagnostic criteria have been proposed for ISD, no precise diagnostic criteria have been identified and agreed upon (Hosker, 2009). These limitations have led some to conclude that the term ISD has limited utility (Smith et al., 2012).

KEY POINT

As knowledge regarding the pathology of SUI evolves, it is increasingly clear that the mechanisms underlying SUI due to urethral hypermobility and SUI due to intrinsic sphincter deficiency are not as distinctly different as previously thought.

ASSESSMENT GUIDELINES

The Sixth International Consultation on Incontinence (ICI) Committee 5 (Diaz et al., 2017) recommended that the following be the components of the initial assessment of all patients presenting with UI, including those with suspected SUI.

History

A complete patient history should be obtained to include the following:

- Presence, duration, and bother of all urinary, bowel, and pelvic organ prolapse (POP) symptoms. Women should be asked about the situations that are typically associated with involuntary urine loss (e.g., coughing, sneezing, laughing, lifting, and exercise for SUI; urgency, on the way to the toilet, running water, and

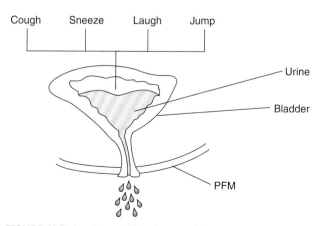

FIGURE 11-2. Involuntary Urine Loss with Sudden Increases in Intra-Abdominal Pressure, for example, Cough. (Brody, L. T., & Hall, C. M. (2010). *Therapeutic exercise*. Philadelphia, PA: Lippincott Williams & Wilkins.)

"key in the door" for UUI; without warning or physical activity; or continuously), the frequency and volume of incontinent episodes, nocturia (including the number of episodes in a typical night), enuresis, urgency, voiding frequency, difficulty emptying their bladder, bladder (lower abdominal) pain, hematuria, dysuria, constipation, fecal incontinence, pelvic discomfort, and dyspareunia. Structured questionnaires such as the International Consultation on Incontinence Modular questionnaires (Bristol Urological Institute, 2014) (https://iciq.net/iciq-modules) are useful tools in screening for pelvic floor problems including UI, prolapse, and fecal incontinence.

- The impact of symptoms on sexual function and quality of life (a variety of validated questionnaires are available for this purpose).
- Symptoms suggestive of neurologic disorders and their severity.
- Previous treatments and their effectiveness.
- Comorbid diseases that can affect lower urinary tract/pelvic floor function, for example, chronic obstructive pulmonary disease, asthma, diabetes mellitus, and neurologic diseases.
- Current medications.
- Obstetric and menstrual history.
- Physical impairments, for example, gait abnormalities or loss of dexterity.
- Environmental issues: physical, social, and cultural.
- Lifestyle: fluid intake (type and amount), alcohol intake, smoking, and exercise.
- Desire for treatment and acceptable treatment options.
- Goals and expectations for treatment.
- Support systems, including caregiver if relevant.
- Cognitive function.
- Depressive symptoms.

Physical Examination
A complete physical examination for SUI should include

- Height and weight (to calculate BMI)
- Physical dexterity and mobility
- Abdominal examination (**Fig. 11-3**)

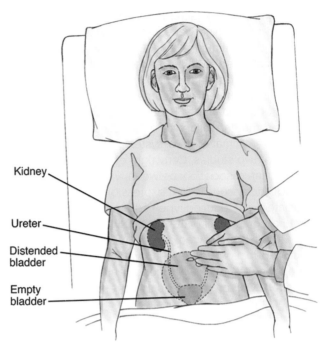

FIGURE 11-3. Abdominal Examination. (Weber, J. R., & Kelley, J. H. (2013). *Health assessment in nursing*. Philadelphia, PA: Lippincott Williams & Wilkins.)

- Pelvic examination, including examination of the perineum and external genitalia for tissue quality and sensation, and vaginal examination for atrophic changes and prolapse. **Figure 11-4** shows insertion of a vaginal speculum. Step one is the technique used for the insertion of a speculum into the vagina to view the cervical opening. The blades are held obliquely on entering the vagina. Half of the speculum can be used to retract the anterior and posterior wall to look for prolapse. (POP is discussed in Chapter 12.) Bimanual pelvic and anorectal examinations should be conducted to assess for pelvic masses or other abnormalities. During inspection of the vaginal mucosa, the examiner should look for atrophic vaginal changes. When these are present, the vaginal mucosa will generally have a thin, pale shiny appearance with a decrease or loss of vaginal rugae (folds).

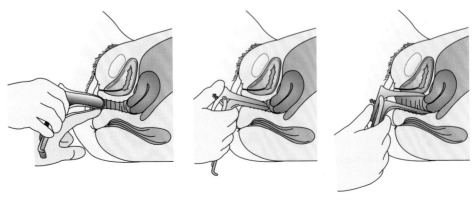

FIGURE 11-4. Pelvic Exam with Speculum. (LifeART image copyright © 2014. Lippincott Williams & Wilkins.)

BOX 11-2	OXFORD SCALE FOR DESCRIBING PELVIC FLOOR MUSCLE STRENGTH

Score	Findings When Patient Is Instructed to Squeeze Tightly around the Examiner's Finger
0	No discernible contraction
1	Barely palpable contraction; flicker
2	Weak but palpable contraction; perceived as slight pressure against the examiner's finger
3	Moderate strength; felt as distinct pressure against the examining finger
4	Good muscle strength with elevation of pelvic floor against light examiner resistance
5	Strong muscle strength; elevation of the examiner's finger against strong resistance

Alternately, there may be diffuse or patchy erythema and/or petechiae. Pelvic floor muscle (PFM) strength should be assessed as part of the pelvic examination. The modified Oxford scale (Box 11-2) is a clinically useful method for quantifying PFM strength during vaginal palpation. One or two fingers are inserted into the vagina and the woman is told to squeeze tightly around the examiner's finger(s). The modified Oxford scale has been shown to have moderate interrater reliability (Frawley et al., 2006) and good agreement with perineometic measure of PFM contraction strength (**Fig. 11-5**) (Isherwood & Rane, 2000).

• Conduct a cough stress test with the bladder comfortably full to look for involuntary urine loss. Have the patient cough deeply or bear down while observing the urethral meatus for involuntary urine loss (Wooldridge, 2017). A positive cough stress test has high sensitivity and specificity for detecting SUI on urodynamic testing (Kobashi et al., 2017).

• Focused neurologic examination (perineal sensation, anal wink, bulbocavernosus reflex, anal sphincter tone, lower extremity neuromuscular function, general mental status, and mobility) (Wooldridge, 2017).

• Postvoid residual (PVR) should always be performed in the geriatric population, if reduced bladder emptying or retention is suspected (Diaz et al., 2017). Accuracy of PVR is enhanced if measurement is taken following voiding completion (see **Fig. 11-6**).

• Request a 3-day bladder diary prior to continence evaluation if possible, to collect objective urinary storage and voiding information and representative of the patient's observations regarding their bladder dysfunction (see **Fig. 11-7**) (Diaz et al., 2017). The bladder diary optimally should incorporate the following: (1) voiding time and volume if possible; (2) urinary leakage episodes and approximate volume; (3) associated activities with leakage; (4) presence of urge sensation; (5) fluid amount and type; and (4) some diaries include type and number of body worn absorbent products (BWAPs) and level of saturation.

• Pad test (optional) may also be obtained prior to clinical evaluation to objectively quantify the volume of urinary leakage (Khullar et al., 2017). Ask the patient to collect wet BWAPs for a full 24-hour period and place in a sealed plastic bag. Patient is instructed to bring one unused BWAP and the plastic bag of wet

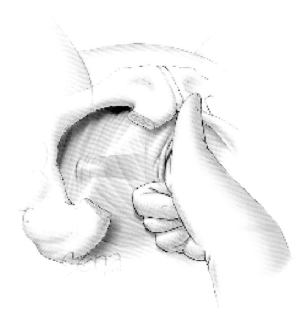

FIGURE 11-5. Assessment of Pelvic Muscle Tone and Contraction During Pelvic Exam. (Used with permission from Marie Sena, Electric Eye & Restorative Tattooing, Medical Illustrator).

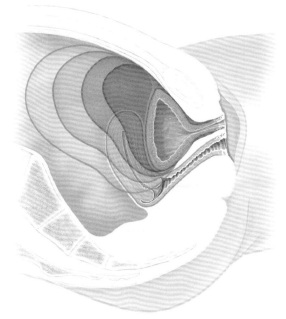

FIGURE 11-6. Contours of the Bladder with Progressive Filling. (Stephenson, S. R. (2012). *Diagnostic medical sonography.* Philadelphia, PA: Lippincott Williams & Wilkins.)

Column # Directions

      1 Urination in toilet: check, measure, or count # of seconds.

      2 Make a check if a urine leak occurs, note small or large.

      3 Note the reason for the accident (jump, sneeze, lift, water, urge).

      4 Note type and amount of fluid intake.

Fill in the day and date at the top of each column.

Name_____   Acct.#_____

DAY												
	toilet	leak	reason	fluid	toilet	leak	reason	fluid	toilet	leak	reason	fluid
6 am												
7 am												
8 am												
9 am												
10 am												
11 am												
12 am												
1 pm												
2 pm												
3 pm												
4 pm												
5 pm												
6 pm												
7 pm												
8 pm												
9 pm												
10 pm												
11 pm												
12 pm												
1 am												
2 am												
3 am												
4 am												
5 am												
TOTAL												
# of pads												

Stop Test Results_____   Patient's Signature_____

Type of pad used _____

FIGURE 11-7. Voiding Diary. (Brody, L. T., & Hall, C. M. (2010). *Therapeutic exercise*. Philadelphia, PA: Lippincott Williams & Wilkins.)

BWAPs to the appointment. The continence specialist will count and weigh wet BWAPs to determine total weight in grams of urine loss and dry weight of the unused BWAP. Dry BWAP weight is multiplied by the number of wet pads then subtracted from the total urine weight to obtain the total weight of all wet pads (Wooldridge, 2017). It is recommended to keep a bladder diary during pad testing as described previously. The bladder diary provides additional objective data to ascertain the pattern and severity of urine leakage along with pad weight testing.

- Chapter 4 discusses the comprehensive patient assessment in greater detail.

KEY POINT

The physical examination for a woman with stress incontinence should include assessment for signs and symptoms of decreased estrogen levels in vaginal tissues, assessment of pelvic muscle contractility, endurance, and the ability to isolate PFM as well as relax upon request and a cough stress test to determine if there is involuntary urine loss.

Urinalysis

Laboratory evaluation should consist of dipstick test or complete urinalysis. Although the ICI committee recommended routine urinalysis or dipstick as part of the initial evaluation of patients with UI, they reported that the level of evidence supporting this recommendation was based on expert opinion rather than research findings.

Bladder Voiding Diary

Figure 11-7 shows an example of a patient-recorded voiding diary, which is used to assess lower urinary tract symptoms (severity of UI, situations associated with UI, timing and frequency of voiding) and fluid intake. Although bladder diaries are recommended, concerns about their use include patient burden, optimal duration, and optimal content and format. Bright et al. (2011) reviewed English language literature on bladder diaries and concluded that the duration needed to reliably provide information on incontinence and voiding habits is unknown, though most authors recommend that data be collected for at least 3 days. Bright and colleagues also reported that there is no research addressing optimal diary content or format. Given the patient burden associated with keeping a bladder diary, Bradley et al. (2011) examined the agreement between self-report UI questions and a 7-day bladder diary. Using the bladder diary diagnosis of SUI as the gold standard, the self-report questionnaires had a sensitivity of 0.79 to 0.82 and a specificity of 0.76 to 0.77; this means that self-report correctly identified 79% to 82% of the women with SUI based on their bladder diary data and correctly identified 76% to 77% of those without SUI. Agreement between self-report and bladder diary in regard to voiding frequency

and frequency of incontinent episodes was good to moderate, respectively ($r = 0.61$ to 0.65; $r = 0.41$ to 0.56). These findings suggest that the use of self-report is an adequate method for diagnosis of SUI and measurement of UI and voiding frequency when the use of bladder diaries is not feasible.

Shamliyan et al. (2012) conducted an Agency for Healthcare Research and Quality (AHRQ) comparative effectiveness review focusing on the diagnosis and non-surgical management of urinary incontinence in women. Based on their extensive review of diagnostic studies, the authors concluded that there was a high level of evidence that in clinic settings, women can be accurately diagnosed with UI based on a clinical history and evaluation, a bladder diary to determine the predominate type of incontinence, and a cough stress test. In this review, a high level of evidence was defined as, "High confidence that the evidence reflects the true effect. Further research is very unlikely to change our confidence in the estimated effect" (p. 10).

KEY POINT

A 3-day bladder diary is a valuable tool to collect objective urinary storage and voiding information and representative of the patient's observations regarding their bladder dysfunction.

For most women with SUI, basic evaluations are sufficient to initiate noninvasive treatment. Additional testing is recommended for women with more complex symptoms such as recurrent or persistent UI despite initial treatment, bladder (lower abdominal) pain, hematuria, recurrent UTI, symptoms suggesting impaired bladder emptying, history of pelvic irradiation or radical pelvic surgery, suspected fistula, or severe pelvic prolapse (Diaz et al., 2017; Kobashi et al., 2017). Depending on the nature of the woman's presentation, the following specialized assessments may be appropriate:

- Uroflowmetry: women with symptoms of voiding dysfunction, physical signs of POP, evidence of bladder distention on abdominal examination, or elevated PVR.
- Lower urinary tract/pelvic imaging (e.g., ultrasound): hematuria, severe POP, or pain.
- Lower urinary tract cystoscopy: hematuria, pain, or suspected fistula.
- Urodynamic testing: when the diagnosis is unclear, there are concerns about lower urinary tract dysfunction, unresponsive to treatment modalities, or signs of neurological abnormalities (Rosier et al., 2017) (see Chapter 5, Box 5-1).

The role of urodynamic testing and postvoid residual in the assessment and management of uncomplicated SUI is controversial (Dillon & Zimmern, 2012; Nager,

2012). While routine assessment of PVR is standard in many practices, it is questionable if it is always necessary in straightforward cases of UI. Staskin et al. (2009) state that "Female patients who present with storage specific symptoms, with normal sensation and no complaints of decreased bladder emptying, and no anatomical, neurological, organ-specific, or comorbid risk factors for retention may be assessed for bladder emptying by history and physical examination alone, depending on the potential morbidity of the failure to diagnose and the nature of the intended therapy" (p. 338). The value of routine urodynamic testing is also questionable, even when surgical intervention is planned. In a randomized controlled trial (RCT) examining whether women with SUI who had urodynamic testing prior to stress incontinence procedures had better outcomes than those who did not, there were no differences in outcomes for the two groups of women (Nager et al., 2012). The author concluded that for most women, an office-based cough stress test can be used instead of urodynamics to confirm the diagnosis of SUI. The test should be performed with a full bladder (instruct women to come to the evaluation with a comfortably full bladder). It can initially be performed with patient supine and the urethral meatus visible, but if negative should be repeated with the woman in a standing position. The woman is asked to cough deeply. If there is no urine loss during the cough, the Valsalva maneuver can be performed. Urine loss during the cough or Valsalva maneuver is a positive stress test and an objective indicator of SUI (**Fig. 11-8**). Consistent with this, the 2017 American Urological Association and Society of Urodynamics, Female Pelvic Medicine and Urogenital Reconstruction guidelines on the surgical treatment of SUI states that urodynamics can be omitted as part of the evaluation of patients when SUI is demonstrated during the physical examination (Kobashi et al., 2017).

> **KEY POINT**
>
> Urodynamic studies are not routinely indicated for women with stress urinary incontinence; urine loss during cough or Valsalva is a positive stress test.

MANAGEMENT OPTIONS

First-line (initial) management options for SUI include lifestyle interventions and PFM training (Bettez et al., 2012; Domoulin et al., 2017; Moore et al., 2013). Additional options include pessaries, vaginal cones, electrical stimulation, urethral inserts, pharmacotherapy, urethral bulking agents, and surgery. Each option will be described along with current evidence regarding its effectiveness in treating SUI. Systematic reviews are generally considered to provide the highest level of evidence to support clinical decision-making. Consequently, where such evidence is available, it will be presented.

Lifestyle Interventions

Although clinicians often recommend alterations in lifestyle in the treatment of UI, research examining the effect of lifestyle interventions is limited. A 2015 Cochrane review examined the effects of commonly recommended lifestyle interventions on UI; randomized or quasi-experimental two-group intervention studies were eligible for inclusion (Imamura et al., 2015). In most of these studies, participants had mixed UI (stress and urge).

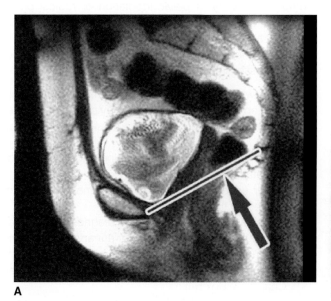

A

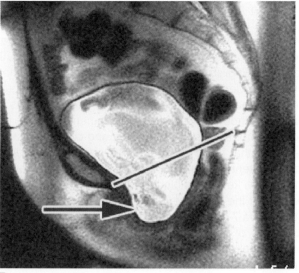

B

FIGURE 11-8. Dynamic Imaging of Pelvic Floor Relaxation Shows the Position of the Bladder Base above the Sacrococcygeal to Inferior Pubic Line (*arrow*) at Rest **(A)**, with Subsequent Descent during Valsalva Maneuver **(B)**. (Leyendecker, J. R., & Brown, J. J. (2004). *Practical guide to abdominal and pelvic MRI.* Philadelphia, PA: Lippincott Williams & Wilkins.)

Among the lifestyle interventions commonly recommended for women, the intervention with the most evidence to support it is weight loss in overweight women. The authors of this systematic review identified four studies examining the effect of weight loss on UI (in two of the studies all participants had UI while this was not the case in the other two) and concluded that weight loss may reduce UI in women who are overweight. Based on this and evidence on the negative effects of overweight and obesity on health, women who are overweight or obese should be educated about the impact of obesity on the risk for UI and the potential benefit of weight loss in improving incontinence. They should be advised to lose weight and provided with specific recommendations or referral to a nutritionist to help them achieve this goal. Women with high baseline fluid intake may benefit from reducing their fluid intake. Authors of the Cochrane review concluded that limited (three studies) and low-quality evidence suggests that reducing fluid intake may improve symptoms of UI although some participants in these studies reported headaches, constipation, and thirst. It is, however, important to advise women to drink sufficient fluid to prevent dehydration (generally about 1,500 mL/day). Given the weak evidence to support the impact of caffeine on SUI, women can be advised to reduce their caffeine intake and monitor its impact on their incontinence. If there is no impact, normal caffeine intake can be resumed. Women with high baseline caffeine intake should be advised to gradually reduce their caffeine intake to reduce the likelihood of caffeine withdrawal symptoms. While lifestyle interventions generally have the advantage of being relatively free of adverse effects, additional evidence is needed to reliably inform clinicians about their helpfulness in the treatment of SUI (Imamura et al., 2015). Chapter 6 further explores lifestyle modifications to promote a healthy bladder.

Pelvic Floor Muscle Training

There is evidence to support pelvic floor muscle training (PFMT) as first-line treatment in motivated women with uncomplicated SUI. Physiologically, there are reasons to expect PFMT to be beneficial. First, during a strong PFM contraction, the levator ani muscles are lifted upward and forward, which compresses the urethra and increases urethral closure pressure. Secondly, toned PFMs provide support for the bladder neck and proximal urethra; a well-supported urethra remains essentially in position with limited descent during activities that increase intra-abdominal pressure, which helps to prevent urine leakage. There is research evidence demonstrating that, compared to continent women, women with SUI have lower PFM tone and strength (Dumoulin et al., 2018). In a study of women with SUI, ultrasound imaging was used to compare changes in urethral morphology in women randomly assigned to a PFMT group (12 weekly physiotherapy sessions plus home PFM exercise

practice) or a no-intervention control group. In women in the PFMT group, urethral cross-sectional area increased following the 12 treatment sessions while it appeared smaller in the control group. The authors postulated that the PFMT caused hypertrophy of the urethral striated muscle, which, in turn, improved sphincter function (McLean et al., 2013). Indeed, there is strong evidence to support the effectiveness of PFMT in reducing SUI. In a systematic review prepared for the AHRQ, Shamliyan et al. (2012) concluded that there was a high level of evidence to support the benefits of PFMT for women with SUI. The findings of a 2018 Cochrane review comparing PFMT to no treatment or an inactive control treatment also support the effectiveness of PFMT in treating SUI (Dumoulin et al., 2018). Women in the PFMT groups of the included studies (4 studies and 165 women) were eight times more likely to report being continent postintervention (56% in PFMT vs. 6% in control group; RR = 8.38, 95% CI 3.68 to 19.07) than women in the control groups. They were six times more likely to report that their UI was either cured (continent) or improved (three studies with 242 women) (74% vs. 11%; RR=6.33, 95% CI 3.88, 10.33). In seven studies (n = 432 women) measuring differences in the number of UI episodes, there was a mean of 1.23 fewer UI episodes per day among women receiving PFMT compared to those in the control group.

> **KEY POINT**
>
> Lifestyle interventions (e.g., weight loss) and pelvic floor muscle training represent first-line treatment for women with stress incontinence.

One question about PFMT that remains unanswered is the specific components of an optimal training regimen. PFMT programs can be designed to

1. Increase PFM strength (the maximal force of contraction)
2. Increase PFM endurance (the time that a contraction can be sustained)
3. Improve PFM coordination (contraction prior to or during activities associated with leaking) (Dumoulin et al., 2011)

However, there are no evidence-based guidelines that clinicians can use in developing a PFMT protocol. Training can be provided on a one-to-one basis or in a group setting (see Box 11-3 for an example of a consumer-focused PFMT brochure); the frequency and duration of treatment visits can vary; and instructions on how to perform the PFM exercises can be verbal, written, taught during the pelvic examination, or taught using biofeedback. The prescribed type of PFM contractions (strength and/or duration focused), the number and frequency of exercises, the positions in which

BOX 11-3	PATIENT EDUCATION: PELVIC FLOOR MUSCLE KEGEL EXERCISES

Purpose: To strengthen and maintain the tone of the pubo-coccygeal muscle, which supports the pelvic organs, reduce or prevent stress incontinence and uterine prolapse, enhance sensation during sexual intercourse, and hasten postpartum healing.

1. Become aware of pelvic floor muscle function by "drawing in" the perivaginal muscles and anal sphincter as if to control urine or defecation, but not contracting the abdominal, buttock, or inner thigh muscles.
2. Sustain contraction of the muscles for up to 10 seconds, followed by at least 10 seconds of relaxation. Another variation is to include several sets of rapid contraction and relaxation each day.
3. Perform these exercises 30 to 80 times daily in supine, sitting, and standing positions.
4. As these exercises can be done inconspicuously, perform them with other daily activities (e.g., brushing teeth, in a car or bus, talking on the telephone, standing in line) as well as before rising from bed and after retiring at night.

Training and exercise should be individualized for each patient.

---

women are taught to perform the exercises, and the addition of resistance to training also vary. In the studies included in systematic reviews, the characteristics of the PFMT intervention varied considerably, and yet, in most of the studies, the majority of women reported continence or reduced SUI (Dumoulin et al., 2018; Shamliyan et al., 2012). One approach is to recommend 40 to 45 PFM exercises per day in three or four sets (either 15 or 10 exercises per set); to suggest that exercises be done in the supine, sitting, and standing positions; to advise patients to avoid use of their abdominal and buttocks muscles during PFM contractions; and to instruct patients to gradually increase the contraction and relaxation time with an end goal of contracting and relaxing the PFM for 10 seconds with each exercise. (The initial time is based on the baseline assessment of the woman's PFM strength, which is reassessed at each treatment visit.) Some clinicians also ask women to perform repeated unsustained maximal force contractions (quick flicks) as part of the exercise regimen. Most exercise protocols include instruction in a stress strategy also known as the "knack"; that is, the patient is taught to contract her PFM strongly before and during activities associated with involuntary urine loss (Miller et al., 2001). Chapter 6 provides additional guidance to PFMT (see Chapter 6, Table 6-5).

Approach to PFMT varies among clinicians treating women with UI. In a Cochrane systematic review, Hay-Smith et al. (2011) compared approaches to PFMT in relation to improvements in UI. They included RCTs and two-group quasi-experimental trials; the women

enrolled in the trials had SUI, UUI, or mixed UI. Each study included at least two groups that received PFMT, with variations in the training protocol between the groups that included one or more of the following: (1) direct versus indirect approach to pelvic muscle contraction; in the direct approach, women were asked to focus specifically on contracting their PFMs, and in the indirect approach, women were instructed to perform PFM contractions along with co-contractions of another related muscle group, for example, the abdominal, hip, or gluteal muscles; (2) differences in exercise parameters (strength of contractions; inclusion of the "knack"; the position during exercises; the number of exercises per set, day, or week; and the duration of contractions); (3) the addition of a resistance factor to contractions (e.g., intravaginal resistance device); (4) approach used for instruction (e.g., verbal, written, individual, or group); (5) differences in the type and amount of health care provider supervision; or (6) the addition of measures (e.g., alarms or text messages) to enhance adherence. Based on the 21 studies included in the review, the authors concluded that there "was insufficient evidence to make strong recommendations about the best approach to PFMT" (p. 2). They did state, however, that based on the limited data available, regular supervision of PFMT (e.g., weekly) was better than little or no supervision. It was not clear, however, whether individual or group supervision was better. The authors also noted a number of limitations in this area: the limited number of studies; the fact that, in a number of the studies, there were multiple differences in the two approaches being compared; the risk of reporting bias due to inability to blind the participants; and the incomplete description of the interventions being compared. Additional research is needed in order to identify the best approach to PFMT.

Biofeedback

Biofeedback is a method of teaching women that incorporates visual and/or auditory feedback to the woman as she attempts to contract and relax her pelvic floor muscles (PFM). Pelvic floor muscle contractions are often measured using surface electrodes placed at 3 and 9 o'clock adjacent to the anus (to measure EMG activity) but can also be measured by a sensor inserted into the vagina (measures EMG activity or pressure during contractions). Surface electrodes placed on the lower abdomen measure abdominal muscle activity. Depending on the biofeedback machine, the patient may be able to see a graph on a computer screen that shows if (1) she is contracting the correct muscles (i.e., the PFM and not the abdominal muscles); (2) how strongly she is contracting her PFM; and (3) how long she can contract her muscles (duration of contraction). The Hay-Smith et al. (2011) review did not examine the impact of biofeedback on outcomes of PFMT. However, a separate Cochrane review (Herderschee et al., 2011) compared

PFMT with and without biofeedback to determine if biofeedback improved outcomes in women being treated for SUI and/or UUI. Twenty-four RCTs or quasi-experimental studies were included and nine compared self-reported improvement or cure of UI among women who received PFMT plus biofeedback versus women who received PFMT alone. Those who received PFMT alone were significantly less likely to report that their UI was improved or cured (RR = 0.75, 95% CI 0.66 to 0.86). The authors concluded that, based on the findings of this review, use of biofeedback to teach PFMT may have added benefit in reducing UI; however, they noted that other differences in the treatment regimens (e.g., more contact with the health care provider) could have also accounted for the greater improvement in the biofeedback group (Herderschee et al., 2011). In contrast to the findings in the Cochrane review, the AHRQ comparative effectiveness review compared the impact of PFMT with and without vaginal EMG probe biofeedback on incontinence and found no significant difference in outcomes (Shamliyan et al., 2012). Based on the studies included in their review, Shamliyan and colleagues concluded that there was a high level of evidence to indicate no differences in outcomes in the PFMT groups with and without biofeedback. The differences in findings may have been related to differences in eligibility criteria used in the two reviews; specifically, the Cochrane review included studies that were not included in the AHRQ review. An RCT conducted in Japan and published after these two reviews compared PFMT with and without biofeedback in women with SUI and found no significant differences between the groups in posttreatment reduction in incontinent episodes as measured by bladder diary (Hirakawa et al., 2013). **Figure 11-9** provides an example of a physical therapist conducting a biofeedback session for PFMT.

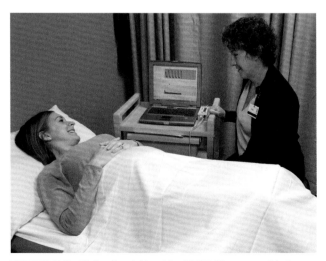

FIGURE 11-9. Biofeedback Used for PMFT. (Courtesy of JoAnn Ermer-Seltun, ARNP, CWOCN.)

Alternate Exercises for SUI

Several other exercise regimens have been proposed as treatments for SUI. In a systematic review (Bø & Herbert, 2013), several alternative exercise programs for SUI were identified. One involves deep abdominal muscle training; the theoretical basis for this approach is that deep abdominal muscle contraction will cause the PFMs to co-contract and that combined PFM and deep abdominal muscle contraction is more effective than PFMT alone in promoting continence. Bø and Herbert concluded that the evidence from RCTs is currently mixed and does not provide strong support for this training method. Another alternative is the Paula method (contraction of the muscles of the mouth and eyes), which is based on the theory that all sphincters in the body work simultaneously and that exercising the ring muscles of the mouth, eyes, or nose will cause co-contraction and strengthening of the PFMs (Liebergall-Wischnitzer et al., 2005). Two studies, however, failed to demonstrate co-contraction of the PFMs during contraction of the mouth or eyes, and two trials comparing Paula therapy to PFMT found no evidence to support the efficacy of the Paula method.

More recent research has examined other nonspecific exercises such as Pilates, yoga, and belly dancing in the treatment of UI. Pilates focuses on a range of movements that strengthen and increase flexibility of the whole body especially core musculature (Pilates & Miller, 1945). Modified Pilates avoids intense abdominal contractions, breath holding, or straining, which can put pressure on the pelvic floor. A small pilot RCT study examined the effect of combining PFMT and modified Pilates to PFMT alone in relation to quality of life in women with stress or mixed UI and found no significant group differences. No data on incontinent episodes were reported (Lausen et al., 2018). In another small pilot study (single arm, noncontrolled), women (n = 18) with self-reported SUI (45 to 65 years of age) participated in a twice weekly 12-week community-based Pilates class focusing on PFM strengthening (Hein et al., 2020). The women completed the International Consultation on Incontinence Short form (ICIQ-SF), which measures self-reported (1) urinary frequency (higher scores represent more frequent incontinence); (2) severity (higher scores represent larger urinary accidents); and (3) impact of incontinence on quality of life (QoL) (higher scores represent a great impact of QoL) at baseline, after 12 weeks and 6 months post-Pilates program. At the end of the intervention (12 weeks), there was a significant reduction in the total ICIQ-SF total score as well the urinary frequency, severity of incontinence, and impact on QoL scores. At 6 months, all scores remained significantly lower than they had been at baseline. The authors concluded a community-based Pilates program to increase PFM strength appeared to effectively reduce SUI and improved QoL in this small sample but recommended further testing in a larger RCT (Hein et al., 2020).

Yoga is a mind–body exercise that included relaxation, meditation, breathing exercises, and body postures that has been used as an intervention in the treatment of a variety of health problems (Sha et al., 2019). Yoga may help improve general body alignment as well as flexibility, strength, and control and these, in turn, are thought to assist in strengthening PFM (Wieland et al., 2019). Weiland and colleagues conducted a systematic review of RCTs comparing yoga to other interventions or to a no-treatment control group in women with UI. Two studies (total of 49 women) were eligible for inclusion in the review. One study compared yoga to a waitlist control (no active treatment) group ($n = 19$ women) and one compared it to a mindfulness stress reduction intervention ($n = 30$). Based on the very small sample sizes and issues with the study methods, Wieland and colleagues concluded that the available evidence was insufficient to judge whether yoga is a useful intervention for women with UI. Subsequent to the review, Huang et al. (2019) published the findings of a small RCT comparing a yoga intervention ($n = 28$) to a nonspecific muscle stretching and strengthening control intervention ($n = 28$) in women with stress, urge, or mixed UI. SUI frequency decreased significantly more in the yoga group (average of 61%) than in the control group (35%, $p = 0.045$) (see Box 11-1 for an explanation p-values). When only women who completed the protocol were included in the analysis, the percent reduction in SUI frequency was no longer significantly different in the two groups ($p = 0.06$).

Only one study was identified that examined the effect of belly dancing in women with UI. Women were randomized to an intervention ($n = 12$) or control group ($n = 12$). The intervention was a belly dancing program focusing on pelvic moves and the outcome measured was maximal pelvic floor muscle contraction and contraction duration. There was a significant increase in maximal PFM contraction pressure (from a mean of 18.7 to 32.5 mm Hg, $p < 0.001$) as well as a mean duration of maximal contractions (from 3.9 to 6.6 seconds, $p < 0.001$) in the intervention group. There were no significant changes in the control group (An et al., 2017). The effect on UI episodes was not reported.

Electrical Stimulation

Electrical stimulation (EStim) has been theorized to be effective in treating SUI by causing passive PFM contraction and increasing the number of muscle fibers recruited during rapid contractions (Schreiner et al., 2013), thereby improving proprioception (awareness of PFM position and movement) and function of a weak PFM. It is postulated that electrical impulses stimulate sensory (afferent) pudendal nerve fibers that cause reflex activation of sympathetic and pudendal motor (efferent) nerve fibers triggering contraction of smooth and striated muscle fibers of the urethral sphincter mechanism and pelvic floor as well as reflex inhibition of the bladder leading to detrusor relaxation (Ozdemir & Surmeli, 2017). It is of

no surprise that nerve pathways must be intact between the sacral cord and pelvic floor for EStim to be therapeutic (Birder et al., 2017; Vo & kielb, 2018). EStim is like biofeedback and often used in conjunction with PFM exercises in women who have great difficulty in identifying and isolating their PFM or in activating very weak muscles. Traditionally, EStim is delivered by a biofeedback trained continence nurse specialist or physical therapist specializing in pelvic floor rehabilitation in a clinic setting optimally three times per week using a vaginal or anal sensor (probe). If pelvic pain exists or there is an aversion to using an internal device, external electrodes may be used. Typically, EStim is delivered with high frequencies (50 to 100 Hz) to engage nerve fibers that supply the striated PFM fast and slow twitch fibers and the urethral sphincters (Ozdemir & Surmeli, 2017). In contrast, lower frequencies of 10 to 20 Hz are generally used to treat overactive bladder and urge incontinence. Women who suffer from mixed incontinence (stress and urge) tend to be treated with something between these two parameters, 20 and 50 Hz. Stimulation parameters from a physical therapist perspective include intensity sufficient to stimulate nerve fibers without causing discomfort as described previously; it must be intermittent such as 2 seconds stimulation followed by 5 seconds of rest period to avoid muscle fatigue, and using an alternating or biphasic current (Ozdemir & Surmeli, 2017). Of interest, there has been a dramatic increase in the sales of portable home units with various modes of EStim delivery including the recent development of wearable "compression like" shorts that delivers an electrical pulse that contracts the PFM 180 times in 30 minutes (Dmochowski, 2018). To add to the confusion, protocols used by clinicians greatly differ and are not well established possible due to the lack of understanding of the physiological principles of electrostimulation making it difficult to determine effectiveness of the modality (Ozdemir & Surmeli, 2017). Hence, variability between clinicians and types of EStim systems along with various techniques in the delivery of waveforms, frequencies, intensities, and the use of intravaginal or anal sensors versus surface electrodes leads to poor study designs, methods, and inability to recommend a standardized protocol for EStim in SUI (Stewart et al., 2017).

Schreiner et al. (2013) published a systematic review of studies examining the impact of transvaginal electrical stimulation (E-stim) on UI in women. Ten studies on E-stim in the treatment of SUI met eligibility criteria. Both the E-stim intervention protocols and the control conditions varied from study to study. Outcome measures also varied and included pad tests, self-report, bladder diaries, and quality of life. Across these studies, findings were mixed in relation to SUI. In contrast, in the AHRQ review, Shamliyan et al. (2012) concluded that there was a high level of evidence to indicate that E-stim increases continence rates and improves SUI compared to sham stimulation. They also concluded that there was a moderate level of evidence indicating no difference between E-stim and PFMT in relation to continence outcomes among women with SUI. In this review, the strength of evidence was graded as moderate defined as "when RCTs with a medium risk of bias reported consistent treatment effects or large observational studies reported consistent associations" and there was "moderate confidence that the evidence reflects the true effect. Future research may change our confidence in the estimate of effect and may change the estimate" (p. 10). A recent (2017) Cochrane review found 56 RCTs (*n* = 3781 women with SUI) comparing EStim to sham (no treatment) or to other available treatment. The authors concluded that the quality of evidence was too low to provide reliable results about the effectiveness of EStim in relation to other active treatments for SUI. However, results of the review suggest that EStim may be more effective than no treatment for SUI (Stewart et al., 2017).

The AHRQ review also examined evidence related to magnetic stimulation (MStim) in the treatment of UI. Five RCTs compared MStim with sham stimulation in women with UI (*n* = 1), SUI (*n* = 2), mixed UI (*n* = 1), and predominant UUI (*n* = 1). Based on the review, Shamliyan et al. (2012) concluded that there was a moderate level of evidence that magnetic stimulation did not improve urinary continence more than sham stimulation. Recently, the 6th ICS Committee (2017) reported a total of 11 studies that compared MStim in women with UI to no active treatment (sham) with 4 studies looking predominantly at SUI. Overall, MStim may be more effective than no active treatment in women with SUI but more rigorous studies are needed for an ICS recommendation due to conflicting evidence and low quality of data (Dumoulin et al., 2017).

Vaginal Cones

Weighted vaginal cones have been recommended as a method to assist women to strengthen their PFMs (see **Fig. 11-10**). Women are instructed to insert the heaviest cone that they can retain while in an upright position

and to leave it in place for 15 minutes twice a day while up and moving around. Over a period of time (usually 1 month or more), they gradually increase the weight of the cone inserted. Theoretically, holding the cone in place requires PFM contraction, and slippage of the cones may provide a form of biofeedback, which may promote both contraction and coordination of the PFMs (Herbison & Dean, 2013). Herbison and Dean conducted a systematic review of RCTs and quasi-experimental studies comparing cones to a control condition; the control condition did not include active PFMT (*n* = 5 studies). The outcome in relation to continence was based on self-report and involved failure to cure or improve UI. Failure to cure was significantly less likely in the cone group (RR = 0.84, 95% CI 0.76 to 0.94), as was failure to improve UI (RR = 0.72, CI 0.52 to 0.99), compared to the control condition. The authors also included studies comparing cone therapy to active PFMT (*n* = 13 studies) and found no significant difference in the two groups in (1) self-reported cure or improvement in UI (RR = 0.97, 95% CI 0.75 to 1.20 in 6 studies); (2) self-reported cure (*n* = 5 studies; RR = 1.10, 95% CI 0.91 to 1.13); (3) UI episodes per day (*n* = 4 studies; mean difference = 0.00, 95% CI −0.20 to 0.20); (4) pad test results (*n* = 6 studies; RR = 1.00, 95% CI 0.76 to 1.31); or (5) PFM strength (mean difference = 0.61, 95% CI −2.49 to 1.27). Overall, this review found that weighted vaginal cones were better than no active treatment and equivalent to PFMT in treating UI in women.

Continence Pessaries

Continence pessaries are usually round with a knob and may or may not have a supporting diaphragm in the center (e.g., the ring or dish; **Fig. 11-11**). Since the goal is to stabilize and support the bladder neck and to compress the urethra to prevent urine leakage during increased intra-abdominal pressure, the pessary should be inserted with the knob positioned against the anterior vaginal

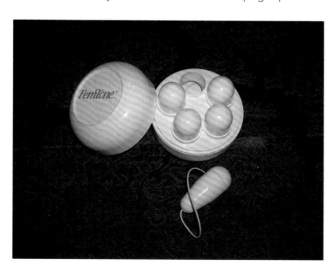

FIGURE 11-10. Weighted Vaginal Cones. (Courtesy of JoAnn Ermer-Seltun, ARNP, CWOCN.)

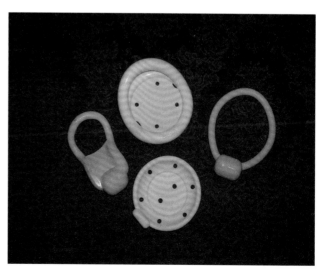

FIGURE 11-11. Image of Pessaries Used for SUI with and Without Support. (Courtesy of JoAnn Ermer-Seltun, ARNP, CWOCN.)

wall, behind the symphysis pubis, and ideally at the level of the urethrovesical junction (Keyock & Newman, 2011) **(Fig. 11-11)**. There is limited research examining the effectiveness of incontinence pessaries in treating SUI. Richter et al. (2010) compared self-reported improvement as measured by the Patient Global Impression of Improvement scale (much or very much better) and the stress incontinence subscale of the Urogenital Distress Inventory (absence of bothersome SUI symptoms) in women treated with a ring or dish pessary, behavioral therapy (PFMT and stress and urge strategies), or combination therapy at 3 and 12 months posttreatment. Using intention-to-treat when analyzing the outcomes, at 3 months, significantly more women in the combination group (53.3%) reported that they were much or very much better than in the pessary only group (39.6%, $p = 0.02$). There were no significant differences between the pessary and behavioral (49.3%) therapy only groups. Significantly more women in the combined treatment group (44.0%) and in the behavioral therapy only group (48.6%) reported no bothersome SUI symptoms at 3 months than those in the pessary only group (32.9%, $p = 0.05$ and 0.006, respectively). At 12 months, there were no significant group differences for either outcome. When the outcomes were analyzed only for those women who completed the interventions (per protocol analysis), there were no significant group differences at either 3 or 12 months. There is a need for additional research examining the effectiveness of pessaries in the treatment of SUI.

Urethral Inserts

There is currently one urethral insert available in the United States (Keyock & Newman, 2011). It is the Fem-Soft, a sterile disposable, single use, intraurethral device. It consists of a narrow, silicone tube encased entirely in a soft, thin, mineral oil-filled sleeve that forms a balloon at the internal tip and comes with a disposable applicator for insertion. It comes in various sizes and is prescribed by a health care provider. It is easily removed for voiding and should be removed at least once every 6 hours (Keyock & Newman, 2011). One single group, quasi-experimental study examining the long-term safety, efficacy, and acceptability of the device in women with SUI was identified (Sirls et al., 2002). One hundred fifty ($n = 150$) women were enrolled in the study. Of these women, 77 (51%) withdrew by the 12-month follow-up visit. The reasons for withdrawal were variable with 33 (43%) doing so for reasons not related to the device. Based on intention-to-treat analysis, 57% of the 112 women had a >50% reduction in total weekly incontinent episodes and did not withdraw secondary to adverse events or dissatisfaction. The most common adverse events were bacteriuria ($n = 58$ women, 38.7%) and symptomatic UTI (31.3%). Additional research is needed to examine the effectiveness of intraurethral inserts on SUI-related outcomes.

Pharmacotherapy

In the United States, there are currently no FDA-approved drugs to treat SUI. There are, however, recent systematic reviews examining the clinical effectiveness of estrogen therapy and duloxetine in treating SUI. Estrogen receptors have been identified in tissues of the vagina, bladder, urethra, and PFMs. Estrogen deficiency may play a role in the development of UI, and estrogen has been used in the treatment of UI including SUI (Cody et al., 2012). The Cochrane review (Cody et al., 2012) included studies examining both systemic and topical estrogen while the AHRQ review (Shamliyan et al., 2012) focused on topical administration. Seventeen of the studies (RCTs or quasi-experimental studies) in the Cochrane review focused on SUI although findings were not reported separately for SUI. The authors concluded that systemic estrogen may actually worsen UI. In contrast, topical estrogen treatment may improve UI. The long-term effects and the impact of discontinuing treatment are currently unknown. In the AHRQ review of pharmacotherapy for SUI, Shamliyan et al. (2012) reported that, "Evidence from individual RCTs indicates greater continence and improvement in UI with vaginal estrogen formulations and worsening UI with transdermal patches" and "Evidence was insufficient to draw conclusions about the clinical efficacy of different topical estrogen treatments for UI" (p. 44). Duloxetine is classified as an SNRI (serotonin and norepinephrine reuptake inhibitor) and has been shown in cat studies to suppress parasympathetic activity and increase sympathetic and somatic neural activity in the lower urinary tract. These effects are thought to increase rhabdosphincter activity and, consequently, urethral closure pressure (Mariappan et al., 2005). In the AHRQ report published in 2012, Shamliyan and colleagues concluded that there was (1) a low level of evidence indicating that it was worse than placebo in resolving UI; (2) a high level of evidence that UI was improved; and (3) a high level of evidence indicating significantly higher adverse event rates relative to placebo, resulting in discontinuation of treatment due to nausea, dizziness, headache, fatigue, diarrhea, and constipation. The authors concluded that, "Duloxetine has an unfavorable balance between improvement in stress UI and treatment discontinuation due to adverse effects" (p. 121). These conclusions are supported by the results of 2016 meta-analysis of randomized controlled clinical trials comparing duloxetine ($n = 958$) to placebo ($n = 955$) in women with SUI (Maund et al., 2016). When findings were combined across the four studies, there were small but statistically significant differences in the percent change in the frequency of incontinent episodes between the duloxetine and placebo groups. There was no significant difference in QoL scores. When adverse effects were examined, the risk of most of harm-related events examined was significantly greater in the duloxetine group than in the placebo group with many more of the patients in the duloxetine group discontinuing it due to adverse events. The authors concluded that potential harm associated with duloxetine outweighed the benefits of treatment. They also noted that the UK National Institute for Health and Care Excellence guidelines state that duloxetine should not be used as a first-line treatment for SUI or routinely offered as a second-line treatment.

Urethral Bulking Agents

Surgical intervention or urethral bulking agents are treatment options for women with SUI. Intra- or periurethral injection of bulking agents is used to plump up the urethral mucosa; this creates artificial urethral cushions that can improve urethral coaptation and restore continence (Kirchin et al., 2012). Agents used for urethral bulking in the United States include carbon beads, copolymers, and polyacrylamide hydrogels (Chapple & Dmochowski, 2019; Keyock & Newman, 2011; Rovner et al., 2017). Kirchin et al. (2012) conducted a systematic review of RCTs and quasi-experimental studies where at least one study arm involved urethral injection therapy. The authors concluded that evidence is insufficient to guide clinical practice. In the AHRQ review, Shamliyan et al. (2012) concluded that a low level of evidence suggests that urethral bulking agents do not result in improvement in UI compared to placebo (low level of evidence means low confidence that current evidence reflects the true effect and an acknowledgment that additional research is likely to change the conclusions). Evidence from uncontrolled studies reported high improvement rates, but also adverse events. The AUA/SUFU 2017 guideline on the surgical treatment of SUI state that bulking agents are viable treatments for SUI, although they acknowledge that there is little long-term data on their effectiveness and note that patients should be counseled on the expected need for repeat injections (Kobashi et al., 2017).

Surgical Procedures

There are a number of different surgical procedures used to treat SUI. The two most common are colposuspension (Burch colposuspension) and midurethral sling procedures (**Fig. 11-12**). Colposuspension, done either as an open lower abdominal procedure or laparoscopically, lifts and stabilizes the bladder neck, which enhances urethral sphincter function during increases in intra-abdominal pressure (Keyock & Newman, 2011; Rovner et al., 2017). While this was considered the gold standard in the past, the midurethral sling has become much more common and is now considered by many to be the gold standard surgery for SUI (Geller & Wu, 2013). Multiple entry techniques (retropubic, suprapubic, and transobturator) have been utilized for insertion of the sling, which is permanently implanted to support the urethra at midpoint between the bladder neck and the urethral meatus. Both retropubic and

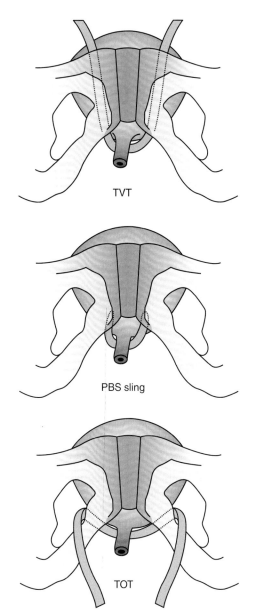

FIGURE 11-12. Mid-Urethral Slings. TVT, tension-free vaginal tape; PBS, public bone stabilization sling; TOT, transobturator tape. (Robert Kovac, S. (2012). *Advances in reconstructive vaginal surgery*. Philadelphia, PA: Lippincott Williams & Wilkins.)

transobturator slings are widely used today. There are a number of sling materials used, including cadaver fascia lata and various synthetic materials including mesh slings (e.g., tension-free vaginal tape) (Lue & Tanagho, 2014). Mesh slings consist of lightweight macroporous polypropylene mesh designed to maximize urethral support while minimizing the risk of erosion. While surgical advances have improved outcomes and allowed surgery to be performed in a shorter period of time, under local anesthetic, and as an outpatient procedure, there are still treatment failures and surgical complications, including voiding dysfunction, bladder injuries, mesh erosion, and pain. In 2008, the FDA released a

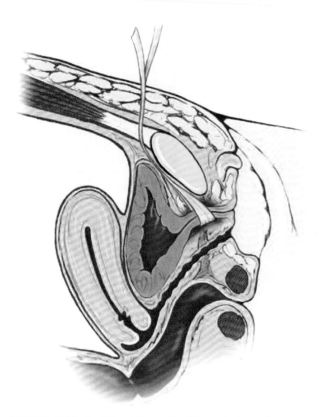

FIGURE 11-13. Traditional Suburethral Sling. Redrawn from original by Jasmine Tan.

Safety Communication describing over 1,000 cases of mesh-related complications; the report was updated in 2011 (Geller & Wu, 2013). A Cochrane review published in 2009 compared procedures involving the traditional suburethral sling (**Fig. 11-13**) and the minimally invasive sling and concluded that they were equally effective and there were fewer adverse events with the minimally invasive sling (Ogah et al., 2009). According to Geller and Wu (2013), the most recent innovation in the mid-urethral sling is the introduction of the mini-sling; the newer adjustable mini-slings can be tightened in the office during postoperative visits. Data on the long-term outcomes are needed (Rovner et al., 2017; Zhang et al., 2015). Box 11-4 summarizes postoperative teaching for women who have had SUI surgery.

KEY POINT

The mid-urethral sling is currently considered by many to be the gold standard for surgical treatment of SUI. The mini-sling is the most recent innovation that can be adjusted at a post-operative office visit; long-term outcomes are unknown.

BOX 11-4 **POSTOPERATIVE TEACHING FOR WOMEN WHO HAVE HAD STRESS URINARY INCONTINENCE SURGERY**

- Although specific postoperative instructions may vary, they often include
  - Resume normal diet.
  - Administer prescribed pain medications as needed to control pain.
  - Most women can resume normal physical activity including walking and going up and down steps once home.
  - Lifting should be restricted to light objects.
  - Avoid strenuous physical activity and heavy lifting for 4 to 8 weeks.
  - Avoid sexual intercourse for 4 to 6 weeks.
  - Depending on the nature of woman's job, work can generally be resumed in 2 to 6 weeks.
- Notify health care provider if having
  - Difficulty voiding or unable to empty bladder
  - Excessive or recurrent vaginal bleeding
  - Malodorous vaginal discharge
  - Pain or burning on urination
  - Blood in urine

CONCLUSION

Stress UI is a common problem among women. SUI generally presents as involuntary loss of small amounts of urine occurring during activities associated with sudden increases in intra-abdominal pressure. Unless the initial evaluation suggests complicated SUI, initial treatment can be initiated following a limited baseline evaluation (history, focused physical examination, cough stress test, and, where feasible, a 3-day bladder diary). PFMT is the best initial treatment option for most women with SUI. A history, focused physical examination (abdominal, pelvic, and neurological), cough stress test, and 3-day bladder diary provide an adequate basis for treating SUI in most women.

There is a high level of research to support the effectiveness of PFMT in treating SUI in women. The ideal method of teaching PFMT and the optimal training regimen are, however, yet to be determined. While a variety of training approaches have been shown to be effective, more frequent continence specialist contact is probably beneficial. The continence nurse plays a vital role in the assessment, evaluation, and management of woman suffering from SUI to reduce or cure symptoms and may ultimately improve the woman's quality of life.

REFERENCES

Altman, D. J., Ekström, A., Forsgren, C., et al. (2007a). Symptoms of anal and urinary incontinence following cesarean section or spontaneous vaginal delivery. *American Journal of Obstetrics and Gynecology, 197*(5), 512.e1–512.e7. doi: 10.1016/j.ajog.2007.03.083.

Altman, D. J., Ekstrom, A., Gustafsson, C., et al. (2006). Risk of urinary incontinence after childbirth. *Obstetrics and Gynecology, 108*(4), 873–878.

Altman, D., Forsman, M., Falconer, C., et al. (2008). Genetic influence on stress urinary incontinence and pelvic organ prolapse. *European Urology, 54*(4), 918–922. doi: 10.1016/j.eururo.2007.12.004.

Altman, D., Granath, F., Cnattingius, S., et al. (2007b). Hysterectomy and risk of stress-urinary-incontinence surgery: Nationwide cohort study. *Lancet, 370*(9597), 1494–1499. doi: 10.1016/S0140-6736(07)61635-3.

An, S. Y., Kim, S. S., Han, G. (2017). Effect of belly dancing on urinary incontinence-related muscles and vaginal pressure in middle-aged women. *Journal of Physical Therapy Science, 29*, 384–386. doi: 10.1589/jpts.29.384.

Aune, D., Mahamet-Saleh, Y., Norat, T., et al. (2019). Body mass index, abdominal fatness, weight gain and the risk of incontinence: A systematic review and dose-response meta-analysis of prospective studies. *BJOG, 126*, 1424–1433. doi: 10.1111/1471-0528.15897.

Bettez, M., Tu, L. M., Carlson, K., et al. (2012). 2012 update: Guidelines for adult urinary incontinence collaborative consensus document for the Canadian urological association. *Canadian Urological Association Journal, 6*(5), 354–363.

Birder, L., Blok, B., Burnstock, G., et al. (2017). Neural control. In P. Abrams, L. Cardozo, A. Wagg, et al. (Eds.), *Incontinence* (6th ed., pp. 259–363). Bristol, UK: ICI-ICS. International Continence Society.

Bø, K., & Herbert, R. D. (2013). There is not yet strong evidence that exercise regimens other than pelvic floor muscle training can reduce stress urinary incontinence in women: a systematic review. *Journal of Physiotherapy, 59*(3), 159–168. doi: 10.1016/S1836-9553(13)70180-2.

Bradley, C. S., Brown, J. S., Van Den Eeden, S. K., et al. (2011). Urinary incontinence self-report questions: Reproducibility and agreement with bladder diary. *International Urogynecology Journal, 22*(12), 1565–1571. doi: 10.1007/s00192-011-1503-3.

Bright, E., Drake, M. J., & Abrams, P. (2011). Urinary diaries: Evidence for the development and validation of diary content, format, and duration. *Neurourology and Urodynamics, 352*, 348–352. doi: 10.1002/nau.

Bristol Urological Institute. (2014). International Consultation on Incontinence Modular Questionnaire (ICIQ). Retrieved from https://iciq.net/iciq-modules

Brown, J. S., Sawaya, G., Thom, D. H., et al. (2000). Hysterectomy and urinary incontinence: A systematic review. *Lancet, 356*(9229), 535–539. doi: 10.1016/S0140-6736(00)02577-0.

Buckley, B. S., & Lapitan, M. C. M. (2010). Prevalence of urinary incontinence in men, women, and children—current evidence: Findings of the Fourth International Consultation on Incontinence. *Urology, 76*(2), 265–270. doi: 10.1016/j.urology.2009.11.078.

Cartwright, R., Kirby, A. C., Tikkinen, M. K. A. O., et al. (2015). Systematic review and metaanalysis of genetic association studies of urinary symptoms and prolapse in women. *American Journal of Obstetrics and Gynecology, 212*(2), 199.e1–199.e24. doi: 10.1016/j.ajog.2014.08.005.

Chang, S. R., Chen, K. H., Lin, H. H., et al. (2014). Association of mode of delivery with urinary incontinence and changes in urinary incontinence over the first year postpartum. *Obstetrics & Gynecology, 123*(3), 568–577.

Chapple, C., & Dmochowski, R. (2019). Particulate versus non-particulate bulking agents in the treatment of stress urinary incontinence. *Research and Reports in Urology, 11*, 299–310. doi.org/10.2147/RRU.S220216.

Cody, J. D., Jacobs, M. L., Richardson, K., et al. (2012). Oestrogen therapy for urinary incontinence in post-menopausal women. *Cochrane Database of Systematic Reviews, 10*, CD001405. doi: 10.1002/14651858.CD001405.pub3.

De Tayrac, R., Chevalier, N., Chauveaud-Lambling, A., et al. (2007). Is vaginal hysterectomy a risk factor for urinary incontinence at long-term follow-up? *European Journal of Obstetrics, Gynecology, and Reproductive Biology, 130*(2), 258–261. doi: 10.1016/j.ejogrb.2006.01.032.

Delancey, J. O. (2010). Why do women have stress urinary incontinence? *Neurourology and Urodynamics, 29*, S13–S17. doi: 10.1002/nau.

Diaz, D. C., Robinson, D., Bosch, R., et al. (2017). Initial assessment of urinary incontinence in adult male and female patients. In P. Abrams, L. Cardozo, A. Wagg, et al. (Eds.), *Incontinence* (6th ed., pp. 497–540). Bristol UK: ICI-ICS. International Continence Society.

Dillon, B. E., & Zimmern, P. E. (2012). When are urodynamics indicated in patients with stress urinary incontinence? *Current Urology Reports, 13*(5), 379–384. doi: 10.1007/s11934-012-0270-0

Diokno, A. C. (2003). Incidence and prevalence of stress urinary incontinence. *Advanced Studies in Medicine, 3*, 824–828.

Dmochowski, R. (2018). Novel external electrical muscle stimulation device for the treatment of female stress urinary incontinence: Randomized controlled noninferiority trial versus intravaginal electrical stimulation. ICS Conference.

Dumoulin, C. Adewuyi, T., Booth, J. (2017). Adult conservative management. In P. Abrams, L. Cardozo, A. Wagg, et al. (Eds.), *Incontinence* (6th ed., pp. 1443–1628). Bristol, UK: ICI-ICS. International Continence Society.

Dumoulin, C., Cacciari, L. P., Hay-Smith, E. J. C. (2018). Pelvic floor muscle training verses no treatment, or inactive control treatments, for urinary incontinence in women. *Cochrane Database of Systematic Reviews*, (10), CD005654. doi: 10.1002/14651858.

Dumoulin, C., Glazener, C., & Jenkinson, D. (2011). Determining the optimal pelvic floor muscle training regimen for women with stress urinary incontinence. *Neurourology and Urodynamics, 30*, 746–753. doi: 10.1002/nau.

Forsgren, C., Lundholm, C., Johansson, A. L. V., et al. (2012). Vaginal hysterectomy and risk of pelvic organ prolapse and stress urinary incontinence surgery. *International Urogynecology Journal, 23*(1), 43–48. doi: 10.1007/s00192-011-1523-z.

Frawley, H. C., Galea, M. P., Phillips, B. A., et al. (2006). Reliability of pelvic floor muscle strength assessment using different test positions and tools. *Neurourology and Urodynamics, 25*(3), 236–242. doi: 10.1002/nau.20201.

Geller, E. J., & Wu, J. M. (2013). Changing trends in surgery for stress urinary incontinence. *Current Opinion in Obstetrics & Gynecology, 25*(5), 404–409. doi: 10.1097/GCO.0b013e3283648cdd.

Gleason, J. L., Richter, H. E., Redden, D. T., et al. (2013). Caffeine and urinary incontinence in US women. *International Urogynecology Journal, 24*(2), 295–302. doi: 10.1007/s00192-012-1829-5.

Gustafsson, C., Ekström, A., Brismar, S., et al. (2006). Urinary incontinence after hysterectomy—three-year observational study. *Urology, 68*(4), 769–774. doi: 10.1016/j.urology.2006.04.001.

Gyhagen, M., Bullarbo, M., Nielsen, T. F., et al. (2013). A comparison of the long-term consequences of vaginal delivery versus caesarean section on the prevalence, severity and bothersomeness of urinary incontinence subtypes: a national cohort study in primiparous women. *BJOG, 120*(12), 1548–1555. doi: 10.1111/1471-0528.12367.

Hannestad, Y. S., Rortveit, G., Daltveit, A. K., et al. (2003). Are smoking and other lifestyle factors associated with female urinary incontinence? The Norwegian EPINCONT Study. *BJOG, 110*, 247–254. doi: 10.10161/S1470-0328(02)02927-0.

Haylen, B. T., Ridder, D. D., Freeman, R. M., et al. (2010). An International Urogynecological Association (IUGA)/International Continence Society (ICS) joint report on the terminology for female pelvic floor dysfunction. *International Urogynecology Journal, 20*, 4–20. doi:10.1002/nau.

Hay-Smith, E. J. C., Herderschee, R., Dumoulin, C., et al. (2011). Comparisons of approaches to pelvic floor muscle training for urinary incontinence in women. *Cochrane Database of Systematic Reviews,* (12), CD009508. doi: 10.1002/14651858.CD009508.

Hein, J. T., Rieck, T. M., Dunfee, H. A., et al. (2020). Effect of a 12-week Pilates pelvic floor-strengthening program on short-term measures of stress urinary incontinence in women: A pilot study. *Journal of Alternative and Complementary Medicine, 26*(2), 158–161. doi. org/10.1089/acm.2019.0330

Herbison, G. P., & Dean, N. (2013). Weighted vaginal cones for urinary incontinence. *Cochrane Database of Systematic Reviews, 7,* CD002114. doi: 10.1002/14651858.CD002114.pub2.

Herderschee, R., Hay-Smith, E. J. C., Herbison, G. P., et al. (2011). Feedback or biofeedback to augment pelvic floor muscle training for urinary incontinence in women. *Cochrane Database of Systematic Reviews, 7,* CD009252. doi: 10.1002/14651858.CD009252.

Hirakawa, T., Suzuki, S., Kato, K., et al. (2013). Randomized controlled trial of pelvic floor muscle training with or without biofeedback for urinary incontinence. *International Urogynecology Journal, 24*(8), 1347–1354. doi: 10.1007/s00192-012-2012-8.

Hosker, G. (2009). Is it possible to diagnose intrinsic sphincter deficiency in women? *Current Opinion in Urology, 19(4),* 342–346. doi: 10.1097/MOU.0b013e32832ae1cb.

Huang, A. J., Chesney, M., Lisha, N., et al. (2019). A group-based yoga program for urinary incontinence in ambulatory women: feasibility, tolerability, and change in incontinence frequency over 3 months in a single-center randomized trial. *American Journal of Obstetrics and Gynecology, 87,* e1–e87. doi: 10.1016/j.ajog.2018.10.031.

Imamura, M., Williams, K., Wells, M., et al. (2015). Lifestyle interventions for the treatment of urinary incontinence in adults (review). *Cochrane Database of Systematic Reviews,* (12), CD003505. doi: 10.1002/14651858.CD003505.pub5.

Isherwood, P. J., & Rane, A. (2000). Comparative assessment of pelvic floor strength using a perineometer and digital examination. *British Journal of Obstetrics and Gynaecology, 107,* 1007–1011. doi: 10.1111/j.1471-0528.2000.tb10404.x.

Jura, Y. H., Townsend, M. K., Curhan, G. C., et al. (2011). Caffeine intake, and the risk of stress, urgency and mixed urinary incontinence. *Journal of Urology, 185*(5), 1775–1780. doi: 10.1016/j.juro.2011.01.003.

Keyock, K. L., & Newman, D. K. (2011). Understanding stress urinary incontinence. *Nurse Practitioner, 36*(10), 24–36; quiz 36–37. doi: 10.1097/01.NPR.0000405281.55881.7a.

Khullar, V., Amarenco, G., Derpapas, A., et al. (2017). Imaging, neurophysiological testing and other tests. In P. Abrams, L. Cardozo, A. Wagg, et al. (Eds.), *Incontinence* (6th ed., pp. 671–804). ICUD-EAU.

Kirchin, V., Page, T., Keegan, P. E., et al. (2012). Urethral injection therapy for urinary incontinence in women. *Cochrane Database of Systematic Reviews, 2,* CD003881. doi: 10.1002/14651858. CD003881.pub3.

Kobashi, K. C., Albo, M. E., Dmochowski, R. R., et al. (2017). Surgical treatment of female stress urinary incontinence: AUA/SUFA Guideline. *Journal of Urology, 298,* 875–883. doi.org/10.1016/j.juro.2017.06.061.

Koelb, H., Igawa, T., Salvatore, S., et al. (2013). Pathophysiology of urinary incontinence, faecal incontinence and pelvic organ prolapse. In A. Abrams, L. Cardozo, S. Khoury, et al. (Eds.), *Incontinence* (5th ed., pp. 263–359). Paris, France: ICUD-EAU. International Continence Society.

Lamerton, T. J., Torquati, L., Brown, W. J. (2018). Overweight and obesity as major modifiable risk factors for urinary incontinence in young to mid-aged women: A systematic review and meta-analysis. *Obesity Reviews, 19*(12), 1735–1745. doi: 10.1111/obr.12756.

Lausen, A., Marsland, L., Head, S., et al. (2018). Modified Pilates as an adjunct to standard physiotherapy care for urinary incontinence: A mixed methods pilot for a randomized controlled trial. *BMC Women's Health, 18,* 16. doi: 10.1186/s12905-017-0503-y.

Leijonhufvud, A., Lundholm, C., Cnattingius, S., et al. (2011). Risks of stress urinary incontinence and pelvic organ prolapse surgery in relation to mode of childbirth. *American Journal of Obstetrics and Gynecology, 204*(1), 70.e1–70.e7. doi: 10.1016/j.ajog.2010.08.034.

Liebergall-Wischnitzer, M., Hochner-Celnikier, D., Lavy, Y., et al. (2005). Paula method of circular muscle exercises for urinary stress incontinence—A clinical trial. *International Urogynecology Journal and Pelvic Floor Dysfunction, 16,* 345–351.

Lue, T. F., & Tanagho, E. A. (2014). Urinary incontinence. In J. W. McAninch, & T. F. Lue (Eds.), *Smith & Tanagho's General Urology* (18th ed., pp. 1–28). New York, NY: McGraw-Hill Companies, Inc.

Madhu, C., Enki, D., Drake, M. J., et al. (2015). The functional effects of cigarette smoking in women on the lower urinary tract. *Urologia Internationalis, 95*(4), 478–482. doi: 10.1016/j.ejogrb.2019.02.003.

Mariappan, P., Alhasso, A. A., Grant, A., et al. (2005). Serotonin and noradrenaline reuptake inhibitors (SNRI) for stress urinary incontinence in adults. *Cochrane Database of Systematic Reviews, 3,* CD004742. doi: 10.1002/14651858.CD004742.pub2.

Markland, A. D., Richter, H. E., Fwu, C.-W., et al. (2011). Prevalence and trends of urinary incontinence in adults in the United States, 2001 to 2008. *Journal of Urology, 186*(2), 589–593. doi: 10.1016/j.juro.2011.03.114.

Maund, E., Guski, L. S., & Gotzsche, P. C. (2016). Considering benefits and harms of duloxetine for treatment of stress urinary incontinence: A meta-analysis of clinical study reports. *CMAJ, 189*(5), E194–E203. doi: 10.1503/cmaj.151104.

McGuire, E. J. (1981). Urodynamic findings in patients after failure of stress incontinence operations. *Progress in Clinical and Biological Research, 78,* 351–360.

McKenzie, P., Rohozinski, J., & Badlani, G. (2010). Genetic influences on stress urinary incontinence. *Current Opinion in Urology, 20*(4), 291–295. doi: 10.1097/MOU.0b013e32833a4436.

McLean, L., Varette, K., Gentilcore-Saulnier, E., et al. (2013). Pelvic floor muscle training in women with stress urinary incontinence causes hypertrophy of the urethral sphincters and reduces bladder neck mobility during coughing. *Neurourology and Urodynamics, 32*(8), 1096–1102.

Miller, J. J. R., Botros, S. M., Beaumont, J. L., et al. (2008). Impact of hysterectomy on stress urinary incontinence: An identical twin study. *American Journal of Obstetrics and Gynecology, 198*(5), 565.e1–565.e4. doi: 10.1016/j.ajog.2008.01.046.

Miller, J. M., Perucchini, D., Carchidi, L. T., et al. (2001). Pelvic floor muscle contraction during a cough and decreased vesical neck mobility. *Obstetrics and Gynecology, 97*(2), 255–260. doi: 10.1016/s0029-7844(00)01132-7.

Minassian, V. A., Stewart, W. F., & Hirsch, A. G. (2008). Why do stress and urge incontinence co-occur much more often than expected? *International Urogynecology Journal and Pelvic Floor Dysfunction, 19*(10), 1429–1440. doi: 10.1007/s00192-008-0647-2.

Moore, K. N., Dumoulin, C., Bradley, C., et al. (2013). Committee 12: Adult conservative management. In A. Abrams, L. Cardozo, S. Khoury, et al. (Eds). *Incontinence* (5th ed., pp. 263–359). Paris, France: ICUD-EAU. International Continence Society.

Nager, C. W. (2012). The urethra is a reliable witness: Simplifying the diagnosis of stress urinary incontinence. *International Urogynecology Journal, 23*(12), 1649–1651. doi: 10.1007/s00192-012-1892-y.

Nager, C. W., Brubaker, L., Litman, H. J., et al.; The Urinary Incontinence Treatment Network. (2012). A randomized trial of urodynamic testing before stress-incontinence surgery. *New England Journal of Medicine, 366,* 1987–1997. doi: 10.1016/j.juro.2012.12.078.

Nygaard, I. E., & Heit, M. (2004). Stress urinary incontinence. *Obstetrics and Gynecology, 104(3),* 607–620. doi: 10.1097/01. AOG.0000137874.84862.94.

Ogah, J., Cody, J. D., Rogerson, L. (2009). Minimally invasive synthetic suburethral sling operations for stress urinary incontinence in women. *Cochrane Database of Systematic Reviews, 4*, CD006375. doi: 10.1002/14651858.CD006375.pub2.

Ozdemir, O. C., & Surmeli, M. (2017). Physiotherapy in women with urinary incontinence. Retrieved from https://www.intechopen.com/books/synopsis-in-the-management-of-urinary-incontinence/physiotherapy-in-women-with-urinary-incontinence

Pilates, J. H., Miller, W. J. (1945). *Return to life through contrology*. New York, NY: J.J. Augustin.

Press, J. Z., Klein, M. C., Kaczorowski, J., et al. (2007). Does cesarean section reduce postpartum urinary incontinence? A systematic review. *Birth, 34(3)*, 228–237. doi: 10.1111/j.1523-536X.2007.00175.x.

Richter, H. E., Burgio, K. L., Brubaker, L., et al. (2010). Behavioral therapy or combined therapy: A randomized controlled trial. *Obstetrics and Gynecology, 115(3)*, 609–617.

Rortveit, G., Daltveit, A. K., Hannestad, Y. S., et al. (2003). Vaginal delivery parameters and urinary incontinence: The Norwegian EPINCONT study. *American Journal of Obstetrics and Gynecology, 189*(5), 1268–1274. doi: 10.1067/S0002-9378(03)00588-X.

Rosier, P. F. W. M., Kuo, H. C., Finazzi, E., et al. (2017). Urodynamic testing. In P. Abrams, L. Cardozo, A. Wagg, et al. (Eds.), *Incontinence* (6th ed., pp. 599–670). Bristol, UK: ICI-ICS. International Continence Society.

Rovner, E., Athanasiou, S., Choo, M. S., et al. (2017). Surgery for urinary incontinence in women. In P. Abrams, L. Cardozo, A. Wagg, et al. (Eds.), *Incontinence* (6th ed., pp. 1741–1854). Bristol, UK: ICI-ICS. International Continence Society.

Sangsawang, B., & Sangsawang, N. (2013). Stress urinary incontinence in pregnant women: A review of prevalence, pathophysiology, and treatment. *International Urogynecology Journal, 24*(6), 901–912. doi: 10.1007/s00192-013-2061-7.

Schreiner, L., Guimarães, T., Borba, A., et al. (2013). Electrical stimulation for urinary incontinence in women: A systematic review. *International Brazilian Journal of Urology, 39*(4), 454–464. doi: 10.1590/S1677-5538.IBJU.2013.04.02.

Sha, K., Palmer, M. H., Yeo, S. (2019). Yoga's biophysiological effects on lower urinary tract symptoms: A scoping review. *The Journal of Alternative and Complementary Medicine, 25*(3), 279–287. doi: 10.1089/acm.2018.0382.

Shamliyan, T., Wyman, J., & Kane, R. L. (2012). Nonsurgical treatments for urinary incontinence in adult women: Diagnosis and comparative effectiveness. Comparative Effectiveness Review No. 36. (Prepared by the University of Minnesota Evidence-based Practice Center under Contract No. HHSA 290-2007-10064-I.) AHRQ Publication No. 11(12)-EHC074- EF. Rockville, MD: Agency for Healthcare Research and Quality. Retrieved from www.effectivehealthcare.ahrq.gov/reports/final.cfm

Sirls, L. T., Foote, J. E., Kaufman, J. M., et al. (2002). Original article long-term results of the FemSoft 1 urethral insert for the management of female stress urinary incontinence. *International Urogynecology Journal, 13*, 88–95.

Smith, P. P., van Leijsen, S. A. L., Heesakkers, J. P. F., et al. (2012). Can we, and do we need to, define bladder neck hypermobility and intrinsic sphincteric deficiency? ICI-RS 2011. *Neurourology and Urodynamics, 312*, 309–312. doi: 10.1002/nau.

Staskin, D., Kelleher, C., Bosch, R., et al. (2009). Initial assessment of urinary and faecal incontinence in adult male and female patients. In P. Abrams, L. Cardozo, S. Khoury, et al. (Eds.), *4th International Consultation on Incontinence*. Paris, France: Health Publications Ltd.

Stewart, F., Berghmans, B., Bø, K., et al. (2017). Electrical stimulation with non-implanted devices for stress urinary incontinence in women. *Cochrane Database of Systematic Reviews*, (12), CD012390. doi: 10.1002/14651858.CD012390.pub2.

Subak, L. L., Richter, H. E., & Hunskaar, S. (2009). Obesity and urinary incontinence: Epidemiology and clinical research update. *Journal of Urology, 182*(6 Suppl), S2–S7. doi: 10.1016/j.juro.2009.08.071.

Swithinbank, L., Hashim, H., & Abrams, P. (2005). The effect of fluid intake on urinary symptoms in women. *Journal of Urology, 174*(1), 187–189. doi: 10.1097/01.ju.0000162020.10447.31.

Tahtinen, R. M., Auvinen, A., Cartwright, R., et al. (2011). Smoking and bladder symptoms in women. *Obstetrics and Gynecology, 118*(3), 643–648. doi: 10.1097/AOG.0b013e318227b7ac.

Thomason, A. D., Miller, J. M., & Delancey, J. O. (2007). Urinary incontinence symptoms during and after pregnancy in continent and incontinent primiparas. *International Urogynecology Journal and Pelvic Floor Dysfunction, 18*(2), 147–151. doi: 10.1007/s00192-006-0124-8.

Van der Vaart, C., van der Bom, J., de Leeuw, J. R., et al. (2002). The contribution of hysterectomy to the occurrence of urge and stress urinary incontinence symptoms. *BJOG, 109*(2), 149–154. Retrieved from http://www.sciencedirect.com/science/article/pii/S1470032802013320

Van Geelen, H., Ostergard, D., Sand, P. (2018). A review of the impact of pregnancy and childbirth on pelvic floor function as assessed by objective measurement techniques. *International Urogynecology Journal, 29*, 327–338. doi: 10.1007/s00192-017-3540-z.

Vo, A., & Kielb, S. J. (2018). Female voiding dysfunction and urinary incontinence. *Medical Clinics of North America, 102*(2), 313–324. https://doi.org/10.1016/j.mcna.2017.10.006

Wieland, L. S., Shrestha, N., Lassi, Z. S., et al. (2019). Yoga for treating urinary incontinence in women (review). *Cochrane Database of Systematic Reviews*, (2), CD012668. doi: 10.1002/14651858.CD012668.pub2.

Wilson, T. S., Lemack, G. E., & Zimmern, P. E. (2003). Management of intrinsic sphincteric deficiency in women. *Journal of Urology, 169*(5), 1662–1669. doi: 10.1097/01.ju.0000058020.37744.aa.

Wooldridge, L. S. (2017). Urinary incontinence. In D. K. Newman, J. F. Wyman, V. W. Welch (Eds.). *SUNA Core Curriculum for Urologic Nursing* (pp. 467–485). Pittman, NJ: A.J. Jannetti.

Yang, X. J., & Sun, Y. (2019). Comparison of caesarean section and vaginal delivery for pelvic floor function of parturients: A meta-analysis. *European Journal of Obstetrics & Gynecology and Reproductive Biology, 235*, 42–48. doi: 10.1016/j.ejogrb.2019.02.003.

Zhang, P., Fan, B., Zhang, P., et al. (2015). Meta-analysis of female stress urinary incontinence treatments with adjustable single-incision mini-slings and transobturator tension-free vaginal tape surgeries. *BMC Urology, 15*, 64. doi: 10.1186/s12894-015-0060-3.

Zhu, L., Li, L., Lang, J. H., et al. (2012). Prevalence and risk factors for peri- and postpartum urinary incontinence in primiparous women in China: A prospective longitudinal study. *International Urogynecology Journal, 23*(5), 563–572.

Mrs. J, a 51-year-old white female, presents with urinary incontinence. Her history reveals that she leaks urine when she coughs and sneezes or if she lifts something heavy. She does not exercise regularly but denies leaking with ordinary physical activities such as walking or changing position. She admits to occasional urgency, but this is not associated with involuntary urine loss. Typically, accidents are small, usually "a few drops," and occur one to two times a day. She only wears a pad if she is going out for an extended period of time or if she has a cold and is coughing a lot. She has had occasional incontinent episodes for the past 3 to 4 years, but they have increased in frequency over the past year, which is what prompted her to seek treatment at this time. She does not believe that the incontinence is having a major impact on the quality of her life at present but would like to treat it before it "gets worse." She is sexually active with her husband and denies UI having any negative impact. She has had no previous treatment for UI. She voids six to seven times a day and usually does not get up at night to urinate unless she has coffee or drinks a lot of fluid in the late evening; she has no enuresis. She typically drinks three to four cups of regular coffee per day, one can of diet Coke, and one to two glasses of water or milk; she has an occasional glass of wine or beer when out or has guests. She denies difficulty emptying her bladder, dysuria, lower abdominal or pelvic pain or pressure, hematuria, and dyspareunia. Her bowels usually move daily. She has occasional "dietary-related" constipation and denies fecal incontinence. History includes three uncomplicated vaginal deliveries; the babies weighed 6.1, 7.5, and 8.2 pounds, respectively. She does recall having occasional leakage during her last pregnancy, which subsided by the 8th week postpartum. She is having menopausal symptoms with hot flashes and irregular, but heavy, menstrual periods; her last menstrual period was 3 months ago. Her husband uses condoms during sexual intercourse; she denies the possibility of pregnancy.

She describes herself as generally healthy without any physical limitations. Her only medical problem other than "needing to lose some weight" is hypertension. She takes hydrochlorothiazide daily and BP is "usually good." She denies smoking. Her past medical history is negative for urinary tract infections, arthritis, diabetes mellitus, asthma, chronic pulmonary disease, neurologic disorders, or depression.

The physical examination reveals overweight, but healthy-looking, alert, cognitively intact middle-aged woman without any obvious functional limitations. Her vital signs are as follows: BP 138/82, HR 76, and BMI 30.2. Her abdomen is obese but soft and nontender without masses or organomegaly and no suprapubic dullness on percussion. On neurologic examination, her gait is normal, cranial nerves are intact, and deep tendon reflexes are normal; she has full range of motion and no sensory deficits. On pelvic examination, there is a stage 1 pelvic prolapse of the anterior vaginal wall. The vaginal mucosa is pink and moist, her ovaries are not palpable, and the uterus is midline, mobile, nontender, and normal in size. She is able to voluntarily contract and isolate her PFMs with verbal instructions and the strength is moderate with slight retraction of the examiner's fingers; she is able to hold the contraction for 3 to 4 seconds times 3 attempts. The rectal examination is negative for masses and stool. The cough stress test, done in a supine position, is positive for involuntary urine loss.

Diagnosis: SUI by history and confirmed by cough stress test and mild, asymptomatic cystocele

Following the visit, the patient completed a 3-day bladder diary in which she documented three UI episodes associated with coughing or sneezing, an average of six voids per day, and no nocturia or enuresis. Average fluid intake was 48 ounce per day with 32 of those being caffeinated beverages (coffee or diet coke). At the second visit, the treatment plan was discussed including recommendations for weight loss with review of dietary and physical activity recommendations, reducing caffeine intake and PFMT. During digital vaginal examination, the patient was taught to perform PFM contractions. The patient was instructed to perform three sets of 15 exercises each day, one set supine and two sitting, and instructed to contract her PFMs for 3 seconds followed by 3 seconds of relaxation for each repetition, to breathe normally, and to avoid contracting her abdominal or buttock muscles. She was told that once she could comfortably contract and relax her PFMs for 3 seconds for all 15 exercises per set, the duration of the contraction and relaxation period could be increased to 4 seconds and then 5 seconds with each exercise. Given that her POP was only stage 1 and she was asymptomatic, no additional treatment (other than the PFMT) was deemed necessary. She was instructed to complete a bladder diary for the 3 days prior to her next scheduled visit in 2 weeks. Progress was assessed at that visit. She reported adhering to the exercise regimen and being able to contract and relax her PFMs for 5 seconds; she documented two SUI episodes in the 3-day diary. She had reduced her caffeine intake to 1 cup per day without any noted impact on her incontinence. She was instructed to continue to do three sets of exercises per day but to do one set standing, one sitting, and one supine. She was told to gradually increase her contraction and relaxation time with a goal of 10 seconds each; she was taught the "knack"— to contract her PFM when she coughed or sneezed and prior to and while lifting heavy objects. Caffeine intake was no longer restricted. She completed three additional visits over the next 8 weeks and reported that her incontinence was much improved with rare urinary accidents. Weight loss strategies were reinforced at each visit, but she only lost 2 pounds. She was referred for nutritional counseling. Follow-up visits will be scheduled on an as-needed basis.

1. A 54-year-old female patient tells the continence nurse: "Every time I take my exercise class, I leak urine." What condition would the WOC nurse expect?
A. Stress urinary incontinence
B. Reduced bladder capacity
C. Urinary tract infection
D. Pelvic organ prolapse

2. When a patient has only SUI, which of the following symptoms would you _not_ expect to be present?
A. Small urinary accidents
B. Involuntary urine loss occurring when coughing
C. Urgency
D. Involuntary urine loss when lifting something heavy

3. Which of the following scenarios demonstrate a true statement regarding SUI risk factors?
A. C-section eliminates the risk for SUI
B. Caffeine is a known risk factor for SUI
C. Vaginal delivery increases the risk for SUI
D. Genetics are unlikely to play a role in the risk for SUI

4. A continence nurse is counseling a female patient diagnosed with stress urinary incontinence. What is a recommended first-line management option for this condition?
A. Vaginal cone
B. Pelvic floor muscle training
C. Urethral bulking agents
D. Pharmacotherapy

5. The continence nurse is explaining treatment options to a female patient diagnosed with stress urinary incontinence. Which statement by the nurse accurately describes current therapeutic options?
A. There is a great deal of research to support the use of urethral inserts for SUI.
B. Based on currently available evidence, the Paula method and deep abdominal muscle training should not be utilized in the treatment of SUI.
C. There are FDA-approved medications that can be prescribed for the treatment of SUI.
D. While there are a variety of treatment options for SUI, for most women, the best initial treatment is vaginal cones or/and incontinence pessary.

6. Which of the following lifestyle interventions is most likely, based on current research, to benefit women with SUI?
A. Weight loss
B. Eliminating caffeine
C. Decreasing fluid intake
D. Stopping smoking

7. For an otherwise healthy woman presenting with symptoms suggesting SUI, which of the following diagnostic tests should be part of the routine evaluation?
A. Postvoid residual urine
B. Cystoscopy
C. Urodynamic testing
D. Cough stress test

8. Based on current evidence, which of the following is true in relation to pelvic floor muscle (PFM) training for SUI?
A. To increase the likelihood of benefit, women need to do at least 40 pelvic floor muscle exercises per day.
B. To achieve maximal benefit, it is important for the exercise regimen to include both sustained contraction and maximal contraction exercises.
C. Using biofeedback to teach women how to perform PFM exercises increased the likelihood of benefit.
D. Regular health care provider supervision increases the likelihood of benefit.

9. A patient with SUI tells you that she has heard that yoga is as beneficial as PFM training in treating SUI. Based on current knowledge, which of the following responses is most appropriate?
A. While yoga has been shown to an effective treatment for a number of health problems, there is not enough evidence to know if it is beneficial for urinary incontinence.
B. Studies show that yoga is as effective as pelvic floor muscle exercises in reducing urinary incontinence.
C. While yoga will not help incontinence as much as pelvic floor muscle training, more research is needed to explore the benefit of alternative exercise programs that may engage the pelvic floor muscles, that is, Pilates, belly dancing.
D. While we are not sure yet whether yoga is as effective as pelvic floor muscle exercises in decreasing urinary incontinence, we do know that it increases pelvic floor muscle strength so should be effective in decreasing involuntary urine loss.

10. A patient tells you that she finds PFM exercises difficult to do and wants to discussion other noninvasive treatment options. Which of the following treatment options currently have research evidence support their potential effectiveness in SUI?
A. Oral estrogen
B. Urethral inserts
C. Duloxetine
D. Vaginal cones

ANSWERS AND RATIONALES

1. A. Rationale: Urine leakage associated with exertional activities that increase intra-abdominal pressure is most likely stress urinary incontinence (SUI).

2. C. Rationale: Urgency is a sign of overactive bladder and is associated with urge urinary incontinence, not stress urinary incontinence.

3. C. Rationale: There is strong evidence to support vaginal delivery as a risk factor for SUI. Vaginal delivery, particularly the first vaginal delivery, can stretch pelvic floor connective tissues beyond their physiologic limit, damage the levator ani muscles, and/or result in neurologic damage, all of which can impair pelvic floor function and lead to post-partum SUI. In most women, subsequent healing of the delivery-related injury and muscle hypertrophy will compensate for the injury and limit the duration of the SUI.

4. B. Rationale: Numerous research studies including well-designed systematic reviews with meta-analysis (considered the highest level of evidence for clinical practice) have shown that compared to usual care (including no intervention) pelvic floor muscle training (PFMT) is associated with both a statistically and clinically significantly higher likelihood of improving or eliminating SUI. In addition to their established efficacy, the low risk of adverse effects makes PFMT the first-line intervention for most women with SUI.

5. B. Rationale: Current research does not support the Paula method (contraction of the muscles of the mouth and eyes based on the theory that all sphincters in the body work simultaneously and that exercising the ring muscles of the mouth, eyes, or nose will cause co-contraction and strengthening of the PFMs) having any benefit is women with SUI. None of the other statements are true:

- There are currently no FDA-approved medications for SUI.
- Research on urethra inserts is too limited to conclude that they are effective.
- While vaginal cones or continence pessary may be beneficial treatment options for some women, research evidence supports PFMT as the initial treatment options for the majority of women with SUI.

6. A. Rationale: Being overweight or obese has been identified as a risk factor for SUI in most studies with the risk increasing linearly as weight increases. In addition, research suggests that weight loss is associated with improvement in continence. While the other lifestyle interventions listed (eliminating caffeine, decreasing fluid intake or not smoking) may improve SUI in some women, the research supporting these interventions is either much more limited or findings are not consistent.

7. D. Rationale: The stress test should be performed as part of the assessment of women with SUI. With a comfortably full bladder, the woman is asked to cough deeply (or to bear down) while the clinician observes the urethral meatus for involuntary urine loss. A positive stress test is considered diagnostic of SUI. The other tests listed (postvoid residual urine, cystoscopy, and urodynamic testing) may be indicated for select women presenting with possible SUI but are not routinely recommended.

8. D. Rationale: In a well-designed systematic review that included studies comparing the effectiveness of various approaches to PFMT, the only variation shown to be associated with greater benefit was regular supervision of the training (provider contact) compared to little or no provider contact.

9. A. Rationale: There are too few studies examining the effect of yoga on urinary incontinence to know if it is an effective intervention for SUI. Well-designed clinical trials are needed before we can conclude that it is or is not effective. Yoga has not been compared to other nonpelvic floor muscle exercise programs and its possible mechanism of action relative to pelvic floor muscle function has not been examined.

10. D. Rationale: Of the intervention options listed in this question, vaginal cones are the only option with adequate evidence to support their effectiveness in treating SUI. In a well-designed systematic review, they were more effective than usual care in improving or eliminating UI and equivalent to PFMT.

CHAPTER 12

ADVANCE PELVIC HEALTH CONSIDERATIONS FOR WOMEN: *(PART A)* CHRONIC PELVIC PAIN SYNDROMES *(PART B)* PELVIC ORGAN PROLAPSE AND VESICOVAGINAL FISTULA

Amy Hull (Part A),
JoAnn M. Ermer-Seltun and Sandra Engberg (Part B)

OBJECTIVES

1. Discuss the prevalence and etiologies of chronic pelvic pain, pelvic organ prolapse, and vesicovaginal fistula in women.

2. Describe the physical examination and applicable diagnostics of the female with chronic pelvic pain, pelvic organ prolapse, and vesicovaginal fistula.

3. Identify treatment options and appropriate referrals to aide in the care of the woman with chronic pelvic pain, pelvic organ prolapse, and vesicovaginal fistula.

TOPIC OUTLINE

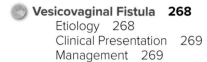
(PART A) ADVANCE PELVIC HEALTH CONSIDERATIONS FOR WOMEN: CHRONIC PELVIC PAIN SYNDROMES

Amy Hull

INTRODUCTION

Chronic pelvic pain (CPP) in women is a common but serious complaint that can be difficult to treat. Given the severity, intensity, and frequency of pain, it can be a debilitating and life altering condition with no known conclusion or cure (Ayorinde et al., 2015). Understanding the condition requires further comprehension of several key concepts: (1) the very word, chronic, denotes pain that is of a longer-term duration; (2) the chronicity of the problem implies it is typically nonemergent or nonacute; (3) even in the absence of a nonemergent illness, CPP is a significant and serious health concern; (4) symptoms of CPP can be caused by multiple etiologies and are often multifactorial (Bruckenthal, 2011). An understanding of these concepts, as well as general education of causes, prevalence, evaluation, and management, will be the focus of this chapter for the Advanced Practice Registered Nurse (APRN) and continence nurse specialist.

DEFINITION

The International Association for the Study of Pain (IASP) (2018) describes pain as an unpleasant sensation that creates a negative emotional response, irrespective of real or possible tissue damage. Pain can be further classified into primary or secondary pain. Primary pain includes conditions without a discernable pain source and include irritable bowel syndrome (IBS) and primary headache. Secondary pain can be attributed to a specific source of concern, such as the pain from cancer, surgery, inflammation, or neuropathy (Lyons & Koneti, 2019).

The American College of Obstetricians and Gynecologists (ACOG) defines CPP as noncyclic pain of 6 or more months' duration that is localized to the pelvis, anterior abdominal wall at or below the umbilicus, the lumbosacral back, or the buttocks, and is of such severity that it may cause functional disability or lead one to seek treatment (ACOG Practice Bulletin No. 51, 2004). Other academic societies, such as the European Association of Urology (EAU), have defined the condition as a syndrome, adopting the terminology of Chronic Pelvic Pain Syndrome (CPPS) (Sutcliffe et al., 2019). EAU states that

CPPS is "chronic or persistent pain perceived in structures related to the pelvis without proven infection or other obvious local pathology that may account for the pain, and it is often associated with negative cognitive, behavioral, sexual, and emotional consequences, as well as with symptoms suggestive of lower urinary tract, sexual, bowel, pelvic floor, or gynecological dysfunction" (Fall et al., 2010).

ACUTE VERSUS CHRONIC PAIN

Delineation between acute and chronic pain must be made as a patient who presents with the complaint of pain of acute onset and without a prior history of pain may require a different, emergent workup (Humes-Goff & Klima, 2015). While discussion of acute pelvic pain is not the focus of this chapter, it is important for the provider to distinguish types of pain that may be acute. See **Table 12-1** for a list of sources of acute and CPP. It is also important to know that many chronic sources of pelvic pain can have acute crisis or flares, which may require an emergent evaluation and management (Humes-Goff & Klima, 2015; Sutcliffe et al., 2019).

TABLE 12-1 ACUTE AND CHRONIC SOURCES OF PELVIC PAIN	
ACUTE	**CHRONIC**
Urinary tract infection or pyelonephritis	Endometriosis
Ovarian cysts and abscesses	Irritable bowel syndrome
Appendicitis	Interstitial cystitis/bladder pain syndrome
Ovarian torsion	Vulvodynia
Pelvic inflammatory disease	Pelvic floor myofascial pain
Bowel obstruction	Pudendal neuralgia
Ectopic pregnancy	Urethral syndrome
Renal and bladder calculi	Adenomyosis and/or uterine leiomyomas
Bartholin gland abscess	Anorectal pain
Vulvovaginitis and contact dermatitis	Depression
Urethral diverticulum	Pelvic congestion syndrome
Acute crises of inflammatory bowel disease: Crohn's, ulcerative colitis, diverticular disease	Inflammatory bowel disease
Endometritis	Ovarian remnant syndrome

PREVALENCE OF CPP

Absolute numbers of women suffering from CPP remain difficult to quantify. Recent epidemiological studies have attempted to determine the prevalence of the issue but, admittedly, there has been a wide range of reported cases, from a very small and narrowly defined segment of the population to a much larger and more general number. Ayorinde et al. (2015) report on these discrepancies, noting two population-based studies from Mexico and New Zealand that attempted to determine the prevalence of women who experience CPP. These studies showed prevalence ranges of 6.4% to 25.4%, respectively, and the review authors note that there are several differences in study design, sample size, and methodology that may have contributed to the wide variation of incidence (Ayorinde et al., 2015; Garcia-Perez et al., 2010; Zondervan et al., 2001).

Attempts to determine the prevalence of CPP among U.S. and UK women have yielded similar variability. Mathias et al. (1996) determined that 14.7% of women, aged 18 to 50, experienced CPP. No other, more recent, U.S. prevalence studies exist to further define and characterize these numbers. Zondervan et al. (2001) determined a prevalence of CPP among UK women to be 24%. Both studies were similarly designed with the means of determination of prevalence via administration of telephone and postal questionnaires and both studies attained strong numbers for evaluation. Yet, as discussed, large contradictions among these prevalence studies may be explained by differences in study design or, possibly, these variations persist due to the lack of a concise definition and understanding of CPP.

PATHOPHYSIOLOGY OF CPP

CHRONIC OVERLAPPING PAIN CONDITIONS

CPP is most often a multifactorial problem and remains poorly understood and a difficult condition to treat. Yet, it is not an uncommon or rare condition. If the number of CPP sufferers is accurate, as determined via past prevalence studies, Gunter (2003) concludes researchers and health care providers can infer a patient population of 9 million reproductive-aged women in the United States alone with the problem. From these numbers, one may determine the direct cost of evaluation and treatment to be 2.8 billion U.S. dollars (Gunter, 2003).

To further compound the problem, researchers have recognized a coalescence of other comorbid conditions frequently seen in patients who have CPP. These clustering disorders, called chronic overlapping pain conditions (COPC), include "temporomandibular disorder, fibromyalgia, irritable bowel syndrome (IBS), vulvodynia, chronic fatigue syndrome, interstitial cystitis/painful bladder syndrome, endometriosis, chronic tension-type headaches, migraine headaches, and chronic lower back pain" (Carey & Moore, 2019). (See **Table 12-2** for the listing of etiologies by system of CPP.) The authors note the greatest predictor for development of another COPC is the presence of any other chronic pain concern and, the more COPCs a person has, the greater the risk other chronic pain disorders may evolve (Carey & Moore, 2019).

Common sources of CPP in women with discussion of the pathophysiology are as follows:

1. **Endometriosis:** This syndrome is characterized by growth of endometrial tissue outside the endometrium of the uterus. Prevalence studies estimate a 10% rate among reproductive-aged women with a high prevalence (25% to 50%) among women who are infertile. The etiology is not well understood but several theories predominate including, retrograde menstruation, genetic factors, immune dysfunction, coelomic metaplasia (endometrium outside the uterus), stress and resulting inflammation, and stem cells (As-Sanie et al., 2019). Signs and symptoms may include dysmenorrhea, dyspareunia, painful defecation, bladder pain, heavy menstrual cycles, and infertility (Perkins, 2019).

2. **Interstitial Cystitis/Bladder Pain Syndrome:** Prevalence of this condition ranges from 2.7% to 6.5% of the U.S. population (Malde et al., 2018). The etiology of this pain syndrome is not well understood

TABLE 12-2 COMMON ETIOLOGIES OF CPP BY AFFECTED SYSTEM				
GYNECOLOGIC	UROLOGIC	GASTROINTESTINAL	NEUROLOGIC	MUSCULOSKELETAL
Endometriosis	Interstitial cystitis/painful bladder syndrome	Irritable bowel syndrome	Vulvodynia	Pelvic floor myofascial pain
Uterine leiomyomas	Urethral syndrome	Anorectal pain	Pudendal neuralgia	Pelvic adhesive disease
Adenomyosis		Chronic, functional constipation	Nerve entrapment	Piriformis syndrome
Pelvic congestion syndrome				
Ovarian remnant syndrome				

with few diagnostic tests to conclusively diagnose the disorder. Therefore, diagnosis is maintained by the presence of symptoms such as low pelvic pain or pressure with urgency, frequency, and nocturia (Ackerman et al., 2018; Birder, 2019).

3. **Irritable Bowel Syndrome:** This condition is classified into three subdivisions: IBS—constipation predominant (IBS-C), IBS—diarrhea predominant (IBS-D), and IBS—mixed (IBS-M). It is believed that up to 45% of the U.S. population is affected and symptoms include abdominal pain with altered bowel consistency including diarrhea, constipation, or both (Pimental, 2016). See Chapter 21 for further discussion of IBS.

4. **Pudendal Neuralgia:** Pudendal neuralgia (PN) is a poorly understood and very likely under diagnosed condition with a reported incidence of 1/100,000 people with women more likely to be affected than men (Hibner et al., 2010). Diagnosis is largely based on clinical findings with little information in the literature to guide the clinician, leading to an underreported and under diagnosed condition. It is believed the source of the pain occurs from injury to the pudendal nerve, which carries motor, sensory, and autonomic fibers. Thus, injury can affect both afferent (sensory) and efferent (motor) pathways. The three branches of the pudendal nerve include the dorsal nerve of the clitoris (penis in men), the perineal nerve, and the inferior anal nerve. Therefore, pain may be described as burning and can be felt along the sacral nerve dermatomes in the vulva, clitoris, perineum, rectum, or vagina, either unilaterally or bilaterally (**Fig. 12-1**). Patients may express discomfort when sitting, worsening of the pain throughout the day, and a relief of the pain when standing (Hibner et al., 2010).

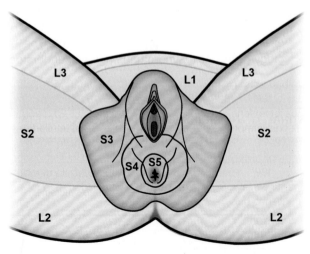

FIGURE 12-1. Sacral Nerve Dermatomes. (Reprinted with Permission from Diane K. Newman, DNP; SUNA Core Curriculum for Urologic Nursing.)

5. **Vulvodynia:** This highly prevalent condition accounts for 12% of women who experience dyspareunia. Pain from this condition is defined by vulvar pain with characteristics to describe the source by the location and localization, provocation versus no provocation, or a combination of characteristics, called mixed. Thus, it may be classified as vestibulodynia or clitorodynia, provoked or unprovoked, generalized or mixed, spontaneous or mixed, intermittent, persistent, constant, immediate, or delayed (Bornstein et al., 2019). Theories on development of vulvodynia include immune dysfunction, hormonal dysfunction, genetic factors, embryological developmental abnormalities, and neuropathic causes (Pereira et al., 2018). There is some thought that the pain of vulvodynia may be a manifestation of PN from pudendal nerve injury, but scholars recognize the need for greater investigation (Labat et al., 2008).

6. **Pelvic Floor Myofascial Pain:** In a retrospective chart review of 1,106 female subjects, Bedaiwy et al. (2013) determined a prevalence of 13.2% of the subjects experienced pelvic floor myofascial pain (PFMP). Pain in the pelvic muscles, the levator ani (LA) and the pelvic wall muscles, may be a primary source or a secondary cause of CPP due to other visceral or musculoskeletal sources. PFMP is specifically characterized by the development of trigger points (TrP), which can be latent or active. Pain from these TrPs can be difficult to discern due to the referral patterns often experienced by patients (Gyang et al., 2013). Examination with palpation of the TrPs remains the most appropriate means of diagnosis as the pain is reproduced upon palpation of the pelvic muscles.

CPP, DEPRESSION, AND TRAUMA

CPP and depression are frequently intertwined, and one concern may exacerbate the other (Ishak et al., 2018). Prevalence rates of depression among patients with chronic pain range from 30% to 54%, and this represents a marked elevation over the baseline general population rates of 5% to 17% (Gunter, 2003). While research indicates a correlation between depression, anxiety, physical and psychological traumas, and chronic pain, it is important the clinician recognize depression is not the sole cause of CPP (Carey & Moore, 2019; Ishak et al., 2018). Research has shown that the long-standing suffering from chronic pain does increase the risk for psychological distress, and adequate treatment programs for chronic pain must address treatment options for depression and anxiety (Till et al., 2019).

VISCERAL AND VISCEROSOMATIC CONVERGENCE

CPP is not a disease in isolation, as evidenced by observation of COPCs as well as the depression and anxiety connections seen among CPP sufferers. An important point of understanding, there can be an identifiable and initiating source or insult to the organ system(s) within the pelvis: the genitourinary tract system, the gastrointestinal system, or the musculoskeletal system that may trigger the causation of CPP and COPCs. Appropriate healing of these structures may occur, but it is believed that the chronicity of the pain develops when the central processing of the body's pain is abnormal (El-Nashar, 2019). This understanding represents a shift away from the traditional thinking that CPP is an end-organ disease with the current research defining CPP as neurogenic (Bruckenthal, 2011).

Pain can be either somatic, visceral, or neurogenic. Somatic sources of CPP include pain in the muscles of the pelvic floor (the LA) and the pelvic wall, fascia, ligaments, and tendons (Corton, 2005). (Discussion of the pelvic floor and pelvic wall musculature will be discussed later in this chapter). Patients may describe somatic pain as being sharp, stabbing, burning, tingling, or cutting (Gorniak & King, 2016). Visceral sources of pain arise from the organ systems in the pelvis and include the uterus, fallopian tubes, and ovaries; the bladder and urethra; and the colon and rectum (Bruckenthal, 2011). Patients may describe this type of pain as a dull, aching sensation or a throbbing, and tight or pressure like sensation (Gorniak & King, 2016). Pain of a neurogenic or neuropathic nature stems from injury to the central or peripheral nervous system and may be described as a lancing, burning pain that may also result in paresthesia, hyperalgesia, or allodynia (Ayorinde et al, 2015; Gunter, 2003).

The complexity of CPP arises from the intricate innervation of the pelvic region. To better understand the complex nature of pelvic pain, it is important to understand the concept of visceral and viscerosomatic convergence, as this concept may explain the referral patterns often seen with chronic visceral pain (Cervero, 1993). Visceral pain fibers and sympathetic nerve fibers converge with the somatic nerve fibers leading to a viscerosomatic convergence at the level of the spinal cord where noxious stimuli from the viscera converge with the somatic afferents (Carey & Moore, 2019). This convergence may allow for the muscle pain and spasms often seen with such conditions as endometriosis and provide a greater understanding of the somatic pain resulting from a visceral source (Carey & Moore, 2019; Cervero, 1993).

Bruckenthal (2011) provides greater understanding of the neurophysiology of the pelvis via further discussion of the innervation of the region. The pelvis and pelvic structures receive innervation from the spine at the level of T10–S4, with T10–L1 innervating the mid-pelvic region and S2–S4 innervating the structures deeper and more lateral within the pelvis. These extensions join into the superior hypogastric plexus to innervate the bladder. The inferior hypogastric plexus innervates the bladder

as well as the rectum, uterus, ovaries, and upper part of the vagina. Additionally, the inferior hypogastric plexus receives input at the level of sacral spinal cord, and this converging may also contribute to sensations of referred pain (Bruckenthal, 2011). See Chapter 2, Figure 2-9 Neural control of voiding.

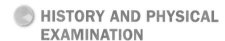 HISTORY AND PHYSICAL EXAMINATION

THE HISTORY

Determination of the source or sources of pain is crucial when working to improve the quality of life (QoL) of one experiencing CPP. Therefore, a thorough history and physical examination are crucial. Much information can be gleaned by taking a detailed and concise history as often this information may guide the progress or direction of the examination. Questions to ask include specific characteristics of the pain. Thoroughness of the query may be enhanced with use of such pain assessment mnemonics as OLDCART or OPQRST (Brooker, 2006; Friese, 2012) (**Table 12-3**). Use of comprehensive pain questionnaires may also prove helpful when obtaining an initial history and is often best completed by the patient prior to an initial appointment and discussion. Many of the commonly used questionnaires are validated for reliability and reproducibility and are good tools to assess severity or sources of pain through use of scoring systems. Furthermore, use of pain questionnaires may provide greater determination of more complex pain syndromes which may necessitate additional specialty provider care (Passavanti et al., 2017). A list of possible questionnaires including Web site locations are listed in **Table 12-3**.

Consideration of all the potential sources of pain (gynecologic, gastrointestinal, urinary, musculoskeletal, and neurologic) is paramount when initiating a discussion with the patient (**Table 12-2**). Therefore, a detailed past medical history should be completed and may help identify pain triggers, exacerbating factors, cyclical sources, and possible primary and secondary sources of pain. Discuss past surgical history and obtain information

TABLE 12-3 PAIN ASSESSMENT MNEMONICS	
OLDCART	OPQRST
O: Onset	O: Onset, gradual or sudden
L: Location	P: Provokes or Palliates
D: Duration	Q: Quality
C: Characteristics	R: Radiates
A: Aggravating factors	S: Severity
R: Relieving factors	T: Time
T: Temperature and other signs	

TABLE 12-4 PATIENT QUESTIONNAIRES AND FOOD AND ELIMINATION DIARIES AND WEB SITES	
The International Pelvic Pain Society Pelvic Health History Form	www.pelvicpain.org
Pelvic Pain and Urgency/Frequency Patient Symptom Scale (PUF) Questionnaire	www.ichelp.org
Irritable Bowel Syndrome-Specific Symptom Questionnaire: Development and Validation	www.astrazeneca.com
Patient Health Questionnaire (PHQ-9)	www.uspreventiveservicestaskforce.org
The Pelvic Pain Impact Questionnaire	https://download.lww.com/wolterskluwer_vitalstream_com/PermaLink/PAIN/A/PAIN_2016_12_02_CHALMERS_PAIN-D-14-15298_SDC2.pdf
Bowel and Bladder Diary	https://myhealth.alberta.ca/Alberta/AlbertaDocuments/bladder-bowel-diary-printable.pdf
3-Day Food Diary	https://www.ichelp.org/living-with-ic/interstitial-cystitis-and-diet/elimination-diet/food-diaries/
Menstrual Diary	http://www.pms.org.uk/assets/files/Menstrual_Chart.pdf

about any surgeries that may have been undertaken as evaluations for the pain, as means for treatment, or as potential triggers for the development of the pain. Obtain a list of current medications and ask the patient to recall any past use, as well as current use, of medications to treat the pain. Query the patient regarding these past surgical and medical interventions regarding what was beneficial and what did not prove helpful. Obtain a detailed gynecologic history to include menstrual history, obstetric history, fertility concerns, sexual pain, including insertional or deeper pain with penile penetration, or vaginal dryness. Discuss bowel and bladder function and discern if pain is increased with fecal or urinary urgency, during defecation or urination, or after elimination and evacuation. Determine if elimination of bowel or bladder contents reduces the pain. Ask the patient about frequency of bowel movements and consistency of stools. Determine day and nighttime urinary patterns. Request any records of past treatments from other providers including operative reports as these may help guide the clinician and yield further clues for causes. Ask the patient to complete a 3-day bowel or bladder diary, a food diary, or a menstrual diary. Information gleaned from these documents may provide more data and address patterns and sources of pain (**Table 12-4**).

THE PHYSICAL EXAMINATION

CPP causes are often multifactorial and physical assessment of the patient with CPP should be thorough with attention to this multifactorial nature. Any red flag or emergent findings on physical examination should be evaluated quickly and concisely (Speer et al., 2016). The examination of the patient begins at first introduction. Observe the patient's gait and posture. Is the patient leaning forward when walking, as if to shield the painful pelvic region? Does the patient ambulate slowly and carefully? Are there any abnormalities with the patient's gait? How does the patient sit? Does she lean to one side or the other while in the seated position? This may indicate a myofascial or neurologic source of the pain (Simons & Travell, 1999).

Tools needed for the physical examination should be prepared ahead of time to allow of completeness and fluidity of the examination. Such items include a split speculum, small and large cotton tipped swabs, saline, and a container to hold the saline and vaginal secretions should a microscopic examination of vaginal discharge be warranted. Other items needed may include 2% lidocaine for patients who have a pain response to the examination. Use latex free gloves and appropriate lubricant to ease the examination. See **Figure 12-2**, Tools for examination.

Abdominal Examination

Evaluate the abdomen with the patient in the supine position. Begin the examination with an initial inspection for scars or other observable signs such as distension and swelling of the bowels or bladder. Palpate for any masses, organomegaly, guarding, and tenderness to

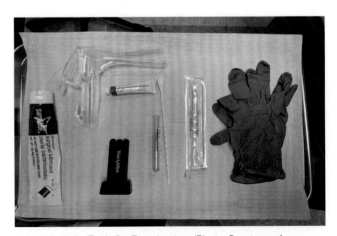

FIGURE 12-2. Tools for Examination. (Photo Courtesy of Margaret A. Hull.)

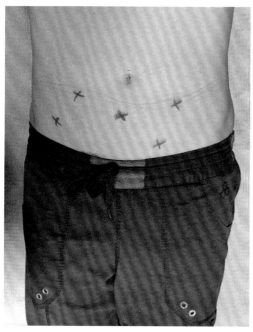

FIGURE 12-3. Abdominal Examination with TrPs Identified. (Photo courtesy of Elizabeth H. Smith.)

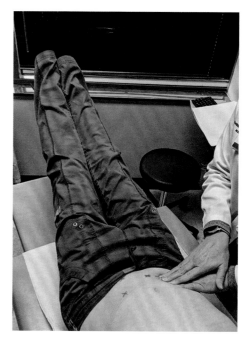

FIGURE 12-4. Carnett Test. (Photo courtesy of Elizabeth H. Smith.)

both light and deeper pressure. Palpation of the abdomen may reveal painful tender points and TrPs which are localized areas of tenderness within a tight or spasming band of muscle and are commonly found in one with PFMP (Gunter, 2003; Simons & Travell, 1999; Wolff et al., 2019). Marking the TrPs may help to guide treatment with TrP injections which will be discussed in greater detail in the treatment section of this chapter (**Fig. 12-3**).

The Carnett test may yield additional clues and help the clinician differentiate between abdominal wall or visceral pain. This test is completed with the patient in the supine position. Ask the patient to raise her legs or head; place a finger on the identified area of pain. With tension of the muscles while lifting the head or legs, TrPs may be activated to reveal a myofascial origin of pain. Pain of a visceral origin may not be as severe when performing this test (Speer et al., 2016) (**Fig. 12-4**).

Examination of the External Genitalia
This portion of the examination is completed with the patient in the lithotomy position. Begin with a general inspection for the presence or absence of pubic hair and distribution. Look for areas of scarring, erythema, rash, lesions, skin discoloration, or loss of architecture. Evaluate the vestibule and introitus of the vagina. Inspect the urethra for the presence of a urethral caruncle or other lesions or irritation. Visible changes may be associated with vulvar dermatoses, genitourinary syndrome of menopause (GSM), or inflammation and irritation from product use (Hull, 2017; Kellogg-Spadt & Albaugh, 2003). Examination of the external genitalia may reveal an absence of any visual or structural abnormalities, a

common finding among patients with vulvodynia and PN. Therefore, a neurosensory examination may yield additional information. Use of a cotton-tipped swab with application of light touch to the skin may help provide a mapping of the locations of pain. This cotton-tipped swab may also yield clues for allodynia, the experience of pain when a nonpainful stimulus is applied, which is often seen in vulvodynia (O'Dell, 2017). This same cotton-tipped swab can be used to asses for pudendal nerve injury by evaluating for areas of paresthesia or hypoesthesia (Gunter, 2003). Evaluation of the reflexes can be done by using the cotton-tipped swab and gently running it across the bilateral labia majora. The subtle movement of the skin is known as the bulbocavernosus reflex. The anal wink reflex can be seen by running the swab on either side of the anal meatus and seeing the movement or puckering of the anus and the skin around the anus (Hull & Corton, 2009; O'Dell, 2017).

Digital Examination
Using one finger, palpate the urethra to assess for pain and discharge by milking the distal portion of the urethra. This technique is completed by inserting the index finger into the vagina and applying pressure to the ventral portion of the urethra while removing the finger from the vagina. Discharge noted from the urethral meatus may indicate a urethral diverticulum or Skene gland abscess. Insertion of the finger deeper into the vagina, with the finger pointed upward and along the anterior vaginal wall, the examiner can the palpate the bladder base. Pain elicited from this and the urethral palpation portion of the examination may be indicative of interstitial cystitis/painful

bladder syndrome (IC/BPS) or urethral syndrome (Hull, 2017). Next, use the index finger and thumb to gently palpate for a mass or discomfort in the area of the Bartholin glands. Perform this part of the examination by inserting the index finger into the most distal part of the opening of the vagina and, at the 5 and 7 o'clock positions, press the thumb against the labia majora. A mass here indicates a Bartholin gland cyst, abscess, or cancer and appropriate referrals should be made.

Attention to the pelvic floor muscle (PFM) examination is paramount as muscle or myofascial pain can be an often overlooked and underevaluated source of CPP. Given the close juxtaposition of the pelvic floor and pelvic wall muscles to the pelvic viscera, speculation that muscle pain may create irritative voiding symptoms and defecatory dysfunction predominates (Meister et al., 2019; Oyama et al., 2004).

The PFMs, also called the LA, support the pelvic viscera and maintain a steady state of contraction helping the urogenital hiatus remain narrowed while drawing the distal portions of the urethra, vagina, and rectum toward the pubic bone (Hull & Corton, 2009). The LA includes the pubococcygeus, iliococcygeus, and puborectalis muscles. The pelvic wall muscles include the coccygeus, piriformis, and obturator internus (OI) muscles. While not involved in support, these muscles are important as they may be sources of CPP (Meister et al., 2019; Oyama et al., 2004). Chapter 2 provides a thorough discussion of the PFMs. See **Figures 12-5** and **12-6**.

With firm but gentle pressure, the examiner inserts one well-lubricated gloved finger into the vagina and systematically palpates each muscle layer to discern any reproduction of pain and location of the pain elicited. Palpation may reveal TrPs within the muscles and, once triggered, may create referred pain, urinary, or bowel pain (Moldwin & Fariello, 2013; Peters et al., 2007). Meister et al. (2019) have devised a standardized system of examination of the PFM and pelvic wall

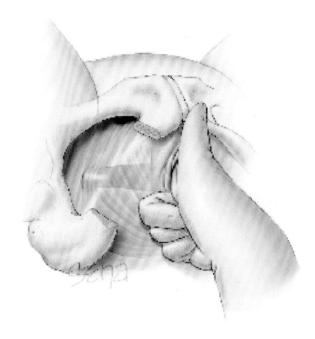

FIGURE 12-6. Digital Examination of the LA and Pelvic Wall Muscles. (Used with permission from Marie Sena, Electric Eye & Restorative Tattooing, Medical Illustrator.)

muscles. The authors recommend the examiner begin by inserting one finger into the vagina and, in a counterclockwise fashion, evaluate the muscles beginning with the right OI and ending with the left OI. With gentle pressure, the examiner sweeps the finger along the length of the muscle to determine the level of pain experienced, as noted on a visual analog scale of 0 to 10, and location of the sensation of the pain (Meister et al., 2019; Wolff et al., 2019).

The Speculum Examination

Visualization of the vaginal epithelium and cervix is important and may yield further details. This portion of the examination utilizes the split speculum to retract the vagina for visualization of these organs. Observance of abnormal vaginal or cervical discharge may warrant further testing to rule out sexually transmitted infections (STI). Inspect the vaginal epithelium for thinning and loss of rugation; observe for friable vaginal epithelium when the speculum blades open the vagina for these findings may be consistent with GSM (Gandhi et al., 2016).

The Bimanual Examination

The examiner assesses the uterus, ovaries, and adnexa by inserting two gloved fingers into the vagina, placing the tips of the fingers on the posterior aspect of the cervix and pressing against the cervix in an upward fashion. With the external hand, the examiner then palpates the uterine fundus by applying downward pressure and "cupping" the fundus with the external hand. Palpation of the ovaries is achieved by moving the vaginal fingers

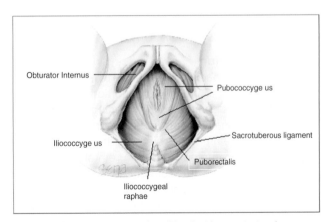

Obturator Internus

Pubococcyge us

Iliococcyge us

Sacrotuberous ligament

Puborectalis

Iliococcygeal raphae

FIGURE 12-5. The Levator Ani. (Used with permission from Marie Sena, Electric Eye & Restorative Tattooing, Medical Illustrator.)

into the right and the left of the sides of the cervix at the deepest portion of the vagina. The examiner then sweeps the external hand downward against the gloved fingers, attempting to palpate each ovary with the intravaginal finger. Pain noted during this part of the examination may indicate adenomyosis, uterine leiomyomas, ovarian cysts, and endometriosis.

The Rectal Examination

Examination of the anus and rectum can be an uncomfortable experience for a patient. For the patient who suffers from CPP, the rectal examination can be potentially more difficult. Clear discussion with permission from the patient must first occur before the examiner begins this portion of the evaluation. Gently separate the buttocks and observe for any lesions, masses, or hemorrhoids. Insert a well-lubricated gloved finger into the anal canal and palpate for any internal masses. Evaluate the tone and strength of the anal sphincter as well as the strength of contraction.

DIAGNOSTIC TESTING AND REFERRALS

Evaluation of acute, curative concerns should be undertaken with appropriate referrals for emergent sources of pain. Urine culture with a microscopic analysis should be obtained with careful attention to specimen collection to avoid contamination (Fletcher & Zimmern, 2009). Obtain additional cultures, including gonorrhea, chlamydia, mycoplasma, and ureaplasma. Obtain a vaginal wet mount specimen for microscopic examination for trichomoniasis, candidiasis, bacterial vaginosis, desquamative inflammatory vaginitis (DIV), and GSM. Among reproductive-aged women, the clinician should obtain information on the last menstrual period (LMP) and obtain a urine pregnancy test (Bruckenthal, 2011). If the clinician suspects the source of pain to be gynecologic, a pelvic ultrasound for further evaluation of the uterus, cervix, and ovaries should be considered. Use of this imaging modality may yield further clues for pelvic congestion syndrome, ovarian cysts, and uterine leiomyomas (Tjong & Oppenheimer, 2019). While this test is not diagnostic for endometriosis, the presence of endometriomas or "chocolate cysts" on the ovaries may be indicative for endometriosis, warranting further evaluation (Nisenblat et al., 2016).

No consistent tests exist for diagnosis of IC/BPS. Recognition of the poor reliability of cystoscopy in the diagnosis of IC/BPS has helped to transition the diagnostic plan for IC/BPS to a symptom-based approach (Fletcher & Zimmern, 2009). However, computerized tomography (CT) scan of the abdomen and pelvis, with and without contrast, may provide confirmation of other visceral abnormalities such as carcinomas, renal calculi, inflammatory bowel diseases, hernias, and abscesses. Consider a referral for urology or urogynecology evaluation

with cystourethroscopy and video urodynamics to further characterize the bladder anatomy and function and to rule out urothelial cancers (Fletcher & Zimmern, 2009). If gastrointestinal concerns (GI) predominate, consider a consult to a GI specialist for further evaluation of inflammatory bowel disease or GI cancers.

MANAGEMENT OPTIONS

Given the difficulty of diagnosis of CPP, it is not uncommon that many patients are left untreated or inadequately treated, often receiving a psychiatric diagnosis as the source of the pain. As stated previously, patients who experience CPP may have coexisting psychiatric illnesses that require treatment. However, this should not be considered the only issue requiring management.

Management of CPP must include a discussion on goal setting as this is a key concept to help the patient understand treatment options are not curative. Goals for a reduction of pain or greater pain free days may be more achievable for the patient. Reinforce with the patient the chronicity of the problem and, while effective, treatment options may take time before beneficial effects are seen. Review the benefits of the establishment of a multidisciplinary team of caregivers to provide the best opportunity for success.

CONSERVATIVE THERAPIES

Behavioral Therapy

Recent research has described as many as 90% of women with IC/BPS have dietary sensitivies, and avoidance of these bladder irritants may prove helpful at mitigating painful flares (Hayden et al., 2019). See **Table 12-5** for a listing of IC/BPS high-risk foods. Patients who have CPP from resulting functional GI disturbances, such as IBS, may benefit from supplementation of dietary fiber, such as psyllium husk, and a daily probiotic (Fukudo et al., 2015). Reduction of specific sugars including fermentable oligosaccharides, disaccharides, monosaccharides, and polyols (FODMAPS), and increased water intake may provide greater consistency and frequency of bowel movements and reduction of painful bloating (Catassi et al., 2017); see **Table 12-6** for a listing of IBS high-risk foods. While elimination of gluten is important for one with celiac disease, or nonceliac gluten sensitivities (NCGS), recent research postulates elimination of gluten from the diet may reduce both IC/BPS and IBS flares (Catassi et al., 2017; Chao et al., 2015).

Patients who suffer from the vulvo-vaginal pain of vulvodynia or PFMP may benefit from perineal care and reduction of provocative agents that increase pain. Such lifestyle modifications may include the use of cotton undergarments, avoidance of constrictive clothing, cessation of skin products in the perineal area, and application of cool compresses or use of sitz baths during painful flares.

TABLE 12-5 THE IC/BPS DIET
HIGHEST RISK FOODS AND CONDIMENTS
Citrus: oranges, grapefruit, lemons, limes
Pineapple
Strawberries
Tomato and tomato-based foods
Yogurt
Soy and soy sauce
Processed meats
Pickles
Spicy foods/chili peppers/chili powder
Ketchup
Salad dressings
Vinegar
Artificial sweeteners
MSG
HIGHEST RISK BEVERAGES
Alcohol
Grapefruit juice
Orange juice
Coffee
Tea
Carbonated sodas
Artificially sweetened/flavored fruit drinks

TABLE 12-6 THE IBS FODMAP ELIMINATION DIET	
FRUCTOSE RICH FOODS: MONOSACCHARIDES	**LACTOSE RICH FOODS: DISACCHARIDES**
Apples	Cow's milk
Pears	Yogurt
Peaches	Ice cream
Cherries	Cottage and ricotta cheese
Mangoes	Puddings and custards
Watermelon	
Honey	
Food containing high fructose corn syrup	
FRUCTANS AND GOS: OLIGOSACCHARIDES	**POLYOLS: SORBITOL AND MANNITOL**
Asparagus	Cauliflower
Brussels sprouts	Mushrooms
Broccoli	Snow peas
Onions	Sweeteners found in sugar free
Artichokes	Gum, cough mints, cough medicines
Wheat	
Rye	
Chickpeas	
Lentils	
Kidney beans	
Soy products	

Other therapeutic behavioral treatments for CPP may include timed voiding, bladder or bowel training, therapeutic massage, yoga, cognitive therapy with a cognitive/behavioral therapist, meditation, guided imagery, and acupuncture (Huang et al., 2017; Malde et al., 2018; Nezhat et al., 2019).

Physical Therapy

Pelvic floor physical therapy (PFPT) has been shown to improve many of the inciting sources of CPP (Hibner et al., 2010). Given the strong viscerosomatic connections of CPP, it is important to offer PFPT to all patients with CPP (Bruckenthal, 2011; Carey & Moore, 2019). It is also important to educate patients to the benefits of PFPT. While strengthening of the PFM is very important for treatment of urinary and fecal incontinence, the goals of PFPT for CPP due to PFMP emphasizes muscle relaxation or "down-training," stretching, postural corrections, and improvement of range of motion of the hips, pelvis, and back (Hibner et al., 2010; O'Dell, 2017). Other therapeutic modalities may include Thiele's massage, TrP release or massage, ischemic compression, biofeedback, electrical stimulation, ultrasound therapy or diathermy, abdominal core strengthening, deep breathing exercises, and mindfulness (Hull & Corton, 2009; O'Dell, 2017).

Pharmacologic Management

Pharmacologic management comprises a wide range of options, such as topical agents, over-the-counter and prescriptive oral (PO) agents, injectables, and instillations. Discussion will begin with a review of the PO agents most frequently recommended and will transition to non-PO agents. For a listing of medications, see **Table 12-7**.

Over-the-counter (OTC) analgesics are considered first-line options for the management of CPP. Acetaminophen and nonsteroidal anti-inflammatory medicines (NSAIDs), such as ibuprofen or naproxen, may prove beneficial for mild to moderate pain (Bruckenthal, 2011). Interestingly, basic science research on rat prostates showed greater penetration of NSAIDs into the tissue. While this is research based on a male animal model, it is reasonable to assume women with CPP may benefit from NSAID use as well (Santharam et al., 2019). However, evidence reveals that these medications may not be as effective in the treatment of pain resulting from endometriosis prevails. Medication management for CPP that is suspected to be originating from endometriosis includes combined oral contraceptives (COC), progestin-only pills, such as

TABLE 12-7 PHARMACOLOGIC TREATMENT OPTIONS

AGENT	INDICATIONS	MECHANISM OF ACTION	SIDE EFFECTS	APRN CONSIDERATIONS
Acetaminophen	Mild to moderate pain	Central acting; Inhibits prostaglandin	GI upset; pruritus	Monitor liver function—especially with liver impairment; monitor for Stevens-Johnson syndrome
OTC NSAIDs: Ibuprofen, Naproxen	Mild to moderate pain; arthritis; dysmenorrhea	Anti-inflammatory; inhibits prostaglandin	GI upset	Caution in older adults; GI upset; blood thinner. Black Box Warning
Prescriptive NSAIDs: Meloxicam	Moderate to severe pain. Arthritic pain	Anti-inflammatory; inhibits prostaglandin	GI upset	Caution in older adults; GI upset; blood thinner. Black Box Warning
Capsaicin cream	Musculoskeletal pain; neuralgia/neuropathic pain	Topical	Burning pain	OTC: Caution regarding burning pain—typically improves after several days of use
Lidocaine ointment, gel; Lidoderm patch	Local acting pain control; neuralgia	Topical	Skin irritation	May cause local skin irritation, daily or PRN use
Tricyclic antidepressant: Amitriptyline, Nortriptyline	FDA approval for depression. Useful for neuropathic pain	Inhibits reuptake of norepinephrine and serotonin	Somnolence; Dry mouth; anticholinergic side effects	Nonaddictive; reduced anxiety; improved sleep; monitor depressive symptoms
Anticonvulsant: Gabapentin, Pregabalin	Neuropathic pain	Interrupts calcium ion channels at postsynaptic dorsal horns to reduce neuropathic pain	Somnolence	Renal failure cautions; must titrate dose
Antihistamines: Hydroxyzine	May reduce pain of IC/BPS; vulvodynia	Blocks H1 histamine receptor	Somnolence; dizziness; dry mouth	Monitor slurring of speech: may cause paradoxical reactions
Pentosan polysulfate	FDA approved for IC/BPS	Binds to bladder urothelium replenish GAG layer; may stabilize mast cells	Diarrhea; hair loss	Mild blood thinner; may take 2-6 months to be effective; TID dosing on empty stomach

Micronor, implantable progestin-only intrauterine devices (Mirena®, Skyla®, Kyleena®), gonadal-releasing hormone (GnRH) agonists, antagonists, and aromatase inhibitors (Nezhat et al., 2019).

Additional pharmacologic options include tricyclic antidepressants such as amitriptyline, imipramine, or nortriptyline with the recommendation to begin with the lowest dose and gradually titrate upward. While not approved by the Food and Drug Administration for CPP, these drugs may reduce the sensation of pain through action on the descending inhibitory neuro pathways to effectively alter the pain response (O'Dell, 2017). Amitriptyline, the most commonly used drug of the tricyclics, has a grade A or B recommendation for use in treatment of IC/BPS (Malde et al., 2018). Use of tricyclic antidepressants may also reduce the pain associated with IBS, PN, and vulvodynia; however, evidence is lacking with few studies with small numbers yielding inconclusive results and high placebo effects (Gunter, 2003; Hoffstetter & Shah, 2015).

Pentosan polysulfate (PPS) is the only FDA-approved medication for the treatment of IC/BPS. However, use of this medication can be cost prohibitive for many patients with realization of therapeutic effects possibly delayed up to six months (O'Dell, 2017). PPS is a mild anticoagulant, therefore it is important to counsel patients with coagulopathies who may be on other blood-thinning medications about this. It is also advisable to collaborate with the patient's other providers to minimize risks of bleeding.

Anticonvulsant medications may help reduce the pain with CPP and are considered first-line therapies for the treatment of PN (Hibner et al., 2010). However, much like research for tricyclic antidepressants, most studies are observational and limited by few numbers. A recent randomized, crossover, placebo-controlled trial of 89 women (45 were randomized to gabapentin first and 44 were randomized to placebo first) showed no reduction of pain among study participants when compared to placebo, prompting the investigators to discourage use of gabapentin for the treatment of vulvodynia (Brown et al., 2018). Pregabalin in a titrated dose, along with muscle relaxant medications, such as cyclobenzaprine HCL, may prove beneficial for treatment of PN (Hibner et al., 2010).

After extensive safety trials, the selective serotonin-4 agonist (5-HT$_4$), tegaserod, was reapproved by the US Food and Drug Administration (USFDA) for the treatment of IBS-C and in late 2019, tenapanor, sodium/hydrogen exchanger 3 (NHE3) inhibitor, was approved for use in adults (Chey et al., 2020; Pharmacy Times, 2019; Prichard & Bharucha, 2018). These medications work by reducing pain and bloating and improving stool consistency and frequency by decreasing colonic transit time. Other approved medications for IBS-C include linaclotide, plecanatide, and lubiprostone (Pimental, 2016; Prichard & Bharucha, 2018). 5-HT$_3$ receptor antagonists for the treatment of IBS-D can be highly effective. Alosetron is indicated for use in women only and carries a black box warning with advisement to discontinue use if constipation develops. Emergent evaluation is required if the constipation does not resolve with discontinuation due to the increased risk for ischemic colitis. Other FDA-approved drugs for IBS-D include a short course of rifaximin (an antibiotic that alters gut microbiota) and eluxadoline (a mu- and kappa-opioid receptor agonist and a delta-opioid receptor antagonist) that slows gut transit time (Cash et al., 2016; Fragkos, 2017). Eluxadoline is contraindicated in individuals without a gallbladder due to the risk of pancreatitis and sphincter of Oddi spasms (Levio & Cash, 2017). The latter two agents should be considered first-line therapy for IBS-D if lifestyle modification and OTC medications proved to be ineffectual (Levio & Cash, 2017). It is advised to exhaust all other therapies before considering initiation of alosetron (Friedel et al., 2001; Levio & Cash, 2017).

Frequent or consistent use of narcotic pain medications for the treatment of CPP is discouraged with recommendations for limited use during crisis only or in collaboration with prescription drug monitoring programs (PDMP). Recommendations to follow include use of these medications for the shortest duration possible in the lowest dose available to achieve adequate relief (American Urological Association Position Statement: Opioid Use, 2019).

Topical Medications, Intramuscular Injections, and Intravesical Instillations

Administration of topical, intramuscular, or intravesical medications may prove helpful with greater tolerability over oral agents. Pain from vulvodynia may be reduced with application of topical analgesics such as lidocaine gel, with most studies recommending use in the 5% dose, or low dose corticosteroids such as 0.5% hydrocortisone cream. If using high-potency corticosteroids, such as clobetasol ointment, recommendations are cautious, with advisement to follow a short-term regimen. Though data are lacking, there are some reports of application and benefits of topical estradiol 0.01% and testosterone 0.1%. Capsaicin cream may provide benefit through desensitization and may be a possible option if the first-line topical options fail (Goldstein et al., 2016). Providers may choose to consider topical compounded options of amitriptyline and gabapentin by working with a trusted compounding pharmacist to enable patients avoid the unsatisfactory

side effects of dry mouth, constipation, and drowsiness that are so common with these medications. However, there are very minimal data to support this practice.

Intravesical instillations can include administration of various cocktails of agents via a small or pediatric catheter. These medications include heparin, steroids (triamcinolone or Solu-Cortef), and analgesics (lidocaine or bupivacaine) (American Urological Association & Society of Urologic Nurses and Associate Joint Statement on Intravesical Administration of Therapeutic Medication, 2015). The European Urological Association (EAU) has given a grade A level recommendation to the intravesical administration of lidocaine, sodium bicarbonate, and pentosan polysulfate for treatment of IC/BPS (Malde et al., 2018). Little evidence exists on timing or duration of a treatment series. Many practices may choose to provide weekly instillations up to 8 weeks duration.

While evidence is limited, TrP injections into the LA or pelvic wall muscles may provide temporary benefit by providing a numbing effect and may be helpful prior to PFPT (O'Dell, 2017). Cocktails for TrP injections may include any combination of lidocaine 1%, bupivacaine 25%, and triamcinolone and can be provided in multiple sites of the LA and pelvic wall muscles. Medication dosages can vary, with reports of as little as 1 to 2 milliliters (mL) into each affected muscle up to 5 to 10 mL per muscle (Langford et al., 2007).

SURGICAL MANAGEMENT

Laparoscopic identification and removal of extra-endometrial implants with histologic confirmation remains the primary diagnostic tool as well as a common endometriosis treatment modality for women who have failed or received inadequate benefits from medical management or when the clinician has a high suspicion for disease based on history and examination findings (Gunter, 2003; Mahnert, 2019).

Cystoscopy with hydrodistention, with or without transurethral fulguration of Hunner lesions, is a third-line option that may provide diagnostic and symptom relief for patients with IC/BPS. However, there is limited evidence for the efficacy of this procedure (Malde et al., 2018).

Recent evidence of benefits of intradetrusor onabotulinum toxin A (BTX-A) has prompted the American Urologic Association (AUA) to amend the IC/BPS guideline to include this therapy using the 100-unit BTX-A dose under cystoscopic guidance and in combination with hydrodistension (Hanno et al., 2015). It is important to educate patients of the life span of BTX-A and a clear discussion of need for retreatments is necessary. Use of BTX-A in the LA has not been shown to be superior to placebo at reduction of pain symptoms. However, it does remain a possible treatment option for a select group (Dessie et al., 2019).

A pudendal nerve block under CT guidance may prove to be both a diagnostic as well as a therapeutic treatment option for PN. Little definitive guidance is available, but nerve blocks can be offered in a series up to three, typically six weeks apart, and can be unilateral or bilateral. Cocktails may include bupivacaine and triamcinolone (Hibner et al., 2010).

Vestibulectomy is considered a last line option for treatment of nonresponsive or poorly responsive vulvodynia, yet this procedure is considered the most effective available treatment option (Goldstein et al., 2016). In a recent study of 22 patients who underwent modified vestibulectomy, Das et al. (2020) noted 94% of patients experienced a reduction of pain and 79% reported satisfaction with the surgery. Despite the small number of subjects, the authors note this is consistent with prior reports of successful treatment.

Light amplification by stimulated emission of radiation (LASER) may show promise for treatment of some vulvar diseases, specifically GSM. However, this therapy has not been shown to be effective for the treatment of vulvodynia and is not recommended at this time (Preti et al., 2019).

NURSING CONSIDERATIONS

APRNs and continence specialists have a unique opportunity to guide the evaluation and management of patients with CPP. Debilitating flares can be frequent and significantly impacting of patients' QoL and care from expert nursing management is vital as these patients require multiple specialty appointments and frequent visits for routine management to achieve success. It is also important to remember the psychological and sexual treatment needs of this patient population, and ongoing assessment should be maintained as patients progress through the different treatment phases. With greater research and multispecialty collaboration, greater beneficial treatments may positively impact this difficult to treat population.

REFERENCES

Ackerman, A. L., Lai, H. H., Parameshwar, P. S., et al. (2018). Symptomatic overlap in overactive bladder and interstitial cystitis/bladder pain syndrome: Development of a new algorithm. *BJU International, 123*(4), 682–893.

ACOG Committee on Practice Bulletin. (2004). ACOG practice bulletin No. 51: Chronic pelvic pain. *Obstetrics & Gynecology, 103*(3), 589–605.

American Urological Association Board of Directors. (2019). AUA position statement: Opioid use. Retrieved from www:auanet.org/guidelines/opioid-use

American Urological Association and Society of Urologic Nurses and Associates Joint Statement on Intravesical Administration of Therapeutic Medication. (2015). Retrieved from www.suna.org/resources/intravesicalMedAdminStatement.pdf

As-Sanie, S., Black, R., Giudice, L. C., et al. (2019). Assessing research gaps and unmet needs in endometriosis. *American Journal of Obstetrics and Gynecology, 221*(2), 86–94. doi: 10.1016/j.ajog.2019.02.033.

Ayorinde, A. A., Macfarlane, G. J., Saraswat, L., et al. (2015). Chronic pelvic pain in women: An epidemiological perspective. *Future Medicine, 11*(6), 851–864. doi.org/10.2217/whe.15.30.

Bedaiwy, M. A., Patterson, B., & Mahajan, S. (2013). Prevalence of myofascial chronic pelvic pain and the effectiveness of pelvic floor physical therapy. *The Journal of Reproductive Medicine, 58*(11), 504–510.

Birder, L. A. (2019). Pathophysiology of interstitial cystitis. *International Journal of Urology, 26*(Suppl 1), 12–15. doi: 10.1111/iju.13985.

Bornstein, J., Preti, M., Simon, J. A., et al. (2019). Descriptors of vulvodynia: A multisocietal definition consensus (International Society for the Study of Vulvovaginal Disease, the International Society for the Study of Women Sexual Health, and the International Pelvic Pain Society). *Journal of Lower Genital Tract Disease, 23*(2), 161–163. doi.org/10.1097/LGT.000000000000461.

Brooker, E. (2006). Acute abdominal pain assessment. *Nursing Standard, 21*(12), 59.

Brown, C. S., Bachmann, G. A., Wan, J., et al. (2018). Gabapentin for the treatment of vulvodynia: A randomized controlled trial. *Obstetrics & Gynecology, 131*, 1000–1007.

Bruckenthal, P. (2011). Chronic pelvic pain: Approaches to diagnosis and treatment. *Pain Management Nursing, 12*(1), S4–S10. doi.org/10.1016/j.pmn.2010.11.004.

Carey, E. T., & Moore, K. (2019). Updates in the approach to chronic pelvic pain: What the treating gynecologist should know. *Clinical Obstetrics and Gynecology, 62*(4), 666–676.

Cash, B. D., Lacy, B. E., Rao, T., et al. (2016). Rifaximin and eluxadoline—Newly approved treatments for diarrhea-predominant irritable bowel syndrome: What is their role in clinical practice alongside alosetron? *Expert Opinion on Pharmacotherapy, 17*(3), 311–322. doi.org/10.1517/14656566.2016.1118052.

Catassi, C., Alaedini, A., Bojarski, C., et al. (2017). The overlapping area of non-celiac gluten sensitivity (NCGS) and wheat-sensitive irritable bowel syndrome (IBS): An Update. *Nutrients, 9*(11), 1–16. doi.org/10.3390/nu9111268.

Cervero, F. (1993). Viscerosomatic convergence. *American Physical Society Journal, 2*(4), 2520255.

Chao, M. T., Abercrombie, P. D., Nakagawa, S., et al. (2015). Prevalence and use of complementary health approaches among women with chronic pelvic pain in a prospective cohort study. *Pain Medicine, 16*(2), 328–340. doi.org/10.1111/pme.12585.

Chey, W. D., Lembo, A. J., & Rosenbaum, D. P. (2020). Efficacy of tenapanor in treating patients with irritable bowel syndrome with constipation: A 12-week, placebo-controlled phase 3 trial ((T3MP)-1). *American Journal of Gastroenterology, 115*(2), 281–293. doi.org/10.14309/ajg.0000000000000516.

Corton, M. M. (2005). Anatomy of the pelvis: Howe the pelvis is built for support. *Clinical Obstetrics and Gynecology, 48*(3), 611–626.

Das, D., Davidson, E. R. W., Walters, M., et al. (2020). Patient-centered outcomes after modified vestibulectomy. *Obstetrics & Gynecology, 135*(1), 113–121. doi.org/10.1097/AOG.0000000000003596.

Dessie, S. G., Von Bargen, E., Hacker, M. R., et al. (2019). A randomized, double-blind, placebo-controlled trial of onabotulinumtoxin A trigger point injections for myofascial pelvic pain. *American Journal of Obstetrics & Gynecology, 221*(5), 517.e1–517.e9. doi: 10.1016/j.ajog.2019.06.044.

El-Nashar, S. A. (2019). What is new in chronic pelvic pain research: Best articles from the past year. *Obstetrics & Gynecology, 134*(2), 413–415. doi: 10.1097/AOG. 0000000000003387.

Fall, M., Baranowski, A. P., Elneil, S., et al. (2010). EAU guidelines on chronic pelvic pain. *European Urology, 57*(1), 35–48. doi.org/10.1016/j.eururo.2009.08.020.

Fletcher, S. G., & Zimmern, P. E. (2009). Differential diagnosis of chronic pelvic pain in women: The urologist's approach. *Nature Reviews Urology, 6*, 557–562. doi.org/10.1038/nrurol.2009.178.

Fragkos, K. C. (2017). Spotlight on eluxadoline for the treatment of patients with irritable bowel syndrome with diarrhea. *Clinical and Experimental Gastroenterology, 10*, 229–240. doi.org/10.2147/CEG.S12362120.

Friedel, D., Thomas, R., & Fisher, R. S. (2001). Ischemic colitis during treatment with alosetron. *Gastroenterology, 120*(2), 557–560. doi.org/10/1053/gast.2001.21177.

Friese, G. (2012). OPQRST: A mnemonic for pain assessment. Retrieved from https://everydayemstips.com/opqrst-a-mnemonic-for-pain-assessment

Fukudo, S., Kaneko, H., Akiho, H., et al. (2015). Evidence-based clinical practice guidelines for irritable bowel syndrome. *Journal of Gastroenterology, 50*(1), 11–30. doi.org/10.1007/s00535-014-1016-1.

Gandhi, J., Chen, A., Dagur, G., et al. (2016). Genitourinary syndrome of menopause: An overview of clinical manifestations, pathophysiology, etiology, evaluation, and management. *American Journal of Obstetrics & Gynecology, 215*(6), 704–711. doi.org/10.1016/j.ajog.2016.07.045.

Garcia-Perez, H., Harlow, S. D., Erdmann, C. A., et al. (2010). Pelvic pain and associated characteristics among women in northern Mexico. *International Perspectives on Sexual and Reproductive Health, 36*(2), 90–98.

Goldstein, A. T., Pukall, C. F., Brown, C., et al. (2016). Vulvodynia: Assessment and treatment. *The Journal of Sexual Medicine, 13*, 572–590. doi.org/10.1016/j.jsxm.2016.01.020.

Gorniak, G., & King P. M. (2016). The peripheral neuroanatomy of the pelvic floor. *Journal of Women's Health Physical Therapy, 40*(1), 3–14. doi.org/10.1097/JWH.0000000000000044.

Gunter, J. (2003). Chronic pelvic pain: An integrated approach to diagnosis and treatment. *Obstetrical and Gynecological Survey, 58*(9), 615–623.

Gyang, A., Hartman, M., & Lamvu, G. (2013). Musculoskeletal causes of chronic pelvic pain: What every gynecologist should know. *Obstetrics & Gynecology, 121*(3), 645–650. doi:10.1097/AOG.0b013e318283ffea.

Hanno, P., Erickson, D., Moldwin, R., et al. (2015). Diagnosis and treatment of interstitial cystitis/bladder pain syndrome: AUA guideline amendment. *The Journal of Urology, 193*(5), 1545–1552. doi:10.1016/j.juro.2015.01.086.

Hayden, C. L., Gilbert, K. L., & Bryden, P. A. (2019). Factors influencing interstitial cystitis flares in women. *Urologic Nursing, 39*(3), 119–132. doi.org/10.7257/1053-816X.2019.39.3.119.

Hibner, M., Desai, N., Robertson, L. J., et al. (2010). Pudendal neuralgia. *The Journal of Minimally Invasive Gynecology, 17*, 148–153. doi.org/10.1016/j.jmig.2009.11.003.

Hoffstetter, S., & Shah, M. (2015). Vulvodynia. *Clinical Obstetrics and Gynecology, 58*(3), 536–545.

Huang, A. J., Rowen, T. S., Abercrombie, P., et al. (2017). Development and feasibility of a group-based therapeutic yoga program for women with chronic pelvic pain. *Pain Medicine, 18*(10), 1864–1872. doi:10.1093/pm/pnw306.

Hull, M. A. (2017). Assessment of women. In V. W. Welch (Ed.), *Core curriculum for urologic nursing* (pp. 235–246). Pittman, NJ: Anthony J. Jannetti, Inc.

Hull, M. A., & Corton, M. M. (2009). Evaluation of the levator ani and pelvic wall muscles in levator ani syndrome. *Urologic Nursing, 29*(4), 225–231.

Humes-Goff, D., & Klima, C. (2015). The effect of a clinical practice guideline for acute pelvic pain on length of stay in the emergency department. *Advanced Emergency Nursing Journal, 37*(3), 223–232. doi:10.1097/TME.0000000000000070.

International Association for the Study of Pain. (2018). IASP terminology. Retrieved from www.iasp-pain.org/terminology?navItemNumber=576#Pain

Ishak, W. W., Wen, R. Y., Naghdechi, L., et al. (2018). Pain and depression: A systematic review. *Harvard Review of Psychiatry, 26*(6), 352–363.

Kellogg-Spadt, S., & Albaugh, J. (2003). External genital and dermatologic examination part 1: The female patient. *Urologic Nursing, 23*(4), 305–306.

Labat, J. J., Riant, T., Robert, R., et al. (2008). Diagnostic criteria for pudendal neuralgia by pudendal nerve entrapment (Nantes Criteria). *Neurourology and Urodynamics, 27*(4), 306–310. doi.org/10.1002/nau.

Langford, C. F., Udvari, S. U., & Ghoniem, G. M. (2007). Levator ani trigger point injections: An underutilized treatment for chronic pelvic pain. *Neurourology and Urodynamics, 26*, 59–62.

Levio, S., & Cash, B. D. (2017). The place of eluxadoline in the management of irritable bowel syndrome with diarrhea. *Therapeutic Advances in Gastroenterology, 10*(9), 715–725. doi.org/10.1177/1756283X17721152.

Lyons, R., & Koneti, K. (2019). Surgical management for chronic pain. *Surgery, 37*(8), 472–477.

Mahnert, N. (2019). Video cafes: Surgical assessment of chronic pelvic pain. *American Journal of Obstetrics & Gynecology, Supplement*, S781.

Malde, S., Palmisani, S., Al-Kaisy, A., et al. (2018). Guideline of guidelines: Bladder pain syndrome. *BJU International, 122*(5), 729–743. doi:10.1111/bju.14399.

Mathias, S. D., Kuppermann, M., Liberman, R. F., et al. (1996). Chronic pelvic pain: Prevalence, health-related quality of like, and economic correlates. *Obstetrics & Gynecology, 87*(3), 321–327.

Meister, M. R., Sutcliffe, S., Badu, A., et al. (2019). Pelvic floor myofascial pain severity and pelvic floor disorder symptom bother: Is there a correlation? *American Journal of Obstetrics & Gynecology, 235*, e1–e15. doi.org/10.1016/j.ajog.2019.07.020.

Moldwin, R. M., & Fariello, J. Y. (2013). Myofascial trigger points of the pelvic floor: Associations with urological pain syndromes and treatment strategies including injection therapy. *Current Urology Reports, 14*, 409–417. doi.org/10.1007/s11934-013-0360-7.

Nezhat, C., Vang, N., Tanaka, P. P., et al. (2019). Optimal management of endometriosis and pain. *Obstetrics & Gynecology, 134*(4), 834–839. doi.org/10.1097/AOG.0000000000003461.

Nisenblat, V., Bossuyt, P. M. M., Farquhar, C., et al. (2016). Imaging modalities for the non-invasive diagnosis of endometriosis. *Cochrane Database of Systematic Reviews, 2*(2), CD009591. doi.org/10.1002/14651858.CD009591.pub2.

O'Dell, K. K. (2017). Bladder and pelvic pain syndromes. In V. W. Welch (Ed.), *Core curriculum for urologic nursing* (pp. 545–562). Pittman, NJ: Anthony J. Jannetti, Inc.

Oyama, I. A., Rejba, A., Lukban, J. C., et al. (2004). Modified Thiele massage as therapeutic intervention for female patients with interstitial cystitis and high-tone pelvic floor dysfunction. *Adult Urology, 64*, 862–865. doi.org/10.1016/j.urolgy.2004.06.65.

Passavanti, M. B., Pota, V., Sansone, P., et al. (2017). Chronic pelvic pain: Assessment, evaluation, and objectivation. *Pain Research and Treatment, 2017*, 1–15. doi.org/10/1155/2017/9472925.

Pereira, G. M., Marcolino, M. S., Reis, Z. M., et al. (2018). A systematic review of drug treatment of vulvodynia: Evidence of a strong placebo effect. *British Journal of Obstetrics & Gynaecology, 125*(10), 1216–1224. doi:10.1111/1471-0528.15223.

Perkins, A. (2019). The silent pain of endometriosis. *Nursing Made Incredibly Easy, 17*(3), 26–33. doi.org/10.1097/01.NME.0000554597.81822.03.

Peters, K. M., Carrico, D. J., Kalinowski, S. E., et al. (2007). Prevalence of pelvic floor dysfunction in patients with interstitial cystitis. *Urology, 70*(1), 16–18. doi.org/10.1016/j.urology.2007.02.067.

Pharmacy Times. (2019). Drug treatment for irritable bowel syndrome with constipation granted FDA approval. Retrieved from https://www.pharmacytimes.com/news/drug-treatment-for-irritable-bowel-syndrome-with-constipation-granted-fda-approval

Pimental, M. (2016). Clinical update: Advances in irritable bowel syndrome. *Gastroenterology & Hepatology, 12*(7), 442–445.

Preti, M., Vieira-Baptista, M. D., Digesu, G. A., et al. (2019). The clinical role of LASER for vulvar and vaginal treatments in gynecology and female urology: An ICS/ISSVD best practice consensus document. *Journal of Lower Genital Tract Disease, 23*(2), 151–160. doi.org/10.1097/LGT.000000000000462.

Prichard, D. O., & Bharucha, A. E. (2018). Recent advances in understanding and managing chronic constipation. *F1000Research, 7,* F1000 Faculty Rev-1640. doi.org/10.12688/f1000research.15900.1.

Santharam, M. A., Khan, F. U., Naveed, M., et al. (2019). Interventions to chronic prostatitis/chronic pelvic pain syndrome treatment. Where are we standing and what's next? *European Journal of Pharmacology, 857,* 1–13.

Simons, D. G., & Travell, J. G. (1999). Pelvic floor muscles. In J. P. Butler (Ed.), *Myofascial pain and dysfunction: The trigger point manual* (1st ed., pp. 110–131). Philadelphia, PA: Lippincott Williams & Wilkins.

Speer, L. M., Mushkbar, S., & Erberle, T. (2016). Chronic pelvic pain in women. *American Family Physician, 93*(5), 380–387.

Sutcliffe, S., Gallop, R., Hing-Hung, H. L., et al. (2019). A longitudinal analysis of urological chronic pelvic pain syndrome flares in the multidisciplinary approach to the study of chronic pelvic pain (MAPP) research network. *British Journal of Urology International, 124,* 522–531.

Till, S. R., As-Sanie, S., & Schrepf, A. (2019). Psychology of chronic pelvic pain: Prevalence, neurobiological, vulnerabilities, and treatment. *Clinical Obstetrics and Gynecology, 62*(1), 22–36.

Tjong, W., & Oppenheimer, D. C. (2019). Imaging of venous diseases in the abdomen and pelvis. *Contemporary Diagnostic Radiology, 42*(8), 1–8.

Wolff, B. J., Joyce, C. J., Brincat, C. A., et al. (2019). Pelvic floor myofascial pain in patients with symptoms of urinary tract infection. *International Journal of Gynecology and Obstetrics, 145,* 205–211. doi.org/10.1002/ilgo.12784

Zondervan, K. T., Yudkin, P. L., Vessey, M. P., et al. (2001). Chronic pelvic pain in the community-Symptoms, investigations, and diagnoses. *American Journal of Obstetrics and Gynecology, 184*(6), 1149–1155.

QUESTIONS

1. Palpation of these tender spots within a muscle indicates a myofascial nature of chronic pelvic pain. What are these tender spots called?
A. Sebaceous cysts
B. Trigger points
C. Muscle spasms
D. Tender points

2. Chronic overlapping pain conditions and other comorbid conditions frequently seen in patients who have CPP include the following except
A. Temporomandibular disorder
B. Urinary tract infections
C. Migraine headaches
D. Chronic fatigue syndrome

3. Which physical examination technique may help differentiate between visceral pain and abdominal wall pain?
A. Carnett sign
B. Palpation
C. Murphy sign
D. McBurney sign

4. Endometriosis causes which of the following?
A. Regular, heavy, but painless menstrual cycles
B. Amenorrhea
C. Painful menstrual cycles
D. Consistently irregular and heavy menstrual cycles

5. Medications for treatment of diarrhea predominant irritable bowel syndrome include the following:
A. Eluxadoline
B. Pentosan polysulfate
C. Micronor
D. Lubiprostone

6. Common sources of chronic pelvic pain include
A. Endometritis
B. Ectopic pregnancy
C. Interstitial cystitis/bladder pain syndrome
D. Bowel obstruction

7. Bladder instillations can be used to treat
A. Urinary tract infections
B. Interstitial cystitis/bladder pain syndrome
C. Bladder cancer
D. Overactive bladder

8. Pharmacologic therapies for chronic pelvic pain include which of the following therapeutic options?
A. Pelvic floor physical therapy and bladder irritant reduction
B. Bladder instillations and suppressive antibiotics
C. Pessary and trigger point injections
D. Amitriptyline and bladder instillations

9. First-line therapy for chronic pelvic pain includes
A. Cystoscopy with hydrodistension.
B. Dietary modifications
C. As needed use of opioids during crisis flares
D. Trigger point injections

10. The common pain assessment mnemonic OLDCART stands for
A. Onset, location, duration, characteristics, alleviation, relieving factors, temperature, and other signs
B. Onset, long-term, duration, chronic, aggravating factors, relieving factors, temperature, and other signs
C. Onset, location, duration, characteristics, aggravating factors, relieving factors, temperature, and other signs
D. Onset, location, duration, characteristics, aggravating factors, relieving factors, and time to resolve

ANSWERS AND RATIONALES

1. B. Rationale: Trigger points can be active or latent. Pain can be felt when these points are palpated.

2. B. Rationale: Urinary tract infections are common among women, are not chronically managed, and do not increase the risk for other, chronic conditions. Treatment success is often realized with antibiotic, palliative care management, and behavioral modifications.

3. A. Rationale: Performance of this test creates tension of the muscles when the patient lifts his or her head or legs, trigger points may be activated, and reveal a myofascial origin of pain. Pain of a visceral origin may not be as severe when performing this test.

4. C. Rationale: With the extra-uterine growth responding to estrogen and progesterone production, inflammation creates pain during the menstrual cycle, bleeding irregularities, urinary or bowel dysfunction, dyspareunia, and infertility.

5. A. Rationale: Pentosan polysulfate treats interstitial cystitis/bladder pain syndrome. Micronor, a progestin only birth control pill, may provide relief with the dysmenorrhea of endometriosis. Lubiprostone is used for constipation-predominant irritable bowel syndrome. Eluxadoline is an FDA-approved drug that slows gut transit time.

6. C. Rationale: Many conditions may create pain. Endometritis, bowel obstructions, and ectopic pregnancies create acute onset of pain and require immediate medical or surgical attention.

7. B. Rationale: Both the American Urologic Association and the European Urologic Association recommend bladder instillations for interstitial cystitis/bladder pain syndrome, with a grade-level recommendation of A.

8. D. Rationale: Physical therapy and bladder irritant reduction can improve chronic pelvic pain symptoms but are not part of the pharmacologic options for treatment. Suppressive antibiotics and pessaries are not recommended options for chronic pelvic pain.

9. B. Rationale: Evidence has shown effectiveness for treatment of chronic pelvic pain when first-line therapies are initiated, helping patients avoid potentially invasive therapies.

10. C. Rationale: This is a commonly used tool when assessing pain.

(PART B) ADVANCE PELVIC HEALTH CONSIDERATIONS FOR WOMEN: PELVIC ORGAN PROLAPSE AND VESICOVAGINAL FISTULA

JoAnn M. Ermer-Seltun and Sandra Engberg

PELVIC ORGAN PROLAPSE

Pelvic organ prolapse (POP) is the herniation or abnormal descent of a pelvic organ toward or through the vaginal introitus (opening) (**Fig. 12-7**). The prolapse can include the vaginal anterior, posterior, or apical walls or compartments (Haylen et al., 2016; Lazarou, 2019). The most common prolapse occurs in the vaginal anterior compartment, usually includes descent of the bladder (cystocele) and less common, the urethra (urethrocele) which can arise alone or more often accompany with a cystocele (cystourethrocele). Posterior compartment prolapse can include the decent of the rectum (rectocele) or small intestine (enterocele), while an apical prolapse entails either the uterus and cervix (uterine prolapse), or posthysterectomy vaginal cuff (vaginal vault prolapse), and is often associated with the descent of the small intestine (enterocele) (Rogers & Fashokun, 2019). Noteworthy, over 50% of the anterior vaginal wall prolapses can be contributed to an apical prolapse (Summers et al., 2006). POP of all three compartments through the vaginal introitus is known as procidentia (Madhu et al., 2018).

> **KEY POINT**
>
> The most common type of POP occurs in the anterior vaginal compartment causing a cystocele or herniation of the bladder into the vagina.

PREVALENCE

Prevalence of POP is difficult to establish precisely for three reasons: (1) dissimilar criteria to identify POP; (2) varied methods in identifying the rate of POP, that is, self-report of symptoms versus vaginal examination; (3) POP is under-recognized or underreported; therefore, the number of women who do not seek medical evaluation is unknown (Milsom et al., 2017; Rogers & Fashokun, 2019). Wu et al. (2014b) used the National Health and Nutrition Examination Survey to examine the prevalence of pelvic floor disorders including POP. Self-reported data on a validated questionnaire—*"Do you see or feel a bulge in the vaginal area?"*—were available for 7,071 nonpregnant women (age 20 years or older). Women with an affirmative response were classified as having a prolapse.

Overall, 2.9% of women had POP. Since POP is often asymptomatic, this estimate likely underestimates the prevalence without a pelvic examination. Using the International Incontinence Society (ICS) definition of POP as any prolapse even if asymptomatic, the prevalence rates have been estimated between 27% and 98% (Abed & Rogers, 2008). The Wu-reported prevalence of 2.9% (2014) is consistent with previously reported prevalence rates for bothersome POP, typically a prolapse extending beyond the hymen (Abed & Rogers, 2008). In contrast, the Women's Health Initiative study examined over 27,342 postmenopausal women (aged 50 to 79 years) with a standardized pelvic examination. In this study, the global rate for POP was 41% in women with a uterus and 38% without uterus (Hendrix et al., 2002). Still the overall rates may have been higher since women who had previous surgical prolapse repair were not identified. Estimated lifetime risk for an 80-year-old woman undergoing a single surgical intervention for POP reconstructive or urinary incontinence (UI) repair is reported as 11.6% to 30% (Olsen et al., 1997; Wu & Welk, 2019; Wu et al., 2014a). Noteworthy, in the United States alone, over 200,000 pelvic repair surgeries for POP are performed annually (Boyles et al., 2003).

> **KEY POINT**
>
> Prevalence of POP is difficult to determine due to study design variability but appears to be more prevalent in older women. It is believed to affect nearly 50% of women who have given birth, whether asymptomatic or symptomatic.

PATHOPHYSIOLOGY AND RISK FACTORS

POP occurs due to weakening of the pelvic floor support structures as a result of direct damage (e.g., tears or breaks) to the supporting structures and/or to neuromuscular dysfunction (Gleason et al., 2012). Chapter 2 provides a detailed discussion of key pelvic floor support structures that provide vital reinforcement to the pelvic soft organs. Specifically, the levator ani muscle, endopelvic fascia, and perineum (perineal body, perineal membrane, superficial and deep perineal muscles) are a system of three integrated levels that provides optimal vaginal support as described by DeLancey (1998). Levator ani muscles (pubococcygeus, puborectalis, and iliococcygeus) and the connective tissue attachments to the bony pelvis provide anatomical support for the pelvic organs. The levator ani muscles are normally tonically contracted at rest, closing the genital hiatus and acting as a platform to support the pelvic organs. The endopelvic fascia envelops the pelvic organs, holding the vagina and uterus in their normal

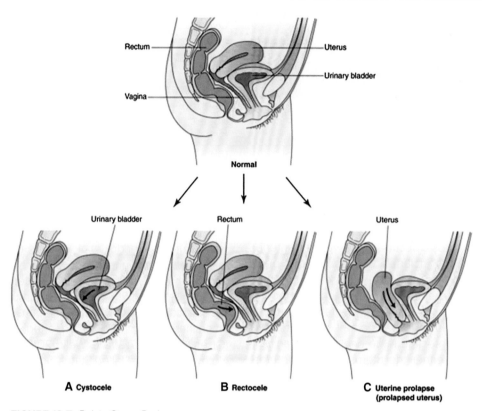

FIGURE 12-7. Pelvic Organ Prolapse.

anatomical position while allowing for enough mobility to permit storage of urine and feces, coitus, parturition (childbirth), and defecation (Stepp & Walters, 2015). The perineum contains structures that support the distal one third of the vagina. The perineal body or "central tendon" of the perineum has multiple attachments that strengthen and maintain pelvic floor integrity especially in women (Siccardi & Bordoni, 2018). Innervation of the pelvic floor structures including the external anal and urethral sphincters are derived from the S-2, S-3, and S-4 spinal nerve fibers that ultimately unite to create the pudendal nerve. Damage or dysfunction of any or all of these components can eventually lead to POP. A variety of pathological changes have been identified as potential causative factors for POP including denervation or direct damage to the levator ani muscles, neuropathic injuries (e.g., related to vaginal delivery or chronic straining), disruption or stretching of the endopelvic fascia attachments, connective tissue abnormalities, smooth muscle abnormalities, and variations in the orientation and shape of the bony pelvis (Rogers & Fashokun, 2019). **Figure 12-8** further depicts three support levels that are interconnected and interdependent through the envelopment of the endopelvic fascia that provides critical support to the female pelvic organs: Level I support is provided by the uterosacral/cardinal ligament complex that attaches the upper vagina, cervix and lower uterus to the sacrum and lateral pelvic walls. Level II support consists of lateral vagina and endopelvic fascia condensations that create a suspension-type bridge with four cable-like attachments to the arcus tendineus fasciae pelvic, also known as the "white line" and superior fascia of the levator ani muscles. Level III support is provided to the distal vagina by fusing with the perineal membrane/perineal body to maintain normal anatomic position. Damage to a level often produces a predictable type of POP For instance, damage to Level I leads to uterine and vaginal prolapses, Level II damage often causes a cystocele and rectocele, and Level III damage may cause significant perineal descent and rectocele if perineal body is injured. In addition, if an individual suffers from weak pelvic floor muscles (PFMs) through nerve damage or mechanical tear, the endopelvic fascia takes on the primary role of support. After a period of stress, the endopelvic fascia attachments lengthen or tear resulting in loss of proper anatomical position or POP (Stepp & Walters, 2015).

Risk factors for POP include age (Awwad et al., 2012; Hendrix et al., 2002; Miedel et al., 2009; Swift et al., 2005; Wu et al., 2014b), vaginal delivery (Awwad et al., 2012; Elenskaia et al., 2013; Gyhagen & Bullar, 2013; Hendrix et al., 2002; Rortveit et al., 2007), high BMI (Awwad et al., 2012; Giri et al., 2017; Gyhagen et al., 2013; Hendrix et al., 2002; Miedel et al., 2009; Swift

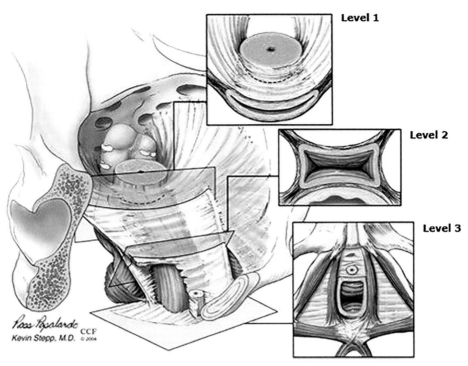

FIGURE 12-8. DeLancey Levels of Vaginal Support. (From Stepp, K. J., & Walters, M. D. (2015). Anatomy of the lower urinary tract, rectum, and pelvic floor. In M. Walters, & M. Karram (Eds.), *Urogynecology and reconstructive pelvic surgery* (4th ed., p. 29). Philadelphia, PA: Elsevier.)

et al., 2005), vaginal hysterectomy (Dallas et al., 2018; Forsgren et al., 2012), parity (Hendrix et al., 2002; Mant et al., 1997; Miedel et al., 2009), family history (Allen-Brady et al., 2011; Chiaffarino et al., 1999; Jack et al., 2006; McLennan et al., 2008; Miedel et al., 2009; Mothes et al., 2016), race (Dietz, 2003; Hendrix et al., 2002; Kim et al., 2005), an occupation involving heavy lifting (Chiaffarino et al., 1999; Jorgensen et al., 1994; Miedel et al., 2009; Woodman et al., 2006), and chronic constipation (Miedel et al., 2009; Rortveit et al., 2007). Of all these risk factors, parity, advancing age, and obesity are well established for the development of POP (de Sam Lazaro et al., 2016; Delancey et al., 2017; Giri et al., 2017; Jelovsek et al., 2018; Vergeldt et al., 2015). In addition, current studies demonstrate a strong scientific influence of genetics including race, ethnicity, and collagen abnormality for the development of POP (Altman et al., 2008; Delancey et al., 2017; Jack et al., 2006). Risk factors for recurrence of POP following surgical reconstruction (25%) includes levator ani avulsion, advance prolapse severity (i.e., Stage 4), and genetics (Friedman et al., 2018). See **Box 12-1**, Risk factors for POP.

Figure 12-9 shows the tension placed on the pelvic organs with prolapse.

KEY POINT

The levator ani muscle, endopelvic fascia, and perineum are a system of three integrated levels that provide optimal vaginal support.

CLINICAL PRESENTATION

Women with POP can present with a range of symptoms directly related to the prolapse including bulging sensation, feeling or seeing a bulge, pelvic pressure, or heaviness and low back discomfort that tend to worsen in the upright position especially at the end of the day. Women may also describe symptoms related to coexisting bladder, bowel, or pelvic floor dysfunction: UI, frequency, urgency, weak or slow urine stream, hesitancy, sensation of incomplete bladder emptying, or the need to shift positions or manually reduce the prolapse (splinting) in order to void. Bowel symptoms can include fecal incontinence, sensation of incomplete bowel emptying, straining in order to defecate, bowel urgency, and need for digital evacuations or maneuvers to manually reduce the prolapse in order to complete defecation. Women may also experience sexual dysfunction including dyspareunia (pain/discomfort during sexual intercourse) and avoidance behaviors owing to fear of discomfort or embarrassment especially if sexual activity leads to urinary or fecal incontinence (Barber et al., 2002; Lowder et al., 2011; Novi et al., 2005). Body image can be greatly affected with the presence of a prolapse that generate feelings of "being different," less womanlike, less good-looking which once again affects sexual intimacy, and partner relationship (Lowder et al., 2011). The symptomatic presentation of POP varies from relatively minor to having a major effect on quality of life (QoL) (Cheung et al., 2016; de Albuquerque Coelho et al.,

BOX 12-1   RISK FACTORS FOR PELVIC PROLAPSE

Established risk factors
- Vaginal birth
- Higher parity
- Advancing age
- Obesity
- Genetics: inheritance and collagen disorders (Marfan, Ehlers-Danlos syndrome)
- Race and ethnicity
- Hysterectomy
- Forceps usage with childbirth

Other possible risk factors
- Constipation
- Pelvic floor muscle weakness
- Increase abdominal pressure
- Hormonal changes (menopause)
- Intrapartum variables (i.e., long second stage of labor, episiotomy)

References: Delancey et al. (2017); Wang and Smith (2017); Rogers and Fashokun (2019).

2016). Several investigators have examined the prevalence of specific symptoms and the association between the extent of prolapse and the presence of symptoms. Ellerkmann et al. (2001) examined self-reported symptoms (measured by questionnaire) in women who subsequently underwent urogynecologic examination (*n* = 237) and found a weak to moderate

association between the severity of prolapse and specific symptoms related to bowel and bladder function. The correlations were moderate for prolapse-specific symptoms (visualized bulging and pelvic discomfort). In another study examining the relationship between the degree of prolapse and symptoms (*n* = 296 women), investigators found that prolapse of 0.5 cm distal to the hymen was sensitive and specific for bulging and protrusion symptoms; however, they were unable to identify a prolapse severity threshold for other symptoms (Gutman et al., 2008). Finally, Swift et al. (2003) examined the association between symptoms and the degree of POP in 477 women. As the POP stage increased, the average number of symptoms increased; however, the increase was not statistically significant (*p* = 0.22 for reported symptoms and *p* = 0.23 for bothersome symptoms).

KEY POINT

The clinical impact of POP varies from minimal to major impact on QoL.

KEY POINT

Symptomatic POP may cause bladder, bowel, or sexual dysfunction.

ASSESSMENT: HISTORY AND FOCUS PHYSICAL EXAMINATION

Upon initial evaluation of a women with suspected POP, a detail symptom assessment should be performed, including the amount of bother affecting the woman's QoL in addition to a thorough medical, surgical, OB/GYN history (ACOG, 2019). Clinical presentation of symptoms was described previously with a focus on lower urinary tract, bowel, and sexual function. Numerous standardized questionnaires such as Pelvic Floor Distress Inventory-short form 20, Pelvic Floor Impact Questionnaire-short form 7, and Pelvic Organ Prolapse/Urinary Incontinence Sexual Function Questionnaire-PISQ12 exist to assist in quantifying the severity of the symptoms to determine appropriate management (Lazarou, 2019).

The pelvic examination is the gold standard for the diagnosis of POP. The basic examination is done with the patient in a supine position and the head of the bed at 45 degrees (Abed & Rogers, 2008). The bladder should be empty; in addition to being uncomfortable for the patient when examined, a full bladder has been shown to restrict the degree of descent and may result in underestimation of the severity of the prolapse (Haylen et al., 2016). While observing the vaginal

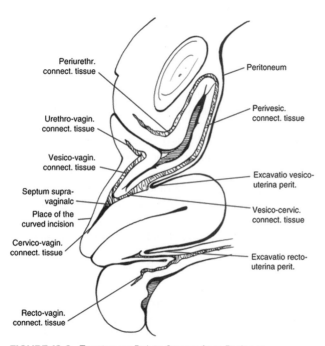

FIGURE 12-9. Traction on Pelvic Organs from Prolapse.

Periurethr. connect. tissue
Urethro-vagin. connect. tissue
Vesico-vagin. connect. tissue
Septum supra-vaginalc
Place of the curved incision
Cervico-vagin. connect. tissue
Recto-vagin. connect. tissue
Peritoneum
Perivesic. connect. tissue
Excavatio vesico-uterina perit.
Vesico-cervic. connect. tissue
Excavatio recto-uterina perit.

introitus, the examiner should ask the woman to perform a Valsalva maneuver and observe for bulging. To determine which compartment of the vagina is involved (anterior, posterior, or apical), a split speculum (one blade) is inserted to retract the posterior and then anterior wall and to observe each portion of the vagina sequentially. If the observed prolapse is not consistent with the degree of protrusion the woman reports experiencing, the examiner should have her stand so the maximum descent can be observed. If prolapse is found, it should be graded as described below. Cough stress test in the lying and standing position is warranted in patients with an anterior or apical compartment prolapse since stress incontinence often accompanies these defects (Lazarou, 2019). Pelvic muscle strength, tone, and endurance should be assessed (ACOG, 2019) using the Oxford grading scale described in Chapter 4 and is an opportunity to coach the patient in correctly performing a pelvic muscle contraction.

Figure 12-10 shows progressive stages of prolapse.

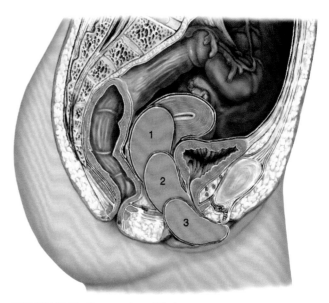

FIGURE 12-10. Progression of Prolapse.

KEY POINT

The pelvic examination is the gold standard in diagnosing POP. It should be performed with an empty bladder so the prolapse is better visualized for severity and less uncomfortable to the woman.

Although there are a number of grading systems for POP, the only system that is internationally acceptable with high interexaminer reliability and reproducibility is the Pelvic Organ Prolapse Quantitative Examination (POP-Q) (Barber et al., 1999; Persu et al., 2011; Stark et al., 2010). This staging system was developed by a multidisciplinary committee of the ICS, the Society of Gynecologic Surgeons, and the American Urogynecologic Society (AUGS). The goal was to establish a standardized system for evaluating and describing POP (Castro Diaz et al., 2017). It describes the topographic positions of six vaginal sites and provides information about perineal descent and changes in the axis of the levator plate based on increases in genital hiatus and perineal body measurements creating a total of nine measurements (Auwad et al., 2004; Castro Diaz et al., 2017) (**Fig. 12-11**). While the POP-Q was developed to provide an objective and reproducible tool for describing and staging POP, it is not widely used in clinical practice owing to the time and training required to execute properly (Castro Diaz et al., 2017). Auwad et al. (2004) conducted a web-based survey of 667 ICS and AUGS members to determine their use of the POP-Q. Of the 380 surveys that were completed, 373 members answered the question about the use of POP-Q in clinical practice. Only 150

(40.2%) reported that they routinely used it; 147 (39.2%) did not use it. The second question asked participants if they used POP-Q for research; 251 (67.1%) of those who responded (*n* = 374) reported that they routinely used it in research. The most common reasons that participants reported not using POP-Q were that it was too time consuming (24.2%), colleagues did not use it (20%), and it was too confusing (17.9%). In 2002, Swift developed a simplified version of the POP-Q by reducing staging ordinal measurement sites to four instead of nine. **Figure 12-12** depicts the Simplified POP-Q.

Another straightforward system to measure degree of POP is the Bayden and Walker Halfway Scoring System. It measures the grade of POP with respect to the hymen therefore does not require the utilization of a ruler.

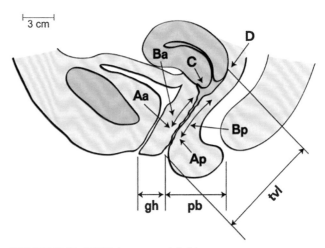

FIGURE 12-11. POPQ Assessment Guide.

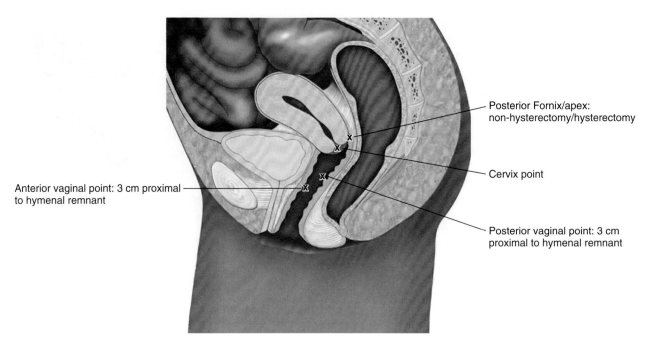

Posterior Fornix/apex:
non-hysterectomy/hysterectomy

Cervix point

Anterior vaginal point: 3 cm proximal
to hymenal remnant

Posterior vaginal point: 3 cm
proximal to hymenal remnant

FIGURE 12-12. Simplified POP-Q.

See Table 4-2, Baden-Walker Halfway Scoring system. The Women's Health Initiative study, where over 27,342 women underwent a pelvic examination, employed an even simpler version to grade POP with the following visual description: none (no evidence of prolapse), grade 1 (prolapse within the vagina), grade 2 (prolapse to introitus), and grade 3 (prolapse outside of the vagina) (Wang & Smith, 2017).

The most recent International Urogynecological Association (IUGA) and ICS report on terminology for pelvic floor dysfunction in women uses the following method for staging POP (Haylen et al., 2016):

KEY POINT

The Pelvic Organ Prolapse Quantitative Examination (POP-Q) is the only system that is internationally acceptable with high interexaminer reliability and reproducibility.

Stage 0: No prolapse is demonstrated.
Stage 1: Most distal portion of the prolapse is more than 1 cm above the level of the hymen.
Stage 2: Most distal portion of the prolapse is 1 cm or less proximal to or distal to the plane of the hymen.
Stage 3: The most distal portion of the prolapse is more than 1 cm below the plane of the hymen.
Stage 4: Complete eversion of the total length of the lower genital tract is demonstrated.

MANAGEMENT

It is generally accepted that approximately 50% of parous women have some degree of POP whether asymptomatic or symptomatic (Awwad et al., 2012; Hendrix et al., 2002). Treatment of asymptomatic POP is normally not indicated except for observation for symptomatology. Current recommended management options for POP include observation, PFMT, pessary support, or surgery (Wu & Welk, 2019). Conservative management is considered a first-line option for POP since it is safe, low-cost, minimally invasive, potential for high patient satisfaction and management of bothersome symptoms (ACOG, 2019). In contrast, surgical reconstruction is associated with potential morbidity and mortality, expense, and risk of complications. A thorough discussion of risks and benefits of conservative to the most invasive treatment option, surgical repair, should be completed. Patient-centered goal setting needs to be explored so the woman can make an informed decision that is best for her based upon symptoms and QoL impact (Hooper, 2018).

Observation

Clinical observation is a viable treatment option for many women with POP who don't experience symptoms or bother. Observation is warranted in asymptomatic women with stage 1 or 2 prolapse and with regular evaluation to monitor for development or worsening of urinary or bowel symptoms. It is also an option for those with stage 3 or 4 POP who experience minimal bother (Abed & Rogers, 2008). Handa et al. (2004) conducted a longitudinal observational study to describe the natural history of POP in postmenopausal women. The study cohort was 412 women with grade 1 (in the vagina), grade 2 (to the introitus), or grade 3 (outside the vagina) prolapses who completed two to eight annual pelvic examinations (mean = 5.7). In this study, regression of the prolapse was common, particularly for grade 1 POP, where the probability of regression was greater than for progression of the prolapse. In contrast, Gilchrist et al. (2013) found minimal changes in POP in a sample of 64 women who selected observation as the primary treatment of the prolapse. Most of the women had stage 2 (48%) or 3 (48%) POP. Over the observation period (medium = 16 months; range, 6 to 91 months), 78% of patients had no change in the leading edge of their prolapse, 3% demonstrated regression (2 cm reduction), and 19% had progression (≥2 cm increase in the leading edge). Implementing lifestyle modifications to promote pelvic health and potentially avert prolapse progression during 'watchful waiting' may be prudent through patient education to prevent constipation, avoidance of heavy lifting, promote proper perineal hygiene, toileting, weight loss, smoking cessation, and pelvic muscle exercise (Dumoulin et al., 2017). Raising awareness may improve health-seeking behaviors if the patient becomes symptomatic or prevent POP progression (ACOG, 2019; Handa et al., 2004; Newman et al., 2017). See Chapter 6, Management Fundamentals.

KEY POINT

Observation with an emphasis on lifestyle modification is a viable option in women with asymptomatic POP or who are experiencing minimal bother from more advance POP.

Pelvic Floor Muscle Training

The PFMs provide structural support for the pelvic organs. Consequently, it can be theorized that PFMT, by improving muscle function, could improve this structural support (Bø, 2012; Hagen & Stark, 2011). Research examining the impact of conservative modalities such as pelvic floor muscle training (PFMT) on POP symptoms and severity is expanding and encouraging with an increase of more rigorous randomized control trials (RCTs) (Dumoulin et al., 2017; Wu & Welk, 2019). The International Consultation on Incontinence (ICI) committee on conservative management of POP reported favorable evidence from 13 trials regarding PFMT in secondary prevention or treatment of POP, 7 of which being more recent than a previous review by Moore et al. (2013) (Dumoulin et al., 2017). These studies examined the impact of PFMT on POP secondary prevention, severity, and/or symptoms. The committee concluded that there

was a high level of evidence to support that PFMT can improve POP symptoms but not reduce severity according to POP-Q stage. Of interest, in one of the reviewed multicenter RCT (Hagen et al., 2014a), 447 women (most with a stage 2 or 3 prolapse) were randomly assigned to a PFMT training group (n = 225) or control group (n = 222). The primary outcome was POP symptoms at 6- and 12-months post intervention, and data were analyzed using an intention-to-treat approach. Women in the PFMT group reported a significantly greater reduction in symptoms at 6 and 12 months compared to control subjects and were significantly more likely to report that their prolapse was better. Women in the control group were significantly more likely to report receiving additional treatments at 12 months than those in the PFMT group (50% vs. 24%, respectively). Among women with a follow-up pelvic examination at 6 months, there was not a statistically significant difference in regression or progression of the prolapse in the two groups. Given the low risk of adverse events associated with PFMT, existing evidence supports the use of this intervention for women with POP.

Based on Dumoulin et al.'s (2017) review of RCTs, new recommendations for practice in using PFMT in women with POP consists of the following: (1) PFMT following the first birth of a child does not prevent or treat POP (Bo et al., 2013); however, it does reduce symptoms of prolapse in women who were followed postnatally at 3 months, 6, and 12 years (Hagen et al., 2014a, 2014b); (2) PFMT is effective in reducing prolapse symptoms especially the sensation of pelvic bulge (8 trials) but does not reduce the severity of POP; (3) performing PFMT and surgical repair for vaginal vault prolapse does not improve POP symptoms or stage at 2 years (Barber et al., 2014); and (4) PFMT alone or with pessary should be considered for treatment due to its equal effectiveness in prolapse symptom reduction and pelvic muscle strength enhancement (Cheung et al., 2016; Hagen et al., 2014a, 2014b; Manonai et al., 2012; Wu & Welk, 2019).

KEY POINT

PFMT is a conservative measure that reduces the symptoms of POP but not its severity.

Pessaries

Vaginal pessaries are generally considered the cornerstone of nonsurgical treatment of POP (ACOG, 2019). They have been used to treat women with POP since 400 BC (Powers et al., 2019; Shah et al., 2006). Although new studies regarding pessaries for management of POP is sparse, 49% to 90% of users report good symptom control (Clemons et al., 2004; Fernando et al., 2006). Pessaries are a lifestyle choice. It can be offered as a first-line treatment option for women who prefer nonsurgical treatment, who plan a future pregnancy, who have lower stage or asymptomatic prolapses, who are not surgical candidates, as a means of symptom control prior to future surgical repair, as a prediction tool of surgical effect or as a diagnostic tool to discover occult stress UI (Wang & Smith, 2017). The limited contraindications and risks associated with pessary use make them a viable option for most women with POP. They should not be used in women with an active pelvic infection, ulcerations in the vagina, or exposed vaginal mesh, who are allergic to silicone or other materials in the pessary, or who are nonadherent and unlikely to attend follow-up visits (Clemons, 2020; Wang & Smith, 2017). When pessaries are used in postmenopausal women, clinicians often also prescribe vaginal estrogen therapy to improve health of the vaginal epithelium prior to pessary fitting and help prevent vaginal mechanical injuries (Atnip & O'Dell, 2012; Bulchandani et al., 2015; Wang & Smith, 2017). Studies have reported that menopausal women have little to minimal lactobacilli in the vagina leading to an elevated pH that is conducive to over colonization of microbes such as fungus, Enterobacteriaceae (i.e., *Escherichia coli*) (Freedman, 2008). Research supports that transvaginal estrogen restores intravaginal lactobacilli levels to 60% to 100% (Reid et al., 2004) and reduces genitourinary symptoms of menopause (GSM) such as vaginal dryness and burning, urinary urgency, frequency, dysuria, dyspareunia, and the incidence of cystitis (ACOG, 2018; Beerepoot & Geerlings, 2016; Santoro & Lin, 2018). See Chapter 18 to explore the options and use of transvaginal estrogen. In contrast, findings from a study examining long-term outcomes associated with pessary use in women with POP (n = 429) suggests that topical estrogen cream may not protect women against the occurrence of erosions (Ramsay et al., 2011). Additional research is therefore needed to provide guidance about estrogen use in postmenopausal women fitted for pessaries.

It is the opinion of this advance practice nurse practitioner (APRN) author and others who have a vibrant pessary practice (Atnip & O'Dell, 2012) that intravaginal estrogen should be offered in postmenopausal women using pessaries to prevent and heal mechanical injuries (vaginal abrasions or erosions) and also for one month prior to pessary fitting if vaginal tissues are atrophic or nonelastic to reduce discomfort or pain with initial fitting. Other benefits of low-dose intravaginal estrogen include overall enhancement of vaginal wall thickness and elasticity, normalization of vaginal flora to lessen risk for vaginal and urinary tract infections, as well as reducing over colonization leading to increased or malodorous discharge (Freedman, 2008; Wang & Smith, 2017). Current research reports minimal systemic absorption with properly dosed vaginal estrogen (Wills et al., 2012) and that concomitant use of progestogens is not indicated in women with a uterus (NAMS, 2010). See Table 18-7,

Commonly used vaginal estrogen therapy. ACOG (2018) in a position statement also supports the use of transvaginal estrogen in women even with a past or current history of breast cancer if they have significant urogenital atrophy and have failed nonhormonal therapies. Risk and benefits of vaginal estrogen should be fully explored with the woman, so an informed and shared decision-making is created with the patient's oncologist or APRN continence specialist. For those who cannot tolerate local estrogen or is contraindicated, longer lasting vaginal moisturizers containing polycarbophil may reduce vaginal discharge, odor, and discomfort with pessary insertion although they do not have the same sustained changes as seen with vaginal estrogen (Biglia et al., 2010).

Types of Pessaries

Current pessaries are generally made of medical grade silicone, which does not absorb vaginal secretions or odors, are nonallergenic, pliable, washable, sterilizable, and have a long shelf life (Atnip & O'Dell, 2012; Wang & Smith, 2017). See **Figure 12-13**. When selecting and fitting a pessary, considerations need to include the nature and extent of the prolapse and the patient's cognitive status, manual dexterity, and level of sexual activity (Atnip & O'Dell, 2012; Wang & Smith, 2017). Pessaries are available in many different shapes and sizes, allowing a variety of options depending on the nature and extent of the prolapse as well as the characteristics of the individual patient. Pessaries can be classified as support, space-occupying or incontinence support pessaries. Support pessaries such as the ring sit in the posterior fornix usually resting behind the pubic bone anteriorly and/or the pelvic floor and will fit approximately 70% of women with stage 2 or 3 prolapse and vaginal introitus that is <3 fingerbreadths in width (Clemons, 2020; Clemons et al., 2004). Ring size 3, 4, or 5 will fit most women. Space-occupying pessaries, such as the cube and donut, occupy a larger space than the introitus and are generally used for larger prolapses. The Gellhorn is a combination of support and space-occupying device (Robert et al., 2013). Gellhorn pessary works well for the women with grade/stage 3 or 4 POP, a history of hysterectomy, and a gapping vaginal introitus that is 3 or more fingerbreadths (Clemons, 2020; Clemons et al., 2004). Gellhorn size 2.5, 2.75, and 3 inches are selected most of the time. Ring and Gellhorn pessary can be used in combination to promote optimal support in advance POP (Clemons, 2020). Incontinence support pessaries generally have a knob or bump that sits behind the symphysis pubis to support the urethrovesical junction (bladder neck) especially during activities that increase abdominal pressure. Incontinence pessaries come with or without support. Chapter 11 further describes this type of pessary. In general, support pessaries do not need to be removed for intercourse while space-occupying

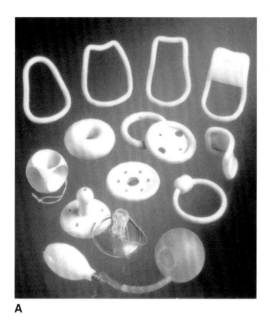

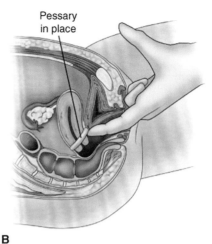

FIGURE 12-13. Examples of pessaries **(A)** and pessary in position **(B)**.

pessaries do (O'Dell & Atnip, 2012). While each type has advantages and disadvantages and there is no consensus about which is optimal, the ring and Gellhorn are popular options in the United States (Dumoulin et al., 2017). Ring pessaries are generally the first-line choice for clinicians because they are easy to insert and remove. Often SUI accompanies POP, therefore a ring with support and knob can stabilize the bladder neck during exertional activities to control leakage as well as prolapse reduction (Lukacz et al., 2017; Wang & Smith, 2017). **Table 12-8** outlines pessary types, classifications, commonly used size, mechanism of action, and APRN considerations.

Insertion of a Pessary

The ring pessary is folded in half and a small amount of lubricant placed on the tip to aid insertion. It is removed by gently pulling and folding it in half. Many women can be taught to manage their own pessary (Atnip & O'Dell, 2012), removing it daily or weekly for cleaning or as infrequently (assuming there are no adverse events) as every 3 months. The Gellhorn is generally the best option for women with more advanced prolapse or in women who are no longer sexually active. It is more difficult to insert and remove so this generally needs to be done by the clinician. According to Atnip & O'Dell (2012), "to insert the Gellhorn, the pessary is folded in half with the use of lubricant on the leading edge to ease insertion. Once the pessary is behind the pubic symphysis, it will expand and rest against the leading edge of prolapse, forming suction. To remove the Gellhorn, the knob is grasped, generally with the help of a ring forceps, while the concave end of the pessary is rotated to release the suction and the pessary is pulled downward, folded and removed" (p. 5).

Size of Pessary

In sizing a pessary, the provider estimates the size of the vagina and then selects the largest pessary that he or she thinks will fit comfortably. Following insertion, the clinician should assure that he or she is able to place a finger between the pessary and the walls of the vagina. After fitting, the woman should be asked to perform various activities (e.g., standing, walking, and bearing down) to make sure she can retain the pessary and that there is no discomfort. It is also critical to ensure that she can void before she leaves the clinic/office. **Table 12-9** provides steps in pessary fitting. **Figure 12-14** demonstrates sizing of a pessary. It should be noted that up to 92% of women can be successfully fitted with a pessary (ACOG, 2019; Cundiff et al., 2007). Risk factors for failed pessary fitting include history of multiple pelvic surgeries, vaginal length <6 cm, inability to retain a single pessary, and onset of occult (hidden) incontinence with the pessary (Nager et al., 2009; Nguyen & Jones, 2005). The woman should be counseled prior to the fitting that finding the "right" pessary may take multiple attempts with the average being 2 to 3 per single session, and at follow-up fittings, it is not unusual for a different size or shape of pessary to be dispensed once she has the chance to perform her usual ADLs. In a recent retrospective study of 8 years, Yang et al. (2018) looked at factors associated with pessary fitting, use, and satisfaction in older females (average 67.8 years) suffering from POP. Three-hundred women underwent pessary fitting with 83% (249) fitted successful with a ring (162) or Gellhorn (87) pessary with 47 women aborting pessary use due to two main factors (1) difficulty in pessary insertion or removal (30.4%) and (2) vaginal erosions (22.8%). Primary reason for pessary fitting failure was advance symptoms with posterior compartment prolapse. Pessary users (162) completed seven validated questionnaires, and 79% were satisfied or very satisfied.

TABLE 12-8 PESSARY TYPES

PESSARY TYPE	CLASSIFICATION	COMMONLY USED SIZE (INCHES)	MECHANISM OF ACTIONS AND APRN CONSIDERATIONS
Ring (with or without support); can be oval in shape	Support pessary	2–5	• Ring (with or without supportive membrane) pessaries are used most often and are the easiest to use • Include a rigid, hinged nylon ring that fits into the length of the vagina, providing support for the anterior, posterior, and apical walls. • Can be folded for ease of insertion. • Positioned similar to a contraceptive diaphragm • Pelvic floor and introitus must provide enough support to contain the pessary. • Comes with or without a supportive membrane or diaphragm, which provides additional support if cystocele or rectocele are present. • Intercourse is possible.
Shaatz	Space-occupying	1.5–3	• Convex shape ensures a snug fit but may change position in the vagina. • More rigid than the ring and may offer firmer support; similar to Gellhorn pessary without knob. • Difficult to remove as it does not fold or have a knob.
Gehrung	Support pessary	2–5	• May be effective in women who have isolated anterior or posterior POP. • Malleable wires incorporated in the edge of the pessary allow the device to be manually shaped to accommodate different anatomies. • Intercourse is possible.
Donut	Space-occupying	2–3	• Requires some introital support. • Can be used if a ring pessary is unsuccessful • Fills vagina more completely, which may increase risk of vaginal epithelial injury and malodorous discharge production. • Adequate lubrication is essential. • Comfortable intercourse with donut pessary is unlikely. • Not easily compressed. • Difficult to remove. • Can deflate the donut pessary with 30- to 50-cc syringe and needle to ease insertion and removal. • More effective for severe POP that extends beyond the hymen than a ring pessary.
Tandem cube (Two cubes fused together)	Space-occupying	1–4	• Retains its position in the vagina by suction of its six concave surfaces on the vaginal wall, but this causes and increased risk of vaginal erosion. • Can support the uterus even with a lack of vaginal tone. • Difficult to remove but has a string on one end to assist removal. • Should be removed and cleaned more often than every 3 months because it is associated with malodorous discharge that is usually trapped within the suction cups (although the cube is available with drainage holes). • Can cause vaginal erosions. • Compressibility will vary by manufacturer. • Can be placed at different depths in the vagina. • More effective for severe POP that extends beyond the hymen than a ring pessary.
Tandem cube (two cubes fused together)	Space-occupying	1–4	• Retains its position in the vagina by suction of its six concave surfaces on the vaginal wall, but this causes an increased risk of vaginal erosion. • Can support the uterus even with a lack of vaginal tone. • Difficult to remove but has a string on one end to assist removal.

TABLE 12-8 PESSARY TYPES (*Continued*)

PESSARY TYPE	CLASSIFICATION	COMMONLY USED SIZE (INCHES)	MECHANISM OF ACTIONS AND APRN CONSIDERATIONS
			• Should be removed and cleaned more often than every 3 months because it is associated with malodorous discharge that is usually trapped within the suction cups (although the cube is available with drainage holes). • Can cause vaginal erosions. • Compress will vary by manufacturer. • Can be placed at different depths in the vagina. • More effective for severe POP that extends beyond the hymen than a ring pessary.
Inflatable donut, silicone Inflato-donut or latex Inflatball	Combination of support and space-occupying	Small to extra large	• Difficult to remove. • Inflatoball material is latex; need to check for latex allergy. • Cannot be autoclaved or boiled. • Should be removed and cleaned with soap and water daily or every other day. • More effective for severe POP that extends beyond the hymen than a ring pessary.
Gellhorn (short or long stem)	Space-occupying	1.75–3	• An option in women who cannot retain a ring pessary due to introital laxity. • Allows the lateral vaginal walls to in-fold under the top dish, while the concave dish itself may create a suction-like action against the proximal vagina, allowing for pessary retention. • Sized by the dish diameter. • May increase risk of mechanical injury. • Difficult to remove due to suction of the dish against apex of the vagina. To remove, consider using a ring or packing self-closing forceps on the base of the stem to apply outward traction, and then use one finger to break the suction and fold the round disc along the stem. • More effective for severe POP that extends beyond the hymen than a ring pessary.
Incontinence dish, incontinence ring with support or knob, Marland	Support pessary for SUI	2–7	• Stabilizes urethra and urethrovesical junction to prevent leakage of urine during times of increased abdominal pressure. • Option to wear only during activity that causes leakage. • Similar to ring pessaries and are fitted similarly, but do not provide as much vaginal support. • Fitting should be performed when the woman has a full bladder to test effectiveness. • Intercourse is possible.
Lever (Hodge, Smith, Risser)	Support pessary	2–4	• Requires vaginal introital integrity. • Smith lever pessary may be more comfortable in women with a narrow vaginal introitus. • Used for mild prolapse in pregnant women with a retroverted uterus. • Intercourse is possible.

Source: © 2017 Society of Urologic Nurses and Associates. Reprinted from the *Core Curriculum for Urologic Nursing*, 2017, p. 535. Used with permission of the publisher, the Society of Urologic Nurses and Associates, Inc.

KEY POINT

The woman should be counseled prior to the fitting that finding the "right" pessary may take multiple attempts at one or more fitting appointments.

KEY POINT

Ring pessaries are best to manage grade 1 and 2 prolapse, while the Gellhorn pessary works well for women who are not sexually active with advance prolapse, grade 3 or 4.

TABLE 12-9 PESSARY FITTING STEPS AND RATIONALE FOR THE APRN

1. Review treatment goals, procedure and expectations. Remind her this is a 'Trial & Error' fitting and common to try several types or sizes of pessaries for the 'Best' fit and symptom control; return visit is required within 1–2 weeks.
   Rationale: Reduces anxiety and sense that somehow her anatomy is "weird." Sets the stage for normalization and adherence.

2. Give permission for a "Time Out" if fitting becomes uncomfortable.
   Rationale: Enhances self-control.

3. Request her to empty bladder and bowels.
   Rationale: Increases ability to identify and stage prolapse.

4. Place the woman in a semi-Fowler position; assure comfort and adjust if needed. Ensure adequate lightening and offer visualization if desirable. Offer chaperone.
   Rationale: Provides physical and emotional comfort, awareness of problem, and promotes a culture of safety.

5. Generously lubricate vagina with water-soluble lubricant and gently reduce any everted POP prior to sizing.
   Rationale: Goal of placing a pessary is to support the prolapse thus reduction must occur in order to place pessary.

6. Digitally assess vagina's length, width, support, and type of prolapse. Observe for any contraindications for pessary fitting, that is, severe atrophy, inelastic tissue, pain, vaginal infection, lesions, or full rectum.
   Rationale: Identifies a starting point for pessary size and type of support required to properly reduce/support prolapse; opportunity to abort fitting and address relative contraindications.

7. Select 1 to 2 types and sizes of pessaries from stock, wash with soap and water; rinse well if not previously sterilized. Place preferred initial pessary at fitting table. Inform patient of pessary placement.
   Rationale: Expedites fitting and normalizes that several attempts maybe required.

8. Apply water-soluble lubricate to leading edge of pessary; insert pessary obliquely (avoids urethral discomfort) with a downward pressure toward the posterior fornix or vaginal wall. Entire pessary should sit behind the symphysis pubis and practitioner is able to place a finger easily between the pessary and vaginal wall. If not, remove pessary gently and reduce size.
   Rationale: Assures comfort, proper size before the woman simulates activities to ascertain proper fit.

9. Ask the patient to cough and Valsalva in both the lying and standing position. Be sure to offer layered paper toweling to place between the legs to capture pessary or de novo SUI. Clinician notes if pessary advances outside of introitus with abdominal pressure or recedes posteriorly with rest. If indicated, adjust size and/or shape of pessary; switch to incontinence type of pessary with support if occult SUI.
   Rationale: Check points occur throughout the fitting to provide opportunity for optimal pessary size, shape, and support.

10. Once appropriate pessary appears to be a viable choice, have the woman mimic usual activities, that is, sitting to standing, walking, bending, squatting, or jumping in place [if able].
    Rationale: Assesses dislodgement or discomfort.

11. Direct the women to use the bathroom to urinate and simulate defecation with a gentle Valsalva. Be sure collection receptacle is placed into toilet to capture pessary if dislodged during simulation. If pessary ventures into toilet, direct not to flush.
    Rationale: Proper fitted pessary should allow and often improves urine flow and emptying if anterior/apical prolapse or facilitates defecation if posterior compartment defect without discomfort or dislodgement.

12. If pessary is successful at this check point, proceed to next step. If not, return to the fitting process, Step 8.
    Rationale: Enhances systematic approach to pessary fitting and opportunity for patient/provider discussion on process.

13. If self-care of pessary is expected, instruct on pessary removal, cleaning, and placement. Ask her to perform a return demo and offer tips if any difficulties, that is, position, adding dental floss to enhance pessary retrieval.
    Rationale: Enhances self-confidence in ability to place and remove pessary independently.

14. Educate and provide educational materials regarding pessary care, removal tips, signs and symptoms to report. Schedule follow-up visit.
    Rationale: Heightens likelihood of adherence to plan of care and timely follow-up.

15. Document size and shape of pessaries utilized during the pessary fitting whether success was achieved.
    Rationale: Expedites subsequent follow-up by avoiding repeat attempts if an alternative pessary warranted.

Follow-up

Generally, the post-fitting visit will focus on adequacy of symptom reduction, presence of pelvic pressure or discomfort, discharge, bleeding, ease and frequency of pessary insertion and removal, presence of elimination dysfunction, sexual and psychosocial health, and lifestyle modification success. The focused physical examination consists of an external genital assessment for rashes or lesions, gentle pessary removal, cleaning with soap and water, careful inspection of the vagina with an appropriate size speculum to detect complications such as odor, discharge, epithelium abrasion, erosion or other lesions, bleeding and discomfort. At this point, the pessary may be left out, replaced or refitted depending upon the results of the examination. Further diagnostics such as vaginal microscopy, urinalysis, and post-void residual maybe

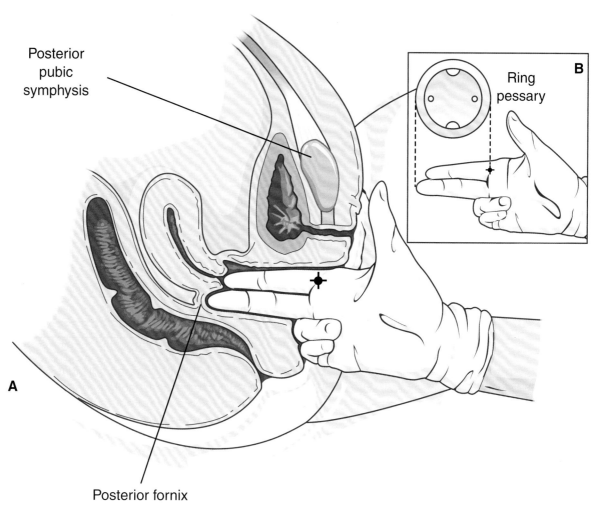

Posterior pubic symphysis

Ring pessary

B

A

Posterior fornix

FIGURE 12-14. Estimating Size of Pessary. **A.** Vaginal length measurement. **B.** Pessary length matches vaginal length measurement. (From Curtis, M., Linares, S. T., & Antoniewicz, L. (2014). *Glass' office gynecology* (7th ed.). Philadelphia, PA: Wolters Kluwer.)

indicated dependent upon findings. Robert et al. recommends a pessary "holiday" for 2 to 4 weeks and considering the use of topical estrogen if there are erosions. If neglected, these can lead to ulcers or fistula formation. Lesions that persist despite treatment should be biopsied. Serious complications such as fistulas are rare and generally seen in women who do not receive regular follow-up care. **Table 12-10** outlines management options for common complications related to pessary use. Currently, there are not any established pessary surveillance guidelines, but expert opinion exists to determine follow-up visit frequency (ACOG, 2019; Lazarou, 2019; O'Dell & Atnip, 2012). Following initial fitting and insertion, the woman should be seen in 2 to 4 weeks to determine if she is satisfied with the pessary or if a different size or style is needed (Robert et al., 2013). If the woman is self-managing, her pessary follow-up visits may be every 3 to 6 months but at least on an annual basis (ACOG, 2019;

Lazarou, 2019). If the woman is unable to self-manage the pessary, it will need to be removed, cleaned, and reinserted by the health care provider, usually every 3 to 4 months (ACOG, 2019; O'Dell & Atnip, 2012; Wang & Smith, 2017). See **Table 12-11**, Pessary: Management Options in Self-Care. Bugge et al. (2013) published a Cochrane review designed to determine the effectiveness of types of pessaries for POP. Only one RCT was found that assessed pessary use for POP, and it compared the ring and Gellhorn pessaries. Both were effective for approximately 60% of the women who completed the study with no significant differences between the two pessaries. The authors concluded that there is currently no consensus on the use of different types of devices, the indications for their use, how often they should be replaced, or how often women require follow-up care. There is a need for well-designed RTCs to address pessary use in comparison to observation, PFMT, and surgery.

TABLE 12-10 PESSARY: TREATMENT OPTIONS OF COMMON PROBLEMS

COMMON PROBLEMS	TREATMENT OPTIONS
Urogenital atrophy and or inelastic vaginal tissue	Treat with intravaginal estrogen for one month prior to pessary fitting, then continue as indicated. See Table 18-7 for dosages. If unable to use estrogen, see vaginal moisturizers.
Pain with pessary removal or difficulty in removing at home	In office: apply 2% lidocaine gel 5 minutes prior to pessary removal; apply generous lubricant to vaginal introitus; ring forceps or tenaculum to retrieve pessary. Self-removal: consider the use of a waxed dental floss loop prior to pessary insertion to expedite self-removal
Split or fissure at introital opening upon removal	Recheck pessary for appropriate size and shape; promote pelvic muscle relaxation with deep breathing; consider use of 2% lidocaine gel prior to removal; consider long-term intravaginal estrogen
Follow-up visit: large amount of discharge noted with absence of pathogens	Place waterproof absorbent pad/toweling under patient, irrigate vagina with Toomey syringe filled with warm water/saline; place towel next to perineum and have patient cough to expel irrigant. May insert applicator full of acidifying gel prior to pessary replacement
Atypical vaginal odor or discharge	Vaginal inspection for erosion; increase frequency of pessary removal and cleaning; microscopic examination for microbial presence, treat infection accordingly; consider vaginal estrogen, moisturizers or acidifying agents; replace malodorous pessary
Vaginal mechanical injuries (abrasions or erosions), bleeding	Consider vaginal estrogen if appropriate; refit with a different size or shape to offload pressure areas; remove pessary at bedtime; pessary holiday for 2–4 weeks with nightly use of vaginal estrogen (0.5 g × 2 weeks) to heal abrasion, then reevaluate; consider biopsy of nonhealing erosions; consider pelvic ultrasound and/or endometrial biopsy in postmenopausal women with uterus
Difficulty with bowel or bladder elimination, pelvic pressure, pain	Pessary refitting to seek resolution of symptoms or abort pessary and discuss alternatives, that is, observation or surgical intervention

---

KEY POINT

Currently, there are not any established pessary surveillance guidelines, but expert opinion exists to determine follow-up visit frequency.

APRN Opportunities

APRNs have a unique opportunity to dramatically improve the QoL for women who suffer from POP (Hull, 2019). Looking at the statistics, POP especially affects older women, many of whom are not surgical candidates or do not want to bear the risks involved in pelvic reconstruction. Based on this, the art and science of a pessary fitting, maintenance, and further research demands attention! Women want lifestyle choices, and with the recent turmoil regarding transvaginal mesh, they want less risk with a sustainable and impermanent option to manage symptoms safely (Powers et al., 2019). APRNs are equipped to lead the charge for pessary management to be a more evidence-based and quality modality that is safe, and an effective lifestyle choice. Studies have demonstrated that practice among gynecologists, other physicians, and nurses vary in pessary management, most likely due to lack of evidence or guidelines (Dwyer et al., 2019; O'Dell et al., 2016; Velzel et al., 2015). Many health care providers do not feel well trained regarding pessary fitting since it appears to be more of a "trial and error" or art form. For instance, Kandadai et al. (2016) reported that 70% of the graduating OBGYN residents did not feel they had the skill set to properly fit and

manage POP with a pessary. Of interest, in order to learn this skill, the resident had to engage in a clinical rotation with an ARNP who provided pessary management. This author also frequently engages as a clinical preceptor to residents and nurses for continence and POP management. ARNPs do possess knowledge and skill that can be shared and influence education of health care providers (Hull, 2019). The development of standards of care and practice guidelines through consensus and research is direly needed to create standardized training opportunities (Hooper et al., 2017). Pessaries may have been around since antiquity, but research is still in its infancy, lacking enlightenment for this modern era. ARNPs are pioneers in pessary care and are in perfect position to trailblaze the paths needed for developing and implementing further studies to establish standards of care and evidence-based guidelines that will promote the culture of safety for colleagues and the millions of women who currently are and will be suffering from POP.

KEY POINT

Practice varies in pessary management among all levels of health care providers. ARNPs are in perfect position to lead the charge in designing and implementing quality research that will lead to practice consensus and guidelines.

Surgery

Current data reveal a woman's lifetime risk for primary surgery for either SUI or POP by the age of 80 years is

TABLE 12-11 PESSARY: MANAGEMENT OPTIONS IN SELF-CARE

Intervals between clinic follow-up visits*	• 1–2 weeks post initial fitting till "ideal" pessary found • Every 3–4 months if clinician removing and cleaning pessary • Every 3 months first year then every 6–12 months if without problems
Self-removal intervals for independent users*	• Nightly, weekly, and at minimum, monthly; replace post-cleaning • Remove at HS, clean and replace AM • Remove in shower, clean, then replace • Periodically remove for cleaning, intercourse if indicated (donut, cube, Gellhorn) or preferred, and discomfort • Incontinence pessary may be used prn with increased activity, that is, workouts, dancing, cleaning
Cleaning of pessary	• Soap, water, rinse, and dry in clean towel* • If protein deposits, discoloration, or mild odor soak in 1:1 white vinegar and water solution for 30 minutes, rinse well, dry in clean towel†
Vaginal moisturizer options	• Commercially available products (creams, gels, inserts) to increase vaginal moisture 2–3 per week. Not to be used as a lubricant prior to intercourse. Consider polycarbophil-based products that can acidify and increase moisture* • Newer products on market with hyaluronic acid, claiming to be iso-osmotic, acidic, and without harsh ingredients† • Naturally occurring moisturizer without scientific support: natural coconut oil, almond oil, vitamin E capsule, Emu oil, Shea butter (will break down condoms)†
Vaginal acidification	• Consider use of low-dose intravaginal cream in menopausal women‡ • Use of acidifying gel from pessary manufacture (Trimosan™); ½ applicator full vaginally 2–3 times weekly.* • Periodic vinegar/water douche only in post-menopausal women. ¼ cup white vinegar to 1 cup water weekly*
Alerts	• Report any abnormal discharge, odor, elimination problems, poor symptom reduction, pessary slippage or dislodgement, discomfort or pain ASAP‡ • Medical alert for women suffering altered cognition*

*Expert opinion.
†No data to support recommendation.
‡Limited studies support recommendation.

20% to 30%, with a 13% risk for POP repair alone (Olsen et al., 1997; Wu et al., 2014a, 2014b). Research reveals that over 200,000 inpatient surgeries for POP occurs annually in the USA with 25% to 30% representing reoperations (Lavelle et al., 2016; Olsen et al., 1997; Shah et al., 2008); costing more than 1 billion in health care dollars (Brown et al., 2002; Shah et al. 2008; Silva et al., 2006). Candidates for surgical pelvic reconstruction are those who have failed or declined conservative measures for symptomatic POP. The goals of POP surgery are to restore normal vaginal anatomy and normal bladder, bowel, and sexual function, ultimately translating into improved QoL (Barber et al., 2009). The ARNP's role in surgical management is to assure the woman has realistic expectations, is fully informed of the risks versus benefits of pelvic surgery especially if there's a presence of multiple comorbidities such as heart and pulmonary disease, diabetes, obesity, anticoagulants therapy, etc. Knowledge of a reputable obstetrical/gynecological referral group where there is collaboration and open communication regarding the patient's health status and journey in POP management is mandatory to facilitate trust and optimal outcomes.

The two main surgical approaches are vaginal and abdominal approaches. Within each of these approaches, there are multiple potential procedures but depend upon location of the compartment defect. For example, vaginal approaches include vaginal hysterectomy and anterior or posterior wall repair; abdominal procedures include hysterectomy, sacral colpopexy, and paravaginal repair and can be performed through an open incision, laparoscopically, or robotically (Maher et al., 2013). According to Rogo-Gupta (2013), there has been a significant evolution in the surgical treatment of POP over the past decade. Historically, the most common procedures were inpatient laparotomy, which included hysterectomy. Since the mid-1990s, minimally invasive ambulatory procedures have become popular. Advances in prolapse repair materials have also resulted in changes in surgical practices with surgical mesh gaining popularity (Chapple et al., 2017; Lazarou, 2019; Mironska et al., 2019). However, adverse event reports associated with the use of mesh have caused elevated concerns, and there has been a significant decline in its use since 2008. A 2013 Cochrane review of surgical procedures for POP (Maher et al., 2013) included RCTs and quasi-experimental studies (*n* = 56) comparing the outcomes of various surgical approaches. There were no trials comparing surgery to other treatment options. After reviewing trials comparing surgical options, the authors concluded that sacral colpopexy has superior outcomes to a variety of vaginal procedures including sacrospinous colpopexy, uterosacral colpopexy, and transvaginal mesh. These benefits must be balanced against a longer operating time, longer time to return to activities of daily living, and increased cost of the abdominal approach. The use of mesh or graft inlays at the time of anterior vaginal wall repair reduces the risk of recurrent anterior wall prolapse on examination. Anterior vaginal polypropylene mesh also reduces awareness of prolapse; however, these benefits must be weighed against increased operating time, blood loss, rate of apical or posterior compartment prolapse, de novo stress UI, and reoperation rate for mesh exposures associated with the use of polypropylene mesh. Posterior vaginal wall repair may be better than transanal repair in the management of rectocele in terms of recurrence of prolapse. The evidence is not supportive of any grafts at the time of posterior vaginal repair. Adequately powered randomized, controlled clinical trials with blinding of assessors are urgently needed on a wide variety of issues, and they particularly need to include women's perceptions of prolapse symptoms using validated instruments. Following the FDA (April 2019) mandate for mesh manufactures to stop selling and withdraw all commercial transvaginal mesh kits from the market for anterior compartment prolapse (cystocele) due to lack of safety and efficacy (Powers et al., 2019), the generalizability of the findings, especially relating to anterior compartment transvaginal mesh, should be interpreted with caution. Noteworthy, this FDA mandate restriction does not include mesh products used for apical prolapses (sacrocolpopexy) or midurethral sling procedures used for SUI (Lazarou, 2019; Mironska et al., 2019). The ICI committee (Baessler et al., 2017) provided conclusions with high-level evidence after reviewing numerous RCT's regarding pelvic reconstruction for POP; a few of these recommendations included the following (1) compared to the use of the women's native tissue, transvaginal mesh operations do not improve anterior compartment prolapse symptoms or anatomy (vaginal bulge, dyspareunia, post-op SUI) and experience a mesh exposure rate of 18% with 9.5% reoperation to remove the mesh (level one, grade A); (2) abdominal sacral colpopexy (ASC) has been found to be superior in outcomes (management of symptoms; less de novo SUI, prolapse recurrence, dyspareunia) to sacrospinous ligament suspensions for apical vaginal prolapse but has a higher rate of complications (longer surgical time, increased length of stay, longer recuperation and costly) (level one, grade A); (3) ASC with the use of polypropylene mesh is superior to native tissue; (4) transvaginal approach for posterior compartment prolapse is superior to transanal approach; (5) women with both vaginal and rectal prolapse experience better outcomes with urogynecologist and colorectal surgeons collaboration; and (6) women must be informed of the safety and potential complications involved with the use of transvaginal meshes including more reoperations than native tissue repairs.

Postoperative care following prolapse surgery is generally similar to the care following surgery for SUI (Chapter 11). Patients may be advised to avoid strenuous exercise and lifting (more than light objects) at least 4 to 6 weeks (Wang & Smith, 2017), and sexual intercourse for a longer period of time (up to 8 weeks following surgery). Detailed discussion regarding methods to avoid constipation is of upmost importance since excessive Valsalva places counterproductive pressure on healing vaginal incisions. Some nonodorous vaginal discharge and spotting are expected but does not resemble the amount found during menses; possible transient urgency and SUI may exist but should be reported if it persists 4 to 6 weeks post-op. Encourage the woman to engage or continue PFMT once pelvic tenderness is minimal to help stabilize the pelvic floor but be sure she is performing correctly since a Valsalva maneuver instead of pelvic muscle contraction is ineffective and possible detrimental following prolapse repair (Wang & Smith, 2017).

> **KEY POINT**
>
> Advances in prolapse repair materials have also resulted in changes in surgical practices with surgical mesh gaining popularity, but adverse event reports have led to removal of transvaginal mesh from the market for cystocele repair.

VESICOVAGINAL FISTULA

Common sites for fistulas are vesicovaginal (bladder to vagina), urethrovaginal (urethra to vagina), vaginoperineal (vagina to the perineum), ureterovaginal (ureter to vagina), and rectovaginal (rectum to vagina) (**Fig. 12-15**).

Vesicovaginal fistula (VVF) is an abnormal tract that forms between the bladder and vagina, allowing urine to continuously drain into the vagina. While most fistulas develop between the bladder and vagina, they can occur between the urethra and vagina as well. The woman with a VVF leaks urine continuously, which can have a devastating impact on QoL (Demirci et al., 2013).

ETIOLOGY

In the developing world, the most common cause of VVF is attempted vaginal delivery in the setting of cephalopelvic disproportion. The prolonged pressure of the fetal head causes ischemia and necrosis, which leads to fistula formation. Young, poorly educated primiparas living in rural areas of the developing world are at highest risk for prolonged (obstructed) labor and, thus, fistula forma-

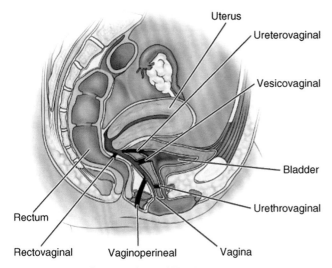

FIGURE 12-15. Common Sites of Fistulas.

tion. In the ICI committee report on fistulas, De Ridder et al. (2017) notes that there are insufficient epidemiological studies on obstetric fistula (OF) but notes the WHO (World Health Organization) estimates 3 per 1,000 women (age 15 to 49 years) from the sub-Saharan African and Asian countries. The effects on young women in these resource poor areas are devastating and often leads to divorce (16% to 92%), social isolation due to family and public ostracism, exacerbating poverty, malnutrition, sexual dysfunction, poor mental and physical health, sense of worthlessness, and suicidal ideations (Cowgill et al., 2015; De Ridder, 2009). Risk factors for OF include marriage at a young age, short stature, delivering of a male child, lack of prenatal care, low socio-economic status and class, unemployment, and illiteracy (Farid et al., 2013; Imoto et al., 2015). The estimated incidence of OFs is low in developed countries; in North America and Europe, it is about 0.01% (McVary & Marshall, 2002). The primary cause of VVF in developed countries is surgical trauma during gynecologic surgery, especially hysterectomy (Demirci et al., 2013; Hadzi-Djokic et al., 2009; Tancer, 1992). The incidence rate following hysterectomy is, however, very low at <1% (Forsgren & Altman, 2010). With radical hysterectomy, the incidence increases to an estimated 1% to 4% (Forsgren & Altman, 2010). Possible mechanisms are direct injury to the bladder or urethra or pressure necrosis secondary to sutures incorporated into the bladder. Data from observational studies have identified a number of characteristics that may increase the risk of hysterectomy-associated VVF. These include older age, laparoscopic or abdominal approaches during the hysterectomy, smoking, and pelvic adhesions (Forsgren & Altman, 2010). Other risk factors include pelvic radiation and, less commonly, destruction of tissue secondary to malignant tumors, ulceration from a foreign body (e.g., pessary), direct trauma, tuberculosis, schistosomiasis, calculi, and endometriosis (McVary & Marshall, 2002).

KEY POINT

VVF although relatively rare in developed countries, the WHO estimates that it may be present in 3 out of 1,000 women in developing African and Asian countries.

CLINICAL PRESENTATION

The diagnosis is obvious in most patients due to the continuous leakage of urine and the observation of urine draining from the vagina. McVary and Marshall (2002) recommend the following diagnostic studies in all patients with VVF: (1) urinalysis, (2) urine culture, (3) intravenous urography, (4) cystoscopy, and (5) vaginoscopy. A noninvasive test that could be done in the office to identify VVF is the ingestion of phenazopyridine, which will stain the urine orange and then place a tampon into the vagina to verify staining in the presence of a fistula (O'Brien & Lynch, 1990). Another simple test is using three proctology swabs line up in the vagina where the most colored orange swab indicates the fistula presumed location (Gannon, 1990). Successful surgical repair is dependent on determining the exact location of the fistula, its size, and the underlying causes. Other tests should be performed as needed, such as a CT scan, MRI, and/or retrograde ureteropyelogram with CT and cystoscopy being the most consistent in detecting fistula (De Ridder et al., 2017). A number of systems exist for classifying VVF although there is currently no universally accepted system (De Ridder, 2011). Frajzyngier et al. (2013) examined the diagnostic performance of five current classification systems and concluded that all of the systems were rather complex, and none had good prognostic value for successful fistula closure. According to the authors, there is a need for a prognostic classification system that is evidence-based, simple, and easy to use.

MANAGEMENT

Patients with VVF leak urine continuously, which places them at high risk for incontinence-associated dermatitis (IAD). Routine cleansing of the perineal area and the application of a moisture barrier product to prevent further damage are an important part of the management during time prior to diagnosis and repair (see Chapter 17) (De Ridder et al., 2017). The use of proper body worn absorbent products (BWAPS) will quickly wick moisture away from the skin and provide dignity and "social continence" (see Chapter 16). Definitive management options for VVF include conservative management, surgical repair, and urinary diversion (De Ridder et al., 2017). While small fistulas are sometimes managed conservatively with prolonged catheter drainage to allow healing and closure, the reported success rate in achieving closure has generally been low (McVary & Marshall, 2002; Narayanan et al., 2009). Currently, surgery is considered the preferred treatment for most patients. According to De Ridder (2011), the surgical approach is dependent on the characteristics of the fistula (e.g., size and location) as well as the expertise of the surgeon (Creanga & Genadry, 2007). In the developed world, a variety of approaches are described. These include vaginal, abdominal, laparoscopic, minimally invasive, and robotic-assisted approaches. Unfortunately, in developing countries, there is a severe shortage of highly skilled urogynecologist, equipment, resources, and skilled nurses. The International Federation for Gynecology and Obstetrics with the International Society of Fistula Surgeons has developed a global competency-based fistula training manual to fill this gap in knowledge and skill (Akhter et al., 2011). Depending on the amount of urethral or bladder damage associated with the fistula, some women will experience persistent SUI despite successful closure (Creanga & Genadry, 2007; de Ridder, 2011). The ICI committee (De Ridder et al., 2017) created several recommendations after rigorous literature review of RCTs regarding VVF; some of the recommendations include (1) tremendous need for local care programs for women who have failed VVF repair; (2) use of only autologous material with fistula repair due to the high risk of infection in synthetic sling materials; (3) SUI repair should be performed no earlier than 6 months post fistula repair; (4) cesarean delivery should be offered in women with history of fistula repair; (5) women experiencing sexual dysfunction due to dyspareunia, constricted vagina should be offered intravaginal estrogen, vaginal dilators, or vaginal flap reconstruction depending on severity; and (6) counseling and psychological rehabilitation is needed to treat mental health issues linked to fistula trauma.

When a fistula cannot be repaired or has failed previous closure attempts, urinary diversion may be indicated. Nursing care needs related to the care of patients with VVF will vary with the type of surgery performed. In the early postoperative period, women will have an indwelling catheter and measures need to be taken to minimize the risk of catheter-associated infection. Women need to be monitored for postoperative complications including infections (urinary tract and wound) and hemorrhage. If a woman experiences SUI following surgical closure of the fistula, PFMT is indicated. Nurses need to be aware of the cultural issues related to UI associated with VVF or occurring for other reasons. For instance, Sange et al. (2008) reported that UI has a more devastating impact on the QoL of Muslim women than for many other women. Muslims have to perform ritual cleansing prior to prayers, which are performed five times a day. If a woman leaks urine, she must perform the cleansing ritual again. This repeated need for cleansing can lead to guilt and perceptions of punishment. As a result of guilt, women may be reluctant to seek treatment for their UI.

KEY POINT

Surgery is a definitive treatment for most women with a vesicovaginal fistula.

 CONCLUSION

POP is a common problem among women and often accompanies SUI. In contrast, VVF is relatively rare; it is a devastating problem for women who experience it. While POP is common, most cases are mild and asymptomatic. Observation and PFMT are viable treatment options for women with lower stage POP and are asymptomatic or experience relatively minimal bother in more advance prolapses. Recently, there is high-level research supporting the effectiveness of PFMT in reducing bothersome POP symptoms but not reducing prolapse severity. Pessaries are the main nonsurgical treatment option for women with POP and should be considered first-line intervention for symptomatic prolapse. The ideal pessary type and size will vary with the severity of the POP as well as other patient characteristics. Surgical reconstruction may be warranted in women with bothersome symptoms and/or advance prolapse. The goal of surgery is to restore normal vaginal anatomy and optimize bladder, bowel, and sexual function to improved QoL. Surgery for POP is common with a 13% lifetime risk and unfortunately, a 25% to 30% risk for reoperation due to POP reoccurrence (Olsen et al., 1997). Although the introduction of synthetic mesh has revolutionized pelvic reconstruction, transvaginal synthetic mesh is no longer recommended in the repair of anterior compartment (cystocele) prolapse due to complications. The role of the ARNP in surgical management is to be a patient advocate, to assure the woman has realistic expectations, and is fully informed of the risks versus benefits of pelvic surgery.

VVF is a rare clinical condition with a major impact on the quality of women's lives. In developing countries, it is usually seen in young primigravidas with obstructed labor due to the fetal head being too large to pass through the pelvis. In the United States, it is generally a surgical complication and occurs most often as a result of a hysterectomy. Women present with continuous leakage of urine from the vagina and skin care is an important consideration. Treatment is usually surgical but depending on the size and location of the fistula and the amount of damage to surrounding tissue, women may continue to experience SUI following surgical correction.

REFERENCES

Abed, H., & Rogers, R. G. (2008). Urinary incontinence and pelvic organ prolapse: Diagnosis and treatment for the primary care physician. *Medical Clinics of North America, 92*(5), 1273–1293, xii. doi: 10.1016/j.mcna.2008.04.004.

ACOG. (2018). *The use of vaginal estrogen in women with a history of estrogen-dependent breast cancer.* ACOG Committee Opinion.

Retrieved from https://www.acog.org/Clinical-Guidance-and-Publications/Committee-Opinions/Committee-on-Gynecologic-Practice/The-Use-of-Vaginal-Estrogen-in-Women-With-a-History-of-Estrogen-Dependent-Breast-Cancer?

ACOG (American College of Obstetrics & Gynecology). (2019). Pelvic organ prolapse: ACOG practice Bulletin, Number 214. *Obstetrics & Gynecology, 134*(5), e126–e142.

Akhter, S., Browing, A., de Bernis, L., et al. (2011). *Global competency-based fistula surgery training manual.* London: FIGO.

Allen-Brady, K., et al. (2011). Identification of six loci associated with pelvic organ prolapse using genome-wide association analysis. *Obstetrics & Gynecology, 118*(6), 1345–1353.

Altman, D., Forsman, M., Falconer, C., et al. (2008). Genetic influence on stress urinary incontinence and pelvic organ prolapse. *European Urology, 54*(4), 918–922. doi: 10.1016/j.eururo.2007.12.004.

Atnip, S., & O'Dell, K. (2012). Vaginal support pessaries; Indications for use and fitting strategies. *Urological Nursing, 32*(3), 114–124.

Auwad, W., Freeman, R. M., & Swift, S. (2004). Is the pelvic organ prolapse quantification system (POPQ) being used? A survey of members of the International Continence Society (ICS) and the American Urogynecologic Society (AUGS). *International Urogynecology Journal and Pelvic Floor Dysfunction, 15*(5), 324–327. doi: 10.1007/s00192-004-1175-3.

Awwad, J., Sayegh, R., Yeretzian, J., et al. (2012). Prevalence, risk factors, and predictors of pelvic organ prolapse: A community-based study. *Menopause, 19*(11), 1235–1241. doi: 10.1097/gme.0b013e31826d2d94.

Baessler, K., Barber, M., Cheon, C., et al. (2017). Surgery for pelvic organ prolapse. In P. Abrams, L. Cardozo, A. Wagg, et al., (Eds.). *Incontinence* (6th ed., p. 1855). Bristol, UK: ICI-ICS. International Continence Society.

Barber, M. D., Brubaker, L., Burgio, K. L., et al. (2014). Comparison of 2 transvaginal surgical approaches and perioperative behavioral therapy for apical vaginal prolapse: The OPTIMAL randomized trial. *JAMA, 311*(10), 1023–1034.

Barber, M. D., Brubaker, L., Nygaard, I., et al. (2009). Defining success after surgery for pelvic organ prolapse. *Obstetrics and Gynecology, 114*(3), 600–609. doi.org/10.1097/AOG.0b013e3181b2b1ae.

Barber, M. D., Cundiff, G. W., Weidner, A. C., et al. (1999). Accuracy of clinical assessment of paravaginal defects in women with anterior vaginal wall prolapse. *American Journal Obstetric Gynecology, 181*(1), 87–90.

Barber, M. D., Visco, A. G., Wyman, J. F., et al. (2002). Sexual function in women with urinary incontinence and pelvic organ prolapse. *Obstetrics & Gynecology, 99*, 281.

Beerepoot, M., & Geerlings, S. (2016). Non-antibiotic prophylaxis for UTI. *Pathogens, 5*, 36. doi: 10.3390/pathogens5020036.

Biglia, N., Peano, E., Sgandurra, P., et al. (2010). Low-dose vaginal estrogens or vaginal moisturizer in breast cancer survivors with urogenital atrophy: A preliminary study. *Gynecologic Endocrinology, 26*(6), 404–412. doi: 10.3109/09513591003632258.

Bø, K. (2012). Pelvic floor muscle training in treatment of female stress urinary incontinence, pelvic organ prolapse and sexual dysfunction. *World Journal of Urology, 30*(4), 437–443. doi: 10.1007/s00345-011-0779-8.

Bo, K., Hilde, G., Tennfjord, M. K., et al. (2013). Randomized controlled trial of pelvic floor muscle training to prevent and treat pelvic organ prolapse in postpartum primiparous women. *Neurourology and Urodynamics, 32*(6), 806–807.

Boyles, S. H., Weber, A. M., & Meyn, L. (2003). Procedures for pelvic organ prolapse in the United States, 1979–1997. *American Journal of Obstetrics and Gynecology, 188*(1), 108–115. doi.org/10.1067/mob.2003.101.

Brown, J. S., Waetjen, L. E., Subak, L. L., et al. (2002). Pelvic organ prolapse surgery in the United States, 1997. *American Journal of Obstetrics and Gynecology, 186*(4), 712–716. doi.org/10.1067/mob.2002.121897.

Bugge, C., Adams, E. J., Gopinath, D., et al. (2013). Pessaries (mechanical devices) for pelvic organ prolapse in women. *Cochrane Database of Systematic Reviews, 2*, CD004010. doi: 10.1002/14651858.CD004010.pub3.

Bulchandani, S., Toozs-Hobson, P., Verghese, T., et al. (2015). Does vaginal estrogen treatment with support pessaries in vaginal prolapse reduce complications? *Post Reproductive Health, 21*(4), 141–145. doi.org/10.1177/2053369115614704.

Castro Diaz, D., Robinson, D., Bosch, R., et al. (2017). Initial assessment of urinary incontinence in adult male and female patients. In P. Abrams, L. Cardozo, A. Wagg, et al. (Eds.), *Incontinence* (6th ed., pp. 497–598). Bristol, UK: ICI-ICS. International Continence Society.

Chapple, C. R., Cruz, F., Deffieux, X., et al. (2017). Consensus Statement of the European Urology Association and the European Urogynaecological Association on the use of implanted materials for treating pelvic organ prolapse and stress urinary incontinence. *European Urology, 72*(3), 424–431. doi.org/10.1016/j.eururo.2017.03.048.

Cheung, R. Y., Lee, J. H., Lee, L. L., et al. (2016). Vaginal pessary in women with symptomatic pelvic organ prolapse: A randomized controlled trial. *Obstetrics and Gynecology, 128*(1), 73–80. doi.org/10.1097/AOG.0000000000001489.

Chiaffarino, F., Chatenoud, L., Dindelli, M., et al. (1999). Reproductive factors, family history, occupation and risk of urogenital prolapse. *European Journal of Obstetrics, Gynecology, & Reproductive Biology, 82*, 63–67.

Clemons, J. L. (2020). Vaginal pessaries: Indications, devices, and approach to selection. In L. Brubaker, & K. Eckler (Eds.), *UpToDate.* Waltham, MA: UpToDate. Retrieved February 11, 2020, from www.uptodate.com/contents/vaginal-pessaries-indications-devices-and-approach-to-selection

Clemons, J. L., Aguilar, V. C., Tillinghast, T. A., et al. (2004). Patient satisfaction and changes in prolapse and urinary symptoms in women who were fitted successfully with a pessary for pelvic organ prolapse. *American Journal of Obstetrics and Gynecology, 190*(4), 1025–1029. doi.org/10.1016/j.ajog.2003.10.711.

Cowgill, K.D., Bishop, J., Norgaard, A. K., et al. (2015). Obstetric fistula in low-re source countries: an under-valued and under studied problem—systematic review of its incidence, prevalence, and association with still birth. *BMC Pregnancy and Childbirth, 215*, 193.

Creanga, A. A., & Genadry, R. R. (2007). Obstetric fistulas: A clinical review. *International Journal of Gynaecology and Obstetrics, 99*(Suppl 1), S40–S46. doi: 10.1016/j.ijgo.2007.06.021.

Cundiff, G. W., Amundsen, C. L., Bent, A. E., et al. (2007). The PESSRI study: Symptom relief outcomes of a randomized crossover trial of the ring and Gellhorn pessaries. *American Journal of Obstetrical Gynecology, 196*, 405.e1–405.e8. (Level II-3).

Dallas, K., Elliott, C.S., Syan, R., et al. (2018). Association between concomitant hysterectomy and repeat surgery for pelvic organ prolapse repair in a cohort of nearly 100,000 women. *Obstetrics & Gynecology, 132*, 1328.

de Albuquerque Coelho, S. C., de Castro, E. B., & Juliato, C. R. (2016). Female pelvic organ prolapse using pessaries: Systematic review. *International Urogynecology Journal, 27*(12), 1797–1803. doi.org/10.1007/s00192-016-2991-y.

De Ridder, D. (2009). Vesicovaginal fistula: A major healthcare problem. *Current Opinion in Urology, 19*(4), 358–361. doi: 10.1097/MOU.0b013e32832ae1b7.

De Ridder, D. (2011). An update on surgery for vesicovaginal and urethrovaginal fistulae. *Current Opinion in Urology, 21*(4), 297–300. doi: 10.1097/MOU.0b013e3283476ec8.

De Ridder, D., Browning, A., Mourad, S., et al. (2017). Fistula. In P. Abrams, L. Cardozo, A. Wagg, et al. (Eds.), *Incontinence* (6th ed., pp. 2143–2185). Bristol, UK: ICI-ICS. International Continence Society.

de Sam Lazaro, S., Nardos, R., & Caughey, A. B. (2016). Obesity and pelvic floor dysfunction: Battling the bulge. *Obstetrical & Gynecological Survey, 71*(2), 114–125. doi.org/10.1097/OGX.0000000000000274.

DeLancey, J. O. (1998). Structural aspects of the extrinsic continence mechanism. *Obstetrics & Gynecology, 72*(3 PT 1), 296–301.

DeLancey, J., Igawa, Y., Koelbl, H., et al. (2017). Pathophysiology of pelvic organ prolapse. In P. Abrams, L. Cardozo, A. Wagg, et al. (Eds.). *Incontinence* (6th ed., pp. 361–409). Bristol, UK: ICI-ICS. International Continence Society.

Demirci, U., Fall, M., Göthe, S., et al. (2013). Urovaginal fistula formation after gynaecological and obstetric surgical procedures: Clinical experiences in a Scandinavian series. *Scandinavian Journal of Urology, 47*(2), 140–144. doi: 10.3109/00365599.2012.711772.

Dietz, H. P. (2003). Do Asian women have less pelvic organ mobility than Caucasians? *International Urogynecology Journal Pelvic Floor Dysfunction, 14*(4), 250–253; discussion 253.

Dumoulin, C., Adewuyi, T., Booth, J., et al. (2017). Adult Conservative management. In P. Abrams, L. Cardozo, A. Wagg, et al. (Eds.). *Incontinence* (6th ed., pp. 1537–1575). Bristol, UK: ICI-ICS. International Continence Society.

Dwyer, L., Kearney, R, Lavender T. (2019). A review of pessary for prolapse practitioner training. *British Journal of Nursing, 28*(9), S18–S24. doi: 10.12968/bjon.2019.28.9.S18.

Elenskaia, K., Thakar, R., Sultan, A. H., et al. (2013). Effect of childbirth on pelvic organ support and quality of life: A longitudinal cohort study. *International Urogynecology Journal, 24*(6), 927–937. doi: 10.1007/s00192-012-1932-7.

Ellerkmann, R. M., Cundiff, G. W., Melick, C. F., et al. (2001). Correlation of symptoms with location and severity of pelvic organ prolapse. *American Journal of Obstetrics and Gynecology, 185*(6), 1332–1337; discussion 1337–1338. doi: 10.1067/mob.2001.119078.

Farid, F. N., Azhar, M., Samnani, S. S., et al. (2013). Psychosocial experiences of women with vesicovaginal fistula: A qualitative approach. *Journal of College Physicians Surgical Pakistan, 23*(10), 828–829.

Fernando, R. J., Thakar, R., Sultan, A. H., et al. (2006). Effect of vaginal pessaries on symptoms associated with pelvic organ prolapse. *Obstetrics and Gynecology, 108*(1), 93–99. doi.org/10.1097/01.AOG.0000222903.38684.cc.

Forsgren, C., & Altman, D. (2010). Risk of pelvic organ fistula in patients undergoing hysterectomy. *Current Opinion in Obstetrics and Gynecology, 22*(5), 404–407. doi: 10.1097/GCO.0b013e32833e49b0.

Forsgren, C., Lundholm, C., Johansson, A. L. V., et al. (2012). Vaginal hysterectomy and risk of pelvic organ prolapse and stress urinary incontinence surgery. *International Urogynecology Journal, 23*(1), 43–48. doi: 10.1007/s00192-011-1523-z.

Frajzyngier, V., Guohua, L., Larson, E., et al. (2013). Development and comparison of prognostic scoring systems for surgical closure of genitourinary fistula. *American Journal of Obstetrics and Gynecology, 208*(2), 112.e1–112.e11. doi: 10.1016/j.ajog.2012.11.040.

Freedman, M. A. (2008). Vaginal pH, estrogen, and genital atrophy. *Menopause Management, 17*(4), 9–13.

Friedman, T., Eslick, G. D., & Dietz, H. P. (2018). Risk factors for prolapse recurrence: Systematic review and meta-analysis. *International Urogynecology Journal, 29*, 13.

Gannon, M. J. (1990). The three-swab test using knots for urovaginal fistula. *Surgery, Gynecology & Obstetrics, 170*(2), 171.

Gilchrist, A. S., Campbell, W., Steele, H., et al. (2013). Outcomes of observation as therapy for pelvic organ prolapse: A study in the natural history of pelvic organ prolapse. *Neurourology and Urodynamics, 32*, 383–386. doi: 10.1002/nau.

Giri, A., Hartmann, K. E., Hellwege, J. N., et al. (2017). Obesity and pelvic organ prolapse: A systematic review and meta-analysis of observational studies. *American Journal of Obstetrics & Gynecology, 184*, 1496.

Gleason, J. L., Richter, H. E., & Varner, R. E. (2012). Pelvic organ prolapse. In J. S. Berek (Ed.), *Berek & Novak's Gynecology* (15th ed., pp. 1–46). Philadelphia, PA: Lippincott Williams & Wilkins.

Gutman, R. E., Ford, D. E., Quiroz, L. H., et al. (2008). Is there a pelvic organ prolapse threshold that predicts pelvic floor symptoms? *American Journal of Obstetrics and Gynecology, 199*(6), 683.e1–683.e7. doi: 10.1016/j.ajog.2008.07.028.

Gyhagen, M., Bullarbo, M., Nielsen, T. F., et al. (2013). Prevalence and risk factors for pelvic organ prolapse 20 years after childbirth: A national cohort study in singleton primiparae after vaginal or caesarean delivery. *BJOG: An International Journal of Obstetrics and Gynaecology, 120*(2), 152–160. doi: 10.1111/1471-0528.12020.

Hadzi-Djokic, J., Pejcic, T. P., & Acimovic, M. (2009). Vesico-vaginal fistula: Report of 220 cases. *International Urology & Nephrology, 41*(2), 299–302.

Hagen, S., Glazener, C., McClurg, D., et al. (2014). A multicenter randomized controlled trial of a pelvic floor muscle training intervention for the prevention of pelvic organ prolapse (PREVPROL). *Neurourology and Urodynamics, 33*(6), 852–853.

Hagen, S., & Stark, D. (2011). Conservative prevention and management of pelvic organ prolapse in women. *Cochrane Database of Systematic Reviews, 12*, CD003882. doi: 10.1002/14651858.CD003882.pub4.

Hagen, S., Stark, D., Glazener, C., et al. (2014). Individualised pelvic floor muscle training in women with pelvic organ prolapse (POPPY): A multicentre randomised controlled trial. *Lancet, 383*(9919), 796–806. doi: 10.1016/S0140-6736(13)61977-7.

Handa, V. L., Garrett, E., Hendrix, S., et al. (2004). Progression and remission of pelvic organ prolapse: A longitudinal study of menopausal women. *American Journal of Obstetrics & Gynecology, 190*, 27.

Haylen, B. T., Maher, C. F., Barber, M. D., et al. (2016). An International Urogynecological Association (IUGA)/International Continence Society (ICS) joint report on the terminology for female pelvic organ prolapse (POP). *International Urogynecology Journal, 27*(2), 165–194. doi.org/10.1007/s00192-015-2932-1.

Hendrix, S. L., Clark, A., Nygaard, I., et al. (2002). Pelvic organ prolapse in the Women's Health Initiative: Gravity and gravidity. *American Journal of Obstetrics and Gynecology, 186*(6), 1160–1166. doi.org/10.1067/mob.2002.123819.

Hooper G. L. (2018). Person-centered care for patients with pessaries. *The Nursing Clinics of North America, 53*(2), 289–301. doi.org/10.1016/j.cnur.2018.01.006.

Hooper, G. L., Atnip, S., & O'Dell, K. (2017). Optimal pessary care: A modified Delphi consensus study. *Journal of Midwifery & Women's Health, 62*(4), 452–462. doi.org/10.1111/jmwh.12624.

Hull, A. (2019). 50 years of pessary use. *Urological Nursing, 39*(5), 265–269.

Imoto, A., Matsuyama, A., Ambauen-Berger, B., et al. (2015). Health-related quality of life among women in rural Bangladesh after surgical repair of obstetric fistula. *International Journal of Gynecology Obstetrics, 130*(1), 79–83.

Jack, G. S., et al. (2006). Familial transmission of genitovaginal prolapse. *International Urogynecology Journal of Pelvic Floor Dysfunction, 17*(5), 498–501.

Jelovsek, J. E., Chagin, K., Gyhagen, M., et al. (2018). Predicting risk of pelvic floor disorders 12 and 20 years after delivery. *American Journal of Obstetrics and Gynecology, 218*(2), 222.e1–222.e19. doi.org/10.1016/j.ajog.2017.10.014

Jorgensen, S., Hein, H. O., & Gyntelberg, F. (1994). Heavy lifting at work and risk of genital prolapse and herniated lumbar disc in assistant nurses. *Occupational Medicine (London), 44*(1), 47–49.

Kandadai, P., Mcvay, S., Larrioux, J. R., et al. (2016). Knowledge and comfort with pessary use: A survey of US obstetrics and genecology residents. *Female Pelvic Medicine & Reconstructive Surgery, 22*(6), 491–496.

Kim, S., Harvey, M. A., & Johnston, S. (2005). A review of the epidemiology and pathophysiology of pelvic floor dysfunction: Do racial differences matter? *Journal of Obstetrics & Gynecology Canada, 27*(3), 251–259.

Lavelle, R. S., Christie, A. L., Alhalabi, F., et al. (2016). Risk of prolapse recurrence after native tissue anterior vaginal suspension procedure with intermediate to long-term follow-up. *Journal of Urology, 195*, 1014.

Lazarou, G. (2019). *Pelvic organ prolapse.* Retrieved March 13, 2020 from emedicine.medscape.com/article/276259-overview#a9

Lowder, J. L., Ghetti, C., Nikolajski, C., et al. (2011). Body image perceptions in women with pelvic organ prolapse: A qualitative study. *American Journal of Obstetrical Gynecology, 204*, 441.e1.

Lukacz, E. S., Santiago-Lastra, Y., Albo, M. E., et al. (2017). Urinary incontinence in women: A review. *JAMA, 318*(16), 1592–1604. doi. org/10.1001/jama.2017.12137.

Madhu, C., Swift, S., Moloney-Geany, S., et al. (2018). How to use the Pelvic Organ Prolapse Quantification (POP-Q) system? *Neurourology. Urodynamics, 37*(S6), S39–S43.

Maher, C., Feiner, B., Baessler, K., et al. (2013). Surgical management of pelvic organ prolapse in women. *Cochrane Database of Systematic Reviews, 4*, CD004014. doi: 10.1002/14651858.CD004014.pub5.

Manonai, J., Harnsomboon, T., Sarit-apirak, S., et al. (2012). Effect of colpexin sphere on pelvic floor muscle strength and quality of life in women with pelvic organ prolapse stage I/II: a randomized controlled trial. *International Urogynecology Journal, 23*(3), 307–312.

Mant, J., Painter, R., & Vessey, M. (1997). Epidemiology of genital prolapse: Observations from the Oxford Family Planning Association Study. *British Journal of Obstetrics & Gynecology, 104*(5), 579–585.

McLennan, M. T., Harris, J. K., Kariuki, B., et al. (2008). Family history as a risk factor for pelvic organ prolapse. *International Urogynecology Journal, 19*(8), 1063–1069. doi: 10.1007/s00192-008-0591-1.

McVary, K. T., & Marshall, F. F. (2002). Vesicovaginal fistula. In J. Y. Gillenwater, J. T. Grayhack, S. S. Howards, et al. (Eds.), *Adult and pediatric urology* (4th ed., pp. 1272–1278). Philadelphia, PA: Lippincott Williams & Wilkins.

Miedel, A., Tegertedt, G., Moehle-Schmidt, M., et al. (2009). Nonobstetric risk factors for symptomatic pelvic organ prolapse. *Obstetrics and Gynecology, 113*(5), 1089–1097.

Milsom, I., Altman, D., Cartwright, R., et al. (2017). Epidemiology of urinary incontinence and other lower urinary tract symptoms, pelvic organ prolapse, and anal incontinence. In P. Abrams, L. Cardozo, A. Wagg, et al. (Eds.), *Incontinence* (6th ed., pp. 67–92). Bristol, UK: ICI-ICS. International Continence Society.

Mironska, E., Chapple, C., & MacNeil, S. (2019). Recent advances in pelvic floor repair. *F1000Research, 8*, F1000 Faculty Rev-778. doi. org/10.12688/f1000research.15046.1

Mothes, A. R., et al. (2016). Risk index for pelvic organ prolapse based on established individual risk factors. *Archives in Gynecology Obstetrics, 293*(3), 617–624.

Nager, C. W., Richter, H. E., Nygaard, I., et al. (2009). Incontinence pessaries: Size, POPQ measures, and successful fitting. *International Urogynecology Journal, 20*(9), 1023–1028. doi.org/10.1007/s00192-009-0866-1.

Narayanan, P., Nobbenhuis, M., Reynolds, K. M., et al. (2009). Fistulas in malignant gynecologic disease: Etiology, imaging, and management. *Radiographics, 29*(4), 1073–1083. doi: 10.1148/rg.294085223.

Newman, D. K., Cockerell, R., Griebling, T. L., et al. (2017). Primary prevention, continence promotion, models of care and education. In P. Abrams, L. Cardozo, A. Wagg, et al. (Eds.), *Incontinence* (6th ed., pp. 2429–2478). Bristol, UK: ICI-ICS. International Continence Society.

Nguyen, J. N., & Jones, C. R. (2005). Pessary treatment of pelvic relaxation: Factors affecting successful fitting and continued use. *Journal of Wound, Ostomy, and Continence Nursing, 32*(4), 255–263. doi.org/10.1097/00152192-200507000-00010.

North American Menopause Society (NAMS). (2010). Position statement: Estrogen and progestogen use in post-menopausal women: 2010 position statement of the NAMS. *Menopause, 17*(2), 242–255.

Novi, J. M., Jeronis, S., Morgan, M. A., et al. (2005). Sexual function in women with pelvic organ prolapse compared to women without pelvic organ prolapse. *Journal of Urology, 173*, 1669.

O'Brien, W. M., & Lynch, J. H. (1990). Simplification of double-dye test to diagnose various types of vaginal fistulas. *Urology, 36*(5), 456.

O'Dell, K., & Atnip, S. (2012). Pessary care: Follow up and management of complications. *Urologic Nursing, 32*(3), 126–136, 145.

O'Dell, K., Atnip, S., Hooper, G., et al. (2016). Pessary practices of nurse-providers in the United States. *Female Pelvic Medicine & Reconstructive Surgery, 22*(4), 261–266. doi.org/10.1097/SPV.0000000000000268

Olsen, A. L., Smith, V. J., Bergstrom, J. O., et al. (1997). Epidemiology of surgically managed pelvic organ prolapse and urinary incontinence. *Obstetrics & Gynecology, 89*(4), 501–506. doi: 10.1016/S0029-7844(97)00058-6.

Persu, C., Chapple, C. R., Cauni, V., et al. (2011). Pelvic organ prolapse quantification system (POP-Q)—A new era in pelvic prolapse staging. *Journal of Medicine and Life, 4*(1), 75–81.

Powers, S. A., Burleson, L. K., & Hannan, J. L. (2019). Managing female pelvic floor disorders: A medical device review and appraisal. *Interface Focus, 9*(4), 20190014. doi.org/10.1098/rsfs.2019.0014.

Ramsay, S., Bouchard, F., & Tu, L. M. (2011). Long term outcomes of pessary use in women with pelvic organ prolapse. *Neurourology and Urodynamics, 30*(6), 1105–1106.

Reid, G., Burton, J., & Devillard, E. (2004). The rationale for probiotics in female urogenital healthcare. *Medscape General Medicine, 6*, 49.

Robert, M., Schulz, J. A., Harvey, M. A., et al. (2013). Technical update on pessary use. *Journal of Obstetrics and Gynaecology Canada, 35*(7), 664–674. Retrieved from http://www.ncbi.nlm.nih.gov/pubmed/23876646

Rogers, R. G., & Fashokun, T. B. (2019). Pelvic organ prolapse in women: Epidemiology, risk factors, clinical manifestations, and management. *UpToDate*. Retrieved February 11, 2020 from https://www.uptodate.com/contents/pelvic-organ-prolapse-in-women-epidemiology-risk-factors-clinical-manifestations-and-management?search=pelvic-organ-prolapse-in%20-women-epidemilogy-riskfactors&source=search_result&selectedTitle=3~111&usage_type=default&display_rank=3

Rogo-Gupta, L. (2013). Current trends in surgical repair of pelvic organ prolapse. *Current Opinion in Obstetrics and Gynecology, 25*(5), 395–398. doi: 10.1097/GCO.0b013e3283648cfb.

Rortveit, G., Brown, J. S., Thom, D. H., et al. (2007). Symptomatic pelvic organ prolapse: Prevalence and risk factors in a population-based, racially diverse cohort. *Obstetrics and Gynecology, 109*(6), 1396–1403.

Sange, C., Thomas, L., Lyons, C., et al. (2008). Urinary incontinence in Muslin women. *Nursing Times, 104*(25), 49–52.

Santoro, N. F., & Lin, I. (2018). Genitourinary syndrome of menopause (GSM): Underdiagnosed & undertreated. *Contemporary OB/GYN, 64*(7). Retrieved March 14, 2020 from https://www.contemporaryobgyn.net/article/genitourinary-syndrome-menopause-underdiagnosed-and-undertreated

Shah, A. D., Kohli, N., Rajan, S. S., et al. (2008). The age distribution, rates, and types of surgery for pelvic organ prolapse in the USA. *International Urogynecology Journal and Pelvic Floor Dysfunction, 19*(3), 421–428. doi.org/10.1007/s00192-007-0457-y.

Shah, S. M., Sultan, A. H., & Thakar, R. (2006). The history and evolution of pessaries for pelvic organ prolapse. *International Urogynecology Journal and Pelvic Floor Dysfunction, 17*(2), 170–175. doi.org/10.1007/s00192-005-1313-6.

Siccardi, M. A., Bordoni, B. (2018). Anatomy, abdomen and pelvis, perineal body. [Updated 2018 December 20]. In: *StatPearls [Internet]*. Treasure Island, FL: StatPearls Publishing. Retrieved from https://www.ncbi.nlm.nih.gov/books/NBK537345/?report=classic

Silva, W. A., Pauls, R. N., Segal, J. L., et al. (2006). Uterosacral ligament vault suspension: Five-year outcomes. *Obstetrics and gynecology, 108*(2), 255–263. doi.org/10.1097/01.AOG.0000224610.83158.23.

Stark, D., Dall, P., Abdel-Fattah, M., et al. (2010). Feasibility, inter- and intra-rater reliability of physiotherapists measuring prolapse using the pelvic organ prolapse quantification system. *International Urogynecology Journal, 21(6)*, 651–656.

Stepp, K. J., & Walters, M. D. (2015). Anatomy of the lower urinary tract, rectum, and pelvic floor. In M. Walters, & M. Karram (Eds.), *Urogynecology and reconstructive pelvic surgery* (4th ed., pp. 19–31). Philadelphia, PA: Elsevier.

Summers, A., Winkel, L. A., Hussain, H., et al. (2006). The relationship between anterior and apical compartment support. *American Journal of Obstetrics & Gynecology, 194*, 1438.

Swift, S. E., Tate, S. B., & Nicholas, J. (2003). Correlation of symptoms with degree of pelvic organ support in a general population of women: What is pelvic organ prolapse? *American Journal of Obstetrics and Gynecology, 189*(2), 372–377. doi: 10.1067/S0002-9378(03)00698-7.

Swift, S., Woodman, P., O'Boyle, A., et al. (2005). Pelvic Organ Support Study (POSST): The distribution, clinical definition, and epidemiologic condition of pelvic organ support defects. *American Journal of Obstetrics and Gynecology, 192*(3), 795–806. doi.org/10.1016/j.ajog.2004.10.602.

Tancer, M. L. (1992). Observations on prevention and management of vesicovaginal fistula after total hysterectomy. *Surgery, Gynecology & Obstetrics, 175*(6), 501–506.

Velzel, J., Roovers, J. P., Van der Vaart, C. H., et al. (2015). A nationwide survey concerning practices in pessary use for pelvic organ prolapse in The Netherlands: Identifying needs for further research. *International Urogynecology Journal, 26*(10), 1453–1458. doi.org/10.1007/s00192-015-2697-6.

Vergeldt, T. F., Weemhoff, M., Inthout, J., et al. (2015). Risk factors for pelvic organ prolapse and its recurrence: A systematic review. *International Urogynecology Journal, 26*, 1559.

Wang, M., & Smith, A. L. (2017). Pelvic organ prolapse. In D. K. Newman, J. F. Wyman, & V. W. Welch (Eds.). *Core curriculum for urological nursing* (pp. 531–543). Pittman, NJ: SUNA.

Wills, S., Ravipatie, A., Venuturumilli, P., et al. (2012). Effects of vaginal estrogens on serum estradiol levels in postmenopausal breast cancer survivors and women at risk of breast cancer taking an aromatase inhibitor or a selective estrogen receptor modulator. *Journal of Oncology Practice, 8*, 144–148.

Woodman, P. J., et al. (2006). Prevalence of severe pelvic organ prolapse in relation to job description and socioeconomic status: A multicenter cross-sectional study. *International Urogynecology Journal Pelvic Floor Dysfunction, 17*(4), 340–345.

Wu, J. M., Matthews, C. A., Conover, M. M., et al. (2014). Lifetime risk of stress urinary incontinence or pelvic organ prolapse surgery. *Obstetrics and Gynecology, 123*(6), 1201–1206. doi.org/10.1097/AOG.0000000000000286.

Wu, J. M., Vaughan, C. P., Goode, P. S., et al. (2014). Prevalence and trends of symptomatic pelvic floor disorders in U.S. women. *Obstetrics and Gynecology, 123*(1), 141–148. doi: 10.1097/AOG.0000000000000057.

Wu, Y. M., & Welk, B. (2019). Revisiting current treatment options for stress urinary incontinence and pelvic organ prolapse: A contemporary literature review. *Research and Reports in Urology, 11*, 179–188. doi.org/10.2147/RRU.S191555.

Yang, J., Han, J., Zhu, F., et al. (2018). Ring and Gellhorn pessaries used in patients with pelvic organ prolapse: A retrospective study of 8 years. *Archives of Gynecology and Obstetrics, 298*(3), 623–629. doi.org/10.1007/s00404-018-4844-z.

QUESTIONS

1. The continence nurse is caring for a female patient diagnosed with a cystocele. Which areas of the pelvic organs are involved in this condition?
   A. Anterior vaginal wall
   B. Posterior vaginal wall
   C. Apex of the vagina
   D. Small or large bowel

2. The continence nurse is providing education regarding POP (pelvic organ prolapse) to future continence nurses. Which of the following statements regarding POP is TRUE?
   A. Least common POP occurs in the anterior vaginal compartment.
   B. It is an uncommon condition in parous women.
   C. POP is underrecognized and underreported.
   D. Advancing age, obesity, and parity are not well-established risk factors.

3. The continence nurse is preparing a patient for a pelvic examination to verify a suspected POP. Which instructions accurately describe a step in the procedure?
   A. The patient should be placed in a prone position.
   B. The patient should be examined with a full bladder.
   C. The patient should be instructed to sit up to observe the prolapse.
   D. The patient should be asked to perform a Valsalva maneuver.

4. You are evaluating a patient with a symptomatic POP. Which of the following clinical presentations is representative of a range of symptoms experienced in patients with POP?
   A. Reduced body image, dyspareunia, and sex avoidance
   B. No change in quality of life, bowel and urinary symptoms
   C. Increase urinary tract infections, loose stools, lack of pelvic pressure
   D. Urinary urgency, frequency, and adequate emptying of bladder/bowel

5. The continence nurse is reading the report of a patient diagnosed with a stage 3 POP via the Bayden and Walker Scoring System. Which findings indicate this level of staging?
   A. The most distal portion of the prolapse is more than 1 cm above the level of the hymen.
   B. The most distal portion of the prolapse is 1 cm or less proximal to or distal to the plane of the hymen.
   C. The most distal portion of the prolapse is more than 1 cm below the plane of the hymen.
   D. Complete eversion of the total length of the lower genital tract is demonstrated.

6. A female patient is diagnosed with stage 2 POP and is asymptomatic. What is the first line of treatment for this condition?
   A. Observation and lifestyle modifications
   B. Vaginal pessary and pelvic muscle exercises
   C. Transvaginal estrogen
   D. Surgical repair

7. Studies have examined the impact of pelvic floor muscle training (PFMT) on POP secondary prevention, severity, and/or symptoms. Which statement reflects the findings of these studies?
   A. PFMT does not reduce the risk of POP development, symptoms, or severity.
   B. PFMT is a conservative measure that reduces the symptoms of POP but not its severity.
   C. PFMT reduces both the symptoms and severity of POP.
   D. PFMT reduces the risk of POP but not symptoms or severity if it exists.

8. You are educating a post-menopausal patient with a symptomatic stage 3 cystocele and stress urinary incontinence regarding treatment options. Which statement accurately describes first-line treatment option in a patient who wants to avoid surgical repair?
   A. Observation and lifestyle modification
   B. Pelvic floor muscle training with a physical therapist
   C. Vaginal estrogen and pessary with a ring, support, and knob
   D. Vagina estrogen and Gellhorn pessary

9. A postpartum 32-year-old female is diagnosed with vesicovaginal fistula (VVF). What is the most common cause of this condition?
   A. Emergency C-section following prolonged labor
   B. Use of high forceps during delivery
   C. Induced labor
   D. Attempted vaginal delivery in the setting of cephalopelvic disproportion

10. What treatment would the continence nurse expect for a patient who is newly diagnosed with vesicovaginal fistula (VVF) due to a surgical complication?
   A. PFMT alone
   B. Surgery to close the fistula
   C. Pharmacological treatment
   D. Hysterectomy

ANSWERS AND RATIONALES

1. A. Rationale: A cystocele is a herniation or prolapse of the bladder into the anterior vaginal compartment, while posterior compartment prolapse can include the decent of the rectum (rectocele) or small intestine (enterocele). Apical prolapse contains either the uterus and cervix, or posthysterectomy vaginal cuff.

2. C. Rationale: OP is under-recognized or underreported; therefore, the number of women who do not seek medical evaluation is unknown. It affects nearly 50% of women who have given birth with the strongest risk factors for development of POP being parity, advancing age, and obesity. Cystocele or prolapse of the anterior vaginal wall is the most common type of POP.

3. D. Rationale: The proper position for a pelvic examine in having the patient assume a supine position with the head of the bed at 45 degrees, an empty bladder to reduce risk of underestimation of POP severity, and asked to perform a Valsalva maneuver to observe for vaginal bulging.

4. A. Rationale: Symptomatic POP may cause bladder, bowel, or sexual dysfunction including poor body image, painful intercourse, and avoidance of sexual intercourse.

5. C. Rationale: Stage 3 POP is demonstrated with the most distal aspect of the prolapse 1 cm below the plane of the hymen.

6. **A. Rationale:** Treatment of asymptomatic POP is normally not indicated except for observation for symptomatology and lifestyle modifications to potentially avert prolapse progressing during "watchful waiting."

7. **B. Rationale:** Based upon study findings, PFMT does not prevent, treat, or reduce severity of POP, but it does reduce symptoms of prolapse especially the sensation of pelvic bulge.

8. **C. Rationale:** Transvaginal estrogen (if not contraindicated) is utilized to prepare vaginal tissues for pessary fitting and reduce risk of pessary complications (abrasion, increase discharge, vaginal/urinary tract infections) and a supportive incontinence ring to address both cystocele and stress incontinence. Incontinence support pessaries have a knob that sits behind the symphysis pubis to support the urethro-vesical junction (bladder neck) especially during activities that increase abdominal pressure.

Gellhorn pessary is difficult to independently manage and may not offer reduction in stress incontinence. Lifestyle modifications and PFMT maybe useful in improving pelvic health but most likely not reduce prolapse severity or progression.

9. **D. Rationale:** The most common cause of VVF is attempted vaginal delivery in the setting of cephalopelvic disproportion. The prolonged pressure of the fetal head causes ischemia and necrosis, which leads to fistula formation. Young, poorly educated primiparas living in rural areas of the developing world are at highest risk for prolonged (obstructed) labor and, thus, fistula formation.

10. **B. Rationale:** Surgery is a definitive treatment for most women with a VVF and possible urinary diversion depending upon the urethral or bladder damage associated with the fistula. Often women may suffer persistent stress urinary incontinence despite successful closure.

CHAPTER 13

UI AND LOWER URINARY TRACT SYMPTOMS IN THE OLDER ADULT

Mary H. Palmer

OBJECTIVES

1. Discuss the impact of incontinence and its implications for continence nurse specialists and other health care providers.

2. Explain how the lower urinary tract functions change with aging and how these changes affect voiding patterns and continence.

3. Discuss current thinking regarding the difference between functional limitations contributing to incontinence and functional incontinence.

4. Describe management options for the patient with functional incontinence.

5. Describe indications and guidelines for toileting programs for management of functional incontinence.

6. Describe factors contributing to transient incontinence and implications for management.

TOPIC OUTLINE

INTRODUCTION: FACTS ABOUT AGING

The portion of the world's population of adults aged 65 years and over is projected to increase from 9.1% in 2019 to 22.6% in 2100 and the number of older adults aged 80 years and over is expected increase from 143 million to 881 million in 2100 (UN, 2019). The United States mirrors this growth in the older adult population; 50.9 million Americans were 65 years and over in 2017 and this number is expected to increase to 94.7 million in 2040. The 85 years and over group is expected to double from 6.5 million in 2017 to 14.4 million in 2040 (Federal Interagency Forum, 2016). The demographic shift is dramatic; there are more middle-aged persons than children in the United States, and by 2035 there will be more older adults than children (US Census Bureau, 2018). **Figure 13-1** depicts changes in the aging population from 1900 to 2060.

This demographic shift impacts health care systems through the increased demand for specialized geriatric acute and long-term care services and supports. Tri-specialty and advance practice tri-specialty nurses, that is, Certified Wound, Ostomy, and Continence Nurse (CWOCN®) and Certified Wound Ostomy Continence Nurse, Advance Practice (CWOCN-AP™), will continue to play a central role in the care of this aging population due to the prevalence of urinary incontinence (UI) and other lower urinary tract symptoms (LUTS). For example, 22% of men between 70 and 79 years of age living in the community and participating in the Health Aging and Body Composition study reported UI and 52% reported nocturia (Bauer et al., 2019). Prevalence of UI in women aged 70 years and over was estimated to be >40% (Milsom & Gyhagen, 2019). According to national estimates published in 2014, 43.8% of older adults living in the community reported urinary leakage, 39% of older adults residing in residential care facilities were reported to have UI in the 7 days preceding the study, 45.4% of home care patients reported difficulty with bladder control, and 46.1% of short-term and 75.8% of long-stay nursing home residents experienced incomplete bladder control in the 14 days preceding the study (Gorina et al., 2014).

CWOCN/CWOCN-AP have in-depth knowledge to screen for, assess, and treat both fecal and urinary incontinence; manage incontinence; contain incontinence with body worn absorbent products (BWAP); and provide skin risk prevention and care (Berke et al., 2019). When working with older adults and frail elders wound, ostomy, continence (WOC) nurses collect and use information about aging-related changes in body systems, consider the impact of multimorbidities (i.e., chronic conditions, functional limitations, and geriatric syndromes) and polypharmacy on lower urinary tract function, and assess the role the environment plays in enhancing and maintaining toileting independence and lower urinary tract health. The lifelong learning process of the WOC nurse must include development and refinement of geriatric competencies that include interdisciplinary collaborations to: (1) foster older adults' function, independence, quality of life, and dignity; (2) consider the needs and preferences of older adults and their family and other caregivers in treatment plans; and (3) help older adults and their families with advance planning and with end-of-life decisions about continence care.

CHANGES IN LOWER URINARY TRACT ASSOCIATED WITH AGING

The major role of the lower urinary tract is storing and emptying urine periodically throughout the day, throughout the life span. Emerging research findings about the urinary microbiome suggest that resident microbiota within the bladder play an important role in urinary health (Govender et al., 2019). Although the prevalence of UI and overactive bladder (OAB) increases with age, *age alone does not cause urinary incontinence.*

> **KEY POINT**
>
> Although the prevalence of urinary incontinence and overactive bladder increases with age, age alone does not cause urinary incontinence.

Age-related changes in the lower urinary tract include decreased urine flow, reduced bladder capacity, reduced detrusor contraction strength, and reduced urethral closure pressure (Mitchell & Waetjen, 2018). Urodynamic changes include increased postvoid residual urine volume, small voided volumes, and increased involuntary detrusor contractions; the ability to empty the bladder efficiently also declines (Wagg et al., 2017).

Age-related differences in young and older women's urinary microbiome have been found. *Lactobacillus*

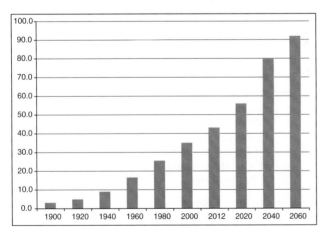

FIGURE 13-1. Number of Persons 65+, 1960 to 2060. (Adapted from Administration on Aging, A Profile of Older Americans: 2013–2014, 06/24, http://www.aoa.gov/Aging_Statistics/Profile/Index.aspx)

tends to be the predominant microbe in younger women's urine, while *Lactobacillus* is not dominant and other bacteria are present in older women's urine. The authors postulated that certain *Lactobacillus* species may play a beneficial role (Govender et al., 2019). More research is needed to determine if diversity of the older women's microbiome is associated with increased LUTS prevalence (Liu et al., 2017). Changes in the lower urinary tract attributed to aging and menopause are variable, and research is still needed to understand the mechanism of these changes. Benign prostatic hypertrophy (BPH) occurs in approximately 80% of men by the age of 70 years, and along with BPH, approximately 50% of men develop prostate enlargement, which in turn can lead to both storage and emptying LUTS (Egan, 2016).

Age-related changes in the neural control include the following. The activation of the brain's neural circuits that control urine storage and emptying declines, which may lessen urine control. Weaker signals to the bladder control network that may be age related could lead to a predisposition for developing OAB symptoms (Suskind, 2017). The use of magnetic resonance imaging (MRI) in research has demonstrated the importance of brain white matter hyperintensities (WMH) on urine control. Researchers found that for each 1% increase in percentage of WMH in the brain, there was a corresponding 1.5 to 2.4 times increased risk for diminished function in voiding, mobility, and cognition (Wakefield et al., 2010). Although associations between WMH and voiding dysfunction have been identified, causal pathways are not understood (Vahabi et al., 2017).

These findings reinforce other research and clinical findings that factors outside the lower urinary tract are important contributors to LUTS in late life. The relationships among factors affecting continence are complex and multifactorial. These factors include age-related changes in central nervous system control and lower urinary tract function; the consequences of life events such as childbirth; the impact of chronic conditions such as diabetes mellitus, obesity, and dementia; and functional limitations, that is, limitations in walking and self-care. Chronological age plays a role in the function of the lower urinary tract and in the development of UI and other LUTS, but other influences such as comorbid conditions and nongenitourinary factors cannot be overlooked. See **Table 13-1**, Nongenitourinary factors associated with UI.

KEY POINT

Factors outside the urinary tract are important contributors to lower urinary tract symptoms in the elderly.

 NOCTURIA

The International Continence Society (ICS) defined nocturia as "the number of times urine is passed during the main sleep period. Having woken to pass urine for the first time, each urination must be followed by sleep or the intention to sleep. This should be quantified using a bladder diary" (Hashim et al., 2019). Nocturia, when using two or more voids at night as a clinical definition, affects approximately 29% to 59.3%

TABLE 13-1 NONGENITOURINARY FACTORS RELATED TO URINARY INCONTINENCE

CHRONIC CONDITIONS	FUNCTIONAL LIMITATIONS	GERIATRIC SYNDROMES	ENVIRONMENT
Diabetes mellitus	Dependent toileting	Physical and cognitive frailty	Cleanliness of toilet facilities
Heart failure	Reduced lower extremity strength	Dementia	Lack of toilet facilities
Depression	Reduced manual dexterity	Polypharmacy	Lack of privacy in toilet facilities
Sleep apnea	Reduced vision	Delirium	Low lighting in bedrooms, bathrooms, hallways
Neurological pathologies: Parkinson disease, cerebrovascular processes, subcortical cerebrovascular white matter lesions	Need for walking aids	Falls	Low or inadequate signage for toilet facilities
Cerebral vascular processes	Communication difficulty	Pressure injuries	Inadequate toilet resources, i.e., handrails, raised toilet seats, toilet paper, running water, paper towels
Bowel symptoms	Self-care deficits	Neglect and abuse	Lack of privacy in toilet facilities
Chronic pulmonary disease		Vertigo	Lack of caregivers to provide timely assistance
Degenerative joint disease		Failure to thrive	
Normal pressure hydrocephalus		Spontaneous bone fractures	

of men and 28.3% to 61.5% women aged 70 years and older (Bliwise et al., 2019), and it is associated with daytime fatigue, mood alterations, dizziness, depression, falls, and mortality. Nocturia is often underreported by older adults, with many assuming waking multiple times at night is a normal part of aging (Bliwise et al., 2019). Evidence exists that causative relationships exist among sleep disruption and pathologies and insomnia and nocturia (Everaert et al., 2019). Besides nocturia, sleep disorders are also associated with daytime LUTS (Fantus et al., 2018).

KEY POINT

Nocturia is a common problem among the elderly and is associated with increased daytime fatigue and falls.

PATHOLOGY

Several underlying mechanisms for nocturia have been identified, including global polyuria and nocturnal polyuria (NP). Global polyuria is defined as "24-hour urine output greater than 40 mL/kg, causing both daytime urinary frequency and nocturia even in the face of normal bladder capacity" (Li et al., 2019). In adults 65 years and older, NP is defined as "excessive production of urine during the individual's main sleep period" (Bliwise et al., 2019). These authors noted that the threshold for excessive should be determined in the clinical and research settings and through the bladder diary. A recent study found that adults with NP have a "unique surge" in diuresis in the early hours of sleep compared to those without NP. For example, individuals with NP had a higher volume and lower urinary osmolarity at 1 AM compared to individuals who do not have NP (Monaghan et al., 2019).

KEY POINT

Nocturia may be caused by excessive 24-hour urine production, excessive nighttime urine production, or inadequate bladder capacity.

Reduced nocturnal bladder capacity may be a symptom of several neurogenic conditions, including Parkinson disease, multiple sclerosis, stroke, or spinal cord injury. Conditions intrinsic to the lower urinary tract that reduce bladder capacity include lower urinary tract cancer and calculi (Cornu et al., 2012). Over 46% of women 70 years and over report nocturia (Daugherty et al., 2018). In older men, benign prostatic enlargement (BPE) can lead to reduced nocturnal bladder capacity (van Doorn et al., 2012). Because nocturia has many causes, assessment and identification of the underlying causes are essential to effective treatment.

ASSESSMENT

Nocturia is a patient-reported symptom; thus, eliciting information from the older adult is essential to a comprehensive assessment. The ICS provides clinicians and researchers a validated and reliable instrument to screen men and women for and assess the impact of nocturia on quality of life. This instrument, ICIQ-Nocturia (https://iciq.net/iciq-n), consists of two items (i.e., frequency and nocturia) and is easy to administer. A bladder diary provides valuable information and helps to differentiate between global polyuria and nocturnal polyuria. Assessment of nocturia in individuals with cognitive or literacy impairments will rely on surrogate report by family members or caregivers. Therefore, health care providers must stress the importance of accurate information to those documenting the episodes of nocturia on the bladder record. See **Table 13-2** for the differential diagnosis of nocturia and **Table 13-3** for nonpharmacological interventions for nocturia.

Because ingestion of fluids influences urine output, obtaining accurate information about fluid volume ingested and types of fluids (i.e., water, alcohol, and caffeinated) is also necessary. Assessing cardiovascular status, the quality of sleep, and the presence of sleep apnea is important since nocturia is closely associated with cardiovascular disease and sleep disorders.

MANAGEMENT

Management of nocturia is determined by the findings from the assessment. More than one issue (e.g., global polyuria, nocturnal polyuria, and/or reduced bladder capacity) may be present, and each condition should be treated. Treatment of sleep disorders and management of chronic medical conditions such as cardiovascular disease, diabetes mellitus, and prostatic enlargement are necessary, and the impact of such treatment on nocturia should be evaluated.

Lifestyle interventions may be helpful in treating nocturia. Some of these lifestyle interventions include restricting fluids, for those who have an excessive fluid intake, about 4 to 6 hours before retiring, limiting evening time consumption of caffeine, and treating insomnia with daytime exercise. For those with lower extremity edema, using compression stocking and elevating legs to promote mobilization of fluid may reduce the need to void at night. Glycemic control for people with diabetes is also important. Evidence shows moving administration of diuretics to 6 hours before bedtime helps to reduce nocturia. Limited evidence, that is, expert opinion, supports weight loss to treat nocturia (Everaert et al., 2019).

The impact of fluid manipulation has been a subject of research, and current data indicate that a 25% reduction in fluid intake can improve nocturia (Hashim & Abrams, 2008). For example, in a study conducted with men experiencing nocturia (ages 53 to 91, mean age 72),

TABLE 13-2 DIFFERENTIAL DIAGNOSIS OF NOCTURIA

CONDITION	DIMINISHED OR REDUCED NOCTURNAL BLADDER CAPACITY	GLOBAL POLYURIA	NOCTURNAL POLYURIA
Presentation	Nocturnal bladder capacity index: (NBCi) = ANV − PNV = ANV − (NUV/MVV) + 1 NBCi > 1.3 nocturia secondary to decreased bladder capacity[*]	24-hour urine production exceeding 40 mL/kg body weight[*]	Nocturnal polyuria index (NPi) is age dependent. NPi = NUV/24-hour urine volume. For adults >65 years, nocturnal urine volumes >33% of total 24-hour volume.[*]
Possible cause	Idiopathic overactive bladder[*] Bladder outlet obstruction,[*] Neurogenic bladder[*] Nocturnal detrusor overactivity[*] Anxiety disorders[*] Bladder calculi[*] Medications[*]	Untreated diabetes/ glycosuria[*] Diabetes insipidus[*] Primary polydipsia[*]	Nephrological: diabetes insipidus, age-related circadian rhythms of the kidney.[†] Sleep: Insomnia, sleep disruption, sleep pathology.[†] Cardiovascular: Hypertension, Metabolic syndrome, heart failure.[†] Lifestyle: Excessive evening fluid/alcohol/ caffeine intake.[†] Medications' side effects.[†] Hormone: sex hormone deficiency.[†]

Source: [*](Li et al., 2019). [†](Everaert et al., 2019).
ANV, actual number of nocturnal voids; PNV, predicted number of nocturnal voids; MVV, maximum voided volume; NUV, nocturnal urine volume.

subjects were instructed to adjust their food and water intake to produce 24-hour urine volumes ≤30 mL/kg. The men were encouraged to reduce the volume of fluid ingested during the day rather than the frequency of fluid ingestion. All men were instructed to drink at least 1 L daily and to drink whenever they felt thirsty. There was significant improvement in nocturia in men who reduced their daytime fluid volume. The authors suggested that daytime, as well as evening, reduction of fluid intake would improve nocturia (Suzuki et al., 2019).

KEY POINT

Lifestyle modifications such as restricting excessive fluid intake 4 to 6 hours prior to bedtime, limiting evening consumption of caffeine, application of compression hose and leg elevation for those with leg edema, and administration of diuretic therapy 6 hours prior to bedtime may help reduce nocturia. Medications (e.g., desmopressin) must be used with caution in older adults.

Medications, especially desmopressin, are used to treat NP (Everaert et al., 2019). Adverse effects of desmopressin include hyponatremia, which can be asymptomatic and requires serologic monitoring (Gordon et al., 2019). Vaginal estrogen used to treat menopausal symptoms also improves nocturia (Bliwise et al., 2019). Pharmacologic treatment, in general, should be used with caution in older adults.

Nocturia can disrupt sleep, an essential component of health. Effective interventions that reduce nocturia, minimize sleep disruption, and improve sleep quality are within the scope of practice for WOC nurses. Collaborating with geriatric specialists is an important role for the WOC nurse to ensure comprehensive assessment of nocturia and implementation of strategies to optimize the quality of sleep for older adults.

FUNCTIONAL URINARY INCONTINENCE

UI can occur as a result of factors outside the genitourinary tract; this is often referred to as functional UI. Over 75% of older adults live with four or more chronic conditions, functional limitations, or geriatric syndromes (Koroukian et al., 2017). In addition to managing chronic conditions, functional limitations, and geriatric syndromes, and following their treatment regimes, older adults often find themselves dealing with symptoms that arise from treatments or interactions among treatments for different diseases and conditions. Older adults also continue to seek preventive health care, such as vaccinations. Yet, many times, older adults do not seek care for UI and other LUTS because of the mistaken belief that these conditions are an unavoidable part of aging (Vethanayagam et al., 2017). For many older adults, especially those living in the community, life is filled with an array of medical appointments, medications, special diets, self-management of untreated conditions, and prescribed treatment regimes. Being in poor physical health, however, has little relevance to life satisfaction in older adults (Puvill et al., 2016).

TABLE 13-3 NONPHARMACOLOGICAL INTERVENTIONS FOR NOCTURIA

CAUSE	SPECIFIC INTERVENTION	SOURCE OF INFORMATION
Lifestyle	Restrict fluid intake, if excessive*	Bladder diary
	Restrict excess calorie intake in weight loss program, especially for individuals who are obese*	History Physical examination Food diary
	Increase physical activity* Physical therapy referral, if applicable	History Physical examination Assess physical activity level and quality of life, i.e., questionnaires Activity log Monitors, i.e., accelerometer

Medications	Review for:
	Medications that may cause leg edema*:
	    Antidepressants
	    Antihypertensives
	    Antivirals
	    Hormones
	    Nonsteroidal anti-inflammatory drugs
	Medications that increase water and osmotic diuresis*
		History
		Physical examination
		Review medical record prescribed and over-the-counter medications and dietary supplements

Sleep	Assess for sleep quality, restless leg syndrome, sleep apnea, insomnia.* Sleep hygiene†	History and physical examination Assess sleep quality and quality of life, i.e., questionnaires Screen for depression Referral for sleep studies
Hormonal	Assess menopausal symptoms	History Physical examination Assess quality of life and quality of sleep, i.e., questionnaires
Urologic, overactive bladder, bladder obstruction	Bladder training Pelvic floor muscle training Physical exercise	History Assess for lower urinary tract symptoms and quality of life, i.e., questionnaires Physical examination Bladder diary
Kidney, nephrological	Salt and protein restriction* Primary prevention of chronic conditions, i.e., diabetes, hypertension, obesity	History Physical examination Food diary Bladder diary
Cardiovascular	Weight loss, if applicable Salt restriction Increase physical activity Leg elevation Compression stockings	History Physical examination Assess quality of life, i.e., questionnaires Assess activity level using questionnaires Screen for depression

Source: *(Everaert et al., 2019). †https://www.cdc.gov/sleep/about_sleep/sleep_hygiene.html

---

KEY POINT

Urinary incontinence and lower urinary tract symptoms are underreported especially in the aging population due to the mistaken belief that urinary dysfunction is an unavoidable consequence of aging.

The older adult population is heterogeneous; people live through different life experiences, have different levels of resources available to them throughout their lives, and respond to life events in multiple ways. Thus, an individualized approach to care for older adults, including those with cognitive impairments, is essential. WOC nurses consult and collaborate with other health care providers who have geriatrics expertise to prevent UI from developing or worsening and to provide effective and dignified care to older adults who experience functional UI.

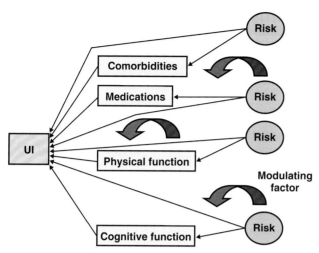

FIGURE 13-2. Incontinence as a Geriatric Syndrome. (Used with permission from Wagg, A., Chen, L. K., Johnson, T., et al. (2017). Incontinence in frail older persons. In P. Abrams, L. Cardozo, A. Wagg, & A. Wein (Eds.), *Incontinence* (pp. 1309–1442). ICI-ICS International Continence Society.)

UI is viewed as a geriatric syndrome in frail older adults largely because of the number of associated morbidities and reduced life expectancy; see **Figure 13-2**.

Because changes in the central nervous system may contribute to urinary urgency, the presence of multimorbidities and the effects of their symptoms can affect older adults' ability to toilet, fully empty their bladders, or recognize and appropriately respond to the sensation of bladder fullness. Many older adults require assistance from another person to use the toilet. This care dependency acts as a risk factor for incontinence (Wagg et al., 2017).

The environment itself can exert an influence on health and health behaviors in people of all ages. The impact of the environment on older adults' toilet access and toileting behaviors should not be underestimated. Older adults who have difficulty carrying out activities of daily living (ADLs), including toileting, may have functional impairments and disabilities. The Centers for Disease Control defined disability as "any condition of the body or mind (impairment) that makes it more difficult for the person with the condition to do certain activities (activity limitation) and interact with the world around them (participation restrictions)" (https://www.cdc.gov/ncbddd/disabilityandhealth/disability.html).

The relationship between disability and UI is complex and can result in different functional pathways. For example, older adults who are frail or who have physical and cognitive impairments that lead to functional decline may, over time, develop toileting and mobility disabilities that result in UI (Coll-Planas et al., 2008). Yet, other older adults may be incontinent of urine and subsequently experience a fall that results in a hip fracture. Functional decline and mobility disability may follow, leading to

intractability of the incontinence. Understanding the nature of the relationship between UI, functional decline, and disability and creating a treatment or management plan that halts or reverses the specific pathway can be challenging and requires interdisciplinary collaboration and consultation.

KEY POINT

Functional urinary incontinence is caused by factors outside the urinary tract as opposed to a problem with bladder function or sphincter function.

Many older adults who are continent but who have chronic conditions, functional impairments, or geriatric syndromes become incontinent during hospitalization. New cases of UI during hospitalization have been reported in older women admitted for hip fracture repair. Risk factors included preadmission use of wheelchair or device for walking, presence of confusion, and admission from a nursing home (Palmer et al., 2002). The use of absorbent products for urine containment during hospitalization with continent older adults increased the risk that the individual will be incontinent of urine at the time of discharge (Zisberg, 2011). Point prevalence of incontinence in hospitalized patients was 26%, and 35.2% of adults aged 85 years and over were incontinent (Condon et al., 2019). Artero-López et al. (2018) found that clinical inertia, defined as "failure to initiate or intensify professional actions," related to UI is prevalent among the hospital nursing staff. Another study found that hospital nursing staff lack knowledge and motivation to provide continence care (Colborne & Dahlke, 2017). For optimal care, however, the nursing staff must provide evidence-based care for incontinence or other LUTS, and be attentive to patients' requests for toileting, have justifications for indwelling urinary catheters, and understand consequences from the use of absorbent products. Evidence-based care is also needed for older adults admitted to home and palliative care and for short- or long-term stays in nursing homes.

Older adults represent 83.5% of the 1,347,600 nursing home residents in the United States. Approximately 89.3% of nursing home residents need assistance with toileting (Harris-Kojetin et al., 2019). Dependency in other ADLs is also prevalent. Percentages for needing any assistance with the following ADLs are 96.7% bathing, 92.7% dressing, 89.3% toileting, 92% walking, 86.8% transferring in and out of bed, and 59.9% eating (Harris-Kojetin et al., 2019). Approximately 75% of residents are incontinent of urine (Gorina et al., 2014). Thus, requisites to effective toileting and continence programs require an adequate number of educated, motivated, and supervised staff and a sufficiently resourced environment that facilitates the provision of evidence-based physical and emotional information and care to older adults, families, and caregivers. CWOCN/CWOCN-AP nurses act as advocates for continence and toileting care planning, delivery, and evaluation.

In summary, the prevalence of UI is high in institutional settings such as hospitals and nursing homes. The increasing number of older adults who have complex care needs resulting from chronic conditions, functional limitations, and geriatric syndromes translates into a demand for attentive health care providers who can provide safe and timely access to toilets or toileting assistance. Dependency on others for toileting assistance often makes a difference between becoming incontinent or remaining continent. Staff education and supervision are important to ensure that toileting assistance and behavioral interventions are being performed as prescribed and evaluated for appropriateness and effectiveness.

COMORBID CONDITIONS

There are several comorbid conditions that increase the risk of incontinence among older adults. Some of the most common are frailty, cognitive impairment, and mobility impairment.

KEY POINT

Comorbid conditions commonly associated with functional incontinence include frailty, cognitive impairment, and mobility impairment.

FRAILTY

Cesari et al. (2017) defined frailty as "a clinical state in which there is an increase in an individual's vulnerability to developing negative health-related events (including disability, hospitalizations, institutionalization, and death) when exposed to endogenous and exogenous stressors" (p. 294). Frailty, a major concept in geriatrics, is the subject of research focus and integration into clinical practice (Walston et al., 2019). Frailty can be measured using validated instruments, including the five-item FRAIL scale that measures fatigue, resistance, aerobic capacity, illnesses, and weight loss (Gleason et al., 2017). Because frailty increases the potential for progressive dependency, it is also associated with increased risk for incontinence. A recent systematic review and meta-analysis reported a wide range of frailty and prefrailty in low-income and middle-income countries. Prevalence ranged from 3.9% in China to 51.4% in Cuba, and prefrailty prevalence ranged from 13.4% in Tanzania to 76.1% in Brazil. Prevalence of frailty increased with age (Siriwardhana et al., 2018).

COGNITIVE IMPAIRMENT

UI is prevalent in older adults who have cognitive impairment. Deterioration in functional, mental, and physical processes is the hallmark of dementia. UI may be due to the older adult not recognizing the need to void, not being able to inhibit urination, not remembering the location of the toilet, or not being able to prepare to toilet. Many older adults with mild cognitive impairment (MCI) and dementia can remain continent if provided adequate toileting cues and assistance with toileting. However, older adults with advanced dementia can react to toileting assistance with distress; thus, caregivers must be able to "read" the behavioral cues of older adults with cognitive impairments who are unable to express their needs (Ostaszkiewicz et al., 2012). It is critical for caregivers to realize that some forms of dementia, such as normal pressure hydrocephalus (NPH), are potentially reversible. Cardinal signs of NPH include gait disturbance (sometimes described as appearing as if the person was walking on a boat), UI, and cognitive decline (Rosseau, 2011). Improvements in LUTS were seen in adults who underwent ventriculoperitoneal shunting for idiopathic NPH (Krzastek, et al., 2017). If NPH is suspected, appropriate referrals must be made, and any newly occurring or suddenly worsening cognitive impairment requires immediate evaluation.

MOBILITY IMPAIRMENT

Impairments in mobility increase the risk for and prevalence of UI (Wagg et al., 2017). Mobility difficulties often accompany chronic conditions such as arthritis, obesity, and cardiovascular diseases; therefore, a screening test to evaluate gait, balance, and walking speed should be part of continence assessments and patient safety programs. In a population-level study, UI was an independent risk factor for falls, but not hip fractures (Schluter et al., 2018).

CHARACTERISTICS OF UI IN THE OLDER ADULT

DIAGNOSTIC STUDIES/GUIDELINES FOR OLDER ADULTS

Primary care providers are recommended to screen older adults for UI because many do not voluntarily report it. A comprehensive geriatric assessment is considered a holistic method to assess continence issues (Aharony et al., 2017). Obtaining history of comorbid conditions, including bowel issues, conducting a medication review for medications that affect urologic function, conducting an assessment of ADLs and use of walking aids, and administering bladder diaries are part of assessment of LUTS. For older adults who have known bladder outlet obstruction or report emptying symptoms, postvoid residual urine volume testing may be indicated.

Implementing a toileting trial is an effective method for determining the potential effectiveness of a behavioral intervention. A toileting trial consists of offering toileting assistance to the older adult every 2 hours over a 3-day period (Rahman et al., 2014). Responsiveness to the trial is determined by a reduction in incontinent episodes; previous research has shown that about 25% to 40% of nursing home residents experience a reduction in incontinent episodes from three to four per day to one or less per day. Rahman et al. (2014) reported that the toileting trial was a stronger predictor of long-term improvement in continence status than was the cognitive and functional status of the older adult.

> **KEY POINT**
>
> A toileting trial provides valuable information regarding the probable benefit of a toileting program; results of the toileting trial are a better predictor of positive results than the individual's cognitive and functional status.

In the long-term care setting, the Minimum Data Set (MDS 3.0) is used to gather information on bladder and bowel function (Section H). The Centers for Medicare and Medicaid Services implemented F-Tag 690 in 2017, which states in part, "Incontinence. §483.25(e)(1) The facility must ensure that a resident who is continent of bladder and bowel on admission receives services and assistance to maintain continence unless his or her clinical condition is or becomes such that continence is not possible to maintain." The F-Tag 690 represents federally mandated guidelines to promote continence restoration of residents in long-term care through structured screening and assessment, development of an individualized bladder/bowel management program, urinary tract infection (UTI) prevention measures and proper UTI treatment in only those with symptoms, appropriate utilization and management of indwelling catheters, and processes to facilitate mobility, toileting, proper hygiene as well as proper use of BWAP. Nursing home state surveyors are given guidance to evaluate long-term care facilities to assure compliance with these mandated guidelines (https://www.cms.gov/Regulations-and-Guidance/Guidance/Manuals/downloads/som107ap_pp_guidelines_ltcf.pdf). If found negligent in implementing measures to optimize bowel and bladder control, the facility risks a financial penalty for each deficiency. The Minimum Data Set, F-tags, and guidance to surveyors undergo periodic revisions; therefore, WOC nurses who work in nursing homes should keep apprised of updated versions and revisions to these important documents. WOC nurses with an entrepreneurial spirit may also have a tremendous opportunity to assist long-term facilities in optimizing residents' quality of life and dignity, and reduce indirect costs through implementation of a bowel and bladder restoration program, measures to reduce UTIs

or catheter-associated UTIs (CAUTI). Consultations may include but not be limited to evaluation of patients with LUTS or incontinence (bowel and/or bladder), educating staff regarding structured incontinence skin care programs, development of skin care or containment product formulary, measures to promote bowel and bladder health, implementing behavioral interventions and toileting programs, and appropriate selection of BWAP etc. (see Table 1-1, Common WOC Proficiencies).

MANAGEMENT OPTIONS/GUIDELINES

Research agendas and consensus reports agree that management of UI is contingent on findings from the assessment (Vaughan et al., 2018; Wagg et al., 2017). Optimizing overall health through chronic disease management and restorative therapies to improve function is an essential element of care. Inclusion of the older adult's preferences for care and personal goals for treatment are cornerstones of the treatment plan. Creating desired end points for the treatment plan is critical to the evaluation of the interventions' effectiveness. Noninvasive behavioral interventions are the first-line treatment option for older adults. See **Figure 13-3** for the management of UI in frail older men and women consensus statement.

> **KEY POINT**
>
> Noninvasive behavioral interventions are the first-line treatment option for older adults.

REVERSIBLE FACTORS/BARRIERS

UI that suddenly occurs or worsens may have been precipitated by a sentinel event or acute health event. Therefore, acute changes in health status, medications, or environment should be assessed. A mnemonic, DIPPERS, can be used to recall factors that contribute to transient (also called acute onset) UI (Wagg et al., 2017). Other mnemonics include TOILETED, DRIP, DIAPPERS, and PPRAISED (Aharony et al., 2017; Resnick & Yalla, 1985; Staskin & Kelleher, 2013).

DELIRIUM

Delirium is an acute worsening of cognitive status, a potentially fatal condition that is often underdetected. It is also called acute brain failure and has multiple risk factors including dementia, functional impairment, visual impairment, history of alcohol misuse, and age over 70 years. Precipitating factors include polypharmacy and the use of psychoactive medications and physical restraints (Inouye et al., 2014). Delirium can present as hyperactive or hypoactive psychomotor disturbances (Marcantonio, 2017). Key diagnostic factors include acute-onset and fluctuating symptoms, inattention, disorientation, memory impairment, and language changes (Inouye et al., 2014). Treatment is dependent on the underlying cause.

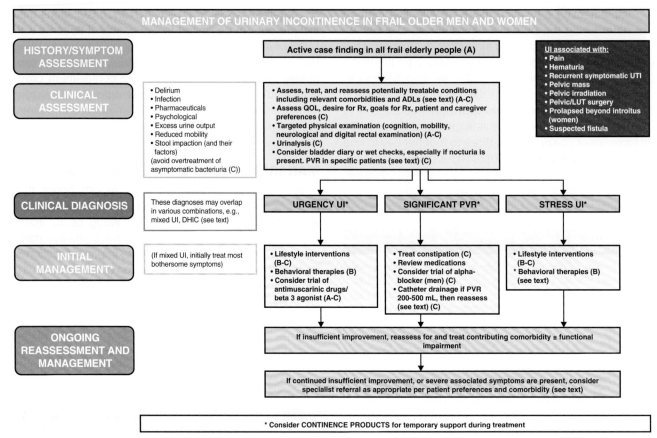

FIGURE 13-3. Management of Urinary Incontinence in Frail Older Men and Women. (Used with permission from Wagg, A., Chen, L. K., Johnson, T., et al. (2017). Incontinence in frail older persons. In P. Abrams, L. Cardozo, A. Wagg, & A. Wein (Eds.), *Incontinence* (6th ed.). Bristol, UK: ICI-ICS.)

Standardized tools are available such as the Confusion Assessment Method (CAM) and the 4AT test for rapid assessment (Shenkin et al., 2019). Some tools are best for use in specific settings, that is, medical units and palliative care settings, and with specific populations, that is, oncology. Patient safety is a paramount concern until delirium is corrected.

INFECTION

Infections can lead to new or worsened UI via several mechanisms. Fatigue and anergia (i.e., lack of energy) often accompany systemic infection, which in turn can make the act of moving to the toilet an effort that requires a great deal of physical and mental exertion. When the older adult recovers from the acute illness and fatigue and anergia recede, the preillness continence level should return. In the case of upper respiratory infections, UI can develop or worsen when the abdominal pressure transmitted to the pelvic floor during coughing exceeds the intraurethral pressure, resulting in urinary leakage. UI can also occur with symptomatic UTIs, especially in older women (Mody & Juthani-Mehta, 2014). Urgency or frequency may worsen and may be accompanied by one or more of the following symptoms: fever, acute

dysuria, suprapubic tenderness, or costovertebral angle pain or tenderness. Older adults with musculoskeletal pain or stiffness that slows walking time or comorbidities that lead to mobility and cognitive impairments are at risk of becoming incontinent in the presence of a symptomatic UTI. According to the Clinical Practice Guideline for Asymptomatic Bacteriuria (ASB), community-dwelling older adults and those living in long-term care facilities should not be screened or treated for ASB (Nicolle et al., 2019). See Chapter 18 regarding ASB and UTI management in adults.

PHARMACEUTICALS

Over half of adults over 65 years old are prescribed three or more daily medications, and nursing home residents receive on average between six to eight oral medications; the risk of adverse drug events and interactions are related with the number of medications ingested (Moore et al., 2018). Polypharmacy is related to the development of frailty, although the mechanism is not understood (Shmuel et al., 2019).

New medications, changed doses of existing medications, and drug–drug interactions can lead to UI. Older adults, especially those with chronic conditions, functional limitations, and geriatric syndromes, are often prescribed multiple medications, including medications added to address symptoms caused by other prescribed medications, also known as a prescribing cascade (Tannenbaum & Johnell, 2014). Diuretics can produce urine volumes that overwhelm the bladder and cause incontinent episodes. Medications that alter consciousness can precipitate incontinent episodes by reducing awareness of the need to void, impairing the ability to communicate the need to void, or impairing the ability to safely navigate to the toilet. Angiotensin-converting enzyme (ACE) inhibitors can cause a cough that precipitates stress UI. Therefore, WOC nurses should conduct medication reviews, consult with geriatric pharmacists, and use resources such as the Beers Criteria for Potentially Inappropriate Medications for Older Adults prior to medication administration. This document is available from the American Geriatrics Society Web site: www.americangeriatrics.org.

KEY POINT

A mnemonic, DIPPERS, can be used to recall common acute (transient) factors that contribute to an acute onset of urinary incontinence: Delirium, Infection, Pharmaceuticals, Psychological Issues, Excess Urine Production, Restricted Mobility, Stool Impaction (constipation).

PSYCHOLOGICAL

Depression is associated with UI. A bidirectional relationship appears to exist. Older adults who experience new-onset UI should be screened for depression.

EXCESS URINE OUTPUT

Excess urine output may overwhelm the bladder and lead to incontinent episodes, especially in older adults with mobility impairments. Excess fluid output could be the result of excessive fluid intake, uncontrolled diabetes mellitus or congested heart failure leading to lower extremity dependent edema where excess fluid returns to the circulatory system when supine, and NP, or global polyuria. Documenting fluid intake and urinary output on the bladder diary will likely help determine the underlying cause of excess urine output.

REDUCED MOBILITY

A sentinel event, such as hip fracture, can abruptly change an older adult's mobility status and, consequently, access to the toilet. Other possible reasons for reduced mobility include exacerbations in arthritis or musculoskeletal pain and stiffness that affect transfer ability. History of a recent fall should be assessed. Consultation or referral to physical therapy to assess gait speed, balance, and transfer ability may be warranted. Pain management to facilitate movement and minimize distress is essential.

STOOL IMPACTION

Constipation is a frequently reported condition among older adults living in nursing homes, with one study reporting 67% prevalence estimates of 30% to 40% in people 65 years and older (Lämås et al., 2017). Another study reported that the prevalence of constipation increased from 46% in 2007 to 59% in 2013. The authors attributed the use of opioid and anticholinergic medications as the reason for the increase (Gustafsson et al., 2019). Of adults admitted to medical wards without constipation, 43% developed it within 3 days of admission (Noiesen et al., 2014). One complication of constipation is stool impaction, which is implicated in the development or worsening of urinary and fecal incontinence. Therefore, prevention and treatment of constipation are recommended. Osmotic rather than bulk-forming laxatives may be appropriate for older adults who are unable to increase or maintain adequate fluid intake (Emmanuel et al., 2017). Privacy during defecation is considered important. Additional preventive measures include adequate intake of dietary fiber, adequate fluid intake, and avoidance of medications with a constipating effect (Wagg et al., 2017).

 ## INTERVENTIONS FOR FUNCTIONAL URINARY INCONTINENCE

SCHEDULED VOIDING/HABIT TRAINING

Habit training/scheduled voiding is a behavioral intervention that is used with older adults who would not benefit from prompted voiding or other interventions designed to restore continence or voiding patterns (Wagg et al., 2017). The goal of scheduled voiding is to preempt an incontinent episode by toileting the older adult on a schedule based on the older adult's current voiding pattern. To be successful in reducing the number of incontinent voids, staff must adhere to the schedule of timely toilet access.

PROMPTED VOIDING

Prompted voiding is a behavioral intervention developed in the 1980s by psychologists for use in nursing homes. The intervention was originally designed as a two-pronged approach. One prong of this intervention was directed toward the nursing staff. Nursing home staff members were given feedback by their supervisor about the number of toiletings they performed and the dryness level of the resident they toileted. The second prong, the prompted voiding protocol, was directed toward the nursing home resident. This protocol involved approaching the older adult and asking if he/she was dry or wet. After a response was obtained, the caregiver physically checked the older adult and gave verbal feedback about the accuracy of the individual's response. The caregiver then assisted the older adult to the toilet and provided praise when the older adult voided in the toilet. In the final step, the caregiver reminds the older adult when the next toileting opportunity will occur after returning the older adult to the same location before toileting.

Prompted voiding is a labor- and time-intensive intervention that was originally intended to increase self-initiated toileting requests and decrease the number of wet episodes (Newman & Butcher, 2019). Evidence exists that prompted voiding results in decreased daytime incontinent episodes in the short term (Wagg et al., 2017). A three-day trial of prompted voiding can indicate a person's success with a prompted voiding intervention (Newman & Butcher, 2019). Caregivers must adhere to the protocol to provide toileting assistance for prompted voiding to be effective in reducing the number of incontinent episodes. One study provided evidence that prompted voiding can be sustained for at least 6 months (Lai & Wan, 2017). Another study applied the use of bladder ultrasound with a prompted voiding protocol and found it effective in reducing incontinent episodes, while not increasing caregiver burden (Suzuki et al., 2019). Prompted voiding is sometimes combined with exercise and food and fluid interventions. Table 6-11 from Chapter 6 discusses toileting programs in depth to promote continence.

ABSORPTIVE PRODUCTS, INDWELLING CATHETERS, AND SKIN CARE

BWAP are in widespread use. One finding from a systematic literature review revealed that 71.6% of nursing home residents in the United States use absorbent products to contain urine on a daily basis (Roe et al., 2011). These products are often necessary for older adults who would not benefit from behavioral or pharmacologic intervention for incontinence or as an adjunct to other interventions to protect skin and promote social interactions with others. Although there is little high-quality evidence in the selection and use of different products, a WOCN® Task Force created recommendations for the selection, use, and evaluation of BWAP for adults with incontinence (Gray et al., 2018). According to this document, factors to use in selection decisions are type and severity of incontinence, gender, timing (day or nighttime), mobility, dexterity and functional status, cognition, patient preferences, waist circumference or body mass index, goals of care, caregiver time and availability, and toileting ability. Products that can be easily removed and reapplied (pull on design), if appropriate, should be used for older adults who are toiletable. There is some evidence that the use of absorbent products by older women who are

continent can increase the risk of becoming incontinent, although the mechanism is not clear. Refer to Chapter 16 for thorough discussion related to BWAP, containment devices, and adaptive aides. An electronic algorithm, WOCN® Body Worn Absorbent Product Guide, may be accessed on any smartphone or electronic device (see Watch & Learn video).

 ## WOCN® BODY WORN ABSORBENT PRODUCT GUIDE

Indwelling urinary catheters are to be avoided unless there is a medical justification for their use. If an indwelling catheter is used, the justification for its use should be regularly reassessed and it should be removed as soon as practicable. See Chapter 19 regarding appropriate use and management of indwelling catheters.

There is limited evidence on effectiveness of topical barriers to prevent incontinence-associated dermatitis (IAD) (Pather et al., 2017). There is evidence, however, that water and soap should be avoided and that a leave-on moisturizer, a protectant, or a combination of both is better than not using these products (Beeckman et al., 2016). WOC nurses must advocate for and participate in high-quality trials to provide evidence for skin care of older adults, and others, who are incontinent of urine. Chapter 17 provides guidelines regarding a structured skin care program to prevent IAD as well as types of skin care products.

CONCLUSION

Interdisciplinary teamwork is at the core of geriatric care. WOC nurses will consult with nurses, physical therapists, physicians, nutritionists, social workers, and others with expertise in geriatrics to provide comprehensive continence care to older adults, especially frail older adults. Integrating geriatric clinical competencies into practice allows the nurse specialist to provide holistic care and draw on the strengths and resources of older adults and their families.

The evidence base for care of older adults who have incontinence and other LUTS is rapidly increasing. WOC nurses must remain abreast of the latest research, especially in prevention of delaying geriatric syndromes, preservation and restoration of cognitive and physical functioning, and palliative care. Specifically, the certified continence nurse specialists play a pivotal role in providing high-quality continence care to older adults and in contributing to the clinical and research evidence for the appropriate and dignified care of older adults.

CASE STUDY

Mrs. Grant is 87 years old and of Irish–German descent. She is widowed and has one daughter who lives out of state. Mrs. Grant was admitted to the Vista View Healthcare, a free-standing rehabilitation facility, 4 days ago after her discharge from the hospital for surgical repair of her left hip fracture. Her medical history reveals that she has arthritis in both of her knees and hands, hypertension, diabetes, history of myocardial infarction 2 years ago, and cataract surgery 3 years ago. She requires the help of one person to transfer from bed to chair and to rise from a chair and toilet. She reluctantly uses a walker saying that she is afraid of falling again, and she walks slowly, taking frequent stops. Lately, she has had a poor appetite, and she has been fretful saying, "I want to go home! What will happen to me?"

Mrs. Grant is distressed by being incontinent, saying that it started in the hospital after surgery and has gotten worse in the past few days. She said that the urine "comes without warning." She said she tried to go to the toilet every hour to prevent accidents. She wears a disposable brief with a seal/reseal tab and insists on having a disposable absorbent pad placed on her bed and chair. She said that she didn't use her call light because "the girls are so busy with people worse off than me." She went on to say that the pain in her knees was "just horrible" and had been worse since the surgery. She also said that at home, she had used a small thin pillow between her knees to sleep, but now, no one could get a pillow for her to use. She also used a topical lotion that helped relieve the pain in her knees at home. She was upset that the nurses "give me sleeping pills, because I feel so fuzzy in my head all morning." She also said that she didn't drink much because "that water (indicating her water container) tastes bad and, maybe, I won't have accidents." When asked what she drank at home, she said she drank hot water with lemon at breakfast, and at meals she drank room temperature tap water with lemon slices, and rarely drank fluids between meals.

There is no mention in the medical record about UI prior to her hip fracture or during hospitalization. An indwelling catheter had been inserted in the emergency department before her surgery and it was removed 48 hours after surgery. Postsurgery she received tramadol for pain until her discharge to Vista View Healthcare.

During the physical examination, Mrs. Grant was not febrile and denied she had pain or burning when voiding. She did not have suprapubic tenderness or costovertebral angle pain or tenderness. Mrs. Grant winced with pain when she turned onto her operative hip. She hesitantly rated her pain at 7, saying, "It's hard to put a number on it." There was no evidence of incontinence-associated dermatitis. The postvoid residual was 110 mL. A digital rectal exam revealed hard stool in the rectum; there was no documentation of a bowel movement in the past 72 hours. Using validated screening tools, there was no evidence of delirium, depression, or dementia.

MEDICATIONS

Hypertension: Hydrochlorothiazide 25 mg, every day

Atenolol 25 mg at bedtime

Constipation: Milk of magnesia 30 m/L at bedtime, prn

Pain: Acetaminophen 650 mg every 4 to 6 hours, prn

Sleep: Diphenhydramine 15 mg at bedtime, prn

A 3-day bladder and fluid intake diary revealed that Mrs. Grant drank about 800 mL/day and voided 10 times/24-hour period, often in small amounts. She was usually incontinent in bed upon awakening and within an hour before or after meals. She was also incontinent in the evening before retiring and once during the night hours. Other voids that were recorded on the bladder diary had been continent and, upon questioning Mrs. Grant, they had been preemptive voids; that is, she voided before feeling the need in order to prevent urine leakage. In reviewing the medication list, the WOC nurse noted that hydrochlorothiazide was given at 10 AM; diphenhydramine was given every night; three doses of acetaminophen had been administered since Mrs. Grant's admission; and no milk of magnesia had been given after admission.

Several factors placed Mrs. Grant at risk for developing incontinence:

1. Impaired mobility

2. Medications that affected urine volume and cognition

3. Pain that caused sleep disruption and reluctance to move

4. Low oral fluid intake

5. Constipation

6. Reluctance to ask for help

7. Psychological factors, that is, fear of falling and concern about an uncertain future

8. Use of an indwelling catheter during hospitalization

9. Use of body worn absorbent products that were difficult to remove for self-toileting

Mrs. Grant was asked about her preferences for care. She stated "Of course, I hate leaking urine and I want to go to the bathroom on my own but..." and her voice drifted off. The WOC nurse asked her if she would like to have a bedside commode in the room for use at night. Mrs. Grant was receptive and the WOC nurse suggested that Mrs. Grant use the toilet according to an individualized schedule, sitting on it until she thought her bladder was empty, and, if she wished, change to a disposable absorbent pad to contain the small volumes of leakage. She also encouraged Mrs. Grant to keep her own bladder diary and share the information with the nursing staff.

The WOC nurse talked with the physical therapist assigned to Mrs. Grant and asked about having a commode near the bed at night and to assess Mrs. Grant's musculoskeletal pain, especially in relation to using the toilet. The physical therapist recommended a set of exercises to help relieve pain and increase lower extremity strength. The physical therapist agreed that the bedside commode would be helpful to Mrs. Grant and also provided a pillow to support Mrs. Grant's legs at night. Since Mrs. Grant found relief from the over-the-counter topical lotion she used at home, the physical therapist suggested that Mrs. Grant resume using it and to take acetaminophen for pain on a regular basis until the pain was under control.

The WOC nurse talked with the nursing staff members who cared for Mrs. Grant and noted Mrs. Grant's reluctance in asking for help. She suggested using a toileting schedule that matched Mrs. Grant's voiding pattern and cueing Mrs. Grant about her exercise regime and about her pain and hydration levels. The WOC nurse talked with the charge nurse and suggested giving the diuretic at 2 PM instead of 10 AM and having Mrs. Grant rest with her feet elevated before her evening meal. She also suggested

discontinuing the use of diphenhydramine as a sleep aid because of its potential to adversely affect Mrs. Grant's cognitive status. She asked the staff to be attentive to Mrs. Grant's increased need to use the toilet after administering her diuretic and to use non-pharmacological measures to facilitate Mrs. Grant's sleep. The WOC nurse also suggested starting and slowly increasing dietary fiber and increasing fluid intake and physical exercise. She recommended an osmotic laxative for constipation for that evening and, when necessary, providing privacy and adequate time when Mrs. Grant was using the toilet. She and Mrs. Grant agreed to establish a regular time to move her bowels following breakfast and a hot liquid to promote regular elimination.

Based on the WOC nurse's recommendation, a dietician visited Mrs. Grant and reviewed her food and fluid likes and dislikes. She talked with Mrs. Grant about the importance of hydration to her overall health and in helping her bowels be regular. She suggested to Mrs. Grant to drink small amounts of fluids throughout the day, and with Mrs. Grant's help the dietician created a daily schedule so that Mrs. Grant was drinking about 1,500 mL/day, with about 200 mL coming from high–water-content foods and with most of the oral fluids ingested during daytime hours. The dietician told Mrs. Grant about the availability of single use packets of crystallized lemon, lime, and orange that could be added to the drinking water to enhance its taste. The dietician also developed a high-fiber diet that included foods with high water content for Mrs. Grant and, because of Mrs. Grant's diabetes and her motivation to increase her oral intake, incorporated a dietary fiber supplement into the food plan to prevent constipation.

In summary, several nongenitourinary factors were associated with Mrs. Grant's incontinence. Mrs. Grant increased her fluid intake and mobility and she had better pain control when the staff initiated the new care plan and Mrs. Grant's incontinence and overall attitude improved.

REFERENCES

Aharony, L., De Cock, J., Nuotio, M. S., et al. (2017). Consensus document on the detection and diagnosis of urinary incontinence in older people. *European Geriatric Medicine, 8*(3), 202–209. doi.org/10.1016/j.eurger.2017.03.012.

Artero-López, C., Márquez-Hernández, V. V., Estevez-Morales, M. T., et al. (2018). Inertia in nursing care of hospitalised patients with urinary incontinence. *Journal of Clinical Nursing, 27*(7–8), 1488–1496. doi.org/10.1111/jocn.14289.

Bauer, S. R., Grimes, B., Suskind, A. M., et al. (2019). Urinary incontinence and nocturia in older men: Associations with body mass, composition and strength in the Health ABC Study. *Journal of Urology, 202*(5), 1015–1021. doi.10.1097/ju.0000000000000378.

Beeckman, D., Van Damme, N., Schoonhoven, L., et al. (2016). Interventions for preventing and treating incontinence-associated dermatitis in adults. *The Cochrane Database of Systematic Reviews, 11*(11), CD011627. https://doi.org/10.1002/14651858.CD011627.pub2

Berke, C., Conley, M. J., Netsch, D., et al. (2019). Role of the wound, ostomy and continence nurse in continence care: 2018 update. *Journal of Wound, Ostomy and Continence Nursing, 46*(3), 221–225. doi.org/10.1097/WON.0000000000000529.

Bliwise, D. L., Wagg, A., & Sand, P. K. (2019). Nocturia: A highly prevalent disorder with multifaceted consequences. *Urology, 133S*, 3–13. doi.org/10.1016/j.urology.2019.07.005.

Cesari, M., Calvani, R., & Marzetti, E. (2017). Frailty in older persons. *Clinics in Geriatric Medicine, 33*(3), 293–303. doi.org/10.1016/j.cger.2017.02.002.

Colborne, M., & Dahlke, S. (2017). Nurses' perceptions and management of urinary incontinence in hospitalized older adults: An integrative review. *Journal of Gerontological Nursing, 43*(10), 46–55. doi.org/10.3928/00989134-20170515-02.

Coll-Planas, L., Denkinger, M. D., & Nikolaus, T. (2008). Relationship of urinary incontinence and late-life disability: Implications for clinical work and research in geriatrics. *Zeitschrift fur Gerontologie Und Geriatrie, 41*(4), 283–290. doi.org/10.1007/s00391-008-0563-6.

Condon, M., Mannion, E., Molloy, D. W., et al. (2019). Urinary and faecal incontinence: Point prevalence and predictors in a university hospital. *International Journal of Environmental Research and Public Health, 16*(2), 194. doi.org/10.3390/ijerph16020194.

Cornu, J. N., Abrams, P., Chapple, C. R., et al. (2012). A contemporary assessment of nocturia: Definition, epidemiology, pathophysiology, and management—A systematic review and meta-analysis. *European Urology, 62*(5), 877–890. doi.org/10.1016/j.eururo.2012.07.004.

Daugherty, M., Ginzburg, N., & Byler, T. (2018). PD32-03 Prevalence of nocturia in us women: Results from NHANES. *Journal of Urology, 199*(4), e645–e646. doi.org/10.1016/j.juro.2018.02.1546.

Egan, K. B. (2016). The epidemiology of benign prostatic hyperplasia associated with lower urinary tract symptoms: Prevalence and incident rates. *Urologic Clinics of North America, 43*(3), 289–297. doi.org/10.1016/j.ucl.2016.04.001.

Emmanuel, A., Mattace-Raso, F., Neri, M. C., et al. (2017). Constipation in older people: A consensus statement. *International Journal of Clinical Practice, 71*(1), 1–9. doi.org/10.1111/ijcp.12920.

Everaert, K., Hervé, F., Bosch, R., et al. (2019). International Continence Society consensus on the diagnosis and treatment of nocturia. *Neurourology and Urodynamics, 38*(2), 478–498. doi.org/10.1002/nau.23939.

Fantus, R. J., Packiam, V. T., Wang, C. H., et al. (2018). The relationship between sleep disorders and lower urinary tract symptoms: Results from the NHANES. *Journal of Urology, 200*(1), 161–166. doi.org/10.1016/j.juro.2018.01.083.

Federal Interagency Forum on Aging-related Statistics. (2016). *Older Americans 2016: Key Indicators of Well-being.* Retrieved from www.agingstats.gov

Gleason, L. J., Benton, E. A., Alvarez-Nebreda, M. L., et al. (2017). FRAIL Questionnaire Screening Tool and Short-Term Outcomes in Geriatric Fracture Patients. *Journal of the American Medical Directors Association, 18*(12), 1082–1086. doi.org/10.1016/j.jamda.2017.07.005.

Gordon, D. J., Emeruwa, C. J., & Weiss, J. P. (2019). Management strategies for nocturia. *Current Urology Reports, 20*(11). doi.org/10.1007/s11934-019-0940-2.

Gorina, Y., Schappert, S., Bercovitz, A., et al. (2014). *Prevalence of Incontinence among Older Americans. Vital & Health Statistics. Series 3, Analytical and Epidemiological Studies.* Retrieved from http://www.ncbi.nlm.nih.gov/pubmed/24964267

Govender, Y., Gabriel, I., Minassian, V., et al. (2019). The current evidence on the association between the urinary microbiome and urinary incontinence in women. *Frontiers in Cellular and Infection Microbiology, 9*, 1–10. doi.org/10.3389/fcimb.2019.00133.

Gray, M., Kent, D., Ermer-Seltun, J., et al. (2018). Assessment, selection, use, and evaluation of body-worn absorbent products for adults with incontinence. *Journal of Wound, Ostomy and Continence Nursing, 45*(3), 243–264. doi.org/10.1097/WON.0000000000000431.

Gustafsson, M., Lämås, K., Isaksson, U., et al. (2019). Constipation and laxative use among people living in nursing homes in 2007 and 2013. *BMC Geriatrics, 19*(1), 1–7. doi.org/10.1186/s12877-019-1054-x.

Harris-Kojetin, L., Sengupta, M., Lendon, J. P., et al. (2019). *Long-Term Care Providers and Services Users in the United States, 2015–2016. Vital and Health Statistics* (Vol. 3). Retrieved from https://www.cdc.gov/nchs/nsltcp/nsltcp_reports.htm

Hashim, H., & Abrams, P. (2008). How should patients with an overactive bladder manipulate their fluid intake? *BJU International, 102*(1), 62–66. doi.org/10.1111/j.1464-410X.2008.07463.x.

Hashim, H., Blanker, M. H., Drake, M. J., et al. (2019). International Continence Society (ICS) report on the terminology for nocturia and nocturnal lower urinary tract function. *Neurourology and Urodynamics, 38*(2), 499–508. doi.org/10.1002/nau.23917.

Inouye, S. K., Westendorp, R. G., & Saczynski, J. S. (2014). Delirium in elderly people. *Lancet, 383*(9920), 911–922. doi.org/10.1016/S0140-6736(13)60688-1.

Koroukian, S. M., Schiltz, N. K., Warner, D. F., et al. (2017). Multimorbidity: Constellations of conditions across subgroups of midlife and older individuals, and related Medicare expenditures. *Journal of Comorbidity, 7*(1), 33–43. doi.org/10.15256/joc.2017.7.91.

Krzastek, S. C., Robinson, S. P., Young, H. F., et al. (2017). Improvement in lower urinary tract symptoms across multiple domains following ventriculoperitoneal shunting for idiopathic normal pressure hydrocephalus. *Neurourology and Urodynamics, 36*(8), 2056–2063. doi.org/10.1002/nau.23235.

Lai, C. K. Y., & Wan, X. (2017). Using prompted voiding to manage urinary incontinence in nursing homes: Can it be sustained? *Journal of the American Medical Directors Association, 18*(6), 509–514. doi.org/10.1016/j.jamda.2016.12.084.

Lämås, K., Karlsson, S., Nolén, A., et al. (2017). Prevalence of constipation among persons living in institutional geriatric-care settings—A cross-sectional study. *Scandinavian Journal of Caring Sciences, 31*(1), 157–163. doi.org/10.1111/scs.12345.

Li, E. S. W., Flores, V. X., & Weiss, J. P. (2019). Current guidelines and treatment paradigms for nocturnal polyuria: A "NEW" disease state for US physicians, patients and payers. *International Journal of Clinical Practice, 73*(8), e13337. doi.org/10.1111/ijcp.13337.

Liu, F., Ling, Z., Xiao, Y., et al. (2017). Characterization of the urinary microbiota of elderly women and the effects of type 2 diabetes and urinary tract infections on the microbiota. *Oncotarget, 8*(59), 100678–100690. doi.org/10.18632/oncotarget.21126.

Marcantonio, E. R. (2017). Delirium in hospitalized older adults HHS public access. *The New England Journal of Medicine, 377*(15), 1456–1466. doi.org/10.1056/NEJMcp1605501.

Milsom, I., & Gyhagen, M. (2019). The prevalence of urinary incontinence. *Climacteric, 22*(3), 217–222. doi.org/10.1080/13697137.2018.1543263.

Mitchell, C. M., & Waetjen, L. E. (2018). Genitourinary changes with aging. *Obstetrics and Gynecology Clinics of North America, 45*(4), 737–750. doi.org/10.1016/j.ogc.2018.07.010.

Mody, L., & Juthani-Mehta, M. (2014). Urinary tract infections in older women. *JAMA: The Journal of the American Medical Association, 311*(8), 844–854. doi.org/10.1001/jama.2014.303.

Monaghan, T. F., Verbalis, J. G., Haddad, R., et al. (2019). Diagnosing nocturnal polyuria from a single nocturnal urine sample. *European Urology Focus, 6*(4), 738–744. doi.org/10.1016/j.euf.2019.10.002.

Moore, K. L., Patel, K., John Boscardin, W., et al. (2018). Medication burden attributable to chronic comorbid conditions in the very old and vulnerable. *PLoS ONE, 13*(4), 1–14. doi.org/10.1371/journal.pone.0196109.

Newman, D., & Butcher, H. (2019). Evidence-based practice guideline: Prompted voiding for individuals with urinary incontinence. *Journal of Gerontological Nursing, 45*(2), 14–26.

Nicolle, L. E., Gupta, K., Bradley, S. F., et al. (2019). Clinical practice guideline for the management of asymptomatic bacteriuria: 2019 update by the Infectious Diseases Society of America. *Clinical Infectious Diseases, 68*(10), e83–e110. doi.org/10.1093/cid/ciz021.

Noiesen, E., Trosborg, I., Bager, L., et al. (2014). Constipation—Prevalence and incidence among medical patients acutely admitted to hospital with a medical condition. *Journal of Clinical Nursing, 23*(15–16), 2295–2302. doi.org/10.1111/jocn.12511.

Ostaszkiewicz, J., O'Connell, B., & Dunning, T. (2012). Residents' perspectives on urinary incontinence: A review of literature. *Scandinavian Journal of Caring Sciences, 26*(4), 761–772. doi.org/10.1111/j.1471-6712.2011.00959.x.

Palmer, M. H., Baumgarten, M., Langenberg, P., et al. (2002). Risk factors for hospital-acquired incontinence in elderly female hip fracture patients. *Journals of Gerontology—Series A Biological Sci-*

ences and Medical Sciences, 57(10), M672–M677. doi.org/10.1093/gerona/57.10.M672.

Pather, P., Hines, S., Kynoch, K., et al. (2017). Effectiveness of topical skin products in the treatment and prevention of incontinence-associated dermatitis: A systematic review. JBI Database of Systematic Reviews and Implementation Reports, 15(5), 1473–1496. doi.org/10.11124/JBISRIR-2016-003015.

Puvill, T., Lindenberg, J., De Craen, A. J. M., et al. (2016). Impact of physical and mental health on life satisfaction in old age: a population based observational study. BMC Geriatrics, 16(1), 1–9. doi.org/10.1186/s12877-016-0365-4.

Rahman, A. N., Schnelle, J. F., & Osterweil, D. (2014). Implementing toileting trials in nursing homes: Evaluation of a dissemination strategy. Geriatric Nursing, 35(4), 283–289. doi.org/10.1016/j.gerinurse.2014.03.002.

Resnick, N. M., & Yalla, S. V. (1985). Management of urinary incontinence in the elderly. The New England Journal of Medicine, 313, 800–804.

Roe, B., Flanagan, L., Jack, B., et al. (2011). Systematic review of the management of incontinence and promotion of continence in older people in care homes: Descriptive studies with urinary incontinence as primary focus. Journal of Advanced Nursing, 67(2), 228–250. doi.org/10.1111/j.1365-2648.2010.05481.x; 10.1111/j.1365-2648.2010.05481.x.

Rosseau, G. (2011). Normal pressure hydrocephalus. Disease-a-Month, 57(3), 615–624.

Schluter, P. J., Arnold, E. P., & Jamieson, H. A. (2018). Falls and hip fractures associated with urinary incontinence among older men and women with complex needs: A national population study. Neurourology and Urodynamics, 37(4), 1336-1343. doi.org/10.1002/nau.23442.

Shenkin, S. D., Fox, C., Godfrey, M., et al. (2019). Delirium detection in older acute medical inpatients: A multicentre prospective comparative diagnostic test accuracy study of the 4AT and the confusion assessment method. BMC Medicine, 17(1), 138. doi.org/10.1186/s12916-019-1367-9.

Shmuel, S., Lund, J. L., Alvarez, C., et al. (2019). Polypharmacy and incident frailty in a longitudinal community-based cohort study. Journal of the American Geriatrics Society, 67(12), 2482–2489. doi.org/10.1111/jgs.16212.

Siriwardhana, D. D., Hardoon, S., Rait, G., et al. (2018). Prevalence of frailty and prefrailty among community-dwelling older adults in low-income and middle-income countries: A systematic review and meta-analysis. BMJ Open, 8(3), 1–17. doi.org/10.1136/bmjopen-2017-018195.

Staskin, D., & Kelleher, C. (Chairs, Committee 5). (2013). Patient-reported outcome assessment. In P. Abrams, L. Cardozo, S. Khoury, A. J. Wein (Eds.), Incontinence: 5th International Consultation on Incontinence (5th ed., pp. 15–107). Paris: ICUD-EAU.68).

Suskind, A. M. (2017). The aging overactive bladder: A review of aging-related changes from the brain to the bladder. Current Bladder Dysfunction Reports, 12(1), 42–47. doi.org/10.1007/s11884-017-0406-7.

Suzuki, M., Miyazaki, H., Kamei, J., et al. (2019). Ultrasound-assisted prompted voiding care for managing urinary incontinence in nursing homes: A randomized clinical trial. Neurourology and Urodynamics, 38(2), 757–763. doi.org/10.1002/nau.23913.

Tannenbaum, C., & Johnell, K. (2014). Managing therapeutic competition in patients with heart failure, lower urinary tract symptoms and incontinence. Drugs and Aging, 31(2), 93–101. doi.org/10.1007/s40266-013-0145-1.

United Nations Department of Economic and Social Affairs (2019). World Population Prospects 2019: Highlights. Retrieved from https://population.un.org/wpp/Publications/Files/WPP2019_10KeyFindings.pdf

US Census Bureau. (2018). Older People Projected to Outnumber Children. Retrieved from https://www.census.gov/newsroom/press-releases/2018/cb18-41-population-projections.html

Vahabi, B., Wagg, A. S., Rosier, P. F. W. M., et al. (2017). Can we define and characterize the aging lower urinary tract?—ICI-RS 2015. Neurourology and Urodynamics, 36(4), 854–858. doi.org/10.1002/nau.23035.

van Doorn, B., Kok, E. T., Blanker, M. H., et al. (2012). Mortality in older men with nocturia. A 15-year follow-up of the Krimpen study. The Journal of Urology, 187(5), 1727–1731. doi.org/10.1016/j.juro.2011.12.078.

Vaughan, C. P., Markland, A. D., Smith, P. P., et al. (2018). Report and Research Agenda of the American Geriatrics Society and National Institute on Aging Bedside-to-Bench Conference on Urinary Incontinence in Older Adults: A Translational Research Agenda for a Complex Geriatric Syndrome. Journal of the American Geriatrics Society, 66(4), 773–782. doi.org/10.1111/jgs.15157.

Vethanayagam, N., Orrell, A., Dahlberg, L., et al. (2017). Understanding help-seeking in older people with urinary incontinence: An interview study. Health and Social Care in the Community, 25(3), 1061–1069. doi.org/10.1111/hsc.12406.

Wagg, A., Chen, L. K., Johnson, T., et al. (2017). Incontinence in frail older persons. In P. Abrams, L. Cardozo, A. Wagg, & A. Wein (Eds.), Incontinence (6th ed., pp. 1309–1442). Bristol, UK: ICI-ICS International Continence Society.

Wakefield, D. B., Moscufo, N., Guttmann, C. R., et al. (2010). White matter hyperintensities predict functional decline in voiding, mobility, and cognition in older adults. Journal of the American Geriatrics Society, 58(2), 275–281. doi.org/10.1111/j.1532-5415.2009.02699.x.

Walston, J., Bandeen-Roche, K., Buta, B., et al. (2019). Moving frailty toward clinical practice: NIA intramural frailty science symposium summary. Journal of the American Geriatrics Society, 67(8), 1559–1564. doi.org/10.1111/jgs.15928.

Zisberg, A. (2011). Incontinence brief use in acute hospitalized patients with no prior incontinence. Journal of Wound, Ostomy, and Continence Nursing: Official Publication of the Wound, Ostomy and Continence Nurses Society/WOCN, 38(5), 559–564. doi.org/10.1097/WON.0b013e31822b3292.

QUESTIONS

1. The continence nurse asked to assess residents in a long-term care facility should consider which age-related change to the bladder when planning care?
   A. Increased urine flow
   B. Reduced bladder capacity
   C. Decreased sensitivity to neurotransmitters
   D. Decreased postvoid residual volumes

2. A newly admitted older adult to a nursing home tells the continence nurse who asks about voiding patterns, "Every night I fall asleep just fine, then I wake up to urinate, and go back to sleep again. This happens two or three times a night and I am getting kind of tired of it." What symptom of overactive bladder would the nurse suspect?
   A. Frequency
   B. Urgency
   C. Urge urinary incontinence
   D. Nocturia

3. A WOC nurse is invited to give a presentation on urinary incontinence to nurses who work on a hospital's medical unit. What nursing actions should the WOC nurse recommend?
   A. Encourage older adults to use absorbent products to promote dignity and prevent falls.
   B. When admitting older adults, ask about their voiding patterns and presence of lower urinary tract symptoms.
   C. Place all older adults on an every two-hour voiding schedule to prevent falls.
   D. Create a habit training schedule for older adults who have dementia.

4. Which older adult should the WOC nurse consider at risk for reduced nocturnal bladder capacity? A person who has
   A. Down syndrome
   B. Rheumatoid arthritis
   C. Parkinson disease
   D. Excess caffeine intake

5. An older adult receiving home care services is experiencing new-onset urinary incontinence. Upon further assessment by the nurse, which patient finding suggests a diagnosis of functional urinary incontinence?
   A. Impaired mobility
   B. Urinary tract infection
   C. Nocturia
   D. BPH

6. The continence nurse assesses an older adult and documents the following: "gait disturbance, urinary incontinence, and cognitive decline." What potentially reversible condition might be causing these findings?
   A. Frailty
   B. Normal pressure hydrocephalus
   C. Alzheimer disease
   D. Spinal cord injury

7. Which assessment should be high priority for a newly admitted resident of a nursing home who is incontinent of urine?
   A. Depression screening
   B. Intake and output monitoring
   C. Dietary consultation
   D. Fall risk assessment

8. A continence nurse is planning care for older adults who are residents in a long-term care facility who are incontinent of urine. What would be a priority intervention for them?
   A. Providing the resident an individual evaluation to select appropriate body worn absorbent products
   B. Keeping the resident's room free from urine odors
   C. Arranging for a toileting schedule based upon each resident's voiding patterns
   D. Reassuring each resident that incontinence is a normal part of aging

9. When using the DIPPERS mnemonic to assess for transient urinary incontinence, the WOC nurse would include an assessment for:
   A. Delirium
   B. Pneumonia
   C. Privacy while using the toilet
   D. Social interactions

10. A continence nurse is initiating a prompted voiding program in a long-term nursing care facility. For which resident would this program be *most* appropriate?
   A. An older adult who does not have dementia and can toilet successfully at least 50% of the time
   B. An older adult who has dementia and can toilet successfully at least 66% of the time
   C. An older adult who does not have dementia and can toilet 66% of the time
   D. An older adult who can achieve 80% more reduction in incontinent episodes during a toileting trial

ANSWERS AND RATIONALES

1. B. Rationale: One of the age-related changes in bladder function is a decrease in bladder capacity. This change is important to consider in recommending a toileting schedule for residence. As a result of reduced bladder capacity, residents generally need be toileted more often than do younger adults to reduce incontinence episodes.

2. D. Rationale: This description is consistent with nocturia, waking up from sleep to urinate and then going (or trying to go) back to sleep.

3. B. Rationale: The first step in planning a bladder management program for patients is to assess their normal voiding pattern and the presence of lower urinary tract symptoms (e.g., urgency, incontinence, bladder management prior to admission). This permits the bladder management program to be patient centered.

4. C. Rationale: Persons with Parkinson disease often experience neurogenic bladder dysfunction, and one of the common symptoms of this dysfunction is nocturia.

5. A. Rationale: Functional urinary incontinence occurs secondary to factors outside the lower urinary tract that impair the individual's ability to recognize the need to toilet and/or get to the toilet and prepare to toilet in sufficient time to prevent involuntary urine loss. Impaired mobility is one example of the many causes of functional urinary incontinence.

6. B. Rationale: Normal pressure hydrocephalus (NPH) is one of the potential reversible causes of incontinence. This patient has the cardinal signs of NPH including a gait disturbance, urinary incontinence, and cognitive decline.

7. D. Rationale: Urinary incontinence is an independent risk factor for falls. Thus, assessment of fall risk is an important component of the assessment of newly admitted nursing home residents. The results of this assessment should help guide the bladder management program if the resident is identified as "at risk" for falling.

8. C. Rationale: Behavioral interventions, specifically toileting programs, should be the first-line intervention for most long-term care residents. While many of these individuals will have age-related reductions in bladder capacity, the frequency with which they will need to be toileted to prevent or reduce urinary incontinence will vary. Matching a resident's toileting schedule to his or her normal voiding pattern will help ensure the effectiveness of the program.

9. A. Rationale: DIPPERS in one of the mnemonics that clinicians can use to recall factors that contribute to potential reversible causes of urinary incontinence. The "D" in this mnemonic stands for delirium, an acute worsening of cognitive function secondary to a variety of potential reversible factors.

10. B. Rationale: Prompted voiding is a scheduled toileting program developed for individuals with dementia. It combines regularly scheduled toileting with measures to increase the individual's awareness of bladder function (asking about wetness and providing feedback on responses) and positive reinforcement for appropriate toileting with the goals of decreasing incontinent episodes and increasing self-initiated toileting. Because it requires more caregiver time than simply toileting the individual, studies have examined the characteristics of individuals with dementia who are most likely to benefit from this intervention and reported that those who voided appropriately in response to prompts at least 66% of the time or experience at least 20% or more reduction in UI episodes following a 3-day toileting trial were most likely to benefit.

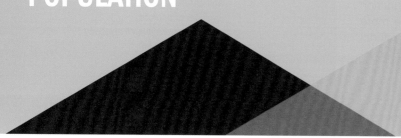

CHAPTER 14

VOIDING DYSFUNCTION AND URINARY INCONTINENCE IN THE PEDIATRIC POPULATION

Valre Welch

OBJECTIVES

1. Identify maturational processes required for the child to achieve urinary continence.

2. Discuss issues and current guidelines related to toilet training.

3. Identify common types of voiding dysfunction and incontinence in the pediatric population.

4. Describe pathology, presentation, assessment, and management of each of the following: nocturnal enuresis, voiding postponement, overactive bladder, and giggle incontinence.

TOPIC OUTLINE

INTRODUCTION

The International Children's Continence Society (ICCS) published an update to their standardized document on bowel and bladder dysfunction (Austin et al., 2014) to promote consistency in the definitions by all providers. The document describes 10 conditions where children can present with bowel and bladder dysfunction (**Box 14-1**). This chapter will discuss some of the more common conditions seen within the bladder dysfunction conditions including overactive bladder (OAB), dysfunctional voiding, bladder, bowel dysfunction (BBD), and voiding postponement. Information on toilet training and the acquisition of continence, vaginal reflux, and giggle incontinence are also reviewed due to the uniqueness in the pediatric population. A more exhaustive differential for conditions causing urologic symptoms is presented in **Table 14-1**.

ACQUISITION OF CONTINENCE/ TOILET TRAINING

Babies begin life with a bladder capacity of only 10 mL. They void often (10 to 15 times/day at 6 to 12 months of age) and do not always empty their bladder completely with each voiding but have multiple small interrupted voids, which eventually empty completely. This pattern changes as the child grows and, in most cases, eventually leads to continence. The mechanisms necessary for the achievement of continence are complex and gradual. The time that this take is also not uniform for every child (Guerra et al., 2014).

PHYSIOLOGIC AND PSYCHOLOGICAL READINESS

As the child grows older, bladder volume increases and voiding frequency decreases. There are also physiologic changes that inhibit overnight bladder contractions and reduce nocturnal urine output. The American Academy of Pediatrics (1999) developed guidelines to help assess a child's readiness for successful toilet training. These include both developmental and behavioral factors. Developmental readiness includes the ability to ambulate to the

TABLE 14-1 CONDITIONS CAUSING UROLOGIC SYMPTOMS	
Bowel and bladder dysfunction	Enuresis (nighttime wetting)
	Overactive bladder
	Voiding postponement
	Dysfunctional voiding
	Vaginal reflux
	Giggle incontinence
	Extraordinary daytime frequency
	Underactive bladder
	Obstruction
	Stress incontinence (rare)
CNS malformations	Myelomeningocele, lipomyelomeningocele
	Tethered cord
	Sacral agenesis
Acquired neurologic conditions	Cerebral palsy
	Multiple sclerosis
	Trauma
	Transverse myelitis
Smooth muscle	Muscular dystrophy
Structural conditions	Bladder/cloacal exstrophy; epispadias
	Cloacal anomalies
	Ectopic ureter
	Prune belly
	Posterior urethral valves

toilet, stability when sitting on the toilet, and the ability to pull clothes up and down. The child should also be able to follow two-step commands and express the need to use the toilet. Behaviorally the child should be able to imitate behaviors, express interest in the toilet, have a desire to please and the independence to say "no," as well decreasing oppositional behaviors and power struggles. They must also physiologically have the ability to store urine for a prolonged period of time.

Parents put significant effort into toilet training their children and are always in search of the fastest and most successful method. Today many parents are also motivated by the requirements of daycare facilities to either accept the child or move them along to be with older children if they are toilet trained—attaining the next level is very important and a definite motivating force to have the child achieve toilet training and continence. Toilet training behaviors are extremely variable, with limited data to support one over another. Some parents begin toilet training at a very early age by recognizing cues in their babies that indicate readiness to void (Sun & Rugolotto, 2004). However, most parents follow a child-centered approach to toilet training described by Brazelton (1962). This involves recognizing when a child is interested in toilet training and possesses the motor skills to void on a toilet, which typically occurs between 18 months of age and 28.5 months. In another, now classic, paper, Foxx and Azrin (1973) discussed child readiness, identified specific tasks to determine readiness,

BOX 14-1	BOWEL AND BLADDER DYSFUNCTION CONDITIONS (ICCS STANDARDIZATION)

Overactive bladder
Voiding postponement
Underactive bladder
Dysfunctional voiding
Bladder outlet dysfunction
Stress incontinence
Vaginal reflux
Giggle incontinence
Extraordinary daytime only urinary frequency
Bladder neck dysfunction

and then described a stepwise process to toilet training. Operant conditioning (OC) has also been proposed as a toilet training strategy; OC uses positive and negative reinforcement to achieve dryness (Sun & Rugolotto, 2004).

KEY POINT

Approaches to toilet training are extremely variable, with limited data to support one over another.

EVIDENCE REGARDING BEST APPROACH TO TOILET TRAINING

There is no evidence to support any method of toilet training over another (Klassen et al., 2006) nor the ideal age at which to begin or complete toilet training, though there is ongoing research to determine how age affects toilet training. The following studies illustrate the challenge of determining best age to begin toilet training. Based on survey questionnaires of parents and follow-up of 3,249 children in the Netherlands, Bakker et al. (2002) suggest that toilet training after 18 months of age places the child at risk for later problems. Joinson et al. (2009) studied 8,000 UK children ages 4.5 to 9 years and reported that toilet training after 24 months could lead to increased risk of daytime wetting and delayed acquisition of daytime control or relapse; Barone et al. (2009), in a case control study of 218 U.S. children aged 4 to 12 (n = 58 symptomatic children; N = 157 asymptomatic controls), suggest that toilet training post-32 months places the child at risk for urge symptoms. On the other hand, in another U.S.-based study, 378 children were followed from 17 months until acquisition of continence (Blum et al., 2004), and the authors found no relationship between age and toilet training outcomes. However, they did find that children who completed training post-42 months of age ("later trainers") were more likely "to have stool toileting refusal, to hide when defecating, to be frequently constipated, and to have lower language score at 18 months" (p. 109). Chen et al. (2009) and Yang et al. (2011), however, found no difference in urinary tract infections (UTIs) or reflux based on age at toilet training, and da Fonseca et al. (2011) indicated that toilet training before or after 24 months did not bear a relationship to voiding dysfunction. De Fonseca's study actually suggests that inappropriate voiding mechanisms may be caused by factors that do not relate to toilet training but to some structural abnormalities, or a maturational delay in either the urinary tract or the nervous system. These studies all illustrate the difficulty in determining both the effect of toilet training and the best age to begin it.

RECOMMENDATIONS

While little evidence exists to support a specific method of toilet training, there is substantial evidence to show

that poor toileting behaviors once toilet trained can result in recurrent UTI and daytime incontinence (Maternik et al., 2014; Sillen et al., 2010; Van Batavia et al., 2013). Stressing to parents the importance of adequate water intake for body weight (50 mL/kg/d up to 2 L), avoidance of caffeinated beverages, increased insoluble dietary fiber to maintain regular soft stools, and regular voiding is likely to be more important to long-term bladder health than the specific age or method of toilet training.

KEY POINT

Stressing to parents the importance of appropriate water intake, avoidance of caffeinated beverages, intake of sufficient fiber to prevent constipation, and regular voiding is probably more important to long-term bladder health than the specific method or age of toilet training.

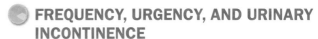 **FREQUENCY, URGENCY, AND URINARY INCONTINENCE**

Urinary frequency, urinary urgency, and daytime and nighttime incontinence are common reasons for children to see a health care provider. Daytime incontinence is found in 6% of girls and 3.8% of boys at age 7 (Schulman, 2004). There has been significant advancement in understanding pediatric voiding dysfunction in recent years due to both research and clinical advancements. The International Children's Continence Society, in an effort to avoid confusion developed a standardized system of nomenclature so that all providers are speaking the same language in relation to the various voiding dysfunctions seen in children (Colaco & Barone, 2014). All of these LUT (lower urinary tract) symptoms can cause a significant impact on the quality of life of children and families (Equit et al., 2014). This can ultimately impact school performance, which can have long-lasting effects. The response of teachers, school counselors, and peers can impact the child's interpersonal and social life with significant detrimental effects (Whale et al., 2017). Simple nighttime incontinence (enuresis), while not as medically alarming, can cause significant psychological distress. However, daytime incontinence has been shown to have more impact on the child's quality of life than enuresis (Deshpande et al., 2011). Research has also shown that if these conditions are not treated appropriately in childhood, they can and will persist into adulthood (Morin et al., 2018). Another situation in which daytime urinary incontinence has been reported is with the adolescent and young adult female athlete. Those involved in higher impact sports tend to be more likely to exhibit daytime stress urinary incontinence (Bauer et al., 2018; Logan et al., 2018).

CLINICAL PRESENTATION

In addition to complaints of frequency, urgency, abdominal pain, nocturia, and incontinence, children may also complain of dysuria or genital pain. Evaluating the child for a possible UTI must always be ruled out first. The dysuria and genital pain could be caused by vaginal or foreskin irritation from chronic wetness or could be the result of referred pain from constipation. BBD (bowel and bladder dysfunction) is a term that encompasses LUTS (lower urinary tract symptoms) and bowel dysfunction in children who do not have any identifiable neurological abnormality (Gaither et al., 2018; Santos et al., 2017). These children have a variety of urinary symptoms as well as constipation and sometimes encopresis. In severe cases, they can develop upper tract abnormalities including hydronephrosis or vesicoureteral reflux (VUR) (Colaco & Barone, 2014). In a large study of children looking at risk for developing UTIs, it was found that girls are more likely to develop BBD than boys (Chen, et al., 2004). Parents who identify the incontinence and are present during toileting may notice a change in the child's urinary stream including hesitancy (difficulty initiating the stream), straining, intermittency (stream that is not continuous), or a weak stream. They may also notice holding behaviors; girls may sit on their heels (often called Wilson curtsey), hold their perineum, or dance around (potty dancing), and boys may hold their penis all in an effort to avoid going to the bathroom. Often when questioned by parents they respond that they "do not have to go to the bathroom."

ASSESSMENT

While all of these symptoms may result from a functional condition, in rare cases, these findings can lead to a serious anatomic condition. As a result, a standard approach should be taken in the evaluation of these children that avoids unnecessary and often traumatic investigations. Most symptoms will be found to relate to symptoms of bladder or bowel dysfunction, and management strategies can be instituted to address this.

KEY POINT

Avoiding unnecessary and often traumatic diagnostic tests in the children is recommended because in most cases these symptoms are the result of a functional condition and not a serious anatomical condition.

History and Voiding Diary/Stool Diary

As in all areas in nursing and medicine, a complete history and physical may be all that is necessary to diagnose and treat children presenting with urologic symptoms. Having children and families complete a voiding/fluid intake and stool diary prior to their clinic visit or as homework prior to the next visit can be very helpful during the evaluation process. The history should focus on voiding behaviors including frequency, episodes of incontinence, voided volumes, presence of urgency, and time

taken to void. Holding behaviors should be discussed as well as dietary habits. Children in today's society frequently do not drink enough water, and often, their only fluid intake is from caffeinated beverages or juice. Dietary fiber intake should be discussed along with bowel movement frequency and stool consistency (see Chapter 23, Box 23-2); the Bristol stool chart (see Chapter 6, Fig. 6-7) (Lewis & Heaton, 1997) is a validated tool that can be used to determine whether constipation is present. It is also helpful to discuss daytime bathroom routines as the school environment can be stressful for children, and often, there is little access to the bathroom. Providing a note for the child to have more frequent access to the bathroom during the school day and to be allowed to have water with them in class is often both helpful and necessary in today's current school environment. Finally, it is important to ask about psychological conditions including anxiety and attention deficit/hyperactivity disorder (ADHD) or major depressive disorder (MDD) as well as learning delays, which have been identified as risk factors for bladder dysfunction (von Gontard & Equit, 2015).

To be successful, management for children with voiding dysfunction must include attention to any psychological or cognitive issues. Questionnaires can be administered to assess the impact the symptoms have on the child's quality of life and to track progress. The two questionnaires that were most commonly used were the Dysfunctional Voiding Symptoms Score (Farhat et al., 2000) and the Pediatric Urinary Incontinence Quality of Life Score (PIN-Q) (Bower et al., 2006). Research has been ongoing to help the clinician and families better evaluate and manage the various aspects of childhood incontinence. New tools have been devised, many of which have been validated, to measure outcomes when treating childhood incontinence. These new tools can be utilized by providers to meet individual patient situations (Chase et al., 2018).

Physical Examination

Physical assessment includes an abdominal exam to palpate for retained stool and for a distended bladder. The back should be examined to rule out sacral dimples (**Fig. 14-1**) or hairy patches, which may suggest a spinal cord pathology. Genital findings to watch for include vaginal redness, labial adhesions, continuous leaking in girls, and meatal or foreskin abnormalities in boys such as balanoposthitis—cellulitis (**Fig. 14-2**) or meatal stenosis. Bladder scanning for pre- and postvoid volumes can be very helpful in the clinic; however, the cost of the machine may prohibit this in smaller centers.

Initial workup for the child with frequency, urgency, and incontinence should focus on voiding and defecation patterns, ruling out constipation, and screening for indicators of neurologic dysfunction. A urinalysis should be performed to eliminate possible infection, renal disease, or metabolic etiologies for incontinence. A renal

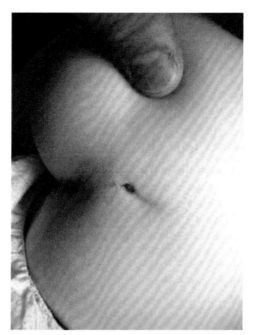

FIGURE 14-1. Sacral Dimple within the Gluteal Cleft. (Courtesy of Paul S. Matz, MD.)

ultrasound is often part of the initial evaluation to be certain that there are no structural abnormalities or abnormalities of the bladder including large postvoid residuals or bladder wall thickening (Colaco & Barone, 2014).

Uroflow

Uroflow is a noninvasive evaluation tool to assess voiding dynamics, whereby children sit on a commode to void and a scale underneath records various measurements. These include voided volume, maximum flow,

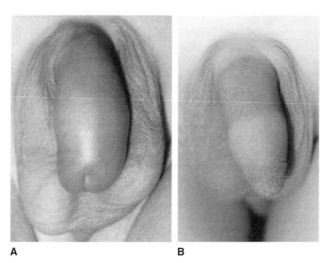

A   **B**

FIGURE 14-2. **A.** Balanoposthitis—cellulitis of normal foreskin with erythema, edema, and tenderness. **B.** Normal foreskin after treatment of balanoposthitis with antibiotics and warm soaks. (From Fleisher, G. R., & Ludwig, S. (2010). *Textbook of pediatric emergency medicine*. Philadelphia, PA: Lippincott Williams & Wilkins.)

and voiding pattern. The addition of an EMG tracing during voiding may be helpful in determining whether the sphincter is active during voiding (dyssynergia), evaluate whether the child is straining or relaxed during voiding, which impacts the ability of empty the bladder. Uroflow can aid in the diagnosis of bladder dysfunction; however, it is not available in many centers.

Imaging Tests

Imaging with ultrasound and abdominal x-ray may be necessary. Ultrasound may be of particular benefit in children who also present with UTI. Anatomic conditions leading to infections may be found; however, it is important to recognize that ultrasound cannot identify all anatomic conditions such as VUR (**Fig. 14-3**) and ectopic ureters (**Fig. 14-4**). Ultrasound imaging should be performed pre- and postvoid to assess for changes with bladder emptying. X-ray may demonstrate a spinal malformation or ureteric calculus. X-ray can also be used to confirm the presence of fecal loading. This can be helpful, or in some cases required, for parents who need evidence of a problem

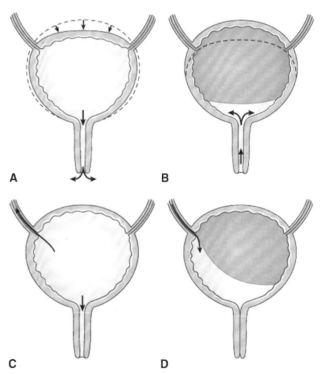

A   **B**

C   **D**

FIGURE 14-3. Urethrovesical and Vesicoureteric Reflux. With coughing and straining, bladder pressure rises, which may force urine from the bladder into the urethra **(A)**. When bladder pressure returns to normal, the urine flows back to the bladder **(B)**, which introduces bacteria from the urethra to the bladder. Vesicoureteric reflux: With failure of the ureterovesical valve, urine moves up the ureters during voiding **(C)** and flows into the bladder when voiding stops **(D)**. This prevents complete emptying of the bladder. It also leads to urinary stasis and contamination of the ureters with bacterium-laden urine. (From Farrell, M., & Dempsey, J. (2010). *Smeltzer and Bare's textbook of medical-surgical nursing*. Philadelphia, PA: Lippincott Williams & Wilkins.)

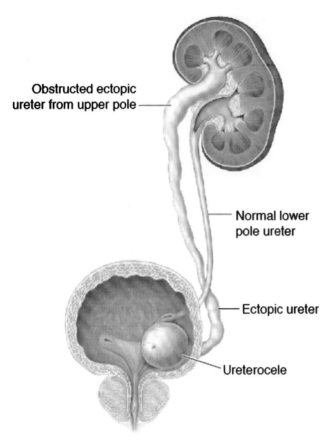

Obstructed ectopic
ureter from upper pole

Normal lower
pole ureter

Ectopic ureter

Ureterocele

FIGURE 14-4. Duplicated Collecting System and Ectopic Ureter.

before they are willing to begin bowel management. **Figure 14-5** demonstrates fecal loading in a child with an impaction, and **Figure 14-6** provides an algorithm for management for pediatric constipation recommended by Constipation Guideline Committee of the North American Society for Pediatric Gastroenterology, Hepatology and Nutrition (2006). In addition, Chapter 23 offers detailed guidance in the assessment and treatment of constipation in the pediatric population.

Video Urodynamics

Children who fail initial management may require further investigation. This typically involves video urodynamics (see also Chapter 5). A urethral catheter, rectal catheter, and EMG pads are placed, the bladder is filled under fluoroscopic imaging, and filling pressures are recorded. If the child is able to voluntarily initiate voiding, he/she is asked to void and emptying pressures are recorded. In older children, the urine during leaks and voids is collected and measured; however, in babies, this may be difficult. Urodynamics may demonstrate abnormal bladder contractions in the child with an overactive or neurogenic bladder. In severe cases, the pressure may increase significantly during filling, which is indicative of poor compliance and implies upper tract involvement. In children who hold off voiding for long periods, the bladder may become atonic; in this case, the bladder can be filled to large volumes with no sensation or contractions.

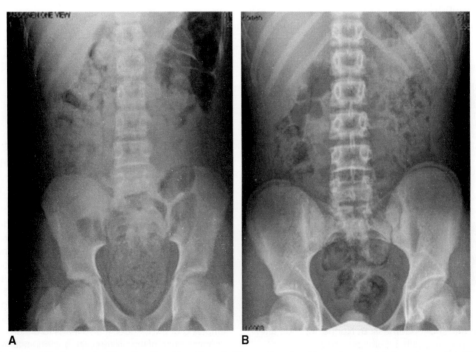

A   **B**

FIGURE 14-5. Abdominal Radiographs Showing Fecal Loading. **A.** The rectum is widened and contains a large fecal impaction. **B.** Rectum is less widened, and the stool is less compacted. (From Fleisher, G. R., & Ludwig, S. (2010). *Textbook of pediatric emergency medicine.* Philadelphia, PA: Lippincott Williams & Wilkins.)

CONSTIPATION, TREATMENT (PEDIATRIC)

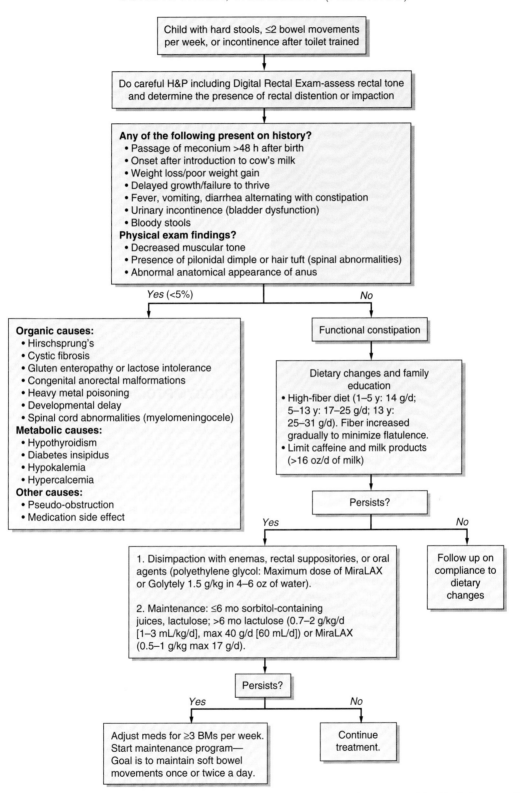

FIGURE 14-6. Algorithm for Management of Constipation. (From Constipation Guideline Committee of the North American Society for Pediatric Gastroenterology, Hepatology and Nutrition. (2006). Evaluation and treatment of constipation in infants and children: Recommendations of the North American Society for Pediatric Gastroenterology, Hepatology and Nutrition. *Journal of Pediatric Gastroenterology and Nutrition*, *43*(3), e1–e13.)

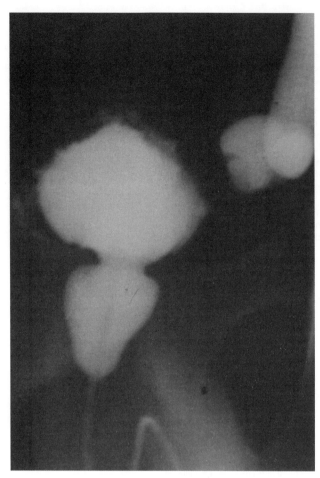

FIGURE 14-7. Spinning-Top Urethra. (From Saxton, H. M., Borzyskowski, M., & Robinson, L. B. (1992). Nonobstructive posterior urethral widening (spinning top urethra) in boys with bladder instability. *Radiology, 182*, 81, with permission.)

In the child with a dysfunctional external sphincter producing obstructed voiding, fluoroscopy can detect VUR, bladder diverticulum, and a "spinning top" urethra (**Fig. 14-7**). The information gleaned from urodynamic testing can be very helpful; however, it does have some drawbacks. First of all, the test can be perceived as very invasive for children and a negative experience may worsen their symptoms. Urodynamic findings have also been shown to have a large interobserver variability (Bael et al., 2009) and may not reflect what is happening during natural bladder filling. This issue may be partly resolved with ambulatory urodynamics; however, there are little data on the reliability of this test, particularly in children (Deshpande et al., 2012).

KEY POINT

Initial workup for the child with frequency, urgency, and incontinence should focus on voiding and defecation patterns, ruling out constipation, and screening for indicators of neurologic dysfunction.

 ENURESIS

The International Children's Continence Society (ICCS) defines enuresis as "intermittent wetting during sleep after organic causes have been ruled out, with a minimum wetting frequency of once/month" (Austin et al., 2014; Franco et al., 2013; Nijman et al., 2013). Enuresis is a common condition affecting approximately 15% of 5 to 6 year olds, 5% of 9 to 10 year olds, and 1% to 3% of children in their late teens. There are estimated to be approximately 5 to 7 million children in the United States who have enuresis. Enuresis is 2 to 3 times more common in boys than girls and approximately 15% of children have their enuresis resolve spontaneously every year. There is a definite familial tendency with enuresis, with a 44% likelihood of the child having enuresis if one parent had enuresis and a 77% incidence if both parents had enuresis (Noto & Berry, 2017). Enuresis has been categorized as monosymptomatic (no LUTS and normal urinalysis) or nonmonosymptomatic (coexisting symptoms of LUT dysfunction) and/or comorbid conditions such as diabetes mellitus (DM), detrusor overactivity (DO), chronic renal failure (CRF), or sleep apnea (OSA). Studies have shown that up to 90% of enuresis is due to genetic predisposition, biological, and developmental factors (Hobbs et al., 2016).

MONOSYMPTOMATIC ENURESIS

Monosymptomatic, this term is used to denote enuresis in children who have no other LUTS and who do not have a history of bladder dysfunction; it may be either primary or secondary (Nevéus et al., 2006). *Primary enuresis* refers to the involuntary passage of urine during sleep in children aged 5 years and older who have never achieved a satisfactory period of nighttime dryness for at least 6 months. *Secondary enuresis* refers to enuresis that develops after a dry period of at least 6 months. It can be related to an unusually stressful event (e.g., parental divorce, birth of a sibling) at a time of vulnerability in a child's life or due to other medical causes such as UTIs, constipation, or voiding dysfunction. However, the exact cause of secondary enuresis remains unknown.

KEY POINT

Enuresis is a common condition affecting approximately 5 to 7 million children in the United States and is 2 to 3 times more common in boys than in girls.

NONMONOSYMPTOMATIC ENURESIS

Nonmonosymptomatic, this term refers to enuresis that is accompanied by any other LUTS such as increased/decreased voiding frequency, daytime incontinence, urgency, hesitancy, straining, a weak stream, intermittency, holding maneuvers, a feeling of incomplete emptying, postmicturition dribble, and genital or LUT pain (Nevéus et al., 2006).

NATURAL HISTORY AND PATHOLOGY

Enuresis has a spontaneous resolution rate of over 15% per year and is typically only diagnosed in children 5 years or older since the acquisition of nighttime continence may take up to 5 years to achieve. However, the need for sensitive care of both the child and parent may be required before age 5 if parents are unrealistic in expecting dry nights and if the enuresis is contributing to child and family stress.

There have been many proposed etiologies and pathophysiology for enuresis including excessive urine output at night due to decrease release of or response to arginine vasopressin, smaller bladder capacity at night due to nocturnal detrusor instability, deep sleep, and an abnormal sleep cycle that prevents awakening to the sensation of a full bladder. Factors that may predispose to nighttime incontinence include constipation (Halachmi & Farhat, 2008), poor daytime voiding habits, and obstructive sleep apnea. Investigations to determine the cause of the nighttime wetting include sleep studies, and stool and voiding diaries. Medical conditions that could cause enuresis must also be excluded such as UTIs, diabetes, diabetes insipidus, and renal disease. Recent studies propose that children with enuresis may have increased sleep fragmentation as compared to children without enuresis, suggesting a central nervous system role in the condition (Dhondt et al., 2014). Enuresis can be correlated with both sleep disorders and psychological problems. In a study reported by Van Herzeele et al. (2016), treatment of enuresis also showed improvement in sleep pattern and some psychological problems. Sleep apnea may cause the same disruption in sleep patterns, and in some studies, enuresis improved after tonsillectomy and adenoidectomy (Jeyakumar et al., 2012).

> **KEY POINT**
>
> Enuresis has been categorized as monosymptomatic (no LUTS and normal urinalysis) or nonmonosymptomatic (coexisting symptoms of lower urinary tract dysfunction) and/or comorbid conditions such as diabetes mellitus (DM), detrusor overactivity (DO), chronic renal failure (CRF), or sleep apnea (OSA).

EVALUATION

Children who present with pure nighttime incontinence do not need extensive testing. A standard history and physical should typically suffice. A detailed voiding and stooling history should be taken with the parent and child. A voiding diary of approximately 2 to 3 weeks can help to determine the frequency and even the number of times the child is wet during the night. Understanding when the wetting occurs, that is, soon after going to bed or closer to morning can also be helpful in planning treatment. It is also important to take a history of fluid intake including what type of fluid and when it is consumed. Discussing with the child and family what are the expectations of treatment and if the child is bothered and ready to stop wetting or is this more a parental expectation. How does the family handle the wetting currently, do the parents feel the child is doing this on purpose or "lazy" and is the child being punished for wetting (physically or psychologically) (Hobbs et al., 2016). In the absence of daytime incontinence, urinary frequency, or UTI, treatment can be implemented immediately.

> **KEY POINT**
>
> Children who present with pure nighttime incontinence do not need extensive testing. A standard history and physical with a detailed voiding and stooling history needs to be included in the comprehensive assessment.

MANAGEMENT

Various management strategies have been employed, based on the proposed pathologic mechanisms (see **Fig. 14-8**). All begin with counseling parents on the age ranges for achieving nighttime dryness, emphasizing that it is not the fault of the child and that punishment will not assist but hinder resolution of the issue. It is also important to determine the child's feelings about being wet and whether they are ready to work with the parents to improve the situation; effective management requires "buy-in" and adherence to management recommendations by both the child and family. Recommendations usually include lifestyle management strategies such as regular voiding during the day, management of constipation, adequate fluid intake during the day, and fluid restriction before going to bed. These changes must be ongoing along with other treatment modalities. The most successful and well-studied medical interventions include the enuresis alarm system and DDAVP (desmopressin).

Enuresis Alarm System

The enuresis alarm may alter neurologic signaling and has a documented success rate of 66% (Glazener et al., 2005). Parent involvement is critical to success as they must wake the child when the alarm sounds if the child does not wake on his/her own. The parent then takes the child to the bathroom to void; this should be done even if the child has already emptied completely in bed. The goal is to teach the child to wake to the sensation of a full bladder. It should be noted that this treatment approach is different from waking the child at set times, which has not proven successful in treating bedwetting (though it may decrease the volume voided). Various factors may

ENURESIS

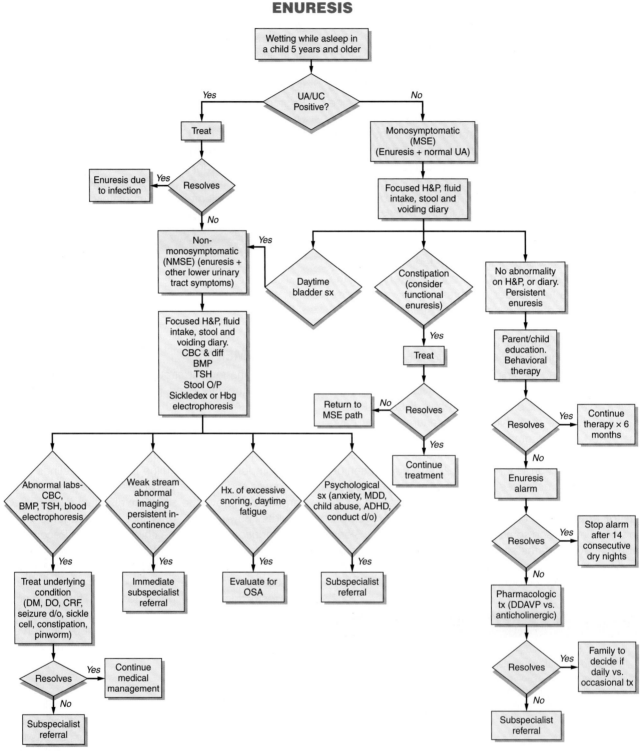

FIGURE 14-8. Algorithm for Management of Enuresis. (From Sweet, M. G., Schmidt-Dalton, T. A., Weiss, P. M., et al. (2012). Evaluation and management of abnormal uterine bleeding in premenopausal women. *American Family Physician*, *85*, 35–43.)

make it difficult for the parents and child to adhere to alarm therapy. For example, during school, the sleep disruption may be harmful to the child's academic performance, and this may stress an already difficult relationship. Siblings may also share a room and parents may not

want the sibling disturbed. Nevertheless, when employed diligently, most children can attain nighttime dryness with this intervention. Parents should be advised effective treatment may take as long as 2 to 3 months of consistent use and they should not be discouraged if they do not see immediate success. Increased bladder capacity with consistent use of the alarm has been achieved (Nield et al., 2018).

DDAVP

The mainstay in pharmacologic treatment of enuresis is DDAVP (desmopressin), a synthetic analogue of the natural pituitary hormone 8-arginine vasopressin (ADH), an antidiuretic hormone that affects renal water conservation. DDAVP acts on the collecting tubule to reabsorb rather than excrete water, thus concentrating the urine and reducing urine volume. It is available in a tablet and melt form. In one study, the melt was found to be more effective than tablet in treating nighttime wetting, especially in the younger child (Juul et al., 2013). Once the medication is discontinued, the child will return to wetting the bed, if they have not started secreting adequate amounts of vasopressin. Usually parents are advised if the medication has affected a cessation of their child's enuresis to try weaning the child off the medication every 3 to 6 months to see if they will now be dry without medication. If the child resumes wetting, then the medication is restarted. This is not an actual cure but a treatment approach which in the child who responds can alleviate the wetting until they no longer need the medication. Tricyclic antidepressant medications have also been used to treat bedwetting and are considered third-line treatment for those who have failed bed alarms and DDAVP (Neveus et al., 2010). Although adverse events are uncommon, very few parents or physicians feel comfortable prescribing this in a healthy, happy child due to potential side effects such as nervousness, personality change, cardiovascular events, or potential risk of death if accidentally overdosed as well as the FDA "Black Box" warning on potential suicide in children and adolescents (US FDA, 2018). Alternative therapies that have been tried for bedwetting include hypnotherapy, acupuncture, chiropractic, and psychotherapy. To date, there is very weak evidence to support any of these for the successful treatment of bedwetting.

Enuresis is a common condition that usually does not require extensive investigation. Children and families should be reassured that there is a high likelihood of cure without intervention and that the condition is not intentional. Reward systems are not helpful given that the children do not have control over the wetting. The anxiety caused by the condition, however, should not be minimized, and treatment is reasonable if the child and parents are willing. **Figure 14-8** provides an algorithm of systematic steps for the management of enuresis. The integration of a variety of professionals—physicians, nurse practitioners, nurses, physical therapists, and urotherapists can bring the slightly different perspective and treatment approach of these various disciplines to the treatment plan, thus often improving outcomes for the child (Caldwell et al., 2018).

OVERACTIVE BLADDER

OAB is defined as urinary urgency, frequency, and often nocturia that is not due to a neurologic cause. It is reported as one of the most frequent LUT urologic conditions in children. Studies have demonstrated that OAB symptoms occur in 16.6% to 17.8% of the general population and up to 57.4% of incontinence children (Colaco & Barone, 2014). This is a disorder of the storage (filling) phase of bladder function (Deshpande et al., 2012). This was previously labeled as "detrusor instability" but is now called DO per the ICCS nomenclature. The pathophysiology of OAB is thought to the overactive, involuntary detrusor contractions during bladder filling. The child will try to counter these contractions by voluntary pelvic floor muscle contractions to postpone voiding and avoid wetting. These detrusor contractions are thought to be due to maturational delay and infantile bladder behaviors. This has also been linked to abnormal toilet training habits though the exact pathophysiology is still being debated (Colaco & Barone, 2014; Noto & Berry, 2017). These children may also have incontinence depending on whether they can reach the toilet on time. The urgency associated with OAB should be differentiated from the normal urgency that occurs when a child postpones voiding while busy and must rush to the bathroom because the bladder is very full. The best way to confirm abnormal frequency and urgency is with a voiding diary; in the absence of a diary, the clinician can ask specific questions about voiding frequency, such as the child's ability to tolerate long car rides or to sit through a movie. Teachers' comments can also help confirm abnormal voiding frequency. Parents may need to advocate for their child if school policy does not allow children to leave the class without permission to use the bathroom. Providing a note for the child to be allowed to use the bathroom at school as needed is often necessary and helpful.

ETIOLOGIC FACTORS

Lifestyle factors can play a significant contributing role in OAB. Consumption of caffeinated beverages may cause increased bladder irritability in addition to its diuretic effect; the combined effects can cause increased frequency and urgency. Many parents do not recognize the impact of caffeine on the bladder and may not realize the need to limit intake of these fluids.

Constipation can also cause urinary frequency and is one of the biggest causes of bladder symptoms in the pediatric population (Veiga et al., 2013); the negative impact of fecal loading on bladder function has been confirmed through urodynamic studies (Panayi et al., 2011). Fecal loading can also cause problems with infrequent voiding, insufficient emptying, and VUR. Anxiety disorders can also play a role in bladder overactivity; in children with OAB and anxiety, stressful situations may amplify the symptoms. An OAB in childhood may predict bladder problems as an adult; however, at this time, there is no evidence that specific interventions can prevent later problems (Fitzgerald et al., 2006; Minassian et al., 2006; Morin et al., 2018). Chapter 6 reviews lifestyle modifications to promote bladder health.

EVALUATION

Initial investigation should focus on the voiding and bowel history as well as a psychological assessment. If the condition is severe and associated with incontinence, the patient may require urodynamics to determine whether a neurologic assessment is necessary. Frequent bladder contractions on urodynamics do support the diagnosis of OAB (**Fig. 14-9**); however, an MRI may be necessary to rule out a spinal cord malformation, especially if initial management is unsuccessful.

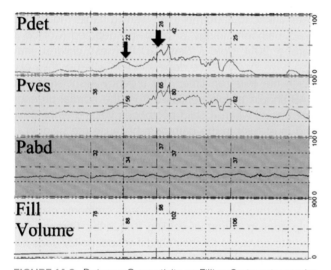

FIGURE 14-9. Detrusor Overactivity on Filling Cystometrography. The patient begins to sense urgency, accompanied by an unstable bladder contraction, when 88 mL of water is instilled into the bladder. The detrusor pressure rises, and when 96 mL of water is instilled, she leaks. Pabd, abdominal pressure; Pves, vesical pressure; Pdet, detrusor pressure. (From Berek, J. S. (2011). *Berek and Novak's gynecology*. Philadelphia, PA: Lippincott Williams & Wilkins.)

MANAGEMENT

Once a diagnosis of OAB is made, management is initiated and should be multimodal. The first step is to ensure that irritating beverages are avoided, and the bowel is under control. An x-ray demonstrating improvement in fecal loading can be helpful though this is not a validated instrument. Bowel management is critically important for children with OAB because the medications used to treat this condition can cause significant constipation. Psychological referral may also be necessary if there is a large component of anxiety, and special consideration should be given to providing support for the child at school.

Many new medications have been introduced to treat adult OAB; these are discussed in detail in Chapter 7. Anticholinergic medications are beneficial in improving OAB symptoms in children as well and fortunately can be used on a long-term basis (Nijman et al., 2007). While short-acting oxybutynin is the only medication with pediatric approval, in reality, pediatric urologists or nurse practitioners will try all adult medications (at pediatric doses), particularly when side effects and practicality become a problem (Ramsay & Bolduc, 2017). Pediatric-friendly formulations include oxybutynin gel and patch and long-acting antimuscarinic medications that retain pharmacokinetics when crushed, such as solifenacin (Nadeau et al., 2014; Ramsay & Bolduc, 2017). Practitioners must remember that most children struggle to swallow pills and short-acting medications are difficult to administer when children are at school.

KEY POINT

Management of OAB in children mirrors OAB management in adults and involves behavioral strategies (e.g., bowel management, elimination caffeinated fluids), antimuscarinic medications if needed, and neuromodulation for refractory cases.

Newer treatment strategies, which have been used less frequently in children, include transcutaneous nerve stimulation (TENS), posterior tibial nerve stimulation (PTNS), sacral neuromodulation via implant (SNM), and Botox injections (De Gennaro et al., 2011; Ramsay & Bolduc, 2017). In a few small studies, TENS has been shown to improve symptoms in up to 73% of patients (Hagstroem et al., 2009; Malm-Buatsi et al., 2007). It has also been shown to improve slow transit constipation, which may help to improve bladder symptoms (Hutson et al., 2015; Ismail et al., 2009). PTNS has shown some success in children with a mean age of 11.7 years and is well tolerated (Capitanucci et al., 2009; De Gennaro et al., 2004; de Wall & Heesakkers, 2017; Hoebeke et al., 2002). SNM has also been shown to improve voiding symptoms; however, there can be up to a 50% risk of reoperation (Dwyer et al., 2014). Botox is an acceptable treatment for children who already perform intermittent catheterization as a result of a neurogenic bladder but is of limited use in children with OAB, because very few children and families will accept the risk of requiring catheterization. However, one study in children did show a significant improvement in symptoms with only 1 of 21 children requiring intermittent catheterization and only for a short period (Hoebeke et al., 2006).

OAB can disrupt a child's life as well as the family dynamics. Investigation should ensure that there is not a neurologic reason for the symptoms. Lifestyle measures should be optimized initially as avoidance of medications is preferable in children. In the absence of improvement, anticholinergic medication has been found beneficial in children and should be prescribed. Neuromodulation and Botox can be considered in refractory cases.

KEY POINT

Overactive bladder can disrupt a child's life as well as the family dynamics. Investigation should ensure that there is not a neurologic reason for the symptoms. Lifestyle measures should be optimized initially as avoidance of medications is preferable in children.

VOIDING POSTPONEMENT AND DYSFUNCTIONAL VOIDING

Children often prefer to play rather than use the toilet on a regular basis. As a result, they may present with urinary incontinence and/or UTI as a result of voiding postponement. These children may also delay defecation, causing bowel dysfunction as well. Parents may notice little girls sitting on their heels, holding their perineum or dancing around (potty dancing), or boys holding their penis, but may not realize there is a problem until the child has an accident while urgently running to the bathroom. If these behaviors are allowed to continue long term, the child may develop dysfunctional voiding, which is defined as voluntary contraction of the urinary sphincter and pelvic floor during voiding (detrusor sphincter dyssynergia). Children with dysfunctional voiding ultimately develop large postvoid residuals and may present with significant incontinence and UTI. **Figure 14-10A** shows discoordination (dyssynergia) between bladder contraction and pelvic floor relaxation (spinning top urethra) that results in incomplete emptying; **Figure 14-10B** shows a chronically distended bladder that empties poorly, resulting from chronic voiding postponement.

KEY POINT

If voiding postponement behaviors are not identified and corrected, they can result in dysfunctional voiding, chronic bladder distention, and frequent UTIs.

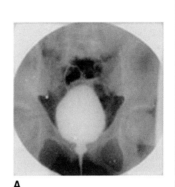 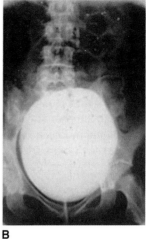

A   **B**

FIGURE 14-10. Video Urodynamics. **A.** Detrusor–sphincter dyssynergia in a child. **B.** Atonic bladder due to chronic urinary holding. (From Schrier, R. W. (2006). *Diseases of the kidney and urinary tract*. Philadelphia, PA: Lippincott Williams & Wilkins.)

EVALUATION

An accurate voiding diary will quickly point to voiding postponement as a cause for the child's urologic symptoms. If available, a uroflow with EMG tracing and a postvoid residual can also help to diagnose dysfunctional voiding; the EMG tracing will demonstrate abnormal sphincter activity during voiding, and the uroflow will reveal an intermittent "staccato" voiding pattern. If the child also presents with UTI, she/he may need a renal bladder ultrasound with particular attention to the postvoid residual. A severe form of dysfunctional voiding called Hinman-Allen syndrome (non-neurogenic neurogenic bladder) can lead to progressive renal disease and renal failure. These children need to be identified and treated before irreversible kidney damage occurs.

MANAGEMENT

Treatment for voiding postponement focuses on timed voiding, relaxation when voiding with proper positioning, increasing water intake, and treating constipation. This becomes critically important with school-aged children, because the child may feel embarrassed to ask to use the bathroom or may only be allowed to go to the bathroom at specific intervals. Vibrating watches can help remind children to void, and the clinician can send letters to the school to ensure teacher cooperation with voiding routines and access to water bottles. PEG 3350 can be used as a stool softener for the child with persistent constipation, and timed bowel elimination attempts are suggested following a meal. It is also critical to treatment success to try to elucidate the child's reasons for postponement, as helping the child with the root cause will greatly improve likelihood of treatment success.

Biofeedback may be of benefit in management of dysfunctional voiding. Biofeedback helps the child to learn how to use their pelvic floor muscles more effectively and allow them to empty their bladder more completely. Biofeedback is just one aspect of "urotherapy" defined by the ICCS as "conservative-based therapy and treatment of LUT dysfunction that rehabilitates the LUT and encompasses a wide field of health care professionals" (Austin et al., 2015, p. e10). Urotherapy may include education regarding LUT dysfunction, lifestyle and behavioral modification, counseling, pelvic floor muscle training with biofeedback, neuromodulation, and intermittent catheterization (Austin et al., 2015).

> **KEY POINT**
>
> "Urotherapy" defined by the ICCS as "conservative-based therapy and treatment of LUT dysfunction that rehabilitates the LUT and encompasses a wide field of health care professionals" including the continence nurse specialist.

Children with voiding postponement may be extremely strong willed and may test the child/parent relationship. If this is the case, a psychologist may be necessary to address the behavioral aspect of care. For the child with dysfunctional voiding who does not empty their bladder completely, alpha blockers such as doxazosin may be part of the treatment plan.

Biofeedback is a time intensive but successful treatment for children as it helps them learn to coordinate pelvic muscle relaxation in order to improve bladder emptying. Improved emptying can also reduce or eliminate incontinence, which improves the child's quality of life (Berry et al., 2014). Patch electrodes are placed on the abdomen and perineal area and connected to a computer software program that looks like a video game. Children learn to properly isolate and relax the pelvic floor muscles. They are educated about healthy bladder and bowel habits. Biofeedback is typically performed weekly for 6 weeks though there is not enough evidence to give definitive advice about length of treatment. Various nonrandomized studies have shown an improvement in UTI (83%) and incontinence (80%) with biofeedback. One randomized trial did not show a statistical difference but did demonstrate an improvement (Desantis et al., 2011).

Biofeedback tends to be favored by parents who prefer a nonmedical approach. Unfortunately, pediatric biofeedback for urological conditions such as dysfunctional voiding is not available in all centers, requires time out of school, time away from work for parents, and may stress a family who must travel a substantial distance. Treatment may not be covered by health insurance, placing a financial strain on the family. In this setting, alpha-blockers can be used to relax the smooth muscle and improve emptying, but behavioral therapy must be incorporated as much as possible. While there is little evidence that alpha-blockers cure dysfunctional voiding, there is a randomized trial that demonstrated subjective improvement as reported

by patients and families (Kramer et al., 2005). Another study demonstrated changes in uroflow parameters with use of the medication (Van Batavia et al., 2010). Alpha-blockers can also be used as adjunctive therapy for the child being managed with biofeedback.

> **KEY POINT**
>
> Management of voiding postponement involves management of constipation, adequate water intake, and timed voiding. Biofeedback may be of benefit in management of dysfunctional voiding. An alpha-blocker may be considered as adjunctive therapy with biofeedback.

Voiding postponement is common in school-aged children and can lead to significant morbidity and voiding dysfunction. Obtaining a reliable voiding history is critical to management. Children and families must be instructed on regular emptying of the bladder and bowel. In more severe situations, biofeedback can be a powerful tool in treating the condition along with other types of urotherapy. Finally, psychological support may be necessary to address behavioral issues and family stress.

 VAGINAL REFLUX

Vaginal voiding or vaginal reflux is a benign condition that can cause troublesome symptoms. It is caused by the passage of urine into the vagina during voiding. With a careful history, the child will describe dribbling after she gets up from the toilet. This can be seen on an ultrasound or a voiding cystourethrogram when urine enters the vagina during voiding. It is important to do a genital exam to be certain that the girl does not have labial adhesions. Girls should be instructed to pull their panties all the way down to their ankles, sit forward on the toilet with their legs spread to ensure that the vagina empties. They should also allow some time before standing up after a void. These simple measures typically cure the condition.

 GIGGLE INCONTINENCE

Giggle incontinence is a unique condition usually only seen in girls, but there have been reported cases in boys (Fernandes et al., 2018) where laughter triggers complete voiding of urine (Glahn, 1979). This can understandably cause a significant amount of anxiety for girls who experience this phenomenon. The pathophysiology is not well understood; girls with this condition are completely dry outside of the giggle episodes and have normal anatomy. If the history and physical do not clearly rule out significant pathology, urodynamics should be considered though the urodynamic study is normal except during laughing episodes. The proposed theory of why this occurs is that the laughing induces sudden detrusor instability and bladder emptying (Colaco & Barone, 2014).

KEY POINT

Giggle incontinence is a poorly understood and highly distressing condition; management involves lifestyle modification (bowel management, avoidance of caffeinated fluids, and scheduled voiding) and sympathomimetic agents to enhance sphincter tone.

Despite the lack of clarity regarding etiology and pathology, treatment to date has focused primarily on improving sphincter tone, timed voiding, biofeedback, and enhancing sympathetic stimulation. Currently recognized treatments include stimulants such as methylphenidate (Berry et al., 2009; Chang et al., 2011) and pseudoephedrine and biofeedback (Richardson & Palmer, 2009). Many parents are reluctant to try methylphenidate due to its association with attention deficit disorder and abuse of the drug. Lifestyle measures such as bowel management, regular voiding, and avoiding caffeine should be encouraged to ensure optimum treatment.

 CONCLUSION

Bladder control is a basic function that many people take for granted. The steps to become toilet trained should occur "naturally," although many parents struggle with this process. Once a child is toilet trained, many things may impact continence. While health care professionals may first think of anatomic factors, in reality, psychological and behavioral factors are responsible for the majority of problems. In this fast-paced world, healthy toileting and dietary habits seem to be forgotten. As such, the investigation and management of children presenting with incontinence should focus on a thorough history and bowel and bladder management. If this fails, children may require more invasive investigation and referral to a pediatric urologist.

REFERENCES

American Academy of Pediatrics. (1999). Toilet training guidelines: Parents-the role of parents in toilet training. *Pediatrics*, *103*(6), 1362–1363.

Austin, P. F., Bauer, S. B., Bower, W., et al. (2014). The standardization of terminology of lower urinary tract function in children and adolescents: Update report from the Standardization Committee of the International Children's Continence Society. *The Journal of Urology*, 191(6), 1863–1865.

Austin, P. F., Bauer, S. B., Bower, W., et al. (2015). The standardization of terminology of lower urinary tract function in children and adolescents: Update report from the standardization committee of the International Children's Continence Society. *Neurourology Urodynamics*, 35, 471–481.

Bael, A., Verhulst, J., Lax, H., et al. (2009). Investigator bias in urodynamic studies for functional urinary incontinence. *The Journal of Urology*, *182*(4 Suppl), 1949–1952.

Bakker, E., Van Gool, J. D., Van Sprundel, M., et al. (2002). Results of a questionnaire evaluating the effects of different methods of toilet training on achieving bladder control. *BJU International*, *90*(4), 456–461.

Barone, J. G., Jasutkar, N., & Schneider, D. (2009). Later toilet training is associated with urge incontinence in children. *Journal of Pediatric Urology*, *5*(6), 458–461.

Bauer, S. B., Vasquez, E., Cendron, M., et al. (2018). Pelvic floor laxity: A not so rare but unrecognized form of daytime urinary incontinence in peripubertal and adolescent girls. *Journal Pediatric Urology*, *14*(6), 544.e1–544.e7. doi: 10.1016/jpurol.2018.04.030.

Berry, A., Rudick, K., Richter, M., et al. (2014). Objective versus subjective outcome measures of biofeedback: What really matters? *Journal of Pediatric Urology*, *10*(4), 620–626. doi: 10.1016/j.jpurol.2014.06.003.

Berry, A. K., Zderic, S., & Carr, M. (2009). Methylphenidate for giggle incontinence. *The Journal of Urology*, *182*(4 Suppl), 2028–2032.

Blum, N. J., Taubman, B., & Nemeth, N. (2004). Why is toilet training occurring at older ages? A study of factors associated with later training. *The Journal of Pediatrics*, *145*(1), 107–111.

Bower, W. F., Wong, E. M., & Yeung, C. K. (2006). Development of a validated quality of life tool specific to children with bladder dysfunction. *Neurourology and Urodynamics*, *25*(3), 221–227.

Brazelton, T. B. (1962). A child-oriented approach to toilet training. *Pediatrics*, *29*, 121–128.

Caldwell, P. H. Y., Lim, M., & Nankivell, G. (2018). An interprofessional approach to managing children with treatment-resistant enuresis: An educational review. *Pediatric Nephrology*, *33*, 1663–1670. doi.org/10.1007/s00467-017-3830-1.

Capitanucci, M. L., Camanni, D., Demelas, F., et al. (2009). Long-term efficacy of percutaneous tibial nerve stimulation for different types of lower urinary tract dysfunction in children. *The Journal of Urology*, *182*(4 Suppl), 2056–2061. doi.org/10.1016/j.juro.2009.03.007.

Chang, J. H., Lee, K. Y., Kim, T. B., et al. (2011). Clinical and urodynamic effect of methylphenidate for the treatment of giggle incontinence (enuresis risoria). *Neurourology and Urodynamics*, *30*(7), 1338–1342.

Chase, J., Bower, W., Gibbs, S., et al. (2018). Diagnostic scores, questionnaires, quality of life, and outcome measures in pediatric continence: A review of available tools from the International Children's Continence Society. *Journal of Pediatric Urology*, *14*(2), 98–107. doi:10.1016/jpurol.2017.12.003.

Chen, J. J., Ahn, H. J., & Steinhardt, G. F. (2009). Is age at toilet training associated with the presence of vesicoureteral reflux or the occurrence of urinary tract infection? *The Journal of Urology*, *182*(1), 268–271.

Chen, J. J., Mao, W., Homayoon, K., et al. (2004). A multivariate analysis of dysfunctional elimination syndrome, and its relationships with gender, urinary tract infection and vesicoureteral reflux in children. *The Journal of Urology*, 171(5), 1907–1910.

Colaco, M., & Barone, J. G. (2014). Evaluation and management of lower urinary tract symptoms in children. *AUA Update Series*, *33*(lesson 39), 393–403.

Constipation Guideline Committee of the North American Society for Pediatric Gastroenterology, Hepatology and Nutrition. (2006). Evaluation and treatment of constipation in infants and children: Recommendations of the North American Society for Pediatric Gastroenterology, Hepatology and Nutrition. *Journal of Pediatric Gastroenterology and Nutrition*, *43*(3), e1–e13.

da Fonseca, E. M., Santana, P. G., Gomes, F. A., et al. (2011). Dysfunction elimination syndrome: Is age at toilet training a determinant? *Journal of Pediatric Urology*, *7*(3), 332–335.

De Gennaro, M., Capitanucci, M. L., Mastracci, P., et al. (2004). Percutaneous tibial nerve neuromodulation is well tolerated in children and effective for treating refractory vesical dysfunction. *The Journal of Urology*, *171*(5), 1911–1913. doi.org/10.1097/01.ju.0000119961.58222.86.

De Gennaro, M., Capitanucci, M. L., Mosiello, G., et al. (2011). Current state of nerve stimulation technique for lower urinary tract dysfunction in children. *The Journal of Urology*, *185*(5), 1571–1577.

de Wall, L. L., & Heesakkers, J. P. (2017). Effectiveness of percutaneous tibial nerve stimulation in the treatment of overactive bladder syndrome. *Research and Reports in Urology*, *9*, 145–157. doi.org/10.2147/RRU.S124981.

Desantis, D. J., Leonard, M. P., Preston, M. A., et al. (2011). Effectiveness of biofeedback for dysfunctional elimination syndrome in pediatrics: A systematic review. *Journal of Pediatric Urology*, *7*(3), 342–348.

Deshpande, A. V., Craig, J. C., Caldwell, P. H., et al. (2012). Ambulatory urodynamic studies (UDS) in children using a Bluetooth-enabled device. *BJU International*, *110*(Suppl 4), 38–45.

Deshpande, A. V., Craig, J., Smith, G. H. H., et al. (2011). Management of daytime urinary incontinence and lower urinary tract symptoms in children. *Journal of Pediatrics and Child Health*, *48*, E44–E52. doi: 10.1111/j.1440-1754.2011.02216.x.

Dhondt, K., Baert, E., Van Herzeele, C., et al. (2014). Sleep fragmentation and increased periodic limb movements are more common in children with nocturnal enuresis. *Acta Paediatrica*, *103*(6), e268–e272.

Dwyer, M. E., Vandersteen, D. R., Hollatz, P., et al. (2014). Sacral neuromodulation for the dysfunctional elimination syndrome: A 10-year single-center experience with 105 consecutive children. *Urology*, *84*(4), 911–918.

Equit, M., Hill, J., Hubner, A., et al. (2014). Health-related quality of life and treatment effects on children with functional incontinence, and their parents. *Journal of Pediatric Urology*, *10*(5), 922–928. doi: 10.1016/j.jpurol.2014.03.002.

Farhat, W., Bagli, D. J., Capolicchio, G., et al. (2000). The dysfunctional voiding scoring system: Quantitative standardization of dysfunctional voiding symptoms in children. *The Journal of Urology*, *164*(3 Pt 2), 1011–1015.

Fernandes, L., Martin, D., & Hum, S. (2018). A case of the giggles—diagnosis and management of giggle incontinence. *Canadian Family Physician*, *64*, 445–447.

Fitzgerald, M. P., Thom, D. H., Wassel-Fyr, C., et al. (2006). Childhood urinary symptoms predict adult overactive bladder symptoms. *The Journal of Urology*, *175*(3 Pt 1), 989–993.

Foxx, R. M., & Azrin, N. H. (1973). Dry pants: A rapid method of toilet training children. *Behavior Research and Therapy*, *11*(4), 435–442.

Franco, I., von Gontard, A., De Gennaro, M., et al. (2013). Evaluation and treatment of non-monosymptomatic nocturnal enuresis: A standardization document from the International Children's Continence Society. *Journal of Pediatric Urology*, *9*, 234–243.

Gaither, T. W., Cooper, C. S., Kornberg, Z., et al. (2018). Risk factors for the development of bladder and bowel dysfunction. *Pediatrics*, *141*(1), 1–6. doi.org/10.1542/peds.2017-2797.

Glahn, B. E. (1979). Giggle incontinence (enuresis risoria). A study and an etiological hypothesis. *British Journal of Urology*, *51*(5), 363–366.

Glazener, C. M., Evans, J. H., & Peto, R. E. (2005). Alarm interventions for nocturnal enuresis in children. *The Cochrane Database of Systematic Reviews*, (2), CD002911.

Guerra, L., Leonard, M., & Castagnetti, M. (2014). Best practice in the assessment of bladder function in infants. *Therapeutic Advances in Urology*, *6*(4), 148–164.

Hagstroem, S., Mahler, B., Madsen, B., et al. (2009). Transcutaneous electrical nerve stimulation for refractory daytime urinary urge incontinence. *The Journal of Urology*, *182*(4 Suppl), 2072–2078.

Halachmi, S., & Farhat, W. A. (2008). The impact of constipation on the urinary tract system. *International Journal of Adolescent Medicine and Health*, *20*(1), 17–22.

Hobbs, A. M., Short, H., & Paul, S. P. (2016). Clinical update: Childhood enuresis. *Community Practitioner*, *89*(9), 30–35.

Hoebeke, P., De Caestecker, K., Vande Walle, J., et al. (2006). The effect of botulinum-A toxin in incontinent children with therapy resistant overactive detrusor. *The Journal of Urology*, *176*(1), 328–330; discussion 330–331.

Hoebeke, P., Renson, C., Petillon, L., et al. (2002). Percutaneous electrical nerve stimulation in children with therapy resistant nonneuropathic bladder sphincter dysfunction: A pilot study. *The Journal of Urology*, *168*(6), 2605–2607; discussion 2607–2608.

Hutson, J. M., Dughetti, L., Stathopoulos, L., et al. (2015). Transabdominal electrical stimulation (TES) for the treatment of slow-transit constipation (STC). *Pediatric Surgery International*, *31*(5), 445–451. doi.org/10.1007/s00383-015-3681-4

Ismail, K. A., Chase, J., Gibb, S., et al. (2009). Daily transabdominal electrical stimulation at home increased defecation in children with slow-transit constipation: A pilot study. *Journal of Pediatric Surgery*, *44*(12), 2388–2392.

Jeyakumar, A., Rahman, S. I., Armbrecht, E. S., et al. (2012). The association between sleep-disordered breathing and enuresis in children. *The Laryngoscope*, *122*(8), 1873–1877.

Joinson, C., Heron, J., von Gontard, A., et al. (2009). A prospective study of age at initiation of toilet training and subsequent daytime bladder control in school-age children. *Journal of Developmental and Behavioral Pediatrics*, *30*(5), 385–393.

Juul, K. V., Van Herzeele, C., De Bruyne, P., et al. (2013). Desmopressin melt improves response and compliance compared with tablet in treatment of primary monosymptomatic nocturnal enuresis. *European Journal of Pediatrics*, *172*(9), 1235–1242.

Klassen, T. P., Kiddoo, D., Lang, M. E., et al. (2006). The effectiveness of different methods of toilet training for bowel and bladder control. *Evidence Report/Technology Assessment*, *147*, 1–57.

Kramer, S. A., Rathbun, S. R., Elkins, D., et al. (2005). Double-blind placebo-controlled study of alpha-adrenergic receptor antagonists (doxazosin) for treatment of voiding dysfunction in the pediatric population. *The Journal of Urology*, *173*(6), 2121–2124; discussion 2124.

Lewis, S. J., & Heaton, K. W. (1997). Stool form scale as a useful guide to intestinal transit time. *Scandinavian Journal of Gastroenterology*, *32*(9), 920–924.

Logan, B. L., Foster-Johnson, L., & Zoto, E. (2018) Urinary incontinence among adolescent female athletes. *Journal Pediatric Urology*, *14*(3), 241.e1–241.e9. doi: 10.1016.jpurol.2017.12.018.

Malm-Buatsi, E., Nepple, K. G., Boyt, M. A., et al. (2007). Efficacy of transcutaneous electrical nerve stimulation in children with overactive bladder refractory to pharmacotherapy. *Urology*, *70*(5), 980–983.

Maternik, M., Krzeminska, K., & Zurowska, A. (2014). The management of childhood urinary incontinence. *Pediatric Nephrology*, *31*(1), 41–50. doi: 10.1007/s00467-014-2791-x.

Minassian, V. A., Lovatsis, D., Pascali, D., et al. (2006). Effect of childhood dysfunctional voiding on urinary incontinence in adult women. *Obstetrics and Gynecology*, *107*(6), 1247–1251.

Morin, F., Akhavizadegan, H., Kavanagh, A., et al. (2018). Dysfunctional voiding: Challenges of disease transition from childhood to adulthood. *Canadian Urological Association*, *12*(4 Suppl 1), S42–S47. doi.org/10.5489/cuaj5230.

Nadeau, G., Schroder, A., Moore, K., et al. (2014). Long-term use of solifenacin in pediatric patients with overactive bladder: Extension of a prospective open-label study. *Canadian Urological Association Journal*, *8*(3–4), 118–123.

Neveus T., Eggert, P., Evans, J., et al.; International Children's Continence Society. (2010). Evaluation of and treatment for monosymptomatic enuresis: A standardization document from the International Children's Continence Society. *Journal of Urology*, *183*(2), 441.

Nevéus, T., von Gontard, A., Hoebeke, P., et al. (2006). The standardization of terminology of lower urinary tract function in children and adolescents: Report from the Committee of the International Children's Continence Society. *Journal of Urology*, *176*(1), 314–324.

Nield, L. S., Nease, E. K., & Grossman, O. K. (2018). Enuresis management in the primary care pediatrics clinic. *Pediatric Annuals*, *47*(10), e390–e395. doi.10.3928/19382359-20180920-01.

Nijman, R. J., Borgstein, N. G., Ellsworth, P., et al. (2007). Long-term tolerability of tolterodine extended release in children 5–11 years of age: Results from a 12-month, open-label study. *European Urology*, *52*(5), 1511–1516.

Nijman, R., Tekgul, S., Chase, J., et al. (2013). Diagnosis and management of urinary incontinence in childhood. In P. Abrams, L. Cardozo, S. Khoury, et al. (Eds.), *5th International Consultation on Incontinence* (pp. 729–825). London, UK: European Association of Urology.

Noto, P., & Berry, A. (2017). Voiding dysfunction and enuresis. In D. K. Newman, J. F. Wyman, & V. W. Welch (Eds.), *Core Curriculum for Urologic Nursing* (1st ed., pp. 167–179). Pitman, NJ: AJ Janetti.

Panayi, D. C., Khullar, V., Digesu, G. A., et al. (2011). Rectal distension: The effect on bladder function. *Neurourology and Urodynamics*, *30*(3), 344–347.

Ramsay, S., & Bolduc, S. (2017). Overactive bladder in children. *Canadian Urological Association journal = Journal de l'Association des urologues du Canada*, *11*(1–2 Suppl 1), S74–S79. doi.org/10.5489/cuaj.4337.

Richardson, I., & Palmer, L. S. (2009). Successful treatment for giggle incontinence with biofeedback. *The Journal of Urology*, *182*(4 Suppl), 2062–2066.

Santos, J. D., Lopes, R. I., & Koyle, M. A. (2017). Bladder and bowel dysfunction in children: An update on the diagnosis and treatment of a common, but underdiagnosed pediatric problem. *Canadian Urological Association Journal, 11*(1–2 Suppl 1), S64–S72. doi.org/10.5489/cuaj.4411.

Schulman, S. L. (2004). Voiding dysfunction in children. *The Urologic Clinics of North America*, *31*(3), 481–490.

Sillen, U., Brandstrom, P., Jodal, U., et al. (2010). The Swedish reflux trial in children: Bladder dysfunction. *The Journal of Urology*, *184*(1), 298–304.

Sun, M., & Rugolotto, S. (2004). Assisted infant toilet training in a Western family setting. *Journal of Developmental and Behavioral Pediatrics*, *25*(2), 99–101.

US FDA. Public Health Advisory. (2018). *Suicidality in children and adolescents being treated with antidepressant medications*. Retrieved April 18, 2020 from https://www.fda.gov/drugs/postmarket-drug-safety-information-patients-and-providers/suicidality-children-and-adolescents-being-treated-antidepressant-medications

Van Batavia, J. P., Ahn, J. J., Fast, A. M., et al. (2013). Prevalence of urinary tract infection and vesicoureteral reflux in children with lower urinary tract dysfunction. *The Journal of Urology*, *190*(4 Suppl), 1495–1499.

Van Batavia, J. P., Combs, A. J., Horowitz, M., et al. (2010). Primary bladder neck dysfunction in children and adolescents III: Results of long-term alpha-blocker therapy. *The Journal of Urology*, *183*(2), 724–730.

Van Herzeele, C., Dhondt, K., Roels, S. P., et al. (2016). Desmopressin (melt) therapy in children with monosymptomatic nocturnal enuresis and nocturnal polyuria results in improved neuropsychological functioning and sleep. *Pediatric Nephrology*, 31, 1477–1484. doi.10.1007/s00467-016-3351-3.

Veiga, M. L., Lordelo, P., Farias, T., et al. (2013). Constipation in children with isolated overactive bladders. *Journal of Pediatric Urology*, *9*(6 Pt A), 945–949.

von Gontard, A., & Equit, M. (2015). Comorbidity of ADHD and incontinence in children. *European Child & Adolescent Psychiatry*, *24*(2), 127–140. doi: 10.1007/s00787-014-0577-0.

Whale, K., Cramer, H., & Joinson, C. (2017). Left behind and left out: The impact of the school environment on young people with continence problems. *British Journal of Health Psychology*, *23*, 253–277. doi: 1010.1111/bjhp.12284.

Yang, S. S., Zhao, L. L., & Chang, S. J. (2011). Early initiation of toilet training for urine was associated with early urinary continence and does not appear to be associated with bladder dysfunction. *Neurourology and Urodynamics*, *30*(7), 1253–1257.

QUESTIONS

1. A continence nurse is taking the history of a 7-year-old girl who comes into the office because of frequent daytime incontinence. She does not have a history of UTIs. Which is an important question to ask?

A. How often does she go to the bathroom at school?

B. Do any of her friends have the same problem?

C. How old was she when she was potty trained?

D. Did her parents have enuresis?

2. Constipation can be a predisposing factor for enuresis. The continence nurse questions the child about his stools. According to the Bristol stool scale, which stool type would be considered constipation?

A. Type 4

B. Type 6

C. Type 2

D. Type 5

3. A 15-year-old girl comes in stating that she has been having incontinence, but this only happens when she is with her friends and laughing. It has been happening more often and she is embarrassed. She is not having any nighttime wetting. Her most likely diagnosis is which of the following?

A. Dysfunctional voiding

B. Vesicoureteral reflux

C. Overactive bladder

D. Giggle incontinence

4. Which can be a predisposing factor for a child having monosymptomatic enuresis?

A. Early potty training

B. Both parents had enuresis

C. Not being circumcised

D. Being in a gifted program at school

5. You have discussed treatment for enuresis and the child and family have opted using an enuresis alarm. Which of the following is a true statement?
A. Children should manage alarm therapy alone
B. If they have accidents then it should be considered a failure
C. Therapy sometimes takes 1 to 2 months to be successful
D. They should drink well before bed

6. Dysfunctional voiding is a condition seen in children. This starts with postponing voiding and often the child has UTIs. When the child does void, they
A. Relax their sphincter and empty their bladder well
B. Void often but do not empty completely
C. They voluntarily contract their urinary sphincter and pelvic floor when voiding
D. Deny having accidents during the day

7. Biofeedback is a treatment approach that can be helpful for children with dysfunctional voiding. When the continence nurse is talking to a parent about biofeedback, which statement is true?
A. This is an invasive procedure.
B. This is an intensive technique that takes at last 6 weeks of treatment with a urotherapy specialist.
C. Parents do not need to be involved in this approach, only the child.
D. The child must take multiple medications during this treatment.

8. A 6-year-old girl is being seen for enuresis. You are trying to determine if she has monosymptomatic enuresis. If this is true, her symptoms would include:
A. Urinary tract infections
B. Daytime incontinence
C. Nighttime wetting without any period of nighttime dryness since potty training
D. Obesity

9. A 10-year-old girl come in for evaluation of incontinence. When taking the history, she states her wetting occurs shortly after she has gone to the bathroom and the volume is small. The cause of her wetting is
A. Vesicoureteral reflux
B. Overactive bladder
C. Giggle incontinence
D. Vaginal reflux

10. In your evaluation of a child for BBD (bowel and bladder dysfunction) you should always obtain
A. Voiding and bowel diary
B. VCUG
C. CBC
D. MRI

ANSWERS AND RATIONALES

1. A. Rationale: The history should focus on voiding behaviors including frequency, episodes of incontinence, voided volumes, presence of urge, and time taken to void. If able, request a bladder and bowel diary before the first visit to obtain higher quality of data.

2. C. Rationale: Type 2 stool on the Bristol stool scale represents a formed, lumpy, sausage-shaped stool representative of a "constipated" type stool.

3. D. Rationale: Giggle incontinence is a unique condition usually only seen in girls where laughter triggers complete voiding of urine. The pathophysiology is not well understood; girls with this condition are completely dry outside of the giggle episodes and have normal anatomy.

4. B. Rationale: There is a definite familial tendency with enuresis, with a 44% likelihood of the child having enuresis if one parent had enuresis and a 77% incidence if both parents had enuresis.

5. C. Rationale: Parent involvement is critical for success in using enuresis alarm to reduce bedwetting. Parents should be advised effective treatment may take as long as 2 to 3 months of consistent use and they should not be discouraged if they do not see immediate success.

6. C. Rationale: If voiding postponement continues long term, the child may develop dysfunctional voiding, which is defined as voluntary contraction of the urinary sphincter and pelvic floor during voiding (detrusor sphincter dyssynergia).

7. B. Rationale: Biofeedback is a time intensive but successful treatment for children as it helps them learn to coordinate pelvic muscle relaxation to improve bladder emptying. Biofeedback is typically performed weekly for 6 weeks with a urotherapy specialist (i.e., physical therapist trained in biofeedback therapy, focusing on pelvic floor muscle relaxation to assist in proper voiding and defecation behaviors).

8. C. Rationale: Monosymptomatic enuresis is used to denote enuresis in children who have no other lower urinary tract symptoms, do not have a history of bladder dysfunction, and suffer nighttime wetting without any period of nighttime dryness since potty training.

9. D. Rationale: Vaginal voiding or vaginal reflux is a benign condition that is caused by the passage of urine into the vagina during voiding. With a careful history, the child will describe dribbling after she gets up from the toilet.

10. A. Rationale: BBD is a term that encompasses LUTS (lower urinary tract symptoms) and bowel dysfunction in children who do not have any identifiable neurological abnormality. These children have a variety of urinary symptoms as well as constipation and sometimes encopresis.

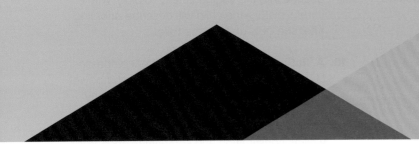

CHAPTER 15

INCONTINENCE AND THE INDIVIDUAL WHO IS OBESE

Susan Gallagher

OBJECTIVES

1. Describe the relationship between BMI, waist circumference, and incontinence.

2. Discuss diagnostic limitations associated with obesity-related incontinence.

3. Describe the impact of obesity on standard care protocols.

4. Recognize the increased risk for sleep apnea among individuals who are obese and how it may increase voiding patterns and continence if left untreated.

5. Explain the role of surgery as a primary treatment modality.

6. Explore weight bias such as discrimination, prejudice, and insensitivity.

TOPIC OUTLINE

INTRODUCTION

RELATIONSHIP BETWEEN OBESITY AND INCONTINENCE

More than 90% of women who are morbidly obese experience some degree of pelvic floor disorder, and 50% of the women indicated to researchers that symptoms were so severe they interfered with activities of daily living (ADLs) and quality of everyday life (Wasserberg et al., 2007). A number of studies suggest that obesity and overweight are directly associated with urinary incontinence (UI). The association with fecal incontinence exists to a lesser extent.

Obesity is one of the most clearly established risk factors for urinary incontinence. Based on the findings from multiple studies, women who are obese are approximately twice as likely to be incontinent of urine (Milsom et al., 2017). In a prospective study of women who participated in the Nurses' Health Study II, the relationship between weight change since age 18 years and the likelihood of developing UI by age 37 to 54 years of age was examined (Townsend et al., 2007). Each 1 kg/m² unit increase in body mass index (BMI) increased the likelihood of frequent UI (defined as UI episodes at least once per week) by 7% and of severe incontinence (at least weekly incontinence of quantities large enough to at least wet underwear) by 9%. Weight gain was associated with an increased likelihood of developing both stress and urge incontinence.

KEY POINT

Obesity is a well-established risk factor for urinary incontinence and as BMI increases the likelihood of developing both stress and urge incontinence increases.

DEMOGRAPHICS OF OBESITY

Obesity and incontinence are both relatively common disorders and the prevalence is increasing in the United States and globally. In order to set a foundation to fully understand weight-related incontinence, it is important to understand standard measurement and definitions associated with obesity. Overweight and obesity are defined as abnormal or excessive fat accumulation. Body mass index (BMI) is simply a mathematical formula that determines relative risk for morbidity and mortality. This weight-for-height formula is commonly used to quantitatively classify overweight and obesity in adults. (**Box 15-1** provides an overview of BMI as it relates to obesity.) It is defined as a person's weight in kilograms divided by the square of their height in meters (kg/m²) (NIH, 2020). According to the World Health Organization (WHO), obesity is classified as class I for a BMI between 30 and 34.9 kg/m², class II for a BMI between 35 and 39.9 kg/m², and class III for a BMI ≥ 40 kg/m² (World Health Organization,

BOX 15-1 BMI CHART	
Weight Categories	**BMI (kg/m²)**
Healthy weight	18.5–24.9
Overweight	25.0–29.9
Obese (Class I)	30.0–34.9
Severely obese (Class II)	35.0–39.9
Morbidly obese (Class III)	40.0–49.9
Super obese (Class IV)	>50

WHO, n.d.). Obesity has become a pandemic problem with increasing prevalence in the United States and worldwide.

There has been a rise of obesity in all populations. Younger populations (18 to 29 years) and women are experiencing increases in the frequency of obesity, while middle aged to older men are experiencing increases in the severity of obesity. In 2018, the Centers for Disease Control (CDC) reported that in 2015–2016, the prevalence of obesity was 39.8% and affected about 93.3 million US adults (Hales et al., 2017).

KEY POINT

The rates of both obesity and incontinence are increasing in the United States and globally.

Hispanics (47.0%) and non-Hispanic blacks (46.8%) had the highest age-adjusted prevalence of obesity, followed by non-Hispanic whites (37.9%) and non-Hispanic Asians (12.7%). The rate of obesity among young adults aged 20- to 39-year-old was 35.7% and 42.8% among middle-aged adults between 40 to 59 years. The prevalence of obesity among adults aged 60 and older was 41%. The prevalence of obesity for those 2- to 19-year-old was 18.5% and affected about 13.7 million children and adolescents. The rate of obesity was 13.9% among 2- to 5-year-olds, 18.4% among 6- to 11-year-olds, and 20.6% among 12- to 19-year-olds. These rates vary somewhat depending on region, gender, demographic, ethnicity, family history, economics, and other criteria. However, most would agree that these rates are high (Hales et al., 2017).

ADIPOSITY-BASED CHRONIC DISEASE

Literature suggests that patients with a high degree of adiposity are at higher risk for a number of well-documented concerns than that of their leaner peers. This risk may be due to the fact that the adipose tissue behaves similarly to an endocrine organ and it influences hormone and cytokine production and secretion. Cytokines such as tumor necrosis factor alpha, leptin, and interleukin-6 are cellular messengers that regulate various inflammatory responses. Dysregulation of cytokines, which is often observed in the presence of excess adiposity, leads to chronic inflammation. This dysregulation affects every organ of the body, including the intestinal tract affecting the risk for fecal incontinence (Gallagher, 2015; Kang et al., 2016).

In 2017, the American Association of Clinical Endocrinologists (AACE) and American College of Endocrinology (ACE) put in place the AACE/ACE blueprint for chronic care associated with excess adiposity (Mechanick et al., 2017). This blueprint makes the argument that many issues associated obesity stem from the dysregulation of cytokines as described above. As a first step to this blueprint, a new term for the condition previously referred to as obesity was identified. Adiposity-based chronic disease (ABCD) was the agreed upon term. The blueprint is a chronic care model that is comprised of an advanced diagnostic framework, clinical practice guidelines, and clinical practice algorithms for the comprehensive management of ABCD. Rather than using BMI as the criteria for care, the AACE/ACE blueprint uses a complication-centric approach to care. Elements to the blueprint include (1) positioning lifestyle medicine in the promotion of overall health; (2) standardizing protocols that address sustained weight loss and management of adiposity-based complications; (3) approaching patient care through contextualization; and (4) developing evidence-based strategies for successful implementation, monitoring, and optimization of patient care over time. The reason this approach is gaining popularity worldwide is because the consequences associated with excess adiposity are chronic in nature. Researchers recognized that these consequences are largely due to the inflammatory nature of adiposity. To that end, fecal and urinary incontinence are arguably a result of ABCD for several reasons and may be best addressed as part of the chronic condition of ABCD.

The number of individuals with excess adiposity is increasing, and incontinence associated with the person of size presents specific challenges. Factors such as diagnosis, treatment, weight management, and weight bias all play a part in the challenge of continence care. Obesity coupled with issues of incontinence impacts ADLs and quality of life (QoL).

The aim of this chapter is not to describe standard protocols of care for urinary and fecal incontinence but instead to describe the nuances of excess adiposity and this impact on continence. Although men and women are equally affected by fecal incontinence, women have an increased risk for weight-related urinary incontinence. Many authors will describe the mechanical and neurogenic elements of both urinary and fecal incontinence; however, it is important to fully understanding the meaning of the term adiposity-based chronic disease in order to fully understand the pathology of weight-related incontinence. For example, the proinflammatory cytokines and adipokines that are associated with the hyperinflammatory state of ABCD effect the intestines and place the individual at risk for diarrhea, cramps, and other gastrointestinal symptoms. And finally, fecal or urinary incontinence among individuals with morbid obesity is remarkable because care and hygiene are more complex. Incontinence in the newly immobile individual who is obese may simply be the result of the inability to self-toilet, more specifically waiting for assistance to the bathroom or bedpan may lead to an incontinent episode and ultimately skin damage, embarrassment, and hygiene challenges. There are diagnostic limitations such as the exam tables, gowns, and equipment. Reasonable accommodation may be limited for the individual with excess weight. Each of these factors impact the understanding of incontinence and the person who is obese.

 INCONTINENCE

PATHOPHYSIOLOGY OF WEIGHT-RELATED INCONTINENCE

The disease of excess weight is associated with numerous adverse health conditions. As mentioned earlier, several professional organizations and professionals suggest that health consequences associated with obesity be described within the context of ABCD. This trend directly relates to the hyperinflammatory state inherent in obesity; however, when considering issues of continence, these cellular changes are exacerbated by the mechanical and neurogenic challenges of weight-related pelvic floor dysfunction.

The relationship between obesity and urinary incontinence is not completely clear. Some studies suggest that excess body weight increases abdominal pressure. This in turn increases bladder pressure and mobility of the urethra. This, then, leads to stress urinary incontinence (SUI) and is thought to cause overactive bladder (Park & Baek, 2018).

Abdominal obesity like in the later stages of pregnancy, which is also often associated with incontinence, can lead to chronic strain, stretching, and weakening of the nerves and muscles of the pelvic area. Iavazzo (2013) notes that the main mechanism causing the development of pelvic floor disorders is chronic increases in abdominal pressure and that this pressure creates structural damage and neurologic dysfunction, which predisposes the individual to prolapse and subsequently increases the risk for fecal and urinary continence. In women, symptoms associated with this pelvic floor disorder include a sensation of vaginal fullness or pressure, uterine descent, sacral back pain with standing, coital difficulty, lower abdominal discomfort, and urinary and fecal difficulties (Iavazzo, 2013). Chapter 12 outlines pelvic floor dysfunction and pathophysiology of pelvic organ prolapse.

KEY POINT

Abdominal or central obesity, which is often associated with incontinence, can lead to mechanical and neurogenic changes such as chronic strain, stretching, and weakening of the nerves and muscles of the pelvic area.

Chen and colleagues reported that pelvic floor disorders were found in 75% of individuals with obesity compared with 44% in nonobese individuals. Compared to nonobese individuals, more obese individuals experienced SUI, urge urinary incontinence, and fecal incontinence. The severity of those symptoms was also higher in individuals with higher BMI (Chen et al., 2009).

In comparison to urinary incontinence, there is less research examining the association between obesity and fecal incontinence. In addition, the mechanism by which obesity contributes to fecal incontinence is not as well understood. However, research suggests that rates of fecal incontinence and diarrhea may be higher in individuals with obesity compared to nonobese individual. One possible explanation for this is the effect of ABCD on inflammatory cytokines in the gastrointestinal tract, rather than structural changes associated with abdominal obesity (Ho & Spiegel, 2008).

KEY POINT

Obesity appears to be associated with higher rates of fecal incontinence and diarrhea and this is thought to be a result of effect of inflammatory cytokines along the gastrointestinal tract, rather than structural changes associated with abdominal obesity.

ABDOMINAL OBESITY—WAIST CIRCUMFERENCE

Central obesity, described as excess fatty tissue in the abdominal area, is one of the most important factors associated with weight-related incontinence (Lambert et al., 2005). Abdominal adiposity is diagnosed by waist circumference or the waist-to-hip ratio. Increasing abdominal obesity is thought to be directly related to SUI but not urge and mixed incontinence. On multivariable analysis of factors associated with urinary incontinence, including BMI, an increasing waist-to-hip ratio was an independent risk factor for stress incontinence but not for urge and mixed incontinence (Brown et al., 1999). In a cohort of Korean women, compared to women in the lowest quartile of waist circumference, the rate for SUI increased significantly in a dose-dependent relationship in the next quartiles after adjusting for BMI (Han et al., 2006). In women in the Nurses' Health Study, there were highly significant trends toward an increasing risk of incontinence with

increasing BMI and waist circumference (Townsend et al., 2008). When BMI and waist circumference were included in models simultaneously, BMI was associated with urge and mixed incontinence but not with stress incontinence. Waist circumference was significantly associated only with stress incontinence.

In the Norwegian Epidemiology of Incontinence in the County of Nord-Trøndelag study of 6,876 incontinent Norwegian women, in multivariate analysis adjusting for age, parity and BMI showed an association between waist-to-hip ratio, and urinary and fecal incontinence (Hannestad, 2005). In the American Boston Area Community Health survey, each 10 cm increase in waist circumference in women was *independently* associated with a higher prevalence of weekly episodes of urinary incontinence (Tennstedt et al., 2008). Based on these findings, an important element of screening for urinary incontinence should include assessment of the waist-to-hip ratio and/or waist circumference (Wesnes, 2014).

KEY POINT

A relationship exists between BMI, waist circumference, and incontinence, suggesting these elements of assessment should be included in the physical exam.

RESPIRATORY CONSIDERATIONS

Obstructive sleep apnea (OSA) is simply described as a condition in which individuals experience apneic episodes during sleep. These apneic episodes lead to hypoxemia and hypercapnia. OSA is a common health issue that is frequently found in individuals with obesity (National Institutes of Health, 2020). For example, population-based studies suggest a relationship exists between OSA and obesity, with over 70% of individuals with OSA considered clinically obese based on BMI (Hargens et al., 2013). A high percentage of individuals with OSA suffer from genitourinary symptoms, such as frequency, nocturia, erectile dysfunction, enuresis, and overactive bladder (Dagur et al., 2015).

Given the association between obesity and both UI and OSA and the potential negative effects of OSA on health (Gottlieb & Punjabi, 2020), during the assessment of UI in obese patients, the continence nurse should ask about symptoms that raise concerns about OSA including snoring, breathing pauses at night, and excessive daytime fatigue or sleepiness. There are short questionnaires available that can be used to screen for OAS risk including the Berlin Questionnaire (https://www.sleepapnea.org/wp-content/uploads/2017/02/berlin-questionnaire.pdf) and the STOP-Bang Questionnaire (http://www.stopbang.ca/osa/screening.php). If OSA is suspected, the patient should be referred for diagnosis and treatment.

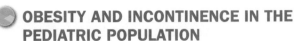

KEY POINT

Given the association between obesity and both UI and OSA and the potential negative effects of OSA on health, during the assessment of UI in obese patients, the continence nurse should ask about symptoms that raise concerns about OSA including snoring, breathing pauses at night, and excessive daytime fatigue or sleepiness.

Having a qualified respiratory care professional, as part of the interdisciplinary team, is helpful in providing a comprehensive respiratory assessment and making recommendations as a strategy to manage the OSA. At home sleep studies are becoming popular for patients who are considered candidates for OSA. Weaver et al. (2014) explain that greater understanding of the physiologic mechanisms associated with OSA has led to a number of all-new options for interventions. Adaptive servoventilation, behavioral interventions to improve adherence with continuous positive airway pressure, and nonsurgical treatments such as oral pressure devices, improved mandibular advancement devices, nasal expiratory positive airway and pressure, and newer approaches to positional therapy are a few options. Recent innovations in surgical interventions have included laser-assisted uvulopalatoplasty, radiofrequency ablation, palatal implants, and electrical stimulation of the upper airway muscles. To date, pharmaceuticals have not specifically been approved to treat OSA, but investigators are evaluating medications that center on increasing ventilatory drive, altering the arousal threshold, modifying loop gain (a dimensionless value quantifying the stability of the ventilatory control system), or preventing airway collapse by affecting the surface tension (Weaver et al., 2014).

Proper management of sleep apnea leads to the regulation of antidiuretic hormone production during sleep. Without regulation of this hormone, the individual may experience frequent episodes of nocturia from increase urine production (Ancoli-Israel, 2011). For example, a number of studies have demonstrated a decrease in nocturic episodes and/or nocturnal urine production when continuous positive airflow pressure therapy treatment for sleep apnea is introduced as a treatment modality (FitzGerald et al., 2006). This applies regardless of patient weight; however, in caring for the person with both obesity and issues of incontinence, it makes sense to explore. Patients using CPAP and other therapy at home should have some provision for pulmonary support when hospitalized in order to prevent an unanticipated pulmonary crisis.

KEY POINT

Obstructive sleep apnea (OSA) is associated with nocturia and urinary incontinence, and therefore, a qualified respiratory care professional should be part of the interdisciplinary team in order to provide a more comprehensive respiratory assessment and make recommendations to manage the OSA.

OBESITY AND INCONTINENCE IN THE PEDIATRIC POPULATION

Wagner et al. (2015) examined the association between urinary and fecal incontinence and BMI among children. Of the children with incontinence (fecal and/or urinary), 17% were obese (≥95th BMI percentile based on age) compared with none of the continent children. The rate of obesity was higher among children with fecal incontinence (24%) than those with urinary incontinence (18.8%). Consistent with Wagner et al.'s findings, Schwartz and colleagues (2009) reported that urinary incontinence was more common in girls who were obese (12.5%) than those who were not obese (none of these girls met the study criteria for urinary incontinence).

Despite data that suggest an association between childhood obesity and incontinence, a causal relationship is still not clearly understood (Saltman et al., 2011). Large population studies in community pediatric populations are needed to assess whether incontinence is more common in the overweight and obese children as compared with the general population. Using a common language to measure and define childhood incontinence is needed in order to be able to compare findings across studies (Austin et al., 2015). In addition, studies examining incontinence and its association with weight in various subpopulations such as teenage girls, children with OSA, and children with stress incontinence are needed.

Experts suggest that when a child who is overweight or obese with incontinence presents in the clinic, regardless the type or the severity, it best serves the child if the clinician does not assume that BMI alone is the underlying pathophysiology. Other potential causes need to be explored as well. In order to best manage needs of the child and family, all of whom may be experiencing quality of life issues; the clinician will want to assess the incontinence holistically and tailor a multifaceted approach to treatment designed to address all factors that may contribute to the child's incontinence (see Chapter 14).

ASSESSMENT OF THE PATIENT WITH OBESITY AND INCONTINENCE

Planning care for diagnostic evaluation of the patient with obesity and incontinence brings with it many size and weight-related concerns, which need to be addressed in order to provide care that is safe, effective, and does not diminish the patient's unique needs. Areas of particular concern include safety, both for the patient and the caregiver; accessibility for the patient, sensitivity of all caregivers and staff; the use of specialized equipment that will work for larger patients; and adequate staffing (Gallagher & Baranoski, 2020; Holsworth & Gallagher, 2017).

Ensuring a facility's readiness to provide for patient safety and comfort can be assessed by performing a survey of the facility, paying specific attention to weight limits of equipment, including chairs in the exam and waiting areas, physical therapy tables, lift/transfer equipment, carts, exam tables, stirrups, wheel chairs, walkers, CT scanner, MRI scanner, and any other equipment needed to provide care for any patient. This is particularly true when performing urodynamic testing. All equipment should be labeled in a way making it easier for staff to be aware of weight restrictions, while not publicizing that it is "bariatric equipment." Subtle methods of labeling include for example, "EC 500" or "U500" for extended capacity to 500 pounds, or under 500 pounds.

Check to see if toilets are floor or wall mounted. Standard wall mounted toilets can be adapted to accommodate patients by using a support that is commercially available. It is important that the weight be distributed evenly when these supports are put in place. A simple post may not support the weight properly and older porcelain toilets have been known to crumble when weight is applied. Additionally, it is necessary to look at the width of doorways, to assure larger equipment will fit into and out of the room. There should be room for a patient to ambulate through the doorway with a larger walker or sit-to-stand device, when appropriate. Consider the width and length and weight limits of elevators. Larger-sized personal items such as gowns, identification bands, and blood pressure cuffs need to be available for patients so that they can be cared for with dignity and safety. Just as we would not put a standard-sized gown on a pediatric patient, it is not acceptable to snap together two standard gowns to fit around a person who is obese. The purpose of ensuring accommodation in diagnostic, treatment and care practices is to control for those common, predictable and preventable complications associated with the failure to provide safe, reasonable care. Preplanning is at the heart of seamless continence care. Conducting simulation exercises with staff members wearing a simulation training suit may be a strategy to better understand some of the frequently misunderstood limitations of diagnostic and support equipment.

KEY POINT

It is important to recognize not only weight limits but functional limitations on diagnostic and support equipment. Consider using a simulation training suit to evaluate size-sensitive equipment.

Caregiver safety is of critical importance, since back injuries can be career ending (American Nurses Association, 2020). Many health care workers are hesitant to care for patients living with obesity in part because of concerns for their own safety. Equipment is available to protect caregivers and must be utilized in all areas of health care in order to provide dignity and help reduce negative perceptions about caring for larger patients. Specially designed diagnostic and support equipment is

thought to add to the expense of caring for patients, but in the long run this equipment is less expensive than worker injuries. Criteria-based protocols for use of equipment and care of patients can make your continence clinic safer for patients and for staff.

KEY POINT

Health care workers may be hesitant to care for patients living with obesity in part because of concerns for their own safety. Equipment that meets the realistic needs of the patient and worker must be in place to protect caregivers and must be utilized in all areas of health care in order to enhance dignity and remove this negative association with larger patients.

 MAINTAINING SKIN HEALTH

BASIC HYGIENE

Providing basic hygiene in order to maintain skin health for patients who are obese may require special considerations, tools, and resources. Consider continence care and hygiene described in Chapter 17 with special considerations to creams and lotion, which the patient may or may not tolerate because of the perceived wetness that is created. Further, powders that accumulate in skin folds can become abrasive and damage fragile skin. Skin deep within skin folds may be difficult to physically reach and from a practical perspective, gloves may not be long enough to protect workers from contamination. Turning and repositioning the patient when providing basic hygiene can predispose the clinician to occupational handling injuries. Consider floor- or ceiling-based lifts with repositioning slings or other in-bed repositioning devices that are designed to reduce compression load on the spine when moving larger patients. Devices that allow for support when standing may protect the provider from injury and reduce the risk of fall-related injury when the patient is standing. An interdisciplinary approach to basic hygiene may best serve the patient and the continence care professional in planning care.

MOISTURE-ASSOCIATED SKIN DAMAGE

Although intertriginous dermatitis (ITD) is considered a category of moisture-associated skin damage (MASD), it is distinctly different from incontinence-associated dermatitis (IAD). It also requires different methods of management.

Intertriginous Dermatitis

Clinicians often find ITD deep within skin folds near the perineal area and this can complicate care. Areas such as underneath the panniculus or deep within skin folds near the upper legs generate and trap excess moisture, which can result in ITD. If not properly clean and dried, the skin will become macerated. Bacterial, viral, and fungal growth often develops. The resultant odor from ITD coupled with odors associated with IAD and urine and fecal stasis is emotionally stressful for the patient. In the author's clinical experience, this combination can lead to social isolation and feelings of hopelessness.

Maintaining skin folds that are clean and dry can be challenging not only for the obese individual but also by the continence nurse who is creating an evidence-based plan of care to manage the ITD. Absorbent fabric, such as soft towels or cloths, or soft absorptive pads such as abdominal pads or sanitary pads are placed within the affected skin folds by the individual as a practical home remedy, however, not supported in the literature as being therapeutic. If these measures are utilized, regular skin assessments should be done at least daily by care givers to make sure the pads, towels, or cloths do not create undue pressure within the skin fold. When proper precautions are in place, these products may absorb moisture and separate the skin folds, thus protecting against frictional forces. Absorptive fabric and pads should be changed frequently to prevent moisture damage and odor. In addition, it may be necessary to find ways to stabilize the absorptive fabric or pad when the patient is out of bed. Disposable net underpants or snug commercially prepared underwear may be used to secure absorptive fabric or pads.

There are products that have been made specifically to wick moisture from the skin surface. This specific category of textile is a polyurethane-coated silver-impregnated fabric. One end of the fabric sheet can be placed at the base of the skin fold, and the other end should extend about 2 to 3 inches beyond the skin fold. This allows for wicking and evaporation of moisture on a continual basis. In some cases, this may separate the skin folds and protect against frictional forces. Because the material is a single layer and thin, it generally remains in place. This intervention allows the person to participate in activities outside of the home setting, such as social events, work, school, and other activities.

Without proper treatment, ITD has been known to deteriorate to cellulitis and sepsis. Be aware of the risks for Fournier gangrene especially among men with obesity, incontinence, ITD, and deep abdominal skin folds (Thwaini et al., 2006).

Incontinence-Associated Dermatitis

Individuals who are obese and incontinent are at risk for IAD and will require prevention measures beyond customary skin cleansing and moisturizing. Use of approved, commercially prepared, moisture-barrier ointments applied to the perineal, genitalia, and buttocks areas provides protection from both moisture and chemical irritants. The ointment should be applied after initial cleaning and reapplied after each toileting or incontinence episode. Patients and providers need to know that it is not necessary to remove barrier ointment after each toileting or incontinent episode; rather, they should

simply wipe away any soiled ointment and replace with additional barrier ointment. A perineal cleanser or disposable wipe can be used to gently remove the ointment once daily to inspect the skin.

Routine protection of the perineal area should be maintained irrespective of practice setting. Patients who do not have incontinence may have difficulty properly cleansing themselves after toileting. The importance of routine cleansing and protection of the skin in the perineal, genitalia, and buttocks should be discussed with the patient prior to transfer from one health care setting to another. If self-application of protective ointments is difficult for the individual, she/he can be instructed to use a three-in-one product that provides cleansing, moisturizing, and protection in a disposable wipe. In addition, consider consulting an occupational therapist to help locate personal hygiene accessories to assist the patient in cleansing and application of ointments to affected areas. Chapter 17 describes the importance of a structured skin care regime based upon the principles of cleanse, protect, and restore to maintain optimal skin health (Beeckman et al., 2015; Gray et al., 2018).

KEY POINT

Intertriginous dermatitis (ITD) is considered a category of moisture-associated skin damage (MASD) and is distinctly different from incontinence-associated dermatitis (IAD). Clinicians often report skin damage associated with ITD deep within skin folds near the perineal area.

BODY WORN ABSORBENT PRODUCTS

Body worn absorbent products (BWAPs) are needed for all incontinent people to manage urine, stool, or both to provide containment, odor control, and dignity. Proper and quality containment with BWAPs for morbidly obese individuals (BMI [kg/m^2] >40) poses a great challenge in that manufacturers of these products do not offer standardized or available sizes to accommodate changes in body habitus that often accompanies morbid obesity such as the potential differences between abdominal girth (pendulous pannus), leg size and skin folds, and length of the absorbent area from front to back. The WOCN° Society developed an evidence and consensus-based electronic tool to assist the continence nurse or other clinicians to properly assess, select, use, and evaluate BWAPs for those suffering UI, FI, or dual incontinence. In the process of developing the electronic tool, WOCN° BWAP Taskforce noted in the review of literature and during conversations with continence specialists across the country at the consensus conference, the lack and dire need for proper absorbent products specifically for morbidly obese individuals. Several of the continence specialists reported urging industry partners who commercially develop and market absorbent products about the need to design BWAPs to meet the unique needs of individuals with this prevalent condition (Gray et al., 2018). During the Consensus Conference (2018), continence specialists also shared stories of individuals using towels, sheets, or bed pads taped or sewn together to manage their incontinence or nothing at all potentially leading to IAD, ITD, perigenital microbial infections, psychosocial issues, mental anguish, and feelings of hopelessness. The WOCN® BWAP Guide found at https://bwap.wocn.org urges continence care nurses to consider the following factors when selecting a BWAP for the morbidly obese person: emotional impact, skin barrier function such as skin pH and microclimate, length of the absorbent area from the front to back (crotch), and the ability to accommodate abdominal girth, leg size as well as skin folds (Gray et al., 2018). Chapter 16 provides further information regarding appropriate use of absorbent products, containment devices, and adaptive aides.

KEY POINT

Continence nurses are challenged in finding containment products that adequately meets the needs of the morbidly obese person and may need to personally encourage manufacturers to design and market quality BWAPs to meet the unique needs of individuals with a BMI (kg/m²) >40.

 FOURNIER GANGRENE

Fournier gangrene, sometimes referred to as necrotizing fasciitis, can be a serious consequence of fecal or urinary incontinence or excess moisture in the perineal, genital, and perianal areas. Fournier gangrene occurs when endarteritis of the subcutaneous arteries results in necrosis of the overlying skin. The condition is relatively rare but can be severe and life threatening. It manifests as a widespread infective necrotizing fasciitis of the external genitalia. Risk factors include male gender, over the age of 50, diabetes, chronic alcohol use, fecal contamination, and high bacterial load to the perineal area (Hagedorm & Wessells, 2017).

"The clinical features of Fournier gangrene include sudden pain and swelling in the scrotum, purulence or wound discharge, crepitation, fluctuance, prostration, pallor and fever greater than 38°C" (Chennamsetty et al., 2015, p. 205). Early diagnosis is imperative as rapid progression of the gangrene can lead to multiorgan failure and death (Huang, 2017). Although diagnosis is straightforward when the lesions are found, failure to examine the genitals, especially in individual with a large abdominal panniculus, can result in delayed diagnosis. Laboratory findings are nonspecific and may show anemia, leukocytosis, thrombocytopenia, electrolyte abnormalities, hyperglycemia, elevated serum creatinine level, azotemia, and hypoalbuminemia. The diagnosis is generally made clinically, although radiography can be helpful when the diagnosis or the extent of the disease is

difficult to discern. The Laboratory Risk Indicator for Necrotizing Fasciitis score (LRINEC) (https://www.mdcalc.com/lrinec-score-necrotizing-soft-tissue-infection) was developed in 2004 to stratify patients into low, moderate, or high risk (Wong et al., 2004). In 2019, Abdullah and colleagues tested the tool for reliability wherein researchers found the LRINEC score continues to be a reliable tool in the clinical diagnosis of necrotizing fasciitis (Abdullah et al., 2019).

The Fournier Gangrene Severity Index (FGSI) can also be used to determine the severity and prognosis of Fournier gangrene. In 1995, Laor and colleagues introduced the FGSI (Laor et al., 1995). The FGSI is based on the following clinical parameters: body temperature, heart rate, respiratory rate, WBC, hematocrit, serum sodium, serum potassium, serum creatinine, and serum bicarbonate. Each of the above listed parameters is assigned a score between 0 and 4, with the higher values indicating greater deviation from normal. The FGSI represents the sum of all the parameters' values, with a FGSI >9 being associated with increased mortality (Yeniyol et al., 2004). In 2010, Yilmazlar updated the FGSI (UFGSI), adding age and extent of disease as two additional parameters to enhance the predictive value of the FGSI (Yilmazlar et al., 2010).

The mainstays of treatment for Fournier gangrene include rapid and aggressive surgical debridement of necrotized tissue, hemodynamic support with fluid resuscitation, and broad-spectrum parental antibiotics. After initial debridement, open wounds are generally managed with sterile dressings and negative pressure wound therapy. In cases of severe perineal involvement, colostomy has been used for fecal diversion. Indications for colostomy include anal sphincter involvement, fecal incontinence, and continued fecal contamination of the wound's margins. After extensive debridement, many patients sustain significant defects of the skin and soft tissue, creating a need for reconstructive surgery for satisfactory functional and cosmetic results.

KEY POINT

Risk factors for Fournier gangrene include male gender, over the age of 50, diabetes, chronic alcohol use, fecal contamination, and high bacterial load to the perineal area.

 THE INTERDISCIPLINARY TEAM

The value of an interdisciplinary team in providing optimal care cannot be overlooked. In addition to the team who is responsible for continence care, the team addressing care of the person who is obese and incontinent may include the continence nurse, occupational therapist, bariatric surgeon, respiratory care professional, safe patient handling professional, and others (Temple et al., 2017). A team of interested, motivated clinicians who engage the patient honestly and are free of judgment contribute to enhance outcomes over time.

SURGICAL TREATMENT

SURGICAL TREATMENT TO ADDRESS STRESS URINARY INCONTINENCE

Surgical procedures targeting incontinence are well described in other chapters. Although risk factors are present with any operative procedure, ABCD poses additional issues. In many cases, obesity prolongs operative time and may thus be a risk factor for short-term complications (Tjeertes et al., 2015). However, literature suggests that obesity may not adversely influence long-term surgical outcomes. In fact, studies suggest that, except for wound infections, complication rates are not increased, unless the person has had a recent weight loss of more than 10% or low serum albumin levels, which are known predictors of postoperative morbidity and mortality. Postoperative immobility associated with obesity may be the greatest predictor of postoperative morbidity and mortality. Therefore, an interdisciplinary plan to provide early, progressive mobility that includes tools and resources to encourage mobility and activity while protecting providers from occupational injury best serves to manage the adverse consequences of care (Holsworth & Gallagher, 2017).

WEIGHT LOSS SURGERY

Subak and colleagues (2009) report that epidemiological studies document overweight and obesity as important risk factors for urinary incontinence. Weight loss by surgical and more conservative approaches is effective to decrease urinary incontinence symptoms (Auwad et al., 2008; Richter et al., 2005). Further, weight loss surgery should be strongly considered a first-line treatment in this patient population (Wasserberg et al., 2007, 2008). Weight loss studies have reported significant reductions in urinary incontinence with both surgical and nonsurgical weight loss (Subak et al., 2009).

In 2017, Alt Said et al. published findings based on 140 patients who had undergone metabolic weight loss surgery. The rate of urinary incontinence was 51% before surgery and decreased to 19% at the 1-year follow-up visit. After metabolic surgery, there was improvement in the rate of SUI from nearly 40% before surgery to 15% at the 1-year follow-up visit. In addition, there was an improvement in the rate of urge urinary incontinence from nearly 40% to 8% at the 1-year follow-up visit. The rate of dysuria also improved from 20% before surgery to 3.4% at the 1-year follow-up visit. There was also a significant improvement in urinary incontinence–specific quality of life. However, at 1-year postoperatively, there was no significant difference in the frequency and/or severity of fecal incontinence (Ait-Said et al., 2017).

In contrast, Burgio and colleagues (2007) reported that the prevalence of fecal incontinence decreased significantly following weight loss surgery (from 19.4% to 9.1% at 6 months and 8.6% at 12 months postsurgery). A systematic review showed that fecal incontinence improved after Roux-en-Y gastric bypass in studies with preoperative data, while the effects of bariatric surgery on diarrhea were unclear (Poylin et al., 2011). It should be mentioned that one of the major disadvantages of the biliopancreatic diversion with duodenal switch operation is diarrhea. Although duodenal switch is associated with more bowel episodes than gastric bypass, the difference is not statistically significant.

Iavazzo (2013) on the other hand, reported that evidence indicated that massive weight loss (45 to 50 kg) after metabolic weight loss surgery improved both fecal and urinary incontinence in morbidly obese women. This study suggests that metabolic weight loss surgery should be considered a primary treatment for the pelvic floor disorders among women struggling with weight and weight issues. Others have made similar claims (Burgio et al., 2007; Wing et al., 2010).

Most recently, Montenegro and colleagues (2019) reported the results of a systemic review of studies examining the prevalence of pelvic floor disorders before and after bariatric surgery. Nineteen studies reporting UI prevalence pre- and postsurgery were included in the meta-analysis, which revealed that bariatric surgery (BS) reduced urinary incontinence by 67%.

The American Society for Metabolic and Bariatric Surgery have set criteria for candidates seeking weight loss surgery, preoperative and postoperative care, credentialing, and more (American Society of Metabolic and Bariatric Surgery, 2020). Continence care professionals best serve patients when weight loss options are provided as a resource and/or intervention.

KEY POINT

While there is evidence to support the beneficial effect of weight loss in decreasing urinary incontinence, there is less evidence in relation to fecal incontinence.

WEIGHT BIAS

Sensitivity to the special needs of individuals who are living with obesity cannot be stressed enough. It is well established that individuals with obesity tend to delay health care intervention for as long as possible for a number of reasons. Loss of control over the physical environment, embarrassment over physical appearance, and fear of failure pose threats to access. Individuals often face humiliation because of their size, and this in turn may prevent timely, appropriate access to health care, which leads to greater emotional and economic expense. This becomes increasingly important in the presence of incontinence. For instance, Fuchs et al. (2018) who looked at the general population reported that the median duration of urinary incontinence before initial access to treatment was 2.7 years. One-third of men experienced a delay of more than 5 years. Older men were found to wait as long as 7 years before intervention (Fuchs et al., 2018). Although no studies were found describing delays among the person who had symptoms of both obesity and incontinence, providers should be sensitive to delays.

Many patients are afraid that they will break equipment, inconvenience staff, or embarrass themselves by asking questions about their care. A number of patients have been taken to loading docks or laundry rooms to be weighed on commercial scales, having been unable to receive treatment because facilities are not equipped with necessary equipment. Worst of all, they are often ignored altogether, treated as if they don't exist, because of other's discomfort with their size. Ongoing sensitivity training for all personnel in a health care facility or clinic should be provided.

KEY POINT

Individuals often face humiliation because of their size, and this in turn may prevent timely, appropriate access to health care, which leads to greater emotional and economic expense. A delay in access is especially problematic in the presence of incontinence, where both men and women typically delay intervention.

Without reasonable accommodation, providers often attempt care without necessary tools and resources. This leads to bias and ultimately insensitivities (Gallagher & Baranoski, 2020; Temple et al., 2017). For instance, phlebotomy, taking a weight, body measurements, collection of urinary specimens, sleep apnea studies, internal abdominal pressure, and more each pose special challenges when the person is either obese or has a maldistribution of weight.

Patients who are obese do not need more care or better care than any other patient. What the patient who is obese and incontinent needs is to receive the *same* quality of care regardless of size, weight, or body habitus. In order to fully understand issues of incontinence, it is imperative to have a collaborative partnership with the patient. Insensitivity threatens a collaborative partnership. Both continence nurse and patient must feel at ease with communication. Patients must be willing to allow a comprehensive physical assessment in order to ensure a differential diagnosis. To that same extent, patients should feel comfortable drawing attention to themselves if they believe there is a change in the nature of their incontinence or misunderstanding relative to same.

 CONCLUSION

The preponderance of clinical evidence suggests a relationship between weight and incontinence irrespective of age, gender, and number of comorbid conditions. Further, the nature of ABCD leads to an imbalance in the inflammatory response. However, the reality is that there are still many uncertainties regarding weight as a risk factor. It must be clarified whether BMI is a better estimate than weight, waist circumference, or waist–hip ratio. It is not completely clear how the distribution of weight affects incontinence. Does being overweight due to heavy muscles, edema, or pregnancy lead to incontinence or only being overweight due to excess adipose tissue? It is unclear for how long a person's excess weight must persist to lead to incontinence. Is there a threshold criterion? We do not know whether weight is an appropriate measure of exposure or whether the association between weight and incontinence is exacerbated by socioeconomic status, medications, nutrition/hydration, OSA, spinal cord damage, weight-related hormonal changes—all conditions that correspond with excess weight (Townsend et al., 2008).

Incontinence concerns among individuals with ABCD have received attention in much of the health care community. Although a causal relationship is in question in some instances, continent care professionals are fully aware of the challenges associated with access, assessment, intervention, and follow-up as it pertains to the individual who is obese.

Professional debate and targeted research are opportunities wherein continence care professionals can best serve the population. Reasonable accommodation in hospitals, clinics, and postacute care enhances access and provides patient dignity. Sensitivity directed toward the individual who struggles with both incontinence and issues of weight is imperative to developing a mutually responsive relationship where patients are willing to share details of their condition in a safe environment.

REFERENCES

Abdullah, M., McWilliams, B., Khan, S. U. (2019). Reliability of the laboratory risk indicator in necrotizing fasciitis (LRINEC) score. *Surgeon, 17*(5):309–318.

Ait-Said, K., Leroux, Y., Menahem, B., et al. (2017). Effect of bariatric surgery on urinary and fecal incontinence: Prospective analysis with 1-year follow-up. *Surgery for Obesity and Related Diseases, 13*(2), 305–312.

American Nurses Association. (2020). *Safe Patient Handling and Mobility Interprofessional National Standards*. Silver Spring, MD: ANA Nursing World.

American Society of Metabolic and Bariatric Surgery. (2020). Retrieved from https://asmbs.org/

Ancoli-Israel, S., Bliwise, D., Norgaard, J. P. (2011). The effect of nocturia on sleep. *Sleep Medicine Reviews, 15*(2), 91–97.

Austin, P. F., Bauer, S. B., Bower, W., et al. (2015). The standardization of terminology of lower urinary tract function in children and adolescents: Update Report from the Standardization Committee of the International Children's Continence Society. *Journal of Urology, 91*(6), 1863–1865.

Auwad, W., Steggles, P., Bombieri, L., et al. (2008). Moderate weight loss in obese women with urinary incontinence: A prospective longitudinal study. *International Urogynecology Journal and Pelvic Floor Dysfunction, 19,* 1251–1259.

Beeckman, D., Campbell, J., Campbell, K., et al. (2015). Incontinence-associated dermatitis: Moving prevention forward. Proceedings of the Global IAD Expert Panel. *Wounds International.* Retrieved from https://www.academia.edu/12441496/Proceedings_of_the_Global_IAD_Expert_Panel._Incontinence_associated_dermatitis_Moving_prevention_forward

Brown, J. S., Grady, D., Ouslander, J. G., et al. (1999). Prevalence of urinary incontinence and associated risk factors in postmenopausal women. Heart and Estrogen/Progestin Replacement Study (HERS) Research Group. *Obstetrics & Gynecology, 94,* 66.

Burgio, K. L., Richter, H. E., Clements, R. H., et al. (2007). Changes in urinary and fecal incontinence symptoms with weight loss surgery in morbidly obese women. *Obstetrics & Gynecology, 110*(5), 1034–1040.

Chen, C. C., Gatmaitan, P., Koepp, S., et al. (2009). Obesity is associated with increased prevalence and severity of pelvic floor disorders in women considering bariatric surgery. *Surgery for Obesity and Related Diseases, 5,* 411–419.

Chennamsetty, A., Khourdaji, I., Burks, F., et al. (2015). Contemporary diagnosis and management of Fournier's gangrene. *Therapeutic Advances in Urology, 7*(4), 203–215.

Dagur, G., Warren, K., Ambroise, S., et al. (2015). Urological manifestations of obstructive sleep apnea syndrome: A review of current literature. *Translational Biomedicine, 6,* 3.

FitzGerald, M. P., Mulligan, M., Parthasarathy, S. (2006). Nocturic frequency is related to severity of obstructive sleep apnea, improves with continuous positive airways treatment. *American Journal of Obstetrics and Gynecology, 194*(5), 1399–1403.

Fuchs, J. S., Shakir, N., McKibben, M. J., et al. (2018). Prolonged duration of incontinence for men before initial anti-incontinence surgery: an opportunity for improvement. *Urology, 119,* 149–154.

Gallagher, S. (2015). *A practical guide to bariatric safe patient handling and mobility: Improving safety and quality for the patient of size* (p. 17). Sarasota, FL: Visioning Publishers.

Gallagher, S. M., & Baranoski, S. (2020). Skin and wound care among the bariatric population. In: E. Ayello, & S. Baranoski (Eds.), *Wound Care Essentials: Practice Principles* (5th ed.). Philadelphia, PA: Lippincott Williams & Wilkins.

Gottlieb, D. J., & Punjabi, N. M. (2020). Diagnosis and management of obstructive sleep apnea: A review. *JAMA, 323*(14), 1389–1400.

Gray, M., Kent, D., Ermer-Seltun, J., et al. (2018). Assessment, selection, use, and evaluation of body-worn absorbent products for adults with incontinence: A WOCN Society Consensus Conference. *Journal of Wound, Ostomy, and Continence Nursing, 45*(3), 243–264.

Hagedorm, J. C., & Wessells, H. (2017). A contemporary update on Fournier's gangrene. *Nature Reviews Urology, 14,* 205–213.

Hales, C. M., Carroll, M. D., Fryar, C. D., et al. (2017). Prevalence of obesity among adults and youth: United States, 2015–2016. Retrieved from https://www.cdc.gov/nchs/data/databriefs. Accessed April 20, 2020.

Han, M. O., Lee, N. Y., & Park, H. S. (2006). Abdominal obesity is associated with stress urinary incontinence in Korean women. *International Urogynecology Journal, 17,* 35–39.

Hannestad, Y. S., & Huskaar, S. (2005). Waist-hip ratio associated with urinary incontinence in women. Presented at annual meeting of International Continence Society, Montreal, Quebec, Canada. August 31, Abstract 168. Retrieved from https://www.ics.org/Abstracts/Publish/43/000168.pdf. Accessed April 20, 2020.

Hargens, T. A., Kaleth, A. S., Edwards, E. S., et al. (2013). Association between sleep disorders, obesity, and exercise: a review. *Nature and Science of Sleep, 5,* 27–35.

Ho, W., & Spiegel, B. M. (2008). The relationship between obesity and functional gastrointestinal disorders: Causation, association, or neither? *Gastroenterology & Hepatology, 4*(8), 572–578.

Holsworth, C., & Gallagher S. M. (2017). Managing care of critically ill bariatric patients. *AACN Advanced Critical Care, 28*(3), 275–283.

Huang, C.- S. (2017). Fournier's gangrene. *New England Journal of Medicine, 376,* 1158.

Iavazzo, C. (2013). Role of bariatric surgery in the pelvic floor disorders. *World Journal of Obstetrics and Gynecology, 2*(2), 16–20.

Kang, Y. E., Kim, J. M., Joung, K. H., et al. (2016). The roles of adipokines, proinflammatory cytokines, and adipose tissue macrophages in obesity-associated insulin resistance in modest obesity and early metabolic dysfunction. *PLoS ONE, 11*(4), e0154003. https://doi.org/10.1371/journal.pone.0154003

Lambert, D. M., Marceau, S., Forse, R. A. (2005). Intra-abdominal pressure in the morbidly obese. *Obesity Surgery,* 15, 1225–1232.

Laor, E., Palmer, L. S., Tolia, B. M., et al. (1995). Outcome prediction in patients with Fournier's gangrene. *Journal of Urology, 154*(1), 89–92.

Mechanick, J. I., Hurley, D. L., Garvey, W. T. (2017). Adiposity-based chronic disease as a new diagnostic term: The Association of Clinical Endocrinologists and American College of Endocrinology position statement. *Endocrine Practice, 23,* 372–378.

Milsom, I., Altman, D., Cartwright, R., et al. (2017). Epidemiology of urinary incontinence (UI) and other urinary tract symptoms (LUTS), pelvic organ prolapse (POP) and anal (AI) incontinence. In P. Abrams, L. Cardozo, A. Wagg, A. Wein (Eds.), *Incontinence* (6th ed.). ICUD-EAU.

Montenegro, M., Slongo, H., Juliato, C. R. T., et al. (2019). The impact of bariatric surgery on pelvic floor dysfunction: A systematic review. *Journal of Minimally Invasive Gynecology, 26,* 816–825.

National Institutes of Health. (2020). *Obstructive Sleep Apnea.* Retrieved from https://ghr.nlm.nih.gov/condition/obstructive-sleep-apnea. Accessed January 3, 2020.

Park S., & Baek K. A. (2018). Association of general obesity and abdominal obesity with the prevalence of urinary incontinence in women: Cross-sectional secondary data analysis. *Iranian Journal of Public Health, 47*(6), 830–837.

Poylin, V., Serrot F. J., Madoff, R. D., et al. (2011). Obesity and bariatric surgery: a systematic review of associations with defecatory dysfunction. *Colorectal Disease, 13,* e92–e103.

Richter, H. E., Burgio, K. L., Clements, R. H., et al. (2005). Urinary and anal incontinence in morbidly obese women considering weight loss surgery. *Obstetrics and Gynecology, 106,* 1272–1277.

Saltman, K., Alexander, S., Caldwell, P. (2011). *Presence and frequency of urinary incontinence associated with childhood overweight and obesity.* Adelaide, Australia: ANZOS.

Schwartz, B., Wyman, J. F., Thomas, W., et al. (2009). Urinary Incontinence in obese adolescent girls. *Journal of Pediatric Urology, 5,* 445–450.

Subak, L. L., Richter, H. E., & Hunskaar, S. (2009). Obesity and urinary incontinence: epidemiology and clinical research update. *The Journal of Urology, 182*(6 Suppl), S2–S7.

Temple, G., Gallagher, S. M., Doms, J., et al. (2017). Bariatric readiness: Clinical and economic implications. *Bariatric Times, 14*(8), 10–16.

Tennstedt, S. L., Link, C. L., Steers, W. D., et al. (2008). Prevalence of and risk factors for urine leakage in a racially and ethnically diverse population of adults: the Boston Area Community Health (BACH) Survey. *American Journal of Epidemiology, 167,* 390.

Thwaini, A., Khan, A., Malik, A., et al. (2006). Fournier's gangrene and its emergency management. *Postgraduate Medical Journal, 82,* 516–519.

Tjeertes, E. K., Hoeks, S. E., Beks, S. B., et al. (2015). Obesity—a risk factor for postoperative complications in general surgery? *BMC Anesthesiology, 15,* 112.

Townsend, M. K., Curhan, G. C., Resnick, N. M., et al. (2008). BMI, waist circumference, and incident urinary incontinence in older women. *Obesity, 16,* 881.

Townsend, M. K., Danforth, K. N., Rosner, B., et al. (2007). Body mass index, weight gain, and incident urinary incontinence in middle-aged women. *Obstetrics & Gynecology, 110*, 346–353.

Wagner, C., Equit, M., Niemczyk, J., et al. (2015). Obesity, overweight, and eating problems in children with incontinence. *Journal of Pediatric Urology, 11*(4), 202–207.

Wasserberg, N., Hamoui, N., Petrone, P., et al. (2008). Bowel habits after gastric bypass versus the duodenal switch operation. *Obesity Surgery, 18*, 1563–1566.

Wasserberg, N., Haney, M., Petrone, P., et al. (2007). Morbid obesity adversely impacts pelvic floor function in females seeking attention for weight loss surgery. *Diseases of the Colon and Rectum, 50*, 2096–2103.

Weaver, T. E., Calik, M. W., Farabi, S. S., et al. (2014). Innovative treatments for adults with obstructive sleep apnea. *Nature and Science of Sleep, 6*, 137–147.

Wesnes, S. L. (2014). Weight and urinary incontinence: the missing links. *International Urogynecology Journal, 25*, 725–729.

Wing, R. R., Creasman, J. M., West, D. S., et al. (2010). Improving urinary incontinence in overweight and obese women through modest weight loss. *Obstetrics & Gynecology, 116*(2 Pt 1), 284–292.

Wong, C. H., Khin, L. W., Heng, K. S., et al. (2004). The LRINEC (Laboratory Risk Indicator for Necrotizing Fasciitis) score: A tool for distinguishing necrotizing fasciitis from other soft tissue infections. *Critical Care Medicine, 32*(7), 1535–1541.

World Health Organization (WHO). (n.d.). *Fact Sheets Obesity and Overweight.* Retrieved from https://www.who.int/news-room/fact-sheets/detail/obesity-and-overweight. Accessed April 20, 2020.

Yeniyol, C. O., Suelozgen, T., Arslan, M., et al. (2004). Fournier's gangrene: Experience with 25 patients and use of Fournier's gangrene severity index score. *Urology, 64*(2), 218–222.

Yilmazlar, T., Ozturk, E., Ozguc, H., et al. (2010). Fournier's gangrene: an analysis of 80 patients and a novel scoring system. *Techniques in Coloproctology, 14*(3), 21–23.

QUESTIONS

1. A continence nurse reports the patient was heard snoring loudly while waiting to be seen in the clinic. What will be an important element specific to the patient's care?
A. Pay close attention to the patient's history.
B. Consider the possibility of OSA and include a respiratory care professional on the team.
C. Determine sleep patterns.
D. Request CO_2 levels to determine etiology of this behavior.

2. The continence nurse is on the telephone with a woman with reported urinary incontinence. The woman weighs 185 kg, she can be brought by private car to the clinic. Today, she is calling to cancel her appointment indicating that at the last visit she developed excruciating knee pain. As the nurse investigates the waiting area, it becomes clear the reason for the cancellation, which is
A. The patient is lazy and looking for a way to cancel the appointment.
B. The rate of health care compliance is low among individuals with obesity.
C. There was no place for the patient to sit because all the chairs were narrow, accommodated about 250 pounds, and had arm rests, all of which forced the woman to stand for the 25 minutes as she waited to be seen.
D. The continence nurse really has no idea for the cancellation.

3. The continence nurse is preparing a treatment plan for a 22-year-old, highly motivated woman who has a BMI 53. What is an important factor to consider when preparing this plan?

A. Ongoing physical assessment will be challenging.
B. Determine the patient's marital status.
C. Explore metabolic weight loss surgery as an option for a long-term treatment plan.
D. Discuss pelvic floor exercises.

4. A 61-year-old woman with a BMI 48 reports to the continence nurse: "I'm so embarrassed that I leak urine every time I pick up my 3-year-old granddaughter." What condition does the continence nurse suspect?
A. Pelvic organ prolapse
B. Constipation
C. Stress urinary incontinence
D. Abdominal obesity

5. The continence nurse is speaking with a young couple who is concerned that their child, whose weight is in the 96th percentile, is experiencing urinary incontinence several times a week. What should be the first step in addressing the couple's concerns?
A. Suggest metabolic weight loss surgery.
B. Suggest an increase in the child's physical activity.
C. Plan holistic assessment consistent with standard diagnostic evaluation.
D. Refer the child to a pulmonologist.

6. Mr. Jones is a 62-year-old retired engineer, with a BMI of 58, blood sugar 328, temperature 101°F, and light perspiration. The clinic assistant reports to the continence nurse that Mr. Jones has a foul odor emanating from beneath his large abdominal panniculus. He is reluctant to allow assessment/care of the perineal area, which includes hygiene as well as basic evaluation for fecal and urinary incontinence. What condition does the continence nurse suspect?

A. Fournier gangrene
B. Intertriginous dermatitis
C. Poor hygiene
D. Inadequate personal care

7. Anne Marie is a 42-year-old woman who weighs 150 kg, she is very compliant in her care but has had persistent incontinence-associated dermatitis (IAD) despite frequent instructions from the continence nurse. What are next steps in Anne Marie's care?

A. Consider an indwelling catheter for 2 weeks.
B. Soak in a warm tub with Epsom salt.
C. Request a consult with an occupational therapist to identify reaching devices.
D. Suggest a stronger soap for cleaning.

8. What skin condition(s) most accurately describe those associated with obesity and urinary incontinence?

A. IAD and ITD
B. ITD only
C. IAD only
D. Fournier gangrene

9. Sharon is a 27-year-old woman with a history of urinary incontinence that has resolved presumably as a result of a 50 kg weight loss since metabolic weight loss surgery (MWLS) over the past 15 months; however, in the past 3 weeks, she has begun to experience fecal incontinence. The continence nurse makes which of the following two recommendations

A. Review pelvic floor strengthening exercises that were taught before MWLS and follow-up with surgeon.
B. Examine for rectal prolapse and refer to an infectious disease practitioner.
C. Provide skin care products and light padding/diaper.
D. Add fiber supplements to the diet and refer for an abdominal x-ray.

10. Caregiver safety is of critical importance, since back injuries associated with handling patients who are obese can be career ending. What steps can the continence nurse take to ensure safety for the patient, colleagues, and the organization?

A. Steps are not necessary because worker injury happens so infrequently.
B. Ask patients to bring their own gowns, socks, or other items because the facility doesn't provide them.
C. Have a policy in place that limits the weight of patients who can be seen.
D. Conduct an environmental assessment that addresses accessibility for the patient, sensitivity of all caregivers and staff, the use of specialized equipment, and adequate staffing.

ANSWERS AND RATIONALES

1. B. Rationale: Obesity is a risk factor for both incontinence and sleep apnea. As a result, the two conditions often coexist in individuals with obesity. Snoring is one sign of sleep apnea when the continence nurse identifies it by history or observation, the patient should be referred to a pulmonary professional for evaluation.

2. C. Rationale: Lack of clinic facilities where the patient can feel comfortable and safe is a barrier to persons with obesity seeking treatment for urinary incontinence.

3. C. Rationale: Research including a recent meta-analysis supports the effectiveness of weight reduction surgery in reducing the prevalence of incontinence in individuals with obesity.

4. C. Rationale: Stress incontinence is characterized by involuntary urine loss associated with activities that increase intra-abdominal pressure. Lifting is one of the activities that is associated with increases in intra-abdominal pressure.

5. C. Rationale: While obesity is a risk factor for urinary incontinence, there are also a variety of other causes that need to be considered. Thus, a holistic evaluation to rule in or out potential factors causing or contributing to incontinence should always precede treatment.

6. A. Rationale: Mr. Jones presented with fever and foul odor (consistent with purulent discharge) that are signs consistent with possible Fournier gangrene. In addition to obesity and a large abdominal panniculus, Mr. Jones has a number of other risk factors for Fournier gangrene including being male, over 50 years of age and poorly controlled diabetes.

7. C. Rationale: Significant obesity can be a barrier to performing adequate self-perineal care following incontinent episodes. When this is the case, as in this example, the continence nurse should consult an occupational therapy provider for recommendations about devices that help the patient effectively complete this self-care.

8. A. Rationale: Individuals with obesity often experience both IAD and ITD.

9. A. Rationale: In contrast to urinary incontinence, where weight loss surgery has been shown to significantly reduce its prevalence, it is unclear whether it decreases the likelihood of fecal incontinence. Behavioral interventions are the recommended first-line treatment for fecal incontinence.

10. D. Rationale: To ensure that individuals with obesity receive high-quality care for their incontinence while protecting staff from injury when providing care, the facility needs to provide adequate staffing and proper equipment to facilitate safe and accessible care.

CHAPTER 16

APPROPRIATE USE OF ABSORBENT PRODUCTS, CONTAINMENT DEVICES, AND ADAPTIVE AIDES

Dea J. Kent and Leah Holderbaum

OBJECTIVES

1. Identify situations in which containment devices or absorbent products are appropriate for management of urinary and/or fecal incontinence.

2. Describe appropriate use of currently available containment devices, to include indications, contraindications, and guidelines for use.

3. Discuss decision-making guidelines related to use of absorbent products.

4. Outline current recommendations for prevention and management of incontinence-associated.

TOPIC OUTLINE

INTRODUCTION

Correct use of continence products can ensure appropriate containment, healthy skin, and user satisfaction. This chapter is aimed primarily at health care professionals seeking to make informed decisions as they choose— or help their patients to choose—between continence product categories and then to select a specific product within the chosen category. The chapter includes a section for each of the major product categories, each section reviewing published data and recommendations for product selection and use. Additionally, intermittent catheterization is highlighted as it pertains to individualizing education, training and use of adaptive equipment in "real life" settings. Prevention of incontinence-associated dermatitis (IAD) is also addressed as it relates to wearing a body-worn absorbent product (BWAP). Chapter 17 features in-depth information on IAD: pathophysiology, risk factors, assessment, and management.

Not all incontinence can be cured completely and even individuals who are ultimately successfully treated may have to live with incontinence for a time (e.g., while waiting for surgery or for pelvic floor muscle training to yield its benefits). Still others, depending on their frailty, severity of incontinence, and/or personal priorities, may not be candidates for treatment or may choose management over attempted cure. For all such people, the challenge is to discover how to address incontinence and minimize its impact on QoL. This usually involves using some type of continence product(s). Managing incontinence successfully with products is often referred to as *contained incontinence, managed incontinence, or social continence,* in recognition of the substantial benefits it can bring to QoL even if cure has not been achieved (Fonda & Abrams, 2006; Öz & Altay, 2018; Wan et al., 2014).

> **KEY POINT**
>
> Incontinence managed successfully with products is often referred to as contained incontinence, managed incontinence, or social continence.

GUIDELINES FOR SELECTING CONTINENCE PRODUCTS

Selecting suitable products is critical for the well-being and QoL of users and caregivers. Urinary incontinence (UI) affects an estimated 200 million people worldwide in some way (Wagg et al., 2019) and the ability to contain and conceal incontinence enables individuals to maintain their public identity as a "continent person" and to avoid the stigma associated with incontinence (Paterson, 2000). Failure to do so can result in limited social and professional opportunities, place relationships in jeopardy, and detrimentally affect emotional and mental well-being, and UI is still considered to be a taboo subject in many cultures (Mitteness & Barker, 1995; Öz & Altay, 2018). The ability to contain and conceal incontinence enables caregivers to feel confident that the person(s) they care for will not be embarrassed publicly and reduces challenges related to hygiene and skin integrity as well as costs and burdens associated with laundry of linens (Paterson et al., 2003).

> **KEY POINT**
>
> The ability to contain and conceal incontinence enables individuals to maintain their public identity as a "continent person" and to avoid the stigma associated with incontinence.

Selecting the best option is a challenge; not only is there a wide diversity of products, but until recently, there has been a gap in the evidence for guidance in their selection (Gray et al., 2018b). Wound Ostomy Continence (WOC) nurses must understand the products available and the indications for proper use of each type of product (Gray et al., 2018). Comprehensive and current information is critical to reduce confusion and stress for both the layperson and the health care professional (Paterson et al., 2003). The intimate and stigmatized nature of incontinence means that issues relating to self-image may also affect user choices.

Product success depends, in part, on the ability to conceal the problem (Shaw et al., 2001), but concealment may involve compromises. For example, the size and bulkiness of a product can create issues in terms of discretion and concealment, even though manufacturers have endeavored to make UI management products more discreet than ever. Fear of leakage is an issue as body image is important to maintenance of social activities and interpersonal relationships (Hocking, 1999; Low, 1996; Wan et al., 2014). Finally, product accessibility may vary enormously between and within countries and even facilities, depending on the funding available, health care policy, and the logistics of supplies, which can include buying contracts (Gibb & Wong, 1994; Paterson et al., 2003; Proudfoot et al., 1994).

PRODUCT CATEGORIES

Continence products can be divided into those that are intended to assist with toileting or provide containment and control as a strategy to manage urinary retention and/or urinary and/or fecal incontinence (FI), which may often also be called "dual," "mixed," or "double" incontinence; "dual" will be the preferred term.

The algorithm provided in **Figure 16-1** provides guidance in determining which product or group of products is likely to be of benefit to a particular person. There are three main questions to be addressed:

1. Are there problems with toilet access (e.g., toilet proximity or toilet design or issues related to mobility and/or urgency)?
2. Is there urinary retention (with or without incontinence)?
3. If the goal is containment and control, is there UI or fecal incontinence or both?

The answers to these questions help to identify the category(ies) of products most likely to help.

PATIENT ASSESSMENT FACTORS

Careful assessment is critical to create the best match between absorbent product and containment device and the user and should take into account a variety of factors (Gray et al., 2018b):

- Gender
- Mobility (ambulatory, assistance with transfers, bedbound)
- Dexterity (ability to apply and remove product/device independently and accurately, including into clothing)
- Cognition
- Incontinence type (UI/FI/Dual), severity, and timing (day/night)
- Care setting (home/hospital/postacute facility, etc.)
- Physical characteristics such as anthropometrics (BMI, waist/hip circumference, general body habitus (underweight/obese/morbidly obese)
- Patient preference (cost, economic impact, design of products/devices, presence of ability to launder items, previous use/experience)
- Perigenital skin health
- Caregiver (availability and ability to apply/remove/manipulate product/device)
- The need for education in use and care of the product at an appropriate level (Wittink & Oosterhaven, 2018)

Volume, frequency, type, and severity of UI, as well as presence of fecal incontinence, along with timing of incontinence is foundational to determining product use for management/containment. Common terms for categories for UI are often discussed as "light" or "moderate/heavy." These terms have some degree of subjectivity but have been defined to assist with product choices, especially in relation to BWAPs. For this discussion, light UI is defined as urinary leakage up to 100 mL, and moderate/heavy UI is defined as urinary leakage of more than 100 mL (Gray et al., 2018b).

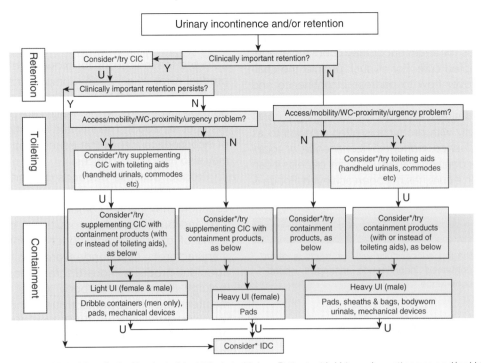

FIGURE 16-1. Algorithm to Help Identify the Products Most Likely to Help a Patient with Urinary Incontinence and/or Urinary Retention. *Consideration should be based on assessment of the patient's physical characteristics, cognitive ability, and personal preferences, as well as the nature of their incontinence. (CIC, clean intermittent self-catheterization; IDC, indwelling catheter; N, no; U, unsatisfactory (considered and deemed unsuitable or tried and found not to work satisfactorily); Y, yes.)

Perigenital skin health cannot be overlooked, and later in this chapter, IAD will be discussed with additional details in Chapter 17.

MAIN USER GROUPS

Dividing users into major groups helps identify the category(ies) of products most likely to benefit them. The following groups have been identified:

- People with urinary retention
- People who need help with toileting/toilet access
- Women with light daytime UI
- Men with light daytime UI
- Ambulatory women and men with light daytime fecal incontinence
- Ambulatory adults with moderate to heavy daytime urinary/fecal/dual incontinence
- Nonambulatory patients with moderate to heavy daytime urinary, fecal, or dual incontinence
- Ambulatory and nonambulatory patients with moderate to heavy nighttime urinary, fecal, or dual incontinence

An individual may belong to more than one group. Each group includes children and young people as well as adults, since the products available for children and adolescents are broadly similar to those for adults.

It is important to remember that the same product will not suit all people, even if assessment parameters are similar, and even if the UI/FI pattern/problem is similar. One product or device will rarely address all issues or is singularly best for all users (Cottenden et al., 2017; Gray et al., 2018b). Often a mix of products from different categories will provide the best solution; for example, needs may vary between day/night and home/away situations, a "wardrobe" of containment products to fit the occasion. This mix may include absorbent products, urinals, male external catheters (also known as condom catheters or sheaths), and bedpans/commodes.

> **KEY POINT**
>
> The same product will not suit all people, even if they have the same clinical issue, because preferences and priorities differ from person to person.

Special and specific considerations must be given to some populations, such as community-dwelling (vs. in a facility), morbidly obese, and/or cognitively impaired individuals. It is very important to normalize the toileting experience for patients with incontinence and dementia, for example. So, individuals who have both incontinence and dementia should be considered for underwear-type products (underwear with pads or a pull-on for example), as a way to enhance the effectiveness of a toileting program, to normalize the toileting experience to reduce

agitation and promote safety (Gray et al., 2018b). The availability and sizing for BWAPs for morbidly obese individuals is limited, and an important feature to consider aside from skin pH are other issues such as the length of absorbent area from front to back where the "landing zone" for urine is located, the ability to accommodate abdominal girth and leg size, and the presence of skin folds (Gray et al., 2018b). Less than good fit can lead to emotional issues and a loss of personal dignity.

ABSORBENT PRODUCTS

Absorbent products are marketed in a wide range of sizes and absorbencies for light to very heavy incontinence and in either disposable or reusable forms. There are multiple product types that include pull-ons, briefs, pads/liners/leaf/shields/guards, and penile wraps. Other absorbent non–body-worn products include underpads.

OVERVIEW

> **KEY POINT**
>
> There are multiple product types that include pull-ons, briefs, pads/liners/leaf/shields/guards, and penile wraps. Other absorbent non–body-worn products include underpads.

Absorbent products have evolved over time. There are multiple options to consider, and as with any product, it is important to recognize the use of the right product at the right time for the patient who is experiencing UI/FI. Not all products are the same structurally and that is reflected in certain features that the products offer, as well as their ability to absorb and contain the urine or feces. Additionally, it is very important to recognize that there are gender-specific physiological features that influence the way that urine is distributed within the absorbent products. Women urinate and the flow lands between the thighs in the pelvic area, while men tend to urinate in a more outward distribution. This influences the "landing zone" where absorbency is most critical. Also, incontinence patterns vary. Persons with UI may "gush" or "dribble" or "flood." Despite features that products can offer; a combination of products may be needed in order to provide confidence and satisfaction simply due to the UI pattern.

Understanding some features of disposable absorbent products may be helpful in order to assist in recommendation of disposable absorbent products, specifically. See **Table 16-1** for definitions of important features.

Reusable absorbent products are often consumer rated on buying sites and may give useful information regarding product fit, bulkiness, laundering, and user perception of the product. Providing guidance to patients/families on which absorbent product to use can

TABLE 16-1 ABSORBENT PRODUCT FEATURES

Absorptive capacity	The maximum capacity of fluid and absorbent product can hold; this value is determined in the laboratory using a standardized technique (MA009-1).
Breathability	Airflow within an absorbent product that allows release of heat, perspiration, and gas in the pelvic girdle region.
Elastication	The ability of elastics that are woven together to maintain fit snugly around the waist or thigh despite repeated movement.
Liquid acquisition rate	The speed at which urine is wicked away from the skin by an absorbent material.
Retention capacity	The maximum volume of fluid an absorbent product can hold without leaking.
Rewet	A measure of an absorbent material's ability to absorb urine with multiple incontinent episodes.

Adapted from Gray et al. (2018).

be daunting. The WOC Nurses Society™ has developed a tool, based on evidence and consensus, called the BWAP Guide, available free of charge, at https://bwap.wocn.org/#home. This user-friendly tool guides the user through a series of questions, to the end point of a recommendation for the patient in relation to a BWAP. This tool was created from a consensus conference on BWAPs and is based on evidence and consensus (Gray et al., 2018a). Consensus statements regarding product selection are highlighted in **Table 16-2**, and others are stated in this chapter. This table provides a summation of product recommendations at a high level.

This BWAP selection tool does not include the use of underpads and is focused on adults with UI/FI/Dual incontinence. Children and adolescents face UI/FI/dual incontinence as well, but their needs may differ slightly from adults. For example, ambulatory children may report better use with the ease of pull-ons with augmentation versus a brief due to ease of use and social issues.

A note of caution: sometimes people are admitted into an acute care facility after a major illness or event occurs. One study found that among patients who voided independently prior to hospitalization, those who used absorbent briefs during hospitalization were more likely to experience a new onset of UI than those who did not use absorbent briefs (Zisberg, 2011). Preserving continence status is patient centric and should be at the forefront of the plan of care for any patient.

TABLE 16-2 BODY-WORN ABSORBENT PRODUCT SELECTION GUIDE

Women with Light Daytime Urinary Incontinence
- Disposable pads designed for urine are a first-line containment recommendation.
- Based on patient preference and acceptability, disposable menstrual pads are an alternative.

Men with Light Daytime Urinary Incontinence
- Disposable menstrual pads are NOT recommended.
- Disposable pads (guards and shields) for urine are a first-line recommendation.

Ambulatory Women and Men with Light Daytime Fecal Incontinence
- Disposable absorbent products positioned over anus and between the buttocks are a first-line recommendation.
- If absorbent products become inadequate, consider use of absorbent brief or pull-on.

Ambulatory Adults with Moderate to Heavy Daytime Urinary, Fecal, or Dual Incontinence
- Disposable pull-ons, including superabsorbent polymer technology are a first-line recommendation.
- In ambulatory women with moderate/heavy daytime UI disposable-shaped pads including SAP technology worn with close-fitting underwear are an alternative first-line recommendation.
- In ambulatory men with moderate/heavy daytime UI/FI/dual incontinence, disposable absorptive briefs including SAP technology are an alternative recommendation.

Ambulatory and Nonambulatory Patients with Moderate to Heavy *Nighttime* UI/FI/Dual Incontinence
- In nonambulatory women, the use of disposable briefs including SAP technology is a first-line recommendation.
- In ambulatory women, first-line recommendation: Disposable pull-ons with SAP technology designed for nighttime use; close-fitting underwear with integral pads (urinary only), designed for nighttime use is an acceptable alternative.
- In ambulatory and nonambulatory men, the use of a nighttime disposable brief including SAP technology is a first-line recommendation.

Nonambulatory Patients with Moderate/Heavy *Daytime* UI/FI/Dual Incontinence
- In nonambulatory nontoiletable women, disposable briefs including SAP technology are recommended. Use of pull-ons are *not* recommended in individuals who are bed-bound and nontoiletable.
- In nonambulatory toiletable women with moderate/heavy daytime UI, disposable pull-ons including SAP technology are a first-line recommendation.
- In nonambulatory toiletable women with moderate/heavy daytime UI, the use of disposable pad with close-fitting underwear is an acceptable cost-effective alternative.
- In nonambulatory men, disposable briefs including SAP technology are a first-line recommendation.
- In nonambulatory, toiletable men, close-fitting underwear with integral pads or pull-ons is an alternative recommendation.

Adapted from Gray et al. (2018).

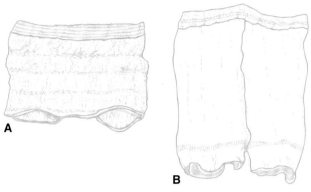

FIGURE 16-2. Mesh Pants with (**B**) and without (**A**) Legs, for Securing Incontinence Pads in Position.

KEY POINT

The Wound Ostomy Continence Nurses Society™ has developed an electronic tool, based on evidence and consensus, called the Body-Worn Absorbent Product Guide, available free of charge, at https://bwap.wocn.org/#home to guide the user in proper assessment, selection, and evaluation of a BWAP for people suffering from UI.

BODY-WORN PRODUCTS

Body-worn absorbent products can be divided into five main design groups: inserts, briefs, pull-ons, guards, and containment augmentation.

Inserts

Inserts (sometimes called liners or, in the case of small pads, shields) are held in place by close-fitting underwear or stretch mesh briefs (**Fig. 16-2**). Many disposable inserts (**Figs. 16-3** and **16-4**) have an adhesive strip on the back to help secure them to the underwear, and some have an indicator that changes color when the pad is wet to signal the need for a change. Longitudinal, elasticated gathers of hydrophobic material help impede lateral leakage of urine and feces and usually fit snugly against the body. Inserts range in absorptive capacity from very light to light and possibly moderate incontinence per manufacturers claims. Some men try

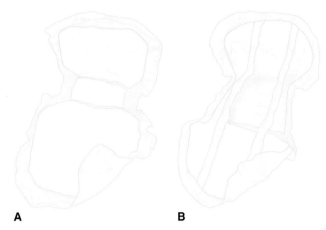

A   **B**

FIGURE 16-4. Disposable Inserts with (**A**) and without (**B**) Standing Gathers, for Moderate/Heavy Incontinence.

disposable menstrual pads in the front of undergarments as an alternative to an insert. However, these pads are *not* designed for the management of either urinary or fecal incontinence in men (Gray et al., 2018b).

Washable inserts are usually more simply designed than disposable ones, with no elastication; they are typically either shaped or a simple rectangle (**Fig. 16-5**).

Briefs

Briefs (sometimes called all-in-ones or diapers) are adult size versions of infant diapers. Disposable briefs (**Fig. 16-6**) usually have elasticated waist and legs and self-adhesive tabs (usually resealable); they may also provide a wetness indicator and standing leg gathers. More recently, modified briefs have been introduced that fasten around the waist before the front is pulled into position and secured, which enables users to apply the brief while standing (**Fig. 16-7**). Washable briefs are usually elasticated at the waist and legs and are secured with Velcro or press studs (**Fig. 16-8**). Briefs are intended for moderate to very heavy UI/FI/dual incontinence. **Table 16-3** describes the anatomy of most absorbent products: top sheet layer, acquisition layer, absorbent core, and backsheet.

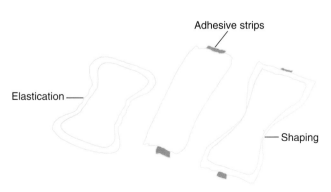

Adhesive strips

Elastication ———

——— Shaping

FIGURE 16-3. Disposable Inserts for Light Incontinence.

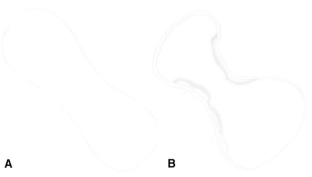

A   **B**

FIGURE 16-5. Reusable Inserts for Light (**A**) and Moderate/Heavy (**B**) Incontinence.

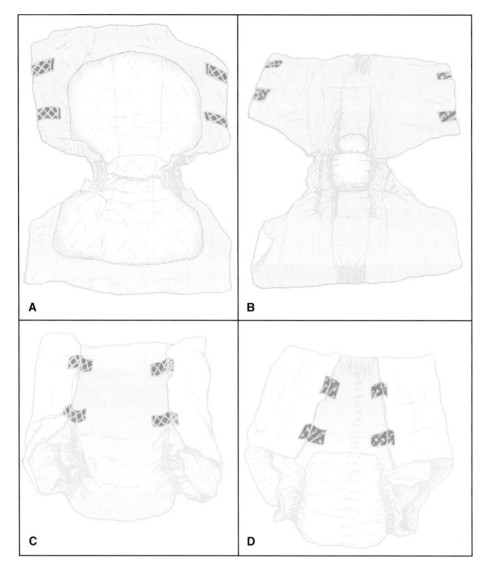

FIGURE 16-6. Disposable Briefs (Diapers) with (**B, D**) and without (**A, C**) Standing Gathers, for Moderate/Heavy Incontinence. Briefs are shown open (**A, B**) and with the tabs secured (**C, D**).

KEY POINT

Inserts are pads or liners that are worn with snug underwear or mesh briefs; they range in absorptive capacity from very light to light and possibly moderate incontinence. Briefs (also known as diapers) are intended for moderate to very heavy incontinence.

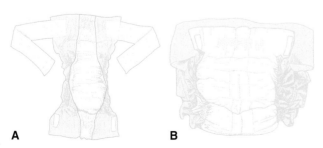

FIGURE 16-7. Modified (T-shaped) Brief. The waistband (**A**) is secured first and then the front pulled up and secured in position (**B**).

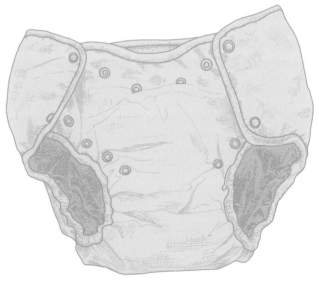

FIGURE 16-8. Reusable Brief.

TABLE 16-3 ANATOMY OF ABSORBENT PRODUCTS

Characteristics of Absorbent Products

Top sheet layer	Web or plastic film with holes enable absorption of moisture
Acquisition layer	Nonwoven synthetic fibers or modified cellulose fiber used to rapidly transport moisture from skin to absorbent core
Absorbent core	Cellulose fluff pulp ± superabsorbent polymers must store and retain moisture away from skin
Backing (containment layer)	Usually a plastic form, designed with variable levels of breathability influence microclimate between absorbent product and skin

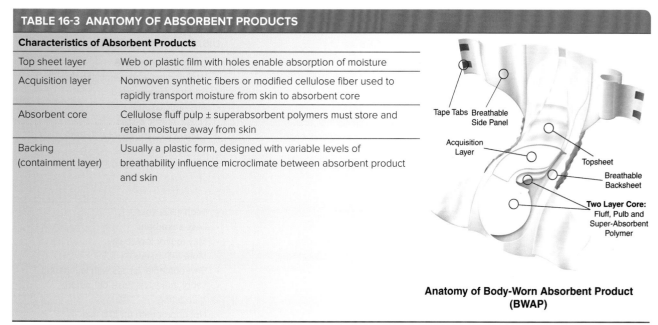

Anatomy of Body-Worn Absorbent Product (BWAP)

Adapted from White (2003); Gray et al. (2018). (Image: Used with permission from Domtar.)

Pull-Ons

Pull-ons are similar in construction to trainer pants for toddlers. The absorbent material is built into a pull-on pant and is either limited to the crotch area or distributed throughout the pant (**Figs. 16-9** and **16-10**). Disposable pull-ons (**Fig. 16-9**) are usually elasticated throughout the pants to give a close fit. Many designs of this type of BWAP are available, with popular styles resembling details of regular adult underwear. Both disposable and washable pull-ons have versions designed for different levels of incontinence. Washable pull-ons for light incontinence are often known as pants with integral pads (**Fig. 16-10**). **Table 16-4** compares advantages and disadvantages of disposable versus reusable BWAP products.

Male Guards

Male guards (sometimes called shields, leafs, pouches) for men with low-volume incontinence are designed to fit around the penis and sometimes the scrotum and typically have an adhesive back (**Figs. 16-11** and **16-12**). They are worn with close-fitting underwear or stretch mesh briefs.

KEY POINT

Male guards fit around the penis (and sometimes the scrotum); they are designed to be worn with snugly fitting underwear or stretch mesh briefs and are intended for low-volume leakage.

Containment Augmentation

Booster pads and other products have been used, especially in infants and children, to enhance the absorbency of BWAPs. They can be used to help remedy inadequate containment when implemented with other products. Booster pads differ from traditional inserted pads in that

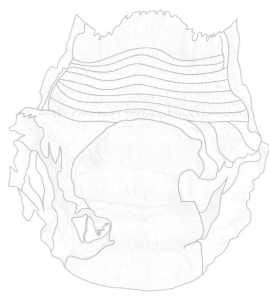

FIGURE 16-9. Disposable Pull-On.

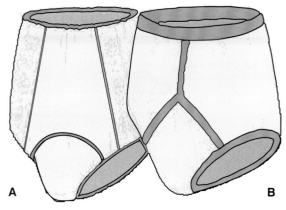

FIGURE 16-10. Reusable Pull-On Pants (Also Known as Pants with Integral pad) for Lightly Incontinent Women (**A**) and Men (**B**).

TABLE 16-4 DISPOSABLE VERSUS REUSABLE FEATURES

PRODUCT TYPE	ADVANTAGES	DISADVANTAGES
Disposable 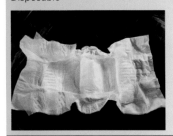	• Less $ initially • Convenient, great for travel • Ease of use • Better for heavy UI • May have wetness indicator • May use for fecal incontinence • Less IAD issues • Caretaker ease	• Long-term more $$$ • Environmental concerns, landfills • Storage area needed • Aesthetic issues • Noise, elastic edges • Lack of industry standardization
Reusable 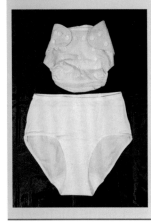	• Less cost over time • Softer on skin • Looks more like underwear • Best for light to intermittent UI • Best for home use	• High initial cost • Less absorbent • May feel or look bulky • More IAD issues • Environmental issues with laundering • Labor intensive; rinse out before laundering • Not appropriate for LTC use • Not recommended for heavy incontinence • Not recommend for FI

Courtesy WEB WOC® Nursing Education Programs.

they have "flow through" technology, lacking the plastic and adhesive backing. When used, often the absorbent capacity is enhanced, and the primary product is used for a longer period of time, which can allow for undisturbed sleep, for example. Traditional booster pads are available, but there are also penile wraps that are more novel. These wraps can be applied to encase the penis, adding extra protection against leakage for males. Additionally, due the design of the product, which has some containment features, sometimes the penile wrap can be changed, while the larger BWAP such as a pull-on or brief can remain in place (Gray et al., 2018b). While these types of products are attractive to extend the wear time of BWAPs, it should be noted that containment augmentation should never be utilized for caregiver or staff convenience (Gray et al., 2018b).

> **KEY POINT**
>
> Body-worn absorbent products can be divided into five main design groups: inserts, briefs, pull-ons, guards, and containment augmentation.

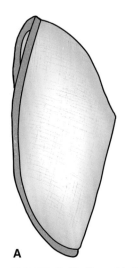
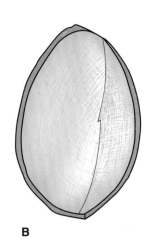

A **B**

FIGURE 16-12. Reusable Pouches/Guards for Men: Side View (**A**) and Front View (**B**).

Pouch for penis ⎯

Adhesive strip helps positioning

FIGURE 16-11. Disposable Pouch for Men.

Absorbent Products for Women with Light Incontinence

The main product designs for women with light incontinence are disposable inserts, washable inserts, and washable pants. Menstrual pads are often used although they are not designed to hold urine. There is robust evidence that disposable inserts are more effective in terms of leakage and more acceptable than menstrual pads, washable pants, and washable inserts (Gray et al., 2018b). However, menstrual pads are cheaper and washable pants are the least expensive option (on a per-use basis), and these products are acceptable to many, particularly those with lighter incontinence and particularly when used at home. Washable inserts are not acceptable to most women.

Absorbent Products for Men with Light Incontinence

Product designs in this category include disposable and washable inserts, disposable and washable guards, and washable pull-ons. However, disposable and washable insert pads are often unappealing to men as they are frequently marketed specifically for women and bear a strong resemblance to menstrual pads. Anatomical differences are also likely to mean that they are less effective for men. Pouch, shield, guard, or leaf products (**Figs. 16-11** and **16-12**) are more suitable for men because they contain the penis or penis and scrotum. Pouches are an absorbent pocket that fits over the penis and absorb a minimal amount of urine (1 to 2 ounces of urine) thus best used for post-void dribbling (see Chapter 10). They can be used with other products. Guards, shields, and leafs are interchangeable terms depending upon geographical location and are an insert absorbent product that covers the penis and scrotum that can be used with close-fitting underwear to absorb urine in the front of the garment (Gray et al., 2018b). Disposable guards (male shield or leaf) are recommended as the most acceptable and effective design for men with light incontinence; simple insert pads are cheaper and may be acceptable to some men; and washable pants with integral pads are likely to be most suitable for men with very light incontinence who have difficulties keeping an inserted guard or pouch in place (Gray et al., 2018b).

Products for Moderate to Heavy Incontinence

For men and women with moderate–heavy UI, there are at least 12 absorbent products. The most commonly used are disposable body-worn inserts, pull-ons, and briefs (Figs. 12-3 to 12-7). Men leak substantially higher volumes of urine usually at a faster rate (gushers) than women, and a brief with superabsorbent polymers (SAP) is the most cost-effective design for men (Gray et al., 2018b). For women, pull-ons are better overall than the other designs, though they are more expensive; the one exception is nighttime management of women living in nursing homes (Gray et al., 2018b). There is evidence that pads containing SAPs leak less, are more comfortable, and keep the skin drier than those without.

DISPOSABLE UNDERPAD

Absorbent underpads are frequently the first-line product used by nurses in acute care to manage patients with urinary/fecal incontinence. These products are designed to be used on the bed or chair and come in various sizes and shapes (**Fig. 16-13**). Disposable underpads, sometimes called "blue pads," are not designed for management of incontinence, as they lack an absorbent filling and allow pooling of urine on the thin plastic surface.

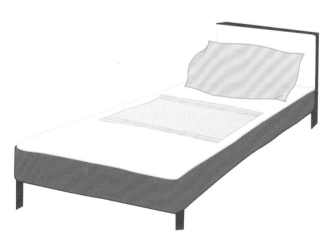

FIGURE 16-13. Disposable Underpad.

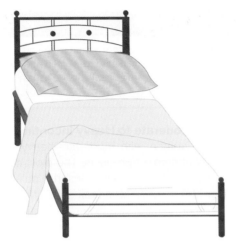

FIGURE 16-14. Reusable Underpad.

This places the patient at risk for skin wetness and breakdown. Washable/reusable underpads (**Fig. 16-14**) may have a waterproof polyvinyl chloride backing with a quilted design for absorbency. Some may have "wings" for tucking beneath the mattress of single beds to help keep them in place. Disposable underpads contain a super absorbent core material that wicks away incontinence moisture and has a breathable backsheet. Both reusable and disposable underpads vary widely in absorbency; less absorbent products may be used as "backup" products (in conjunction with body-worn products), and more absorbent products may be used as sole protection on the bed at night.

KEY POINT

Absorbent underpads are frequently the first-line product used by nurses in acute care to manage patients with urinary/ fecal incontinence. These products are designed to be used on the bed or chair and come in various sizes and shapes.

ABSORBENT PRODUCT CAPACITY

Underpads come in a range of absorbencies to meet the needs of users with different levels of UI. In addressing a system-wide skin and pressure injury prevention and treatment program, WOC nurses in collaboration with purchasing managers wish to know how much urine the various pads will hold. There are three commonly used industry standards for determining the absorbent capacity for disposable underpads. The *re-wet test* measures a product's ability to retain moisture under pressure. The *absorptive capacity test* measures how quickly an absorbent product acquires a given amount of fluid, and the *total absorbent capacity test* (International Organization for Standardization [ISO] standard 11948–1) measures how much fluid a product can absorb. These results can help to differentiate between light, moderate, and heavy absorbent products (Leander, 2019).

Unfortunately, there is no simple answer; pads do not have a volume of urine below which they are guaranteed not to leak. Rather, the probability of success decreases as the volume of the urine increases and the position of the user changes. For example, a bed-bound individual places continuous pressure on the product, which increases the risk that they will "squeeze" urine out of the pad. In contrast, the same pad worn by a mobile individual may not leak. Body weight also affects pad capacity. However, for higher-absorbency pads, the performance falls away more slowly with increasing urine volume than it does for lower absorbency products. See **Table 16-1** for characteristics of absorbent products.

Product Standardization

In response to lack of standardization of all types of absorbent products, the National Association for Continence (NAFC) formed a counsel of experts and key stakeholders and created nine specific recommendations for minimum performance standards *beyond* the total absorption capacity in hopes to standardize features of disposable products since it is difficult to compare brands without established baseline standards (Muller & McInnis, 2013). The Taskforce believe that minimum performance standards may reduce opportunities for fraud, waste, and abuse by suppliers, as well as establish a benchmark for quality and performance of absorbent products manufactures. Another case in point for standardization is that payors (consumers, buying groups, care facilities, Medicaid programs) for absorbent products do not know which products to purchase and if they are receiving value for dollars spent (Muller & McInnis, 2013).

- Recommendations for *minimum* performance standards include the following:
  1. Re-wet rate—ability to withstand multiple UI episodes between changes
  2. Rate of acquisition—speed at which urine is drawn away from the skin by a product
  3. Product retention capacity—product's capacity to hold fluid without rewetting the skin
  4. Sizing options
  5. Absorbency levels
  6. Product safety
  7. Closure technology
  8. Breathable zones—air permeability across a textile-like fabric
  9. Elasticity

KEY POINT

Three commonly used industry standards for determining the absorbent capacity for disposable underpads includes rewet, absorptive capacity, and total absorbency capacity tests. However, there is a lack of national minimum performance standards that goes *beyond* the total absorption capacity, which makes it difficult for consumers to compare brands and if they are receiving value and quality for their purchase.

Washable/Reusable versus Disposable

The decision to use washable/reusable underpads versus disposable underpads can be confusing for many. Concerns related to the environment and the cost of disposable products have led to an increase in the number of available products that are washable/reusable. In 2017, Francis et al. conducted a randomized controlled trial (RCT) to determine the incidence of pressure injury development as well as IAD using disposable versus reusable absorptive underpads. The results showed hospital-acquired pressure injuries were significantly lower in the disposable underpads group versus the reusable group. Rates of hospital-acquired IAD were not significantly different between the two groups. While this study indicates a benefit to using disposable underpads, an important consideration in the comparison of washable and disposable designs is the relative environmental cost, particularly landfill costs of disposable designs versus energy costs associated with laundering the washables, whether an underpad or BWAP.

If washable underpads are the only absorbent product being used (i.e., without a BWAP), the individual will need to be naked below the waist. Aspects of assessment that are particularly important regarding washable underpads are patient acceptability and preference, particularly with regard to willingness to be naked below the waist (if sole use intended) and availability of laundry and drying facilities (see **Table 16-4**).

Technological Advances

Over the past decade, technological advances have been made in the design and efficacy of underpads. Manufacturers have designed disposable underpads with embedded technology to alert care providers to episodes of UI in patients unable or unwilling to signal for assistance. Washable/reusable underpads have also seen design advances with the 2014 ruling from the FDA approving the first ever medical grade silk-like bed linen system (including underpads) for patients with UI. These silk-like linens have a low coefficient of friction (CoF) to reduce the risk of skin damage in patients with UI (Hasler, 2019).

KEY POINT

Technological advances in absorbent products include disposable underpads with embedded technology to alert care providers to episodes of urinary incontinence in patients unable or unwilling to signal for assistance and silk-like linens possessing low coefficient of friction to reduce risk of skin damage in patients with UI.

Pads for Light Fecal Incontinence

There are very few quality products available for mild or moderate fecal incontinence; this is an area where improved products are desperately needed. For mild

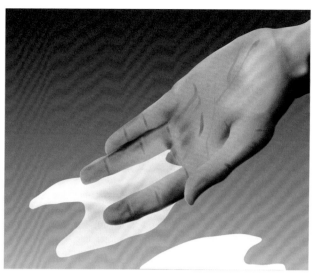

FIGURE 16-15. Insert for Light Fecal Incontinence. It is positioned against the anus and held in place by the cheeks of the buttocks.

fecal incontinence (e.g., stool that remains trapped between the buttocks without soiling underwear), the only real option at this time is to place a soft pad (insert) or gauze between the buttocks. For light fecal incontinence, the insert may be a small cotton gauze dressing placed against the anus and held in place by the cheeks of the buttocks (**Fig. 16-15**). Additionally, there is a soft woven insert that can fit between the cheeks of the buttock and has light adhesive strips on it to hold into place that is characterized as a butterfly shape.

EXTERNAL COLLECTION DEVICES

External collection devices (ECDs) are a group of devices that adhere to the external genitalia or pubic area and collect urinary output; they are further divided into the following categories: condom catheters, reusable body-worn urinals, nonsheath glans adherent, penile compression devices, and female suction devices (Gray et al., 2016).

MALE CONDOM CATHETERS

Condom catheters (also known as external catheters or sheaths) are typically used in combination with a urine drainage bag and are suitable for men experiencing moderate to heavy urine loss and for men who have limited mobility and are experiencing frequency and urgency, who are unable to engage in a toileting program, who require an adjunct to a toileting program, or who may require monitoring of urine output (Gray et al., 2020). These devices may also be considered for use in combination with intermittent catheterization (IC). They are *not* recommended for those with cognitive impairment, men who are considered psychologically vulnerable, or men

TABLE 16-5 APPLICATION GUIDELINES FOR EXTERNAL COLLECTION DEVICES FOR MEN

Condom Catheter
- Inspect the skin of the glans penis and penile shaft for inflammation and integrity prior to initial application or device change.
- Select an appropriately sized device based on manufacturer's sizing tool and recommendations.
- Avoid use of condom external collection devices in patients with spina bifida of a history of hypersensitivity or allergy to latex.
- Cleanse and dry the skin before application.
- Apply liquid barrier skin protectant to penile skin if needed; let dry.
- Apply adhesive or securement mechanism based on manufacturer's recommendations.
- Do not apply additional adhesive securement products to the penis.
- Expected wear time is 1–2 days.

Retracted Penis Pouch
- Inspect the penile and suprapubic skin adjacent to the penis for inflammation and integrity.
- Clip hair as needed; do not shave hair.
- Cleanse and dry the skin before application.
- Apply liquid barrier skin protectant to suprapubic skin if needed, let dry.
- Place the penis through the pouch opening. Hold the adherent surface in place using gentle, warming hand pressure to activate the adhesive.
- Do not apply additional adhesive or securement products to the penis or suprapubic skin.
- The expected wear time is 1–2 days.

Nonsheath Glans-adherent Devices
- Inspect the glans penis and skin of the penile shaft for inflammation and integrity prior to initial application or device change.
- Cleanse and pat dry before application or device change.
- Follow manufacturer recommendations; gentle, warming hand pressure is essential to activate the adhesive.
- Do not apply additional adhesive or securement products to the penis.
- Expected wear time is 2–3 days.

with decreased genital sensation (Golji, 1981; Pemberton et al., 2006; Potter, 2007).

Proper size and fit of the condom catheter is critical to its effectiveness, and the care provider or user needs instruction in correct application of the device, followed by return demonstration of correct technique. **Table 16-5** provides the guidelines for ECD for men. Failure to follow the manufacturer's instructions may result in serious penile trauma, impaired penile skin integrity, and leakage. An effective male external catheter is one that stays securely

in place for an acceptable period of time; is leak-free, comfortable to wear, and easy to apply and remove; avoids skin damage; and channels the urine effectively into a urine drainage bag. **Figure 16-16** illustrates the principal design features of condom catheters, which must be considered when assisting an individual to select an appropriate product. Consider a condom catheter in males with

- Intact penile skin
- Adequate penile shaft length to accommodate device (at least 1 inch of persistent penile protrusion)

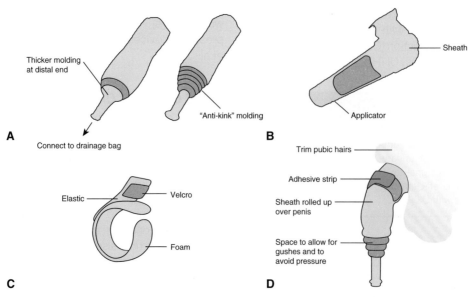

FIGURE 16-16. Various Sheaths (**A, D**), a Sheath Applicator (**B**), and an External Fixation Strip (**C**).

- Consider a nonsheath glans adherent device or penis pouch in males with:
  - Buried or retracted penis
  - Shorter penile shaft length

Do not use external female collection devices in males (Gray et al., 2020).

In addition to the widely available adhesive condom catheters, there are also nonadhesive sheaths secured with a strap, and penile cups secured with snugly fitting underwear.

> **KEY POINT**
>
> Proper size and fit of a condom catheter is *critical* to its effectiveness; sizing guides are available from manufacturers free of charge.

FEATURES

Condom catheters vary in terms of material, size, adhesive design, availability of applicator, anti-twist and anti-blow-off features, connection features, durability, and appropriateness for use with a retracted penis:

- Material: Condom catheters may be constructed of latex, silicone rubber, or other synthetic polymers. Some men are allergic to latex, and queries regarding allergies are an important component of assessment. In addition, regular users should be routinely checked as latex allergy status can change over time and with prolonged exposure.
- Size: Most companies supply condom catheters in various lengths, with diameters ranging from about 20- to 40-mm, in 5- to 10-mm increments. It is critical for the product to be accurately sized, and most companies provide simple and disposable sizing guides free of charge, while others provide actual products to assure correct fit.
- Adhesive: The adhesive may be integrated into the condom (one-piece systems) or may be provided as a separate strip or spray (two-piece systems). Some men are allergic to selected adhesives. Products with integral adhesive are popular and easier to apply than those with the separate adhesive strip.
- Applicator: Some devices come with an applicator intended to help users and carers to put the sheath on.
- Anti-kinking/Twisting Features: Some devices promote improved drainage by reducing kinking and twisting at the distal end, near the connection to the drainage bag tube. There is the risk of leakage (or urinary retention) if the condom twists or the external band is too tight, impairing drainage to the urine bag.
- Anti-blow-off/Falloff Feature: This feature is intended to reduce the likelihood of the external catheter coming off at high urine flow rates, for example, at

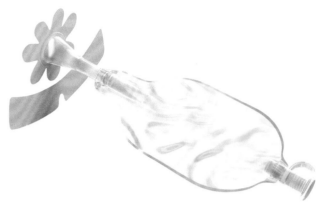

FIGURE 16-17. BioDerm Liberty Male External Catheter. (Courtesy of BioDerm®, Inc.)

the beginning of a void. This feature may involve a thickened and bulbous area at the distal end of the sheath that maintains sheath patency between voids.

- Connection Features: Some condom catheters include features designed to increase the ease and security of connection to the drainage tube (e.g., a push ring or ridge at the end of the outlet tubing).
- Retracted Penis Features: Some sheaths are designed with specific features intended to accommodate a retracted penis (e.g., a shorter sheath or a wider adhesive seal). In addition, there are selected products now available with hydrocolloid adhesive designed to safely adhere to the glans; these products are indicated for men with persistent or episodic retraction that prevents adherence of a condom catheter (see **Fig. 16-17**).
- Durability: Some condom catheters are intended for use over a limited time period (e.g., 24 hours), while other (generally more robust) designs are intended for extended wear.
- Transparency: Some condom catheters are transparent allowing for observation of the condition of the skin along the shaft and glans of the penis.

> **KEY POINT**
>
> Condom catheters come with an integrated adhesive feature (1-piece) or with an adhesive strip (2-piece); the 1-piece systems are easier to apply and generally preferred.

PENILE COMPRESSION DEVICES

Penile compression devices (penile clamps) are mechanical devices designed to prevent urine leakage by compressing the penis. Various designs are available, but occlusion is usually achieved with either a clamp or a peri-penile strap (**Fig. 16-18**). Such devices have the potential advantages of low cost and simplicity

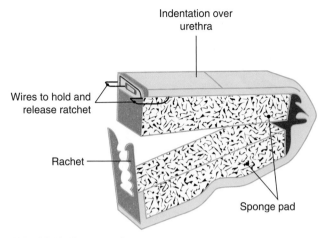

FIGURE 16-18. Penile Clamp.

compared with a sheath and drainage bag and evidence of improvement in stress incontinent symptoms and QoL was demonstrated in a small study (Barnard & Westenberg, 2014). However, there is potential for tissue damage, and these devices should be used with caution (Lemmens et al., 2019).

These devices must be used with caution to prevent ischemic damage to the penis (due to restricted blood flow) causing device-related pressure injuries, urethral erosion, stricture, or diverticulum (Barnard & Westenberg, 2014; Kalra et al., 2015; Moore et al., 2004). Penile clamps should be fitted by a trained health professional and subject to regular review. The continence nurse needs to provide clear verbal and written instructions to prevent potential complications (see **Box 16-1**, Considerations for penile compression device use). Moore et al. (2004) evaluated three different devices (Timms C3 penile compression device, Cunningham clamp, and U-Tex male adjustable tension band) in a crossover study in which 12 men with stress UI following radical prostatectomy tried each device in turn. Each of the devices significantly ($p < 0.05$) reduced mean urine loss (measured using 4-hour pad tests), as compared to baseline measurements of urine loss. There was some objective or subjective improvement in continence for each of the 12 men with at least one of the devices, although none completely eliminated urine loss when applied at a comfortable pressure. Ten of the 12 men rated the Cunningham clamp positively; 2, the C3; and none, the U-Tex.

BOX 16-1   CONSIDERATIONS IN USE OF PENILE COMPRESSION DEVICES

CONSIDERATIONS	PRECAUTIONS
Candidates: Men suffering stress incontinence only, that is, post-radical prostatectomy, alert without cognitive decline, intact genital sensation, and good dexterity	
1. Inspect and clean genitals with soap and water or incontinence skin cleanser. Dry well, apply skin protectant if needed.	If any skin discoloration or open skin noted, do not use clamp device.
2. Open clamp, place around penis midway down the shaft, squeeze shut but avoid too much pressure. It should not hurt. Follow manufacture's guidelines if using a compression device that does not open with a hinge or is disposable.	Too tight will cause poor circulation to the penile skin and cause tissue death.
3. Release clamp every 1–3 hours to urinate even if you do not feel like you need to pass urine. Observe condition of penile skin; if red or broken skin, do not replace clamp.	Less risk of skin trauma and penile ischemia; Insufficient evidence to determine the safety of using device. Reduced blood flow noted with recent study after wearing 50 minutes (Lemmens et al., 2019).
4. Use only during the daytime intermittently when being dry or less wet is important, that is, if going outside of home.	Less risk of skin integrity issues.
5. *Never* use during sleeping hours.	Damage may occur without realization during sleeping hours; prevents risk for penile ischemia and loss.
6. Be aware that the use of compression devices does not completely prevent urine leakage. Consider use of BWAP, that is, guard.	Proper BWAP product selection for light incontinence, that is, guard. Reconsider use if leakage is significant even with compression device.
7. Device maintenance: if reusable device, wash with soap and water and air dry daily. Replace if evidence of damage.	Reduce risk of microbial skin infections or UTIs.
8. Contact continence nurse or doctor to report: • Any skin disruptions or discolorations that do not improve within 24 hours. • Any discharge from penis, pain, burning with urination. • Unable to urinate even after compression device released.	Early interventions will prevent significant complications including penile loss.

Source: Lemmens, J. M., Broadbridge, J., Macaulay, M., et al. (2019). Tissue response to applied loading using different designs of penile compression clamps. *Medical Devices (Auckland, N.Z.), 12,* 235–243. doi: 10.2147/MDER.S188888.

However, the C3 and U-Tex maintained good cavernosal artery blood flow, while the Cunningham clamp caused a significant reduction in arterial flow. Overall, Moore and colleagues concluded that, used correctly, the Cunningham clamp can be an effective method of controlling UI in men with stress UI who are cognitively intact and aware of bladder filling and have normal genital sensation, intact penile skin, and sufficient manual dexterity to open and close the device. However, it should be noted that these devices do not totally eliminate leakage.

Expert opinion and anecdotal reports suggest that penile clamps may be more successful when used for short periods (e.g., while attending meetings or engaging in activities such as swimming or jogging) (Lemmens et al., 2019). Such activities may not only exacerbate incontinence but also preclude the use of bulky and/or absorbent products.

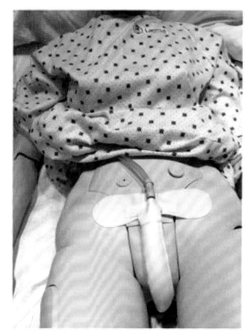

FIGURE 16-19. Female External Collection Device. (From Beeson, T., & Davis, C. (2018). Urinary management with an external female collection device. *Journal of Wound Ostomy and Continence Nursing 45*(2), 187–189.)

KEY POINT

Penile compression devices (penile clamps) should be used only for men with stress incontinence who are cognitively intact and aware of bladder filling and have intact sensation and the ability to open and close the device. Incorrect use can result in ischemic damage and penile loss.

FEMALE EXTERNAL COLLECTION DEVICES

Options for ECD for females have been limited in the past. However, there is new technology available, which is quite novel. This technology shows promise as alternatives for internal urinary catheters (IUC), which are associated with catheter associated urinary tract infection (CAUTI) rates for all settings and provides an option for urine catching that may be safer for patients from a physical standpoint as well. The literature is just evolving for this type of ECD, and currently, just two products in this category are commercially available in the United States (see **Fig. 16-19**).

The ECD for females in this case, is a powered device, in that it must be connected to suction to work effectively. The device itself does not require any electricity to work. The device is somewhat flexible to fit the contour of the female anatomy. After placement, this device is then connected to low suction, which allows for diversion and containment of the urine, thus preserving the perineal area (and buttocks) from erosion from urine wetness and dampness and assisting in prevention of skin breakdown. This device allows for at least some measure of urinary output and provides opportunity for getting out of bed. It is not to be used during transfers or ambulation, but it can be used while the patient is in bed or chair. This breakthrough device is important because the most important risk factor for CAUTI is prolonged use of an indwelling urinary catheter (Centers for Disease Control & Prevention [CDC], 2015). For those patients who need urinary output monitoring, or continued urine containment and diversion, this type of device may be a suitable alternative to the indwelling device.

A literature review found that these types of ECD for females have a 99.9% efficacy of urine capture, and also verified that no further skin breakdown or irritation occurred in patients who used these devices (Glover et al., 2019). One study of 300 reported that use of the ECD in females improved CAUTI rates and found strong evidence supporting integration of the female ECD as a CAUTI bundle element (Dublynn & Episcopia, 2019). Another larger study of 394 patients verified that device decreased the number of IUCs in females, leading to a decrease in CAUTI rates (Mueller, 2019). Lastly, the female ECD has an economic implication to both patients and organizations. In a pilot study of 12 patients, the potential cost savings to patients who used this ECD versus and indwelling urinary catheter was $994, and the total savings to the organization was $1018 per patient (Tran & Rodrique, 2018). A large metropolitan hospital found that patients reported less pain and reported feelings of improved dignity and cleanliness. Additionally, the bedside nurses reported increased satisfaction with the use of a female ECD (Beeson & Davis, 2018). This team also reported that the female ECD was used in female patients successfully, without regard to body habitus, which is encouraging (Beeson & Davis, 2018).

This female ECD does have some clear boundaries for patient selection (**Boxes 16-2** and **16-3**), and it should not be assumed that the device is a reasonable solution for total elimination of indwelling urinary catheters. However, it is also evident that this device has a place in the toolbox of the continence nurse specialist, as well as in the repertoire of the bedside clinician.

Implementation of this type of device should include the reasons to not use the device, the indications for use, along with practical tips for securement, and placement. It is suggested that using a video to educate staff about this information may be a streamlined and efficient way to share the information. It is important for the continence nurse to remember to educate not just nursing colleagues but also all colleagues who may need to understand this device and its utilization, such as physical and occupational therapists, respiratory therapists, and others who may need to move/reposition the patient, or who may assist with basic hygienic needs. Also, family education is important. This device has no barrier to use along the health care continuum, so long as the suction component is available in some form. Additionally, to be noted, a bowel management system can be used for stool containment/management simultaneously with use of the female ECD.

HANDHELD URINALS

Handheld urinals are portable devices designed to allow a person to empty their bladder when access to a toilet is not possible or convenient, due most commonly to mobility, hip abduction, or flexibility limitations. They can be especially helpful for those suffering from frequency and/or urgency. An effective handheld urinal must enable its user to empty the bladder in comfort, require limited physical effort, and be easy to use with no spillage.

Before recommending a handheld urinal, the continence nurse should assess the potential user in terms of the following:

- User postures for voiding (in bed, on side of bed, back in chair, on edge of chair, standing/crouching/ kneeling)
- Leg abduction
- Approach to urinal (from front, side, behind, above)
- Ability to initiate void
- Dexterity and ability to position and remove urinal
- Level and availability of assistance
- User preference

Female Handheld Urinals

Female handheld urinals come in various shapes and sizes (**Fig. 16-20**). Most are molded plastic, but they may be made from metal or single-use cardboard. Some are designed for use in particular postures, like standing, sitting, or lying down. Some have handles to facilitate grip and positioning, and some are designed for use with a drainage bag either during use or immediately after use.

Although female handheld urinals are often described and discussed in general nursing articles on continence products, they have only been the subject of one published crossover evaluation. Fader et al. (1999) carried out a multicenter study in which 37 community-based women (age range of 33 to 89 years; mean age of 61 years) were invited to evaluate all 13 products on the UK market in 1997. No product suited everybody, but each was successful for at least some of the subjects. The key requirements for success were that the user should be able to position the urinal easily and feel confident that it would catch urine without spilling. Many products were successful when used in the standing/crouching position or when sitting on the edge of a chair/bed/wheelchair. Fewer worked well for users sitting in a chair/wheelchair.

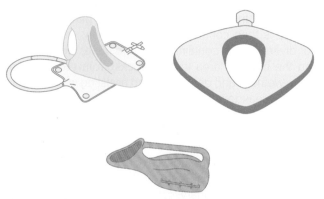

FIGURE 16-20. Various Female Handheld Urinals.

Only one worked even reasonably well when users were lying/semilying (Suba-Seal). In general, subjects with higher levels of dependency found fewer suitable urinals. Future developments may include a powered urinal designed to pump urine into a reservoir (Macaulay et al., 2007). One small study found that female urinals may be helpful in palliative care patients (Farrington et al., 2016).

Male Handheld Urinals

Most handheld urinals for men have a narrowed neck opening into which the penis is placed. Some products come with a detachable or integral nonspill adaptor containing a flutter valve to impede backflow of urine from the urinal. There are no published trials of such products. Recommendations for selecting suitable urinals for men include flat bottom, which may be more stable (and less likely to spill) for those using a urinal in bed; soft plastic jug style or with a funnel for easier grip; lighter weight devices, especially for those with poor manual dexterity; and drainage bag attachment to simplify emptying the urinal for men living at home with limited support. Vickerman (2006) also suggests that homemade devices, such as empty wide-mouthed containers with a handle and lid (e.g., those used for clothes washing liquid or conditioner), might be a practical (and inexpensive) option; however, care would be required to avoid sharp edges if modifying a plastic container. For those with a retracted penis, female urinals may be easier to use than male products.

Effective Use of Urinals

Successful use of urinals depends on many factors (Macaulay et al., 2006; McIntosh, 2001; Vickerman, 2003, 2006):

- Experimentation is often needed to find the optimum urinal. A "library" of urinals (i.e., a collection of different types of urinals to be lent out to users for experimentation) has therefore been recommended, but rigorous cleaning methods are needed.
- Clothing alterations can aid quick and easy use of a urinal. For men, extending the fly opening of trousers or replacing zippers with *Velcro* can be helpful, as can boxer shorts. For women, drop front pants may be needed, particularly if mobility is limited.
- Disposable and reusable "travel" handheld urinals are available for both men and women. These urinals fold away to fit into a pocket and may therefore be more discreetly portable than conventional urinals. They are available at many camping suppliers.
- Some disposable urinals include superabsorbent polymer in their reservoirs, which turn urine into a gel and help to prevent spillage. Sachets of superabsorbent polymer may also be added to reusable urinals.
- Use of a urinal is not always free from leakage, and provision of absorbent chair or bed pads to protect bedding, clothes, and furniture (particularly when testing out urinals) may be necessary.

- The limited range of urinal options in acute settings, where often only bedpans are available, has been criticized, and the process of introducing handheld urinals to hospital services is recommended.
- When used by one individual in the home, urinals can be cleaned with soap and water between uses. If a library of urinals is used, then robust methods are necessary and must be compliant with local infection control procedures.

KEY POINT

Successful selection and use of urinals depends on many factors: user postures for voiding, leg abduction, approach to urinal, ability to initiate void, dexterity and ability to position and remove urinal, level and availability of assistance, user preference, clothing adaptations, reusable or disposable, and care setting.

COMMODES AND BEDPANS

Toilet adaptations such as raised toilet seats, padded seats, and grab rails can be very helpful in enabling individuals with mobility issues to access the toilet easily and comfortably. Bottom wipers and bidets can also be useful. However, if access to the toilet is impossible, commodes and other toileting receptacles should be considered. Nurses should be aware that there are major defects in most of the current commode designs: poor aesthetics, poor trunk support, instability (i.e., a tendency to tip over easily), poor comfort, difficult cleansing, and poor pressure relief.

Defecation on a bedpan or other portable receptacle presents problems with safety and unacceptability to users and should be avoided if possible. A sani-chair/shower chair is usually preferable to a commode if direct transfer to a toilet is impossible or unsafe. The main user concerns about commodes and bedpans are lack of privacy; embarrassment related to noise and odor associated with stool and gas elimination, poor aesthetics, poor perineal cleansing accessibility, and inadequate facilities for cleaning the devices in the home.

If a commode is used, the nurse should assure that good trunk support is provided, the chair is stable, and methods are offered to manage concerns regarding noise and odor. Moreover, with commodes and sani-chairs/shower chairs, the user's buttocks should never be visible to others, and transportation to the toilet and use of the toilet or commode should be carried out with due regard to privacy and dignity. Patients at risk for pressure injuries should not sit on a commode/sani-chair/shower chair for prolonged periods. The person should be provided privacy whenever possible and given a direct method of calling for assistance when left on the toilet/commode/sani-chair/shower chair. Cleaning of bedpans and commodes should be carried out after each use following local infection control policies (in institutional settings).

URINE DRAINAGE BAGS AND ACCESSORIES

Urinary drainage bags are attached to an indwelling catheter or condom catheter to collect and store urine. Features of effective drainage bag systems include ease of operation of all components (connectors, taps, and support devices), comfort, and discreetness. Aspects of assessment that are particularly important regarding urine drainage bags are patient/carer dexterity (Pomfret, 1996, 2006) and eyesight. Both are necessary to manage the drainage bag system, including the outlet tap used to empty the drainage bag. It is also important to assess the patient's preferred and usual mode of dress (Pomfret, 1996, 2006); for example, a male who prefers shorts will want a drainage system that is not visible and allows easy access for emptying urine drainage bags fall into two major categories: leg/body-worn bags for daytime use and large capacity body-free bags for nighttime use (night drainage bags), which are suspended from a stand or bed hook.

LEG-WORN/BODY-WORN BAGS

Leg-worn/body-worn bags come with various features, of which the following are the most important:

- Volume: Most bags have a volume in the range of 350 to 750 mL, but some are larger.
- Material: Most bags are made from transparent PVC (polyvinyl chloride), but PVDF (polyvinylidene fluoride) bags are also available and are associated with less noise from rustling; polyethylene or rubber/latex may be used as well.
- Sterility: Bags may or may not be supplied sterile.
- Wear Position: Bags may be designed to be worn over the knee, across or down the thigh, down the calf, or against the abdomen.
- Attachment/Suspension System: Most leg bags are attached to the leg with straps, which are usually made from latex or an elasticized fabric. Various hooks, loops, buttons/buttonholes, and Velcro may be used to secure straps and to attach bags to straps. Some bags are designed to be suspended around the waist. Some straps and suspension devices can be bought separately from bags, but they are generally not suitable for use with all bags (**Fig. 16-21**).
- Connecting Tube: Leg bags come with various connecting tube lengths, which may impact on selection; for example, the length required for a bag to be worn on the calf will be greater than that for a bag to be worn on the thigh. Some tubes can be cut to the preferred length.
- Drainage Tap: Drainage tap designs vary widely and can be easy or difficult to manage depending on cognition and manual dexterity (**Fig. 16-22**).

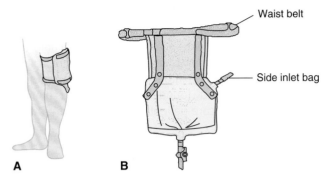

FIGURE 16-21. Body-Worn Urine Drainage Bags Held in Place Using Leg Straps (**A**) and a Waistband Suspension System (**B**).

- Sampling Port: Bags may or may not have a sampling port (for obtaining urine specimens).
- Comfort Backing: Some leg bags have a fabric backing against the skin to reduce sweating and increase comfort.
- Discretion: Some leg bags come with features intended to increase discretion—most commonly, internal welds/folds between the front and back faces to reduce bulging and/or noise caused by a large volume of liquid moving about as the user mobilizes.
- Anti-kinking/Twisting Feature: Some bags come with features intended to improve drainage by reducing kinking and twisting in the connecting tube.
- Infection Reduction Features: The risk of infection may be reduced with a nonreturn valve that reduces reflux of urine up the tubing when the bag is moved, a sampling port, and/or a tap with an outlet sleeve to allow attachment of the overnight bag to the body-worn bag. However, although convenient, there is no evidence that these features reduce UTI incidence. Presealed drainage systems to prevent breaking the closed system are also available, and these could be beneficial in reducing time to bacteriuria (Hooton et al., 2010).

KEY POINT

Urinary drainage bags are available in body-worn (leg bag) and bedside drainage versions; body-worn bags may be designed to be worn over the knee, down the thigh or calf, or against the abdomen.

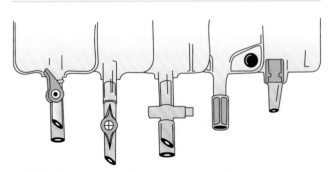

FIGURE 16-22. Various Urine Drainage Bag Tap Designs.

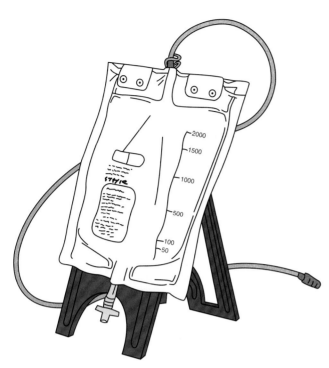

FIGURE 16-23. Night Urine Drainage Bag on a Stand.

NIGHT DRAINAGE BAGS

These bags are also known as "bedside bags" and are usually attached to a suspension system on the bed frame (**Fig. 16-23**). They may be connected directly to the catheter, or they may be connected to the drainage tap of the leg-worn/body-worn bag. They usually have a capacity of 2,000 to 4,000 mL and have various design features, many of which are similar to those for leg-worn/body-worn bags. Night drainage bags are available without a tap (for single use) and with various drainage tap designs for emptying and reuse.

Current standard drainage tubing/bag designs may evacuate the bladder suboptimally, leading to residual urine. Outflow obstruction can be caused by the development of airlocks in the dependent curls or loops of tubing; thus, it is important to avoid dependent loops and to keep the tubing straight and patent in order to assure continuous drainage. Dependent loops permit pooling of urine and require increased bladder pressure to move urine into the drainage bag. In addition, there is no anti-reflux valve between the tubing and the bladder; if the drainage bag is lifted above the bladder, urine in the tubing will drain freely back into the bladder. New drainage tubing designs may incorporate a coiled downward spiral-shaped configuration to eliminate airlock obstruction.

> **KEY POINT**
>
> Dependent loops of drainage tubing create outflow obstruction, and all caregivers must be taught to manage the tubing to prevent dependent loops.

There is little research to support the common practice of changing drainage bags every 5 to 7 days (or any other particular change regime) and little to no guidance on solutions to clean the overnight bag except with soap and water (Royal College of Nursing). These practices appear to be based upon expert opinion, anecdotal evidence, and manufacturers' recommendations.

> **KEY POINT**
>
> The drainage bag should never be lifted above the level of the bladder as this permits urine to drain back into the bladder, increasing the risk of UTI.

INTERMITTENT CATHETERIZATION

The goal of bladder management is to maintain and preserve a functional, infection-free genitourinary system through prevention of upper and lower tract complications with a management system compatible with an injury-free lifestyle (Lisenmeyer et al., 2006). There is no "gold standard" for bladder management (Clinical Practice Guidelines); the implemented strategy must be patient specific and adhere to their QoL. The ideal model is interdisciplinary, responsive, and reality-based in meeting the individual's needs.

There are two techniques for intermittent catheterization: sterile technique and clean technique. Sterile technique was introduced in 1954 by Sir Ludwig Guttman and was described as a way of reducing infection; however, this method is typically utilized only for a restricted period of time by nursing staff, in institutional settings, and is not intended to be a long-term method of bladder management unless the individual has had two documented UTIs in the past year while performing clean intermittent self-catheterization (CISC). CISC accommodates for the difficulty of completing sterile technique in a "real life," normal living environment, preventing high residual volumes, and reducing the risk of UTI. Intermittent self-catheterization (ISC) results in a lower rate of infection compared to indwelling catheters. In order to optimally complete ISC, hands should be washed or aseptic towelettes should be used before and after catheterization. The penis or labia should be cleansed prior to catheter insertion using appropriate wipes, or soap and water. It is important to note that for women, the labia and urethral orifice must be cleaned front to back, to reduce infection risk. See **Box 16-4** for a summary of the technique for male and female catheterization.

Some benefits of ISC are that it can be performed by the individual, caregiver, or health care professional. Intermittent catheterization is the best solution for bladder decompression of motivated individuals who can physically and cognitively participate in their own care (Gill, 2018; Lamin & Newman, 2016). This technique is

---

BOX 16-4 MALE AND FEMALE CATHETERIZATION TECHNIQUE

General Instructions: Catheterize four times per day and before bed or as directed by health care provider. Volumes should not exceed 400 to 500 mL. If this consistently occurs, then catheterize more often or adjust fluid intake.

Preparation: Gather supplies for easy access, position self and arrange clothing for ease of access. Cleanse genitals with soap and water. Wash hands with soap and water or hand sanitizer.

The technique for ISC for males is as follows:

- Extend penis upward at a 90-degree angle (urethra is "S" shaped)
- Insert the catheter until you meet resistance. Relax. Breathe.
- Use coude tip if BPH history; curve or olive tip in the upright position when inserting.
- Apply mild gentle pressure (do not force) until the catheter passes freely and urine begins to flow; pass catheter another 1 to 2 inches once urine flows.
- Once urine stops flowing, pull the catheter back slowly to empty residual urine.

The technique for ISC for females is as follows:

- Separate labia with nondominate hand using first and third fingers; identify clitoris with second finger. Below clitoris is the urethra. Use mirror if necessary, to locate.
- Hold catheter like a pencil about 2 inches from the end; insert the catheter upward into the urethra until urine begins to flow. Relax. Breathe.
- Once urine stops flowing, pull the catheter back slowly to empty residual urine.
- If the catheter is accidentally inserted into vagina/rectum, which is not an uncommon occurrence—It happens!! Do *NOT* reinsert the same catheter into the urethra! Start procedure again with another clean or sterile catheter.

Instructions after catheterizing:

If performing clean technique: Wash catheter with soap and hot water, rinse with hot water; place catheter in paper towel to air dry. Store dried catheters in clean plastic container or plastic bag. Replace catheter weekly and if damaged.

Source: Newman and Willson (2011).

---

preferred by men and women, over indwelling catheters, as a healthy alternative for bladder management. ISC may be performed anywhere there is privacy. It promotes patient autonomy through freedom from indwelling catheters, tubes, and collection bags. Individuals may have unimpeded sexual relations, as ISC provides a means of complete bladder emptying without an indwelling catheter. ISC preserves function of upper tract, while preventing over-distention of the bladder. Moreover, it decreases the risk of UTI and urethral trauma and increases independence in self care as it simulates a normal voiding schedule and maintains continence (Dorsher & McIntosh, 2012).

Just as before the injury or diagnoses, the bladder must be drained on a regular basis at timed intervals (every 4, 6, or 8 hours), depending on bladder volume

(Taweel & Seyam, 2015). The average adult bladder holds approximately 300 to 500 mL of urine. In a clinical setting, postvoid residual (PVR) volumes may be monitored to assess need for ISC: <50 mL is "normal," >50 to 100 is abnormal and may be managed with IC depending upon the residual volume (Ballstaedt & Woodbury, 2019). Ideally, the amount drained should not exceed 400 to 500 mL. If the volume is regularly more or less, fluid intake and frequency of catheterization will need to be reassessed.

In regard to pediatric ISC, the primary consideration is who will be performing ISC: parent, school nurse, caregiver, or the individual. It is important to understand that when the child shows interest in ISC, and has the functional capacity to learn, they can be taught. However, supervision for optimal technique is important for prevention of incontinence and UTIs.

KEY POINT

The pediatric patient should be catheterized every 4 hours, and schedule maintenance is key.

EDUCATION AND TRAINING

The first step for a successful bladder management program is to educate and inform the individual. Review anatomy (Do NOT assume!). Provide input regarding effectiveness of a bladder program relative to their daily routines. Clinicians must have a full understanding of the individual's bladder needs, in order to promote independence, compliance, and QoL.

Catheter selection is dictated somewhat by insurance coverage. However, the clinician and the patient will work together to determine an appropriate product based on the individual's hand function, body habitus, balance, strength, environment for ISC, and routines, as well as assessing the type of preferred lubricant, rigidity of catheter, length, and circumference (French) in promoting compliance and independence.

There are a multitude of factors to assess when determining best practice for ISC (Yates, 2013):

- Consideration of feasibility of the bladder management program integration within the individual's life
- Physical abilities
- Dexterity
- Core flexibility
- Strength
- Balance/posture
- Cognitive function
- Sensation
- Tone
- Willingness to learn/anxiety
- Personal factors
- Environmental factors
- Cultural and spiritual beliefs

- Roles
- Routines
- Bowel function
- Support of family/caregivers
- Financial considerations

ENVIRONMENTAL FACTORS

ISC is more dynamic than bladder drainage. It is important to consider the patient, as well as where they will be performing ISC (bed, power wheelchair, manual wheelchair, over the commode, public restroom, etc). As clinicians, it is easy to become desensitized on how much we facilitate success in the hospital setting; however, the real world is not as conducive to the ease of ISC. It is also crucial to trial strategies and techniques for clothing management, including the implementation of adaptive equipment. Is the individual more successful managing their clothes in their wheelchair or over the commode? When is the individual going to assume proper positioning for ISC, before or after their clothes are managed? Are they ambulatory?

POSITIONING

As previously stated, it is important to note that not every individual will perform ISC in a bed, nor will they have access to hospital bed functions (elevating head, bed rails). To set patients up for success, they must perform ISC in various real-life settings and positions that will be most common for their lifestyle (see Appendix 16-A at the end of chapter).

ISC has been proven to be an effective method of bladder emptying and infection prevention when proper technique is followed. Transitioning from sterile technique to clean technique is less cumbersome and more adequate for implementation into "real-life." ISC is dynamic and requires input from the interdisciplinary team for patient success, independence, and QoL. Referrals to occupational therapists can provide further insight in developing adaptations to the procedure with additional assistant aides and individualized positions to facilitate successful bladder management program.

ADAPTIVE EQUIPMENT

Depending on the patient's functional ability and the circumstances under which they will be performing ISC, there is a variety of adaptive equipment available that can facilitate an individual's ability to self-catheterize (Holderbaum, 2019). See **Box 16-5** and **Appendix 16-A** and **B** at the end of this chapter.

 ## INCONTINENCE-ASSOCIATED DERMATITIS

The skin of an incontinent individual will be regularly exposed to contact with urine and/or feces, which places the individual at high risk for skin damage. Skin irritation within the pad occlusion area is usually termed diaper

BOX 16-5	**ADAPTIVE EQUIPMENT TO FACILITATE INTERMITTENT SELF-CATHETERIZATION (ISC)**

- Mirrors
  - Great tool for initial education during ISC (anatomy, technique/strategies) or long-term use for females
  - Individuals who need visual feedback during ISC
- Pants holder, Betty hook, Bungee
  - Keeps clothing out of the way during ISC
    - *Top hook goes into the waistband of pants, bottom bar is inserted between wheelchair cushion and seat
  - Males performing ISC
- Catheter inserter
  - Maintains grip and coordinated insertion of catheter
    - *Easy clamp allows for independent use
  - Individuals with impaired hand function who have difficulty grasping catheter
- Penis stabilizer
  - Keeps the penis stable and in proper position for ISC. Allows for hands-free approach during ISC management.
  - Males with impaired hand function.
- Asta-Cath
  - When inserted into the vaginal canal, the urethral opening will coincide with one of the holes, guiding the catheter and promoting independence.
  - Females performing ISC.

*See Appendices 16A & B.

dermatitis in infants. In adults, the more accurate term is *incontinence-associated dermatitis (IAD)*; this is a better term because the affected skin areas are not confined to the perineum (Gray et al., 2007) but frequently extend to involve the buttocks, hips, and sacrum. These areas are very high risk for damage because they are exposed to pressure, shear, and friction as well as stool and urine. IAD is one of four types of moisture-associated skin damage (MASD). MASD is the result of prolonged exposure of the skin to wetness such as with urine, stool, wound drainage, saliva, or mucus (Beekman, 2017; Black et al., 2011; Gray et al., 2012). Chapter 17 provides a thorough discussion to this topic, but for the purpose of this chapter, IAD will be discussed as it relates to BWAPs.

KEY POINT

The most accurate term for skin damage caused by prolonged or recurrent contact with stool and/or urine is *incontinence-associated dermatitis*

KEY POINT

The major mechanisms of damage in IAD include changes in pH and wetness.

PREVENTION AND MANAGEMENT OF IAD

Measures to maintain or restore skin health are a critical element of care for individuals with incontinence who require use of absorbent products. These measures include product selection, frequent hygienic care, and protective skin products.

Superabsorbent Polymers and Shaped Fibers

The characteristics of BWAPs are important in the prevention of IAD. In the 1980s, product manufacturers introduced diapers with SAP, which were designed to reduce skin wetness, buffer pH, and reduce skin contact with urine and stool. The effectiveness of SAP in reducing skin wetness (measured by TEWL), reducing pH, and reducing severity of diaper dermatitis was demonstrated in infants. Only one study, now 20 years old (Brown, 1993, 1994; Brown et al., 1995), has been conducted on adults with UI. The authors reported better skin scores in those who were assigned to SAP products indicating skin health benefits of SAP. Other studies have produced insufficient evidence in relation to SAPs versus other absorbent materials in BWAPs (Brazzelli et al., 1999), and further research with well-controlled studies is required to better understand the full benefit of SAP.

In recent years, advances in product technology have results in improved skin protection. Shaped fibers have been added into the layers of diapers, just under the top layer of the diaper that goes against the skin. The fibers have added even more absorbency to the polymer layers and result in positive effects on the skin. For example, a design change that incorporated spiral shaped fibers was studied. One study found that the use of absorbent products that contained these spiral-shaped fibers decreased the pH of the skin in elderly (Bliss et al., 2017). Curly-shaped fibers were used in briefs, and breathable side panels were also added. This design led to both a decrease in pH in the adult skin, as well as decreased the maceration of the skin by allowing more air exchange secondary to the breathable side panels (Beguin et al., 2010), thus favoring a healthier microclimate for skin health.

> **KEY POINT**
>
> Evidence about enhancing diaper design is favorable and use of briefs to prevent IAD may be very reasonable in some patients.

Frequent Checks and Prompt Change for Wet or Soiled Products

Prompt replacement of a wet or soiled BWAP also reduces skin wetness and may therefore benefit skin health (Berg, 1987). In the inpatient setting, current recommendations also include leaving absorbent products open underneath the patient whenever he or she is in bed; this keeps the perineal skin cooler and drier and thus more resistant to both IAD and friction damage (Gray et al., 2012). However, change times of absorptive products should be patient centered, based on skin health, odor control, sleep, and elimination patterns and dignity, and should also consider product properties (Gray et al., 2018b). Additionally, especially for fecal incontinence, products should be changed as soon as possible to preserve skin health and promote odor control and dignity. Change times for BWAPs should never be based on routine or caregiver convenience (Gray et al., 2018b).

> **KEY POINT**
>
> Prompt replacement of a wet or soiled product with a dry BWAP reduces skin wetness and may therefore benefit skin health. For individuals experiencing fecal incontinence, products should be changed as soon as possible to preserve skin health and promote odor control and dignity. Change times for BWAPs should *never* be based on routine or caregiver convenience.

Preventive Skin Care and the Use of Body-Worn Absorbent Products

There are no data to indicate that one skin protectant is superior to another; however, there are much data indicating that any standardized protocol that addresses the two key elements of cleansing and using a moisture barrier product consistently significantly reduces the incidence of IAD (McNichol et al., 2018). Also, there is evidence that some leave-on skin products may clog absorbent products and impair liquid acquisition into the product, but the findings are mixed and do not provide clear guidance for use of barrier products in combination with BWAPs (Dykes & Bradbury, 2016; Fleming et al., 2014).

> **KEY POINT**
>
> There are no data to indicate that one barrier product is superior to another; however, there are much data indicating that any standardized skin care protocol that addresses the key elements of cleansing and using a moisture barrier product consistently and significantly reduces the incidence of IAD.

CONCLUSION

Evidence-based product choices remain problematic because of the lack of RCTs in the area of containment. The challenge for researchers is that products are continually improved or modified, so trial results can become outdated quickly. More important perhaps is the user's evaluation of product designs—for example, in men, comparisons of penile clamps, condom catheters, and/

or incontinence pads and exploring the subjective aspects of product use. A patient-centered, collaborative approach to choose the best product for the individual is required because choices differ between users, degree of incontinence, and length of use.

Teaching the individual or the caregiver about skin care is critical as IAD is a common problem among absorbent product users and skin wetness overhydrates skin, potentiates the effects of other irritants, and increases the risk of friction, abrasive damage, and pressure injury development (Gray & Giuliano, 2018). Those individuals with both urinary and fecal incontinence (especially liquid stool) are in a very high-risk group for skin issues since fecal matter is more irritating than urine, and preventative measures must be taken to protect the vulnerable skin. Although most hospitals have a skin care protocol with appropriate products, individuals cared for at home may be using less optimal regimens, which may negatively affect skin health and pH. Caregivers and individuals with incontinence may require guidance on a regular and structured skin care regimen using appropriate cleansers, or moisture barrier creams with a particular focus on skin folds and those areas of the perigenital skin in direct contact with urine and stool.

The continence care nurse performs a fundamental role in assisting individuals in proper containment choices that is individualized, effective, ascetically pleasing, cost-effective and supports personal dignity. Product choices, patient teaching, and ongoing follow-up are critical for effective and dignified continence control, maintaining a safe bladder emptying program and promoting skin health in the care of an individual with urinary and fecal incontinence.

ACKNOWLEDGMENT

Special thanks to Dianne Mackey for her contribution to this chapter regarding underpads: their evolution and use.

REFERENCES

Ballstaedt, L., & Woodbury, B. (March 31, 2019). *Bladder post void residual volume*. Treasure Island, FL: StatPearls Publishing.

Barnard, J., & Westenberg, A. M. (2014). The penile clamp: Medieval pain or makeshift gain? *Neurourology Urodynamics, 34*, 115–16. doi: 10.1002/nau.22597.

Beekman, D. (2017). A decade of research on Incontinence-Associated Dermatitis (IAD): Evidence, knowledge gaps and next steps. *Journal of Tissue Viability, 26*(1), 47–56.

Beeson, T., & Davis, C. (2018). Urinary management with an external female collection device. *Journal of Wound Ostomy & Continence Nursing, 45*(2), 187–189.

Beguin, A. M., Malaquin-Pavan, E., Guihaire, C., et al. (2010). Improving diaper design to address incontinence associated dermatitis. *Biomed Central Geriatrics, 10*(86), 1–10.

Berg, R. W. (1987). Etiologic factors in diaper dermatitis: A model for development of improved diapers. *Pediatrician, 14*(1), 27–33.

Black, J. M., Gray, M., Bliss, D. Z., et al. (2011). MASD Part 2: Incontinence-associated dermatitis and intertriginous dermatitis, a

consensus. *Journal of Wound Ostomy & Continence Nursing, 38*(4), 359–170.

Bliss, D. Z., Bland, P., Wiltzen, K., et al. (2017). Incontinence briefs containing spiral-shaped fiber acidify skin pH of older nursing home residents at risk for incontinence-associated dermatitis. *Journal of Wound Ostomy & Continence Nursing, 44*(5), 475–480.

Brazzelli, M., Shirran, E. E. A. S., Vale, L. (1999). Absorbent products for containing urinary and/or faecal incontinence in adults. *Cochrane Database of Systematic Reviews*, (3), CD001406.

Brown, D. S. (1993). Perineal dermatitis: Can we measure it? *Ostomy Wound Management, 39*(7), 28–32.

Brown, D. S. (1994). Diapers and underpads, Part 1: Skin integrity outcomes. *Ostomy Wound Management, 40*(9), 20–22, 24–26, 28 passim.

Brown, D. S., Small, S., & Jones, D. (1995). Standardizing skin care across settings. *Ostomy Wound Management, 41*(10), 40–43.

Centers for Disease Control and Prevention (2015). *Catheter-associated urinary tract infections (CAUTI)*. Retrieved April 29, 2020 from https://www.cdc.gov/hai/ca_uti/uti.html

Cottenden, A., Fader, M., Beeckman, D., et al. (2017). Management using continence products. In P. Abrams, L. Cardozo, A. Wagg, et al., (Eds.), *Incontinence* (6th ed., pp. 2303–2426). Bristol, UK: International Continence Society.

Dorsher, P. T., & McIntosh, P. M. (2012). Neurogenic bladder. *Advances in Urology, 2012*. Retrieved from https://www.hindawi.com/journals/au/2012/816274/

Dublynn, T., & Episcopia, B. (2019). Female external catheter use: A new bundle element to reduce CAUTI. *American Journal of Infection Control, 47*(6), S39–S40.

Dykes, P., & Bradbury, S. (2016). Incontinence and absorption and skin barrier creams: A non-patients study. *British Journal of Nursing, 25*(22), 1244–1248.

Fader, M., Pettersson, L., Dean, G., et al. (1999). The selection of female urinals: Results of a multicentre evaluation. *British Journal of Nursing, 8*(14), 918–5.

Farrington, N., Hill, T., Fader, M., et al. (2016). Supporting women with toileting in palliative care: Use of the female urinal for bladder management. *International Journal of Palliative Nursing, 22*(11), 524–533.

Fleming, L., Zala, K., & Ousey, K. (2014). Investigating the absorbency of LBF barrier cream. *Wounds UK, 10*(2), 24–30.

Fonda, D., & Abrams, P. (2006). Cure sometimes, help always—a "continence paradigm" for all ages and conditions. *Neurourology and Urodynamics, 25*(3), 290–292.

Francis, K., Pang, S. M., Cohen, B., et al. (2017). Disposable versus reusable absorbent underpads for prevention of hospital-acquired incontinence-associated dermatitis and pressure injuries. *Journal of Wound Ostomy Continence Nursing, 44*(4), 374–379.

Gibb, H., & Wong, G. (1994). How to choose: Nurses' judgements of the effectiveness of a range of currently marketed continence aids. *Journal of Clinical Nursing, 3*(2), 77–86.

Gill, B. C. (2018). What is intermittent catheterization for the treatment of neurogenic bladder? *Medscape*. Retrieved from https://www.medscape.com/answers/453539-51618/what-is-intermittent-catheterization-for-the-treatment-of-neurogenic-bladder

Glover, E., Bleeker, E., Bauermeister, A., et al. (2019). External catheters and reducing adverse effects in the female inpatient. Northwestern College, Department of Nursing. Retrieved April 29, 2020 from https://nwcommons.nwciowa.edu/cgi/viewcontent.cgi?article=1026&context=celebrationofresearch

Golji, H. (1981). Complications of external condom drainage. *Paraplegia, 19*(3), 189–197.

Gray, M., Beeckman, D., Bliss, D. Z., et al. (2012). Incontinence-associated dermatitis: A comprehensive review and update. *Journal of Wound Ostomy & Continence Nursing, 39*(1), 61–74.

Gray, M., Beeson, T., Kent, D., et al. (2020). Interventions post catheter removal (iPCaRe) in the acute care setting. *Journal of Wound, Ostomy and Continence Nursing, 47*(6), 601–618.

Gray, M., Bliss, D. Z., Doughty, D. B., et al. (2007). Incontinence-associated dermatitis: A consensus. *Journal of Wound, Ostomy, and Continence Nursing, 34*(1), 45–54.

Gray, M., Ermer-Seltun, J., Kent, D., et al. (2018a). Setting the standard for body worn absorbent products: Results of the WOCN Consensus Conference, Lecture, June 3, Powerpoint slides.

Gray, M., & Giuliano, K. (2018). Incontinence-associated dermatitis, characteristics, and relationship to pressure injury: A multisite epidemiologic analysis. *Journal of Wound, Ostomy, and Continence Nursing, 45*(1), 63–67.

Gray, M., Kent, D., Ermer-Seltun, J., et al. (2018b). Assessment, selection, use and evaluation of body-worn absorbent products for adults with incontinence. *Journal of Wound, Ostomy, and Continence Nursing, 45*(3), 243–264.

Gray, M., Skinner, C., & Kaler, W. (2016). External collection devices as an alternative to the indwelling urinary catheter. *Journal of Wound Ostomy Continence Nursing, 43*(3), 301–307.

Hasler, E., (Ed.). (2019). European Pressure Injury Advisory Panel, National Pressure Injury Advisory Panel and Pan Pacific Pressure Injury Alliance. Prevention and treatment of pressure injury/injuries: Quick reference guide.

Hocking, C. (1999). Function or feelings: Factors in abandonment of assistive devices. *Technology and Disability*, (11), 3–11.

Holderbaum, L. (September, 2019). Clean intermittent catheterization: Guidelines for healthcare professionals. Presented at WOCN Iowa Affiliate Fall Conference. Johnson, Iowa, United States.

Hooton, T. M., Bradley, S. F., Cardenas, D. et al. (2010). Diagnosis, prevention, and treatment of catheter-associated urinary tract infection in adults: 2009 International Clinical Practice Guidelines from the Infectious Diseases Society of America. Clinical Infectious Diseases: *An Official Publication of the Infectious Diseases Society of America, 50*(5), 625–663. https://doi.org/10.1086/650482

International Organization for Standardization (ISO). (2017). Urine-Absorbing Aids—General Guidelines on Evaluation ISO/FDIS 15621: 2017. Retrieved from https://www.iso.org/standard/65740.html. Accessed April 26, 2020.

Kalra, S., Srinivas, P. R., Manikandan, R., et al. (2015). Urethral diverticulum: A potential hazard of penile clamp application for male urinary incontinence. *BMJ case reports, 2015*, bcr2015209957. doi: 10.1136/bcr-2015-209957.

Lamin, E., & Newman, D. (2016). Clean intermittent catheterization revisited. *International Urology and Nephrology, 48*, 931–939.

Leander, H. (2019). Standards for incontinence management products. *Proceedings of the Institution of Mechanical Engineers. Part H, Journal of Engineering in Medicine, 233*(1), 19–22.

Lemmens, J. M., Broadbridge, J., Macaulay, M., et al. (2019). Tissue response to applied loading using different designs of penile compression clamps. *Medical devices (Auckland, N.Z.), 12*, 235–243. doi: 10.2147/MDER.S188888.

Lisenmeyer, T. A., Bodner, D. R., Creasey, G. H., et al. (2006). Consortium for spinal cord medicine. bladder management for adults with spinal cord injury: A clinical practice guideline for health-care providers. *Journal of Spinal Cord Medicine, 29*(5), 527–573.

Low, J. (1996). Negotiating identities, negotiating environments: An interpretation of the experiences of students with disabilities. *Disability and society, 11*(2), 235–248.

Macaulay, M., Clarke-O'Neill, S., Cottenden, A., et al. (2006). Female urinals for women with impaired mobility. *Nursing Times, 102*(42), 42–43, 45, 47.

Macaulay, M., van den, H. E., Jowitt, F., et al. (2007). A noninvasive continence management system: Development and evaluation of a novel toileting device for women. *Journal of Wound, Ostomy, & Continence Nursing, 34*(6), 641–648.

McIntosh, J. (2001). A guide to female urinals. *Nursing Times, 97*(6), VII–VIX.

McNichol, L., Ayello, E. A., Phearman, L. A., et al. (2018). Incontinence-associated dermatitis: State of the science and knowledge translation. *Advances in Skin & Wound Care, 31*(11), 501–513.

Mitteness, L. S., & Barker, J. C. (1995). Stigmatizing a "normal" condition: Urinary incontinence in late life. *Medical Anthropology Quarterly, 9*(2), 188–210.

Moore, K. N., Schieman, S., Ackerman, T., et al. (2004). Assessing comfort, safety, and patient satisfaction with three commonly used penile compression devices. *Urology, 63*(1), 150–154.

Mueller, C. (2019). Finally! An external female catheter device for women! *American Journal of Infection Control, 47*(6), S13. doi: 10.1016/j.ajic.2019.04.164.

Muller, C., & McInnis, E. (2013). The development of national quality performance standards for disposable absorbent products for adult incontinence. *Ostomy Wound Management, 59*(9), 40–45.

Newman, D., & Willson, M. (2011). Review of intermittent catheterization and current best practices. *Urologic Nursing*, (1), 12–28, 48.

Öz, Ö., & Altay, B. (2018). Relationships among use of complementary and alternative interventions, urinary incontinence, quality of life, and self-esteem in women with urinary incontinence. *Journal of Wound, Ostomy & Continence Nursing, 45*(2), 174–178.

Paterson, J. (2000). Stigma associated with post-prostatectomy urinary incontinence. *Journal of Wound, Ostomy & Continence Nursing, 27*(3), 168–173.

Paterson, J., Dunn, S., Kowanko, I., et al. (2003). Selection of continence products: Perspectives of people who have incontinence and their carers. *Disability and Rehabilitation, 25*(17), 955–963.

Pemberton, P., Brooks, A., Eriksen, C. M., et al. (2006). A comparative study of two types of urinary sheath. *Nursing Times, 102*(7), 36–41.

Pomfret, I. J. (1996). Catheters: Design, selection and management. *British Journal of Nursing, 5*(4), 245–251.

Pomfret, I. (2006). Penile sheaths: A guide to selection and fitting. *Journal of Community Nursing, 20*(11), 14–18.

Potter, J. (2007). Male urinary incontinence-could penile sheaths be the answer? *Journal of Community Nursing, 21*(5), 4042.

Proudfoot, L. M., Farmer, E. S., & McIntosh, J. B. (1994). Testing incontinence pads using single-case research designs. *British Journal of Nursing, 3*(7), 316, 318–320, 322.

Shaw, C., Tansey, R., Jackson, C., et al. (2001). Barriers to help seeking in people with urinary symptoms. *Family Practice, 18*(1), 48–52.

Taweel, W., & Seyam, R. (2015). Neurogenic bladder in spinal cord injury patients. *Research and Reports in Urology, 7*, 85–99.

Tran, C., & Rodrique, D. (2018). An Alternative to the Indwelling Foley Catheter in Incontinent Female Patients [Poster presentation]. NACNS National Conference, Austin, TX, United States. Retrieved April 29, 2020 from http://www.nacns.org/wp-content/uploads/2018/02/Poster-58-Tran.pdf

Vickerman, J. (2003). The benefits of a lending library for female urinals. *Nursing Times, 99*(44), 56–57.

Vickerman, J. (2006). Selecting urinals for male patients. *Nursing Times, 102*(19), 47–48.

Wagg, A., Gove, D., Leichsenring, K., et al. (2019). Development of quality outcome indicators to improve the quality of urinary and faecal continence care. *International Urogynecology Journal, 30*(1), 23–32.

Wan, X., Wang, C., Xu, D., et al. (2014). Disease stigma and its mediating effect on the relationship between symptom severity and quality of life among community-dwelling women with stress urinary incontinence: A study from a Chinese city. *Journal of Clinical Nursing, 23*(15–16), 2170–2179.

White, C. F. (2003). Proceedings of the institution of mechanical engineers. *Part H—Journal of Engineering in Medicine, 217*(4), 243–251.

Wittink, H., & Oosterhaven, J. (2018). Patient education and health literacy. *Musculoskeletal Science and Practice, 38*, 120–127.

Yates, A. (2013). Teaching Intermittent catheterization: barriers. *Nursing Times, 109*(44), 22–25.

Zisberg, A. (2011). Incontinence brief use in acute hospitalized patients with no prior incontinence. *Journal of Wound Ostomy Continence Nursing, 38*(5), 559–564.

QUESTIONS

1. The continence nurse is considering a product to use for a female patient who has very light urinary incontinence. What would be an appropriate recommendation?
   A. Menstrual pad
   B. Guard product
   C. Disposable brief
   D. Disposable underpants

2. A male patient complains of light fecal incontinence. What product would the incontinence nurse recommend for this patient?
   A. Disposable underpants
   B. Washable underpants
   C. Absorbent disposable pad
   D. Soft pad or gauze between the buttocks

3. For which patient experiencing heavy urine loss would a male condom catheter be the most appropriate continence product?
   A. A patient who has failed clean intermittent catheterization
   B. A patient with limited mobility and who is experiencing frequency
   C. A patient who is considered psychologically vulnerable
   D. A patient with decreased genital sensation

4. Your patient is a 24-year-old male with T3 paraplegia after a dirt bike accident. What is the first step toward independent ISC?
   A. Review his insurance and provide him with products that will be covered.
   B. Provide education on anatomy, and the process for independent ISC.
   C. Provide him with adaptive equipment and discuss clothing management.
   D. Do nothing; this is outside your scope of practice and is the responsibility of nursing.

5. The Continence care nurse is teaching intermittent self-catheterization (ISC) to an individual with paraplegia. Which of the following is NOT an example of an adaptive equipment used for ISC?
   A. Penis stabilizer
   B. Asta-Cath
   C. Bungee cord
   D. Penile compression device

6. The continence nurse is assisting a male patient who has urge incontinence to choose a handheld urinal. Which of the following is a recommended guideline?
   A. Choose a urinal with a curved bottom.
   B. Do not use a handheld urinal if penis is retracted.
   C. Choose a lighter-weight urinal device.
   D. Avoid using homemade urinal devices such as empty detergent bottles.

7. Which of the following is the primary user concern when using commodes and bedpans for defecation?
   A. Safety
   B. User friendliness
   C. Device design
   D. Lack of privacy

8. Which of the following is the most appropriate intervention for a nonambulatory 52-year-old female with neurogenic bladder, who is a heavy gusher?
   A. Indwelling urinary catheter
   B. Booster pad with brief
   C. External female collection (suction) device
   D. Superabsorbent underpad

9. The continence nurse is teaching a patient how to use a urinary drainage bag. Which teaching point follows recommended practice for use of this device?
   A. Most bags have a volume in the range of 350 to 750 mL.
   B. All drainage bags are supplied sterile.
   C. Nonreturn valves on the devices are proven to reduce UTIs.
   D. The drainage bag should be lifted above the level of the bladder.

10. A physician calls for your advice about which type of incontinence product his or her patient needs. Your actions may include which of the following?
    A. E-mail the doctor a copy of your product formulary.
    B. Refer to the PSAG tool.
    C. Educate the MD about the electronic BWAP Guide and work the problem together.
    D. Refer the MD to the urologist for assistance.

ANSWERS AND RATIONALES

1. A. Rationale: A menstrual pad is an appropriate option for a woman with very light UI and has the advantage of being less costly than incontinence-specific products.

2. D. Rationale: Products for light fecal incontinence are limited and placing a soft pad or gauze between the buttocks is often the best option.

3. B. Rationale: A male condom catheter is a good option for a man with urinary frequency and limited mobility that makes regular toileting difficult.

4. B. Rationale: The first step in preparing patients to perform ISC is to educate them about lower urinary tract anatomy and teach the self-catheterization technique.

5. D. Rationale: A penile compression device is used to reduce symptoms of stress incontinence in cognitively intact men. All the other options listed are adaptive equipment for individuals who have functional limitations that make it difficult for them to self-catheterize.

6. C. Rationale: Selecting a lightweight urinal device will make it easier for patients to handle without risk of spills. Some patients will need to try several different types of urinals to find the one that works best for them.

7. D. Rationale: Lack of privacy during defecation is often an issue when a patient must use a portable commode or bedpan.

8. B. Rationale: Adding a booster pad to a brief increases its absorptive capacity and will decrease the chance of the brief leaking.

9. A. Rationale: It is important to educate the patient of the volume of urine that the bag he or she is using.

10. C. Rationale: The Wound Ostomy Continence Nurses Society™ electronic BWAP Guide is an excellent resource that you can share with your colleague.

BEST PRACTICE

Clean intermittent self-catheterization (CISC) or intermittent self-catheterization (ISC) is more dynamic than just bladder drainage. It is important to consider the patient, as well as where the patient will be performing ISC (bed, power wheelchair, manual wheelchair, over the commode, public restroom, etc). ISC can be performed anywhere, and promotes the individual's autonomy as it provides greater freedom from alternatives such as catheters, tubes, or bags.

As clinicians, it is easy to become desensitized on how much we facilitate success in the hospital setting; however, the real world is not as conducive to the ease of ISC.

It is also crucial to trial strategies and techniques for clothing management, including the implementation of adaptive equipment. Is the individual more successful managing his or her clothes in the wheelchair or over the commode? When is the individual going to assume proper positioning for ISC, before or after his or her clothes are managed? Is he or she ambulatory?

POSITIONING

As previously stated, it's important to note that not every individual will perform ISC in a bed, nor will they have access to hospital bed functions (elevating head, bed-rails). To set patients up for success, they must perform ISC in various, real-life settings and in positions that will be most common for their lifestyle.

FACTORS TO CONSIDER

1. *Is the individual more successful managing the clothes in the wheelchair or over the commode?*

2. *When is the individual going to assume proper positioning for ISC, before or after the clothes are managed?*
3. *Is the individual ambulatory?*

Males

Intermittent catheterization can be completed in bed, in the wheelchair, or standing, if able, the goal being complete bladder emptying. It is important to note that the patient is in a position in which he can achieve independence, so as not to restrict urinary flow. Therefore, a somewhat extended truncal position is ideal.

He may choose to drain into a urinal, directly into the commode, or using a closed system catheter with a bag attached, if insurance permits.

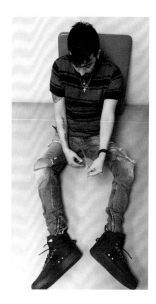

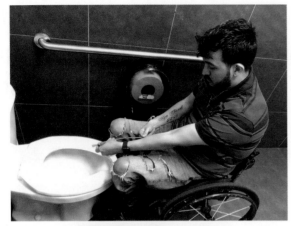

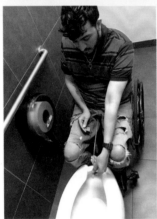

- Posterior pelvic tilt
- Truncal extension
- Lower extremities externally rotated, if able

Optimal positioning in wheelchair:

- Posterior pelvic tilt
- Truncal extension
- Lower extremities externally rotated, if able
- To achieve this, the first step is scooting to the edge of the seat cushion

Tip: This can be scary, and it's common for ladies to not scoot forward far enough to achieve urethral access. Once on the edge of the cushion, if she looks between her legs and sees her cushion, she is most likely not far enough forward for adequate posterior pelvic tilt.

- The photo below exhibits no cushion visibility, which will facilitate urethral access and bladder emptying.

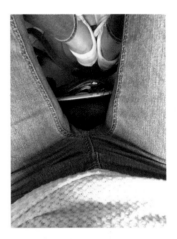

Females

Intermittent catheterization can be completed in bed, in the wheelchair, or sitting on the commode; the goal is complete bladder emptying. For independent completion of intermittent catheterization in any setting, a significant posterior pelvic tilt is crucial for optimal urethral accessibility.

Depending on the circumstances in which she chooses to perform intermittent catheterization, she may drain into a urinal, directly into the commode (using a male-length catheter, an extended-length catheter, or an extension tub attachment), or using a closed system catheter with a bag attached, if insurance permits.

Optimal positioning in bed:

She may choose to put one or both legs on top of the commode. Functional skills and factors to consider are body habitus, strength, balance, and energy conservation, as well as clothing management. It is also important to determine when and how she will manage all supplies for intermittent cathing, as once she is in position for completion, it may be difficult for her to reach, depending on the setup.

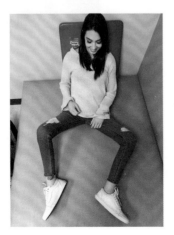

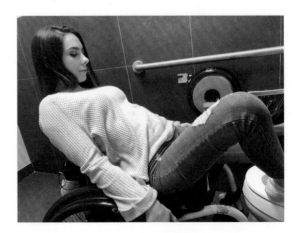

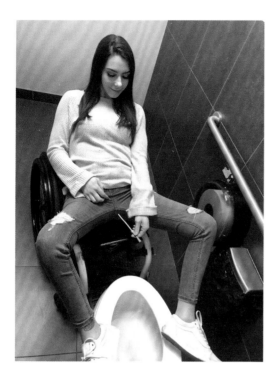

Optimal positioning over the commode:

- Posterior pelvic tilt
- Truncal extension
- Lower extremities externally rotated, if able

Important considerations:

- Will she manage her clothing before, or after she transfers?
- Where will she store her supplies for accessible reach?
- Does she require use of a grab bar for balance?

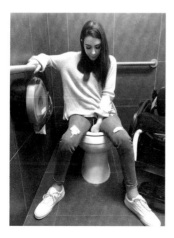

CONCLUSION

In conclusion, the benefits of ISC as a means of promoting bladder health and management, by reducing the incidence of UTI, are vital to enable individuals to participate in everyday life.

The clinician and the patient work together as a team to determine and implement an ideal method. Determination of the most appropriate techniques and strategies will be based on factors such as the individual's hand function, body habitus, balance, strength, environment for ISC, lifestyle, and routines.

ISC is dynamic and requires input from the interdisciplinary team for patient success, independence, and quality of life.

MODELS

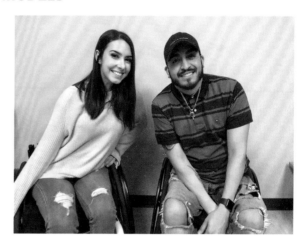

Anthony Sanchez

Anthony Sanchez is a T4 complete paraplegic, from a motorcycle accident in 2014. He enjoys spending time with his daughter Mya, working out, partying with friends, and attending sporting events and concerts.

#AISC
Ant Can, I CAN!

Kathryn Georgiou

Kathryn Georgiou has a complete T10 and an incomplete C5 spinal cord injury, and is also a Registered Nurse. She loves making art, riding her hand-cycle, and watching bad reality television.

Special "Thank You" to photographer Leah Holderbaum and ISC models, Anthony Sanchez and Kathryn Georgiou, in creating a visual learning opportunity in positioning for independent ISC.

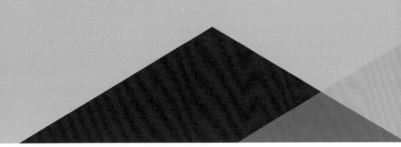

APPENDIX 16B
ADAPTIVE EQUIPMENT TO PROMOTE ISC INDEPENDENCE

INTRODUCTION

The goal of bladder management is to maintain and preserve a functional, infection-free genitourinary system through prevention of upper and lower tract complications with a management system compatible with an injury-free lifestyle (Lisenmeyer, 2006).

There is no "gold standard" for bladder management (Clinical Practice Guidelines); the implemented strategy must be specific to the individual, and enhance his or her quality of life. The ideal model is interdisciplinary, responsive, and reality based in proactively meeting the individual's needs.

Clean intermittent self-catheterization (CISC) or intermittent self-catheterization (ISC) can be performed by the individual, caregiver, or health care professional. ISC is the best solution for bladder decompression for motivated individuals who can physically and cognitively participate in their own care (Gill, 2018). In addition, this technique is preferred by men and women, over the use of an indwelling catheter, as a healthy alternative for bladder management.

Based on the individual's diagnosis, some barriers to independent ISC may be present. Adaptive equipment and modified strategies may be implemented to facilitate the patient's goals (see **Table 16B-1**).

TABLE 16B-1 ADAPTIVE EQUIPMENT AND MODIFIED STRATEGIES

EQUIPMENT	DESCRIPTION	PATIENT NEED	PHOTOGRAPH
Mirror	Great tool for initial education during CIC (anatomy, technique/strategies), or long-term use for females. Optimal positioning for females is an extreme posterior pelvic tilt to facilitate access to urethra. Males with a rotund body habitus or other anatomical barriers may also benefit from use of a mirror.	Individuals who need visual feedback during CIC	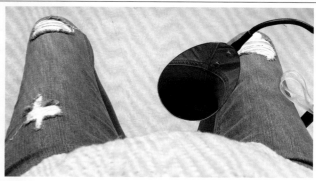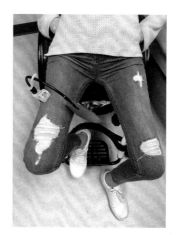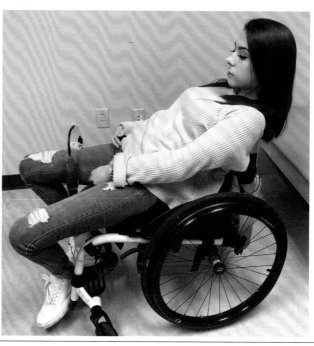

(Continued)

TABLE 16B-1 ADAPTIVE EQUIPMENT AND MODIFIED STRATEGIES (*Continued*)

EQUIPMENT	DESCRIPTION	PATIENT NEED	PHOTOGRAPH
Catheter inserter	Maintains grip and coordinated insertion of catheter Easy clamp allows for independent use	Individuals with impaired hand and finger function, who have difficulty grasping and manipulating the catheter	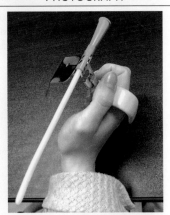
Pants holder, Betty hook, Bungee cord	Keeps clothing out of the way during CIC, allowing a hands-free approach for access. *Pants holder/Betty hook* Top hook goes into the waistband of pants; bottom bar is inserted between wheelchair cushion and seat *Bungee cord* One end of the cord is tied around the frame of the wheelchair. The individual manipulates the other end of the cord into the waistband of pants. The resistance of the cord holds clothing out of the way.	Males performing CIC	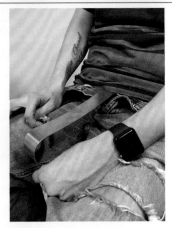 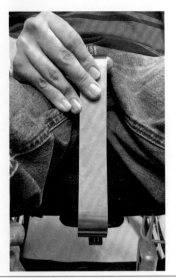

TABLE 16B-1 ADAPTIVE EQUIPMENT AND MODIFIED STRATEGIES (*Continued*)

EQUIPMENT	DESCRIPTION	PATIENT NEED	PHOTOGRAPH
Pants holder, Betty hook, Bungee cord (*Continued*)			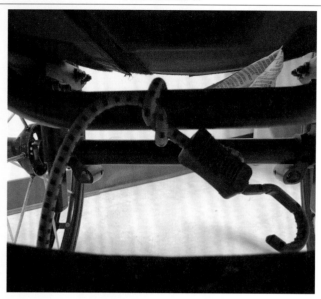 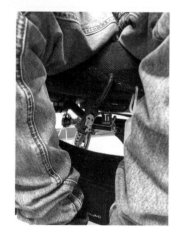 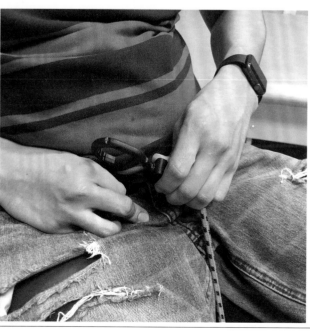

TABLE 16B-1 ADAPTIVE EQUIPMENT AND MODIFIED STRATEGIES (*Continued*)

EQUIPMENT	DESCRIPTION	PATIENT NEED	PHOTOGRAPH
Penis stabilizer, Household	Keeps the penis stable and in proper position for CIC Allows for hands-free approach	Males with impaired hand function	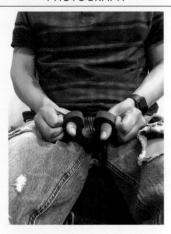 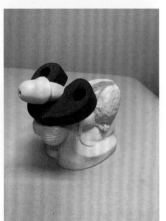 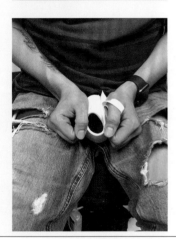

TABLE 16B-1 ADAPTIVE EQUIPMENT AND MODIFIED STRATEGIES (*Continued*)

EQUIPMENT	DESCRIPTION	PATIENT NEED	PHOTOGRAPH
Penis stabilizer, Household (*Continued*)			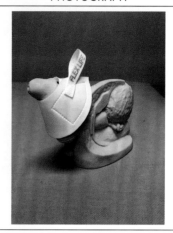
Asta-Cath	Designed by nurse, Linda Asta When inserted into the vaginal canal, the urethral opening will coincide with one of the holes, guiding the catheter into the urethra, facilitating independence.	Females performing CIC	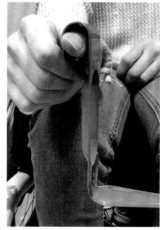 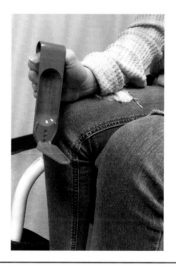

CHAPTER 17

INCONTINENCE-ASSOCIATED DERMATITIS

Debra Thayer and Denise Nix

OBJECTIVES

1. Explain the pathology and clinical presentation of incontinence-associated dermatitis (IAD).

2. Describe strategies for prevention and management of incontinence-associated dermatitis (IAD).

TOPIC OUTLINE

DEFINITION

Incontinence-associated dermatitis (IAD) is a type of top-down injury and the most common form of moisture-associated skin damage (MASD). IAD is characterized by erythema and edema of the surface of the skin, sometimes accompanied by serous exudate, erosion, or secondary cutaneous infection (Beeckman et al., 2016; Gray et al., 2012). See **Figure 17-1**.

The term dermatitis denotes inflammation and erythema with or without erosion or denudation. The term IAD specifically identifies the source of the irritant (urine or fecal incontinence) and acknowledges that the area of the skin affected commonly extends beyond the perineum (Bryant, 2012). Further, the term is not limited to an anatomical location (e.g., perineum) or persons using body worn absorbent products (BWAPs) such as diapers or briefs (Gray et al., 2007).

KEY POINT

Incontinence-associated dermatitis (IAD) is characterized by erythema and edema of the surface of the skin, sometimes accompanied by serous exudate, erosion, or secondary cutaneous infection. It involves only the superficial layers of the skin, thereby reflecting a "top-down" injury.

SIGNIFICANCE

IAD can result in pain, discomfort, infection, pressure injuries, depression, loss of independence, disruption in

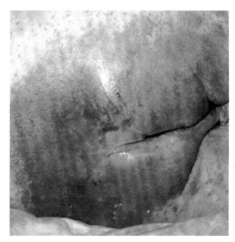

FIGURE 17-1. Incontinence-Associated Dermatitis (IAD). Note diffuse erythema, patchy areas of denudation, and coexisting candidiasis. (Courtesy of KDS Consulting.)

activities and/or sleep, reduced quality of life, and undue burden of care (Beeckman et al., 2015; Campbell et al., 2016; Demarre et al., 2015; Minassian et al., 2013). The prevalence and clinical relevance of IAD has been measured in a variety of health care settings.

In a large sample of 5,342 adults in *acute care* facilities in 36 states in the United States, 46.6% of patients were incontinent of urine, stool, or both. In that sample, the prevalence of IAD was 45.7% with 14.8% of the patients with IAD also presented with secondary fungal infections (Gray & Giuliano, 2018). In *long-term care,* researchers combined data from two electronic databases, the MDS and practitioners' orders, and reported a 5.5% incidence of IAD in a group of 10,713 nursing home residents newly diagnosed with incontinence (Bliss et al., 2017). A large study (*N* = 3,406) of residents in German nursing homes reported a 5.2% point prevalence for individuals with incontinence (Boronat-Garrido et al., 2016). A *long-term acute care* setting in the United States reported a 22.8% point prevalence of IAD and a 7.6% incidence based on direct observation of 171 patients (Long et al., 2012). In a study of 189 *community-dwelling* individuals with fecal or fecal and urinary incontinence (dual), more than half (52.5%) reported recurring episodes of IAD (Rohwer et al., 2013).

IAD was identified as an independent risk factor for pressure injuries (*p* = 0.001) in a secondary analysis of a randomized clinical trial with 610 patients with incontinence (Demarre et al., 2015). A meta-analysis of 58 studies showed a statistically significant association between incontinence and pressure injuries and a statistically significant (*p* < 0.05) relationship between IAD and full-thickness pressure injuries (Beeckman et al., 2014). Data from a study of 176,689 patients cared for in predominately acute care facilities over 2 years showed a 53% prevalence of incontinence. The likelihood of developing pressure injuries among incontinent patients was

higher (6.3%) compared to patients without incontinence (4.1%). Of the subjects with facility-acquired pressure injuries, 6% had incontinence while 1.6% did not (Lachenbruch et al., 2016). Similarly, in the large sample of acute care patients (*N* = 2,492) mentioned earlier, Gray and Giuliano (2018) reported that the patients with IAD were also more likely to experience a facility-acquired sacral area pressure injury (32.3%) compared to only 6.3% of patients without IAD (*p* < 0.001). Further, the subjects with IAD were more likely to develop a facility-acquired full-thickness sacral pressure injury (6.4%) compared to 1.5% of patients without IAD (*p* < 0.001). Not surprisingly, occurrence of pressure injuries has been positively related to the severity of IAD (Park & Kim, 2014).

> **KEY POINT**
>
> IAD is quite a prevalent condition especially in acute care facilities; it is an *independent risk factor* for pressure injury development.

PATHOLOGY

Overhydration of the stratum corneum compromises the brick-and-mortar configuration of the epidermal layer and permits penetration by irritants found in urine and stool, which results in inflammation and impaired tensile strength. As urea in urine breaks down, highly alkaline ammonia is produced and changes pH from acid to alkaline compromising the protective acidic mantle of the skin. Gray and Giuliano (2018) demonstrated that individuals exposed to urine and stool or liquid stool are at higher risk for IAD than those exposed to formed stool (*p* < 0.001). The pH properties of formed stool are more neutral and have fewer active enzymes than liquid stool.

> **KEY POINT**
>
> Overhydration of the stratum corneum compromises the brick-and-mortar configuration of the epidermal layer and permits penetration by irritants found in urine and stool; urine urea changes into ammonia causing elevated skin pH creating a conducive environment for microbial growth.

Friction is the resistance to motion in a parallel direction relative to the common boundary of two surfaces. Skin injury by friction initially appears as erythema and progresses to an abrasion. Friction primarily affects superficial layers and thus does not result in tissue necrosis (Bryant, 2012). Incontinence care involves the use of friction for skin cleansing. Forces of friction, shear, or drag against an underlying surface (bed, chair, linen, containment garments) facilitate deformation of tissue layers and injure the skin allowing pathogens such as *Candida* and *Staphylococcus* to invade and cause secondary infections (Voegeli, 2012).

RISK FACTORS

Risk factors for developing IAD include incontinence, frequent episodes of incontinence, poor skin condition, compromised mobility, diminished cognitive awareness, inability to perform personal hygiene, pain, raised body temperature, select medications, poor nutritional status, and critical illness (Beeckman et al., 2015). Dual fecal and urinary incontinence, loose stools, and diarrhea increase the likelihood of IAD. Although increased age is associated with higher prevalence of incontinence, age does not appear to be an independent risk factor for IAD (Kottner et al., 2014). Raised body temperature causes the body to sweat and store heat longer impairing moisture evaporation or transepidermal water loss (TEWL). Environmental humidity also impairs TEWL. When environmental humidity decreases, TEWL is likely to increase (Gray et al., 2011). As previously described, exposure to urine and stool or liquid stool are at greater risk for IAD due the more neutral pH properties and fewer active enzymes in formed stool (see **Fig. 17-2**).

RISK

Pressure injury risk assessment tools are not designed to predict the risk for IAD. Risk assessment tools for IAD have been developed and tested for validity and reliability (Li et al., 2019; Nix, 2002; Shiu et al., 2013). IAD risk assessment tools, however, are not widely used in clinical practice. Much like pressure injury risk assessment tools, IAD risk assessment tools do not capture all known risk factors.

CLINICAL PRESENTATION AND SKIN ASSESSMENT

IAD appears initially as erythema ranging from pink to red. Darker skin tones may present with paler, yellow, or dark discoloration (Bliss et al., 2014). Affected skin can look patchy with nondistinct edges. IAD can be located at any anatomical location exposed to urine and/or stool. Vesicles, papules, or pustules may be present, or the epidermis may be eroded exposing moist, weeping dermis (see **Fig. 17-3**). IAD-affected skin may be warm or firm on palpation due to the underlying inflammation. Whether the IAD presents as intact erythema or severely eroded skin, patients often complain of burning, itching, tingling, or pain. A red rash with pinpoint satellite lesions (papules or pustules) indicative of a candidiasis (a secondary infection) is not uncommon (Beeckman et al., 2015). Bacterial infections secondary to IAD are not commonly reported in peer review literature.

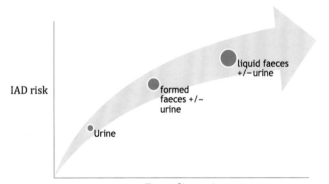

FIGURE 17-2. IAD Risk. (Beeckman, D. et al. (2015). Proceedings of the Global IAD Expert Panel. Incontinence-associated dermatitis: Moving prevention forward. *Wounds International.* Reproduced with kind permission of Wounds International, London, UK.)

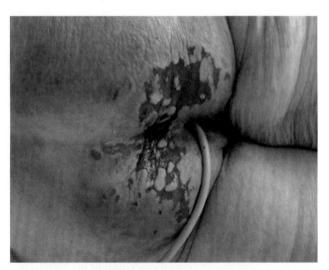

FIGURE 17-3. Severe IAD-Note Areas of Denudement Surrounded by Erythema. (Beeckman, D., et al. (2015). Proceedings of the Global IAD Expert Panel. Incontinence-associated dermatitis: Moving prevention forward. *Wounds International.* Reproduced with kind permission of Wounds International, London, UK.)

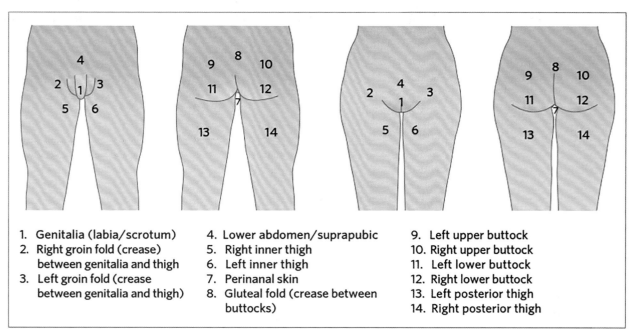

1. Genitalia (labia/scrotum)
2. Right groin fold (crease) between genitalia and thigh
3. Left groin fold (crease between genitalia and thigh)
4. Lower abdomen/suprapubic
5. Right inner thigh
6. Left inner thigh
7. Perinanal skin
8. Gluteal fold (crease between buttocks)
9. Left upper buttock
10. Right upper buttock
11. Left lower buttock
12. Right lower buttock
13. Left posterior thigh
14. Right posterior thigh

FIGURE 17-4. Anatomic Locations Susceptible to IAD. (Beeckman, D., et al. (2015). Proceedings of the Global IAD Expert Panel. Incontinence-associated dermatitis: Moving prevention forward. *Wounds International*. Reproduced with kind permission of Wounds International, London, UK.)

All patients with urinary and/or fecal incontinence should have their skin assessed regularly to check for signs of IAD. This should be done at least once daily but may be indicated more often based on contributing factors such as frequent or loose stools. In a critical care population, Coyer et al. (2017) observed that IAD developed rapidly and resulted in moderate to severe skin damage. IAD can develop in any anatomical location exposed to urine and feces such as anus, vulva, scrotum, labia, groin folds, lower abdomen, thighs, gluteal folds, gluteal cleft, buttocks, and the sacrococcygeal region (see **Fig. 17-4**).

Decision-making for managing IAD is dependent on visual skin assessment and determination of the severity of skin damage. Tools have been developed to guide visual assessment of IAD and have various degrees of validity and reliability testing (Beeckman et al., 2015, 2018; Borchert et al., 2010). However, they are not yet routinely used in clinical practice.

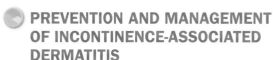 **DIFFERENTIAL DIAGNOSIS**

IAD, moisture lesions, stage 2 pressure injuries, and friction injury are superficial "top down" wounds. Full-thickness wounds from pressure and shear are considered "bottom up" (Sibbald et al., 2011). These types of wounds can occur alone or in combination on or near the perineal, perianal, sacral, and buttocks region making differential assessment a challenge. Careful attention must be paid to exact anatomical location, pain descriptions, patterns, distribution of lesions, and risk factors not only for IAD and pressure but also other skin conditions that may occur near the perineal, perianal, sacral, and buttocks region (see **Table 17-1**).

PREVENTION AND MANAGEMENT OF INCONTINENCE-ASSOCIATED DERMATITIS

All patients who are incontinent are at risk for developing skin damage. Because of the adverse clinical outcomes associated with IAD (pressure injury development, secondary infection, and pain), the continence nurse specialist needs to create and implement a robust prevention strategy. This includes establishing guidance for care, creating a product formulary and educating of bedside caregivers to recognize risk, assess skin condition, and consistently implement relevant interventions.

A guideline for IAD prevention and treatment has not been developed but a set of best practice principles has been established (Beeckman et al., 2015). Key interventions include risk assessment, continence management, skin assessment, and skin care.

As discussed previously, risk for IAD is primarily driven by the type of incontinence with patients who have fecal and dual incontinence at higher risk than those incontinent of urine alone. In their study, Park and Kim (2014) reported that all patients with fecal incontinence had some evidence of IAD. More recently, intensive prevention efforts for catheter-associated urinary tract infection (CAUTI), especially in the acute care setting, have led to reduced usage of indwelling catheters.

TABLE 17-1 DIFFERENTIAL DIAGNOSIS OF PERINEAL/PERIANAL SKIN CONDITIONS

	IAD	CANDIDIASIS	HERPES ZOSTER	PRESSURE
Location	Perineum Buttocks Inner thighs Groin Lower abdominal skin folds	Perineum Buttocks Inner thighs Groin Lower abdominal skin folds	Perianal Buttocks Genitals	Near bony prominences Coccyx, sacrum, ischium Under device/tube
Confirmed Risk Factors	Urinary and/or fecal incontinence	Moisture Antibiotics Immunosuppression	Immunosuppression Elderly Stress	Limited mobility or activity Dependent on others for repositioning, transferring, etc.
Blisters	Yes	No	Initially vesicles then pustules	Sometimes (stage II)
Distribution Pattern	Confluent or patchy Irregular edges with erythema Shallow denudement and/or maceration Fleshy part of buttocks	Confluent or patchy rash Small round pustules, plaques, and/or satellite lesions	Grouped unilateral distribution of rash or ulcerations along dermatome Pustules erode into ulcerations Clusters or isolated individual shallow lesions or blisters	Isolated individual lesions on or near bony prominence or pressure-causing device Damage ranges from intact discoloration to partial- or full-thickness wounds
Color	Pink/red	Pink/red	Initial: Pink/red Ulcer may have yellow slough Later: Crust Severe cases: Necrosis	Pink, red, yellow, tan, gray, brown, black
Discomfort	Pain may be mild to severe	Itching, burning	Tingling sometimes noted initially Often very painful	Pain may be absent to severe
Diagnostic Tests	None	Potassium hydroxide preparation scraping (KOH)	DNA polymerase chain reaction assay and direct immunofluorescent stain of skin scraping for VZV antigen Tzanck preparation Tissue culture	None

With permission from Bryant, R. A. (2012). Types of skin damage and differential diagnosis. In R. A. Bryant & D. P. Nix (Eds.), *Acute and chronic wounds: Current management concepts* (5th ed.). St Louis, MO: Mosby Elsevier.

As a result, dual incontinence is more common and places patients at higher risk of skin damage.

> **KEY POINT**
>
> People who suffer dual incontinence (urine and stool) are at higher risk for IAD, especially with liquid stool.

The most effective way to prevent IAD is to eliminate or reduce incontinent episodes. This removes the primary factors (moisture, irritants, friction) that contribute to skin injury. In any setting, the continence nurse should be able to perform a basic continence evaluation and implement a plan of care to address reversible problems such as urinary retention, urinary tract infection, and fecal impaction. Additionally, identification of problematic medications that are continence–disruptive can be accomplished through collaboration with a pharmacist; alternatives can be identified and suggested to the primary care provider. For patients in acute care who are nonambulant but able to toilet, toileting schedules and equipment (e.g., commodes) should be built into the plan of care in order to formalize incontinence as a health care problem and continence as a goal.

> **KEY POINT**
>
> The most effective way to prevent IAD is to eliminate or reduce incontinent episodes. This removes the primary factors (moisture, irritants, friction) that contribute to skin injury.

In postacute settings, more comprehensive continence management programs can be undertaken. Behavioral programs including bowel and/or bladder training programs should be considered for patients with the potential for bladder or bowel rehabilitation. Attention to mobility improvement and dietary modifications can also be implemented. Refer to Chapter 6 for more information on bladder and bowel health measures and conservative continence management.

During continence restoration or whenever continence is intractable, containment or diversion should be used to protect skin from stool or urine. Use of body worn absorbent products (BWAPs) remains the most common approach to containment (Gray et al., 2018). Briefs, pull-ons, and pads comprise the most common designs with products typically composed of four layers. The "cover-stock" is the layer contacting skin, an "acquisition" layer facilitates fluid movement, the absorbent core sequesters fluid, and an outer barrier layer prevents egress of fluid from the product into the environment. Modern absorbent cores contain superabsorbent polymers (SAPs), molecules that are designed to absorb many times their weight and retain fluid away from the skin. Increasingly, products are designed with a breathable outer barrier to improve moisture and heat transfer.

Concern over the effect of occlusive absorbent products on skin began with observations regarding the effect of infant diapers (Berg, 1988). While absorbent products do not cause IAD, product composition and construction can contribute to altered microclimate and skin damage (Falloon et al., 2018). Adult products with poorly absorbent core material such as fluff or pulp do not sequester liquid, resulting in skin contact with moisture. Occlusive outer layers have been shown to trap moisture and increase heat at the product–skin interface. The practice of leaving briefs unfastened and the skin "open to air" evolved from concerns that brief trapped moisture. Many clinicians believe that this is beneficial for skin health, but no evidence exists to support this assumption. This practice is of questionable value when BWAPs containing materials that support normal microclimate are used. Additionally, a brief that is not positioned on the patient as designed nor fastened can move and bunch potentially creating a source of friction or pressure.

KEY POINT

Absorbent products do not cause IAD, product composition, and construction can contribute to altered microclimate and skin damage.

Layering of pads and linens under the patient has been identified not only as a risk factor for pressure injuries but also for IAD (Kayser et al., 2019). As with occlusive body worn products, normal microclimate is compromised by heat and excessive hydration. Increasing from 1 to 6 layers has been shown to double the risk of pressure injury development (Schwartz et al., 2018).

KEY POINT

Layering of pads and linens under the patient has been identified not only as a risk factor for pressure injuries but also for IAD.

With the reduction in indwelling catheter use, use of female external urinary containment devices has grown. See **Figure 17-5**. Intended for bed and chair-bound individuals, these devices are positioned over the urethral meatus and labia and connected to suction. Urine moves across the absorbent interface and is absorbed into material within the device. Two devices have been commercialized, one with a latex outer covering and the

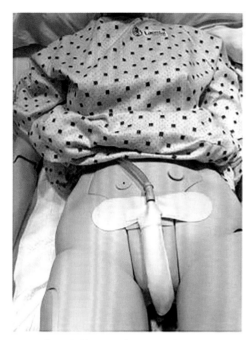

FIGURE 17-5. Female External Collection Device. (Beeson, T., & Davis, C. (2018). Urinary management with an external female collection device. *Journal of Wound Ostomy and Continence Nursing, 45*(2), 187–189.)

other covered in silicone. Early published experience (Beeson & Davis, 2018) suggests benefits not only for skin but also in minimizing the sleep disruptive effects of incontinence. As with any device with rigid components, patients are at risk for medical device–related pressure injury.

Based on available published evidence and expert opinion, external collection devices (ECDs) can be safely used for urine diversion in males (Gray et al., 2016). ECDs include latex and nonlatex sheath devices (i.e., "condom" catheters). Sheath devices should be available in a range of sizes and staff should be trained in principles and techniques of application and removal in order to prevent medical adhesive–related skin injury (MARSI). Other ECD options include a retracted penile pouch and a glans-adherent device (see Chapter 16).

Options for stool diversion and containment remain limited with BWAPs engineered to primarily manage urine (i.e., fluid). Fecal management systems are used for diversion of liquid stool in non- or minimally ambulant patients. A silicone catheter with a soft inflatable cuff is retained in the rectum and connected to bedside drainage. These devices offer the advantage of stool diversion and containment providing benefits for both skin health and infection control. Benoit and Watts (2007) reported a 30.5% reduction in prevalence and incidence of pressure injuries when a fecal management system was used as part of a comprehensive pressure ulcer prevention program. Echols et al. (2007) reported fewer UTIs and skin and soft tissue infections in a burn population. Because leakage can occur around the catheter, skin protection is an essential intervention (see Fig. 22-3, Chapter 22).

A fecal pouch applied to the perianal area can provide an alternative to an indwelling fecal management device (see Fig. 22-2, Chapter 22). While a noninvasive approach, application can be difficult due to anatomic contours and available space between the vagina/scrotum and the anus. The pouch can also be easily disrupted with patient movement or repositioning. Devices are most successful when connected to bedside drainage. As with female urinary devices, attention to prevention of device-related pressure injury is required.

SKIN CARE

Recent data have identified a relationship between IAD and pressure injury (Barakat-Johnson et al., 2018; Demarre et al., 2015; Gray & Giuliano, 2018). Considering this, it is important to think of skin care not merely as a tool for IAD prevention, but rather as an essential and complementary component of a successful PI prevention bundle.

First described by Lyder et al. (1992), a "structured skin care regimen" is still considered a best practice approach to prevention *and* treatment of IAD (Beeckman et al., 2009; Park & Kim, 2014). This term describes a standardized approach to care and product selection based on skin condition. A protocol or algorithm guides care while simplifying decision-making for bedside staff and helping to ensure compliance with best practice (Beeckman et al., 2015). Cleansing and protection comprise the two key interventions within a structured skin care regimen (Beeckman et al., 2015). Product choice for these interventions is primarily based on clinician preference and increasingly, contractual agreements. Unlike other medical products or even a consumer product like sunscreen, there are no accepted standards or criteria by which to evaluate and compare efficacy of cleansers, moisturizers, or protective products. From a regulatory perspective, most skin care products used for IAD prevention and treatment fall into one of three FDA categories: (1) over-the-counter ("OTC") products (many moisture barriers, antifungals, and some multifunctional products); (2) cosmetics (moisturizers, some moisture barriers, and cleansers); or (3) medical devices (barrier films and skin protectants). Rules for labeling and claims differ for each category. For both OTC drugs and cosmetics, efficacy is primarily based on composition. Only OTC drugs are required to identify an "active" ingredient.

KEY POINT

Think of "structured skin care regimen" not merely as a tool for IAD prevention and treatment, but rather as an essential and complementary component of a successful pressure injury prevention bundle.

Two recent reviews have evaluated the quality of evidence for incontinence-related skin care. A total of 18 papers were included in final analyses with 5 studies included in both reviews. Prather and colleagues (2017) reported on 10 studies, noting significant deficiencies including weak methodologies, wide variation in "comparators [and] outcomes," ambiguous or incomplete data, and a range of measurement tools. A 2016 Cochrane review by Beekman and colleagues set out to "assess and compare the effectiveness of various products and procedures to prevent and treat incontinence-associated dermatitis in adults." Authors reported that the majority of trials suffered from small sample size and lack of blinding. Based on these limitations, pooling of data and meta-analysis was not possible in either review and the Cochrane review concluded that "there is little evidence of very low to moderate quality, on the effectiveness of interventions for preventing and treating IAD in adults" (Beeckman et al., 2016, p. 34).

Best practice guidance for cleansing advocates use of no-rinse, "pH balanced" liquid cleansers. Similar in principle to cosmetic facial cleansers, cleansers for incontinence are water-based solutions that contain ingredients ("surfactants") to reduce surface tension and allow cleansing with a minimum of friction. "Gentleness" has consistently been identified as an important criterion for cleanser selection and the term while somewhat vague is generally interpreted to mean lack of potential to induce irritation. While the category of surfactant (anionic, cationic, nonionic) has been often cited as an important decision criterion, product safety should be assessed based on the *overall formulation*.

KEY POINT

Cleansing the skin following an incontinence episode is the *first* step in a structured skin care program. Cleansers for incontinence should be pH balanced, contain surfactants to reduce surface tension and friction with incontinence skin cleansing practices.

While the benefit of these products for incontinence cleansing is widely accepted, this is largely based on formulation science and expert opinion. A small crossover trial (Byers et al., 1995) evaluated 10 nursing home patients comparing a no-rinse liquid cleanser to (1) liquid soap; (2) liquid cleanser plus skin protectant; (3) soap and water plus skin protectant; and (4) soap and water. No skin breakdown was observed in any group, but in the cleanser group, positive effects were noted for the parameters of pH and TEWL. In their systematic review, Prather et al. evaluated two studies that compared foam cleansers to soap and water (Cooper & Gray, 2001; Park & Kim, 2014). They concluded that the foam cleanser appeared to be "slightly more effective than soap in water in preventing IAD or skin breakdown that may lead to pressure ulcers."

Cleansers are typically classified as cosmetics. Suitability for use on damaged skin should not be assumed and should be evaluated using manufacturer's data.

Cleansers are delivered as sprays, foams, or in premoistened wipes. For liquids and foams, use with soft, nonlinting cloths is recommended. In settings where concentrated formulations are used, it is critical that staff understand and follow instructions for dilution. From an ease of use perspective, cleansers and multifunctional products are convenient and reduce nursing time required as opposed to basins and cloths (Beeckman et al., 2015; Lewis-Byers et al., 2002; Warshaw et al., 2002).

In settings where cleansers are not available, a liquid soap formulated for sensitive skin can be an option. No published trials have compared sensitive skin formulation soaps (liquid or bar) to liquid cleansers. Plain water can be an acceptable alternative for cleansing (Beeckman et al., 2015). When skin is denuded and pain is present, water gently delivered by syringe may be better tolerated than a spray cleanser or wipes. Use of standard bath bar soaps is discouraged as they are considered to be pH disruptive, drying, and irritating based on their formulation.

Evidence to support routine use of antiseptics for incontinence cleansing has not been published. The continence nurse should carefully evaluate cleansers promoted as antimicrobial or antibacterial. This labeling may be referencing ingredients (e.g., benzalkonium hydrochloride, benzethonium hydrochloride) that are incorporated to preserve the formulation and that do not provide an antimicrobial therapeutic benefit.

KEY POINT

Plain water can be an acceptable alternative for cleansing especially if the skin is denuded, water gently delivered by syringe may be better tolerated than a spray cleanser or wipes. Use of standard bath bar soaps is discouraged as they are pH disruptive, drying, and irritating based on their formulation.

Bedside staff should understand that patients experiencing incontinence are at risk for *preventable* skin injury and intervene accordingly. Recent evidence has shown that exposure to synthetic urine rapidly creates adverse changes to barrier function, even with the presence of a wicking absorbent pad (Phipps et al., 2019). When stool and especially liquid stool is present, removal of irritants is even more critical, reinforcing the importance of prompt cleansing.

KEY POINT

Bedside staff should understand that patients experiencing incontinence are at risk for *preventable* skin injury and need to intervene with prompt cleansing. Research reports that exposure to synthetic urine rapidly creates adverse changes to barrier function, even with the presence of a wicking absorbent pad and more so with liquid stool.

Protection of skin is the *second* critical step in a structured skin care regimen. For a product to provide protection, *minimally* it must repel moisture (i.e., be waterproof) and remain in place over the affected area. Protection from liquid stool or dual stool and urine requires a substantive barrier that is capable of protecting skin from an irritant (i.e., fecal enzymes) in addition to moisture remaining in place over the affected area.

The terms skin protectant, moisture barrier, and skin barrier are used interchangeably to describe these products. Recently, the term "leave-on" (as opposed to products that are rinsed off) has been applied to moisture barriers (Kottner & Surber, 2016).

KEY POINT

Protection of the skin with a "leave-on" moisture barrier is the *second* critical step in a structured skin care regimen. Several terms are used to describe skin barrier products: moisture barrier, skin barrier, and skin protectant, but "moisture barrier" is the preferred term.

Several characteristics are desirable for a protective product (see **Table 17-2**). Beyond barrier capability, the ability to allow evaporation from the skin surface, often referred to as breathability is critical for normal stratum corneum function. Skin is constantly transpiring moisture vapor and occlusive materials have been shown to trap moisture within hours of application. This results in an impaired epidermal barrier and reduced skin breaking strength. Additionally, frictional forces are increased when skin is wet (Gerhardt et al., 2008; Schaefer et al., 2002; Zhai & Maibach, 2002). Increased friction can not only result in superficial injury but also contributes to shear strain.

Polymer-based liquids, creams, ointments, and pastes are the most common forms of barrier products. Because standard measures of barrier performance have not been established, comparisons of different forms are difficult at best (Beeckman, 2017). In this chapter, the term *moisture barrier* will be used as a generic descriptor to describe protective products.

KEY POINT

The term "skin protectant" may be used as a generic descriptor or may refer to a specific FDA category of over-the-counter (OTC) drugs. Only OTC skin protectants designate an "active" ingredient and a document called a "monograph" recognizes 21 ingredients that may be identified as an "active." Specific guidance for labeling and claims based on the ingredient(s) used are provided for manufacturers. Creams, ointments, and pastes not labeled as OTC drug skin protectants are typically cosmetics; cosmetics are not considered to have active ingredients.

TABLE 17-2 DESIRABLE MOISTURE BARRIER PRODUCT CHARACTERISTICS

DESIRABLE MOISTURE BARRIER PRODUCT CHARACTERISTICS	RATIONALE
Provides durable protection	Minimally should be waterproof, should be capable of protection from fecal enzymes if used for protection from liquid stool
Breathable	To allow normal moisture–vapor transmission from skin
Close to skin pH	Note—pH value not relevant to chemistry of most polymeric films
Low irritant potential	Previously referred to as "hypoallergenic," dye-free, fragrance-free
Nonstinging and/or comfortable during wear	Promotes patient comfort
Transparent	Allows skin inspection
Does not require removal or easily removed	Minimizes friction required for cleansing, promotes patient comfort ease of use
Does not contribute to skin damage (e.g., does not increase friction)	Minimizing friction at skin surface will reduce risk of tissue deformation associated with shear strain
Does not interfere with absorption of incontinence products	Enables function of BWAPs or external female devices

Modified from General characteristics of the ideal product for prevention and treatment of IAD (Beeckman et al., 2015).

Liquid barriers include barrier films and skin protectants. Modern barrier films contain polymers (large molecules composed of monomers) dissolved in a nonstinging, alcohol-free solvent delivered via an applicator or spray. The solvent acts as a carrier to deliver the polymer and then evaporates, leaving a thin, transparent waterproof coating on the skin. Products are similar in appearance but vary in protective ability. Film products that are described by the manufacturer as "easy to remove" with soap and water are not waterproof and will fail to form a durable barrier.

KEY POINT

While the term "skin sealant" is often used to describe barrier films, it more accurately describes early formulations containing copolymers and alcohol primarily used for ostomy care.

Barrier films do not readily attach to wet surfaces. When using the product to protect a damaged surface that is also wet, many Wound Ostomy Continence (WOC) nurses employ a technique called "crusting." Ostomy powder is dusted onto the damaged surface to create a dry platform. Excess powder is removed, and the barrier film is then sprayed or blotted onto the powder and allowed to dry creating a protective barrier. The process is then repeated two or more times depending on preference. Anecdotally, the technique is reported to be effective but can be labor-intensive and difficult for bedside staff to replicate. Data evaluating the efficacy of crusting versus other forms of moisture barriers have not been reported.

Film-forming liquid skin protectants differ from barrier films. Two products are commercially available: a cyanoacrylate monomer and a polymer–cyanoacrylate complex. Long available as tissue sealants, cyanoacrylates impart the ability to attach to wet, surfaces. As such, they offer an option for protection of severely damaged skin where weeping is present. A nonrandomized prospective study (Brennan et al., 2017) evaluated the polymer–cyanoacrylate formulation in 16 patients with IAD. Skin condition improved in 13 of 16 patients. Pain reduction was noted in those patients able to self-report. In a randomized, prospective trial of 21 healthy volunteers (Mathisen et al., 2018), the polymer–cyanoacrylate product showed superior durability to repeated washing as compared to two commercially available barrier films and the cyanoacrylate monomer product.

KEY POINT

Film-forming liquid skin protectants differ from traditional barrier films. Two products are commercially available: a cyanoacrylate monomer and a polymer–cyanoacrylate complex that adhere well to weeping skin and resist washing off.

Traditional moisture barrier formulations used for skin protection include nonmedicated creams, ointments, and pastes. The term cream describes an emulsion of water in oil, or oil in water. Creams may be a vehicle for moisturizers, barriers, or combination products. Barrier function is achieved by adding common ingredients such as zinc oxide, petrolatum, and dimethicone alone or in combination. Formulations may vary from thin liquids to extremely thick semisolids. Some liquid creams are formulated to be breathable. Creams can also be made to vanish into the epidermis as opposed to remaining on the skin surface; this provides the benefit of visualization of the underlying surface. Because creams contain water, they require preservatives to prevent microbial growth during their shelf-life.

The term cream describes an emulsion of water in oil, or oil in water; may be a vehicle for moisturizers, barriers (zinc oxide, petrolatum, dimethicone), or combination products. Dimethicone is a cream moisture barrier that is breathable.

Ointments are moderately thick, semi-solids formed from a "base," often petrolatum. As such, they typically have an oilier feel than creams. Ointments are *always* occlusive. Formulations for incontinence skin protection are intended to sit on the skin and do not vanish. Ointments do not contain water and some products are formulated without preservatives.

Ointments are moderately thick, semi-solids formed from a "base," often petrolatum and are *always* occlusive, altering TEWL of the skin.

Pastes emerged from the early practice of clinicians compounded mixtures of zinc oxide and ostomy powder in an effort to create a material that would attach to and protect moist, denuded skin. Today, "bedside compounding" is discouraged; not only it is outside the scope of nursing practice but it yields a product of unknown safety and stability. Pastes are now commercially manufactured semi-solids (typically an ointment) to which an absorbent (e.g., carboxymethylcellulose) has been added. The absorbent can impart a gritty texture to the finished product, making it uncomfortable for application to damaged skin. Pastes are intended to be applied in a thick layer in order to provide a physical barrier to irritants. The degree to which the coating remains intact during wear varies by formulation. Some products can dry and crack yet remain firmly adherent to the underlying surface. This creates an ineffective barrier, yet one that is difficult to remove.

Difficulty in removing moisture barriers can negatively impact the burden of care for bedside staff particularly when caring for patients with acute fecal incontinence with diarrhea (AFID). In the FIRST study (Bayon-Garcia et al., 2012), 60% of clinicians estimated that management of a single episode of AFID required between 10 and 20 minutes. Heidegger et al. (2016) reported the average time needed for management of an AFID episode was 17 minutes, 33 seconds and involved an average of 1.4 nurses and 0.8 aides. In both studies, the majority of time was required by the cleansing and removal of thick barriers.

To mitigate the challenges associated with removal of semi-solid barriers, clinicians resort to "work-around" practices such as applying products in a thin layer (i.e., less than the recommended amount) and/or attempting to wipe only stool from the surface in order to avoid damage to the underlying injured skin. Neither practice has been studied for effectiveness or infection control implications.

Pastes are intended to be applied to damaged skin in a thick layer to provide a physical barrier to irritants; they adhere to the skin and are difficult and time consuming to remove. Inappropriate use of pastes can further skin damage.

Clinical efficacy of barrier products should not be assumed based on labeling or ingredients. Viscosity (i.e., thickness) and visibility do not correlate to protective ability. Unfortunately, no well-designed comparative study has demonstrated the superiority of any barrier cream, ointment, or paste. In the absence of published evidence, the continence nurse should request manufacturer's data demonstrating barrier capability. At a minimum, testing in healthy volunteers should show that the material is waterproof and resistant to removal with soap and water. Protection from diarrhea requires a substantive barrier that can hold up to fecal enzymes as well as wetness. Products that are intended for protection (i.e., "treatment") of denuded skin should be non- or minimally cytotoxic.

No well-designed comparative study has demonstrated the superiority of any barrier cream, ointment, or paste. The continence care nurse should request manufacturer's data demonstrating barrier capability.

Additional important considerations when selecting a moisture barrier include impact on BWAPs and effect on friction. Ointments, pastes, and nonvanishing barrier creams sit on the surface of the skin and can transfer off, interfering with the coverstock of the absorbent product. Impaired wicking and functionality of absorbent products has been shown with use of these types of moisture barriers (Zehrer et al., 2005) although in three other studies that acknowledged some product transfer to the coverstock but no major effect on absorption (Bolton et al., 2004; Dykes & Bradbury, 2016; Fleming et al., 2014). All four studies were performed in a nonclinical setting and deemed to be of low quality thus, more research is needed to verify if ointments reduce product absorption in a clinical setting (Gray et al., 2018). At this time, vanishing barrier creams and polymer-based barriers attach to the skin and appear to not transfer to other surfaces, maintaining functionality of BWAP.

Many incontinent patients are also at risk for pressure injury. Emerging data from a laboratory model suggest that some ointments and pastes have the potential to increase friction (Asmus et al., 2018). With friction being an important contributor to shear strain and tissue deformation, use of a barrier that does not increase friction is desirable.

While moisturization has long been advocated as an essential second step in incontinence skin care, the relative contribution of moisturizers to IAD prevention has not been studied. As with barriers, guidance regarding moisturizers in the incontinence care literature can be confusing with the terms moisturizer and emollient used interchangeably. Moisturizers are typically formulated as lotions and creams, both of which contain water. Based on their ingredients, they function by (1) retaining available moisture in the epidermis-through incorporation of humectants such as glycerin or urea or (2) softening and improving the appearance and feel of the epidermis through inclusion of ingredients called emollients. Occlusive skin conditioners comprise another category of ingredients sometimes used for moisturization; they retard evaporative loss by laying down a greasy film on the skin.

KEY POINT

Ingredients can be confusing: Urea is a humectant whereas diazolidinyl urea, which is a preservative. Humectants should be avoided in incontinence skin care products since they draw moisture into the skin that is already compromised from moisture (urine).

By design, moisturizers are intended to work on the epidermis. *Excessive wetness* is known to be a key contributing factor for IAD development and places IAD within the moisture-associated skin damage framework. When the epidermis is excessively hydrated or absent (i.e., denuded) moisturizers provide *no benefit* and have the potential to add *undesirable* hydration. While stratum corneum (SC) lipid replenishment (also referred to as "restoration") has been advocated (Beeckman et al., 2015) and may be beneficial to aid barrier repair, not all moisturizers and specifically emollients are capable of this. Lipid replenishment requires a formulation that incorporates relevant SC lipids (e.g., ceramides) and is capable of epidermal permeation. This should be supported by manufacturer's data, minimally with data from healthy volunteers.

KEY POINT

Not all moisturizers are able to provide lipid replenishment (restoration). Restoration requires a formulation that incorporates relevant SC lipids (e.g., ceramides) and is capable of epidermal permeation. *Principles of a structured skin care therefore include cleansing, protecting, and restoring as needed to promote perigenital skin health.*

Multifunction products (also referred to as "3-in-1" products) gained attention in the 1990s. These products are intended to cleanse, moisturize, and protect the skin in a single step, replacing the early and confusing practice of using three separate products. Initially delivered in the form of spray-on lotions, premoistened wipes are now the most common delivery format. Dimethicone is commonly used to provide barrier function; other ingredients will include one or more surfactants and skin conditioning ingredients. Driver (2007) reported that IAD developed in 19% of a group that received a 3-in-1 wipe as compared to 50% of subjects treated with a no rinse cleanser and a zinc oxide ointment with menthol. Beeckman et al. (2011) observed superior skin outcomes when a "3-in-1" wipe was compared to soap and water for incontinence care. No barrier was used for the soap and water group. After 120 days, there was a 27.1% incidence of IAD in the soap and water group compared to an 8.1% incidence in the intervention group. Another study (Brunner et al., 2012) compared a 3-in-1 wipe to a no-rinse cleanser and barrier film. In this study, the wipe group did not demonstrate superior outcomes with 27.3% of subjects developing IAD as compared to 22.6% in the cleanser/barrier film group. Additionally, patients in the cleanser/barrier film group took longer to develop IAD (213.3 vs. 91.1 hours). As with other skin care products, effectiveness should not be judged based on ingredients alone. Because the product is delivered by wiping across the skin, data on barrier retention is needed to evaluate effectiveness.

KEY POINT

Products that cleanse and protect are often combined to provide an effective but simplified structured skin care program.

TREATMENT OF IAD AND SECONDARY INFECTIONS

As with prevention, care should be focused on prompt removal of irritants and protection of the affected area to promote healing. Use of nonirritating and noncytotoxic products is important when skin is damaged even if the epidermis is intact. Unlike treatment for other forms of irritant contact dermatitis, use of topical corticosteroids for management of IAD is rare. Reasons for this may include clinician's lack of familiarity with potency of various steroids and/or lack of prescriptive authority. Pain from IAD has not been studied but clinician experience validates that it is a significant concern. Application of topical barriers may mitigate discomfort, but analgesics should be considered when skin injury is severe.

Guidance for management of concomitant fungal infections is based on expert opinion and information extrapolated from the skin and nail care literature. Topical antifungal medications are common first-line treatments for candidiasis. They are available as a prescription formulation (nystatin) or OTC preparations. Miconazole is a broad-spectrum antifungal and the most common active ingredient incorporated into OTC medications. Systemic antifungals are preferred by some providers.

Some general guidance for application of topical antifungals can be considered: an antifungal powder may be helpful in reducing moisture if the affected area is wet. The powder should be applied or "dusted" on in a thin coating to cover the entire affected area. Creams and lotions contain water and can add undesirable moisture when skin is wet or macerated. When the affected area is dry, a cream or ointment can be used. Ointments may provide some barrier function, but additional protection should be considered especially where ongoing exposure to liquid stool is likely. The common practice of "sealing in" antifungal powders under a barrier film or semi-solid moisture barrier ointment or paste is a long-standing practice based on expert opinion as opposed to manufacturer's recommendation. It is important to understand that this may constitute "off-label" use of both products. The ideal duration of treatment for IAD-related fungal infections has not been established. In women, vaginal infection may accompany cutaneous infection and should be evaluated. If initial treatment was based on clinical assessment and the patient is not improving, an appropriate skin specimen should be obtained for culture. Referral to a provider skilled in dermatology may be indicated. While bacterial infections have been anecdotally described as associated with IAD, incidence is not known, and best practice guidance has not been established.

KEY POINT

Some general guidance for application of topical antifungals includes the "dusting" of prescription antifungal powder in a thin coating and covered with a liquid skin barrier or cream or ointment formulation. OTC antifungal barrier products containing miconazole are available as well.

INFECTION CONTROL CONSIDERATIONS

Collaboration with infection prevention colleagues is essential to identify how goals for skin integrity can align to or be balanced with infection control requirements. With the emphasis on CAUTI prevention, use of antiseptic agents for "catheter care" is becoming more common and the compatibility of antiseptics and skin care products must be considered. In settings where chlorhexidine gluconate (CHG) bathing is routine and includes application of CHG in the perineal/buttocks region, the compatibility of "leave-on" protective products with CHG should be determined. Additionally, all antiseptics are cytotoxic to some degree; use on damaged skin can potentially interfere with repair.

Environmental contamination is another consideration. Most products used for skin care are multiuse. During incontinence care and especially when diarrhea is present, there is potential for micro- and macrocontamination

of tubes or bottles with fecal material. This can raise the risk of spreading pathogens to other surfaces in the patient room and beyond. Consideration of product packaging that minimizes the risk of cross contamination is desirable and especially in settings where pathogens like *Clostridium difficile* have been problematic.

 ## PROFESSIONAL PRACTICE CONSIDERATIONS

In many organizations, the WOC nurse is responsible for outcomes related to skin integrity. With this in mind, it is important to monitor incidence of IAD. Frequent consults for severe IAD (GLOBIAD Category 2/2A, Beeckman et al., 2018) should trigger a review of incontinence skin care practice and products.

A number of quality improvement projects have demonstrated improvement in IAD outcomes. Gates et al. (2019) implemented a skin care algorithm in a surgical intensive care unit. Seventy-nine and 132 patients were included in the pre- and postassessment, respectively. They reported a 24% decrease in IAD over a 4-month period. Prather and Hines (2016) implemented nursing education and product standardization. Improvements included a 40% increase of staff ability to differentiate IAD from PI and a 41% increase in correct application of skin protectants. When the project was initiated, 100% of staff were using multiple products. Following implementation, 70% of staff were using the standard protocol. Skin outcomes were not reported. Hall and Clark (2015) implemented an on-line education program on IAD and HAPIs along with a one-step product for skin care. Preintervention, 29.4% of incontinent patients (*n* = 5) developed IAD with all developing a HAPI. Postintervention, no patients developed either IAD or a PI (*p* = 0.017).

Additional important information on process elements was provided by Nix and Ermer-Seltun (2004). They asked staff nurses to identify factors contributing to the development of IAD. Participants responded that absence of, or incomplete protocols, inadequate product knowledge and lack of convenient access to products were felt to be precursors to IAD. These data support the creation of facility-relevant protocols or algorithms for IAD prevention and treatment. The continence nurse should consider type and patterns of incontinence in order to create population-appropriate interventions. Processes and products should be clearly identified and understood by all levels of staff providing care.

Additionally, the continence nurse must create and maintain a formulary of products to support care delivery. This requires knowledge of products used for IAD care. In many organizations, this also involves collaborative work with business buyers including health value analysts. In the absence of published evidence on efficacy, product decisions can be based on a well-designed product evaluation. Performance criteria should be specific and measurable and consistent with indications for

---

BOX 17-1 IAD PREVENTION CHECK LIST

Does my facility have a written protocol for IAD prevention?
Does the staff know what it says and what is required of them?
Does the staff understand how to use the products specified in the protocol?
Can bedside staff access products 24 hours per day, 7 days per week?

---

use. If bedside staff participate, they should have clinical assessment expertise and be trained on product use.

The Institute for Healthcare Improvement (2011) has identified that *bedside accessible* skin care supplies are key to prevention efforts for pressure injuries. Within the four principles of health care ethics (Beauchamp & Childress, 2001), the concept of beneficence states that "health care providers must do all they can to benefit the patient in each situation." When applied to IAD prevention and treatment, this thinking calls for products to be available to staff whenever patient need arises. **Box 17-1** calls the continence care nurse to evaluate current "State of Affairs" in their care setting if they have the protocols, product formulary, accessible products, and knowledgeable staff to implement and optimize an IAD prevention program.

Beyond skin care, the acquisition of basic continence care knowledge and skills can be a valuable addition to the consultative services that the continence nurse provides. In addition to improved patient outcomes and satisfaction, the continence nurse may be able to show improved resource utilization and potential cost savings.

 ## CONCLUSION

IAD is an avoidable and preventable health care-associated skin injury that impacts quality of care often leading to pain, infection, pressure injuries, and patient dissatisfaction. Health care organizations need to acknowledge that all patients with incontinence are at risk for IAD and know the incidence of IAD in their organizations. Caregivers require education and infrastructure support that facilitates understanding of etiology, risk, and differential diagnosis for IAD. Structured protocols are critical to decreasing IAD in health care. Protocols must address reversible causes of incontinence, skin cleansing, application of a moisture barrier, and if indicated, treatment of secondary infection. As with most clinical challenges, patient and family education and engagement must be included with any care plan to prevent and manage IAD.

REFERENCES

Asmus, R., Bodkhe, R., Ekholm, B., et al. (November 2018; March 2019). The effect of a high endurance polymeric skin protectant on friction and shear stress. Poster presentation at 2018 Symposium on Advanced Wound Care Las Vegas NV and 2019 National Pressure Ulcer Advisory Panel Annual Conference St Louis MO.

Barakat-Johnson, M., Barnett, C., Lai, M., et al. (2018). Incontinence, incontinence-associated dermatitis, and pressure injuries in a health district in Australia: A mixed-methods study. *Journal of Wound, Ostomy, and Continence Nursing, 45*(4), 349–355.

Bayon-Garcia, C., Binks, R. M., DeLuca, E., et al. (2012). Prevalence, management and financial challenges associated with acute fecal incontinence in the ICU and critical care settings: The FIRST™ cross-sectional descriptive survey. *Intensive & Critical Care Nursing, 28*, 242–250.

Beauchamp, T. L., & Childress, J. F. (2001). *Principles of biomedical ethics* (5th ed.). New York, NY: Oxford University Press.

Beeckman, D. (2017). A decade of research on Incontinence-associated Dermatitis (IAD): Evidence, knowledge gaps and next steps. *Journal of Tissue Viability, 26*, 47–56.

Beeckman, D., Campbell, J., Campbell, K., et al. (2015). Incontinence-associated dermatitis: Moving prevention forward. Proceedings of the Global IAD Expert Panel. *Wounds International*. Retrieved October 21, 2019, from https://www.academia.edu/12441496/Proceedings_of_the_Global_IAD_Expert_Panel._Incontinence_associated_dermatitis_Moving_prevention_forward

Beeckman, D., Schoonhoven, L., Verhaeghe, S., et al. (2009). Prevention and treatment of incontinence-associated dermatitis: Literature review. *Journal of Advanced Nursing, 65*(6), 1141–1154.

Beeckman, D., Van Damme, N., Schoonhoven, L., et al. (2016). Interventions for preventing and treating incontinence associated dermatitis in adults. *The Cochrane Database of Systematic Reviews*, (11), CD011627.

Beeckman, D., Van den Bussche, K., Alves, P., et al. (2018). Towards an international language for incontinence-associated dermatitis (IAD): Design and evaluation of psychometric properties of the Ghent Global IAD Categorization Tool (GLOBIAD) in 30 countries. *The British Journal of Dermatology, 178*(6), 1331–1340.

Beeckman, D., Van Lancker, A., Van Hecke, A., et al. (2014). A systematic review and meta-analysis of incontinence-associated dermatitis, incontinence, and moisture as risk factors for pressure ulcer development. *Research in Nursing and Health, 37*(3), 204–218.

Beeckman, D., Woodward, S., Rajpaul, K., et al. (2011). Clinical challenges of preventing incontinence-associated dermatitis. *British Journal of Nursing, 20*(13), 784–786, 788, 790.

Beeson, T., & Davis, C. (2018). Urinary management with an external female collection device. *Journal of Wound, Ostomy, and Continence Nursing, 45*(2), 187–189.

Benoit, R. A. Jr, & Watts, C. (2007). The effect of a pressure ulcer prevention program and the bowel management system in reducing pressure ulcer prevalence in an ICU setting. *Journal of Wound, Ostomy, and Continence Nursing, 34*(2), 163–175.

Berg, R. W. (1988). Etiology and pathophysiology of diaper dermatitis. *Advances in Dermatology, 3*, 75–98.

Bliss, D. Z., Hurlow, J., Defalu, J., et al. (2014). Refinement of an instrument for assessing incontinent-associated dermatitis and its severity for use with darker-toned skin. *Journal of Wound, Ostomy, and Continence Nursing, 41*(4), 365–370.

Bliss, D. Z., Mathiason, M. A., Gurvich, O., et al. (2017). Incidence and predictors of incontinence associated skin damage in nursing home residents with new onset incontinence. *Journal of Wound, Ostomy, and Continence Nursing, 44*(2), 165–171.

Bolton, C., Flynn, R., Harvey, E., et al. (2004). Assessment of pad clogging. *Journal of Community Nursing, 18*(6), 18–20.

Borchert, K., Bliss, D. Z., Savik, K., et al. (2010). The incontinence-associated dermatitis and its severity instrument: Development and validation. *Journal of Wound, Ostomy, and Continence Nursing, 37*(5), 527–535.

Boronat-Garrido, X., Kottner, J., Schmitz, G., et al. (2016). Incontinence-associated dermatitis in nursing homes: Prevalence, severity, and risk factors in residents with urinary and/or fecal incontinence. *Journal of Wound, Ostomy, and Continence Nursing, 43*(6), 630–635.

Brennan, M. R., Milne, C. T., Agrell-Kann, M., et al. (2017). Clinical evaluation of a skin protectant for the management of incontinence-associated dermatitis: An open-label, nonrandomized, prospective study. *Journal of Wound, Ostomy, and Continence Nursing, 44*(2), 172–180.

Brunner, M., Droegemueller, C., Rivers, S., et al. (2012). Prevention of incontinence-related skin breakdown for acute and critical care patients: Comparison of two products. *Urologic Nursing, 32*(4), 214–219.

Bryant, R. A. (2012). Types of skin damage and differential diagnosis. In R. A. Bryant & D. P. Nix (Eds.), *Acute and chronic wounds: Current management concepts* (pp. 83–107). St Louis, MO: Mosby Elsevier.

Byers, P. H., Ryan, P. A., Regan, M. B., et al. (1995). Effects of incontinence care cleansing regimens on skin integrity. *Journal of Wound, Ostomy, and Continence Nursing, 22*(4), 188–192.

Campbell, J. L., Coyer, F. M., & Osborne, S. R. (2016). Incontinence-associated dermatitis: A cross-sectional prevalence study in the Australian acute care hospital setting. *International Wound Journal, 13*(3), 403–411.

Cooper, P., & Gray, D. (2001). Comparison of two skin care regimes for incontinence. *British Journal of Nursing, 10*(6), S7–S20.

Coyer, F., Gardner, A., & Doubrovsky, A. (2017). An interventional skin care protocol (InSPIRE) to reduce incontinence-associated dermatitis in critically ill patients in the intensive care unit. *Intensive & Critical Care Nursing, 40*, 1–10.

Demarre, L., Verhaeghe, S., Van Hecke, A., et al. (2015). Factors predicting the development of pressure ulcers in an at-risk population who receive standardized preventive care: Secondary analyses of a multicenter randomized controlled trial. *Journal of Advanced Nursing, 71*(2), 391–403.

Driver, D. S. (2007). Perineal dermatitis in critical care patients. *Critical Care Nurse, 27*, 42–46.

Dykes, P., & Bradbury, S. (2016). Incontinence pad absorption and skin barrier creams: A non-patients study. *British Journal of Nursing, 25*(22), 1244–1248.

Echols, J., Friedman, B. C., Mullins, R. F., et al. (2007). Clinical utility and economic impact of introducing a bowel management system. *Journal of Wound, Ostomy, and Continence Nursing, 34*(6), 664–670.

Falloon, S. S., Abbas, S., Stridfeldt, C., et al. (2018). The impact of microclimate on skin health with absorbent incontinence product use: An integrative review. *Journal of Wound, Ostomy, and Continence Nursing, 45*(4), 341–348. doi.org/10.1097/WON.0000000000000449.

Fleming, L., Zala, K., & Ousey, K. (2014). Investigating the absorbency of LBF barrier cream. *Wounds UK, 10*(2), 24–30.

Gates, B. P., Vess, J., Long, M. A., et al. (2019). Decreasing incontinence-associated dermatitis in the surgical intensive care unit. *Journal of Wound, Ostomy, and Continence Nursing, 46*(4), 327–331.

Gerhardt, L. C., Strassle, V., Lenz, A., et al. (2008). Influence of epidermal hydration on the friction of human skin against textiles. *Journal of the Royal Society Interface, 5*, 12.

Gray, M., Beeckman, D., Bliss, D. Z., et al. (2012). Incontinence associated dermatitis: A comprehensive review and update. *Journal of Wound, Ostomy, and Continence Nursing, 39*(1), 61–74.

Gray, M., Black, J., Baharestani, M., et al. (2011). Moisture-associated skin damage: Overview and pathophysiology. *Journal of Wound, Ostomy, and Continence Nursing, 38*(3), 233–241.

Gray, M., Bliss, D., Doughty, D., et al. (2007). Incontinence-associated dermatitis: A consensus. *Journal of Wound, Ostomy, and Continence Nursing, 34*(1), 45–54.

Gray, M., & Giuliano, K. K. (2018). Incontinence-associated dermatitis, characteristics and relationship to pressure injury: A multisite epidemiologic analysis. *Journal of Wound, Ostomy, and Continence Nursing, 45*(1), 63–67.

Gray, M., Kent, D., Ermer-Seltun, J., et al. (2018). Assessment, selection, use, and evaluation of body-worn absorbent products for adults with incontinence: A WOCN® Society Consensus Conference. *Journal of Wound, Ostomy, and Continence Nursing, 45*(3), 243–264.

Gray, M., Skinner, C., & Kaler, W. (2016). External collection devices as an alternative to the indwelling urinary catheter: Evidence-based review and expert clinical panel deliberations. *Journal of Wound, Ostomy, and Continence Nursing, 43*(3), 301–307.

Hall, K., & Clark, R. A. (2015). Prospective, descriptive, quality improvement study to decrease incontinence-associated dermatitis and hospital-acquired pressure ulcers. *Ostomy/Wound Management, 61*(7), 26–30.

Heidegger, P., Graf, S., Perneger, T., et al. (2016). The burden of diarrhea in the intensive care unit (ICU-BD). A survey and observational study of the caregivers opinions and workload. *International Journal of Nursing Studies, 59*, 163–168.

Institute for Healthcare Improvement. (2011). *How-to guide: Prevent pressure ulcers*. Cambridge, MA: Institute for Healthcare Improvement . Retrieved November 14, 2019, from www.ihi.org.

Kayser, S. A., Phipps, L., VanGilder, C. A., et al. (2019). Examining prevalence and risk factors of incontinence-associated dermatitis using the international pressure ulcer prevalence survey. *Journal of Wound, Ostomy, and Continence Nursing, 46*(4), 285–290.

Kottner, J., Blume-Peytavi, U., Lohrmann, C., et al. (2014). Associations between individual characteristics and incontinence-associated dermatitis: A secondary data analysis of a multi-center prevalence study. *International Journal of Nursing Studies, 51*, 1372–1380.

Kottner, J., & Surber, C. (2016). Skin care in nursing; a critical discussion of nursing practice and research. *International Journal of Nursing Studies, 61*, 20–28.

Lachenbruch, C., Ribble, D., Emmons, K., et al. (2016). Pressure ulcer risk in the incontinent patient: analysis of incontinence and hospital-acquired pressure ulcers from the International Pressure Ulcer Prevalence™ Survey. *Journal of Wound, Ostomy, and Continence Nursing, 43*(3), 235–241.

Lewis-Byers, K., Thayer, D., & Kahl, A. M. (2002). An evaluation of two incontinence skin care protocols in a long-term care setting. *Ostomy/Wound Management, 48*(12), 44–51.

Li, Y., Lee, H., Lo, Y. et al. (2019). Perineal assessment tool (pat-c): Validation of a Chinese language version and identification of a clinically validated cut point using roc curve analysis. *Journal of Wound, Ostomy, and Continence Nursing, 46*, 150–153.

Long, M. A., Reed, L. A., Dunning, K., et al. (2012). Incontinence-associated dermatitis in a long-term acute care facility. *Journal of Wound, Ostomy, and Continence Nursing, 39*(3), 318–327.

Lyder, C. H., Clemes-Lowrance, C., Davis, A., et al. (1992). Structured skin care regimen to prevent perineal dermatitis in the elderly. *Journal of ET Nursing, 19*, 12–16.

Mathisen, M., Grove, G., Houser, T., et al. (2018). Durability of an advanced skin protectant compared with other commercially available products in healthy human volunteers. *Wounds, 30*(9), 269–274.

Minassian, V., Devore, E., Hagan, K., et al. (2013). Severity of urinary incontinence and effect on quality of life in women, by incontinence type. *Obstetrics and Gynecology, 121*(5), 1083–1090.

Nix, D., & Ermer-Seltun, J. (2004). A review of perineal skin care protocols and skin barrier product use. *Ostomy/Wound Management, 50*(12), 59–67.

Nix, D. H. (2002). Validity and reliability of the perineal assessment tool. *Ostomy/Wound Management, 48*(2), 43–49.

Park, K. H., & Kim, K. S. (2014). Effect of a structured skin care regimen on patients with fecal incontinence: Comparison cohort study. *Journal of Wound, Ostomy, and Continence Nursing, 41*(2), 161–167.

Phipps, L., Gray, M., & Call, E. (2019). Time of onset to changes in skin condition during exposure to synthetic urine: A prospective study. *Journal of Wound, Ostomy, and Continence Nursing, 46*(4), 315–320.

Prather, P., & Hines, S. (2016). Best practice nursing care for ICU patients with incontinence-associated dermatitis and skin complications resulting from faecal incontinence and diarrhea. *International Journal of Evidence-Based Healthcare, 14*(1), 15–23.

Prather, P., Hines, S., Kynoch, K., et al. (2017). Effectiveness of topical skin products in the treatment and prevention of incontinence-associated dermatitis: A systematic review. *JBI Database Systematic Reviews and Implementation Reports, 15*(5), 1473–1496.

Rohwer, K., Bliss, D. Z., & Savik, K. (2013). Incontinence-associated dermatitis in community-dwelling individuals with fecal incontinence. *Journal of Wound, Ostomy, and Continence Nursing, 40*(2), 181–184.

Schaefer, P., Berwick-Sonntag, C., Capri, M. G., et al. (2002). Physiological changes in skin barrier function in relation to occlusion level, exposure time and climactic conditions. *Skin Pharmacology and Applied Skin Physiology, 15,* 7–19.

Schwartz, D., Magen, Y. K., Levy, A., et al. (2018). Effects of humidity on skin friction against medical textiles as related to prevention of pressure injuries. *International Wound Journal, 15*(6), 1–9.

Shiu, S. R., Hsu, M. Y., Chang, S. C., et al. (2013). Prevalence and predicting factors of incontinence-associated dermatitis among intensive care patients. *Journal of Nursing & Healthcare Research, 9*(3), 210.

Sibbald, G., Krasner, D., & Woo, K. (2011). Pressure ulcer staging revisited: Superficial skin changes and deep pressure ulcer framework. *Advances in Skin & Wound Care, 24*(12), 571–580.

Voegeli, D. (2012). Moisture-associated skin damage: Etiology, prevention and treatment. *British Journal of Nursing, 21*(9), 517–521.

Warshaw, E., Nix, D., Kula, J., et al. (2002). Clinical and cost effectiveness of a cleanser protectant lotion for treatment of perineal skin breakdown in low-risk patients with incontinence. *Ostomy/Wound Management, 48*(6), 44–51.

Zehrer, C., Grove, G., Newman, D., et al. (2005). Assessment of diaper-clogging potential of petrolatum moisture barriers. *Ostomy/Wound Management, 51*(12), 54–58. Retrieved from http://www.o-wm.com/content/assessmentdiaper-clogging-potential-petrolatum-moisture-barriers

Zhai, H., & Maibach, H. (2002). Occlusion versus skin barrier function. *Skin Research and Technology, 8,* 1–6.

CASE STUDY

Mr. Jones is an 80-year-old male who was admitted to home health care services following a recent hospitalization for pneumonia. Mr. Jones lives at home with his wife who is his primary caregiver. Mr. Jones' medical history includes Parkinson disease and hypertension. He has occasional fecal incontinence with episodes of loose stool. He wears a pull-on BWAP. In addition to his prehospitalization medication regimen, he was prescribed an oral antibiotic for 7 days.

Mr. Jones had been ambulatory in his home prior to this illness but now requires assistance to stand and transfer from his bed to the chair or commode. He sits in a recliner chair when up. His appetite is poor, but he has adequate fluid intake. He drinks one can of liquid nutritional supplement daily. He has had a 5-pound weight loss since his recent illness. Mrs. Jones provides daily hygiene and incontinence care. Personal care is often difficult for her to provide due to his weakness and limited mobility.

The home health nurse visits Mr. Jones twice a week. Upon assessment, the nurse observed that the scrotum was erythemic. The skin was moist and shiny, and Mr. Jones reported this area was sore. It was noted that the buttocks and intergluteal area were also reddened and moist, with scattered superficial lesions present. The home health care nurse requested a consultation from the Wound Ostomy Continence (WOC) nurse to determine the etiology of the skin breakdown and develop a plan to manage incontinence and skin care.

CASE STUDY QUESTIONS

1. What are the key factors contributing to skin breakdown?

    The key factors contributing to Mr. Jones skin breakdown include the following:
    - The skin is exposed to moisture and irritants from liquid stool. Stool may contain enzymes as well as other irritants that are damaging to the skin. Alteration in normal skin pH (change from acidic to alkaline) is also common. The presence of microbes can trigger a secondary infection.
    - Decreased mobility makes toileting difficult and incontinence care a challenge for his caregiver.
    - Friction from aggressive cleansing, moist or soiled incontinence garments, and transferring from a sitting to standing position contributes to skin breakdown. Moist skin is more prone to damage.

2. What are the clinical characteristics that will help the WOC Nurse determine that this is IAD versus a pressure injury?

    The characteristics most critical to differential assessment include location, depth and distribution of the damage, and patient history. Mr. Jones' breakdown involved areas exposed to urine and stool, the lesions were superficial and scattered, and his history includes multiple episodes of fecal incontinence; all of these findings are consistent with IAD. Pressure injuries are generally distinct open lesions that are located over and localized to a bony prominence.

3. What interventions must be included in the WOC Nurse's management plan?
    - Gentle cleansing with pH-balanced no-rinse cleanser
    - Protect skin with:
      - A polymer–cyanoacrylate skin protectant or
      - Pectin powder followed with an alcohol-free barrier film ("crusting") or
      - A moisture barrier ointment or
      - A moisture barrier paste

A pH-balanced no-rinse cleanser and disposable soft cloth would be appropriate. Application of a polymer–cyanoacrylate skin protectant provides a durable barrier that is easy to clean and does not require removal, easing the caregiver burden. "Crusting" is an alternative but may be difficult for home health staff to replicate. A moisture barrier ointment or paste may also be used but will require family to remove and reapply periodically.

Additional measures would include the following:
- Establish cause of diarrhea: perform basic continence assessment including gentle rectal exam to rule out impaction

- Review findings with primary care provider
- Use of a polymer-based absorptive product that wicks liquid away from the skin
- Bedside commode to facilitate toileting; scheduled toileting if indicated
- Consider physical therapy consult to provide strengthening exercises
- Nutritional assessment and modifications as indicated

QUESTIONS

1. Which of the following statement is true?
- A. IAD and MASD are used interchangeably.
- B. IAD is nonblanchable erythema.
- C. IAD is incontinence associated inflammation and erythema with or without erosion or denudation.
- D. IAD will become infected without antibiotics.

2. Pathophysiology of IAD includes:
- A. Overhydration of the stratum corneum
- B. Penetration by environmental irritants
- C. pH changes from alkaline to acid
- D. Presence of friction

3. What role does friction play in the development of IAD?
- A. Friction is associated with pressure injuries, not IAD
- B. IAD causes friction
- C. Incontinence skin cleansing causes friction
- D. All moisture barrier skin protectants cause friction

4. How does IAD present differently depending on skin tone?
- A. IAD appears initially as erythema in lighter skin while darker skin tones may present with paler, yellow, or dark discoloration.
- B. IAD appears patchy on lighter skin while darker skin tones present with distinct edges.
- C. IAD presents as partial-thickness skin breakdown with lighter skin while darker skin tones can have full-thickness IAD.
- D. None of the above.

5. On a patient with IAD, a red rash with pinpoint satellite lesions (papules or pustules) in the perineal region is most likely indicative of:
- A. *Staphylococcus aureus*
- B. Herpes zoster
- C. Candidiasis
- D. Tinea pedis

6. The WOC nurse is preparing a teaching plan for prevention and treatment of incontinence-associated dermatitis (IAD) in long-term care facilities. What teaching point should the nurse include?
- A. Cleanse the skin vigorously twice per day using a soft cloth and antibacterial soap.
- B. Apply a moisturizer to any skin that is red.
- C. Always leave briefs open to air.
- D. Use a moisture barrier to protect skin from urine and stool.

7. A WOC nurse is preparing a treatment plan for a patient with IAD and denuded skin. Which intervention is not recommended for this patient?
- A. Using an ointment containing glycerin and petrolatum on denuded skin
- B. Leaving the area open to air
- C. Using a moisture barrier paste
- D. Using a polymer–cyanoacrylate skin protectant

8. Desirable characteristics for a moisture barrier include:
- A. Durable, breathable and transparent
- B. Transparent, antifungal and antibacterial
- C. pH balanced, breathable and vanishing
- D. Noncytotoxic, pH balanced and visible

9. For IAD prevention, multifunction ("3-in-1") products are used to:
   A. Cleanse, disinfect, and protect
   B. Cleanse, protect, and restore if needed
   C. Cleanse, moisturize, and treat
   D. Cleanse, protect, and soothe

10. When designing a program for IAD prevention and treatment, the continence care nurse should incorporate which of the following elements:
   A. Staff autonomy in determining skin care protocol for each patient
   B. Formulary with at least 3 cleansers and 3 moisture barriers
   C. Structured skin care regimen (protocol) and bedside accessible supplies
   D. Engagement of medical staff for guidance

ANSWERS AND RATIONALES

1. C. Rationale: IAD is a type of top-down injury and the most common form of moisture-associated skin damage (MASD). IAD is characterized by erythema and edema of the surface of the skin, sometimes accompanied by serous exudate, erosion, or secondary cutaneous infection.

2. A. Rationale: Overhydration of the stratum corneum compromises the brick-and-mortar configuration of the epidermal layer and permits penetration by irritants found in urine and stool, which results in inflammation and impaired tensile strength. As urea in urine breaks down, highly alkaline ammonia is produced and changes pH from acid to alkaline and compromised the protective acidic mantle of the skin.

3. C. Rationale: Incontinence care involves the use of friction for skin cleansing. Forces of friction and shear against an underlying surface (bed, chair, linen, containment garments) wound the skin and allow pathogens such as *Candida* and *Staphylococcus* to enter, invade, and cause secondary infections.

4. A. Rationale: IAD appears initially as erythema ranging from pink to red. Darker skin tones may present with paler, yellow, or dark discoloration. All skin effected by IAD can look patchy with nondistinct edges. Current evidence suggests that IAD is limited to partial-thickness skin breakdown.

5. C. Rationale: A red rash with pinpoint satellite lesions (papules or pustules) is indicative of a candidiasis (a secondary infection) and is not uncommon. Bacterial infections secondary to IAD are not commonly reported in peer review literature. Herpes zoster is an important differential diagnosis for IAD but presents without satellite lesions and are generally grouped unilaterally along dermatomes.

6. D. Rationale: Cleansing skin vigorously is never appropriate. When skin is red, IAD is already present and a moisture barrier versus moisturizer is indicated. The practice of leaving briefs open to air may provide some benefit but would not be a recommendation for all residents. All incontinent patients are at risk for IAD so use of a moisture barrier to protect skin is always advisable.

7. B. Rationale: Once IAD has been observed and especially if denudement is present, the objective of care is to protect the skin from further exposure to stool and/or urine and create an environment that promotes healing. This is accomplished with application of a moisture barrier. Leaving the area open to air will not provide skin protection.

8. A. Rationale: Important characteristics for a moisture barrier include durability (to assure protection over time), breathability (to allow moisture vapor transmission from the skin), and transparency (allows for skin assessment). The presence of an antifungal or antibacterial is not necessary unless an infection is present. While visible barriers are desired by some clinicians, visible barriers can interfere with skin assessment.

9. B. Rationale: Multifunction products contain ingredients "to cleanse" and "to protect" by utilization of a moister barrier skin protectant, and some products contain ceramides to help replace lipids lost to the skin thus "restoring" barrier function. They do not contain antifungals or antibacterials. Because of formulation characteristics, they are best used for prevention of IAD. When used in patients at *high risk* for IAD (i.e., frequent or continuous liquid stool), skin should be observed often as a more protective barrier may be required.

10. C. Rationale: A structured skin care regimen and bedside accessible supplies are considered essential to effective IAD prevention efforts.

Improved outcomes have been demonstrated when staff follows an established protocol for skin care, individualizing a care plan can then occur as needed. Stocking multiple products within a single category can prove confusing to staff and can add unnecessary cost. While support of the medical staff is always desirable, the wound care nurse can provide valuable guidance on IAD prevention and treatment *to* physician colleagues.

CHAPTER 18

URINARY TRACT INFECTION (UTI) PREVENTION AND MANAGEMENT IN ADULTS

Kelly Nelles and JoAnn M. Ermer-Seltun

OBJECTIVES

1. Distinguish the types of UTI and demonstrate correct terminology.
2. Describe the pathophysiology of UTIs including risk factors.
3. Implement evidence-based prevention and treatment of UTIs in adults.

TOPIC OUTLINE

OVERVIEW AND PREVALENCE

In adults, urinary tract infections (UTIs) are one of the most common bacterial infections, occurring second in frequency only to respiratory infections. Adult UTIs account for almost 25% of all infections presenting across patient care settings including primary care, specialty clinics, the emergency department and, when complicating factors are present, often results in acute hospitalization. *Escherichia coli (E. coli)* is the bacteria that most commonly causes UTI and is responsible for 85% of community-acquired UTIs and 50% of hospital-acquired UTIs.

Women are more likely than men to experience UTI (Geerlings, 2016; Stapleton, 2014). Sixty percent of U.S. women have at least one symptomatic UTI during their lifetime with approximately 10% also having one or more episodes of symptomatic UTIs each year (Lee & Le, 2018; Medina & Castillo-Pino, 2019). By age 24, one in three women will have experienced a UTI. The prevalence of UTI in men is significantly less than women with only about 20% of all UTIs occurring in men. After the age of 50, UTI in men occurs most commonly as this is when urologic structural abnormalities including enlarged prostate or bladder outlet obstruction are more likely to occur (McLellan & Hunstad, 2016). As both men and women age, it is important to note that the risk for cystitis gradually increases for both genders after the age of 35 until age 65 when the incidence for both becomes similar. No racial or ethnic difference in UTI prevalence has been found.

KEY POINT

UTIs are the most common bacterial infection, and women are at a higher risk for development compared to men.

TERMINOLOGY AND CLASSIFICATION

Urinary tract infection or *UTI* is the broad term used to describe a bacterial infection or invasion of microbial uropathogens occurring in the lower or upper urinary tract or both. Microbial infection can occur in any part of the urinary tract including the urethra, bladder, ureters, and kidneys (see **Fig. 18-1**). Anatomically, UTIs are typically identified as lower urinary tract (LUT) or upper urinary tract (UUT) infection based on their site of origin. Infections of the LUT are typically found in the bladder (cystitis)

or urethra (urethritis), while UUT infection is found in the ureter or kidney (pyelonephritis). Determining the origin of the UTI is important in correlating potential health risk and management options. Patients often use the term "bladder infection" to refer to all UTIs, and determining the site of the infection aids the nurse in assessing risk and monitoring for related health problems.

In addition to identification of the UTI by anatomic origin, UTIs can also be further categorized as simple, complicated, and recurrent. See **Box 18-1** for UTI terminology and definitions. Simple UTIs are also referred to as uncomplicated UTIs and occur in young, healthy, nonpregnant women with normal anatomy. Complicated UTIs occurs in patients with factors that increase the risk of bacterial colonization and decrease the efficacy of therapy (Stapleton, 2014). Risk factors associated with complicated UTI include the following: involvement of the UUT; male anatomy; pregnancy; anatomic abnormalities; urolithiasis; the presence of catheters, stents, or tubes; malignancy; chemotherapy and immunosuppression; failure of antibiotics; and hospital or health care exposure (Dubbs & Sommerkamp, 2019).

KEY POINT

UTIs are categorized as simple, complicated, and recurrent. Simple UTIs occur in healthy, young, nonpregnant females with a normal genitourinary system.

KEY POINT

Risk factors for a complicated UTI include pregnancy, male anatomy, structural or functional abnormalities, presence of foreign objects, immunosuppression, disease of the renal system, antibiotic failure, and health care exposure.

Recurrent UTI (rUTI) is defined as having two or more infections within 6 months of completion of treatment of the initial infection or three or more infections in 12 months with either reinfection with a previously isolated organism or persistence of bacteria (Freeman et al., 2017). Recurrent UTIs are more likely to occur in women with 20% to 30% experiencing a reinfection within 6 months from the completion of their initial

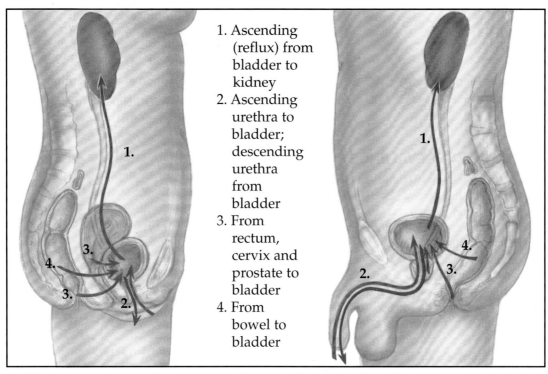

1. Ascending (reflux) from bladder to kidney
2. Ascending urethra to bladder; descending urethra from bladder
3. From rectum, cervix and prostate to bladder
4. From bowel to bladder

Routes of Infection in the Urinary Tract

FIGURE 18-1. Lower and Upper Urinary Tract. (Anatomical Chart Company. (2000). *Urinary tract anatomical chart*. Philadelphia, PA: Wolters Kluwer Health, Inc.)

BOX 18-1 UTI TERMINOLOGY AND DEFINITIONS

TERM	DEFINITION
Urinary tract infection (UTI)	Broadly describes the presence of pathogenic bacteria within the urinary tract in combination with clinical symptoms and/or inflammation in response to the pathogen.
Lower UTI	The presence of clinical symptoms and pathogenic bacteria affecting the urethra (urethritis) or bladder (cystitis).
Upper UTI	The presence of clinical symptoms and pathogenic bacteria affecting the ureter and kidneys (pyelonephritis).
Simple, uncomplicated UTI	LUT infection in otherwise healthy, nonpregnant women.
Complicated UTI (cUTI)	Occurs in patients with factors that increase the risk of bacterial colonization and decrease the efficacy of therapy including pregnant women; all men with obstruction; immunosuppression; renal failure; renal transplantation; urinary retention from neurologic disease and individuals with risk factors that predispose to persistent or relapsing infection (e.g., calculi, indwelling catheters or other drainage devices); health care associated.
Recurrent UTI (rUTI)	>2 infections in 6 months or >3 infections in 12 months with either reinfection with a previously isolated organism or persistence of bacteria.
Asymptomatic bacteriuria (ASB)	The presence of bacteria in the urine without signs and symptoms of infection.
Uncomplicated pyelonephritis	Infection involving renal structures limited to healthy individuals and nonpregnant pregnant women.
Complicated pyelonephritis	Infection of the kidney in individuals who are at a higher risk for urosepsis and treatment failure. See risk factors as described under complicated UTI.
Catheter-associated UTI (CAUTI)	UTI in an individual with an indwelling catheter at least 48 hours in place prior to the UTI or day after the catheter was removed (CDC, 2020).
Urosepsis	Life-threatening infection of the urinary tract that causes a systemic inflammatory chain reaction in the body that rapidly leads to tissue damage, organ failure, or death if treatment is delayed.

treatment and approximately 3% experiencing a third UTI (Lee & Le, 2018). Interestingly, there appears to be a genetic predisposition to rUTI. Women with a family history of UTIs have been found to be more susceptible to rUTIs. Recurrent UTIs also occur more frequently in women who have P1 blood phenotype or who are non-secretors of ABO blood group antigens. The expression of *E. coli* receptors and enhanced adherence of *E. coli* have been found to be present in this group (Freeman et al., 2017). Morbidity experienced by women with rUTIs directly impacts quality of life and includes pain, missed work or school, and the need for bed rest. Pregnant women, frail elderly, and those who are immunocompromised are most at risk for mortality associated with rUTIs. Pregnant women are more likely to develop pyelonephritis, experience premature delivery, and fetal mortality. Frail elders and immunocompromised persons are at greater risk for pyelonephritis, urosepsis, and death.

KEY POINT

Recurrent UTI is defined as having two or more episodes of cystitis in 6 months or three UTIs within a 12-month period.

Recurrent UTI is different from asymptomatic bacteriuria (ASB), which is often mistaken as recurrence or reinfection. While bacteriuria is defined as the presence of bacteria in the urine that has not been contaminated from a source outside of the body such as the skin, vagina, or foreskin; ASB is then, the presence of bacteria in the urine *without* signs and symptoms of infection (Bonkat et al., 2019; Nicolle et al., 2019). Factors that influence the likely development of bacterial colonization of the urinary tract without symptom development include incomplete bladder emptying, long-term urinary catheter use, and ureteral stents. Postmenopausal women and frail elders living in community-dwelling settings such as nursing homes are also more likely to demonstrate ASB (Nicolle et al., 2019). It is important to note that there is no evidence of increased mortality or morbidity associated with ASB. Antibiotic therapy for ASB is not indicated in most cases; it is harmful in persons with rUTI because it promotes multidrug-resistant (MDR) organisms, colonization, and potential for drug-related adverse reactions (Bonkat et al., 2019; Kang et al., 2018; Nicolle et al., 2019). Strong evidence does support screening and treatment of ASB in individuals undergoing urological procedures that may disrupt the urethral mucosa, and there is weak evidence to support screening for and treating ASB in pregnant women with appropriate short-course treatment (Bonkat et al., 2019; Kang et al., 2018; Nicolle et al., 2019) (see **Table 18-1**).

TABLE 18-1 SCREENING AND TREATMENT FOR ASYMPTOMATIC BACTERIURIA		
CLINICAL SCENARIO	YES	NO
Individuals with recurrent UTIs		X
Postmenopausal women		X
Residents of assisted living or long-term care		X
Renal transplant patients		X
Individuals with arthroplasty		X
Diabetic patients		X
Women with risk factors for UTIs		X
Individuals with indwelling catheters		X
Individual with ileal conduit, nephrostomy tube, reconstructed, or dysfunctional lower urinary tracts		X
Individuals undergoing urological procedures that may breach genitourinary mucosa	X	
Pregnant women	X	

Adapted from Bonkat et al. (2019).

KEY POINT

ASB is commonly found in older adults who reside in care facilities; patients with an indwelling catheter, stent, or nephrostomy tube; and those who perform intermittent catheterization. Screening and treatment of ASB is not recommended except in pregnancy or prior to urological procedure.

 PATHOPHYSIOLOGY

In healthy adults, urine is sterile throughout the urinary tract from the renal glomerulus to the external sphincter in men and the bladder neck in females (Hickling et al., 2015). The unobstructed forward flow of urine that occurs with normal voiding is the primary way that the urinary tract maintains sterility. Other factors that play a significant role in preventing UTIs include urine acidity, immunologic defenses, and mucosal barriers (Dubbs & Sommerkamp, 2019). In the LUT, cystitis occurs 30% more commonly in women than in men (Foxman, 2002, 2010), primarily due to the anatomic differences that include a shorter urethral length, close proximity of the vagina and anus, and a moist periurethral environment conducive to microbial proliferation (Hickling et al., 2015; Lee & Le, 2018). Both of these factors contribute to the colonization and migration of bacteria from the urethra to the bladder in women. In both men and women, the ability of the bacteria to adhere to the uroepithelium and propel itself is a significant mechanism in the development of cystitis with infection occurring when the virulence of the bacteria overcomes the hosts defense mechanisms. These same mechanisms are also factoring in the development of UUT infections (pyelonephritis) as bacteria ascends to kidneys by the ureters. Risk for

UUT infections is increased with the presence of catheters, kidney, or bladder stones or in incomplete bladder emptying or retention.

Most UTIs are caused by gram-negative bacteria with the most common being *E. coli*. *E. coli* is part of the *Enterobacteriaceae* family, which are found in the GI tract and accounts for 80% to 90% of cystitis and pyelonephritis in young, healthy, sexually active women and 50% of hospital-acquired UTIs (Freeman et al., 2017). In women, the colonization of bacteria from the rectum to the perineum, vagina, and/or distal urethra can ascend into the bladder and is often a precipitating event leading to a UTI. Other gram-negative organisms causing infection include *Klebsiella*, *Proteus*, *Enterobacter*, and *Pseudomonas*. Gram-positive organisms include streptococci, enterococci, and staphylococci (see **Box 18-2**).

KEY POINT

Gram-negative bacteria, especially *E. coli*, are responsible for most lower or upper urinary tract infections.

RISK FACTORS

The risk of developing a UTI is related to a series of factors. Underlying health conditions related to systemic disease, alterations in urinary tract function or structure, instrumentation, the presence of a foreign body, and obstruction have all been shown to significantly increase the risk of UTI. Gender including hormone status in women and health behaviors also increase UTI

BOX 18-2	COMMON ORGANISMS THAT CAN CAUSE URINARY TRACT INFECTION
GRAM-POSITIVE BACTERIA	**GRAM-NEGATIVE BACTERIA**
Streptococcus faecalis	*Escherichia coli (E. coli)*
Streptococcus pneumoniae	*Klebsiella* species
Enterococcus faecalis may have specific affinity for the kidney	Extended-spectrum beta-lactamase-resistant (ESBL) *E. coli/Klebsiella* species
Enterococcus faecium	*Enterobacter* species
Methicillin-sensitive *Staphylococcus aureus* (MSSA)	*Proteus mirabilis*
Staphylococcus aureus (S. aureus): rare	
Methicillin-resistant *Staphylococcus aureus* (MRSA)	*Pseudomonas aeruginosa*
Staphylococcus epidermidis	*Citrobacter*

Source: Newman, D., Wyman, J., & Welch, V. (2017). Chapter 33: Urinary tract infections. In *Core curriculum for urologic nursing* (1st ed.). SUNA.

risk. Diabetes, kidney disease, malignancy, HIV, and immunosuppression are examples of systemic disease states that increase risk of UTI development. Alterations in urinary tract function or structure that increase UTI risk include urethral stricture, urinary stone development or urolithiasis, vesicoureteral reflux in which urine follows backward from the bladder into the kidneys and neurogenic dysfunction of the LUT. The structural changes related to pelvic organ prolapse in women and prostate enlargement in men increase the likelihood of incomplete bladder emptying and risk of UTI. Instrumentation related to urologic procedures and the use of urinary catheters, stents, and nephrostomy tubes also result in increased UTI risk. The presence of a foreign body such as a calculus, enlarged prostate, and bladder neck obstruction also significantly increase risk (see **Box 18-3**).

In women, maternal family history of UTI or UTI before the age of 15 increases overall UTI risk. Women ages 16 to 35 who become sexually active and/or have a new sexual partner within the past year also are more likely to experience UTI. Contraceptive options including spermicides, condoms, or diaphragms may also contribute. Alterations in pregnancy also increase risk for UTI including pyelonephritis. The enlarging uterus can put pressure on the ureters resulting in mechanical obstruction. Normal physiologic changes of pregnancy including bladder enlargement and smooth muscle relaxation can lead to increased capacity and urinary stasis resulting in infection. Estrogen deficiency and its accompanying physiologic alterations of uro-vaginal tissue, structure, and pH result in increased UTI risk (Hickling et al., 2015). Estrogen deficiency is common with menopause, the use of progestin-only contraceptives, and some medications including selective estrogen receptor modulators (SERMs) used to prevent or treat breast cancer. The relaxation of pelvic organs seen with pelvic organ prolapse can result in obstruction or incomplete bladder emptying. Changes in healthy vaginal flora, particularly the lack of H_2O_2 producing lactobacilli, can increase the risk of periurethral colonization with bacteria (most commonly *E. coli*) resulting in UTI (Stapleton et al., 2011).

UTI risk for men increases with anal intercourse, lack of circumcision, and the presence of underlying urologic abnormalities that occur with aging. This includes benign prostate hypertrophy that causes enlargement of the prostate, which in turns can put pressure on the bladder neck resulting in failure to empty the bladder completely and facilitating bacteria growth.

Health behaviors predominately related to UTI risk include hydration, voiding frequency, and hygiene. Poor fluid intake, dehydration, infrequent or incomplete bladder emptying, inadequate personal hygiene, and use of unsanitary urination devices have all been shown to increase UTI risk. Living conditions where there is a lack of privacy or limited showers may make personal hygiene difficult. This is common problem particularly for

BOX 18-3   UTI RISK FACTORS

Underlying health conditions	Diabetes
	Kidney disease
	Malignancy
	HIV
	Immunosuppression
Altered urinary tract function or structures	Urethral stricture
	Urinary stone development (urolithiasis)
	Vesicoureteral reflux (VUR)
	LUT neurogenic dysfunction
	Pelvic organ prolapse
	Enlarged prostate (benign prostatic hypertrophy)
Instrumentation	Urologic procedures
	Urinary catheters
	Stents
	Nephrostomy tubes
Foreign body	Calculus
Young and premenopausal women	Maternal family history
	First UTI before age of 15
	New sexual partner
	Contraceptive use of spermicides and/or diaphragm
	Pregnancy
Postmenopausal and elderly women	History of UTI before menopause
	Estrogen deficiency
	Cystocele
	Urinary incontinence
	Increased postvoid urine volume
	Blood group antigen secretory status
	Urinary catheterization
	Functional or mental decline in elderly institutionalized women
Men	Anal intercourse
	Lack of circumcision
	Benign prostate enlargement
Health behaviors	Poor fluid intake, dehydration
	Infrequent toileting or voiding
	Inadequate personal hygiene
	Use of unsanitary urination devices (e.g., bottles, bags, funnels)

Sources: Bonkat et al. (2019); Lee and Le (2018).

women in the armed services or living in shelter or group situations. There are some jobs where breaks or toileting opportunities are limited or the inconvenience of removing bulky clothing or gear results in workers intentionally limiting their fluid intake or holding their urine for extended periods of time thus increasing their UTI risk.

 ## CLINICAL PRESENTATION

Acute uncomplicated UTIs commonly seen with cystitis are characterized by signs and symptoms of bladder irritation, increased frequency, urgency and dysuria, and occasionally hematuria. Patients may also report suprapubic pressure, tenderness, or pain. The presence of fever, chills, costovertebral angle (CVA) tenderness, nausea, and vomiting suggests a more complicated UTI consistent with pyelonephritis. Malaise, nocturia, urinary incontinence (UI), or complaint of foul-smelling urine is more likely to be experienced by postmenopausal women and the elderly (Freeman et al., 2017). In addition, dizziness, hypotension, and altered mental status may also be experienced more commonly in the elderly. The nursing assessment should assess for all these potential symptoms to determine the severity of the clinical presentation.

KEY POINT

Classic symptoms of uncomplicated cystitis include urinary frequency, urgency, and dysuria and possible hematuria and suprapubic pressure or pain. Fever, chills, CVA tenderness, nausea, or vomiting generally are classic signs of an upper tract infection (pyelonephritis).

 ## FOCUSED PATIENT HISTORY

While Chapter 4—Primary Assessment of Patients with Urinary Incontinence and Voiding Dysfunction—should be referred to for detailed guidance specific to comprehensive assessment, there are key components of the history and physical that should be performed when assessing for UTI.

CHIEF COMPLAINT AND/OR PRESENTING SYMPTOMS

It is important to document in the patient's own words the symptoms they are experiencing. Patient states they are experiencing "burning with urination and going to the bathroom more frequently" is an example of such a statement. Subjective data are helpful in describing the clinical presentation and should be captured in a statement using the patient's own words.

HISTORY OF PRESENT ILLNESS

The nurse should expand on the patient's presenting statement by gathering more information about symptoms. Using the acronym OLDCART provides a nursing prompt to specifically assess the onset, length, duration, characteristics, aggravating factors, relieving factors, and timing of symptoms or self-employed treatment (see Chapter 4, Box 4-1). Symptoms of both cystitis and pyelonephritis should be thoroughly assessed and documented.

MEDICAL/SURGICAL HISTORY

Review of patient history should include past and current history of medical conditions, surgeries, and procedures that could impact overall UTI risk. A history of diabetes, kidney disease, immunocompromised, and recent urologic instrumentation are factors that need to be identified as they complicate the clinical picture. History of UTI and sexually transmitted infection (STI) should also be determined along with a history of prostatitis in men and vaginitis in women.

FAMILY HISTORY

Specifically reviewing maternal history for UTI and rUTI is also helpful in determining the clinical picture related to potential UTI risk.

MEDICATIONS

While all medications should always be reviewed at every visit, recent antibiotic use and the use of immune-modifying drugs should specifically be documented. The use of phenazopyridine (Pyridium) often employed to self-treat symptoms should also be identified as this medication can alter the urinalysis results by causing nitrites to be falsely positive. In 2015, the U.S. Food and Drug Administration (USFDA, 2015) safety assessment lead to additional label warnings on a specific class of type 2 diabetes medicines called sodium–glucose cotransporter-2 (SGLT2) inhibitors regarding the elevated risk for serious urinary tract infections that could result in hospitalization. SGLT2 inhibitors also cause glucosuria due to kidney excretion of glucose to reduce blood sugar levels, which may be reflected in the urinalysis.

KEY POINT

A thorough review of medications is conducted to further explore complicating factors that may affect UTI management including immunosuppressants, recent antibiotic use, and over-the-counter products to ameliorate urogenital symptoms.

GYNECOLOGIC HISTORY

Date of last menstrual period, sexual history including current and new partners, pregnancy risk, and contraceptive use, including spermicide and barrier methods, should be assessed and documented. Vaginal and pelvic symptoms including vaginal discharge, odor, itching, knowledge of vaginal prolapse, perigenital skin health, and low abdominal pain should also be determined. In addition, ask about sensation of incomplete emptying of bladder, the presence of urinary or fecal incontinence, absorptive product use, past urogynecology procedures, douche practices, and last documented UTI if known.

GU HISTORY

In men, sexual history including current and new partners, anal intercourse, history of sexually transmitted diseases (STDs) urethral discharge, knowledge of an enlarged prostate, LUT symptoms, and previous urological interventions should be reviewed.

SOCIAL HISTORY

Living and work situations are important considerations to explore as these may provide clues to potential contributing factors such as hydration, voiding patterns, and hygiene practices that may be related to increased UTI risk.

● FOCUSED PHYSICAL EXAMINATION

GENERAL ASSESSMENT

The patient's overall health status including overall comfort level and hydration status should be described. Vital signs including temperature, blood pressure, and pulse should be collected and documented. Temperature of 38.5°C or 101°F and tachycardia should alert the nurse to a more complicated UTI and possible pyelonephritis. Depending on the clinical presentation, assessment of overall, cognitive, and functional status may be indicated.

ABDOMINAL EXAMINATION

Comprehensive abdominal examination including inspection, auscultation, percussion, and palpation are indicated. Percussion should specifically test for CVA tenderness. This can be performed in either a sitting or lying position. When performing this aspect of the examination, the nurse places one hand over the CVA of the patient's back and provides a percussive thump with the other hand, allowing the kidney to vibrate (see **Fig. 18-2**). The test is positive when either CVA tenderness is elicited or back/flank pain is reproduced. If the patient experiences no pain, then renal involvement is ruled out. In addition, percussion for suprapubic dullness may indicate urinary retention, a risk factor for UTI. Chapter 4 reviews the technique of percussion to define the outline of a distended bladder.

GENITAL EXAMINATION

Vaginal or urethral discharge, excoriations, moisture-associated skin damage (MASD), tenderness, swelling and ulcerations, and poor personal hygiene can be identified on genital and perianal examination. Evidence of pelvic organ prolapse, atrophic vaginal and urethral changes, and Skene gland cyst may be observed in women. Digital rectal examination to assess for hard stool depending upon history and prostate enlargement to tenderness or bogginess may be indicated for men.

KEY POINT

Focus physical examination provides objective findings to confirm potential causal and contributing factors of urogenital symptoms.

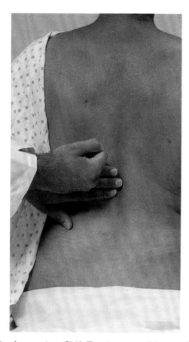

FIGURE 18-2. Assessing CVA Tenderness. (Hogan-Quigley, B., Palm, M. L., & Bickley, L. S. (2016). *Bates' nursing guide to physical examination and history taking*. Philadelphia, PA: Wolters Kluwer Health, Inc.)

LABORATORY AND DIAGNOSTIC STUDIES

URINALYSIS

Urinalysis (UA) is the most important initial test to obtain. The urine sample should be collected using either midstream voided collection or sterile straight catheterization. The clean catch method for obtaining voided specimens is the most common method of sample collection. It involves cleaning the periurethral area with a sterile wipe and collection of midstream urine with the foreskin retracted in uncircumcised males or the labia fully separated in females. In patients who are unable to provide a satisfactory voided sample, sterile urethral catheterization can be performed with either a single-use intermittent catheter or an indwelling catheter, if indicated. Care must be taken during catheterization, as it is possible for bacteria to be introduced into the urinary system during the placement process (Dubbs & Sommerkamp, 2019). The presence of epithelial (skin) cells on microscopic examination is suggestive of a contaminated specimen, and the UA should be repeated (see **Box 18-4**, Urinalysis and Culture).

The urine dipstick is the most common initial step in urine laboratory testing. It can be used in combination with microscopic urine evaluation. The dipstick uses color changes to indicate the presence of leukocyte esterase, nitrite, urobilinogen, protein, blood, ketones, bilirubin, and glucose. It also provides a range of pH and specific gravity. UA obtained in symptomatic individuals should be considered positive in the presence of any of

BOX 18-4   URINALYSIS AND THE URINE CULTURE

Protein in the urine (proteinuria) can usually be detected by dipstick when present in large amounts. Protein may appear constantly or only intermittently in the urine, depending on the cause. Proteinuria may occur normally after strenuous exercise, such as marathon running, but is usually a sign of a kidney disorder. Small amounts of protein in the urine may be an early sign of kidney damage due to diabetes. Such small amounts may not be detected by dipstick. In these cases, urine will need to be collected over a period of 12 or 24 hours and tested by a laboratory.

Glucose in the urine (glucosuria) can be accurately detected by dipstick. The most common cause of glucose in the urine is diabetes mellitus, but absence of glucose does not mean a person does not have diabetes or that the diabetes is well controlled. Also, presence of glucose does not necessarily indicate diabetes or another problem.

Ketones in the urine (ketonuria) can often be detected by dipstick. Ketones are formed when the body breaks down fat. Ketones can appear in the urine as a result of starvation or uncontrolled diabetes mellitus and occasionally after drinking significant amounts of alcohol.

Blood in the urine (hematuria) is detectable by dipstick and confirmed by viewing the urine with a microscope and other tests. Sometimes the urine contains enough blood to be visible, making the urine appear red or brown.

Nitrites in the urine (nitrituria) are also detectable by dipstick. High nitrite levels indicate a UTI.

Leukocyte esterase (an enzyme found in certain white blood cells) in the urine can be detected by dipstick. Leukocyte esterase is a sign of inflammation, which is most commonly caused by a urinary tract infection.

The acidity of urine is measured by dipstick. Certain foods, chemical imbalances, and metabolic disorders may change the acidity of urine.

The concentration of urine (also called the osmolality, roughly indicated by specific gravity) can vary widely depending on whether a person is dehydrated, how much fluid a person has drunk, and other factors. Urine concentration is also sometimes important in diagnosing abnormal kidney function. The kidneys lose their capacity to concentrate urine at an early stage of a disorder that leads to kidney failure. In one special test, a person drinks no water or other fluids for 12 to 14 hours. In another test, a person receives an injection of vasopressin (also called antidiuretic hormone). Afterward, urine concentration is measured. Normally, either test should make the urine highly concentrated. However, in certain kidney disorders (such as nephrogenic diabetes insipidus), the urine cannot be concentrated even though other kidney functions are normal.

Sediment in urine can be examined under a microscope to provide information about a possible kidney or urinary tract disorder. Normally, urine contains a small number of cells and other debris shed from the inside of the urinary tract. A person who has a kidney or urinary tract disorder usually sheds more cells, which form a sediment if urine is spun in a centrifuge (a laboratory instrument that uses centrifugal force to separate components of a liquid) or allowed to settle.

Source: Figler, B. (December 2017). Urinalysis and the urine culture. *Merck Manual*. Retrieved from https://www.merckmanuals.com/home/kidney-and-urinary-tract-disorders/diagnosis-of-kidney-and-urinary-tract-disorders/urinalysis-and-urine-culture

the following: leukocyte esterase, nitrites, occult blood, or bacteria. Positive for leukocyte esterase reflects the presence of white blood cells (WBC). Positive nitrite reflects the presence of urinary nitrite, which is reduced from urinary nitrate produced by some bacteria. Positive nitrites suggest the presence of gram-negative bacteria, which converts urinary nitrates to nitrites. The test will not be positive if gram-positive species are the causative microbes (Freeman et al., 2017). It is important to note that not all bacteria produce nitrite and that not all UTIs are associated with WBCs; however, if both the nitrite and leukocyte esterase tests are positive, then a UTI is present more than 90% of the time (Buttaro et al., 2016; Freeman et al., 2017). In the future, a novel diagnostic may be introduced to better identify UTIs in the frail elderly or pediatric populations who present with vague symptoms through the measurement of serum procalcitonin, a peptide that changes into calcitonin. Serum procalcitonin will rapidly and consistently elevate in the presence of a severe microbial infection thus may serve as a sensitive and specific indicator for UTI diagnosis, but further studies are needed to validate this simple test in UTI diagnosis (Levine et al., 2018; Pescatore et al., 2019).

> **KEY POINT**
>
> Urinalysis is key in the diagnosis of a UTI. Presence of epithelial or skin cells reflects a contaminated sample. Instruct the patient on cleaning of the genitals and obtain another midstream urine sample.

MICROSCOPIC URINALYSIS

Urine can also be examined microscopically, which also allows for easier detection of red blood cells (RBCs), WBCs, bacteria, and WBC casts. Microscopic UA of spun urine is considered indicative of UTI when >5 WBC/HPF, >3 RBC/HPF, and/or bacteria are present (Dubbs & Sommerkamp, 2019; Freeman et al., 2017). Typically, a count higher than 10 WBCs/mm correlates with bacterial concentrations of 100,000 (10^5) colony-forming units (CFU)/mL, which is high enough to meet the definition of UTI on culture. Sheets of numerous crystals suggest calculi, and the presence of WBC casts (a renal cylindrical plug of tightly packed leukocytes) is considered proof positive of kidney involvement of either stones or infection (Buttaro et al., 2016). Abnormalities of pH, protein, and blood are nonspecific for UTI. Blood (hematuria) and WBCs (pyuria) are often indicators of inflammation. When hematuria is present, other causes of bleeding should be ruled out.

URINE CULTURE AND SENSITIVITY

The urine culture is a definitive test that uses urine from the sample to determine bacteria growth over a 24- to 72-hour period in laboratory conditions consistent with body temperature.

Positive growth is described by colony-forming units (CFUs). A colony count of >100,000 (10^5) CFUs of a single organism is definitive of UTI. In symptomatic individuals, a lower CFU between 10^2 and 10^5 may be indicative of UTI (Anger et al., 2019; Freeman et al., 2017). As important as the colony count is the identification of the bacterial species. Identification of the causative organism and its "sensitivity" to antibiotic therapy is determined by the urine sensitivity test. This test is an important diagnostic tool to aid selection of the appropriate antibiotic therapy to treat the UTI.

Urine culture and sensitivity (C&S) is not recommended for managing simple, uncomplicated cystitis. Urine culture is, however, recommended to accurately direct antimicrobial treatment in those with rUTIs, pregnant women, those with fever, who are seriously ill, who have recently been hospitalized, or if treatment failure is suspected. Urine cultures should also be obtained in young men because infections are unusual and may suggest an underlying problem (Bonkat et al., 2019; Buttaro et al., 2016; Lee & Le, 2018). International urological guidelines do not recommend posttreatment urinalysis nor culture in asymptomatic individuals; however, in patients with persistent UTI symptoms following antimicrobial regimen, prescribers should obtain urine cultures to guide further antimicrobial treatment (Anger et al., 2019; Bonkat et al., 2019).

POSTVOID RESIDUAL

Postvoid residual (PVR) volume may be indicated in situations where incomplete bladder emptying is suspected (see Chapter 4).

SERUM STUDIES

Blood work is not indicated in simple, uncomplicated cystitis. However, renal studies may be warranted if patient suffers complicated cystitis to detect altered kidney function. Additional blood tests are needed if suspicious for an acute pyelonephritis including complete blood count with differential, procalcitonin (detects sepsis), creatine, blood cultures if fever, or hypotension (Freeman et al., 2017).

IMAGING STUDIES AND CYSTOSCOPY

Imaging studies such as renal ultrasound, IV pyelography, CT scan, MRI, radiography of kidney, or cystoscopy in women who are younger than 40 years of age with rUTI and no risk factors are not recommended, although may be considered for uncomplicated cystitis in women with febrile infections. Individuals with suspected or history of calculi, ureteral tumor, ureteral stricture, congenital ureteropelvic junction obstruction, previous urologic surgery or instrumentation, diabetes, persistent symptoms despite several days of appropriate antibiotic therapy, rapid recurrence of infection after apparently successful treatment may all be situations in which imaging studies and cystoscopy would be indicated (Bonkat et al., 2019). Renal ultrasound is recommended in acute uncomplicated pyelonephritis, but other imaging studies such as a CT scan are only advocated if the patient does not respond to treatment within 72 hours.

SEXUALLY TRANSMITTED DISEASE CULTURES

Specifically, chlamydia and gonorrhea cultures may be indicated based on patient history and/or clinical presentation.

SEGMENTED URINE

In men in which prostatitis is suspected, segmented urine testing (urine collected before, during, and after prostatic massage) and expressed prostatic secretions may be indicated.

 ## DATA SYNTHESIS: PULLING IT ALL TOGETHER

DIFFERENTIAL DIAGNOSIS

Urinary tract symptoms of dysuria, urinary urgency, frequency, flank, or suprapubic pain can be caused by other infectious or noninfectious conditions. Differential diagnosis for each type of lower or UUT infection includes the following:

- Acute uncomplicated UTI: genitourinary syndrome of menopause (GSM), urethritis, vaginitis, cervicitis, sexually transmitted infections (e.g., *Neisseria Gonorrhea, Chlamydia trachomatis*, herpes simplex), pelvic inflammatory disease, and interstitial cystitis
- Complicated UTI: structural abnormalities, neurologic dysfunction, renal calculi and masses, intrarenal or perirenal abscess, bladder tuberculosis, prostate enlargement, and prostatitis
- Acute pyelonephritis: appendicitis, abdominal abscess, renal calculi, urinary tract obstruction, pancreatitis, pelvic inflammatory disease, and ectopic pregnancy (Belyayeva & Jeong, 2020)

 ## MANAGEMENT OF CYSTITIS

THERAPY GOALS AND OUTCOMES

First, it is imperative that prompt identification, treatment, and/or referral of urological risk factors such as urethral strictures, renal calculi, cystocele, incomplete emptying, etc., is conducted to avoid future UTIs and complications (see **Box 18-1**, definition of complicated UTI). Quick resolution of presented signs and symptoms is the anticipated outcome within 48 hours of antibiotic treatment (Hooten et al., 2019) and within 72 hours of acute uncomplicated pyelonephritis treatment (Hooten & Gupta, 2019).

ANTIMICROBIAL STEWARDSHIP

Prior to prescribing an antimicrobial for a cystitis, the clinician must consider the clinical situation carefully to be sure an antibiotic is truly warranted, as well as to select the correct agent, form, and duration. It is an accepted fact that the overuse and misuse of antibiotics has contributed to MDR organisms and colonization (collateral damage) leading to a dangerous public health crisis (Anger et al., 2019). The goals of antibiotic stewardship programs are twofold, first, adherence to local, national or international infectious disease, or urological guidelines, and secondly, develop ongoing strategies to monitor performance in following the mandated guidance. Guideline-driven education assists the prescriber to use narrow-spectrum agents for empirical therapy, through continued education on best use of antimicrobials (i.e., avoid screening and treatment of ASB in most cases), local antibiograms (usually available from the facility's infectious disease department) regarding pathogen resistance trends, as well as collaboration with infectious disease, pharmacy, clinical microbiologists, availability of rapid diagnostics to reduce delay of treatment, regular audits, and feedback to prescribers regarding antibiotic prescribing practices (Bonkat et al., 2019; Goff et al., 2017; Lajiness & Lajiness, 2019). All prescribers must take ownership of this privilege and partake in local stewardship activities to reduce MDR organisms to diminish the threat of catastrophic consequences to global health.

Prescribing key points for the advance practice continence specialist (**Box 18-5**) highlights important prescribing considerations regarding antimicrobials for cystitis and in special adult populations. Urosepsis and complicated pyelonephritis is beyond the scope of this chapter. Refer to Chapter 19 for the assessment and management for catheter-associated UTI (CAUTI). An overview of common antimicrobials for the treatment of uncomplicated cystitis, rUTIs, complicated UTIs, acute pyelonephritis, and prophylaxis is presented in **Tables 18-2** to **18-5**.

BOX 18-5	**APRN ANTIMICROBIAL PRESCRIBING CONSIDERATIONS**

Periodically review local antibiogram for pathogen resistance especially *E. coli*

⊞ Avoid fluoroquinolones for uncomplicated cystitis

⊞ Avoid fluoroquinolones if *E. coli* resistance >10%

⊞ Potential for severe musculoskeletal, neurological, or mental adverse events and collateral damage causing multidrug resistance (MDR) with fluoroquinolones

Practice antibiotic stewardship: use narrow-spectrum agent, correct form and duration

⊞ Do not screen or treat ASB except in pregnancy or pending urological instrumentation/procedure

⊞ Obtain urine C&S in rUTI and cUTIs; alter treatment based on susceptibilities ASAP

⊞ Posttreatment C&S is not needed if symptoms resolve

⊞ Consult pharmacy for proper dosing in patients with renal disease or potential drug-to-drug interactions

⊞ Consult infectious disease if MDR pathogen identified

Acute uncomplicated UTI considerations

⊞ Use first-line agents when possible, that is, nitrofurantoin

⊞ Fosfomycin covers MDR gram-negative bacteria, has few side effects, one dose convenient but may be expensive

⊞ Beta-lactams are an alternate if allergies or resistance develops: cefdinir, cefaclor, amoxicillin–clavulanate, cefpodoxime

⊞ Avoid TMP-SMX if *E. coli* resistance >20%

⊞ Consider concurrent probiotic to reduce antibiotic-associated diarrhea

⊞ Educate patients, take most antibiotics with food and full glass of fluids until gone

Recurrent UTI considerations

⊞ Educate patient regarding behavioral preventive modalities

⊞ Advocate for nonantimicrobial preventive measures

⊞ If fails behavioral and nonantimicrobial preventive measures consider antibiotic prophylaxis: postcoital, self-diagnosed/treatment, continuous

⊞ Consider transvaginal estrogen to reduce risk of rUTIs in peri- and postmenopausal women

⊞ Refer patient to urology for further evaluation if repetitive microscopic hematuria without infection to r/o stones, bladder cancer, etc.

Complicated UTI considerations

⊞ Acute cystitis in men is complicated until proven otherwise; consider agent with good prostate penetration for empirical treatment until prostatitis is rule out

⊞ Acute cystitis in pregnant women is complicated due to threat to unborn child; consult OB/GYN if any upper tract UTIs suspected

⊞ Avoid fluoroquinolone if patient has had agent in last 6 months or a patient from a urology clinic due to high-resistance rates

⊞ Imaging studies are not warranted in most cases, consider renal ultrasound if renal calculi suspected or uncomplicated pyelonephritis

UNCOMPLICATED CYSTITIS

Women are most likely to suffer from an acute uncomplicated UTI episode. Men who are diagnosed with a UTI often have an infection beyond the bladder as seen in prostatitis therefore fall under a more complicated antimicrobial regimen to penetrate the prostate gland. First-line antimicrobial therapies for acute, uncomplicated UTI include nitrofurantoin (100 mg twice a day for 5 days), TMP-SMX (160 mg trimethoprim and 800 mg sulfamethoxazole [1 double-strength tablet] for 3 days), and fosfomycin trometamol (single dose of 3 g) (Anger et al., 2019; Bonkat et al., 2019; Hooten et al., 2019). These agents are effective and less likely to cause collateral damage than alternative agents (see **Table 18-2**). Trimethoprim/sulfamethoxazole (TMP-SMX) is not recommended in regions where antibiograms report >20% resistance rate (Anger et al., 2019; Bonkat et al., 2019). Beta-lactams are considered a suitable second-line agent even over fluoroquinolones due to adverse drug events. Ampicillin and amoxicillin should not be used for empirical treatment due to the high rate of microbial resistance (Hooten et al., 2019). Fluoroquinolone agents may be selected if allergies or drug resistance is verified. Although quite effective in treating uropathogens, fluoroquinolones (ciprofloxacin, levofloxacin, and ofloxacin) have fallen out of favor due to 2008 FDA black box warnings of adverse side effects including QTc prolongation, increase tendon and aortic rupture, and a greater potential for collateral damage and are thus reserved for individuals with resistant pathogens, allergies, or intolerance to first- or second-line agents (Anger et al., 2019; Hooten et al., 2019). Since 2008, the FDA has issued several news releases to strengthen warnings regarding risks of fluoroquinolone antibiotics to include mental health side effects (disturbance in attention, agitation, nervousness, disorientation, memory impairment, delirium), low blood sugars leading to hypoglycemic coma, and nerve damage (USFDA, 2018). Prudent prescribers certainly must weight risks and benefits in using this modality due to the laundry list of adverse side effects.

KEY POINT

In uncomplicated cystitis, first-line antibiotics are nitrofurantoin, TMP-SMX, and fosfomycin trometamol. Beta-lactams are considered a suitable second-line treatment even over fluoroquinolones.

KEY POINT

Fluoroquinolones should be reserved for complicated UTIs and special populations due to potential adverse events and collateral damage.

RECURRENT UTI

Individuals with recurrent cystitis are treated with a reasonable, short-course antimicrobial regimen (no longer than 7 days) the same as acute uncomplicated UTIs (Anger et al., 2019). Treatment may be empirical but adjusted based upon culture and susceptibility results.

TABLE 18-2 ACUTE UNCOMPLICATED UTI ANTIMICROBIAL MANAGEMENT

DRUG	DOSAGE	DURATION	COMMENTS AND COMMON SIDE EFFECTS
First line			
Nitrofurantoin	100 mg twice daily	5 d	N/V, reduced appetite, headache, diarrhea, stomach pain
Trimethoprim–sulfamethoxazole	160/800 mg twice daily	3 d 7 d for men	Consider if resistance <20% N/V, diarrhea, reduced appetite, rash, swollen tongue, dizziness
Fosfomycin trometamol	3 g	Once	Nausea, diarrhea, upset stomach, headache, dizziness, weakness, vaginal itching
Second line			Consider if allergies or intolerance to first line
Amoxicillin–clavulanate	875/125 mg twice daily	5–7 d	N/V, diarrhea, abdominal pain, rash
Cefpodoxime proxetil	100 mg twice daily	5–7 d	N/V, diarrhea, headache, dizziness, drowsiness, rash, itching, swelling
Cefdinir	300 mg twice daily	5–7 d	Diarrhea, vaginal yeast, nausea, headache, dizziness, stomach pain
Cefadroxil	500 mg twice daily	5–7 d	N/V, diarrhea, upset stomach, stiff muscles, joint pain, unusual taste
Cephalexin	250–500 mg every 6 h	5–7 d	Diarrhea, fatigue, dizziness, headache, vaginal itching, joint pain
Trimethoprim	100 mg bid	3 d	Itching, rash, diarrhea, N/V, reduced appetite, changes in taste
Third line			Consider if local resistance pattern for *E. coli* is <10%
Ciprofloxacin	250 mg twice daily	3 d 7 d for men	Educate on potential musculoskeletal and neurological adverse effects, *C. difficile*, N/V, indigestion, diarrhea, headache
Levofloxacin	250 mg daily	3 d	Educate on potential musculoskeletal and neurological adverse effects, *C. difficile*, N/V, headache, insomnia, dizziness, abdominal pain

Adapted from Hooten et al. (2019); Bonkat et al. (2019); Freeman et al. (2017); Lee and Le (2018).

TABLE 18-3 COMPLICATED UTI AND ASYMPTOMATIC BACTERIURIA MANAGEMENT IN PREGNANT WOMEN

DRUG	DOSAGE	DURATION	COMMENTS
Nitrofurantoin	100 mg twice daily	5–7 d	Avoid in first trimester and end of pregnancy
Trimethoprim–sulfamethoxazole	160/800 mg twice daily	3 d	Avoid in first trimester and end of pregnancy
Trimethoprim	100 mg twice a day	5 d	Avoid in first trimester and end of pregnancy
Fosfomycin trometamol	3 g PO	Once	
Amoxicillin	500 mg every 8 h	3–7 d	
Amoxicillin–clavulanate	500/125 mg twice daily	3–7 d	
Cefpodoxime proxetil	100 mg twice daily	3–7 d	
Cefaclor	750 mg twice daily	3–7 d	RCT reports efficacious and better tolerance than 500 mg three times daily*
Cephalexin	250–500 mg every 6 h	3–7 d	

*Stamatiou, K., Alevizos, A., Tetrakos, G., et al. (2007). Study on the efficacy of cefaclor for the treatment of asymptomatic bacteriuria and lower urinary tract infections in pregnant women with history of hypersensitivity to penicillin. *Clinical and Experimental Obstetrics & Gynecology, 34*(2), 85–87.
Adapted from Hooten et al. (2019); Bonkat et al. (2019); Lee and Le (2018).

TABLE 18-4 COMPLICATED UTI AND ANTIMICROBIAL OUTPATIENT MANAGEMENT

DRUG	DOSAGE	DURATION	COMMENTS
Empirical therapy **Adjust therapy with susceptibility**			
Nitrofurantoin	100 mg twice daily	7 d	Poor prostate penetration
Trimethoprim–sulfamethoxazole	160/800 mg twice daily	7 d	Good prostate penetration, consider if resistance is <20%
Ciprofloxacin	500 twice daily	7 d	Consider if resistance <10%
Levofloxacin	500 mg daily	7 d	Same as above
Alternatives, confirm susceptibility			
Amoxicillin–clavulanate	500/125 mg twice daily	7 d	
Cefpodoxime proxetil	100 mg twice daily	7 d	
Cefdinir	300 mg twice daily	7 d	
Cefadroxil	500 mg twice daily	7 d	

Adapted from Bonkat et al. (2019); Hooten and Gupta (2019); Lee and Le (2018).

Guidelines also support the use of parenteral antibiotics for a short course (no longer than 7 days) in acute rUTIs episodes if urine cultures demonstrate resistance to oral antibiotics (Anger et al., 2019). Some individuals may be candidates for evidence-based prophylactic options if behavioral, nonantimicrobial, and conventional antimicrobial regimens fail to reduce recurrent episodes of cystitis (Anger et al., 2019; Bonkat et al., 2019).

COMPLICATED LOWER UTI

UTIs are considered to be complicated (cUTIs) if there is evidence of systemic symptoms such as fever or delirium *or* if the cystitis occurs in a patient with an elevated risk for a complicated course. In men, all UTIs should be considered cUTIs until underlying factors are excluded (i.e., prostatitis, obstruction). UTIs are also considered cUTIs when they occur during pregnancy; if there are anatomical or functional abnormalities of the upper or lower urinary track (obstruction, renal calculi, instrumentation, indwelling catheter, etc.); in presence of renal diseases (insufficiency, polycystic kidney), DM, immunosuppression (i.e., renal transplant), or incomplete voiding; and they are health care–associated infections (Bonkat et al., 2019; Geerlings, 2016) (see **Box 18-1**). Presenting clinical symptoms may include dysuria, urgency, frequency, flank pain, CVA tenderness, suprapubic pain, and fever. Symptoms

TABLE 18-5 UNCOMPLICATED PYELONEPHRITIS ANTIMICROBIAL OUTPATIENT MANAGEMENT

DRUG	DOSAGE	DURATION	COMMENTS*
First line			
Ciprofloxacin	500 mg twice daily	7 d	If resistance <10%
Ciprofloxacin	1 g ER daily	7 d	Same as above
Levofloxacin	750 mg daily	5 d	Same as above
Ceftriaxone[†] followed by fluoroquinolone	1 g IM once As described above	5–7 d	If more acutely ill but nontoxic or if fluoroquinolone resistance >10%
Ertapenem[†] followed by fluoroquinolone	1 g IM once As described above	5–7 days	Same as above
Alternatives if intolerant to fluoroquinolones; confirm susceptibility			May select long-acting parental agent[†] × 1 if more acutely ill but nontoxic with alternative regimens
Trimethoprim–sulfamethoxazole	160/800 mg twice daily	14 d	Good prostate penetration
Amoxicillin–clavulanate	500/125 mg twice daily	10–14 d	
Cefpodoxime proxetil	200 mg twice daily	10–14 d	
Cefadroxil	1 g twice a day	10–14 d	
Cefdinir	300 mg	10–14 d	

*Consider inpatient treatment if very ill or signs of urosepsis.
[†]Long-acting parental agent.
Adapted from Bonkat et al. (2019); Freeman et al. (2017); Hooten and Gupta (2019); Lee and Le (2018).

can be atypical in some older adults and those with CAUTI or neurogenic bladder complications (Bonkat et al., 2019). Treatment options depend on the severity of the clinical presentation, complicating factor, regional antibiogram, C&S results, and allergies. Initial outpatient treatment for nonpregnant women and men without prostatitis, as well as individuals without evidence of upper tract UTI (pyelonephritis) includes nitrofurantoin, fosfomycin trometamol, TMP-SMX, beta-lactams, and fluoroquinolones for 7 days. Men with cystitis should be treated with TMP-SMX or fluoroquinolones for 7 to 14 days if there is suspicion of prostatitis or upper tract involvement. The optimal duration is unknown, but in one large study of men, longer treatment duration was associated with higher rates of late cystitis recurrence (more than 30 days after the initial treatment) and an elevated risk for *Clostridium difficile* (Drekonja et al., 2013). Currently, a 7-day duration appears be adequate, although this may change when further evidence exists (Germanos et al., 2019; Lee & Le, 2018; Mospan & Wargo, 2016). It should be noted that patients who have been treated with fluoroquinolones in the last 6 months, are followed by urology, or reside in an area where local resistance is >10% should not be empirical prescribed fluoroquinolones due to a high degree of treatment failure (Bonkat et al., 2019). Nitrofurantoin and fosfomycin can be utilized if resistance organisms produce extended-spectrum beta-lactamases (ESBLs) or AmpC-B-lactamase. These resistant organisms produced chemicals or enzymes that prevent inhibition activity by beta-lactam's and clavulanic acid containing antimicrobials. In pregnant women, appropriate antimicrobials for acute UTIs and ASB include cephalexin, cefpodoxime, cefaclor, amoxicillin, amoxicillin/clavulanate in all trimesters, nitrofurantoin, or TMP-SMX except in the first trimester and near term in the third trimester (Bonkat et al., 2019; Lee & Le, 2018; Stamatiou et al., 2007). The Infectious Disease Society of America suggests 4 to 7 days of antibiotic therapy rather than a shorter duration in pregnant women (Nicolle et al., 2019) (see **Tables 18-3 and 18-4**).

KEY POINT

All men with cystitis are considered complicated until underlying factors such as prostatism or obstruction is ruled out. Men should be treated with TMP-SMX or fluoroquinolones for at least 7 days due to good prostate penetration.

KEY POINT

TMP-SMX is a good choice if local antibiograms shows *E. coli* resistance <20%. If resistance is <10%, fluoroquinolones are a viable agent for complicated UTIs.

UNCOMPLICATED UPPER TRACT UTIs: ACUTE PYELONEPHRITIS

Acute pyelonephritis is an infection of the kidney that clinically presents with three classic symptoms: (1) fever, (2) flank pain, and (3) nausea or vomiting; however, all these symptoms need not to be present (Belyayeva & Jeong, 2020). It is a result of an unrecognized or inadequately treated lower tract UTI, which spreads from the bladder to the upper tract or due to vesicoureteral reflux, calculi or urological procedures. Uncomplicated pyelonephritis occurs in healthy individuals without evidence of aforementioned risk factors listed in **Box 18-3**. Gram-negative organisms such as *E. coli* (most common), *Proteus*, *Klebsiella*, and *Enterobacter* are the primary causal pathogens. Urinalysis usually presents with pyuria; nitrates if the causative bacteria is *E. coli*, *Proteus*, or *Klebsiella*; proteinuria; and hematuria. Kidney stones are often the culprit when microscopic hematuria is present (Belyayeva & Jeong, 2020). Urine C&S is mandatory to guide antimicrobial therapy. Serum studies should be considered to look for elevated white blood count, evidence for possible sepsis in patients who present quite ill, and a renal panel to assess kidney function. Recent European guidelines recommend renal ultrasound to rule out obstruction or kidney stone disease, but other image studies (CT scan) are not recommended unless there is no responsive to 72 hours of outpatient treatment or there are complicated risk factors (Bonkat et al., 2019). Outpatient treatment options are listed in **Table 18-5**. Patients with uncomplicated pyelonephritis can generally be treated as outpatients with antimicrobial therapy based on resistance patterns, C&S, and host factors. Oral regimens include fluoroquinolones for 5 to 7 days if <10% local resistance is noted, alternatives include cefpodoxime proxetil or amoxicillin/clavulanate for 10 to 14 days, and TMP-SMX and for 14 days (Bonkat et al., 2019; Hooten & Gupta, 2019; Lee & Le, 2018). European guidelines only recommend oral fluoroquinolones and cephalosporins for oral empirical treatment; however, TMP-SMX or oral beta-lactams maybe utilized if the uropathogen is susceptible (Bonkat et al., 2019; Hooten & Gupta, 2019). In addition to antimicrobial treatment, alert the patient to the benefits of nonsteroidal anti-inflammatory drugs (NSAIDs) to reduce fever and discomfort, fluids to remain hydrated, and antiemetics to manage N/V if present (Lee & Le, 2018). Patients receiving outpatient management should return after 2 days of antimicrobial therapy to monitor treatment efficacy. Patients who appear toxic or have symptoms of sepsis, are unresponsive to outpatient treatment, or present with complicated pyelonephritis require inpatient intravenous antibiotic treatment.

REFERRALS

Frequently, consultation by other specialists (urology, infectious disease, OB/GYN, nephrology, pharmacy) is essential in patients with rUTIs with resistant pathogens, complicated rUTIs including pyelonephritis, as well as patients presenting with microscopic hematuria without infection.

 ## EDUCATION AND RECURRENT UTI PREVENTION

Education of the patient regarding antimicrobial management, potential side effects, and worsening or residual symptoms that need to be reported is mandatory. Furthermore, continence specialists have a timely opportunity to discuss preventative measures to potentially reduce UTI recurrence. Prevention of rUTI includes (1) counseling individuals regarding the avoidance of identifiable behavioral risk factors (see **Box 18-6**), (2) nonantimicrobial modalities (see **Table 18-6**), and (3) administration of antimicrobial prophylactics in carefully selected individuals (see **Table 18-8**) (Bonkat et al., 2019).

 ## BEHAVIORAL MODIFICATION AND RISK MANAGEMENT

Although there is insufficient evidence to support behavioral modification as a means of reducing UTI risk, effective risk reduction counseling that supports bladder health may benefit some patients. Reviewing personal hygiene practices, addressing issues specific to bowel regularity, determining the adequacy of daily fluid intake, voiding patterns, and bladder emptying as well as identification and avoidance of perigenital products and vaginal cleansing practices are some of the behavioral activities that may reduce UTI risk and improve bladder health. See **Box 18-6** and Chapter 6 for further healthy bladder habits and risk reduction tactics.

TABLE 18-6 NONANTIBIOTIC PREVENTION OF RECURRENT UTI

PRODUCT	MECHANISM OF ACTION	COMMENTS
Probiotics—lactobacillus Oral or vaginal suppository	Normalize vaginal flora to discourage colonization of unwanted microbes	Limited quality studies to support or refute its use.
Cranberry Tablet, powder, juice, or cocktail	Antiadherence properties to lower GU tract to prevent bacterial colonization	Numerous studies support reduction in rUTI in younger and perimenopausal women. No available dosage recommendation due to various study designs and formulation.
Vitamin C Tablet, chewable, beverage	Enhance immune system, acidify urine to discourage pathogen colonization	No quality studies available. Low risk may cause loose stools in large doses. Frequently used as a home remedy.
D-Mannose Capsule, powder	Binds to urothelium receptor sites and blocks microbial adherence	Limited evidence supports reduction in rUTI; used frequently in animals to treat UTIs. Safe option for home remedy.
Acupuncture	Unknown by Western medicine; activation of the body's natural healing powers per Eastern culture	Larger well-designed studies needed to verify safety and efficacy in rUTIs reduction.
Methenamine salts Rx needed: 1 g every 12 h	Changes to formaldehyde in acidic urine and acts as a bacteriostatic agent to kill microbes	Frequently taken with vitamin C to encourage acidic environment for metamorphical change to formaldehyde. Do not use in pregnancy or breast-feeding. Side effects: N/V, diarrhea, abdominal pain, loss of appetite.
Transvaginal estrogen Rx needed Forms: cream, tablet, ring, suppository inserts	Fosters lactobacilli growth that reduces vaginal pH discouraging pathogen colonization in postmenopausal women. Reduces genitourinary symptoms of menopause as well	Multiple studies confirm reduced rate of rUTIs; supported in several guidelines. Minimal systemic absorption. Do not use in undiagnosed vaginal bleeding. Side effects: vaginal irritation, burning, itching.

BOX 18-6   RECOMMENDATIONS TO PATIENTS FOR PREVENTING URINARY TRACT INFECTIONS

1. Good personal hygiene
   - Handwashing before and after urinating.
   - At least once each day, genitals should be washed with a gentle soap and thorough cleansing, including the skin around the anus.
     - Women should wipe front to back after voiding and especially after a bowel movement to avoid spreading bacteria from the rectum to the vagina and urethra.
     - Do not wipe from behind because tissues or wipes can pick up fecal bacteria from the anal area.
     - Uncircumcised male should wash under foreskin regularly and after drying, replace foreskin over glans.
   - In women who have rUTIs:
     - Genital area should be cleansed before and after sexual intercourse to minimize urethral contamination from perineal bacteria.
     - Avoid sitting in bath water; rather, shower and spraying perineal area after washing.
     - Avoid Loofahs and all reusable sponges because they can retain bacteria.
     - If menstruating, use of tampons is recommended because feminine hygiene pads can become contaminated with bacteria.
   - Encourage bowel regularity
2. Adequate daily fluid intake
   - Drink enough clear, noncaffeinated, nonalcoholic beverages to keep urine dilute.
3. Promotion of regular and complete bladder emptying
   - Urination should not be put off for long periods of time but should occur shortly after feeling the urge.
   - To ensure complete bladder emptying, double voiding should be encouraged (urinating twice within a few minutes).
   - Voiding should occur before and after sexual intercourse to flush out any bacteria that may have been introduced in the urethra and to ensure bladder emptying.
4. Other considerations
   - Suggest wearing cotton underwear because it absorbs moisture.
   - Avoid soaps, bubble bath, talc powders, or perfumed toilet paper.
   - Educate women who experience urine leakage about the use of incontinence pads for protection and not to use feminine hygiene pads.
   - Prescribe transvaginal estrogen or lactobacilli probiotics for postmenopausal women because these will reestablish vaginal colonization.
   - Sexually active women should avoid contraceptive diaphragms and nonoxynol-9 spermicides intravaginally.

Source: © 2017 Society of Urologic Nurses and Associates. Reprinted from the Newman, D., Wyman, J., & Welch, V. (2017). *Core Curriculum for Urologic Nursing* (p. 428). Used with permission of the publisher, the Society of Urologic Nurses and Associates, Inc.

NONANTIMICROBIAL MANAGEMENT

PROBIOTICS

There are limited quality studies demonstrating the use of probiotics to reduce rUTIs (Schwenger et al., 2015; Stapleton et al., 2011). Probiotics, specifically lactobacillus species, orally or vaginally, are used prophylactically to replenish diminished lactobacillus flora, especially in menopausal women, in the hopes to reduce the rate of vaginal colonization with Enterobacteriaceae (*E. coli*) that often leads to recurrent cystitis. A Cochrane systematic review of nine studies involving over 735 people demonstrated no significant difference in rates of rUTI, but the studies were small with poor methodological reporting. Currently, there is not enough evidence to support or refute the use and safety of probiotics to prevent cystitis in at-risk populations (Anger et al., 2019; Bonkat et al., 2019; Schwenger et al., 2015). It should be noted, however, that recent evidence discourages the use of probiotics for those who are immunosuppressed.

CRANBERRY SUPPLEMENTATION

Cranberries have been used for countless years for the prevention of cystitis due to the potent antiadhesion properties found in anthocyanidins and proanthocyanidins (PACs) that enable uropathogens, like *E. coli*, with type 1 and P fimbriated (linear projections) binding to the uroepithelium of the urethra and bladder. It is thought that microbes cannot adhere to the bladder lining, colonization is then halted, and the bacteria are more likely washed away during urination (Farford, 2018). Numerous studies have been conducted that demonstrate the reduction of rUTI in young and premenopausal women with its use but the form (juice, cocktail, powder, tablets) and dosage is elusive given the variety of study designs and cranberry formulations. Cranberry may be an option offered as prophylaxis in a form that is convenient and tolerable (Anger et al., 2019). Caution should be given to individuals self-administering cranberry supplementation who are on warfarin (may alter INR), and they may promote stone formation in individuals who suffer nephrolithiasis.

VITAMIN C SUPPLEMENTATION

Controversy remains whether vitamin C supplementation actually enhances urine acidity thereby reducing bacterial replication in the LUT. Currently, there are not any well-designed studies to support its use, although it is frequently consumed as a home remedy to discourage cystitis (Anger et al., 2019; Beerepoot & Geerlings, 2016; Bonkat et al., 2019).

D-MANNOSE

D-Mannose shows promising benefit in prophylactic use to reduce the reoccurrence of cystitis. It is a natural occurring, simple sugar that adheres to the uroepithelium receptor site blocking the attachment of invading microbes. Some forms can bind the invading bacteria and facilitate its removal during urination (Bates et al., 2004). D-Mannose has been used extensively in the treatment of UTIs in dogs, cats, and horses (Altarac & Papes, 2014). It is also marketed for human consumption to prevent rUTIs by health food companies and homeopathic practitioners. In a randomized control trial, 308 women who suffered rUTI were randomly assigned to one of three groups with prophylaxis for 6 months with (1) 2 g of D-mannose daily, (2) nitrofurantoin 50 mg daily, (3) no prophylaxis. Results demonstrated a significant reduction in rUTI in the groups receiving D-mannose (15%) and nitrofurantoin (20%) compared to placebo (60%) group (Kranjcec et al., 2014). D-Mannose may be a consideration for women seeking home remedy option to reduce rUTI, although evidence is limited (Bonkat et al., 2019; Farford, 2018; Freeman et al., 2017).

ACUPUNCTURE

Another hopeful alternative method to diminish the rate rUTIs used for centuries and for numerous other health ailments is acupuncture (Beerepoot & Geerlings, 2016). Only two small open trials ($n = 67$ and $n = 94$) demonstrated a reduction in UTIs utilizing acupuncture in comparison to sham acupuncture (Alraek et al., 2002; Aune et al., 1998). Larger well-designed, double-blind randomized control trials are needed before acupuncture can be considered a safe and effective method to reduce cystitis. Furthermore, the mechanism of action is unclear through the eyes of traditional Western medicine, although Eastern medicine notes that acupuncture activates the natural healing power of the body to prevent microbial invasion in the bladder (Aoi, n.d.).

ALTERNATIVES ON THE HORIZON

The use of an oral immunostimulant (OM-89) and a vaginal vaccine (Urovac) use different types of heat-killed uropathogens to stimulate immunity by increasing macrophage phagocytosis and neutrophils to discourage cystitis (McLellan & Hunstad, 2016). Preliminary meta-analysis of studies has shown a significant reduction in rUTIs in women using OM-89 and slight reduce rate using the vaginal vaccine immunization booster; neither products are available in the United States (Beerepoot & Geerlings, 2016). Of interest, fecal microbiota transplantation (donor feces) has also been reported to decolonize the gut for

multidrug-resistant bacteria such as ESBL producing *E. coli* to reduce the risk of complicated upper tract UTIs and rUTIs (Singh et al., 2014; Tariq et al., 2017).

> **KEY POINT**
>
> Cranberry and D-mannose have antiadhesion properties that may reduce the risk of uropathogen colonization leading to rUTIs.

PHARMACOLOGIC MANAGEMENT

TRANSVAGINAL ESTROGEN

GSM (genitourinary syndrome of menopause) describes a collection of vulvovaginal symptoms of the genital, sexual, and urinary changes in the LUT associated with low estrogen levels (Portman & Gass, 2014). It is underdiagnosed and undertreated for symptoms of vaginal dryness, irritation, itching, dyspareunia, reduced lubrication, dysuria, urinary urgency, frequency, and elevated risk for rUTIs (Alperin et al., 2019; Santoro & Lin, 2018). Multiple studies confirm the use of transvaginal (topical) estrogen as an effective modality to reduce this constellation of symptoms including recurrent cystitis in peri- and postmenopausal females and is endorsed by the American College of Obstetricians and Gynecologists menopausal guideline (ACOG, 2014) and international urological guidelines (Anger et al., 2019; Bonkat et al., 2019). Postmenopausal women may have minimal to no lactobacilli in the vagina, but with the use of estrogen replacement therapy, it is reported to increase to levels of 60% to 100% (Reid et al., 2004). It is noted that women without lactobacilli in the vagina have higher pH with both abnormalities potentially fostering over colonization of offending microbes (fungus, Enterobacteriaceae such as *E. coli*) (Hickling et al., 2015). Studies report that intravaginal lactobacilli levels improved and that vaginal pH and colonization with Enterobacteriaceae decreased along with incidence of cystitis with transvaginal estrogen (Beerepoot & Geerlings, 2016). Of interest, an ACOG position statement supports the use of low-dose transvaginal estrogen in women with a history of estrogen-positive breast cancer or who are currently undergoing treatment, who suffer rUTI or other urogenital symptoms that have failed to respond to nonhormonal modalities (ACOG, 2018). Data confirm minimal systemic absorption of estrogen especially with use of an estrogen vaginal ring or tablets (Wills et al., 2012). In addition, research studies demonstrate no elevated risk of breast cancer recurrence in those undergoing current cancer treatment or with a past history of breast cancer using low-dose transvaginal estrogen (Le Ray et al., 2012; O'Meara et al., 2001; Ponzone et al., 2005). Education regarding the risks and benefits of low-dose

TABLE 18-7 COMMONLY USED VAGINAL ESTROGEN THERAPY

FORMULATION	COMPOSITION	STRENGTH AND DOSAGE
Vaginal tablet	Estradiol hemihydrate	10 µg/d for 2 wk, then 10 µg 2–3 times weekly
Vaginal ring	17-βstradiol	2 mg ring released 7.5 µg/d for 3 mo (changed by patient or provider)
Vaginal cream	17-βstradiol	2 g daily for 2 wk, then 1 g 2–3 times per week
	Conjugate equine estrogen	0.5 g daily for 2 wk, then 0.5 g twice weekly
Vaginal insert	17-βstradiol	4 or 10 µg daily for 2 wk, then 2 times per week

vaginal estrogen requires informed and shared decision-making process with the woman's oncologist or APRN continence specialist. Oral estrogens do not provide the same outcomes and are associated with an increased risk for heart disease, stroke, DVTs, and breast cancer and are therefore not recommended in UTI prophylaxis (Beerepoot et al., 2013; Bonkat et al., 2019). Local estrogen comes in many forms such as cream, tablet, ring, suppository; it is typically well tolerated with unpleasant accounts of vaginal irritation, burning, and itching, which may resolve if the form of estrogen is switched (see **Table 18-7**).

METHENAMINE SALTS

Methenamine salts, also known as methenamine hippurate or methenamine mandelate, are another option that has been shown to have favorable benefits in small studies and may be a viable option in rUTI prevention on a short-term basis without any ill effects (Lee et al., 2012). Methenamine salts serve as bacteriostatic agent by changing into formaldehyde in acid urine (pH < 6) that destroys the protein and nucleic acid of bacteria and lack bacterial resistance. The recommended dosage is 1 g twice daily that can be given with vitamin C 500 mg to promote hydrolysis of methenamine (Freeman et al., 2017). This product is contraindicated in pregnancy, renal or liver disease, and should be used with caution until good clinical evidence advocates the use.

KEY POINT

Behavioral and nonantimicrobial modalities for prevention of rUTI should be employed first before considering prophylactic use of antibiotics due to the potential adverse events and MDR organisms.

ANTIBIOTIC PROPHYLAXIS

Currently, guidelines support the use of postcoital, acute self-treatment, and continuous prophylaxis for those who suffer uncomplicated rUTIs if behavioral modification and nonantimicrobial efforts have failed (Anger et al., 2019; Bonkat et al., 2019). The antibiotic option will depend upon regional antibiograms demonstrating local resistance patterns, allergies, adverse effects, previous C&S studies, and availability as well as cost (see **Table 18-8**). Risks, benefits, and alternatives needs to be considered in a shared decision-making process regarding antibiotic prophylaxis to reduce rUTI. In addition, antibiotic stewardship should be a point of discussion with the rising rate of antibiotic resistance and collateral damage described as the ecological adverse effects of antibiotics that create MDR organisms (Goff et al., 2017).

POSTCOITAL PROPHYLAXIS

Postcoital prophylaxis can be recommended if the individual with rUTIs reports that UTI symptoms occur within 48 hours following sexual contact. Recommendations include taking the antibiotic before or after sexual relations with one of the following regimens: single dose of trimethoprim 100 mg, nitrofurantoin 50 or 100 mg, trimethoprim–sulfamethoxazole 40/200 mg to 80/400 mg, or during pregnancy in women who experienced rUTI prior to pregnancy with cephalexin 125 or 250 mg or cefaclor 250 mg (Anger et al., 2019; Bonkat et al., 2019; Farford, 2018; Freeman et al., 2017; Lee & Le, 2018).

SELF-DIAGNOSIS AND SELF-TREATMENT

Studies confirm that women with a history of reliable compliance (trustworthy with communication and self-assessment) can accurately diagnose rUTI most of the time (85% to 95%) (Gupta et al., 2001; Schaeffer & Stuppy, 1999). International guidelines recommend a short course of antibiotics that mirrors the antimicrobial agent chosen for an acute, uncomplicated UTI (Anger et al., 2019; Bonkat et al., 2019). In scenarios where shared decision-making process is employed with knowledgeable patients, a short-course antibiotic is safe, effective, and economical. The individual should be counseled to seek follow-up care if the symptoms do not improve in 48 hours after the initiation of self-treatment. Women can be counseled to utilize a commercially available urine dipstick to check for the presence of nitrates and leukocytes to enhance self-diagnosis and treatment, although studies have not substantiated this recommendation (Farford, 2018).

CONTINUOUS PROPHYLAXIS

If the timing of the rUTI is not related to sexual intercourse, low-dose continuous antibiotics may be suggested before bed and given for up to 6 months, although the optimal duration is unknown (Bonkat et al., 2019; Farford,

TABLE 18-8 RECURRENT UTI PROPHYLAXIS TREATMENT OPTIONS

ANTIBIOTIC	CONTINUOUS	POSTCOITAL	SELF-TREATMENT*
Nitrofurantoin	50 mg once daily OR 100 mg once daily	50 mg once OR 100 mg once	100 mg twice daily × 5 d
Trimethoprim–sulfamethoxazole	40/200 mg OR 80/400 mg	40/200 mg OR 80/400 mg	160/800 mg twice daily × 3 d
Trimethoprim	100 mg once daily	100 mg single dose	100 mg twice daily × 3 d
Cephalexin†	125 mg once daily OR 250 mg once daily	125 mg once OR 250 mg once	250 mg every 6 hours × 5–7 d
Cefaclor†	250 mg once daily	250 mg once	750 mg twice daily × 5–7 d
Fosfomycin trometamol	3 g every 10 d	Not an option	3 g once

*See Table 18-2—Acute Uncomplicated Cystitis for more options.
†Consider in pregnant women who had rUTIs prior to pregnancy.
Adapted from Anger et al. (2019); Bonkat et al. (2019).

2018). Studies have reported up to 95% rate reduction of cystitis with continuous prophylaxis (Freeman et al., 2017). Recommended antibiotics are the same as recommended for postcoital prophylaxis with the additional consideration of fosfomycin trometamol 3 g every 10 days (Anger et al., 2019; Bonkat et al., 2019). Individuals need to be counseled regarding the risks and benefits of continuous intake of antibiotics. Adverse events reported in the use of all antimicrobial agents include candidiasis (oral and vaginal), upset stomach, loss of appetite, soft or loose stools, explosive diarrhea as seen in *C. difficile* infection, nausea, skin rash, or allergic reactions. Current guidelines (AUA/CUA/SUFU) do not recommend ciprofloxacin for prophylaxis due to previously mentioned FDA black box warning of the elevated risk for tendonitis and tendon rupture, as well as QT interval prolongation, seizures, and *C. difficile*–related diarrhea. Nitrofurantoin is not recommended for individuals with a creatinine clearance below 30 mL/min. Noteworthy, is the rare but potential serious risk for lung or liver adverse events with the use of nitrofurantoin. Close monitoring of this agent especially for those with mild renal disease and avoidance in individuals with pulmonary and liver disease is prudent. Currently, there is little evidence to support the benefit of rotating antibiotic agents in continuous prophylaxis (Anger et al., 2019). Careful risk assessment, patient education with shared decision-making, and clinical monitoring will diminish the risk of serious potential adverse events during continuous prophylaxis for rUTI.

KEY POINT

Nitrofurantoin should not be used in patients with renal disease and a creatinine clearance below 30 mL/min, or in advance pulmonary or liver disease.

 HEALTH PROMOTION AND PREVENTION

Continence specialty nurses have an opportunity to provide patient education, anticipatory guidance, and risk reduction counseling that promotes bladder health and emphasizes UTI prevention. Chapter 6 provides a thorough discussion on the fundamental components of a healthy bladder. Although there is insufficient evidence to support behavioral and personal hygiene measures in preventing UTIs, it may help some individuals and essentially risk free for adverse reactions with these measures (Bonkat et al., 2019). Bladder health promotion and prevention focuses on personal hygiene practices, adequate fluid intake, regular and complete bladder emptying, avoidance of perigenital irritants, and early recognition of UTI symptoms (Freeman et al., 2017). Personal hygiene practices that have been shown to be effective in preventing UTI include washing hands before and after toileting, thoroughly cleansing the genital area including the anal area with mild soap at least once daily, and maintaining bowel regularity that includes measures to avoid constipation or loose stools (Freeman et al., 2017). Women should be instructed to wipe from front to back after urinating and after a bowel movement to reduce the risk of bacterial transmission. Women who are prone to UTI related to sexual intercourse benefit from washing the genital area before and after sex to reduce the likelihood of introducing bacteria from the rectum to the vagina and urethra. Uncircumcised males should be advised to wash under the foreskin regularly and after drying, replace the foreskin over the glans (Freeman et al., 2017).

Maintaining an adequate daily fluid intake is an important factor in ensuring the forward flow of urine needed to maintain bladder sterility and may reduce the risk for UTIs (Lean et al., 2019; Scott et al., 2020). Fluid intake includes any beverage drank during the day such as milk and juice as well as water. Caffeinated and alcoholic beverages can act as bladder irritants and should be avoided (Friedlander et al., 2012; Sutcliffe et al., 2018). Adequate fluid intake is described as drinking enough clear, noncaffeinated, nonalcoholic beverages to keep the urine light in color.

Promoting regular and complete bladder emptying includes going to the bathroom shortly after the urge to void is felt and not holding or postponing voiding for long periods of time (Palmer et al., 2018). Double voiding techniques including voiding twice within a few minutes ensure complete bladder emptying. Voiding before and after sexual intercourse is also important in flushing out any bacteria as well as ensuring bladder emptying (Bonkat et al., 2019; Foxman & Chi, 1990; Freeman et al., 2017).

Avoiding the use of scented soaps, perfumes, and powders in the perigenital area as well as rough, scented toilet paper and tight-fitting pants reduces the risk of irritation and discomfort (Freeman et al., 2017). Perigenital moisture is reduced by wearing cotton underwear. Sexually active women using contraceptive diaphragms and/or spermicides containing nonoxynol-9 should be counseled on the potential of perigenital/vaginal irritation and risk of UTI and offered alternative, effective contraceptive options. Women should also be educated that menstrual pads can cause irritation and harbor bacteria and that daily use is not recommended. Menstruating women may opt to use tampons to reduce this risk and if using menstrual pads reminded to change pads frequently and avoid pads with chemicals and deodorants. Women experiencing bladder leaking and urinary incontinence should be counseled to use absorbent products specifically designed for urine as these products pull urine away from the skin thus reducing the risk of incontinence-associated dermatitis and UTI risk.

Patients should also be educated to recognize UTI symptoms and seek care should they experience increased urinary urgency and frequency, urinating in small amounts, sudden urine leakage, feeling that their bladder is not emptying completely even after urinating, any discomfort or unusual sensation when urinating, foul smelling urine, fever or chills or blood in the urine. Remind patients that early intervention is important in reducing further UTI risk (see **Box 18-6**).

CONCLUSION—WOC NURSE PRACTICE CONSIDERATIONS

Wound, ostomy, continence (WOC) nurses are in key positions to partner with patients and their health care team to develop a plan of care for individuals at risk for and experiencing UTI that includes health promotion and prevention, risk reduction strategies, accurate assessment, and treatment interventions. Through shared decision-making,

the WOC nurse can assure that patients experiencing UTI are able to make informed, evidence-based decisions related to their health and treatment options. WOC nurses work in partnership with the patient to develop and implement plans of care that are individualized and represent patient preferences and decisions about their health. The WOC nurse is able to provide ongoing follow up related to patient response to treatment and UTI status and communicate patient status to the health care team. The WOC nurse also has an opportunity to impact health outcomes related to rUTI by practicing antibiotic stewardship and recommending nonmicrobial management. In all situations, the WOC nurse is aware of factors that can complicate UTI and participates in appropriate risk reduction, consultation, and referral.

REFERENCES

Alperin, M., Burnett, L., Lukacz, E., et al. (2019). The mysteries of menopause and urogynecologic health: Clinical and scientific gaps. *Menopause, 26*(1), 103–111.

Alraek, T., Soedal, L. I. F. S., Fagerheim, S. U., et al. (2002). Acupuncture treatment in the prevention of uncomplicated recurrent lower urinary tract infections in adult women. *American Journal of Public Health, 92*(10), 1609–1611.

Altarac, S., & Papes, D. (2014). Use of D-mannose in prophylaxis of recurrent urinary tract infections (UTIs) in women. *BJU International, 113*, 9–10.

American College of Obstetricians and Gynecologists (ACOG). (2014). Practice Bulletin No. 141: Management of menopausal symptoms. *Obstetrics & Gynecology, 123*(1), 202–216. doi: 10.1097/01.AOG.0000441353.20693.78

American College of Obstetricians and Gynecologists (ACOG). (2016, updated 2018). The use of vaginal estrogen in women with a history of estrogen-dependent breast cancer. Committee Opinion No. 659. American College of Obstetricians and Gynecologists. *Obstetric & Gynecology, 127*, e93–e96.

Anger, J., Una, L., & Ackerman, L. A. (2019). *Recurrent uncomplicated urinary tract infections in women: American Urological Association (AUA)/Canadian Urological Association (CUA)/Society of Urodynamics, Female Pelvic Medicine & Urogenital Reconstruction (SUFU) Guideline.* Linthicum, MD: American Urological Association Education and Research, Inc.

Aoi, Y. F. (n.d.). Japanese acupuncture. Retrieved February 3, 2020, from https://www.acupunctureliving.com/how-does-acupuncture-work-for-uti/

Aune A., Alraek T., LiHua H., et al. (1998). Acupuncture in the prophylaxis of recurrent lower urinary tract infection in adult women. *Scandanavian Journal of Primary Health Care, 16*(1), 37–39.

Bates, J. M., Raffi, H. M., Prasadan, K., et al. (2004). Tamm-Horsfall protein knockout mice are more prone to urinary tract infection: Rapid communication. *Kidney International* 65, 791–797.

Beerepoot, M., & Geerlings, S. (2016). Non-antibiotic prophylaxis for Urinary tract infection. *Pathogens, 5*(2), 36. doi: 10.3390/pathogens5020036.

Beerepoot, M. A., Geerlings, S. E., van Haarst, E. P., et al. (2013). Non-antibiotic prophylaxis for recurrent urinary tract infections: A systematic review and meta-analysis of randomized controlled trials. *Journal of Urology, 190*, 1981–1989.

Belyayeva M, & Jeong JM. (2020). Acute pyelonephritis. [Updated 2019 Feb 28]. In *StatPearls [Internet]*. Treasure Island, FL: StatPearls Publishing. Retrieved from https://www.ncbi.nlm.nih.gov/books/NBK519537/

Bonkat, G., Bartoletti, R., Bruyere, T., et al. (2019). *European Association of Urology (EAU) Guidelines on urological infections*. Arnhem, The Netherlands: EAU Guidelines Office. Retrieved from http://uroweb. org/guidelines/compilations-of-all-guidelines/

Buttaro, T., Trybulski, J., Polgar-Bailey, P., et al. (2016). Chapter 153: Urinary tract infections and sexually transmitted diseases. *Primary Care A Collaborative Practice* (5th ed.). St. Louis, MO: Elsevier.

CDC. (2020). Urinary tract infections (catheter-associated UTIs) and non-catheter associated UTI events. Retrieved from https://www. cdc.gov/nhsn/PDFs/pscManual/7pscCAUTIcurrent.pdf

Drekonja, D. M., Rector, T. S., Cutting, A., et al. (2013). Urinary tract infection in male veterans: Treatment patterns and outcomes. *JAMA Internal Medicine, 1*, 62–68.

Dubbs, S. B., & Sommerkamp, S. K. (2019). Evaluation and management of urinary tract infection in the emergency department. *Emergency Medical Clinics of North America, 37*, 707–723. doi.org/10.1016/j. emc.2019.07.007emed.theclinics.com

Farford, B. (2018). Management and prevention of recurrent urinary tract infections in women. *Consultant, 58*(3), 99–103.

Figler, B. (2017). Urinalysis and the urine culture. *Merck Manual*. Retrieved from https://www.merckmanuals.com/home/kidney-and-urinary-tract-disorders/diagnosis-of-kidney-and-urinary-tract-disorders/urinalysis-and-urine-culture

Foxman, B. (2002). Epidemiology of urinary tract infections: Incidence, morbidity, and economic costs. *American Journal of Medicine, 113*(Suppl 1A), 5S–13S.

Foxman, B. (2010). The epidemiology of urinary tract infection. *Nature Reviews. Urology, 7*, 653–660. doi.org/10.1038/nrurol.2010.190

Foxman, B., & Chi, J. W. (1990). Health behavior and urinary tract infection in college-aged women. *Journal of Clinical Epidemiology, 43*(4), 329–337. doi.org/10.1016/0895-4356(90)90119-a

Freeman, J., Martin, K., & Uithoven, R. (2017). Urinary tract infections. In D. K. Newman, J. F. Wyman, & V. W. Welch (Eds.), *SUNA core curriculum for urologic nursing*, (1st ed., pp. 423–437). Pitman, NJ: SUNA.

Friedlander, J. I., Shorter, B., & Moldwin, R. M. (2012). Diet and its role in interstitial cystitis/bladder pain syndrome (IC/BPS) and comorbid conditions. *BJU International, 109*, 1584–1591.

Geerlings S. E. (2016). Clinical presentations and epidemiology of urinary tract infections. *Microbiology Spectrum, 4*(5), doi: 10.1128/ microbiolspec.UTI-0002-2012.

Germanos, G. J., Trautner, B. W., Zoorob, R. J., et al. (2019). No clinical benefit to treating male urinary tract infection longer than seven days: An outpatient database study. *Open Forum Infectious Diseases, 6*(6), ofz216. doi.org/10.1093/ofid/ofz216

Goff, R. K., Goldstein, E. J., Gilchrist, M., et al. (2017). A global call from five countries to collaborate in antibiotic stewardship: United we succeed, divided we might fail. *The Lancet Infectious Diseases, 17*, e56–e63. doi.org/10.1016/S1473-3099(16)30386

Gupta, K., Hooton, T. M., Roberts, P. L., et al. (2001). Patient-initiated treatment of uncomplicated recurrent urinary tract infections in young women. *Annals of Internal Medicine, 135*(1), 9–16.

Hickling, D. R., Sun, T. T., & Wu, X. R. (2015). Anatomy and physiology of the urinary tract: relation to host defense and microbial infection. *Microbiology Spectrum, 3*(4), UTI-0016-2012.

Hooten, T. M. & Gupta, K. (2019). Acute complicated urinary tract infection (including pyelonephritis) in adults. *UpToDate*. Retrieved from https://www.uptodate.com/contents/acute-complicated-urinary-tract-infection-including-pyelonephritis-in-adults

Hooten, T. M., Gupta, K., Calderwood, B., et al. (2019). Acute simple cystitis in women. *UpToDate*. Retrieved from https://www.uptodate. com/contents/acute-simple-cystitis-in-women

Kang, C. I., Kim, J., Park, D. W., et al. (2018). Clinical practice guidelines for the antibiotic treatment of community-acquired urinary tract infections. *Infection & Chemotherapy, 50*(1), 67–100. doi. org/10.3947/ic.2018.50.1.67

Kranjcec, B., Papeš, D., & Altarac, S. (2014). D-mannose powder for prophylaxis of recurrent urinary tract infections in women: A randomized clinical trial. *World Journal of Urology, 32*(1), 79–84. https:// www.ncbi.nlm.nih.gov/pubmed/23633128

Lajiness, B., & Lajiness, M. J. (2019). 50 years of urinary tract infections and treatments—Has much changed? *Urologic Nursing, 39*(5), 235–239. doi: 10.7257/1053-816X.2019.39.5.235

Lean, K., Nawaz, R. F., Jawad, S., et al. (2019). Reducing urinary tract infections in care homes by improving hydration. *BMJ Open Quality, 8*(3), e000563. doi.org/10.1136/bmjoq-2018-000563.

Lee, B. S. B., Bhuta, T., Simpson, J. M., et al. (2012). Methenamine hippurate for preventing urinary tract infections. *The Cochrane Database Systematic Reviews, 10*, CD003265. doi: 10.1002/14651858. CD003265.pub3.

Lee, H. S., & Le, J. (2018). *Urinary tract infections: Pharmacology self-assessment program SAP 2018 Book 1: Infectious Diseases*. ACCP. January; ISBN-13: 978-1-939862-60-0.

Le Ray, I., Dell'Aniello, S., Bonnetain, F., et al. (2012). Local estrogen therapy and risk of breast cancer recurrence among hormone-treated patients: A nested case-control study. *Breast Cancer Research and Treatment, 135*, 603–609.

Levine, A, Tran, M., Naut, E. (2018). The diagnostic value of procalcitonin in urinary tract infections. *Critical Care Medicine, 46*(1), 306. doi: 10.1097/01.ccm.0000528655.81932.99

McLellan, L., & Hunstad, D. (2016). Urinary Tract Infection: Pathogenesis and outlook. *Trends in Molecular Medicine, 22*(11), 946–957. doi: 10.1016/j.molmed.2016.09.003.

Medina, M., & Castillo-Pino, E. (2019). An introduction to the epidemiology and burden of urinary tract infections. *Therapeutic Advances in Urology, 11*, 3–7.

Mospan G. A., & Wargo, K. A. (2016). 5-day versus 10-day course of fluoroquinolones in outpatient males with a urinary tract infection (UTI). *Journal of the American Board of Family Medicine, 29*, 654–662

Nicolle, L. E., Gupta, K., Bradley, S. F., et al. (2019). Clinical practice guideline for the management of asymptomatic bacteriuria: 2019 update by the Infectious Diseases Society of America. *Clinical Infectious Diseases, 68*(10), e83–e110. doi.org/10.1093/cid/ciy1121.

O'Meara, E. S., Rossing M. A., Daling, J. R., et al. (2001). Hormone replacement therapy after a diagnosis of breast cancer in relation to recurrence and mortality. *Journal of the National Cancer Institute, 93*, 754–762.

Palmer, M. H., Willis-Gray, M. G., Zhou, F., et al. (2018). Self-reported toileting behaviors in employed women: Are they associated with lower urinary tract symptoms? *Neurourology and Urodynamics, 37*(2), 735–743.

Pescatore, R., Niforatos, J., & Rezaie, S., et al. (2019). Evidence-informed practice: Diagnostic questions in urinary tract infections in the elderly. *The Western Journal of Emergency Medicine, 20*(4), 573–577. doi: 10.5811/westjem.2019.5.42096.

Ponzone, R., Biglia, N., & Jacomuzzi, M. E. (2005). Vaginal oestrogen therapy after breast cancer: is it safe? *European Journal of Cancer, 41*, 2673–2681.

Portman, D. J., & Gass, M. L. (2014). Genitourinary syndrome of menopause: new terminology for vulvovaginal atrophy from the International Society for the Study of Women's Sexual Health and the North American Menopause Society. *Maturitas, 79*(3), 349–354.

Reid, G., Burton, J., & Devillard, E. (2004). The rationale for probiotics in female urogenital healthcare. *Medscape General Medicine, 6*(1), 49.

Santoro, N. F., & Lin, I. (2018). Genitourinary syndrome of menopause (GSM): Underdiagnosed and undertreated. *Contemporary OB/ GYN, 64*(7). Retrieved from https://www.contemporaryobgyn.net/ article/genitourinary-syndrome-menopause-underdiagnosed-and-undertreated

Schaeffer, A. J., & Stuppy, B. A. (1999). Efficacy and safety of self-start therapy in women with recurrent urinary tract infections. *Journal of Urology, 161*(1), 207–211. https://www.ncbi.nlm.nih.gov/ pubmed/10037399.

Schwenger, E. M., Tejani, A. M., & Loewen, P. S. (2015). Probiotics for preventing urinary tract infections in adults and children. *Cochrane Database of Systematic Reviews, 23*(12), CD008772. https://www.ncbi.nlm.nih.gov/pubmed/26695595

Scott, A. M., Clark, J., Mar, C. D., et al. (2020). Increased fluid intake to prevent urinary tract infections: Systematic review and meta-analysis. *The British Journal of General Practice, 70*(692), e200–e207. doi.org/10.3399/bjgp20X708125.

Singh, R., van Nood, E., Nieuwdorp, M., et al. (2014). Donor feces infusion for eradication of Extended Spectrum beta-lactamase producing *Escherichia coli* in a patient with end stage renal disease. *Clinical Microbiology and Infection, 20*, 977–978.

Stamatiou, K., Alevizos, A., Tetrakos, G., et al. (2007). Study on the efficacy of cefaclor for the treatment of asymptomatic bacteriuria and lower urinary tract infections in pregnant women with history of hypersensitivity to penicillin. *Clinical and Experimental Obstetrics & Gynecology, 34*(2), 85–87.

Stapleton A. E. Au-Yeung M., Hooton T. M., et al. (2011). Randomized, placebo-controlled phase 2 trial of *Lactobacillus crispatus* probiotic given intravaginally for prevention of recurrent urinary tract infection. *Clinical Infectious Diseases, 52*(10), 1212–1217.

Sutcliffe, S., Jemielta, T., Lai, H. H., et al. (2018). A case-crossover study of urologic chronic pelvic pain syndrome flare triggers in the MAPP research network. *Journal of Urology, 199*(5), 1245–1251.

Tariq, R., Pardi, D. S., Tosh, P. K., et al. (2017). Fecal microbiota transplantation for recurrent *Clostridium difficile* infection reduces recurrent urinary tract infection frequency. *Clinical Infectious Diseases, 65*(10), 1745–1747.

United States Food and Drug Association. (2015). FDA Drug Safety Communication. Retrieved from https://www.fda.gov/drugs/drug-safety-and-availability/fda-drug-safety-communication-fda-revises-labels-sglt2-inhibitors-diabetes-include-warnings-about

United States Food and Drug Association. (2018). FDA New release: FDA updates warnings for fluoroquinolone antibiotics on risk for mental health and low blood sugar adverse reactions. Retrieved from https://www.fda.gov/news-events/press-announcements/fda-updates-warnings-fluoroquinolone-antibiotics-risks-mental-health-and-low-blood-sugar-adverse

Wills, S., Ravipati, A., Venuturumilli, P., et al. (2012). Effects of vaginal estrogens on serum estradiol levels in postmenopausal breast cancer survivors and women at risk of breast cancer taking an aromatase inhibitor or a selective estrogen receptor modulator. *Journal of Oncology Practice, 8*(3), 144–148. doi.org/10.1200/JOP.2011.000352.

QUESTIONS

1. Which of the following is the most common bacterial infection in adults?
   A. Pneumonia
   B. Influenza
   C. Urinary tract
   D. Gastritis

2. The continence specialist is educating staff on the definitions of UTIs. Which of the following would be omitted from the presentation to categorize UTIs?
   A. Type of bacteria
   B. Anatomic location
   C. The terms simple or complicated
   D. The term recurrent

3. Which of the following is risk factor for complicated UTIs?
   A. Presence of bacteria in the urine without symptoms
   B. Healthy, nonpregnant female
   C. Male with enlarged prostate
   D. Normal anatomy

4. A continence nurse APRN evaluates patients at the continence clinic for UTIs. Which of the following scenario does not reflect a recurrent UTI definition?
   A. Having two or more episodes of cystitis in 6 months of completion of treatment

   B. Three UTIs within a 12-month period
   C. Reinfection with a previously isolated organism or persistence of bacteria after completion of treatment
   D. Persistent perigenital itching and urethral discharge

5. Screening and treatment for asymptomatic bacteriuria is recommended in which of the following?
   A. Frail elders living in a nursing home
   B. Pregnant women
   C. Patient with an indwelling catheter
   D. Patient with a nephrostomy tube

6. Which of the following gram-negative bacteria is responsible for most lower and upper UTIs?
   A. *Klebsiella*
   B. *E. coli*
   C. *Enterobacter*
   D. *Proteus*

7. Which of the following symptom is *most* clearly associated with a complicated UTI?
   A. Urinary frequency
   B. Dysuria
   C. Suprapubic pressure
   D. CVA tenderness

8. Which of the following is *not* true regarding laboratory and diagnostic testing related to uncomplicated UTI?
   A. Urinalysis is key in the diagnosis of UTI.
   B. Urine culture and sensitivity is recommended for all patients with a positive UA.
   C. Postvoid residual may be recommended in situations where incomplete bladder emptying is suspected.
   D. Chlamydia and gonorrhea cultures may be indicated in sexually active patients.

9. Prescribers are called to be good stewards in utilizing antimicrobial therapy. Which of the following does *not* reflect this concept?

   A. Determining if antibiotic therapy is warranted
   B. Selection of a narrow-spectrum antibiotic
   C. Ensuring that the correct form and duration are prescribed
   D. Standing protocol for over the phone antibiotic therapy

10. Patient education, anticipatory guidance, and risk reduction counseling promote bladder health and emphasize UTI prevention. Which of the following may increase the risk for developing an UTI?
    A. Advising individuals to postpone voiding
    B. Reviewing personal hygiene practices
    C. Encouraging an adequate fluid intake
    D. Early recognition of UTI symptoms

ANSWERS AND RATIONALES

1. **C. Rationale:** Adult UTIs account for almost 25% of all infections presenting across all types of patient care settings.

2. **A. Rationale:** UTIs are categorized by anatomical location, as simple, complicated, and recurrent.

3. **C. Rationale:** UTI risk for men increases with anal intercourse, lack of circumcision, and the presence of benign prostate hypertrophy that results in failure to empty the bladder completely and facilitating bacteria growth.

4. **D. Rationale:** Definition of rUTI includes >2 infections in 6 months or >3 infections in 12 months with either reinfection with a previously isolated organism or persistence of bacteria.

5. **B. Rationale:** Screening and treatment of ASB is not recommended except in pregnancy or prior to urological procedure.

6. **B. Rationale:** Gram-negative bacteria, especially *E. coli*, are responsible for most lower or upper urinary tract infections.

7. **D. Rationale:** The presence of fever, chills, costovertebral angle (CVA) tenderness, nausea, and vomiting suggests a more complicated UTI consistent with pyelonephritis.

8. **B. Rationale:** Urine culture and sensitivity (C&S) is not recommended for managing simple, uncomplicated cystitis.

9. **D. Rationale:** A responsible prescriber will consider if the antibiotic is warranted and if so, whether it is a narrow-spectrum antibiotic, in the correct form and duration with each prescription.

10. **A. Rationale:** Bladder health promotion and prevention focuses on personal hygiene practices, adequate fluid intake, regular and complete bladder emptying, avoidance of perigenital irritants, and early recognition of UTI symptoms.

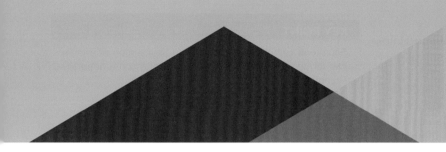

OBJECTIVES

1. Identify indications and contraindications for use of indwelling urinary catheters.

2. Describe guidelines for selection of an indwelling urinary catheter, to include catheter material, catheter size and tip, and balloon size.

3. Describe current guidelines for prevention and management of complications associated with indwelling urinary catheter use: CAUTI, obstruction, and leakage/bypassing.

4. Discuss advantages and disadvantages of urethral versus suprapubic urinary catheters.

5. Describe indications and guidelines for intermittent catheterization.

6. Detail the different types of catheter material use for intermittent catheterization.

TOPIC OUTLINE

INTRODUCTION

A catheter is a hollow flexible tube that is inserted into the bladder either through the urethra or suprapubically to allow continuous flow of urine into an external collection device. Indwelling urinary catheters are used for either short-term or long-term bladder management in patients with nonneurogenic or neurogenic lower urinary tract dysfunction (NLUTD) who have incomplete bladder emptying (urinary retention). Short-term catheterization is defined as insertion of a catheter for up to 1 month (28 days or 4 weeks); long-term catheterization is generally accepted as in situ for 30 days or more.

This chapter will address indications and guidelines for use of indwelling urethral and suprapubic catheters (SPCs) and for intermittent catheterization (IC) as well as provide the most current evidence base for the selection, nursing care, and recommendations for their use.

As the names imply, indwelling urethral catheters (IUCs) are inserted into the bladder via the urethra (referred to as transurethral); indwelling SPCs are inserted into the bladder above the suprapubic bone through the skin and an epithelialized track (see details of insertion in Chapter 8). Indwelling catheters are commonly known as Foley catheters, after a Boston-based American urologist, Dr. Frederic Foley, who designed the first balloon retention catheter. This balloon design (called a retention catheter) allowed for urinary catheters to remain in place (indwelling in the bladder) with a reasonable degree of patient comfort (Newman et al., 2018). He used the catheter for postprostatectomy hemostasis. Although Dr. Foley never held the patent for the catheter (it remains with Davol Company), his design was adopted in the 1930s and manufactured by C.R. Bard, Inc. who named the prototypes in honor of Dr. Foley. While the materials used to construct IUCs have evolved over the years, the original design of the catheter remains practically unchanged.

Indwelling catheters are not recommended for management of individuals with urinary incontinence (UI) and should be considered as a last resort option for UI not amenable to treatment by any other means (Gould et al., 2009, 2010). Short-term use of an indwelling catheter is an option for acute urinary retention for immediate bladder decompression (Billet & Windsor 2019; Sheldon et al., 2018).

 GUIDELINES FOR CATHETER SELECTION: DESIGN AND FEATURES

Continence nurses should be knowledgeable regarding the various design features for indwelling (or intermittent) catheters, in order to select the best catheter for an individual patient. Features to be considered include catheter size, catheter tip, balloon size, and catheter material. The various parts of an IUC and drainage system are shown in **Figure 19-1**. The goal of most catheterizations is to facilitate maximal drainage with minimal discomfort to the patient while minimizing complications (Newman, 2017; Newman et al., 2018).

CATHETER SIZE

Catheter size (gauge) is measured by the outer diameter using a measurement scale known as the French scale. Joseph-Frederic-Benoit Charriere was a 19th century Parisian maker of surgical instruments, and thus, the

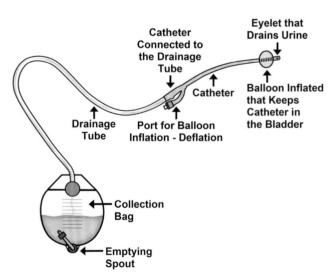

FIGURE 19-1. Closed "Two-Way" Indwelling Catheter System. (Courtesy Diane K. Newman).

TABLE 19-1 CATHETER SIZES

AGE	WEIGHT	FRENCH (FR) SIZES
Premature		5–6
Newborn	Up to 9 kg	5–8
Toddler	10–30 kg	5–8
School-age child 11–12 y		8–10
Adult age >13 y		Female: 12–14 Male: 14–16
Adult: hematuria or clots		18–20
Adult: obstruction		20–24
Adult: with prostatic bleeding		30 with 30 mL balloon

From Wound, Ostomy and Continence Nurses Society. (2016). *Care and management of patients with urinary catheters: A clinical resource guide.* Mt. Laurel, NJ: Author.

term "French (Fr)" size was coined. In adults, the standard size recommended is 14 Fr, unless a larger or smaller size catheter is indicated for specific urologic reasons. The routine use of large-size catheters (16 Fr or larger) is not recommended as larger catheter diameters can cause more erosion of the bladder neck and urethral mucosa, can cause stricture formation, and do not allow adequate drainage of periurethral gland secretions leading to irritation and infection (Newman et al., 2018). Large Fr sizes (e.g., 20 to 24 Fr) are most commonly used for drainage of hematuria or blood clots. The vast majority of IUCs are 41 to 44 cm in length, although there are specialized catheters that are longer and shorter than this (Newman et al., 2018). **Table 19-1** shows the usual sizes for different age groups. **Table 19-2** lists the various types of catheters and their use. **Figure 19-2** depicts the parts of a two-way IUC.

TABLE 19-2 CATHETER TYPES AND USAGE

MATERIAL	DEFINITION	ADVANTAGES	DISADVANTAGES	BEST USE
Silicone elastomer–coated latex	Coated chemically with bonded silicone adhered to a latex catheter	Reduces contact of latex to the urethra Reduces incidence of insertion trauma, urethritis, and encrustation Less expensive than 100% silicone For use with latex sensitivity	Flexibility: >100% silicone; less flexible than 100% latex Elastic coating may dissolve over time exposing patient to latex Balloons may lose fluid filling over time as compared to 100% latex	Short-term usage Use cautiously in patients with latex sensitivity
PTFE or polytetrafluoroethylene	Teflon-coated latex catheters	Absorption of water is reduced due to the Teflon coating smoother than plain latex has good biological compatibility and low friction Developed to protect the urethra against latex Prevent encrustation and irritation	Because these are latex, allergy remains a concern	Use cautiously in patients with latex sensitivity
Hydrogel-coated "Lubricath" latex	Absorbs secretions from the urethra (hydrophilic), causing the catheter to soften and be more comfortable	Produces a slippery (lubricious) outside surface that reduces friction and protects urethra from tissue damage Resists encrustation and bacteria colonization	Because these are latex, allergy remains a concern	Popular catheter in acute care Consider for long-term IUC use as may be better tolerated
Red rubber latex	A latex catheter that is soft and flexible Latex: natural product that is a yellowish brown in color	Flexibility; good for allowing for easy insertion especially for short-term usage Low cost Comfort	Contraindicated in patients with latex allergies Swells with absorption of fluid thereby decreasing diameter of lumen and increasing outside diameter Potential for toxicity with mucosal tissue resulting in stricture and inflammation Prone to encrustations	Short-term usage for urethral dilation and intermittent catheterization For patients without allergies to latex

(Continued)

TABLE 19-2 CATHETER TYPES AND USAGE (Continued)

MATERIAL	DEFINITION	ADVANTAGES	DISADVANTAGES	BEST USE
PVC	A firm catheter made from a plastic polymer that has had plasticizer added to soften and increase flexibility	Becomes soft and pliable with body temperature Has wide internal diameter	Limited utility as indwelling catheters, secondary to encrustation formation increased risk with >1 wk usage Has been debated as to safety with exposure to liquid over long periods of time, that is, may break down Uncomfortable due to stiffness Balloon may be made of latex	Short-term use
Silicone	An inert product that is clear or white in color	Thin-walled tube with larger lumen that may not lead to buildup of protein and mucus (biofilms) Catheters more compatible with lining of the urethra Latex free More lumen stability with bladder irrigation and aspiration	Stiff; uncomfortable for some Balloons tend to become "cuffed" when deflated, thus making removal potentially traumatic Balloon has tendency to lose fluid filling over time leading to inadvertent removal	Long-term usage, patients with allergies to other products Latex free, which allows hospitals to ensure a "latex-reduced" environment Not recommended for SPT usage
Silver alloy/hydrogel coated	Combines a thin layer of silver alloy with antiseptic hydrogel	Antiseptic that inhibits growth of gram-positive and gram-negative bacteria Reduce bacterial adherence/encrustations Minimize biofilm and encrustation formation through release of silver ions, which prevent bacteria from settling on the surface	More expensive than other catheters. Effectiveness is shown only for short-term use (e.g., 2 wk)	Short-term benefit Consider use if CAUTI rate does not decrease after implementing a comprehensive strategy to reduce rates

From Wound, Ostomy and Continence Nurses Society. (2016). *Care and management of patients with urinary catheters: A clinical resource guide.* Mt. Laurel, NJ: Author; Newman, D. K., Cumbee, R. P., & Rovner, E. S. (2018). Indwelling (transurethral and suprapubic) catheters. In: D. K. Newman, E. S. Rovner, A. J. Wein (Eds.), *Clinical application of urologic catheters and products* (pp. 1–45). Switzerland: Springer International Publishing.

CATHETER TIP

KEY POINT

The adult standard IUC size is 14 Fr, unless a larger or smaller size catheter is indicated for specific urologic reasons. The routine use of large-size catheters (16 Fr or larger) is not recommended as larger catheter diameters can cause more erosion of the bladder neck and urethral mucosa, can cause stricture formation, and do not allow adequate drainage of periurethral gland secretions leading to irritation and infection.

The catheter tip extends beyond the balloon at the end of the catheter and may vary depending on intended use. The most common is the straight tip; however, a coudé-tip catheter is frequently useful for men with prostatic benign hyperplasia and urethral obstruction (e.g., urethral stricture) as the curved tip allows for easier passage through the prostatic curve than a straight-tip

catheter (see **Fig. 19-3**). There are one or two eyeholes, also termed eyelets or drainage holes cut into the tube adjacent to the tip. Eyeholes should be smooth as

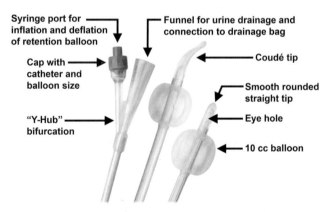

FIGURE 19-2. Indwelling Silicone Balloon-Retention Catheter with Coudé and Straight Tips. (Courtesy Diane K. Newman).

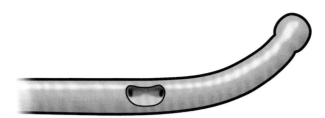

FIGURE 19-3. Coudé-Tip Latex Catheter.

irregularities and surface striations from the manufacturing process can facilitate the initial adhesion of bacterial cells to the catheter (Feneley et al., 2015; Stickler, 2008).

CATHETER BALLOON

The catheter is maintained within the bladder via an inflated balloon at the proximal end that is filled with sterile water. Saline should not be used to inflate the balloon because the fluid may crystallize in the balloon port, clogging it and preventing balloon deflation and catheter removal. The balloon sits at the base of the bladder, obstructing the internal urethral orifice resulting in 10 to 100 mL of urine remaining in the bladder when its flow has ceased (**Fig. 19-4**). This can contribute to urine leakage around the catheter, and this urine stasis may contribute to a CAUTI.

The distal end of an indwelling catheter has two ports (termed "double lumen"), one for filling/inflation of the balloon and the other for drainage of urine; they are occasionally referred to as "two-way catheters." Catheters used for bladder irrigation postoperatively or in management of hemorrhage are called "three-way catheters" because they have an additional lumen to allow fluid influx, mainly for continuous bladder irrigation (CBI). Standard intravenous tubing and an adaptor can be inserted in the third lumen to allow for infusion of irrigant. Catheter balloons come in 10- and 30-mL sizes. In clinical practice, the standard size balloon (both 5 and 10 mL) should be inflated with 10 mL of sterile water, because the balloon itself requires 5 mL for symmetrical inflation, and 5 mL of water is retained along the filling channel, for a total of

10 mL (Newman, 2017; Newman et al., 2018). Only sterile water should be used to inflate the balloon as previously stated, as saline may crystallize in the balloon port, obstructing it, preventing balloon deflation at time of catheter removal. A larger (e.g., 30 mL) balloon size is generally only used to facilitate drainage or provide hemostasis when necessary, especially in the postoperative period. It should *never* be inserted for long-term bladder drainage because of the serious trauma on the bladder neck, and the larger size balloon can increase the amount of undrained urine that pools below the level of the catheter drainage eyelets, thus increasing the risk of infection. Several catheter materials have been found to lose water from the inflated balloon over time with 100% silicone catheters losing as much as 50% of their volume within 3 weeks (Barnes & Malone-Lee, 1986).

> **KEY POINT**
>
> Saline is not used to inflate the balloon because the fluid may crystallize in the balloon port, clogging it and preventing balloon deflation and catheter removal.

CATHETER CONSTRUCTION (MATERIAL)

Indwelling catheters are manufactured from various materials, and the material used has significant implications for clinical use. Latex impregnated with polytef particles and hydrogel-coated latex catheters both reduce fluid absorption into the catheter surface and aid in a smooth insertion; uncoated latex is not used for urethral catheters as there is a high contact sensitivity to the material. Silastic catheters are silicone coated but latex based; in contrast, pure silicone catheters contain no latex and provide the advantage of a thinner wall and wider lumen as compared to latex-based catheters (**Fig. 19-5**). This is advantageous for individuals who require long-term catheterization and who are "mucus producing"; the wider lumen may maintain patency for longer periods

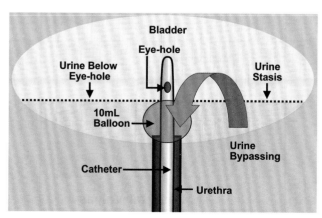

FIGURE 19-4. Residual Urine Bypassing the Catheter Causing Urine Leakage. (Courtesy Diane K. Newman).

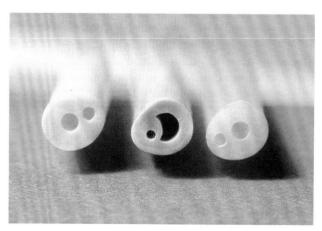

FIGURE 19-5. Comparison of a 16-Fr Silicone Catheter and 16-Fr Latex-Based Catheter. Note the much larger lumen in the silicone (*blue*) catheter.

than other catheter materials. Pure silicone catheters are also an important option for those with latex allergy, a growing problem in clinical practice. Silicone catheters are stiffer, have thinner walls and slightly larger lumens compared to other catheters, and are less likely to kink/bend (Cottenden et al., 2017).

The choice of catheter depends on the circumstances for use. In acute care and for short-term use, coated latex catheters are often used (either polytef or hydrophilic/lubricious), but this is changing because of latex allergies as many institutions are becoming 100% latex-free environments. There are reported increases in allergies and reactions in patients with long-term use of all urinary latex and rubber catheters. Latex has also been implicated in causing toxicity to mucosal tissue, resulting in inflammation and urethral strictures in long-term catheterization. So Silastic and silicone catheters are more frequently used for long-term care. Patients who have asthma and other allergies are at increased risk for these allergies. None of the catheters in this group are designed to reduce bacteriuria or catheter-associated urinary tract infection (CAUTI).

Two different catheters were designed specifically to reduce the risk of CAUTI: antibiotic coated and silver alloy. There are two types of antibiotic-impregnated catheters that have been marketed, nitrofurantoin and a combination of minocycline and rifampicin. In 2012, nitrofurazone-impregnated catheters were taken off the market due to the concern regarding the development of resistance of microbes against these antibiotics. Feneley et al. (2015, pp. 9) noted "if antimicrobials are to be incorporated into catheters to prevent encrustation, they must diffuse from the catheter into the urine and, thus, prevent the bacteria from elevating the urinary pH."

Silver is an antiseptic that inhibits growth of gram-positive and gram-negative bacteria and silver-coated catheters may reduce urinary catheter–related bacteriuria and have a low risk for generating antibiotic resistance (Majeed et al., 2019). A Cochrane group review (Lam et al., 2014) of patients with IUCs in situ short-term (<10 days) concluded that silver alloy catheters prevented asymptomatic bacteriuria (ASB). Silver-coated catheters may also have a low risk for generating antibiotic resistance (Leuck et al., 2012). Silver alloy–impregnated catheters in situ for 14 days or less will reduce the incidence of bacteriuria and thus potentially reduce the risk of CAUTI; beyond 14 days, the benefit is no longer realized as they lose antimicrobial activity over long periods.

> **KEY POINT**
>
> Silver alloy–impregnated catheters in situ for 14 days or less will reduce the incidence of bacteriuria and thus potentially reduce the risk of CAUTI; beyond 14 days, the benefit is no longer realized as they lose antimicrobial activity over long periods.

CATHETER DRAINAGE

An IUC is attached to a drainage tube connected to a drainage bag (**Fig. 19-1**) or to a catheter valve. There are a variety of catheter drainage bags available, and their material is latex, silicone, or vinyl. Drainage bags vary in capacity based on situation and time of use. Large capacity bags (2 L) are convenient for overnight use and in the acute care setting, whereas small capacity (350 to 750 mL), referred to as "leg bags," are used during the day and preferred by mobile patients when at home (Weissbart et al., 2018). There are also catheter valves, tap-like devices that fit into the end of either an IUC or SPC (**Fig. 19-6**). A valve may help maintain bladder function, capacity, and tone by allowing the filling and emptying of the bladder, mimicking normal function. Other advantages include their discreteness and reduce trauma to the bladder neck and meatus as the weight of a drainage bag is eliminated. Catheter valves are more frequently used by patients with short-term SPCs, especially post genitourinary surgery (**Fig. 19-7**) (Newman, 2017; Newman et al., 2018).

INDWELLING CATHETER–RELATED COMPLICATIONS

Indwelling urinary catheters are important adjuncts to patient care. When used on a short-term basis (i.e., for a few days), there are few complications apart from risk of urinary tract infection (UTI) or dislodgement. Conversely, when used on a long-term basis (over 30 days), both urethral catheters and SPCs are associated with

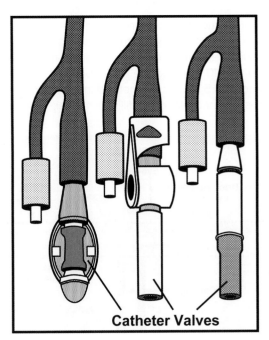

Catheter Valves

FIGURE 19-6. Sample Catheter Valves. (Courtesy Diane K. Newman).

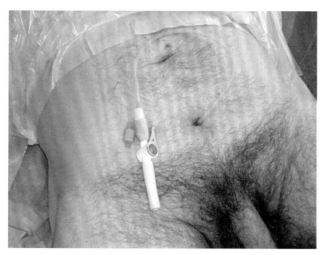

FIGURE 19-7. Flip-Flop Catheter Valve Attached to an SPC. (Courtesy Diane K. Newman).

complications that can be serious. Foremost is CAUTI; additional potential complications of IUCs include bladder calculi and urinary leakage around the catheter. Risks associated with transurethral IUCs include urethral erosion or tearing (iatrogenic hypospadias; **Fig. 19-8**), bladder neck injury, and in men epididymitis or orchitis. Risks specific to SPCs are skin irritation/breakdown at the stoma site or dislodgement and track closure. In addition, the initial insertion of a SPC has been associated with bowel perforation and bladder injury (Hall et al., 2019; Harrison et al., 2011). Long-term use of either a urethral or an SP catheter also increases the risk of squamous cell bladder carcinoma (Groah et al., 2002; Massaro et al., 2014).

Wilde and colleagues (2013) reported on 220 community-based long-term highly disabled IUC patients. Urethral catheters were used slightly more often (56%)

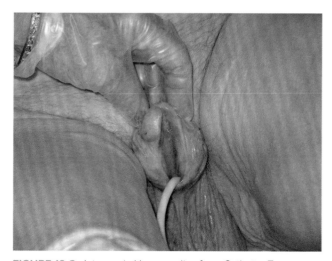

FIGURE 19-8. Iatrogenic Hypospadias from Catheter Trauma. (LeBlanc, K., & Christensen, D. (2005). Addressing the challenge of providing nursing care for elderly men suffering from urethral erosion. *Journal of Wound, Ostomy, and Continence Nursing, 32*(2), 131–134.)

than suprapubic (44%), for a mean of 6 years (SD 7 years). A high percentage of catheter problems were reported including 43% experiencing leakage (bypassing of urine), 31% having had a UTI, 24% with blockage of the catheter, 23% with catheter-associated pain, and 12% with accidental dislodgment of the catheter.

> **KEY POINT**
>
> Risks specific to suprapubic catheters are skin irritation/breakdown at the stoma site or dislodgement and track closure.

CATHETER-ASSOCIATED URINARY TRACT INFECTION

At least 80% of UTIs are associated with an IUC, referred to as "catheter-associated urinary tract infection or CAUTIs" (Lo et al., 2014). A CAUTI is classified as a complicated UTI as the presence of a foreign body in the urinary tract not only predisposes the patient to a UTI but alters the body's ability to eradicate bacteria from the lower urinary tract. It is the most severe and common catheter-associated complication because it can lead to urosepsis and septicemia. Much attention has been paid to CAUTIs, particularly since 2008; at that time, the Centers for Medicare and Medicaid Services (CMS) changed reimbursement regulations, calling a CAUTI "preventable harm" and withholding payment for additional costs related to CAUTI treatment (CMS, 2007; Wald & Kramer, 2007).

The main risk for developing a CAUTI is prolonged catheterization >6 days. Other risk factors include female gender, catheter insertion outside the operating room, urology procedures, diagnosis of diabetes, presence of malnutrition, and azotemia.

All individuals with catheters will develop significant microbial colonization within a few days, a condition known as ASB; ASB does not produce symptoms and does not require treatment. ASB must be differentiated from CAUTI, which does produce symptoms and requires some type of intervention (**Box 19-1**).

Etiology of CAUTI

There are many causes of CAUTIs as bacteria can enter the closed drainage system through extraluminal or intraluminal methods. Intraluminal bacteria are transmitted from the drainage bag through the entire length of the drainage tube and catheter secondary to urinary stasis because of drainage failure, a break in the closed system, or from contamination of the urine collection bag or urine. Extraluminally, bacteria can migrate from the skin surrounding the urethral opening into the urinary tract and ascend into the bladder during catheter manipulation (Newman et al., 2018). Catheterization can cause perimeatal uropathogen introduction into the urethra

| BOX 19-1 | CDC: CATHETER-ASSOCIATED URINARY TRACT INFECTIONS |

CDC-Catheter-Associated Urinary Tract Infection Criteria

- Indwelling urinary catheter was in place for more than 2 days on the date of event, with day of device placement being day 1, and an IUC was in place on the date of event or the day before. If an IUC was in place for more than 2 consecutive days in an inpatient location and then removed, the date of event for the UTI must be the day of device discontinuation or the next day for the UTI to be catheter associated.
- Must have at least one of the following signs or symptoms:
  - Fever with temperature >38°C (if >65 years of age, the IUC needs to be in place for more than 2 consecutive days in an inpatient location on date of event)
  - Suprapubic tenderness
  - Costovertebral angle pain or tenderness
- Patient has a urine culture with no more than two species of organisms identified, at least one of which is a bacterium of more than 10^5 CFU/mL.

Signs not directly associated with a CAUTI:

- Pyuria—not a good indicator as it is common in catheterized individuals
- Odor—the persistent bacteria in the urine of catheterized patients will produce odor

Possible signs in an elderly patient:

- Increased restlessness or altered mental status
- Change in health status not attributable to any other cause (pneumonia, medication side effects)

Treatment of CAUTI once diagnosis is established:

- If possible, remove the catheter and follow bladder management at least until the antibiotic course is completed.
- If not possible to leave the catheter out, change the catheter prior to starting antibiotics so that there is the least amount of biofilm present.
- Start antibiotics—typical course of antibiotics is 7 to 14 days, usually a fluoroquinolone.
- Chart symptom improvement.

Adapted from CDC. Retrieved from https://www.cdc.gov/nhsn/pdfs/pscmanual/7psccauticurrent.pdf.

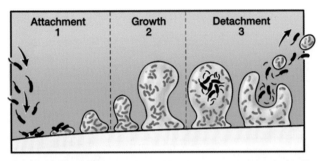

FIGURE 19-9. Biofilm Life Cycle. The three major stages in the life cycle of a biofilm: attachment, growth, and detachment. (Gehrig, J. S., & Willmann, D. E. (2011). *Foundations of periodontics for the dental hygienist.* Philadelphia, PA: Lippincott Williams & Wilkins.)

biofilm development, from initial microbial adherence to an anchored (sessile) community of organisms. Biofilms make treatment difficult, as these communities provide a physical barrier through the incorporation of both host and microbial factors, which reduce antibiotic efficacy.

Biofilms replicate rapidly, as short as 2 weeks in the setting of an IUC. The organisms within the sessile grouping are protected by a matrix of extracellular polymeric substances that, once established, are essentially impenetrable to antibiotics (**Fig. 19-10**) (Donlan & Costerton, 2002). These bacteria within a biofilm are different from bacteria that float in urine (called planktonic bacteria). Bacteria within a biofilm exhibit a greater ability to communicate and exchange genetic information than do free-floating bacteria. This communication is hypothesized to promote antibiotic resistance and spread of the biofilm to other surfaces of the catheter, particularly the balloon, and urinary epithelium (Stickler, 2014; Werneburg

and ascension toward the bladder, and a difficult catheterization can cause damage to the bladder or urethral mucosa; both have been linked to increased incidence of CAUTIs.

A CAUTI can also be caused by a biofilm. Biofilms are complex structures that include bacteria, host cells, and cellular by-products. Biofilm development on the external and internal surfaces of the catheter occurs as early as the first 15 minutes following insertion with the intraluminal and distal aspects showing the greater predominance (Werneburg et al., 2020). The biofilm burden progressively increases the longer the catheter remains in situ (Stickler, 2008). **Figure 19-9** illustrates the cycle of

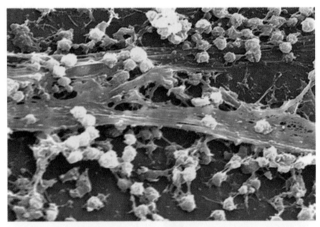

FIGURE 19-10. Electron Micrograph Depicting Large Numbers of *Staphylococcus aureus* Bacteria, Which Were Found on the Luminal Surface of an Indwelling Catheter. Of importance are the sticky-looking substances woven between the round cocci bacteria, which were composed of polysaccharides and are known as biofilm. This biofilm has been found to protect the bacteria that secrete the substance from attacks by antimicrobial agents such as antibiotics (magnified ×2,363). (Centers for Disease Control and Prevention Public Health Images Library. No. 7488. Courtesy of Rodney M. Donlan, Janice Carr.)

et al., 2020). Organisms constituting the biofilm typically originate from the periurethral area (and colonize the external surface of the catheter) or ascend via the catheter drainage tubing (and colonize the internal surface of the catheter); all organisms gain access to the bladder and new organisms are acquired at the rate of 3% to 7% a day (Nicolle, 2014). The most common infecting organism is *Escherichia coli*; *Enterococcus* spp. and *Candida* spp. Other gram-negative and gram-positive organisms are also isolated in the urine of an infected patient, and many of these are resistant to antibiotics.

The microbiologic environment changes with long-term catheterization (more than 30 days); *Proteus mirabilis* is isolated in as many as 40% of samples from individuals requiring long-term catheter use. *Proteus mirabilis* is an important organism, because it is persistent and it produces copious amounts of biofilm, which can actually block the catheter; in addition, the bacteria in the biofilm can be extremely difficult to eradicate. Proteus is also a key urease-producing organism (Stickler et al., 1998). Urease alters the urine pH, which causes hydrolysis of the urea to free ammonia; this in turn raises the pH and promotes precipitation of minerals such as calcium phosphate and magnesium ammonium phosphate (struvite) leading to bladder stones, a common complication in patients with long-term catheters. These minerals deposit on the eyes and lumen of the catheter, forming a "gravel" of mineral encrustation (Donlan & Costerton, 2002; Feneley et al., 2015).

There is no treatment for encrusted catheters except removal and replacement. Care must be taken during removal as large clumps of mineral deposits can form on the exterior of the catheter. Encrustation can also impair deflation of the balloon, thereby making it quite difficult to remove the catheter (Newman, 2017; Newman et al., 2018). In **Figure 19-11**, heavy mineral and mucous deposits have formed around a pubic hair, which was probably inserted (inadvertently) during catheterization. Introduced pubic hair is a more common occurrence in patients performing intermittent self-catheterization (ISC).

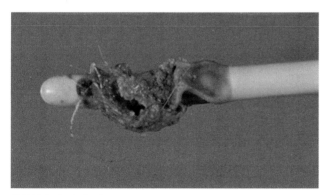

FIGURE 19-11. Biofilm Buildup Around a Hair Nidus at the Tip of an Indwelling Catheter. Note that the eyes of the catheter are completely blocked. (Loiselle, C. G., Profetto-McGrath, J., Polit, D. F., et al. (2010). *Canadian essentials of nursing research*. Philadelphia, PA: Lippincott Williams & Wilkins.)

> **KEY POINT**
>
> Urease (produced by bacteria) alters the urine pH, which causes hydrolysis of the urea to free ammonia; this in turn raises the pH and promotes precipitation of minerals such as calcium phosphate and magnesium ammonium phosphate (struvite) leading to bladder stones and catheter encrustations.

Prevention of Biofilm and CAUTI Development

To date, research attempts to eradicate catheter biofilms have included flushing of catheters with acidic solutions, use of antibiotic meatal ointments, instillation of antibiotics into urine drainage bags, and antibiotic prophylaxis (Wilson et al., 2009), but none have been effective, and bladder irrigation as a CAUTI prevention measure is not recommended (Shepherd et al., 2017). Moreover, no catheter materials have demonstrated the ability to reduce biofilm development (Donlan & Costerton, 2002).

As Méndez-Probst et al. (2012, pp. 188) note, future research on catheter designs to reduce/prevent CAUTI "must include an improved understanding of biofilm formation and ways to avoid their occurrence. This knowledge along with improvements in biomaterials and in drug elution technology will pave the way for the next evolution in urologic device development."

Diagnosis of CAUTI

All individuals with long-term catheters will develop colonization (ASB) as the daily risk of bacteriuria when IUC is present is 3% to 7% and after 1 month, all individuals will have bacteriuria (Lo et al., 2014) but urine cultures are not indicated unless the individual is symptomatic. The Centers for Disease Control and Prevention (CDC) have three criteria for diagnosing a CAUTI and those are listed in Box 19-1. A combination of symptoms within 2 days of catheter placement or removal include fever >38°C (>100.4°F), suprapubic tenderness, and costovertebral angle pain or tenderness. However, especially in the older adult with cognitive impairment, CAUTI can be difficult to diagnose; this is because other disease processes can cause similar symptoms. Thus, diagnosis is usually one of exclusion. It is important for the continence nurse to realize that pyuria is *not* a good indicator of CAUTI because it is common even in the absence of symptoms and occurs because of the inflammatory reaction to the catheter as a foreign body.

> **KEY POINT**
>
> All individuals with long-term catheters will develop colonization (ASB) as the daily risk of bacteriuria when IUC is present is 3% to 7% and after 1 month, all individuals will have bacteriuria but urine cultures are not indicated unless the individual is symptomatic.

Obtaining a Urine Specimen

Before antibiotic therapy is initiated, urine for analysis is obtained via the specimen collection port of the catheter. A mature biofilm with multiple organisms will be established if the catheter has been in situ for longer than 14 days; urine specimens in this case should be obtained from a newly inserted catheter to increase the likelihood of culturing relevant organisms (Hooton et al., 2010).

CATHETER OBSTRUCTION (BLOCKAGE)

A catheter blockage is defined as anything that inhibits or completely stops the drainage of urine from the bladder through the catheter tube. Indwelling catheters may become blocked or obstructed by blood or by precipitates and biofilm, and the management differs based on the obstructing substance. Catheter blockage can result in urine leakage around the catheter ("catheter bypassing") and often leads to accumulation of infected urine in the bladder, and eventual reflux of infected urine to the upper urinary tract and kidneys (Pelling et al., 2019). Obstruction is the most common reason for an after-hours home care nursing visit (Wilde et al., 2017). When the catheter is blocked or draining poorly due to blood clots (e.g., in patients post urologic surgery), catheter irrigation is indicated. This is performed either manually with gentle flushing of the catheter using normal saline and a 60-mL syringe or with a "three-way" catheter system (CBI) (Sturdy, 2017).

Other risk factors include reduced urine flow because of a kinked catheter and/or drainage tube, and external pressure resulting from constipation and/or fecal impaction, suboptimal positioning of the drainage bag or straps, or a full drainage bag resulting in reflux back into the bladder (Newman, 2017; Newman et al., 2018).

In contrast, long-term IUCs blocked by crystals, heavy mucus, or biofilm typically need to be removed and replaced. In this situation, catheter irrigation provides no clear advantage even if done with specifically designed acidic catheter-washout solutions (Chatterjee et al., 2014; Gould et al., 2010; Shepherd et al., 2017). **Box 19-2**

BOX 19-2   URINE NOT DRAINING CAUSE AND NURSING ACTION

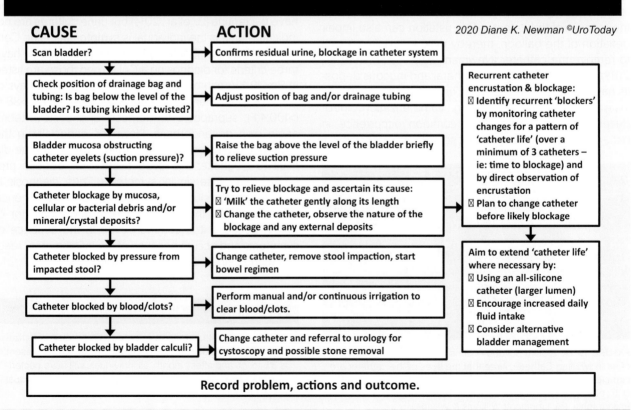

Urine (Catheter) Not Draining

2020 Diane K. Newman ©UroToday

CAUSE	ACTION
Scan bladder?	Confirms residual urine, blockage in catheter system
Check position of drainage bag and tubing: Is bag below the level of the bladder? Is tubing kinked or twisted?	Adjust position of bag and/or drainage tubing
Bladder mucosa obstructing catheter eyelets (suction pressure)?	Raise the bag above the level of the bladder briefly to relieve suction pressure
Catheter blockage by mucosa, cellular or bacterial debris and/or mineral/crystal deposits?	Try to relieve blockage and ascertain its cause: ☒ 'Milk' the catheter gently along its length ☒ Change the catheter, observe the nature of the blockage and any external deposits
Catheter blocked by pressure from impacted stool?	Change catheter, remove stool impaction, start bowel regimen
Catheter blocked by blood/clots?	Perform manual and/or continuous irrigation to clear blood/clots.
Catheter blocked by bladder calculi?	Change catheter and referral to urology for cystoscopy and possible stone removal

Recurrent catheter encrustation & blockage:
☒ Identify recurrent 'blockers' by monitoring catheter changes for a pattern of 'catheter life' (over a minimum of 3 catheters – ie: time to blockage) and by direct observation of encrustation
☒ Plan to change catheter before likely blockage

Aim to extend 'catheter life' where necessary by:
☒ Using an all-silicone catheter (larger lumen)
☒ Encourage increased daily fluid intake
☒ Consider alternative bladder management

Record problem, actions and outcome.

provides causes and nursing actions for IUCs that are not draining. Rather than trying to unblock the catheter, which can be uncomfortable for the individual, time consuming for the nurse, and potentially traumatic to the bladder, the continence nurse should identify a characteristic pattern of catheter life (Palka, 2014). If the individual is a "frequent blocker," it is usually helpful to then establish an anticipatory change schedule; for example, changing every 20 days if blocking occurs by 21 days after last catheter change (Cottenden et al., 2017). This approach can be very helpful in planning follow-up visits and in helping to reduce the risk of recurrent blockage and discomfort. The continence nurse should consult with urology for suggestions on best options for long-term management (Newman, 2017; Newman et al., 2018).

> **KEY POINT**
>
> Irrigation as a method to unblock catheters with crystals or heavy mucus has no clear advantage and is not recommended, even with specifically designed acidic catheter-washout solutions.

LEAKAGE AROUND THE URETHRAL OR SUPRAPUBIC CATHETER

Urine leakage around the catheter, referred to as "bypassing," is caused by the bladder forcing urine around the catheter. For individuals with urethral catheters, leakage places the perineal area at high risk for incontinence-associated dermatitis (IAD); for those with SPCs, in addition to urethral leakage, stoma leakage threatens skin integrity (Hunter et al., 2013). Possible causes include blockage of the drainage holes in the catheter from mucous or encrustations, kinked or crushed (caught in a bedrail) catheter drainage tubing, or blood clots.

If simple care measures are not effective, such as ensuring tube patency and improved catheter securement, the catheter is probably blocked, and the usual next step would be to change the catheter. If the problem continues, then further investigation may be indicated. For example, if ongoing "grit" or "gravel" is felt in the catheter or observed in the tubing or drainage bag, the individual may have a bladder calculus that will require urological intervention such as a cystoscopy. As indicated earlier in this chapter, the practice of inserting a larger catheter size or inflating the balloon with more fluid will not address the underlying problem and should not be done because of the risk of permanent bladder neck damage. **Box 19-3** provides nursing actions for causes of urine leakage around the IUC.

Another cause of catheter bypassing is bladder "spasms" or bladder overactivity. Prescribing an agent (e.g., antimuscarinic or beta-3 adrenergic agonist) used for an overactive bladder to reduce persistent leakage

should be considered once reversible factors and catheter securement have been addressed. If drug therapy is prescribed, the care plan must be updated to address the side effects and include evaluation following 14 days of treatment. If there is no change in leakage after 14 days of drug therapy, it should be discontinued as further improvement is unlikely; consultation with urology should be considered.

> **KEY POINT**
>
> For individuals with urethral catheters, leakage places the perineal area at high risk for incontinence-associated dermatitis; for those with SPCs, in addition to urethral leakage, stoma leakage threatens skin integrity.

PREVENTION OF COMPLICATIONS

Meta-analyses indicate that up to approximately 50% of CAUTIs can be prevented (Meddings et al., 2014; Schreiber et al., 2018). The most important prevention strategy is to avoid or remove the IUC and to consider alternate methods of management such as IC, external (condom [male], pouch or suction collection device [female]) catheter drainage, or incontinence products and toileting. **Figure 19-12** depicts the "best practices" nursing care measures to prevent CAUTIs.

INDWELLING CATHETER USE RESTRICTED TO ACCEPTED "INDICATIONS"

Complication prevention begins with the decision to insert the catheter. Continence nurses should also question the use of an IUC for bladder management in any patient: "Is this catheter really necessary? Can it be removed and alternate bladder management measures instituted?"

The use of IUCs in the acute care setting was detailed in the Agency for Healthcare Research and Quality–funded national initiative (On the CUSP-Stop CAUTI) to reduce CAUTI in acute care hospitals (Greene et al., 2014). Data were collected from five cohorts of hospitals (n = 726) from all regions in the United States. Catheter utilization was 31%, utilization in the ICU (61%) was greater than in the non-ICU (20%). Western U.S. hospitals had the highest utilization in the non-ICU setting (24%), while the South had the highest utilization in the ICU (63%). Approximately 30% to 40% of catheters in the non-ICU setting were placed without an appropriate indication.

The nurse should take into account the Healthcare Infection Control Practice Advisor Committee (HICPAC) Centers of Disease Control (CDC) (Gould et al., 2009, 2010; Meddings et al., 2015) guidelines for appropriate catheter insertion, which can serve as a checklist:

- Postoperative urinary retention (per facility catheter-removal policy)

BOX 19-3   URINE LEAKAGE BYPASSING

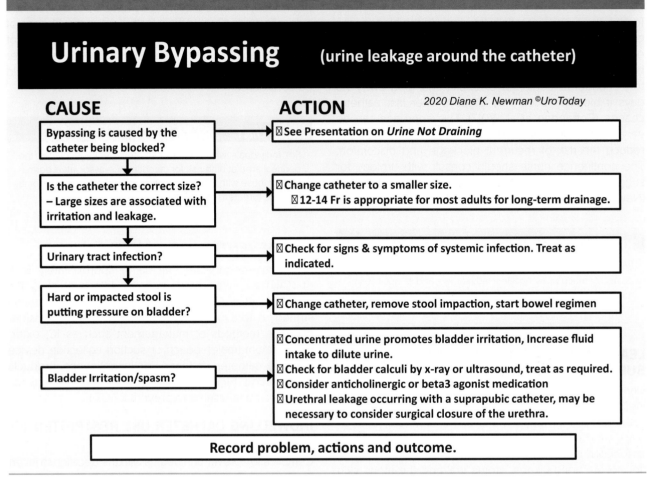

Urinary Bypassing   (urine leakage around the catheter)

CAUSE	ACTION
	2020 Diane K. Newman ©UroToday
Bypassing is caused by the catheter being blocked?	☒ See Presentation on *Urine Not Draining*
Is the catheter the correct size? – Large sizes are associated with irritation and leakage.	☒ Change catheter to a smaller size. ☒ 12-14 Fr is appropriate for most adults for long-term drainage.
Urinary tract infection?	☒ Check for signs & symptoms of systemic infection. Treat as indicated.
Hard or impacted stool is putting pressure on bladder?	☒ Change catheter, remove stool impaction, start bowel regimen
Bladder Irritation/spasm?	☒ Concentrated urine promotes bladder irritation, Increase fluid intake to dilute urine. ☒ Check for bladder calculi by x-ray or ultrasound, treat as required. ☒ Consider anticholinergic or beta3 agonist medication ☒ Urethral leakage occurring with a suprapubic catheter, may be necessary to consider surgical closure of the urethra.

Record problem, actions and outcome.

- Acute urinary retention that requires immediate attention (e.g., bladder outlet obstruction)
- Need for accurate measurements of urinary output in critically ill patients for which urine cannot be measured in another way
- Patients who require prolonged immobilization (e.g., potentially unstable thoracic, or lumbar spine, multiple traumatic injuries such as pelvic fractures)
- Assist in healing of open sacral or perineal wounds in patients with UI
- CBI for clot retention
- Administration of drugs directly into the bladder (e.g., chemotherapeutic medication to treat bladder cancer)
- Palliative care for terminally ill at the end of life
- Perioperative use in selected surgical procedures:
- Urologic/gynecologic/perineal procedure and other surgeries on contiguous structures of GU tract
- Anticipated prolonged duration of surgery (should be removed in PACU once patient is awake)
- Patients anticipated to receive large-volume infusions or diuretics during surgery

- Operative patients with UI
- Need for intraoperative hemodynamic monitoring of fluids

Note that UI is not a valid reason for insertion of an IUC unless there is a perineal wound that is being contaminated or the patient is at the end of life and wishes to have a catheter for comfort.

According to the guidelines, examples of inappropriate catheter insertion are

- For perceived comfort in patients with urinary or fecal incontinence
- To obtain a urine specimen if the individual is able to voluntarily void
- Prolonged postoperative use without appropriate indications

Despite the awareness of CAUTI and other catheter-associated complications, many catheters are inserted for unclear or inappropriate reasons. In one study (Murphy et al., 2014), emergency room staff

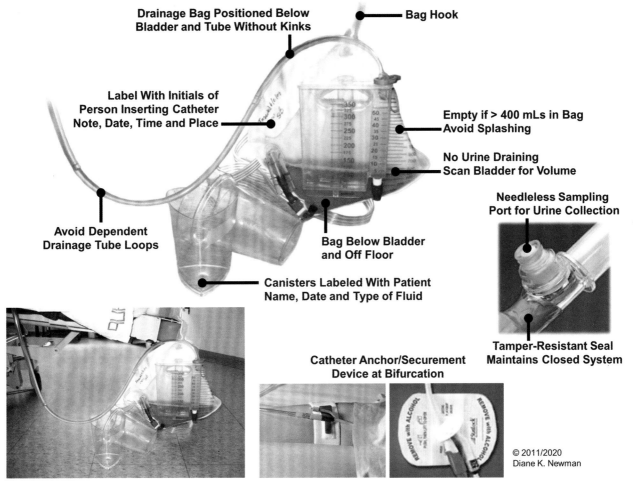

Drainage Bag Positioned Below Bladder and Tube Without Kinks

Bag Hook

Label With Initials of Person Inserting Catheter Note, Date, Time and Place

Empty if > 400 mLs in Bag Avoid Splashing

No Urine Draining Scan Bladder for Volume

Avoid Dependent Drainage Tube Loops

Needleless Sampling Port for Urine Collection

Bag Below Bladder and Off Floor

Canisters Labeled With Patient Name, Date and Type of Fluid

Catheter Anchor/Securement Device at Bifurcation

Tamper-Resistant Seal Maintains Closed System

© 2011/2020
Diane K. Newman

FIGURE 19-12. IUC Best Nursing Care Practices. (Courtesy Diane K. Newman).

indicated high levels of uncertainty over when an IUC should be used, specifically citing concerns about missing a patient in retention. Some stated that insertion of a catheter for monitoring urine output was often a routine decision; some indicated that catheters should be inserted for skin protection, comfort, and dignity; and others stated that catheters should not be used to manage UI in any circumstances, except end-of-life care. Greene and colleagues (2018) reported that a system-based collaboration including recommended guidelines for appropriate IUC placement and promoting adherence through use of clinical champions reduced unnecessary IUC use.

Older people are a particularly vulnerable group in terms of inappropriate catheter insertion. In another emergency-based study (Ma et al., 2014), 63% of catheter insertions occurred in patients ≥65 years old, only 43% had a written order for the IUC, and only 5% had a documented reason for IUC. Using the current CDC guidelines, the research team concluded that only 41% of the catheter insertions were appropriate. Both studies highlight the challenges faced by clinicians in emergency departments when time is limited, and decisions need to be made quickly.

KEY POINT

Prevention of problems starts with the decision to insert the catheter. The nurse should take into account the HICPAC CDC guidelines for appropriate catheter insertion.

ASEPTIC TECHNIQUE FOR INSERTION

Aseptic insertion and maintenance are the standard of practice for catheter insertion in many care settings, including acute care, rehabilitation facilities, and nursing homes (American Nurses Association [ANA], 2014; Meddings et al., 2019).

KEY POINT

Despite the awareness of CAUTI and other catheter-associated complications, many catheters are inserted for unclear reasons; older people are particularly at risk of inappropriate catheter insertion.

BOWEL MANAGEMENT AND CONSTIPATION PREVENTION

In many studies, constipation is noted as a predictor of UI and detrusor overactivity. In one comprehensive review of constipation and bladder function, the authors note that the majority of studies are small with varying outcome measures and most involve children and younger women. Interestingly, none of the studies addressed the impact of constipation on catheter-related outcomes (Averbeck & Madersbacher, 2011). One urodynamic study reported that women with an artificially distended rectum had statistically significant lower bladder volumes at which first and strong desire to void was felt as well as a 26% reduction in bladder capacity, as compared to the group without distention (Panayi et al., 2012).

Consequences of severe impaction are illustrated in case studies involving major rectal impaction resulting in ureteric obstruction and bilateral hydronephrosis in patients with spinal cord injury (SCI) (Downs et al., 2012) or cancer (Gonzalez, 2010). In both situations, the reports indicate that relief of the impaction resulted in gradual resolution of the hydronephrosis.

Individuals at particular risk for constipation and impaction are frail older adults, those with neurogenic bowel and bladder, those with cancer, and those receiving opioid medications. All care plans for individuals with IUCs should include comprehensive bowel assessment and systematic management. Intervention studies on constipation and catheter-related problems are scarce, but clinical judgment would suggest that nonconstipated individuals are at lower risk for straining and therefore less likely to dislodge the catheter from the bladder during a bowel movement.

STRATEGIES TO REDUCE CATHETER TIME IN SITU

Reminders on charts or flags similar to those used for medication reminders and/or ongoing (daily) review of the patient's need for a catheter, coupled with prompt removal when the catheter is no longer necessary, or automatic IUC stop orders are effective methods of promoting appropriate and limited use of IUCs (Meddings et al., 2019; Saint et al., 2016, 2019). There is good evidence that institutions that establish a catheter care bundle of education, catheter insertion/management guidelines, and surveillance can reduce CAUTI (Bernard et al., 2012; Carter et al., 2014; Saint et al., 2009). **Box 19-4** provides an example of such a bundle, the ABCDE BUNDLE that can be followed for CAUTI prevention.

In addition to assuring ongoing surveillance and prompt removal of IUCs, it may be helpful to consider nursing unit policies about time of removal. Nurse-driven CAUTI algorithms with automatic IUC removal (stop) orders in the electronic medical record (EMR) have been instituted in acute care hospitals and shown to decrease the incidence of CAUTIs and catheter use (Russell et al., 2019). The standard of practice is removal of the catheter

---

BOX 19-4   ABCDE CAUTI PREVENTION BUNDLE

Bundle (ABCDE) Checklist for Prevention of CAUTIs

- **A**dherence to infection control principles, standard supplies, procedures, and processes
  - Hand hygiene—most important factor in preventing nosocomial infections
  - Aseptic catheter insertion procedure
  - Proper Foley catheter maintenance, education, and care by nursing staff
  - Foley catheter use surveillance and feedback
- **B**ladder ultrasound use protocol in place to avoid unnecessary catheterizations
- **C**atheter alternatives
  - Intermittent ("in and out") catheterization for incomplete bladder emptying
  - External condom catheter for men with urinary incontinence
  - Absorbent pads and products for men and women with urinary incontinence
- **D**o not use the Foley catheter unless medically appropriate; know appropriate indications
- **E**arly removal of the catheter using a reminder or nurse-initiated (i.e., automatic "stop orders"); removal protocol appears warranted

© 2020 Diane K Newman; Adapted from Saint, S., et al. (2009). Translating health care-associated urinary tract infection prevention research into practice via the bladder bundle. Joint Commission Journal *on Quality and Patient Safety,* 35(9), 449–455. Meddings, J., et al. (2019). A tiered approach for preventing catheter-associated urinary tract infection. *Annals of Internal Medicine,* 171(7 Suppl), S30–S37.
© UroToday CAUTI. http://www.urotoday.com

---

at midnight as this allows time for the bladder to fill resulting in success in early morning voids and consequently, greater initial voided volume, resulting in a faster return to a regular voiding pattern (Newman, 2017).

Successful programs for changes in catheter management policies took into account cultural norms, organizational barriers (context), and practitioner values or beliefs about indwelling catheter use.

KEY POINT

Chart reminders, flags, and automatic "stops" that are reviewed on a daily basis to answer the question "Is this catheter necessary?" are just one measure in a catheter care bundle to reduce inappropriate catheter use and CAUTI.

CATHETER AND BALLOON SIZE

Avoiding long-term catheterization is the ultimate preventative strategy, but if ongoing catheterization is required, the standard catheter size is 14 Fr. Larger size catheters (e.g. 16 to 18 Fr) are often used post genitourinary surgery where bleeding is anticipated as stated previously. Large catheters and balloons are of particular significance for women requiring long-term urethral catheters. Persistent tension on the catheter and the increased weight of large retention balloons can render the bladder neck and sphincter incompetent and cause irreparable bladder neck damage that leaves the patient completely incontinent. Large catheters and large balloons also increase the risk of bladder spasms, which are painful, cause leakage, and may result in the catheter being expelled. The temptation to use a larger catheter and balloon to prevent catheter dislodgement must be avoided since a larger balloon, 30 mL, for example, weighs 30 g and is almost the size of a chicken egg.

For the patient experiencing bladder spasms and leakage around the catheter, treatment with an agent (e.g., antimuscarinic or beta-3 adrenergic agonist) used for an overactive bladder is warranted once other causes of overactivity have been ruled out. Routine use of a catheter-stabilizing device and routine use of a small catheter and balloon will minimize the risk of bladder spasms, leakage, and bladder neck/urethral erosion. **Figure 19-13** illustrates the points at which a catheter exerts pressure on the bladder neck and urethra in a male.

KEY POINT

The temptation to use a larger catheter and balloon must be avoided since a larger balloon—30 mL, for example—weighs 30 g, is almost the size of a chicken egg and will cause irreparable bladder neck damage that renders female patients, in time, completely incontinent.

CATHETER SECUREMENT (ANCHORING)

Catheter securement using a stabilization device is critical for patient comfort and to prevent traction on the bladder neck and urethral trauma and erosion as well as to optimize urine drainage (Holroyd, 2019; Newman, 2017; Newman et al., 2018). Catheters can be secured by medical hydrocolloid adhesive devices or by specially designed devices (Darouiche et al., 2006; Shum et al., 2017); the essential element to positive outcomes is elimination of tension on the catheter, the bladder, or the male urethral meatus. Catheter securement may also contribute to reduced movement of periurethral organisms, thereby delaying the onset of CAUTI, but only limited research has been conducted on the effects of catheter securement on reduction of UTI.

There are a variety of securement devices for ambulatory and bed-restricted individuals, and these include adhesive stays, straps, buttons, and hook and loop closure systems. The goal is to keep tension off the catheter and maintain the tubing and urine drainage bag in a dependent position so that urine will flow freely. Securing the tube at the Y-hub helps to decrease the incidence of bladder irritation and potential traumatic erosion (**Fig. 19-14**).

Catheters for both men and women may be secured to the abdomen or upper thigh as long as tension on the catheter is minimal with both rest and activity. **Figure 19-15** illustrates urethral trauma, edema, and dermatitis from an inadequately secured catheter and persistent leakage around the catheter in a man with reduced genital sensation as a result of stroke. A waist anchor strap is commonly used to secure SPCs (**Fig. 19-16**).

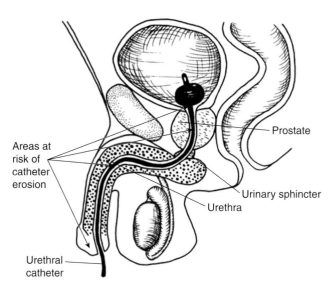

FIGURE 19-13. Pressure Points at Risk of Injury from an Indwelling Catheter in a Male: Bladder Neck, Prostatic Urethra, Bulbous Urethra, Meatus. (Illustration by Janna Linsenmeyer).

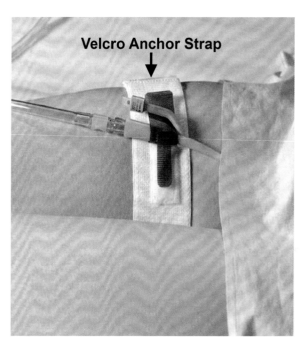

FIGURE 19-14. Properly Supported Catheter with Velcro (Dale) Anchor Strap Positioned at "Y" Hub Catheter Connector. (Courtesy Diane K. Newman).

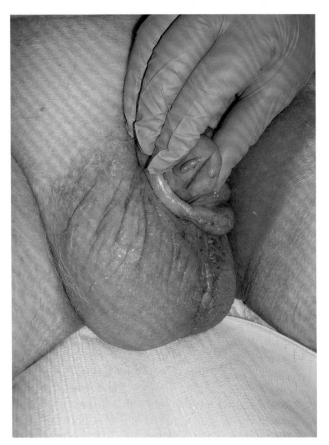

FIGURE 19-15. Improperly Supported Catheter Led to Urethral Injury, Penile and Scrotal Edema, and Incontinence-Associated Dermatitis in a Long-Term Care Patient.

Despite the recommendation to secure all IUCs, Appah and colleagues (2016) found that only 18% (8/44) of IUCs in an urban tertiary hospital in Western Canada were secured; 1 of 17 (6%) on the inpatient medial units and 7 of 27 (26%) on the surgical units. Of the eight catheters that were secured, only seven were secured correctly, six on the upper thigh (7/8; 88%) with sufficient slack to allow movement and one to the abdomen.

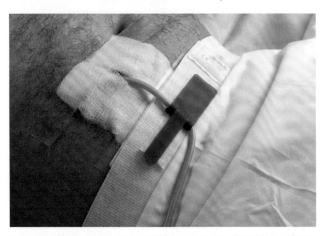

FIGURE 19-16. Securement of SPC with Velcro (Dale) Waist Strap. (Courtesy Diane K. Newman).

PREVENTION-DEPENDENT LOOPS OF DRAINAGE TUBING

For an individual in bed, drainage tubing must be straight, without dependent loops, a configuration of catheter tubing where the drainage tube dips below the entry point into the catheter bag (**Fig. 19-12**). In a laboratory study, it was found that dependent loops greatly increased the bladder pressure required to push urine through the tubing into the drainage bag, increased the length of time it took for urine to travel through the tubing, and increased the risk of backflow of urine into the bladder if the tubing and bag were raised above the bladder (Schwab et al., 2014). They may also play a role in intraluminal bacterial contamination and migration.

Dependent loop has been identified as a significant problem in hospitalized patients (Danek et al., 2015). Wuthier et al. (2016) conducted an observational cross-sectional study to determine the prevalence and nature of IUCs dependent loops in an inpatient hospital setting. Data on 55 of 78 inpatients with IUCs showed dependent loop in 87.3% of cases with 42 (76.4%) of the total showing an established pressure differential across the tubing low point. At the time of the evaluation, 26 catheters (48.1% of the total) demonstrated the characteristic of being at least potentially air-locked due to presence of the dependent loop.

KEY POINT

Dependent loops may increase the bladder pressure required to push urine through the tubing into the drainage bag, increased the length of time it took for urine to travel through the tubing, and increased the risk of backflow of urine into the bladder if the tubing and bag were raised above the bladder.

INITIAL DRAINAGE FOR PATIENT IN RETENTION

Immediate bladder compression for acute urinary retention is performed by inserting a transurethral or suprapubic catheter (Sheldon et al., 2017). When removing the catheter, historically, policies stated that bladder drainage should be done intermittently by draining a certain amount and then clamping the catheter for an unspecified length of time. However, this practice is no longer recommended as evidence to support incremental bladder drainage is lacking. There is no need to clamp the catheter after a certain amount of urine is drained as there is not significant difference between rapid and gradual bladder decompression. Complications of rapid decompression (e.g., hematuria, hypotension) are rare. Suprapubic catheterization may provide for an easier voiding trial and may be the choice in patients undergoing recent urologic or gynecologic surgery and where transurethral catheterization is contraindication.

If drained urine volume exceeds 400 cc, a transurethral IUC is inserted and left in place for 3 to 5 days, after which the patient should undergo a voiding trail. If the patient has a contraindication to urethral catheterization (e.g., recent surgery, urethral stricture disease, large prostate), or fails urethral catheterization, insertion of a SPC may be necessary.

Etafy and colleagues (2017) found no significant differences when comparing rapid versus gradual decompression of the bladder regarding effectiveness and adverse events (e.g., hematuria, hypotension, pain) in 62 male patients with acute urinary retention.

APPROPRIATE MANAGEMENT OF DRAINAGE BAG

A closed urinary drainage system with an integrated anti-reflux valve has long been recognized and is routinely recommended as an important measure in preventing early onset of CAUTI. Minimal disruption of the closed system should be allowed to reduce infection risk, especially in situations of short-term catheter use (e.g., acute care settings). Strict adherence to hand washing prior to any manipulation of the system (such as emptying) should also be maintained.

However, for active individuals living at home with long-term IUCs, there is usually a need to change from a larger night bag to a smaller capacity leg bag, and a closed system is impossible to maintain. One practice has been to connect a night bag to a leg bag, but there is no evidence to support this and many patients find this difficult with current drainage bags.

Most insurance companies provide a limited number of drainage bags per month, usually two, and thus, individuals need to clean their bags to control odor and remove debris. Although some research has been conducted on drainage bag cleaning with vinegar, soap and water, bleach, or hydrogen peroxide, there is no evidence that one solution is significantly better than another in controlling organisms and none that suggests CAUTI is reduced by a particular solution (Wilde et al., 2013). Cleaning is done primarily for control of odor and aesthetic purposes. **Box 19-5** outlines WOCN recommendations for cleaning of leg bags when reuse is indicated.

CATHETER CHANGE FREQUENCY

Traditionally, long-term indwelling catheters have been changed on a prescribed routine basis with the goal of preventing complications. Unfortunately, there is no specific catheter change interval that has been associated with reduced incidence of complications. For convenience, changing routines seem to be every 30 days, but there is no evidence that this improves patient outcomes. Some individuals require much more frequent changing,

---

BOX 19-5   CLEANING DRAINAGE BAGS

Drainage bags should be cleaned prior to reuse, such as after changing from leg to night drainage. Methods include the following steps:

1. Wash hands before and after bag cleansing with soap and water.
2. Disconnect bag from the catheter.
3. Run clear water through the system or use a soft squirt bottle to irrigate with water.
4. Irrigate with cleansing system with either a bleach solution *or* a vinegar solution.
   a. Bleach solution: 1 part bleach to 10 parts water
   b. Vinegar solution: 1 part vinegar to 3 parts water
5. Place solution in bag and tubing, irrigate for 30 seconds, and then drain.
6. Air-dry.

Be aware that bleach solution may discolor surfaces with which it comes in contact.

From Wound, Ostomy and Continence Nurses Society. (2016). *Care and management of patients with urinary catheters: A clinical resource guide.* Mt. Laurel, NJ: Author.

---

and others can manage for 2 months or longer. Why such variation occurs is not well understood although it appears partly related to the health of the individual, amount of fluid intake, and physical activity. Current clinical recommendations are to change the catheter when necessary rather than fixed intervals (Gould et al., 2009); however institutional/organizational policy may require changes every 30 days.

KEY POINT

Current recommendations are that the catheter change frequency should be individualized; evidence demonstrates that changing catheters on a fixed interval does not reduce complications.

CATHETER LUBRICATION AND INSERTION

Indwelling catheter insertion requires lubrication for patient comfort as well as ease of insertion. The research is conflicting on whether topical anesthetic gel is effective for reducing the pain of catheter insertion. The American Urological Association (AUA) White Paper on CAUTIs noted the main benefit of intraurethral anesthetic gel may be from the lubrication it provides rather than the anesthetic effect (Averch et al., 2014). An anesthetic gel provides local anesthesia and may promote sphincter relaxation. In men, it may help to "open" the urethral lumen when the lubricant is held in the urethra using mild compression at the fossa navicularis (just below the glans penis) (Newman et al., 2018; Schede & Thuroff, 2006). For females, water-soluble lubricant is typically used although at least two randomized trials have shown that females report significantly less discomfort with lignocaine gel versus water-soluble lubricant (Chan et al., 2014; Chung et al., 2007). Use of the anesthetic gel may reduce discomfort when catheterizing postmenopausal women with atrophic vaginitis (Newman et al., 2018).

Adequate anesthesia occurs only if inserting the gel into the urethra, not by applying it directly on the catheter. The usual recommendation is to instill the anesthetic gel slowly (over approximately 5 seconds) and to wait at least 5 to 10 minutes before proceeding with instrumentation. An anesthetic gel is not included in closed catheter kits and instilling the gel and waiting for it to take effect while maintaining aseptic catheter insertion technique may be difficult.

SUPRAPUBIC CATHETERS (SEE ALSO CHAPTER 8)

There are some advantages to SPCs as compared to urethral catheters, especially for those who require long-term catheters. SPCs are an alternative to urethral catheters in patients with urethral/pelvic surgery or trauma, men with prostatic obstruction and urethral stricture, and those in whom it is difficult to insert a urethral catheter due to obstruction (Harrison et al., 2011). For short-term use, such as following gynecologic surgery, an SPC allows for a trial of voiding and may be a more acceptable alternative to IC for that group of patients

In the longer term, an SPC provides protection of the bladder neck and urethra from trauma associated with urethral catheters. Although it has been suggested that UTI is lower with SPC, in long-term use, there appears to be no difference in UTI rates (Hunter et al., 2013). Moreover, SPCs offer protection to those individuals with a lack of urethral or perineal sensation or those who are sitting for extended periods in a wheelchair, who are at risk for urethral or bladder neck injury caused by tension on the catheter or for pressure ulcers from sitting on the catheter tubing (Hunter et al., 2013). SPC may also be a better choice for individuals who wish to be sexually active or who experience urethral discomfort related to the urethral catheter. **Figure 19-6** shows an SPC in situ.

Care of the SPC is similar to that of a urethral catheter. The stoma site will need monitoring for skin irritation and urine leakage. Urethral leakage is also a possibility, and the continence nurse will need to ensure good skin care, and supportive user education about care and complications (Chapple et al., 2015).

Contraindications to SPC use include pelvic radiotherapy or surgery resulting in adhesions or scarring, obesity, and hematuria requiring bladder irrigation. The frequency for changing an SPC is based on time frame to blockage (as with a urethral catheter). Prior to removal,

the catheter should be clamped, or instill 60 to 100 mL of sterile water through the existing catheter as having residual urine/fluid in the bladder that drains once catheter is inserted can confirm correct placement. To remove the catheter, the nurse should gently rotate the catheter to loosen it. **Box 19-6** provides causes of undeflating balloon and nursing actions. Once the balloon is deflated, if the catheter does not slip out with gentle traction, the nurse should reinsert some sterile water into the balloon to loosen any attached debris that may be preventing removal. Slight reinflation may also be beneficial for the individual who is being managed with an all-silicone catheter, as the walls of the balloon occasionally have irregularities that are smoothed out with slight reinflation. If, for some reason, the catheter cannot be removed, the patient should be referred to urology as there may be calcification involving the catheter and cystoscopy may be required for removal. If the SPC is no longer required, the catheter should be removed, and a gauze dressing should be placed over the stoma. Closure can occur within a few hours and should require no longer than 1 to 2 days.

INTERMITTENT CATHETERIZATION

IC is the act of inserting and then immediately removing the catheter once urine has drained via the urethra or other catheterizable channel such as a Mitrofanoff continent urinary diversion. According to the International Continence Society report on the terminology for Adult Neurogenic Lower Urinary Tract Dysfunction (Gajewski et al., 2018), IC insertion techniques include aseptic, sterile, clean intermittent catheterization (CIC), or no-touch method (see Goetz et al., 2018; Newman, 2017).

IC mimics normal bladder function, allowing the bladder to fill and periodically to empty completely, thus minimizing the risk of infection (Feneley et al., 2015; Lamin & Newman, 2016; Newman & Willson, 2011; Newman et al., 2018). IC is an accepted method of bladder emptying for individuals with nonneurogenic or neurogenic lower urinary tract dysfunction where bladder emptying is impaired or incomplete, such as SCI or multiple sclerosis, and for those with urinary retention. In acute care, IC is recommended as the preferred alternative to an indwelling catheter (Gould et al., 2009). The benefits of IC are that it can maintain renal function by reducing the pressure in the bladder, make the bladder mucosa more safe against pathogen invasion by improving bladder blood flow, and minimize bladder degeneration due to chronic urinary retention.

In addition to providing regular emptying of the bladder until voiding resumes, IC is the preferred bladder drainage method for acute and chronic urinary retention and treatment of postoperative urinary retention, excluding genitourinary surgery. In addition, IC is used to:

• Obtain urine sample in individuals who cannot provide a clean catch specimen

BOX 19-6   INFLATION BALLOON DOES NOT DEFLATE

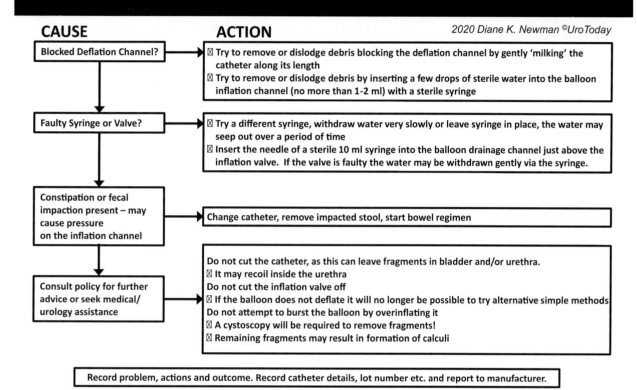

Inflation Balloon Does Not Deflate

CAUSE

ACTION   *2020 Diane K. Newman ©UroToday*

| Blocked Deflation Channel? | ☒ Try to remove or dislodge debris blocking the deflation channel by gently 'milking' the catheter along its length
☒ Try to remove or dislodge debris by inserting a few drops of sterile water into the balloon inflation channel (no more than 1-2 ml) with a sterile syringe |

| Faulty Syringe or Valve? | ☒ Try a different syringe, withdraw water very slowly or leave syringe in place, the water may seep out over a period of time
☒ Insert the needle of a sterile 10 ml syringe into the balloon drainage channel just above the inflation valve. If the valve is faulty the water may be withdrawn gently via the syringe. |

| Constipation or fecal impaction present – may cause pressure on the inflation channel | Change catheter, remove impacted stool, start bowel regimen |

| Consult policy for further advice or seek medical/urology assistance | Do not cut the catheter, as this can leave fragments in bladder and/or urethra.
☒ It may recoil inside the urethra
Do not cut the inflation valve off
☒ If the balloon does not deflate it will no longer be possible to try alternative simple methods
Do not attempt to burst the balloon by overinflating it
☒ A cystoscopy will be required to remove fragments!
☒ Remaining fragments may result in formation of calculi |

Record problem, actions and outcome. Record catheter details, lot number etc. and report to manufacturer.

- Measure residual urine if portable ultrasound is not available
- Instill intravesical medication such as chemotherapy, antibiotics

When the IC is performed by the patient, it is referred to as ISC. ISC is not restricted by age; in fact, young children (such as those with spina bifida) may be able to self-catheterize by age four with parental supervision. Some older individuals may rely on their spouse or caregiver to do IC where this is acceptable to both parties. Motivation and ability to understand and adhere to a catheterization routine are key success indicators. When assessing a patient for IC and preparing to teach him or her the procedure, the nurse must assure that the individual can adequately expose and access the urethra to safely insert the catheter; some individuals use a mirror for visualization of the meatus to guide catheter insertion, while others use meatal palpation (Goetz et al., 2018; Newman & Willson, 2011).

Individualized care plans should identify appropriate catheterization frequency; this decision is based on

functional bladder capacity, postvoid residual urine volumes, the purpose and goals of the IC program, frequency–volume charts, and impact on quality of life. The number of catheterizations per day varies; a general rule for adults is to catheterize frequently enough so bladder urine volume does not exceed 400 to 500 mL as the risk of bacteriuria increases with volumes >400 mL.

In patients with NLUTD, clinical decisions must also take into account urodynamic findings (if available), detrusor filling pressures, the presence of reflux, and renal function. For individuals with SCI who have high detrusor pressures or persistent incontinence due to detrusor overactivity, IC may be augmented with Botox or antimuscarinics.

KEY POINT

Individualized care plans should identify appropriate catheterization frequency based on user goals, impact on quality of life, frequency–volume charts, functional bladder capacity, and postvoid residual urine.

ADVANTAGES

Current Association of French Urologists, European Association of Urology (EAU), American Urological Association (AUA), and the Healthcare Infection Control Practices Advisory Committee (HICPAC) guidelines recommend IC over other catheter-based options (Averch et al., 2014; Gamé et al., 2020; Gould et al., 2009; Groen et al., 2016). Advantages of IC over indwelling catheterization include the following:

- Increased potential for improved quality of life, body image, self-esteem, and peer relationships as it promotes independence and control of bladder function as the catheterization schedule can be tailored to individual lifestyle
- Reduced need for equipment and appliances, for example, drainage bag
- Greater freedom for expression of sexuality
- Reduced risk of symptomatic UTI compared to indwelling or external catheters
- Fewer barriers to intimacy and sexual activity when compared to other catheters

Quality of life is a relative term, and health care professionals must bear in mind and be sensitive to the fact that the individual who must self-catheterize may not perceive his or her quality of life as being "good." Post SCI, most individuals are discharged using IC; however, by 1-year follow-up, it is not uncommon for some to use other options, such as an indwelling catheter, citing personal preference, difficulty with caregiver catheterizing, incontinence, or urethral strictures as main reasons for discontinuing IC (Patel et al., 2020). Perception depends, in part, on what type of bladder management the individual had prior to beginning IC as well as hand function, seating ability for catheterizing, continence status, and whether IC has actually improved the symptoms that precipitated the recommendation for IC (Stillman et al., 2018; Yılmaz et al., 2014). Chapter 16 provides insight into adaptive aides and methods to facilitate ISC in those who have physical limitations.

Another common concern is the lack of accessible and suitable toilets with a shelf on which to place equipment and receptacles to discard catheters. Adherence to an IC program may require collaboration among the individual, nursing, occupational therapists, and physical therapists. Listening to the individual's concerns and providing accessible follow-up is a critical part of assisting people to adapt.

CATHETERS

Catheters for intermittent use come in a variety of designs, including plain uncoated; hydrophilic coated; and nonhydrophilic-coated, prelubricated models (Goetz et al., 2018).

"Choosing the right catheter is a large component in making sure that the patient feels comfortable and is able to easily and successfully catheterize each and every time" (Lamin & Newman, 2016). The continence nurse needs to be knowledgeable on all available catheters as survey research highlighted the nurses' explanations for ISC as having the greatest impact on the patient's choice of the catheter (Hentzen et al., 2020). Patients may need to try multiple different types of catheters before they find one that works best.

Plain Uncoated Catheters

Plain uncoated catheters (typically clear plastic PVC or PVC free) are packed singly in sterile packaging (Lamin & Newman, 2016). As per industry standards, all disposable catheters are labeled for one-time use, and health care professionals recommend that catheters be used once only. Some individuals will reuse the catheter because of cost, limited insurance coverage, or concern about the environment. Most plain uncoated catheters are used with separate lubricant, although this is a matter of personal choice; some IC users prefer not to use lubricant or just to use water. At this time, there is no evidence-based cleaning method for catheters reused for IC, and the cleaning method is dependent on the patient's choice. Laboratory studies to identify specific cleaning solutions are ongoing (Chan et al., 2009; Wilks et al., 2020). Cleansing methods used for catheters vary including washing with antibacterial soap and water, boiling, soaking in aseptic solutions and disinfectant, microwave sterilization, or simply rinsing with water and combinations of these methods. Cleaned catheters are air-dried and then stored in a convenient container (often plastic containers or bags). If the patient is reusing catheters for multiple catheterizations, the catheter should be discarded daily.

Hydrophilic-Coated Catheters

Hydrophilic-coated catheters (HCs) are single use only (discarded after use, cannot be cleaned and reused) with an integral lubricated surface that has been shown to reduce urethral trauma and CAUTIs (Cardenas et al., 2011; DeFoor et al., 2017; Rognoni & Tarricone, 2017; Shamout et al., 2017). Common HC coatings are preactivated and ready to use or not activated requiring the addition of water (sterile water provided in the package or water is added by the user) at the time of use to form a lubricious layer (Goetz et al., 2018). According to HICPAC's 2009 Guideline for Prevention of Catheter-Associated Urinary Tract Infection, HCs might be preferable to standard catheters for patients requiring IC. The 2020 Intermittent catheterization clinical practice guidelines from the Association of French Urology recommend that both men and women use HC for ISC (Gamé et al., 2020).

A meta-analysis reported a 16% reduction in risk of CAUTIs for patients using HCs compared to patients using nonhydrophilic catheters (NHCs) (Rognoni & Tarricone, 2017). Feng et al. (2020) screened 221 articles; 14 studies were included in the final meta-analysis and 8 studies were included in the qualitative analysis and found that the use of HC, in comparison with NHC, reduced the risk of UTIs by about 54% (OR = 0.46, p = 0.002), which was consistent with the reduction in the risk of urethral trauma which was reduced by 55% (OR = 0.45, p = 0.0005). The authors felt that the additional HC cost was offset from savings due to fewer complications in comparison to NHC when considering over a lifetime from the societal perspective. They also felt that the decrease in patient suffering from fewer complications would also add to the quality of life benefits of HC. These authors found that adults reported more satisfaction with HC while children preferred NHC.

Nonhydrophilic, Prelubricated Catheters

Nonhydrophilic, prelubricated catheters are supplied prepacked with an integrated coating of water-soluble gel (Beauchemin et al., 2018; Bermingham et al., 2013; Lamin & Newman, 2016). There are also several prelubricated products with an integrated collection bag (all-in-one), which gives flexibility for the user and are efficient for hospital use (Goetz et al., 2018; Newman, 2017).

Catheter length also varies, and recent introductions on the market include shorter-length portable hydrophilic products that women may fund easier to manipulate and which can be discreetly stored or carried in a handbag/backpack (Lamin & Newman, 2016). These products are all single use and have been rated positively compared to the standard-length HC (Chartier-Kastler et al., 2013). Individuals vary in their preference of catheters for IC. Some find the longer hydrophilic-coated products too slippery to handle, while others enjoy the prelubricated surface and single use. The more compact shorter-length designs may reduce the difficulty with insertion, especially for women. A longer length catheter may be required for individuals with a large pannus, who have difficulty accessing the perineum and meatus, and if catheterizing a stoma. Others prefer PVC with added lubricant. People beginning an IC program should be offered a choice of products to determine the best fit for their lifestyle and personal goals for management.

COMPLICATIONS

The most common complication of ISC is UTI. Other less common problems include urethral irritation, urethral stricture, and epididymitis/orchitis.

Urinary Tract Infection

UTI is the most frequent complication, and catheterization frequency and the avoidance of bladder overfilling are recognized as important prevention measures. Prophylactic antibiotics are indicated only for high-risk individuals

such as children with high-grade reflux. Repeated UTIs are of concern in individuals who perform ISC as "too many urine infections" is one of the most common reasons for discontinuing IC in the SCI patients (Patel et al., 2018). Other reasons cited were inconvenience and urine leakage. Catheters used for IC are manufactured as single-use devices, and international guidelines do not endorse multiple reuse due to lack of research on storage and cleaning procedures (Blok et al., 2018; Gamé et al., 2020; Gould et al., 2010). Although there continues to be environmental and cost concerns, single use of catheters is recommended as multiple reuse poses a potential safety concern for people with NLUTD whose bladder management is IC. Catheter multiple reuse may increase the risk of UTI through microbial colonization (Newman et al., 2020) and has an impact on adherence/acceptance of IC.

Avery and colleagues (2018) conducted qualitative in-depth interviews on a convenience sample of 42 IC users in the United Kingdom to determine their views regarding the advantages and disadvantages of single use or reuse of catheters. The participants included 24 men and 15 women, with a mean age of 67 years (range 23 to 86 years) who had been using IC for a mean length of 8.5 years (range 9 months to 30 years). The majority of participants (n = 34) were using a catheter once and discarding it after use with 30 using HCs. Most appreciated their current catheters as they were convenient, comfortable, and easy to use. Single-use individuals voiced concerns about risk of UTIs, catheter cleaning, storage, and preparation in relation to reused catheters. Some felt that reuse of catheters would save space in the home and reduce waste and cost to the health system.

> **KEY POINT**
>
> UTI is the most frequent complication of IC or ISC, and catheterization frequency and the avoidance of bladder overfilling are recognized as important prevention measures.

Pyelonephritis

Pyelonephritis is a serious consequence of UTI and can cause renal scarring, hydronephrosis, and eventually renal failure. Individuals at risk are those with high-pressure bladders that are not easily controlled with routine IC. Close urology follow-up is necessary in these individuals, who may require other more aggressive management.

Prostatitis

Prostatitis, epididymitis, orchitis, and urethritis are identified risks in men. Epididymitis has been reported in 10% to 29% of patients who perform IC using PVC catheters (Stohrer et al., 2009) and in 6% in patients using low-friction HC catheters.

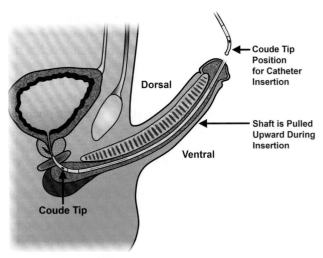

FIGURE 19-17. Catheterization of Men Who Have a History of Bladder Outlet Obstruction Performed Using a Coudé-Tip Catheter; Point the Tip Upward (Toward the Patient's Head/Umbilicus) in the 12 o'clock Position. (Courtesy Diane K. Newman).

Trauma

Trauma secondary to catheterization, as measured by hematuria and difficult catheterization, is reported, but lasting effects appear limited. The recent introduction of hydrophilic-coated or gel-coated catheters is believed to reduce urethral trauma, and laboratory research measuring epithelial cells on coated or uncoated catheters supports this hypothesis. However, longitudinal research studies are required to assess the clinical significance for long-term catheter users. Continence nurses must teach individuals to lubricate their catheters well and to insert without pressure. At-risk people for urethral trauma are those with limited or no sensation. In men, inability to visualize urinary meatal opening can occur when the foreskin cannot be retracted in an uncircumcised man or if a "buried" or retracted penis is present. Catheterization of men who have a history of bladder outlet obstruction (enlarged prostate, urethral strictures) should be performed using a Coudé-tip catheter; point the tip upward (toward the patient's head/umbilicus) in the 12 o'clock position throughout the insertion (see **Fig. 19-17**). An arrow or raised bump on the Foley catheter, on the drainage port, indicates the position of the tip during insertion. Observation of catheter insertion and assessment of the individual's understanding of insertion technique are critical in this group.

Urethral Strictures

Estimates of the prevalence of urethral strictures and false passages increase with longer use of IC and/or with traumatic catheterization. Occurrence is more common in men, occurring either in the anterior (meatus, penile–pendulous urethra, bulbar urethra) or in the posterior portion (membranous urethra and prostatic urethra) of the urethra (**Fig. 19-18**) (Goetz et al., 2018). Urethral strictures are seen more often in patients using latex catheters. This is felt to be related to cellular toxicity due to elutes from rubber causing urethral erosion over time, particularly in males (Bailey & Jaffe, 2017). Patients present with obstructive voiding symptoms (e.g., slow and decreased urinary flow).

Based on clinical opinion, the most important preventative measures appear to be good education and ongoing support for all involved in IC, adherence to the catheterization protocol, healthy lifestyle, and bowel management/avoidance of constipation, although the

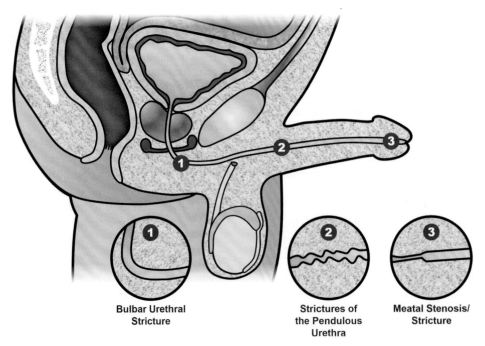

Bulbar Urethral Stricture

Strictures of the Pendulous Urethra

Meatal Stenosis/ Stricture

FIGURE 19-18. Sites of Urethral Strictures. (Courtesy Diane K. Newman).

level of evidence for these clinical opinions is weak (Beauchemin et al., 2018; Goetz et al., 2018).

PATIENT TEACHING

Beginning IC as an ongoing bladder management plan can be a necessary but difficult undertaking for people, and the continence nurse must be prepared to spend time and provide ongoing support and encouragement. The Society of Urology Nurses and Associates (SUNA) is a good resource for continence nurses who teach men and women how to perform ISC.

Frequency of catheterization depends on patient history and the clinical reasons for initiating an IC program. For example, the individual with reflux and symptomatic UTI will require more frequent catheterization than will the person who is using IC to manage leakage caused by incomplete emptying and who has no UTI symptoms. Patients are often instructed to catheterize 2 to 6 times per day, but the frequency of ISC will be determined individually according to the volumes of urine drained. Women often panic when they view the vaginal and perineal area and cannot see the urethral meatus; men recoil at the thought of causing pain by putting something in their penis. Body size, ability to abduct the legs, hand dexterity and vision, mobility, motivation, and support from family/significant others all need to be taken into account. Restrictions in upper extremity (UE) motor function is by far the best predictor for a lack of ISC implementation. To assess if hand dexterity or UE strength are barriers, consider the use of a tool, such as the Pencil and Paper test described by Amarenco et al. (2011). This employs a series of simple tasks using a pencil and paper that mimics the ability to open the packaging and handle a catheter, as well as cognitive strategies required (Goetz et al., 2018; Newman, 2017).

At times, the family member will be responsible for catheterizing; in this situation, all involved need to agree to the treatment plan. It is recommended that teaching for ISC follow a formalized protocol (Gamé et al., 2020). Teaching and support are not "one-time" events but require ongoing follow-up and encouragement from the continence nurse. This is particularly important for individuals with progressive diseases such as multiple sclerosis (Beauchemin et al., 2018; Goetz et al., 2018).

KEY POINT

Initial steps in an IC program should include a bladder diary of fluid intake, voided volumes (if able to void), and postvoid catheterization amount.

Knowledge of cystometric bladder capacity and urodynamic results is helpful but not mandatory, depending on the individual's history. Initial assessment should include a bladder diary of fluid intake, voided volumes

(if able to void), and postvoid catheterization amount. This will assist in planning the number of times a day for catheterizing as well as the best time—for example, early in the day, the individual may be able to void sufficiently to adequately empty the bladder but may be unable to void by evening. Thus, timing the catheterization(s) to coincide with the individual's personal schedule and clinical needs is a useful first step. In time, most individuals progress to catheterizing three to four times a day. Success in an IC program requires regular follow-up in person and by telephone.

It is not unusual for beginning IC users to develop a UTI. Teaching should include signs and symptoms of UTI and when to call the health care practitioner. Some clinicians start individuals with a short course of antibiotics, but a preferred approach is to treat only symptomatic infections and to base treatment on urine culture results.

If the insurance company provides enough catheters for single use, then people need advice on proper and safe disposal of products. If individuals are reusing their PVC catheters, then teaching on cleaning with soap and water, storage, and reuse will be important. Currently, there are no catheters for IC that can be flushed down the toilet.

● CONCLUSION

Indwelling catheters are a necessary option for specific patient populations. Avoidance of long-term use, if possible, is recommended. The preferred bladder management for patients with incomplete bladder emptying is ISC. Yet when an IUC unavoidable, staff and patients need to be educated to ensure that appropriate care and complication minimization is achieved for indwelling catheterization. The continence care nurse plays a vital role in selection of equipment, patient education, and early recognition of problems to improve outcomes and promote a culture of safety for this population.

REFERENCES

Amarenco, G., Guinet, A., Jousse, M., et al. (2011). Pencil and paper test: A new tool to predict the ability of neurological patients to practice clean intermittent self-catheterization. *Journal of Urology, 185*(2), 578–582.

American Nurses Association. (2014). *ANA CAUTI prevention tool*. Retrieved from https://www.nursingworld.org/~4aede8/globalassets/practiceandpolicy/innovation--evidence/clinical-practice-material/cauti-prevention-tool/anacautipreventiontool-final-19dec2014.pdf

Appah, Y., Hunter, K. F., & Moore, K. N. (2016). Securement of the indwelling urinary catheter: A prevalence study. *Journal of Wound, Ostomy, and Continence Nursing, 43*(2), 173–177. doi: 10.1097/WON.0000000000000176.

Averbeck, M. A., & Madersbacher, H. (2011). Constipation and LUTS: How do they affect each other? *International Brazilian Journal of Urology, 37*(1), 16–28. doi: 10.1590/S1677-55382011000100003.

Averch, T. D., Stoffel, J., Goldman, H. B., et al. (2014). AUA white paper on catheter-associated urinary tract infections: definitions and significance in the urologic patient. *Urology Practice, 2*(6), 321–328.

Avery M, Prieto J, Okamoto I, et al. (2018). Reuse of intermittent catheters: a qualitative study of IC users' perspectives. *BMJ Open 8*(8), e021554. doi: 10.1136/bmjopen-2018-021554.

Bailey, L., & Jaffe, W. I. (2017). Obstructive uropathy. In: D. K. Newman, J. F. Wyman, V. W. Welch (Eds.), *Core Curriculum for Urologic Nursing* (pp. 405–421). Pitman, NJ: Society of Urologic Nurses and Associates, Inc.

Barnes K. E., & Malone-Lee J. (1986). Long-term catheter management: minimizing the problem of premature replacement due to balloon deflation. *Journal of Advanced Nursing, 11*, 303–307. doi: 10.1111/j.1365-2648.1986.tb01252.x.

Beauchemin L., Newman D. K., Le Danseur M., et al. (2018). Best practices for clean intermittent catheterization. *Nursing, 48*(9), 49–54. doi: 10.1097/01.NURSE.0000544216.23783.b.

Bermingham S., Hodgkinson S., Wright S., et al. (2013). Intermittent self-catheterization with hydrophilic, gel reservoir, and non-coated catheters: a systematic review and cost effectiveness analysis. *BMJ, 346*, e8639.

Bernard, M. S., Hunter, K. F., & Moore, K. N. (2012). A review of strategies to decrease the duration of indwelling urethral catheters and potentially reduce the incidence of catheter associated urinary tract infections. *Urologic Nursing, 32*(1), 29–37.

Billet, M., & Windsor, T. A. (2019). Urinary retention. *Emergency Medicine Clinics of North America*, 37(4), 649–660. doi: 10.1016/j.emc.2019.07.005.

Blok, B., Pannek, J., Castro-Diaz, D., et al. (2018). Guidelines on neuro-urology. EAU European Association of Urology. Retrieved from https://uroweb.org/wp-content/uploads/EAU-Guidelines-on-Neuro-Urology-2018-large-text.pdf

Cardenas, D. D., Moore, K. N., Voaklander, D. C., et al. (2011). Intermittent catheterization with a hydrophilic-coated catheter delays urinary tract infections in acute spinal cord injury: A prospective, randomized, multicenter trial. *PM & R, 3*(5), 408–417.

Carter, N. M., Reitmeier, L., & Goodloe, L. R. (2014). An evidence-based approach to the prevention of catheter-associated urinary tract infections. *Urologic Nursing, 34*(5), 238–245.

Center for Disease Control and Prevention. (2019). Urinary tract infection (catheter-associated urinary tract infection [CAUTI] and non-catheter-associated urinary tract infection [UTI]) and other urinary system infection [USI]) events. Device-associated Module. UTI. 7.1–7.17 National Healthcare Safety Network (NHSN) Patient Safety Component Manual. Retrieved from https://www.cdc.gov/nhsn/PDFs/pscManual/7pscCAUTIcurrent.pdf 1

Centers for Medicare & Medicaid Services. (2007). Medicare program: changes to the hospital Inpatient Prospective Payment Systems and fiscal year 2008 rates. *Federal Register, 72*(162), 47129–48175.

Chan J. L., Cooney, T. E., & Schober J. M. (2009). Adequacy of sanitization and storage of catheters for intermittent use after washing and microwave sterilization. *Journal of Urology, 182*(4 Suppl), 2085–2089. doi: 10.1016/j.juro.2009.03.019.

Chan, M. F., Tan, H. Y., Lian, X., et al. (2014). A randomized controlled study to compare the 2% lignocaine and aqueous lubricating gels for female urethral catheterization. *Pain Practice, 14*(2), 140–145. doi: 10.1111/papr.12056.

Chatterjee S., Maiti, P., Dey R., et al. (2014). Biofilms on indwelling urologic devices: microbes and antimicrobial management prospect. *Annals of Medical and Health Science Research, 4*, 100–104. doi: 10.4103/2141-9248.126612.

Chapple, A., Prinjha, S., & Feneley, R. (2015). Comparing transurethral and suprapubic catheterization for long-term bladder drainage: A qualitative study of the patients' perspective. *Journal of Wound, Ostomy, and Continence Nursing, 42*(2), 170–175. doi: 10.1097/WON.0000000000000096.

Chartier-Kastler, E., Amarenco, G., Lindbo, L., et al. (2013). A prospective randomized crossover, multicenter study comparing quality of life using compact versus standard catheters for intermittent self-catheterization. *Journal of Urology, 190*(3), 942–947.

Christnsen, J., Ostri, P., Frimodt-moller, C., et al. (1987). Intravesical pressure changes during bladder drainage in patients with acute urinary retention. *Urologia Internationalis, 42*(3), 181–184.

Chung, C., Chu, M., Paoloni, R., et al. (2007). Comparison of lignocaine and water-based lubricating gels for female urethral catheterization: a randomized controlled trial. *Emergency Medicine Australasia: EMA, 19*(4), 315–319.

Cottenden, A., Fader, M., Beeckman, D., et al. (2017). Management using continence products. In: P. Abrams, L. Cardozo, A. Wagg, et al. (Eds), *International Consultation on Incontinence* (6th ed., pp. 2303–2426). Plymouth, UK: Health Publications Ltd.

Danek, G., Gravenstein, N., Lizdas, D.E., et al. (2015). Prevalence of dependent loops in urinary drainage systems in hospitalized patients. *Journal of Wound, Ostomy, and Continence Nursing, 42*(3), 273–278.

Darouiche, R. O., Goetz, L., Kaldis, T., et al. (2006). Impact of StatLock securing device on symptomatic catheter-related urinary tract infection: A prospective, randomized, multicenter clinical trial. *American Journal of Infection Control, 34*(9), 555–560.

DeFoor, W., Reddy, P., Reed M., et al. (2017). Results of a prospective randomized control trial comparing hydrophilic to uncoated catheters in children with neurogenic bladder. *Journal of Pediatric Urology, 13*(4), 373e1–375e5. doi: 10.1016/j.jpurol.2017.06.00.

Donlan, R. M., & Costerton, J. W. (2002). Biofilms: Survival mechanisms of clinically relevant microorganisms. *Clinical Microbiology Reviews, 15*(2), 167–193. doi: 10.1128/CMR.15.2.167-193.2002.

Downs, J., Wolfe, T., & Walker, H. (2012). Development of hydronephrosis secondary to poorly managed neurogenic bowel requiring surgical disimpaction in a patient with spinal cord injury: A case report. *Journal of Spinal Cord Medicine, 37*(6), 795–798.

Etafy, M. H., Saleh F. H., Ortiz-Vanderdys, C., et al. (2017). Rapid versus gradual bladder decompression in acute urinary retention. *Urology Annals, 9*(4), 339–342.

Feneley, R. C., Hopley, I. B., & Wells, P. N. (2015). Urinary catheters: History, current status, adverse events and research agenda. *Journal of Medical Engineering & Technology, 39*, 459–570.

Feng, D., Cheng, L., Bai, Y., et al. (2020). Outcomes comparison of hydrophilic and non-hydrophilic catheters for patients with intermittent catheterization: An updated meta-analysis. *Asian Journal of Surgery, 43*(5), 633–635. doi: 10.1016/j.asjsur.2019.12.009.

Gajewski, J. B., Schurch, B, Hamid, R, et al. (2018). An International Continence Society (ICS) report on the terminology for adult neurogenic lower urinary tract dysfunction (ANLUTD). *Neurourology and Urodynamics, 37*, 1152–1161. https://doi.org/10.1002/nau.23397

Gamé, X., Phé, V., Castel-Lacanal, E., et al. (2020). Intermittent catheterization: Clinical practice guidelines from Association Française d'Urologie (AFU), Groupe de Neuro-urologie de Langue Française (GENULF), Société Française de Médecine Physique et de Réadaptation (SOFMER) and Société Interdisciplinaire Francophone d'UroDynamique et de Pelvi-Périnéologie (SIFUD-PP). *Progrès en Urologie, 30*(5), 232–251. doi: 10.1016/j.purol.2020.02.009.

Goetz, L. L., Droste, L., Klausner, A. P., et al. (2018). Catheters used for intermittent catheterization. In D. K. Newman, E. S. Rovner, A. J. Wein (Eds.), *Clinical Application of Urologic Catheters and Products* (pp. 47–77). Switzerland: Springer International Publishing. doi: 10.1007/978-3-319-14821-2_2.

Gonzalez, F. (2010). Obstructive uropathy caused by fecal impaction: Report of 2 cases and discussion. *The American Journal of Hospice & Palliative Medicine, 27*(8), 557–559. doi: 10.1177/1049909110367784.

Gould, C., Umscheid, C., Agarwal, R., et al. (2009). Healthcare Infection Control Practices Advisory Committee (HICPAC). In *Guideline for prevention of catheter-associated urinary tract infections*. Atlanta, GA: Centers for Disease Control and Prevention (CDC). Retrieved from http://www.cdc.gov/hicpac/pdf/cauti/cautiguideline2009final.pdf

Gould, C. V., Umscheid, C. A., Agarwal, R. K., et al. (2010). Guideline for prevention of catheter-associated urinary tract infections 2009.

Infection Control and Hospital Epidemiology, 31(4), 319–326. doi:10.1086/651091.

Greene, M. T., Fakih, M. G., Fowler, K. E., et al. (2014). Regional variation in urinary catheter use and catheter-associated urinary tract infection: results from a national collaborative. *Infection Control and Hospital Epidemiology, 35*(Suppl 3), S99–S106. doi: 10.1086/677825.

Greene, M. T., Fakih, M. G., Watson S. R., et al. (2018). Reducing inappropriate urinary catheter use in the emergency department: Comparing two collaborative structures. *Infection Control and Hospital Epidemiology, 39*(1), 77–84. doi: 10.1017/ice.2017.256.

Groah, S. L., Weitzenkamp, D. A., Lammertse, D. P., et al. (2002). Excess risk of bladder cancer in spinal cord injury: Evidence for an association between indwelling catheter use and bladder cancer. *Archives of Physical Medicine and Rehabilitation, 83*(3), 346–351.

Groen, J., Pannek, J., Castro Diaz D., et al. (2016). Summary of European Association of Urology (EAU) guidelines on neuro-urology. *European Urology, 69*(2), 324–333. doi: 10.1016/j.eururo.2015.07.071.

Hall, S., Ahmed, S., Reid, S., et al. (2019). A national UK audit of suprapubic catheter insertion practice and rate of bowel injury with comparison to a systematic review and meta-analysis of available research. *Neurourology and Urodynamics, 38*(8), 2194–2199. https://doi: 10.1002/nau.24114

Harrison, S. C. W., Lawrence, W. T., Morley, R., et al. (2011). British Association of Urological Surgeons' suprapubic catheter practice guidelines. *BJU International, 107*(1), 77–85.

Hentzen, C., Turmel, N., Chesnel, C., et al. (2020). What criteria affect a patient's choice of catheter for self-catheterization? *Neurourology and Urodynamics, 39*(1), 412–419. doi: 10.1002/nau.24223.

Holroyd, S. (2019). The importance of indwelling urinary catheter securement. *British Journal of Nursing, 28*(15), 976–977. https://doi: 10.12968/bjon.2019.28

Hooton, T., Bradley, S. F., Cardenas, D., et al. (2010). Diagnosis, prevention and treatment of catheter-associated urinary tract infection in adults: 2009 international clinical practice guidelines from the Infectious Diseases Society of America. *Clinical Infectious Diseases, 50*(5), 625–663.

Hunter, K. F., Bharmal, B., & Moore, K. N. (2013). Long-term bladder drainage: Suprapubic catheter versus other methods: A scoping review. *Neurourology and Urodynamics, 32*(7), 944–951. doi: 10.1002/nau.22356.

Lam, T. B. L., Omar, M. I., Fisher, E., et al. (2014). Types of indwelling urethral catheters for short-term catheterisation in hospitalised adults. *Cochrane Database of Systematic Reviews,* (9), CD004013. doi: 10.1002/14651858.CD004013.pub4.

Lamin, E., & Newman, D. K. (2016). Clean intermittent catheterization revisited. *International Urology and Nephrology, 48*(6), 931–939. doi: 10.1007/s11255-016-1236-9.

Leuck, A. M., Wright, D., Ellingson, L., et al. (2012). Complications of Foley catheters—Is infection the greatest risk? *Journal of Urology, 187*(5), 1662–1666.

Lo, E., Nicolle, L., Coffin, S. E., et al. (2014). Strategies to prevent catheter-associated urinary tract infections in acute care hospitals: 2014 update. *Infection Control and Hospital Epidemiology, 35*(3), 464–479, S41–S50. doi: 10.1086/675718.

Ma, A. Y., Hunter, K. F., Rowe, B., et al. (2014). Appropriateness of indwelling urethral catheter insertions in the emergency department (Abstract 317). *Neurourology and Urodynamics, 33*(6), 756–757.

Majeed, A., Sagar, F., Latif, A., et al. (2019). Does antimicrobial coating and impregnation of urinary catheters prevent catheter-associated urinary tract infection? A review of clinical and preclinical studies. *Expert Review of Medical Devices, 16*(9), 809–820. doi: 10.1080/17434440.2019.1661774.

Massaro, P. A., Moore, J., Rahmeh, T., et al. (2014). Squamous cell carcinoma of the suprapubic tract: A rare presentation in patients with chronic indwelling urinary catheters. *Canadian Urological Association Journal, 8*(7–8), E510–E514. doi: 10.5489/cuaj.1637.

Meddings, J., Manojlovich, M., Fowler, K.E., et al. (2019). A tiered approach for preventing catheter-associated urinary tract infection. *Annals of Internal Medicine, 171*(7 Suppl), S30–S37. doi: 10.7326/M18-3471.

Meddings, J., Rogers, M. A., Krein, S.L., et al. (2014). Reducing unnecessary urinary catheter use and other strategies to prevent catheter-associated urinary tract infection: An integrative review. *BMJ Quality & Safety, 23*, 277–289. doi: 10.1136/bmjqs-2012-001774 8.

Meddings, J., Saint, S., Fowler, K. E., et al. (2015). The Ann arbor criteria for appropriate urinary catheter use in hospitalized medical patients: results obtained by using the RAND/UCLA appropriateness method. *Annals of Internal Medicine, 162*(9 Suppl), S1–S34.

Méndez-Probst, C. E., Razvi, H. R., & Denstedt, J. D. (2012). Fundamentals of instrumentation and urinary tract drainage. In A. J. Wein, L. R. Kavoussi, A. C. Novick, et al. (Eds.), *Campbell-Walsh urology* (pp. 177–191.e4). Philadelphia, PA: Elsevier.

Murphy, C., Fader, M., & Prieto, J. A. (2014). Interventions to minimise the initial use of indwelling urinary catheters in acute care: A systematic review. *International Journal of Nursing Studies, 51*(1), 4–13.

Newman, D. K. (2017). Devices, products, catheters, and catheter-associated urinary tract infections. In: D. K. Newman, J. F. Wyman, V. W. Welch (Eds.), *Core Curriculum for Urologic Nursing* (pp. 429–466). Pitman, NJ: Society of Urologic Nurses and Associates, Inc.

Newman, D. K., New, P. W., Heriseanu, R. et al. (2020). Intermittent catheterization with single- or multiple-reuse catheters: Clinical study on safety and impact on quality of life. *International Urology and Nephrology, 52*(8), 1443–1451. https://doi.org/10.1007/s11255-020-02435-9

Newman, D. K., Cumbee, R. P., & Rovner, E. S. (2018). Indwelling (transurethral and suprapubic) catheters. In: D. K. Newman, E. S. Rovner, A. J. Wein (Eds.), *Clinical Application of Urologic Catheters and Products* (pp. 1–45). Switzerland: Springer International Publishing.

Newman, D. K., & Willson, M. M. (2011). Review of intermittent catheterization and current best practices. *Urologic Nursing, 31*(1), 12–28, 48; quiz 29.

Nicolle, L. E. (2014). Catheter associated urinary tract infections. *Antimicrobial Resistance and Infection Control, 3*(23), 1–8. doi: 10.1186/2047-2994-3-23.

Palka, M. A. (2014). Evidenced based review of recommendations addressing the frequency of changing long-term indwelling urinary catheters in older adults. *Geriatric Nursing, 35*(5), 357–363. doi: 10.1016/j.gerinurse.2014.04.010.

Panayi, D. D., Khullar, V., Digesu, G. A., et al. (2012). Rectal distention: The effect on bladder function. *Neurourology and Urodynamics, 30*(3), 344–347.

Patel, D. N., Alabastro, C. G., & Anger, J.T. (2018). Prevalence and cost of catheters to manage neurogenic bladder. *Current Bladder Dysfunction Reports, 13*, 215–223. doi: 10.1007/s11884-018-0483-2.

Patel, D. P., Herrick, J. S., Stoffel, J. T., et al. (2020). Validation of upper extremity motor function as a key predictor of bladder management after spinal cord injury. *Neurourology and Urodynamics, 39*(1), 211–219. doi: 10.1002/nau.24172.

Pelling, H., Nzakizwanayo, J., Milo, S., et al. (2019). Bacterial biofilm formation on indwelling urethral catheters. *Letters in Applied Microbiology, 68*(4), 277–293. doi: 10.1111/lam.13144.

Rognoni, C., & Tarricone, R. (2017). Intermittent catheterisation with hydrophilic and non-hydrophilic urinary catheters: systematic literature review and meta-analyses. *BMC Urology, 17*(1), 4. doi: 10.1186/s12894-016-0191-1.

Russell, J. A., Leming-Lee, T., Watters, R. (2019). Implementation of a nurse-driven CAUTI prevention algorithm. *The Nursing Clinics of North America, 54*(1), 81–96. doi: 10.1016/j.cnur.2018.11.001.

Saint, S., Greene, M. T., Fowler, K. E., et al. (2019). What US hospitals are currently doing to prevent common device-associated infections: results from a national survey. *BMJ Quality & Safety, 28*(9), 741–749. doi: 10.1136/bmjqs-2018-009111.

Saint, S. J., Olmsted, R. N., Forman, J., et al. (2009). Translating health care–associated urinary tract infection prevention research into practice via the bladder bundle. *Joint Commission Journal on Quality and Patient Safety, 35*(9), 449–455.

Saint, S., Greene, M. T., Krein, S. L., et al. (2016). A program to prevent catheter-associated urinary tract infection in acute care. *The New England Journal of Medicine, 374*, 2111–2119.

Schede, J., & Thuroff, J. W. (2006). Effects of intra-urethral injection of anaesthetic gel for transurethral instrumentation. *BJU International, 97*(6), 1165–1167. doi: 10.1111/j.1464-410X.2006.06199.x.

Schreiber P. W., Sax, H., Wolfensberger, A. (2018). The preventable proportion of healthcare-associated infections 2005-2016: Systematic review and meta-analysis. *Infection Control and Hospital Epidemiology, 39*(11), 1277–1295. doi: 10.1017/ice.2018.183.

Schwab, W. K., Lizdas, D. E., Granvenstein, N., et al. (2014). Foley drainage tubing configuration affects bladder pressure: A bench model study. *Urologic Nursing, 34*(1), 33–37.

Shamout, S., Biardeau, X., Corcos, J., et al. (2017). Outcome comparison of different approaches to self-intermittent catheterization in neurogenic patients: a systematic review. *Spinal Cord, 55*(7), 629–643. doi: 10.1038/sc.2016.192.

Sheldon, P., Wyman, J. F., & Newman, D. K. (2017). Neurogenic lower urinary tract dysfunction. In: D. K. Newman, J. F. Wyman, & V. W. Welch (Eds.), *Core curriculum for urologic nursing* (pp. 675–687). Pitman, New Jersey: Society of Urologic Nurses and Associates, Inc.

Shepherd, A. J., Mackay, W. G., & Hagen, S. (2017). Washout policies in long-term indwelling urinary catheterisation in adults. *Cochrane Database of Systematic Reviews*, (3), CD004012. doi: 10.1002/14651858.CD004012.pub5.

Shum, A., Wong, K.S., Sankaran, K., et al. (2017). Securement of the indwelling urinary catheter for adult patients: A best practice implementation. *International Journal of Evidence-Based Healthcare, 15*(1), 3–12. doi: 10.1097/XEB.0000000000000084.

Stickler, D. J. (2008). Bacterial biofilms in patients with indwelling urinary catheters. *Nature Clinical Practice. Urology, 5*(11), 598–608.

Stickler, D., Morris, N., Moreno, M. C., et al. (1998). Studies on the formation of crystalline bacterial biofilms on urethral catheters. *European Journal of Clinical Microbiology and Infectious Diseases, 17*(9), 649–652.

Stickler, D. J. (2014). Clinical complications of urinary catheters caused by crystalline biofilms: Something needs to be done. *Journal of Internal Medicine, 276*, 120–129. doi: 10.1111/joim.12220.

Stillman, M. D., Hoffman, J. M., Barber, J. K., et al. (2018). Urinary tract infections and bladder management over the first year after discharge from inpatient rehabilitation. *Spinal Cord Series and Cases, 19*(4), 92. doi: 10.1038/s41394-018-0125-0.

Stohrer, M., Blok, B., Castro-Diaz, D., et al. (2009). EAU guidelines on neurogenic lower urinary tract dysfunction. *European Urology, 56*, 81–88. doi: 10.1016/j.eururo.2009.04.028.

Sturdy, S. (2017). Post-operative care. In: D. K. Newman, J. F. Wyman, V. W. Welch (Eds.), *Core Curriculum for Urologic Nursing* (pp. 678–679). Pitman, NJ: Society of Urologic Nurses and Associates, Inc.

Wald, H. L., & Kramer, A. M. (2007). Nonpayment for harms resulting from medical care: Catheter-associated urinary tract infections. *JAMA, 298*(23), 2782–2784. doi: 10.1001/jama.298.23.2782.

Weissbart, S., Kaschak, C. B., & Newman, D. K. (2018). Urinary drainage bags. In: D. K. Newman, E. S. Rovner, A. J. Wein (Eds.), *Clinical Application of Urologic Catheters and Products* (pp. 133–147). Switzerland: Springer International Publishing.

Werneburg, G. T., Nguyen, A., Henderson, N. S., et al. (2020). The natural history and composition of urinary catheter biofilms: Early uropathogen colonization with intraluminal and distal predominance. *Journal of Urology, 203*(2), 357–364. doi: 10.1097/JU.0000000000000492.

Wilde, M. H., Fader, M., Ostaszkiewicz, J., et al. (2013). A systematic review of urinary bag decontamination for long-term use. *Journal of Wound, Ostomy, and Continence Nursing, 40*(3), 299–308. doi: 10.1097/WON.0b013e3182800305.

Wilde, M. H., McMahon, J. M., Crean, H. F., et al. (2017). Exploring relationships of catheter-associated urinary tract infection and blockage in people with long-term indwelling urinary catheters. *Journal of Clinical Nursing, 26*(17–18), 2558–2571. doi: 10.1111/jocn.13626.

Wilks, S. A., Morris, N. S., Thompson, R., et al. (2020). An effective evidence-based cleaning method for the safe reuse of intermittent urinary catheters: In vitro testing. *Neurourology and Urodynamics, 39*(3), 907–915. doi: 10.1002/nau.24296.

Wilson, M., Wilde, M., Webb, M. L., et al. (2009). Nursing interventions to reduce the risk of catheter-associated urinary tract infection. Part 2: Staff education, monitoring, and care techniques. *Journal of Wound, Ostomy, and Continence Nursing, 36*(2), 137–154.

Wuthier, P., Sublett, K., & Riehl, L. (2016). Urinary catheter dependent loops as a potential contributing cause of bacteriuria: An observational study. *Urologic Nursing, 36*(1), 7–16. doi: 10.7257/1053-816X.2016.36.1.7.

Yılmaz, B., Akkoç, Y., Alaca, R., et al. (2014). Intermittent catheterization in patients with traumatic spinal cord injury: Obstacles, worries, level of satisfaction. *Spinal Cord, 52*(2), 826–830. doi: 10.1038/sc.2014.134.

ADDITIONAL RESOURCES

American Nurses Association, (2016). Streamlined Evidence-Based RN Tool: Catheter Associated Urinary Tract Infection (CAUTI) Prevention. Available at https://www.nursingworld.org/practice-policy/work-environment/health-safety/infection-prevention/ana-cauti-prevention-tool/

Wound, Ostomy and Continence Nurses Society. (2016). *Care and management of patients with urinary catheters: A clinical resource guide*. Mt. Laurel, NJ: Author. Retrieved from https://cdn.ymaws.com/www.wocn.org/resource/resmgr/publications/Care_&_Mgmt_Pts_w_Urinary_Ca.pdf

QUESTIONS

1. For which patient would an indwelling catheter be considered an appropriate management measure?
   A. A patient who is diagnosed with incontinence
   B. A patient who is experiencing urinary retention for the first time
   C. A critically ill patient who requires ongoing monitoring of urine output
   D. Any postoperative patient until normal urinary functioning returns

2. The continence nurse is choosing a catheter for a patient who requires bladder irrigation postoperatively. Which catheter would be the best choice?
   A. Three-way catheter
   B. Two-way catheter
   C. One-piece catheter set
   D. Catheter with a balloon that is 30 mL or larger

3. The continence nurse chooses a coudé-tip catheter for a patient. What is a usual condition warranting this choice of tips?
   A. Neurogenic bladder
   B. Condition resulting in "mucous production"
   C. Bladder infection
   D. Prostatic hypertrophy

4. The continence nurse is choosing a short-term catheter for a patient who is in an acute care unit. Which catheter is the norm?
   A. Coated hydrogel latex
   B. Silicone
   C. Antibiotic coated
   D. Silicone coated (Silastic)

5. Which potential complication is associated specifically with the use of a suprapubic catheter?
   A. CAUTI
   B. Track closure
   C. Bladder neck injury
   D. Bladder calculi

6. The continence nurse is caring for a patient who presents with asymptomatic bacteriuria (ASB). What treatment would the nurse recommend?
   A. Use of antibiotic meatal ointments
   B. Flushing of the catheter with acidic solutions
   C. Instillation of antibiotic into urine drainage bag
   D. No treatment is required

7. The continence nurse is caring for a patient whose indwelling catheter has become blocked with blood. What is the initial intervention recommended for this patient?

   A. Remove catheter and call primary care provider.
   B. Remove and replace catheter.
   C. Perform manual catheter irrigation.
   D. No intervention is required as blood clots pass spontaneously.

8. What question should be prompted when a continence nurse assesses leakage around the catheter?
   A. "Am I using the correct catheter?"
   B. "Is this catheter really necessary?"
   C. "Should this catheter be replaced on a regular schedule?"
   D. "Should this catheter be irrigated on a regular basis?"

9. Which of the following is a recommended guideline for inserting and changing indwelling catheters?
   A. Catheters should be changed as necessary, not at fixed intervals.
   B. Anesthetic gel is not effective for reducing the pain of catheter insertion.
   C. For an individual in bed, drainage tubing must contain dependent loops.
   D. Using a larger catheter helps prevent irreparable bladder neck damage.

10. For which patient would a suprapubic catheter be contraindicated?
   A. A patient with diabetes mellitus
   B. An obese patient
   C. An elderly patient
   D. A pediatric patient

11. What is the most common complication of intermittent catheterization?
   A. Pyelonephritis
   B. Prostatitis
   C. Trauma from catheterization
   D. Urinary tract infection

12. The continence nurse recommends an IC program for a patient choosing to use intermittent catheterization to manage leaking caused by incomplete emptying. What is the initial step when instituting an IC program?
   A. Teaching the patient clean technique
   B. Choosing a catheter size
   C. Keeping a diary to determine fluid intake and catheterization volumes
   D. Learning cystometric bladder capacity and urodynamic results

ANSWERS AND RATIONALES

1. C. Rationale: The only option listed that makes patients appropriate candidates for an indwelling catheter is being critically ill and needing ongoing monitoring of urine output.

2. A. Rationale: A three-way catheter has a port for instillation of bladder irrigations.

3. D. Rationale: A coudé-tip catheter's curved tip allows it to pass more easily through the prostate curve than a straight-tip catheter. It should be inserted with the point tipped upward (toward the patient's head/umbilicus) in the 12 o'clock position throughout the insertion.

4. A. Rationale: Currently, in acute care and for short-term use coated latex catheters are often used, but this is changing because of latex allergies as many institutions are becoming 100% latex-free environments.

5. B. Rationale: The potential complication that is specific to use of a suprapubic catheter is track closure; the remaining complications are also seen with indwelling urethral catheters.

6. D. Rationale: Asymptomatic bacteriuria does not produce symptoms and does not require treatment. Prescribing antibiotics for individuals without symptoms is representative of poor antibiotic stewardship and may lead to multidrug-resistant organisms (MDRO) and potential for adverse side effects.

7. C. Rationale: When the catheter is blocked or draining poorly due to blood clots, catheter irrigation is indicated.

8. B. Rationale: One possible explanation for leakage around the catheter is that the bladder is starting to contract adequately and if so, the catheter may no longer be needed.

9. A. Rationale: There is no specific catheter change interval that has been associated with reduced incidence of complications. Consequently, current clinical recommendations are to change the catheter when necessary rather than at fixed intervals. The exception is if the individual is a "frequent blocker"; it is usually helpful to then establish an anticipatory change schedule, for example, changing every 20 days if blocking occurs by 21 days after last catheter change.

10. B. Rationale: Abdominal obesity is one of the contraindications to insertion of a suprapubic catheter.

11. D. Rationale: The most common complication associated with intermittent catheterization is urinary tract infections.

12. C. Rationale: Bladder diary data documenting fluid intake and catheterization will help the continence nurse develop a patient-centered catheterization schedule.

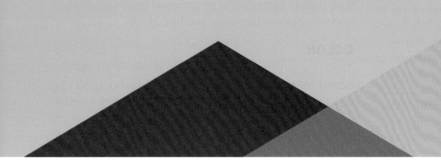

CHAPTER 20
PHYSIOLOGY OF NORMAL DEFECATION

JoAnn M. Ermer-Seltun

OBJECTIVES

1. Explain how each of the following contributes to normal bowel function and fecal continence: normal peristalsis; sensory awareness of rectal distention and ability to distinguish between solid, liquid, and gaseous contents; internal anal sphincter function; external anal sphincter function; and rectal capacity and compliance.

2. Describe the roles of each of the following in regulation of motility and fecal continence: enteric

nervous system, autonomic nervous system, and somatic nervous system.

3. Describe intrinsic and extrinsic factors affecting continence.

4. Describe the normal process of controlled defecation.

TOPIC OUTLINE

INTRODUCTION

Fecal continence is defined as the ability to control stool elimination, that is, defecation that occurs at a socially appropriate place and time. In contrast, fecal *incontinence* refers to the accidental passage of formed or liquid stool, while anal incontinence includes loss of gas at an undesirable time or place (Milson et al., 2017). Functional bowel disorders, such as constipation, diarrhea, irritable bowel syndrome, fecal or anal incontinence, or obstructed defecation syndrome, can all result in significant psychosocial morbidity and economic burden (Damon et al., 2006; Gorina et al., 2014; Wagner et al., 2017). In order to properly evaluate and manage functional bowel disorders, the continence specialist must have a fundamental understanding of the anatomical structures and physiologic processes controlling bowel function and stool elimination. This chapter will provide an overview of the basic structures and function of the small intestine, colon, anorectal unit, anal sphincters, and neural structures critical to normal function and continence and will also provide a discussion of environmental and social factors that impact bowel function.

KEY POINT

To evaluate and manage functional bowel disorders, the continence specialist must have a fundamental understanding of the anatomical structures and physiologic processes controlling bowel function and fecal continence.

 GI TRACT: CRITICAL STRUCTURES AND FUNCTIONS

KEY POINT

Gastrointestinal tract function has a major impact on the volume and consistency of the stool and is therefore a critical determinant of bowel function and continence.

SMALL INTESTINE

The small intestine measures approximately 16.5 to 20 feet (5 to 6 m) and is subdivided into three functional segments: the duodenum, jejunum, and ileum (Huether, 2019). The primary function of the small bowel is to digest and absorb life-sustaining nutrients and fluids. It is noteworthy that the terminal ileum (distal 100 cm of ileum) is the only site in the bowel where bile salts and vitamin B_{12}–intrinsic factor complex can be reabsorbed.

ILEOCECAL VALVE

The ileocecal valve is a one-way valve that is located at the junction of the ileum and cecum (the pouch-like structure that is the first segment of the colon and from which the appendix originates). The ileocecal valve controls passage of liquid stool from the small bowel into the colon and prevents retrograde (backward) flow of stool from the colon into the small intestine; this "one-way" flow pattern protects the small bowel against contamination with colonic bacteria (Huether, 2019).

COLON

The large intestine (colon) is much shorter than the small bowel, measuring approximately 4 to 5 feet or 1.2 to 1.5 m; anatomically, it is seen to "bracket" the small intestine. The colon is divided into the following sections: cecum with attached appendix, colon (ascending, transverse, descending, and sigmoid), rectum, and anal canal. **Figures 20-1 and 20-7** depict the sections of the large intestine and its blood supply (Huether, 2019).

The cecum is located on the lower right side of the abdomen and is the entry point into the large intestine, accepting 500 to 1,500 mL daily from the ileum (Boutros & Gordon, 2017). The cecum in turn drains into the ascending colon, which travels vertically upward on the right side of the abdomen to the hepatic flexure; the colon then makes a left turn to travel transversely across the abdomen along the inferior border of the liver, stomach, and spleen to the splenic flexure (transverse colon). The transverse colon is the primary site for mixing and storage of the fecal mass (Huether, 2019); the semifluid stool is reduced to a mush-like consistency. The transverse colon is very mobile because it has only two fixation points: one at the hepatic flexure and the other at the splenic flexure. The greater omentum (a vital, fatty intraperitoneal structure) hangs like an apron over the transverse colon and covers the intestinal surface down to the posterior abdominal wall. Once the transverse colon reaches the splenic flexure, it makes a sharp 180-degree turn down and backward to become the descending colon. This section of the colon begins just below the stomach and spleen and continues vertically down the left side of the abdomen until it reaches the level of the iliac crest; at this point, it becomes the sigmoid colon (Boutros & Gordon, 2017; Huether, 2019).

As the stool passes from the transverse colon to the sigmoid colon, it is converted from semimushy consistency to a more solid state. The sigmoid colon begins at the iliac crest and extends to the rectum. It resembles an "S-shaped" curvature because it bends more to the left at the distal portion and then curves back around to reach the rectum. This left curvature is the rationale for placing a patient on their left side for digital rectal or endoscopic examination and for giving an enema. Both the descending and sigmoid colon act as a conduit to deliver stool from the transverse colon to the rectum prior to defecation (Boutros & Gordon, 2017; Huether, 2019).

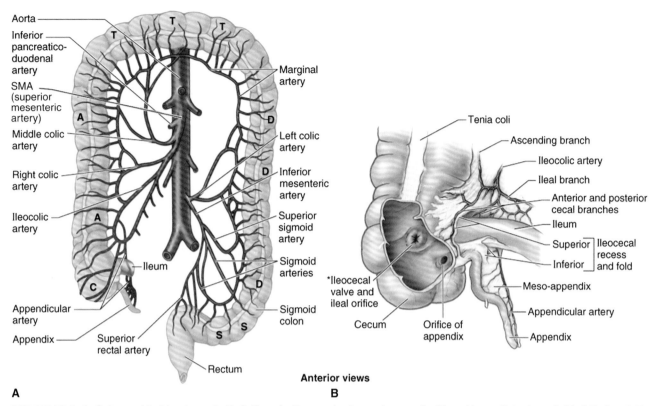

FIGURE 20-1. A. Colon and its blood supply. **B.** Orifices for ileocecal valve and appendix. (From Moore, K. L., Agur, A. M., & Dalley, A. F. (2014). *Essential clinical anatomy*. Philadelphia, PA: Lippincott Williams & Wilkins.)

RECTUM AND ANAL CANAL

The rectum is a hollow, expandable, and angulated structure that is approximately 5 to 6 inches (12 to 15 cm) in length and slightly wider in diameter than the sigmoid colon, which allows it to accommodate stool for temporary storage. There are three folds of rectal mucosa, known as the *valves of Houston*, located within the rectum: the superior (left), middle (right), and inferior (left) rectal valves (Boutros & Gordon, 2017; Huether, 2019).

The rectum empties into the anal canal, which begins where the rectum passes through the levator ani muscle and ends at the anal verge (anus); the anal canal measures 1 to 1.5 inches (approximately 3 to 4 cm) in length. The anal canal is normally closed at rest in order to maintain fecal continence. This airtight seal is accomplished through the tonic activity of the anal sphincter complex (internal and external sphincters) and the compressive effect of the anal vascular cushions (venous hemorrhoidal plexus); these structures and their functions will be described in greater detail later in the chapter. (See **Fig. 20-2** for illustrations of the sphincters and venous

hemorrhoidal plexus.) In addition, the puborectalis muscle loops around the anal canal and creates a 90-degree anorectal angle that assists in preservation of continence (Boutros & Gordon, 2017; Rao, 2010) (**Fig. 20-3**).

An important point of reference is a sawtooth pattern at the epithelial junction, the *dentate line*, located at midpoint in the anal canal. To assist in identification of this midpoint, vertical folds of the mucosa create pillar-like structures called the columns of Morgagni that are located just above the dentate line. Anal glands (4 to 10) are located in crypts that lie in the lower part and between the columns. Obstruction of these glands may lead to infection or abscess formation (Boutros & Gordon, 2017). The significance of the dentate line is as follows: above this line, the anal canal is lined with columnar epithelium, and distal to the dentate line, it is lined with squamous epithelium, which is richly innervated with sensory

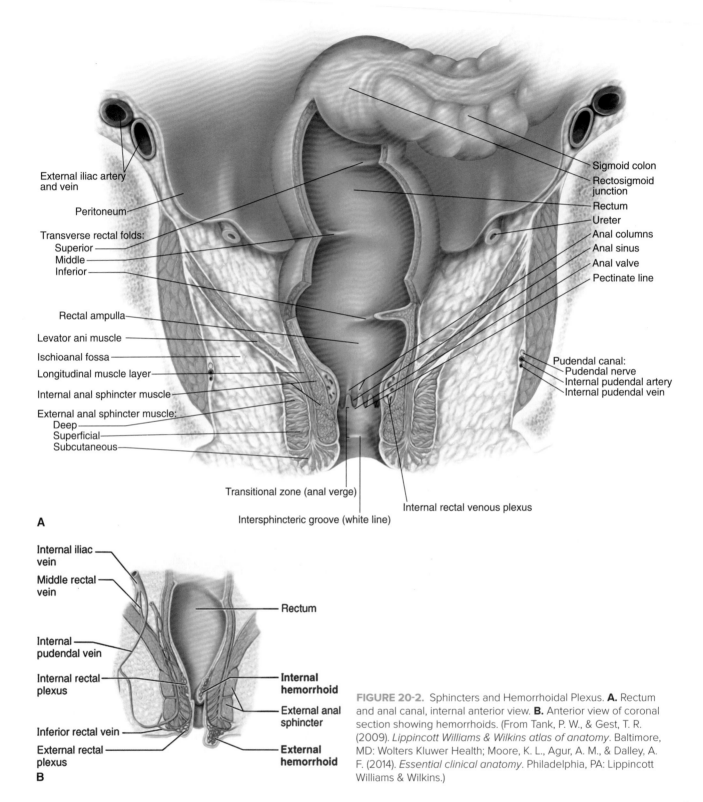

A

B

FIGURE 20-2. Sphincters and Hemorrhoidal Plexus. **A.** Rectum and anal canal, internal anterior view. **B.** Anterior view of coronal section showing hemorrhoids. (From Tank, P. W., & Gest, T. R. (2009). *Lippincott Williams & Wilkins atlas of anatomy*. Baltimore, MD: Wolters Kluwer Health; Moore, K. L., Agur, A. M., & Dalley, A. F. (2014). *Essential clinical anatomy*. Philadelphia, PA: Lippincott Williams & Wilkins.)

receptors. The conversion from columnar to squamous epithelium occurs gradually in the area proximal to the dentate line, and this area is therefore known as the transitional zone (Yu & Rao, 2014). As noted, the squamous epithelium possesses a skin-like structure and sensory nerve fibers and is therefore very sensitive to pain, touch, hot, and cold. In addition, the sensory receptors

in the distal anal canal permit differentiation between solid, liquid, and gaseous rectal contents, which is important to continence. This richly innervated area between the dentate line and the anal verge is often called the anoderm (Boutros & Gordon, 2017). The dividing line between the anoderm and the perianal skin is known as the anal verge, which is located at the anus. The perianal

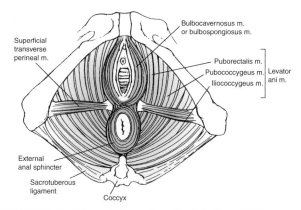

FIGURE 20-3. Puborectalis and Levator Ani. (From Pfeifer, S. M. (2011). *NMS obstetrics and gynecology.* Philadelphia, PA: Lippincott Williams & Wilkins.)

skin begins at the anal verge featuring skin-like structures such as hair follicles and glands (Boutros & Gordon, 2017) (**Fig. 20-4**).

KEY POINT

The sensory receptors in the distal anal canal (also known as the anoderm) are able to differentiate between solid, liquid, and gaseous rectal contents.

ANAL SPHINCTERS

The anal canal is encircled by the internal and external anal sphincters (EAS). The internal anal sphincter (IAS) is composed of a thick band of smooth muscle within the anal canal that is actually an extension of the circular muscle layer of the rectum. It is about 2.5 to 5 cm long and encloses the anorectal junction and the upper 2 cm of the anal canal (Barleben & Mills, 2010). The IAS chiefly controls continence at rest and is best suited to this momentous task by its composition of slow-twitch, fatigue-resistant smooth muscle fibers (Palit et al., 2012).

Because the IAS is a condensation of the circular muscle, it is primarily innervated by the myenteric plexus; it is also innervated by branches of the autonomic nervous system (ANS) and is therefore under involuntary control (Huether, 2019). In contrast, the EAS is composed of both striated skeletal and smooth muscle and overlaps the IAS. The longitudinal muscle of the rectum comprises the smooth muscle portion of the EAS, while the striated skeletal portion fuses with the puborectalis muscle to form a functional unit. The striated muscle of the EAS can be voluntarily contracted or relaxed; these fibers are innervated by the somatic fibers of the pudendal nerve, which exits the spinal cord at S2, S3, and S4 (Boutros & Gordon, 2017) (**Fig. 20-2**).

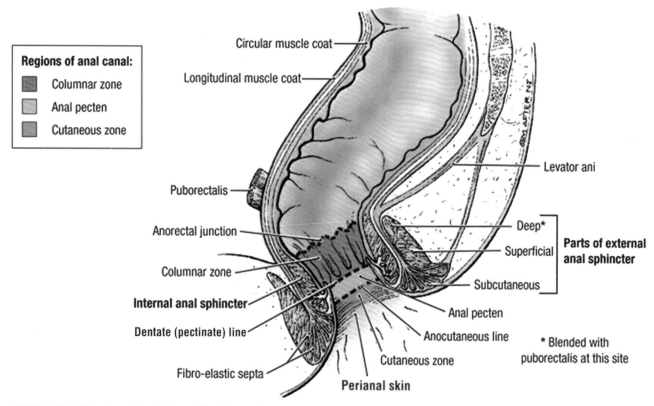

FIGURE 20-4. Rectal and Anal Mucosa/Epithelium. (From Agur, A. M., & Dalley, A. F. (2012). *Grant's atlas of anatomy.* Philadelphia, PA: Lippincott Williams & Wilkins.)

BLOOD SUPPLY

Blood supply to the cecum and the ascending and transverse colon is supplied by the superior mesenteric artery, while blood supply to the descending and sigmoid colon and proximal rectum is provided by the inferior mesenteric artery. Blood supply to the distal rectum is provided by the middle and inferior rectal (hemorrhoidal) arteries. Venous and lymphatic drainage closely mirror the arterial blood supply (Boutros & Gordon, 2017; Huether, 2019) (**Fig. 20-1**).

FUNCTIONS OF COLON

The primary functions of the colon are (1) to absorb water and electrolytes (primarily sodium, chloride), converting the liquid stool into a soft but solid fecal mass containing the waste products of digestion (food residue, unabsorbed GI secretions, shed epithelial cells, and bacteria) and (2) to serve as a reservoir for feces until a suitable time and place for elimination is found. Additional colonic functions are the responsibility of the colonic bacteria or microbiota, which rise in concentration from the proximal colon to the distal colon. These bacteria play a vital role in functions such as metabolism of bile salts, estrogens, androgens, lipids, and various drugs, the synthesis of vitamin K and B vitamins, promoting angiogenesis and enteric nerve function and the conversion of unabsorbed carbohydrates to absorbable short chain fatty acids (SCFAs), (Bharucha & Camilleri, 2019; Greenwood-Van Meerveld et al., 2017; Huether, 2019). Noteworthy, SCFAs are the preferred fuel for colonocytes (epithelial cells of the colon), boost sodium, chloride, and water absorption and may enhance immune function, weight loss as well as wound healing within the colon. Diets rich in fiber, beans, resistant starches, and complex carbohydrates increase the production of SCFAs (Alexander et al., 2019; Bharucha & Camilleri, 2019).

Currently, there has been an explosion of research regarding the gut microbiota, its role in immunity, and preservation of optimal health. The disturbance of the microbiota balance, called dysbiosis, has been associated with functional bowel disorders, inflammatory bowel disease, obesity, diabetes, allergies, autism, and even cancer (Castaner et al., 2018; Kasubuchi et al., 2015; Parthasarathy et al., 2016; Pickard et al., 2017). Moreover, some research has postulated that an individual's unique microbiome may determine their risk for certain diseases (Akaza, 2012; Scott et al., 2019; Toor et al., 2019); nonetheless, great caution is encouraged to use a critical eye in extrapolating correlations with causative results (Hanage, 2014).

The bacterial action on unabsorbed carbohydrates (dietary fiber) is the primary source of the odorous, flammable gas characteristic of the large bowel; swallowed air and the process of blood diffusion contribute lesser volumes of gas. Most of the colonic ecosystem comes from three main bacterial divisions: Firmicutes (gram positive, i.e., Clostridia species, lactobacillus), Bacteroidetes (gram negative, rod shaped, i.e., *B. fragilis*), and Actinobacteria (gram positive, i.e., *Bifidobacterium bifidum, Collinsella*) (Bharucha & Camilleri, 2019; Zhang et al., 2015). It is postulated that the microflora can affect gastrointestinal motility by releasing bacterial substances or end products of bacterial fermentation. Of interest, fecal microbiota from individuals who have longer transit times as seen in constipation was predominately from the Bacteroidetes species, while individuals with faster transit time, the Firmicutes species were more abundant (Parthasarathy et al., 2016). Evidence demonstrates that each individual has their own unique microbiome composition that can be negatively influenced by illness, stress, aging, and antibiotics, as well as lifestyle choices such as dietary habits (Zhang et al., 2015). Indubitably more research is needed to explore the relationships of the colonic microbiome and human health as well as investigate the potential use of gut bacteria in the prevention and treatment of chronic diseases (Zhang et al., 2015).

⬤ PELVIC FLOOR

KEY STRUCTURES OF THE PELVIC FLOOR TO PROMOTE BOWEL CONTINENCE

The pelvic floor is a complex network of fascia, ligaments, and muscles that support the pelvic organs and oppose downward displacement to maintain continence. Currently, pelvic floor dysfunctions are common and on the rise, predominately affect older women and leads to pelvic or anal pain, constipation, rectocele, rectal prolapse, and fecal incontinence with anal triangle defects (Bordoni et al., 2019; Nygaard et al., 2008;

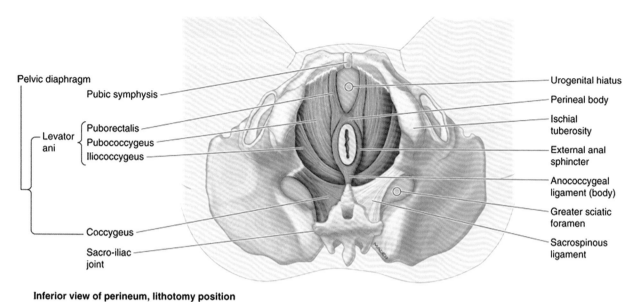

Inferior view of perineum, lithotomy position

FIGURE 20-5. Structures of the Pelvic Floor. (From Moore, K. L., Agur, A. M. R., & Dalley, A. F. (2013). *Clinically oriented anatomy.* Philadelphia, PA: Lippincott Williams & Wilkins.)

Salvator et al., 2017; Schey et al., 2012). Although the pelvic floor is made of several complex layers, key structures within those layers play a pivotal role in maintaining fecal continence such as the endopelvic fascia, perineal membrane, perineal body, anal sphincters, and levator ani (Bordoni et al., 2019) (see **Figs. 20-3 and 20-5**). For the purpose of this chapter, a brief discussion of the pelvic floor muscle as it relates to defecation and fecal continence is provided to assist the reader's understanding of pelvic floor disorders that lead to disordered defecation discussed in Chapters 21 and 22. Refer to Chapter 2 for an in-depth synopsis of the three layers of the pelvic floor, structures residing in each of the layers and their functions.

ENDOPELVIC FASCIA

The pelvic floor layers must be anchored to the bony structures of the pelvis in order to provide optimal support. The endopelvic fascia, connective tissue which is unique in that it is composed of collagen, elastin, and smooth muscle, provides a confluent suspensory apparatus for the pelvic organs by connecting them to the bony pelvis. It is intimately linked or encapsulates the pelvic viscera (soft organs within the pelvis including the urethra, vagina, bladder, uterus, and prostate) and with the third layer of the pelvic floor (pelvic diaphragm), which creates a secondary source of support for the cervix, vagina, and upper uterus plus indirect support for the bladder and rectum (Bordoni et al., 2019).

PERINEAL MEMBRANE, PERINEAL BODY, AND ANAL SPHINCTER

The perineal membrane, perineal body, and anal sphincter comprise an inferior supportive layer of the pelvic floor.

The perineal membrane is a triangular fibrous structure that spans the anterior pelvis (urogenital triangle, see Fig. 2-7B); the vagina and urethra pass through a central hole in this supportive membrane. The primary function of the perineal membrane is to limit descent of the pelvic organs by attaching the perineal body (PB) to the pubic bones. The perineal membrane provides secondary support by limiting descent of the perineal body and vagina when the levator ani is relaxed during the processes of defecation, urination, and birth (Sampselle & DeLancey, 1998). Damage to the perineal membrane may lead to vaginal/uterine/urethral prolapse and urinary incontinence. The perineal body also plays a vital role in maintaining pelvic floor integrity especially in women (Siccardi & Bordoni, 2018). Injury of the perineal body as seen in labor and delivery may lead to muscle or fascial defects such as rectocele or enterocele and bowel dysfunction. The anal sphincter resides in the anal triangle (see Fig. 2-7B); its role in providing bowel continence is discussed later in the chapter.

LEVATOR ANI

The innermost layer and the principal source of support for the pelvic floor is the levator ani located above the perineum and urogenital triangle (Ashton-Miller & DeLancey, 2007; Bordoni et al., 2019; Sampselle & DeLancey, 1998). The levator ani is a group of smaller muscles including the iliococcygeus, pubococcygeus, and puborectalis muscles, all of which function as a single unit (**Figs. 20-3 and 20-5**). The pubococcygeus muscle is a thick U-shaped muscle that arises from the pubic bones, extends around the posterior rectum, and attaches to the lateral walls of the vagina and rectum. It's fibers also wrap around the vagina (pubovaginalis), urethra (pubourethralis), and anus (puborectalis). This

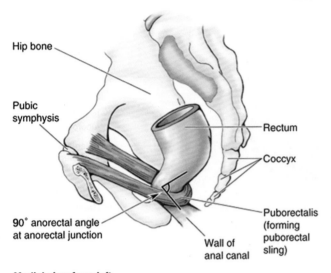

Hip bone

Pubic symphysis

Rectum

Coccyx

Puborectalis (forming puborectal sling)

90° anorectal angle at anorectal junction

Wall of anal canal

Medial view from left

FIGURE 20-6. The Anorectal Angle. (From Moore, K. L., Dalley, A. F., & Agur, A. M. (2009). *Clinically oriented anatomy*. Philadelphia, PA: Lippincott Williams & Wilkins.)

association and attachments with the midline viscera lend reason for this muscle to be also referred as the pubovisceralis. The puborectalis muscle blends with the upper end of the external anal sphincter and pubococcygeus muscle and creates a U-shaped configuration around the anorectal junction (Bordoni et al., 2019).

The primary function of the pubococcygeus (including the puborectalis) muscle is to lift the anus, vagina, and urethra and to pull them forward; this anterior pull creates a compressive force against the lumen of these organs that promotes closure through increased intra-urethral, intravaginal, and intra-anal pressures (Bordoni et al., 2019; Sampselle & DeLancey, 1998). Some anatomists specifically label the section of the levator ani muscle complex that creates a U-shaped configuration around the anorectal junction as the puborectalis muscle. This muscle acts as a "sling" around the anorectal junction; at rest, the passive contraction of this muscle creates a 90-degree angle between the rectum and the anal canal that promotes bowel continence (**Fig. 20-6**). However, with straining (Valsalva) and relaxation of the pelvic floor, this angle straightens to approximately 135 degrees to promote stool elimination (Yu & Rao, 2014). The iliococcygeus is a thinner muscle that attaches to the pelvic side walls (arcus tendineus) and covers the midplane of the pelvis with a sheet-like layer. In order for the levator ani to function normally and to provide optimal support for pelvic organs, there must be adequate attachment to the arcus tendineus and to the lateral walls of the vagina, rectum, and anus (Pradidarcheep et al., 2011; Sampselle & DeLancey, 1998). Detachment of the levator ani from the arcus tendinous may lead to pelvic floor dysfunction such as prolapse, urinary incontinence, and fecal incontinence (Ashton-miller & DeLancey, 2007; Salvator et al., 2017).

The levator ani is innervated by the pudendal and levator ani nerve branches of the sacral plexus (Pradidarcheep et al., 2011); these nerves are prone to damage due to stretch injury during vaginal delivery or pelvic surgery (Pradidarcheep et al., 2011). The levator ani complex is composed of both type 1 (slow-twitch) and type 2 (fast-twitch) muscle fibers, with a predominance of Type 1 (70%). This predominance of Type 1 (slow-twitch) muscle fibers provides sustained muscle tone over prolonged periods of time, such as is needed by an individual in the standing position. In contrast, type 2 (fast-twitch) muscle fibers provide rapid, strong contractions of the pelvic muscles that are maintained for only a short period of time; these fibers provide the support needed to offset abrupt increases in intra-abdominal pressures that develop when an individual coughs, sneezes, or lifts something heavy (Bordoni et al., 2019).

HISTOLOGY OF COLON WALL

The GI tract consists of four basic layers: mucosa, submucosa, muscularis, and serosa. It is innervated by nerve fibers from the intrinsic (also known as enteric, or within the intestine) and extrinsic (outside of the intestine) nervous systems. There are some unique differences between the histology of the small and large intestines. This chapter will focus on large intestinal histology as it relates more to the elimination process (Heitkemper, 2006; Huether, 2019) (**Fig. 20-7**).

MUCOSA

The colonic mucosal layer is the innermost layer that comes in contact with fecal contents. It is composed of columnar epithelial cells, which assist in absorbing water, electrolytes (chloride and sodium), glucose, and urea. Intestinal glands known as Lieberkuhn's crypts extend into the deeper mucosa; along with mucus-secreting goblet cells, these glands produce secretions that neutralize acids produced by bacteria, lubricate the feces to aid in transport, and protect the mucosa from injury by intraluminal substances. The pH of the stool is alkaline (approximately 7.8) due to the bicarbonate in these secretions. Of interest, stress and anxiety reduce mucus

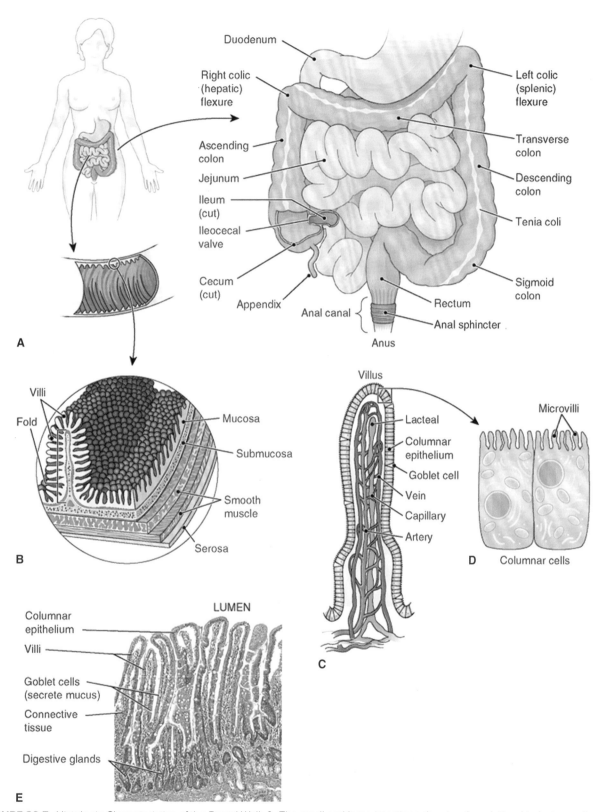

FIGURE 20-7. Histologic Characteristics of the Bowel Wall. **A.** The small and large intestines showing the relationship between them. The small intestine has three sections: the duodenum, jejunum, and ileum. The colon is the main portion of the large intestine. **B.** The wall of the small intestine showing folds in the lining and multiple small villi. **C.** Drawing of a villus showing blood vessels, a lacteal of the lymphatic system, and goblet cells that secrete mucus. **D.** Columnar epithelial cells of the intestine with microvilli, folds of the plasma membrane. **E.** Micrograph of intestinal villi. (Reprinted with permission from Cormack, D. H. (2001). *Essential histology* (2nd ed.). Philadelphia, PA: Lippincott Williams & Wilkins.)

production while bacterial, mechanical, or chemical irritants increase secretion (Huether, 2019).

SUBMUCOSA

The submucosal layer aids in attachment of the muscularis to the mucosal layer. It contains blood and lymphatic vessels, connective tissue, and nerve fibers called Meissner's (or submucosal) plexus.

MUSCULARIS

The muscularis consists of two types of smooth muscle: longitudinal and circular. The longitudinal muscle is gathered into three distinct bands known as the taeniae coli that begin in the ascending colon and continue through the descending colon; at the rectosigmoid junction, these muscle bands fan out to form a complete outer longitudinal layer. The taeniae coli produce a "gathered" appearance because the length of the muscle bands is shorter than the actual colon; the circular muscles act to separate the "gathers" and to create outpouchings called haustra. The haustra become more prominent with circular muscle contraction and less prominent during relaxation. The circular and longitudinal muscles produce rhythmic patterns of muscle contraction that promote mixing and fluid/electrolyte absorption as well as transport of stool from the cecum to the anal canal; mixing contractions are known as haustral contractions and propulsive contractions are known as peristaltic waves. The *Auerbach's* or myenteric plexus lies between the two muscle layers and plays the primary role in regulating colonic motility (Palit et al., 2012; Rodriguez et al., 2011).

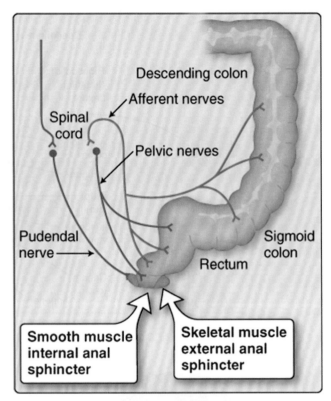

FIGURE 20-8. Innervation of Colon, Sphincters, and Pelvic Floor. (From Preston, R. R., & Wilson, T. (2012). *Physiology*. Philadelphia, PA: Lippincott Williams & Wilkins.)

the somatic system controls the voluntary muscles and thereby plays a vital role in maintenance of continence and normal defecation (Rodriguez et al., 2011).

> **KEY POINT**
>
> The circular and longitudinal muscle layers work together to mix and dehydrate the stool and to propel the stool distally; mixing contractions are known as haustral contractions and propulsive contractions are known as peristaltic waves.

> **KEY POINT**
>
> There are three nervous systems that work to provide integrated regulation of colonic motility, sphincter function, and fecal continence: the central nervous system, the enteric nervous system, and the peripheral nervous system.

SEROSA

The outermost layer is the serosa. It is made of simple squamous epithelial tissue and is continuous with the mesentery and visceral peritoneum. It secretes a watery serous fluid to reduce friction between the visceral organs and the large intestine.

INNERVATION OF THE COLON, SPHINCTERS, AND PELVIC FLOOR

The bowel has three nervous systems that provide an extremely organized, complex, and integrated regulation of colonic motility, sphincter function, and fecal continence. Innervation involves the central nervous system (CNS) (brain and spinal cord), the sympathetic and parasympathetic branches of the ANS, and the enteric nervous system (ENS) (**Figs. 2-8 and 20-8**). In addition,

ENTERIC NERVOUS SYSTEM

The ENS and the ANS control sensory and motor function of the GI tract. The ENS is the intraintestinal (local) nervous system and the primary mediator in colonic motility. It consists of interstitial cells of Cajal (ICC), neurons (sensory, motor), and interneurons that are situated in two primary plexuses: the submucosal (Meissner's) plexus and the myenteric (Auerbach's) plexus, located between the circular and longitudinal muscle layers. The primary function of the submucosal plexus is to detect intraluminal substances (such as irritants), control GI blood flow, and regulate epithelial cell function; the myenteric plexus exerts primary control over colonic motility. Myenteric ICC serve as an electrical pacemaker to produce slow phasic wave contractions of smooth muscle with a frequency of 2 to 4 per minute (Bharucha & Camilleri, 2019; Huizinga,

2018). ICC also augment neuronal activity, generates a measurable response to mechanical stimulation, and sets smooth muscle action potential (Bharucha & Camilleri, 2019). Nerve cell clusters or ganglia comprise these intramural nerve plexuses, which are interconnected to allow integration and processing of data and communication between the bowel wall and the ganglia along the entire length of the colon. Sensory neurons process thermal, chemical, osmotic, or mechanical stimuli transmitted by sensory receptors in the mucosa and muscle. For example, chemoreceptors respond to luminal contents by, in essence, "tasting" luminal substances; in contrast, mechanoreceptors within the muscle react to stretch and tension. Motor neurons control gut motility, secretion, and absorption by acting upon smooth muscle and secretory and endocrine cells. Interneurons provide a conduit between sensory neuron information and motor neurons; they "present" sensory information to motor neurons, which often leads to an action or response. For instance, messages from sensory receptors responding to stretch and tension within the bowel wall are relayed through the interneurons to motor neurons, which initiate smooth muscle contraction (peristalsis) (Palit et al., 2012).

KEY POINT

The enteric nervous system is contained within the bowel wall and contains ICC that act as an electrical pacemaker, sensory neurons, motor neurons, and interneurons; the ENS responds to thermal, chemical, osmotic, and mechanical stimuli transmitted by receptors in the mucosal and muscle layers that generates peristalsis.

OVERVIEW OF CENTRAL NERVOUS SYSTEM AND PERIPHERAL NERVOUS SYSTEM

CNS consists of the brain and spinal cord. Its primary role is to integrate sensory information received from the peripheral nervous system (PNS) then coordinate voluntary or involuntary activities such as elimination (micturition and defecation). The PNS consists of all other types of nervous tissue outside of the CNS. Its principle role is to present sensory impulses from different parts of the body to the brain and follow its commands via motor impulses to the body's organs, glands, and muscles. The spinal cord acts as a conduit between the brain and body as well as controls musculoskeletal reflexes. The PNS is divided into the autonomic and somatic nervous systems. The somatic system is composed of consciously (voluntary) controlled nerves that accept sensory stimuli from the CNS and deliver motor input (efferent) to striated muscles, while the autonomic system regulates involuntary (unconscious) bodily functions such as internal secretions, digestion, gut motility, storage, and elimination processes involving smooth muscle (Huether, 2019) (**Fig. 2-8**).

CENTRAL NERVOUS SYSTEM

In reference to the defecation process, the awareness of the "call to stool" occurs in the prefrontal cortex, specifically the superior frontal gyrus and anterior cingulate gyrus (Poggio et al., 2019) as a result of sensory (afferent) stimuli presented from mechanoreceptors (tension) in a rectum filling with stool. Impulses to initiate socially acceptable defecation or inhibit or "to hold" on are relayed from the cerebral cortex, spinal cord then to the PNS (autonomic and somatic divisions), and to colon, rectum, anal sphincters, and pelvic floor muscles.

AUTONOMIC NERVOUS SYSTEM

As stated, the ENS is the primary mediator for colonic motility (peristalsis), but it is augmented by the extrinsic ANS. The sympathetic and parasympathetic nerve fibers from the ANS terminate on the nerve cells of the myenteric and submucosal plexus to modulate colonic motility, by stimulating or inhibiting peristaltic activity. The sympathetic nervous system (SNS) arises from T10 to L2 of the spinal cord and acts to reduce intestinal secretion and motility. In contrast, the parasympathetic nervous system (PSNS) arises primarily from S2 to S4 of the spinal cord and acts to promote peristaltic activity, especially in the descending and sigmoid colon (branches of the vagus nerve provide parasympathetic stimulation to the proximal colon, i.e., ascending and transverse colon).

Mass movements (series of peristaltic waves) propel stool into the sigmoid colon or rectum; when the amount of stool is sufficient to trigger rectal distention and the defecation reflex, the elevated intrarectal pressure stimulates reflexive contraction of the rectosigmoid, relaxation of the IAS, and contraction of the EAS. It is hypothesized that this reflexive activity is mediated by the sacral PSNS and its outflow tracts. Increased pressure in the rectum stimulates afferent (sensory) fibers to send messages *from* the rectum *to* the spinal cord and brain, which triggers parasympathetic efferent (motor) activity that sends messages *from* the brain *to* the distal bowel to stimulate reflex contractions in the sigmoid and rectum (Huether, 2019; Palit et al., 2012).

This defecation reflex does not lead to the act of defecation in itself but produces a strong urge or "call to stool." This urge "to go" can be deferred with conscious contraction of the EAS and pelvic floor muscles, which interrupts peristalsis and causes rectal wall relaxation; this results in reduced intrarectal pressure and reduced sense of the need to defecate. The rectum may also displace the stool into the sigmoid by retrograde contraction until a more convenient time for elimination. Interestingly, pain or the fear of pain related to defecation (e.g., patient with fissures, hemorrhoids, or history of severe constipation) may also inhibit the defecation reflex (Huether, 2019).

SOMATIC NERVOUS SYSTEM

Somatic nerves that exit the lower sacral region (S2–S4) innervate skeletal muscles of the pelvic floor and external anal sphincter to consciously contract or relax depending upon the decision to defecate or defer to an appropriate time. Sacral reflexes such as the anal wink or bulbocavernosus reflex can be stimulated to ascertain the function of the pudendal nerve which innervates these muscles and sphincter.

IMPLICATIONS

Although the ENS is the primary mediator for colonic motility, the impact of ANS modulation should not be underestimated. For instance, the individual with an S2 spinal cord lesion loses not only their ability to sense rectal distention but also parasympathetic-induced peristalsis of the distal colon; this leads to profound constipation and increased risk for impaction. These individuals also lose voluntary control of the EAS, which is innervated by the pudendal nerve; however, they retain normal innervation of the IAS, which is controlled by the ENS, specifically the myenteric plexus. This is because the ENS is not affected by spinal cord injury.

 ## FACTORS AFFECTING/PROMOTING CONTINENCE

Multiple factors may influence GI function, the evacuation process, and fecal continence. The most critical "control" factors include the following:

1. Colonic transit, stool volume, and consistency
2. Sensory awareness
3. Sphincter competence
4. Rectal compliance and capacity
5. Extrinsic factors, such as posture for defecation and cultural norms

Intrinsic factors such as age and comorbidities can also influence bowel function and continence.

Factors critical to bowel function and control include normal transit time resulting in stool of normal consistency, sensory awareness of rectal filling, normal sphincter function, adequate rectal capacity and compliance, and intrinsic and extrinsic factors such as posture for defecation (Boutros & Gordon, 2017; Palit et al., 2012).

COLONIC TRANSIT AND STOOL VOLUME AND CONSISTENCY

Colonic transit time is defined as the amount of time it takes for food that enters the gut to be digested and absorbed and for the waste products to be evacuated through the anus. Stool transit time is determined by peristaltic activity, the coordinated colonic contractions that propel stool along the length of the colon and into the rectum; transit time profoundly impacts stool volume and consistency (Degen & Phillips, 1996a). Colonic motor activity demonstrates a predictable pattern: it increases after waking (Bharucha & Camilleri, 2019; Rao et al., 2001), is higher during the day than at night (Dinning et al., 2010; Narducci et al., 1987; Rao et al., 2001), and is significantly increased by eating (Bampton et al., 2001; Bharucha & Camilleri, 2019; Dinning et al., 2010; Rao et al., 2001), especially after a fatty meal (Bharucha & Camilleri, 2019; Rao et al., 2000; Renny et al., 1983). The upper limit for normal transit time is around 72 hours in adults (Spanish Group for the Study of Digestive Motility, 1998), whereas in children, it is faster, around 57 hours (Weaver, 1988). Of interest, transit time is reduced (i.e., faster) by coffee consumption (with effects equal to that of a meal) (Rao et al., 1998), fatty meals (Rao et al., 2000; Renny et al., 1983), and fecal contents with a high osmotic load (e.g., as occurs with bile salt malabsorption or lactose intolerance) (Rao, 2004), and increased (i.e., slower) with protein-rich meals (Battle et al., 1980; Wright et al., 1980) and alcohol (Berenson & Avner, 1981; Bouchoucha et al., 1991). Men have faster transit time than women (Meier et al., 1995; Stewart et al., 1999), and individuals over 65 usually have slower transit time and increased risk of constipation due to a multitude of factors (Chatoor & Emmnauel, 2009).

Intuitively, loose stools are usually associated with reduced (faster) transit time, due to the reduction in time for water absorption; this perception has been confirmed by some studies. In contrast, constipation is usually associated with slow gut motility and increased (slower) transit time; this provides increased time for water absorption, which results in smaller caliber and drier stools, both of which are risk factors for disordered defecation (Palit et al., 2012). Certainly, individuals with diarrhea have a greater potential for fecal incontinence since the rapid delivery of loose and large-volume stool may overwhelm the continence mechanism. However, frequency of stool elimination is poorly correlated with colonic transit time, possibly because individuals with constipation may make several attempts to evacuate stool (Dinning et al., 2011; Saad et al., 2010), passing only small amounts each time; in contrast, the individual with soft bulky stool may report less frequent but higher-volume bowel movements.

Interestingly, Bannister et al. (1987a) demonstrated that stool size and the amount of time needed for stool evacuation are inversely related; more time and effort are required for defecation of small, hard stools (pellet-like) as compared to soft formed stools. Although not well studied, the postulated "ideal" stool for facilitation of defecation is about 2 cm in diameter and is formed but not dry (Heitkemper, 2006) (see Chapter 6, Fig. 6-7, Bristol Stool Scale, Types 3 and 4). In general, the frequency of normal defecation ranges anywhere from three stools per day to three stools per week as long as there is no discomfort and no excessive straining, and continence is preserved (Schaefer & Cheskin, 1998).

> **KEY POINT**
>
> The postulated "ideal" stool in terms of facilitated defecation is about 2 cm in diameter and is formed but not dry.

SENSORY AWARENESS

The ability to recognize rectal filling promptly and to determine the type of rectal contents accurately is critical to the normal defecation process and the maintenance of continence. This perception of rectal distention and correct classification of rectal contents (gas, liquid, or solid) is provided by stretch receptors in the rectum and pelvic floor and sensory receptors in the anal canal. As previously discussed, colonic distention triggers afferent sensory (stretch) receptors in the rectum and pelvic floor muscles, which transmit the message to the spinal cord; it is then passed to the cerebral cortex, where it elicits conscious recognition of the distention and the "call to stool." The anal canal distal to the dentate line contains numerous epithelial sensory receptors that are able to distinguish between gas (flatus), liquid, and solid stool; this is known as the sampling reflex. (The sampling reflex occurs when rectal distention causes brief relaxation of the internal sphincter, which allows rectal contents to pass into the anal canal; the receptors in the distal anal canal then "sample" the contents and provide feedback to the individual as to type.)

Any damage to the stretch receptors, sensory receptors in the anoderm, neurologic pathways, or cognition will alter sensory awareness of rectal distention and type of contents and may compromise continence. For instance, if a person repeatedly defers the "call to stool," over time, their sensory awareness of rectal distention becomes blunted (limited). In fact, it may lead to a vicious cycle of chronic rectal distention (megarectum), constipation, and even fecal impaction. Habitually ignoring the urge "to go" may also alter or reduce cognitive processing of the urge sensation (Scott et al., 2011). This "conditioning" behavior can occur in children (as is seen in retentive encopresis) (see Chapter 23) as well as adults (Richards et al., 2010); the end results are reduced stool frequency and volume and increased rectosigmoid transit time. This supports the concept that constipation can be a "learned" behavior (Klauser et al., 1990). Other causes of reduced sensory awareness of the "call to stool" include neurologic conditions (e.g., diabetic neuropathy, MS, SCI, myelomeningocele), cognitive impairment (inability to appropriately interpret sensory messages to the CNS), and anorectal lesions (e.g., large hemorrhoids or rectal prolapse).

> **KEY POINT**
>
> Sensory awareness of rectal distention is provided by stretch receptors in the rectal wall and pelvic floor muscles; accurate differentiation among gas, liquid, and solid stool is provided by the sensory receptors in the anal canal.

SPHINCTER COMPETENCE: IAS AND EAS

Normal sphincter function is essential to continence and involves both the IAS, which is under involuntary control, and the EAS, which can be voluntarily contracted.

Internal Anal Sphincter

The IAS is responsible for up to 85% of anal tone and predominantly responsible for continence at rest (Frenckner, 1975; Heitkemper, 2006). It is composed of slow-twitch, fatigue-resistant smooth muscle fibers, and "at rest," it is tonically contracted. The IAS relaxes in response to rectal distention. This involuntary, reflexive response is known as the rectoanal inhibitory reflex. This reflex also allows the sensory receptors in the anal canal to "sense" (or "taste") the rectal contents and to determine consistency (gas, liquid, or solid stool); this is called the sampling reflex, as already explained. In healthy individuals, it has been determined that the sampling reflex occurs seven times per hour (Miller et al., 1988b); it occurs less often in those who suffer from fecal incontinence (Miller et al., 1988a). The function of the IAS (and thus the sampling reflex) is primarily controlled by the ENS, specifically the myenteric plexus; as already explained, the branches of the ANS also contribute to innervation of the IAS. There is no sensorimotor innervation of the IAS; it is therefore under involuntary control (Frenckner, 1975; Huether, 2019; Meunier & Mollard, 1977). Sympathetic stimulation, which occurs via the hypogastric plexus that exits the cord at T10–L2, causes release of norepinephrine and contraction of the IAS. In contrast, parasympathetic stimulation (via the pelvic plexus that exits the cord at S2–S4) causes release of acetylcholine and reflexive relaxation of the IAS (Huether, 2019).

> **KEY POINT**
>
> The IAS relaxes in response to rectal distention (rectoanal inhibitory reflex); this permits contact between the anoderm and the rectal contents and the "sampling reflex."

External Anal Sphincter

The EAS is composed of both striated and smooth muscle and is innervated primarily by the somatic fibers of the pudendal nerve, which exits the spinal cord at S2, S3, and S4. A gentle stroke with a finger or cotton swab at the 3 and 9 o'clock position will elicit an observable quick contraction of the EAS, known as the "anal wink"; this assures pudendal innervation is intact. The EAS is also in a state of constant tonic contraction at rest, producing up to 30% of the resting anal tone (Lestar et al., 1989). The anal vascular cushions (hemorrhoidal plexus) also contribute to resting tone; more importantly, they provide the airtight seal that cannot be obtained by sphincteric tone alone (Lestar et al., 1989; Palit et al., 2012). One of the unique characteristics of the EAS is the tonic contraction provided by the sacral reflex. This sacral reflex activity is enhanced during activities that increase intra-abdominal and intrarectal pressure (e.g., coughing, lifting, and standing). In addition, the skeletal muscle components of the EAS can be voluntarily contracted, which doubles the anal canal pressure; this typically elevates anal canal pressure to a level that exceeds intrarectal pressures, thus maintaining continence until the individual reaches an appropriate time and place for defecation. Maximum voluntary contraction of the EAS can be maintained for a limited time (1 to 3 minutes maximally); thus, adequate rectal capacity and compliance are required to maintain continence past the point at which the EAS begins to fatigue and anal canal pressures begin to decrease (Heitkemper, 2006). Because the EAS plays a critical role in maintaining continence during periods of rectal distention, any injury to the muscle itself or to the nerves innervating the muscle is likely to cause some level of fecal incontinence.

KEY POINT

The EAS has both reflex tone and voluntary contractility; strong contraction of the EAS and pelvic floor doubles the pressure in the anal canal and permits the individual to delay defecation until a socially appropriate time and place.

Impact of Sphincter Damage/Denervation

Damage to the IAS is likely to result in incontinence of gas and liquid stool, while injuries to or denervation of the EAS is commonly associated with "urge incontinence," that is, inability to maintain anal canal closure and continence during periods of rectal distention and fecal urgency. (Individuals with EAS damage or denervation report knowing when they have stool in the rectum, but being unable to "hold it," especially if the stool is mushy or liquid). If the EAS is severely denervated or totally disrupted, the individual may experience complete fecal incontinence, that is, involuntary passage of formed stool (Rao, 2004; Salvator et al., 2017).

RECTAL CAPACITY AND COMPLIANCE

The rectum is a distensible organ that has the ability to act as a storage reservoir when defecation needs to be delayed. The reservoir is normally compliant, which enables it to store stool at relatively low pressure. Once the EAS returns to a resting state, the intrarectal pressure must drop to a level lower than that of the anal canal if continence is to be preserved; this requires both compliance (stretch) and capacity. The mechanisms responsible for normal compliance and capacity are complex and not well understood. Sensory awareness of rectal filling may occur at volumes as low as 11 to 68 mL, and rectal capacity usually ranges from 250 to 510 mL; once capacity is reached, intrarectal pressures rise significantly and defecation becomes imminent.

On average, rectal pressure begins to increase at about 300 mL; when capacity is approached and rectal pressures rise significantly, the defecation reflex is activated as explained previously (i.e., the IAS opens and there is increased peristaltic activity in the rectosigmoid that results in stool elimination unless the individual voluntarily contracts the EAS to delay defecation) (Heitkemper, 2006). Any increase or decrease in rectal capacity and compliance places the individual at risk for bowel dysfunction or fecal incontinence; that is, increased rectal capacity and compliance are seen in those who habitually ignore the defecation urge, while reduced rectal capacity and compliance are experienced by those who suffer from inflammatory bowel disease or other inflammatory conditions of the anorectum. Individuals with inflammatory anorectal conditions experience intense fecal urgency and frequency and possibly incontinence due to loss of rectal capacity and compliance; they typically report that they can "hold it" only briefly and that if they cannot get to the bathroom quickly, they experience incontinence (Bharucha, 2006). Chapters 21 and 22 provide an in-depth discussion of bowel dysfunction and fecal incontinence.

KEY POINT

Normally, the rectum is a distensible compliant organ, allowing it to store stool at low intrarectal pressures.

EXTRINSIC AND INTRINSIC FACTORS

Additional factors that affect defecation and continence include posture, cultural norms, gender, and age (Huether, 2019; Palit et al., 2012; Yu & Rao, 2014). Posture is of particular importance and is determined primarily by cultural norms. To facilitate defecation, the anorectal angle must straighten from 90 to 135 degrees; this occurs when the sphincter and pelvic floor are voluntarily relaxed and the individual contracts the abdominal muscles via straining (**Fig. 20-9**). Research involving

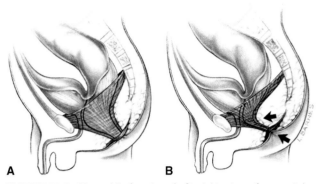

FIGURE 20-9. Normal Defecation. **A.** Straightening of anorectal angle during defecation. **B.** Increased anorectal angulation during sphincter contraction (*arrows*). (From Corman, M., Nicholls, R. J., Fazio, V. W., et al. (2012). *Corman's colon and rectal surgery.* Philadelphia, PA: Lippincott Williams & Wilkins.)

defecography (simulation of defecation with a stool-like substitute under fluoroscopic screening) has shown that a squat position facilitates straightening of the anorectal angle and promotes movement of stool from the rectum into the anal canal (Sikirov, 2003; Tagart, 1966). One could appreciate the importance of this position if asked to pass stool on a bed pan while in a supine position.

The position for defecation is most often dictated by cultural factors. For instance, in Africa and Asia, a squatting position is standard, because defecation occurs over a hole or low-lying receptacle on the floor; in contrast, in Western countries, sitting on a standard toilet/commode is the norm. In a study comparing a Western style commode to a standard toilet with a 10-cm footstool and to the squatting position, the squatting position offered the fastest and most complete stool evacuation, while the standard toilet without the stool provided the least optimal evacuation (Sikirov, 2003). Moreover, and not surprisingly, studies that compared defecation in a sitting to lying down position demonstrated better evacuation in the sitting position (Barnes & Lennard-Jones, 1985; Rao et al., 2006). Other extrinsic factors have been reported to affect bowel habits and GI function, including psychobehavioral factors such as psychological impairment (Dykes et al., 2001; Nehra et al., 2000; Wald et al., 1989), history of traumatic life events including sexual and physical abuse (Drossman et al., 1995; Leroi et al., 1995), coercive toilet training (Palit et al., 2012), stress and anxiety (Palit et al., 2012), lack of privacy or toilet substitute (Kamm, 2006), and dietary intake and pharmaceuticals that reduce gut motility.

KEY POINT

Squatting is reported to be the best posture for defecation because it promotes straightening of the anorectal angle and movement of stool from the rectum to the anal canal.

Intrinsic factors such as age and gender may also impact defecation and continence (Greenwood-Van Meerveld et al., 2017; Palit et al., 2012: Yu & Rao, 2014). Epidemiological studies report several spikes in the occurrence of constipation; the first occurs during infancy, with the transition from breast milk to formula, the second during early childhood (between 3 and 5 years of age) (Del Ciampo et al., 2002), and the third after the age of 60 to 65 (Sandler et al., 1990; Sonnenberg & Koch, 1989). Minimal functional changes have been documented within the GI tract purely as a result of aging; however, loss of tissue elasticity within the rectoanal unit (Bannister et al., 1987b), pelvic floor weakness and laxity (Ryhammer et al., 1996), prolonged intestinal transit time (Huether, 2019), increased occurrence of neuropathy (Bartolo et al., 1983, Yu & Rao, 2014), reduced rectal sensation, compliance, capacity (Yu & Rao, 2014) changes in mobility and/or cognition, and polypharmacy (Chatoor & Emmnauel, 2009) may negatively impact evacuation of stool. In animal models, the effects of advanced aging on the gut appears to alter intestinal barrier function, immune system, ENS, and ANS innervation (Greenwood-Van Meerveld et al., 2017). In summary, there is a growing body of knowledge regarding the effects of aging which is extremely important in light of the steady growth of people over age 65 (Greenwood-Van Meerveld et al., 2017).

With regard to gender, constipation is reported to be higher in women. It is postulated that this preponderance of female constipation may be related to slower colonic transit time in comparison to men (Degen & Phillips, 1996b; Meier et al., 1995), the influence of female hormones (Heaton et al., 1992) and the menstrual cycle (Celik et al., 2001; Fukuda et al., 2005), and the effects of pregnancy and childbirth on pelvic floor function (Kepenekci et al., 2011; Ryhammer et al., 1996; van Ginkel et al., 2003). Some studies confirm that aging women are at higher risks for altered anorectal function including thinning of the internal and external anal sphincter muscle leading to reduced resting tone and squeeze pressures (Gundling et al., 2010; Yu & Rao, 2014). Of note, Gorina et al. (2014) studied fecal incontinence in noninstitutionalized individuals age 65 or over and found no statistical difference in the incidence of bowel leakage related to age, gender, or race.

PROCESS OF NORMAL DEFECATION

In the process of normal defecation (**Fig. 20-10**), the liquid stool that enters the cecum from the small bowel undergoes a gradual change to solid consistency as the colonic contents are mixed and slowly propelled from the proximal to the distal colon. Complex colonic motility patterns facilitate this transition and transport; haustral contractions provide mixing and absorption of water, thus converting the stool from liquid to solid, and peristaltic waves provide progressive slow movement from the ascending to

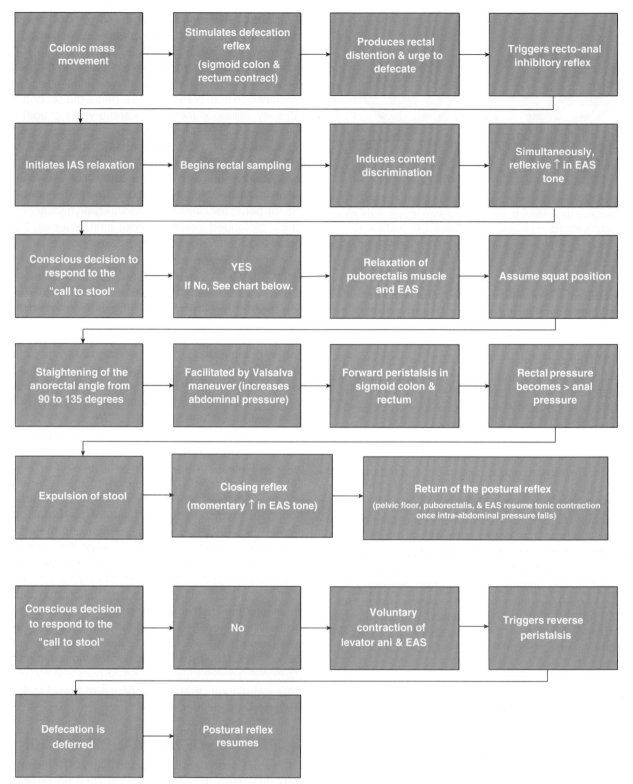

FIGURE 20-10. The Process of Defecation.

the transverse colon. As noted, stool is primarily stored in the transverse colon until just prior to defecation, at which point a series of peristaltic contractions known as mass movements rapidly propel the stool from the transverse colon to the sigmoid colon and rectum triggering

the defecation reflex (Huether, 2019). The sudden rectal distention causes the urge to defecate (i.e., the "call to stool"). (The stretch receptors in the rectal wall and surrounding muscles are considered the source of this sensory awareness of the need to defecate.) At the same time, the rectoanal inhibitory reflex causes relaxation of the IAS, which permits "sampling" of rectal contents by the receptors in the anoderm and differentiation between gaseous, liquid, and solid rectal contents (Thiruppathy et al., 2017). While the IAS is relaxing to permit "sampling," there is a reflex increase in EAS tone; if the individual is cognitively intact and defecation is not socially appropriate, this reflex increase in EAS tone is further augmented by voluntary contraction of the EAS, which doubles anal canal pressure and prevents distal propulsion of the stool (Mawer & Alhawaj, 2019; Palit et al., 2012).

With limited levels of rectal distention, the relaxation of the IAS and intense urge to defecate are transient; with high levels of distention, the relaxation is persistent, and defecation becomes imminent. When the individual reaches an appropriate place for stool elimination, he/she assumes a squatting or sitting position, voluntarily relaxes the sphincter, and contracts the abdominal muscles via straining (Valsalva). The sitting/squatting position and straining maneuver result in straightening of the anorectal angle, which facilitates evacuation, and increased intrarectal pressure (to a level exceeding anal canal pressure); this permits passage of stool (Palit et al., 2012; Rodriguez et al., 2011).

Once evacuation is complete, there is a brief increase in EAS activity, which triggers anal canal closure; this is known as the "closing reflex" (Brookes et al., 2009; Mawer & Alhawaj, 2019). Once straining and Valsalva cease, the pelvic floor muscles, puborectalis, and EAS resume tonic contraction (postural reflex), and the anorectal angle returns to 90 degrees; thus, the anorectal unit is returned to a "storage/continence" condition (Porter, 1962).

KEY POINT

Stool is stored in the transverse colon until just prior to defecation, at which point mass movements rapidly propel the stool into the rectum initiating the defecation reflex; this causes sudden distention, sensory awareness of the need to defecate, relaxation of the IAS, and contraction of the EAS.

 CONCLUSION

Normal defecation and fecal continence require the integrated function of a variety of structures and processes. Specifically, the individual must have sensory awareness of rectal distention, the ability to control stool elimination via sphincter control, and the ability to store stool temporarily, which requires normal rectal capacity and compliance. These functions are orchestrated by voluntary and involuntary neural pathways that control peristalsis, the sphincters, and the pelvic floor musculature; critical structures and pathways include the CNS, ANS, and ENS. Any intrinsic or extrinsic factor causing dysfunction of the GI system can dramatically alter bowel function, continence,

and ultimately quality of life. It is imperative for the continence specialist to understand the factors affecting GI tract function and defecation in order to accurately assess and manage any dysfunction or incontinence.

REFERENCES

Alexander, C., Swanson, K., Fahey, G., et al. (2019). Perspective: Physiologic importance of short-chain fatty acids from nondigestible carbohydrate fermentation. *Advances in Nutrition, 10*(4), 576–589.

Akaza, H. (2012). Prostate cancer chemoprevention by soy isoflavones: Role of intestinal bacteria as the "second human genome". *Cancer Science, 103*, 969–975.

Ashton-Miller, J. A., & DeLancey, J. O. (2007). Functional anatomy of the female pelvic floor. *Annals of the New York Academy of Sciences, 1101*, 266–296. doi: 10.1196/annals.1389.034.

Bampton, P., Dinning, P., Kennedy, M., et al. (2001). Prolonged multipoint recording of colonic manometry in the unprepared human colon: Providing insight into potentially relevant pressure wave parameters. *American Journal of Gastroenterology, 96*(6), 1838–1848. doi: 10.1111/j.1572-0241.2001.03924.x.

Bannister, J. J., Abouzekry, L., & Read, N. W. (1987a). Effect of aging on ano-rectal function. *Gut, 28*(3), 353–357. doi: 10.1136/gut.28.3.353.

Bannister, J. J., Davison, P., Timms, J. M., et al. (1987b). Effect of stool size and consistency on defecation. *Gut, 28*(10), 1246–1250. doi: 10.1136/gut.28.10.1246.

Barleben, A., & Mills, S. (2010). Anorectal anatomy and physiology. *Surgical Clinics of North America, 90*(1), 1–15. doi: 10.1016/j.suc.2009.09.001.

Barnes, P. R., & Lennard-Jones, J. E. (1985). Balloon expulsion from the rectum in constipation of different types. *Gut, 26*(10), 1049–1052. doi: 10.1136/gut.26.10.1049.

Bartolo, D. C., Jarratt, J. A., Read, M. G., et al. (1983). The role of partial denervation of the puborectalis in idiopathic fecal incontinence. *British Journal of Surgery, 70*(11), 664–667.

Battle, W. M., Cohen, S., & Snape, W. J., Jr. (1980). Inhibition of postprandial colonic motility after ingestion of an amino acid mixture. *Digestive Diseases and Sciences, 25*(9), 647–652. doi: 10.1007/BF01308322.

Berenson, M. M., & Avner, D. L. (1981). Alcohol inhibition of rectosigmoid motility in humans. *Digestion, 20*(4), 210–215.

Bharucha, A. E. (2006). Update of tests of colon and rectal structure and function. *Journal of Clinical Gastroenterology, 40*(2), 96–103.

Bharucha, A., & Camilleri, M. (2019). Physiology of the colon and its measurement. In C. Yeo (Ed.), *Shackelford's surgery of the alimentary tract* (8th ed., pp. 1676–1688). Philadelphia, PA: Elsevier.

Bordoni, B., Sugumar, K., & Leslie, S. W. (2019). Anatomy, abdomen and pelvis, pelvic floor [Updated April 25, 2019]. In *StatPearls [Internet]*. Treasure Island, FL: StatPearls Publishing. Retrieved from https://www.ncbi.nlm.nih.gov/books/NBK482200/

Bouchoucha, M., Nalpas, B., Berger, M., et al. (1991). Recovery from disturbed colonic transit time after alcohol withdrawal. *Diseases of the Colon and Rectum, 34*(2), 111–114. doi: 10.1007/BF02049982.

Boutros, M., & Gordon, P. H. (2017). Anatomy and physiology of the colon, rectum, and anal canal. In V. Fazio, J. Church, C. Delaney, et al. (Eds.), *Current therapy in colon and rectal surgery* (3rd ed., pp. 3–11). St. Louis, MO: Elsevier.

Brookes, S. J., Dinning, P. G., & Gladman, M. A. (2009). Neuroanatomy and physiology of colorectal function and defaecation: From basic science to human clinical studies. *Neurogastroenterology and Motility, 21*(Suppl 2), 9–19. doi: 10.1111/j.1365-2982.2009.01400.x.

Celik, A. F., Turna, H., Pamuk, G. E., et al. (2001). How prevalent are alterations in bowel habits during menses? *Diseases of the Colon and Rectum, 44*(2), 300–301. doi: 10.1007/BF02234310.

Castaner, O., Goday, A., Park, Y. M., et al. (2018). The gut microbiome profile in obesity: A systematic review. *International Journal of Endocrinology, 2018*, 9. doi: 10.1155/2018/4095789.

Chatoor, D., & Emmnauel, A. (2009). Constipation and evacuation disorders. *Best Practice & Research Clinical Gastroenterology, 23*(4), 517–530. doi: 10.1016/j.bpg.2009.05.001.

Damon, H., Guye, O., Seigneurin, A., et al. (2006). Prevalence of anal incontinence in adults and impact on quality-of-life. *Gastroenterology Clinique et Biologique, 30*(1), 37–43.

Degen, L. P., & Phillips, S. F. (1996a). How well does stool form reflect colonic transit? *Gut, 39*(1), 109–113. doi: 10.1136/gut.39.1.109.

Degen, L. P., & Phillips, S. F. (1996b). Variability of gastrointestinal transit in healthy women and men. *Gut, 39*(2), 299–305. doi: 10.1136/gut.39.2.299.

Del Ciampo, I. R., Galvao, L. C., Del Ciampo, L. A., et al. (2002). Prevalence of chronic constipation in children at a primary health care unit. *Jornal de Pediatria (Rio J), 78*(6), 497–502. doi: 10.2223/JPED.906.

Dinning, P. G., Hunt, L., Lubowski, D. Z., et al. (2011). The impact of laxative use upon symptoms in patients with proven slow transit constipation. *BMC Gastroenterology, 11*(1), 121–127. doi: 10.1186/ 1471-230X-11-121.

Dinning, P. G., Zarate, N., Szczeniak, M. M., et al. (2010). Bowel preparation affects the amplitude and spatiotemporal organization of colonic propagating sequences. *Neurogastroenterology and Motility, 22*(6), 633–e176. doi: 10.1111/j.1365-2982.2010.01480.x.

Drossman, D. A., Talley, N. J., Leserman, J., et al. (1995). Sexual and physical abuse and gastrointestinal illness. Review and recommendations. *Annals of Internal Medicine, 123*(10), 782–794.

Dykes, S., Smilgin-Humphreys, S., & Bass, C. (2001). Chronic idiopathic constipation: A psychological enquiry. European *Journal of Gastroenterology & Hepatology, 13*(1), 39–44.

Frenckner, B. (1975). Function of the anal sphincters in spinal man. *Gut, 16*(8), 638–644. doi: 10.1136/gut.16.8.638.

Fukuda, S., Matsuzaka, M., Takahashi, I, et al. (2005). Bowel habits before and during menses in Japanese women of climacteric age: A population based study. *The Tohoku Journal of Experimental Medicine, 206*(2), 99–104. doi: 10.1620/tjem.206.99.

Gorina, Y., Schappert, S., Bercovitz, A., et al. (2014). Prevalence of incontinence among older Americans. *Vital Health Statistics*. Series 3, # 36. Washington, DC: National Center for Health Statistics, Department of Health and Human Services.

Greenwood-Van Meerveld, B., Johnson, A. C., & Grundy, D. (2017). Gastrointestinal physiology and function. In B. Greenwood-Van Meerveld (Eds.), *Gastrointestinal pharmacology. Handbook of experimental pharmacology* (Vol. 239). Cham, Switzerland: Springer. doi: 10.1007/164_2016_118.

Gundling, F., et al. (2010). Influence of gender and age on anorectal function: Normal values from anorectal manometry in a large caucasian population. *Digestion, 81*(4), 207–213.

Hanage, W. (2014). Microbiology: Microbiome science needs a healthy dose of skepticism. *Nature, 512*, 247–248. doi: 10.1038/512247a.

Heaton, K. W., Radvan, J., Cripps, H., et al. (1992). Defecation frequency and timing, and stool form in the general population: A prospective study. *Gut, 33*(6), 818–824. doi: 10.1136/gut.33.6.818.

Heitkemper, M. M. (2006). Physiology of bowel function. In D. B. Doughty (Ed.), *Urinary & fecal incontinence: Current management concepts* (3rd ed., pp. 413–434). St. Louis, MO: Mosby.

Huether, S. E. (2019). Structure and function of the digestive system. In K. L. McCance & S. E. Huether (Eds.), *Pathophysiology: The biologic basis for disease in adults and children* (8th ed., pp. 1294–1315). St. Louis, MO: Elsevier.

Huizinga, J. (2018). The physiology and pathophysiology of interstitial cells of cajal: Pacemaking, innervation, and stretch sensation. In J. D. Huizinga (Ed.), *Physiology of the gastrointestinal tract* (pp. 305–335). St. Louis, MO: Elsevier. doi: 10.1016/B978-0-12-809954-4.00013-X.

Kamm, M. A. (2006). Clinical case: Chronic constipation. *Gastroenterology, 131*(1), 233–239. doi: 10.1053/j.gastro.2006.05.027.

Kasubuchi, M., Hasegawa, S., Hiramatsu, T., et al. (2015). Dietary gut microbial metabolites, short-chain fatty acids, and host metabolic regulation. *Nutrients, 7*, 2839–2849.

Kepenekci, I., Keskinkilic, B., Akinsu, F., et al. (2011). Prevalence of pelvic floor disorders in the female population and the impact of age, mode of delivery, and parity. *Diseases of the Colon & Rectum, 54*(1), 85–94.

Klauser, A. G., Voderholzer, W. A., Heinrich, C. A., et al. (1990). Behavioral modification of colonic function. Can constipation be learned? *Digestive Diseases and Sciences, 35*(10), 1271–1275. doi: 10.1007/BF01536418.

Leroi, A. M., Bernier, C., Watier, A., et al. (1995). Prevalence of sexual abuse among patients with functional disorders of the lower gastrointestinal tract. *International Journal of Colorectal Disease, 10*(4), 200–206. doi: 10.1007/BF00346219.

Lestar, B., Penninckx, F., & Kerremans, R. (1989). The composition of anal basal pressure. An in vivo and in vitro study in man. *International Journal of Colorectal Disease, 4*(2), 118–122. doi: 10.1007/BF01646870.

Mawer, S., & Alhawaj, A. F. (March 16, 2019). Physiology, defecation. In *StatPearls [Internet]*. Treasure Island, FL: StatPearls Publishing. Retrieved from http://www.ncbi.nlm.nih.gov/books/NBK539732/PubMed.

Meier, R., Beglinger, C., Dederding, J., et al. (1995). Influence of age, gender, hormonal status and smoking habits on colonic transit time. *Neurogastroenterology and Motility, 7*(4), 235–238. doi: 10.1111/j.1365-2982.1995.tb00231.x.

Meunier, P., & Mollard, P. (1977). Control of the internal anal sphincter (manometric study with human subjects). *Pflügers Archive: European Journal of Physiology, 370*(3), 233–239. doi: 10.1007/BF00585532.

Miller, R., Bartolo, D. C., Cervero, F., et al. (1988a). Anorectal sampling: A comparison of normal and incontinent patients. *British Journal of Surgery, 75*(1), 44–47. doi: 10.1002/bjs.1800750116.

Miller, R., Lewis, G. T., Bartolo, D. C., et al. (1988b). Sensory discrimination and dynamic activity in the anorectum: Evidence using a new ambulatory technique. *British Journal of Surgery, 75*(10), 1003–1007. doi: 10.1002/bjs.1800751018.

Milson, I., Altman, D., Lapitan, M. C., et al. (2017). UI, other LUTS, POP and anal incontinence. In P. Abrams, L. Cardozo, A. Wagg, et al. (Eds.), *Incontinence* (6th ed.). Bristol, UK: International Continence Society. ISBN: 978–0956960733.

Narducci, F., Bassotti, G., Gaburri, M., et al. (1987). Twenty four hour manometric recording of colonic motor activity in healthy man. *Gut, 28*(1), 17–25. doi: 10.1136/gut.28.1.17.

Nehra, V., Bruce, B. K., Rath-Harvey, D. M., et al. (2000). Psychological disorders in patients with evacuation disorders and constipation in a tertiary practice. *American Journal of Gastroenterology, 95*(7), 1755–1758. doi: 10.1111/j.1572-0241.2000.02184.x.

Nygaard, I., Barber, M. D., Burgio, K. L., et al.; Pelvic Floor Disorders Network. (2008). Prevalence of symptomatic pelvic floor disorders in US women. *JAMA, 300*(11), 1311–1316. doi: 10.1001/jama.300.11.1311.

Parthasarathy, G., Chen, J., Chen, X., et al. (2016). Relationship between microbiota of the colonic mucosa vs feces and symptoms, colonic transit, and methane production in female patients with chronic constipation. *Gastroenterology, 150*, 367–379, e361.

Palit, S., Lunniss, P. J., & Scott, S. M. (2012). The physiology of human defecation. *Digestive Diseases and Sciences, 57*(6), 1445–1464. doi: 10.1007/s10620-012-2071-1.

Pickard, J. M., Zeng, M. Y., Caruso, R., et al. (2017). Gut microbiota: Role in pathogen colonization, immune responses, and inflammatory disease. *Immunological reviews, 279*(1), 70–89. doi: 10.1111/imr.12567.

Poggio, J. L., Grossman, J., Kucejko, R., et al. (2019). *Neurogenic bowel dysfunction*. Retrieved October 26, 2019 from https://emedicine.medscape.com/article/321172

Porter, N. H. (1962). A physiological study of the pelvic floor in rectal prolapse. *Annals of the Royal College of Surgeons of England, 31*(6), 379–404.

Pradidarcheep, W., Wallner, C., Dabhoiwala, N. F., et al. (2011). Anatomy and histology of the lower urinary tract. In K. E. Andersson & M. C. Michel (Eds.), *Urinary tract, handbook of experimental pharmacology* (pp. 117–148). Berlin, Heidelberg, Germany: Springer-Verlag.

Rao, S. S. (2004). Pathophysiology of adult fecal incontinence. *Gastroenterology, 126*(1 Suppl 1), S14–S22. doi: 10.1053/j.gastro.2003.10.013.

Rao, S. S. (2010). Advances in diagnostic assessment of fecal incontinence and dyssynergic defecation. *Clinical Gastroenterology Hepatology, 8*(11), 910–919.

Rao, S. S., Kavlock, R., Beaty, J., et al. (2000). Effects of fat and carbohydrate meals on colonic motor response. *Gut, 46*(2), 205–211. doi: 10.1136/gut.46.2.205.

Rao, S. S., Kavlock, R., & Rao, S. (2006). Influence of body position and stool characteristics on defecation in humans. *The American Journal of Gastroenterology, 101*(12), 2790–2796. doi: 10.1111/j.1572-0241.2006.00827.x.

Rao, S. S., Sadeghi, P., Beaty, J., et al. (2001). Ambulatory 24-h colonic manometry in healthy humans. *American Journal of Physiology. Gastrointestinal and Liver Physiology, 280*(4), G629–G639.

Rao, S. S., Welcher, L., Zimmerman, B., et al. (1998). Is coffee a colonic stimulant? *European Journal of Gastroenterology & Hepatology, 10*(2), 113–118.

Renny, A., Snape, W. J. Jr., Sun, E. A., et al. (1983). Role of cholecystokinin in the gastrocolonic response to a fat meal. *Gastroenterology, 85*(1), 17–21.

Richards, M. M., Banez, G. A., Dohil, R., et al. (2010). Chronic constipation, atypical eating pattern, weight loss, and anxiety in a 19-year-old youth. *Journal of Developmental and Behavioral Pediatrics, 31*(3 Suppl), S83–S85.

Rodriguez, G., King, J. C., & Stiens, S. A. (2011). Neurogenic bowel: Dysfunction and rehabilitation. In R. L. Braddom (Ed.), *Physical medicine and rehabilitation* (4th ed., pp. 619–640). Philadelphia, PA: Saunders.

Ryhammer, A. M., Laurberg, S., & Hermann, A. P. (1996). Long term effect of vaginal deliveries on anorectal function in normal perimenopausal women. *Diseases of the Colon & Rectum, 39*(8), 852–859. doi: 10.1007/BF02053982.

Saad, R. J., Rao, S. S., Koch, K. L., et al. (2010). Do stool form and frequency correlate with whole-gut and colonic transit? Results from a multicenter study in constipated individuals and healthy controls. *The American Journal of Gastroenterology, 105*(2), 403–411. doi: 10.1038/ajg.2009.612.

Salvator, S., Delancey, J., Igawa, H., et al. (2017). Pathophysiology of urinary and fecal incontinence and pelvic organ prolapse. In P. Abrams, L. Cardozo, A. Wagg, et al. (Eds.), *Incontinence* (6th ed.). Bristol, UK: International Continence Society. ISBN: 978–0956960733.

Sampselle, C. A., & DeLancey, O. L. (1998). Anatomy of female continence. *Journal of Wound, Ostomy, and Continence Nursing, 25*(2), 63–74.

Sandler, R. S., Jordan, M. C., & Shelton, B. J. (1990). Demographic and dietary determinants of constipation in the US population. *American Journal of Public Health, 80*(2), 185–189.

Schaefer, D. C., & Cheskin, L. J. (1998). Constipation in the elderly. *American Family Physician, 58*(4), 907–914.

Schey, R., Cromwell, J., & Rao, S. S. (2012). Medical and surgical management of pelvic floor disorders affecting defecation. *The American journal of gastroenterology, 107*(11), 1624–1634. doi: 10.1038/ajg.2012.247.

Scott, A. J., Alexander, J. L., Merrifield, C. A., et al. (2019). International Cancer Microbiome Consortium consensus statement on the role of the human microbiome in carcinogenesis. *Gut, 68*, 1624–1632. Accessed December 07, 2019. doi: 10.1136/gutjnl-2019-318556.

Scott, S. M., van den Berg, M. M., & Benninga, M. A. (2011). Rectal sensorimotor dysfunction in constipation. *Best Practice & Research Clinical Gastroenterology, 25*(1), 103–118. doi: 10.1016/j.bpg.2011.01.001.

Sikirov, D. (2003). Comparison of straining during defecation in three positions: Results and the implications for human health. *Digestive Diseases and Sciences, 48*(7), 1201–1205. doi: 10.1023/A:1024180319005.

Siccardi, M. A., & Bordoni, B. (2018). Anatomy, abdomen and pelvis, perineal body [Updated December 20, 2018]. In *StatPearls [Internet]*. Treasure Island, FL: StatPearls Publishing. Retrieved from www.ncbi.nlm.nih.gov/books/NBK537345/?report=classic.

Sonnenberg, A., & Koch, T. R. (1989). Epidemiology of constipation in the United States. *Diseases of the Colon & Rectum, 32*(1), 1–8. doi: 10.1007/BF02554713.

Spanish Group for the Study of Digestive Motility. (1998). Measurement of colonic transit time (total and segmental) with radiopaque markers. National reference values obtained in 192 subjects. *Gastroenterology and Hepatology, 21*, 71–75.

Stewart, W. F., Liberman, J. N., Sandler, R. S., et al. (1999). Epidemiology of constipation (EPOC) study in the United States: Relation of clinical subtypes to sociodemographic features. *American Journal of Gastroenterology, 94*(12), 3530–3540. doi: 10.1111/j.1572-0241.1999.01642.x.

Tagart, R. E. (1966). The anal canal and rectum: Their varying relationship and its effect on anal continence. *Diseases of the Colon and Rectum, 9*(6), 449–452.

Thiruppathy, K., Mason, J., Akbari, K., et al. (2017). Physiological study of the anorectal reflex in patients with functional anorectal and defecation disorders. *Journal of Digestive Diseases, 18*(4), 222–228.

Toor, D., Wsson, M. K., Kumar, P., et al. (2019). Dysbiosis disrupts gut immune homeostasis and promotes gastric diseases. *International Journal of Molecular Sciences, 20*, 2432.

van Ginkel, R., Reitsma, J. B., Buller, H. A., et al. (2003). Childhood constipation: Longitudinal follow-up beyond puberty. *Gastroenterology, 125*(2), 357–363. doi: 10.1016/S0016-5085(03)00888-6.

Wagner, T. H., Moore, K. H., Subak, L. L. (2017). Economics of urinary, fecal incontinence and pelvic organ prolapse. In P. Abrams, L. Cardozo, A. Wagg, et al. (Eds.), *Incontinence* (6th ed.). Bristol, UK: International Continence Society. ISBN: 978–0956960733.

Wald, A., Hinds, J. P., & Caruana, B. J. (1989). Psychological and physiological characteristics of patients with severe idiopathic constipation. *Gastroenterology, 9*, 932–937.

Weaver, L. T. (1988). Bowel habit from birth to old age. *Journal of Pediatric Gastroenterology and Nutrition, 7(5)*, 637–640.

Wright, S. H., Snape, W. J., Battle, W., et al. (1980). Effect of dietary components on gastrocolonic response. *American Journal of Physiology, 238*(3), G228–G232.

Yu, S. W., & Rao S. S. (2014). Anorectal physiology and pathophysiology in the elderly. *Clinics in Geriatric Medicine, 30*(1), 95–106.

Zhang, Y. J., Li, S., Gan, R. Y., et al. (2015). Impacts of gut bacteria on human health and diseases. *International Journal of Molecular Sciences, 16*(4), 7493–7519. doi: 10.3390/ijms16047493.

QUESTIONS

1. Which structure of the GI tract is responsible for the absorption of the vitamin B_{12}–intrinsic factor complex?
A. Distal small intestine
B. Ileocecal valve
C. Colon
D. Anal canal

2. What is the rationale for placing a patient on his or her left side for a digital rectal or endoscopic examination or for giving an enema?
A. The location of the internal and external sphincter
B. To better reference the *dentate line*
C. To facilitate blood supply to the cecum
D. To accommodate the left curvature of the sigmoid colon

3. Which structure of the GI tract is responsible for converting liquid stool to solid and serving as a reservoir for feces until it is expelled?
A. Anal canal
B. Colon
C. Anal sphincters
D. Pelvic floor

4. Which layer of the pelvic floor is the principal source of support for pelvic organs?
A. Levator ani
B. Endopelvic fascia
C. Perineal membrane
D. Anal sphincter

5. Which layer of the colon wall promotes mixing and peristalsis?
A. Serosa
B. Mucosa
C. Muscularis
D. Submucosa

6. Which nervous system is the primary mediator for colonic motility (peristalsis)?
A. Central nervous system (CNS)
B. Autonomic nervous system (ANS)
C. Enteric nervous system (ENS)
D. Somatic system

7. The continence nurse is counseling a patient with a sacral-level spinal cord injury (SCI). For what GI condition is this patient at risk?
A. Constipation
B. Diarrhea
C. Flatulence
D. Bowel perforation

8. Sensory awareness of rectal distention is provided by
A. Sensory receptor in the anal canal
B. Sensorimotor innervation of the IAS
C. Innervation of the somatic fibers of the pudendal nerve
D. Stretch receptors in the rectal wall and pelvic floor muscles

9. A patient experiencing fecal incontinence complains that he "cannot get to the bathroom in time" when he feels the urge to defecate. Which structure helps delay defecation until a socially appropriate time and place?
A. Rectum
B. External anal sphincter (EAS) and pelvic floor
C. Internal anal sphincter (IAS)
D. Colon

10. Which position is the best posture for defecation?
A. Squatting
B. Sitting
C. Supine
D. Position has no effect on defecation.

ANSWERS AND RATIONALES

1. A. Rationale: Intrinsic factor (produce in the stomach) combined with B_{12} is absorbed by the distal ileum.

2. D. Rationale: Sigmoid colon resembles an "S-shaped" curvature because it bends more to the left at the distal portion and then curves back around to reach the rectum. This left curvature is the rationale for placing a patient on their left side accesses the left curvature for anal exams or procedures.

3. B. Rationale: The large intestines role is to convert liquid stool into a soft but solid fecal mass containing the waste products of digestion and to serve as a reservoir for feces until a suitable time and place for defecation.

4. A. Rationale: The levator ani is a group of muscles that act as a single unit to provide the primary support to the pelvic organs (anus, vagina, urethra) to promote closure especially during activities that cause increase abdominal pressures.

5. C. Rationale: The circular and longitudinal muscles of the muscularis produces rhythmic patterns of muscle contraction that promote mixing and fluid/electrolyte absorption as well as transport of stool from the cecum to the anal canal.

6. C. Rationale: The ENS is contained within the bowel wall and responds to thermal, chemical, osmotic, and mechanical stimuli transmitted by receptors in the mucosal and muscle layers that generates peristalsis.

7. A. Rationale: Parasympathetic nerve fibers exit at the S2–S4 level and stimulates peristalsis in the distal colon. SCI in this region prevents parasympathetic activation of peristalsis.

8. D. Rationale: Perception of rectal distention and correct classification of rectal contents (gas, liquid, or solid) is provided by stretch receptors in the rectum and pelvic floor and sensory receptors in the anal canal.

9. B. Rationale: Voluntary contraction of the external anal sphincter and pelvic floor doubles anal canal pressure and prevents distal propulsion of the stool.

10. A. Rationale: Squatting position facilitates straightening of the anorectal angle and promotes movement of stool from the rectum to the anal canal.

Kendra Kamp and Margaret Heitkemper

OBJECTIVES

1. Discuss the impact of bowel dysfunction or fecal incontinence on lifestyle and quality of life and implications for psychosocial support and counseling.

   a. Explain how each of the following contributes to normal bowel function and fecal continence: normal peristalsis; sensory awareness of rectal distention and ability to distinguish between solid, liquid, and gaseous contents; internal anal sphincter function; external anal sphincter function; and rectal capacity and compliance.

   b. Describe criteria and guidelines for use of anorectal pouching systems and internal drainage/bowel management systems.

2. Describe the etiology, pathology, clinical presentation, and management options for acute and chronic diarrhea.

   a. Differentiate the pathology, presentation, and management of normal-transit constipation, slow-transit constipation, and obstructed defecation.

3. Describe the pathology and clinical presentation of irritable bowel syndrome.

4. Describe the critical components of assessment and management for the individual with irritable bowel syndrome.

TOPIC OUTLINE

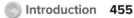
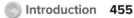
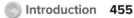

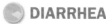
INTRODUCTION

Functional gastrointestinal (GI) disorders, such as diarrhea, constipation, and irritable bowel syndrome (IBS), cause considerable distress for both young and old. Transient episodes involving a change in stool consistency, frequency, or painful defecation are often self-diagnosed and treated through dietary modification and over-the-counter (OTC) remedies. Persistent changes in bowel function, however, usually prompt consultation with a health care professional. Altered defecation patterns negatively affect quality of life due to the combination of physical symptoms, anxiety, and negative emotions arising from the symptoms (e.g., embarrassment). The emotional response to the physical symptoms may amplify the symptoms and cause further GI distress (Midenfjord et al., 2019).

> **KEY POINT**
>
> Functional GI disorders negatively affect quality of life due to the combination of physical symptoms, anxiety, and negative emotions such as embarrassment.

In this chapter, alterations in bowel motility are defined as a deviation from a "normal" bowel pattern of regularly timed passage of soft, formed stools, without any difficulty or discomfort. Comprehensive management of bowel elimination problems by the continence nurse is described with a focus on reducing symptomatology and improving quality of life. Specific topics include pathology and clinical presentation of common motility disorders, guidelines for comprehensive nursing assessment, management options to include implications for patient-focused education and counseling, and indications and guidance for referrals to specialists.

A lack of clear definitions for terms such as *constipation* and *diarrhea* has hampered evidence-based practice in the treatment of bowel irregularity. Client perceptions of bowel symptoms vary greatly; some individuals focus solely on stool consistency or frequency, while others are more concerned about associated symptoms, such as pain with defecation and flatulence. Effective

management of any disorder is dependent in large part on identifying and correcting the physiologic or structural source of the presenting symptoms; however, many common bowel problems are *functional* disorders, meaning that no structural or tissue abnormality can be detected that explains the symptoms (Lacy et al., 2016).

> **KEY POINT**
>
> Many bowel problems are functional disorders, meaning that no structural or tissue abnormality can be detected that explains the symptoms.

Bowel motility may be conceptualized as a continuum as seen in **Table 21-1**. One extreme is slow-transit constipation, with marked reduction in peristaltic activity, while the other extreme is diarrhea, with rapid transit of stool and water through the colon. The definition of "normal" bowel function lacks precision and in fact "normal" function varies from person to person and is affected by that individual's perceptions of normal. For example, intermittent constipation with no additional symptoms is considered acceptable and normal by many, especially during events that disrupt normal daily routines, such as travel.

> **KEY POINT**
>
> The definition of normal bowel function lacks precision, and in fact normal function varies from person to person and is affected by that individual's perceptions of normal.

DIARRHEA

Diarrhea originated from the ancient Greek term *diarrhein*, meaning "flow through" (Oxford English Dictionary, 2019). For the individual suffering from diarrhea, it may indeed seem as though everything ingested flows immediately through the GI tract. Left untreated, diarrhea may result in dehydration, electrolyte imbalance, and death. It is frequently associated with perianal and perineal skin irritation that may range from mild erythema to epidermal erosion and ulceration. The previously toilet-trained

TABLE 21-1 THE BOWEL MOTILITY CONTINUUM

	NO GO	SLOW-GO	GO	GO-GO-GO!
Clinical condition	Obstructed defecation	Constipation IBS-C	"Normal" bowel pattern	Diarrhea IBS-D
Description	No bowel output	Stools hard, dry, difficult to pass without pain, strain, or discomfort. May be at less frequent intervals than usual bowel pattern	Stools soft, formed, passed at approximately regular intervals without pain, strain, or discomfort	Stools unformed or liquid, passed more frequently than normal bowel pattern (or >3 times/d) and often accompanied by cramping abdominal pain or tenesmus
Symbol	Stop sign	Sloth	Clock	Roadrunner

child or adult client may experience fecal incontinence during an acute diarrheal illness, as the rapid filling of the rectum and large volume of stool may overwhelm rectal capacity and sphincter contractility and endurance.

DEFINITION

Inconsistencies in both clinical and research literature demonstrate that there is no globally accepted definition for diarrhea. In addition, there are wide variations in individuals' normal stool volume and consistency. For research purposes, diarrhea is often operationally defined as ≥3 loose or liquid stools within a 24-hour period or passage of >200 g of stool in a 24-hour period. It should also be noted that research definitions often disregard the impact of the symptom experience of diarrhea on the client (i.e., physical and emotional distress) even though symptom distress usually prompts the individual to seek medical attention. In clinical practice, measurement of stool mass is rarely possible, and clinicians typically rely upon client reports regarding frequency and consistency of stooling and the impact of the diarrhea. Clinicians should also be alert to the fact that some individuals with fecal incontinence come to the provider with complaints of "diarrhea."

The World Health Organization (WHO) defines diarrhea as "the passage of three or more loose or liquid stools per day, or more frequently than is normal for the individual" (World Health Organization, 2017) NANDA International, Inc. simply defines diarrhea as "passage of loose, unformed stool" (Makic & Ackley, 2017). The Oncology Nursing Society has defined chemotherapy-induced diarrhea as "an abnormal increase in stool liquidity and frequency that may be accompanied by abdominal cramping" (Thorpe et al., 2017). Each definition addresses stool consistency, two definitions include an increase in stool frequency, only one definition addresses related symptomatology, and no definitions address symptom-related quality-of-life issues or distress.

In this chapter, diarrhea is defined as an alteration in bowel elimination characterized by increased frequency and volume of stools and decreased stool consistency, compared to the bowel elimination pattern that is normal for the individual. Diarrhea is often accompanied by abdominal cramping, a persistent sensation of stool in the rectum (tenesmus), and related psychosocial distress that may amplify the physical distress.

EPIDEMIOLOGY

The WHO estimates that 1.7 billion cases of diarrhea occur globally each year (World Health Organization, 2017), and the most serious consequences are experienced by children under the age of 5. Estimates of disease burden due to diarrhea are difficult to determine due to lack of accurate surveillance and the variability in outcomes reported in epidemiologic studies (Arnold et al., 2011). However, a prospective study conducted in Asia and sub-Saharan Africa reported that children in these areas are 8.5 times more likely to die if they develop moderate-to-severe diarrhea before age 5 (Kotloff et al., 2013). It is estimated that improvements in water and sanitation can decrease diarrheal disability-adjusted life-years lost by 13% (GBD Diarrhoeal Disease Collaborators, 2017).

> **KEY POINT**
>
> The most serious consequences of diarrhea are experienced by children under 5 years of age.

ASSESSMENT

Diarrhea should be considered both a symptom and a sign. Some clients use the term "diarrhea" to describe loose bowel movements, regardless of stool frequency. It is important to seek subjective information about associated symptoms such as cramping, abdominal pain, tenesmus, bowel urgency, fecal incontinence, fatigue, and symptom severity when collecting assessment data for the client with complaints of diarrhea. Objective data collection should include inspection for perianal or peristomal skin breakdown and auscultation for hyperactive bowel sounds. Complaints of fatigue should trigger an assessment of functional status and safety, as well as clinical and laboratory assessment of fluid and electrolyte balance. In general, acute-onset diarrhea is caused by an infectious process, and workup includes a careful history to determine potential sources of exposure (e.g., travel history), clinical and laboratory assessment of fluid electrolyte balance, and stool analysis for bacteria, ova, and parasites. In contrast, chronic diarrhea is likely to be caused by an underlying disease process (e.g., malabsorption syndrome, motility disorder, or inflammatory bowel disease [IBD]); these individuals frequently require a gastroenterology referral and workup. **Table 21-2** lists factors to include in a comprehensive assessment of bowel function.

KEY POINT

When assessing the individual with diarrhea, it is important to obtain information about cramping, abdominal pain, tenesmus, fecal urgency, fecal frequency, episodes of incontinence, the presence of blood in the stool, and symptoms of fluid and electrolyte imbalance and fatigue.

The continence nurse can provide valuable contributions to the assessment data and may identify associated problems, such as skin irritation, that might be overlooked by providers focused primarily on identifying the underlying cause of diarrhea as a basis for medical and/or surgical treatment. In particular, the continence nurse can play a unique role in identifying the amount of GI symptom distress experienced by the client and his/her specific concerns.

CLASSIFICATION OF DIARRHEA

KEY POINT

Diarrhea is classified according to duration of illness, etiology and pathology (infectious vs. noninfectious), and characteristics of stool.

TABLE 21-2 COMPREHENSIVE COLLABORATIVE ASSESSMENT OF DIARRHEA

PROVIDER LEVEL	SUBJECTIVE DATA	OBJECTIVE DATA

Specialist WOC Nurse	Focused history
	  Duration of diarrhea
	  Stool frequency
	  Stool form, using standardized pictorial tool
	  Stool color
	  Abdominal pain
	  Travel history
	  OTC and prescribed medications
	  Episodes of fecal incontinence
	  Associated symptoms
	    Bloating
	    Tenesmus
	    Change in stool odor
	  Distress
	    Anxiety/hypervigilance
	    Fatigue
	    Fear of serious problems
	    Embarrassment
	    Loss of control
		Vital signs
		Presence of blood in stool
		Stool frequency
		Stool form, using standardized pictorial tool
		Stool color
		Stool odor
		Abdominal distention
		Bowel sounds
		Blood in stool
		Fluid balance
		  Skin turgor
		  Mucus membranes
		  Vital signs
		Perineal, perianal, or peristomal skin integrity

Advanced Registered Nurse Practitioner or Physician	Complete history
	  Recent travel
	  Self-care attempted
	    OTC drugs
	    Dietary changes
	    Alternative therapy
	  Diet recall
	  Antibiotic usage
	  Chronic illnesses (diabetes, HIV, hyperthyroidism)
	  Associated symptoms
	    Fever
	    Nausea
	    Vomiting
		Laboratory and diagnostic testing
		  Stool examinations
		    Fecal leukocytes
		    Ova and parasites
		    Bacterial stool culture
		    Giardia antigen
		    C. difficile toxin
		    Fecal analysis, including occult blood and fecal fat
		  CBC
		  Hct and Hgb
		  C-reactive protein
		  Fecal calprotectin
		  Lactose tolerance
		  Flexible sigmoidoscopy or colonoscopy with intestinal biopsy
		  Flat plate of abdomen

Acute versus Chronic Diarrhea

Acute diarrhea is diarrhea which lasts <14 days (Barr & Smith, 2014). Diarrhea that has been present for 14 to 30 days is considered persistent, and diarrhea longer than 30 days is termed chronic (Ochoa & Surawicz, 2012).

Chronic diarrhea is usually noninfectious and may be caused by medications (such as those containing magnesium), artificial sweeteners such as sorbitol (an osmotic laxative), malabsorption syndromes (such as lactose intolerance or celiac disease), motility disorders (such as diabetes gastroenteropathy), inflammatory conditions (such as Crohn disease or ulcerative colitis), short bowel syndrome resulting from surgical resection of large portions of the small bowel, or bile salt–induced diarrhea caused by resection of the terminal ileum. Diarrhea may also occur following initiation of enteral feedings in individuals who have had very limited oral/enteral intake for a number of days, due to temporary flattening of the villi with resultant loss of absorptive surface.

Infectious versus Noninfectious Diarrhea

Acute diarrhea is most often caused by infectious disease via the fecal–oral route through contaminated food or water containing pathogens such as viruses, bacteria, and parasites. Infectious diarrhea is a leading cause of death in the developing world due to fluid and electrolyte imbalance. In 2011, 35% of hospitalizations was due to nontyphoidal *Salmonella* spp. (Sell & Dolan, 2018). Other common causes include norovirus (26%), *Campylobacter* spp. (15%), and *Toxoplasma gondii* (8%). In a review of global and regional health burden, it was estimated that *Salmonella* results in the largest diarrheal disease burden (Kirk et al., 2015).

Within the United States, rotaviruses comprise the majority of infectious diarrhea in infants and children, while Norwalk virus (also known as Norovirus) comprises the majority of infectious diarrhea in adults. Foodborne illnesses play a significant role in acute infectious diarrhea and are continually monitored within the United States by the Centers for Disease Control and Prevention (CDC). Data from 2017 monitoring indicate the most common bacterial infections are *Salmonella, Clostridium perfringens, Campylobacter, E. coli,* and *Vibrio* (CDC, 2019). Detailed information about surveillance procedures and data can be found at the CDC Web site https://www.cdc.gov/foodborneburden/index.html.

KEY POINT

Acute episodes of diarrhea are usually caused by infectious processes, while chronic diarrhea is more commonly due to noninfectious factors such as medications, malabsorption syndromes, motility disorders, inflammatory bowel disease, or short bowel syndrome.

The term *traveler's diarrhea* is used to designate a nonspecific infectious diarrhea, typically bacterial. High-risk areas are Central and South America, Africa, and Asia (Chen et al., 2018). Approximately 22% of travel-related illnesses in the United States are due to traveler's diarrhea (Sell & Dolan, 2018).

Of particular concern within health care organizations and group living facilities is diarrhea caused by the spore-forming bacterium *Clostridium difficile*. Although previously associated with advanced age, immunosuppression, and prior use of broad-spectrum antibiotics, recent outbreaks have involved more serious and possibly evolving strains that can affect previously healthy individuals (Dayananda & Wilcox, 2019). Because *C. difficile* spores can survive in the environment for prolonged periods of time, person-to-person transmission can easily occur. Extremely virulent strains may result in a condition called pseudomembranous colitis, which is potentially fatal.

KEY POINT

Traveler's diarrhea is a nonspecific infectious diarrhea that is typically bacterial and frequently associated with travels to an area with poor sanitation.

Characteristics of Stool

Diarrhea is also classified by type of stool. *Bloody stools* (hematochezia) are associated with inflammation. These patients commonly exhibit leukocytosis as well, due to the underlying inflammatory process. Bloody stools may result from an invasive infection, such as *C. difficile*, or may be the result of chronic inflammation, such as IBD, cancer, or radiation proctitis. In all of these conditions, the intestinal mucosa is damaged, resulting in the visible blood within the diarrheal stools.

Fatty diarrhea occurs due to malabsorption. One of the most common causes malabsorption is lactose intolerance, which frequently becomes a chronic condition requiring diet modification. Surgical procedures, such as short bowel syndrome, bowel resection, and gastric bypass, as well as pancreatic disease may be associated with malabsorption and fatty diarrhea. Various medications can also contribute to malabsorption, including orlistat and acarbose. Malabsorption is also the mechanism for diarrhea caused by the parasite *Giardia*.

Watery diarrhea is the most common type of diarrhea and is typically further classified as secretory, osmotic, or functional based on the underlying pathology. *Secretory* diarrhea occurs when the epithelial cells in the intestinal mucosa are damaged by an infectious organism or intestinal toxin, resulting in an inability to absorb water and electrolytes *from* the lumen of the bowel and abnormal secretion of fluid *into* the lumen of the bowel. Secretory diarrhea is usually high volume and unaffected by reduced oral/enteral intake. Irritant laxatives, serious enteric infections (such as *C. difficile*), and chemotherapy are potential causes of secretory diarrhea (Thorpe et al., 2017). In contrast, osmotic diarrhea is caused by the presence of high-osmolarity substances within the lumen of the bowel, which pull water from the blood stream into the gut. Osmotic diarrhea responds rapidly to reduced oral/enteral intake. Food additives, such as high-fructose corn syrup, sorbitol, and xylitol, osmotic laxatives (polyethylene glycol [PEG], milk of magnesia, lactulose), and celiac disease are associated with *osmotic diarrhea*. The final category, chronic watery diarrhea (also known as *functional diarrhea*) occurs when the diarrhea cannot be associated with a disease, medication, or structural problem. Functional diarrhea often overlaps with IBS.

KEY POINT

Watery diarrhea may be classified as secretory, osmotic, or functional; secretory diarrhea is high volume and unaffected by oral intake, while osmotic diarrhea responds rapidly to reduced oral or enteral intake. Functional diarrhea is often chronic and not associated with a disease, medication, or structural problem.

TREATMENT

Treatment for diarrhea is based upon management of the underlying etiology and supportive care to prevent complications.

Management of Underlying Pathology

Management of the underlying disease process is extremely variable, reflecting the wide variety of conditions causing diarrhea, but commonly involves antibiotic therapy (for infectious diarrhea), medical management of inflammatory conditions and motility disorders, and dietary modifications for individuals with malabsorption syndromes.

Supportive Care

Both adult and pediatric clients with diarrhea are at risk for fluid volume deficit and electrolyte imbalance, but the most vulnerable are the elderly and the very young (i.e., infants and young children). Nursing care involves careful monitoring of intake and output and identifying signs of dehydration. Dry mouth, decreased urinary output, skin tenting, hypotension, lethargy, tachycardia, and elevated temperature should arouse suspicion of dehydration with the potential for shock, especially in the pediatric client.

For clients who develop an actual fluid volume deficit, rehydration is essential. Oral rehydration is the route of choice, but intravenous fluids may be required for more rapid fluid resuscitation in the critically ill client. The WHO advocates making oral rehydration salts readily available, particularly in the developing world, so that early rehydration can be provided in the home setting. This is particularly important in management of diseases such as cholera, which can quickly lead to mortality due to dehydration (Pietroni, 2019).

Dietary modifications are also recommended. Although the BRAT diet (bananas, rice, applesauce, and toast) is frequently recommended by clinicians, there is little evidence to support this level of dietary restriction. Avoidance of highly spiced or fatty foods and increased intake of foods with significant amounts of soluble fiber are recommended and anecdotally reported as helpful. The WHO advocates zinc supplementation for young children with diarrhea at a rate of 10 mg/day for infants under 6 months and 20 mg/day for children over 6 months for a duration of 10 to 14 days (World Health Organization, 2019).

KEY POINT

Management of diarrhea involves treatment of the underlying pathology, supportive care to maintain fluid and electrolyte balance and to reduce symptomatology, and skin care and containment when needed.

Pharmacologic Therapy

Antibiotics are typically prescribed for infectious diarrhea and should be based on identification of the specific organism and the agents to which it is sensitive (culture-based therapy). Antimotility agents are not recommended, because the goal is to eliminate the causative organism from the body as rapidly as possible. However, for diarrhea caused by chemotherapy, antimotility agents such as loperamide are frequently considered first-line therapy with progression to octreotide for persistent diarrhea (Thorpe et al., 2017). For traveler's diarrhea, bismuth subsalicylate is frequently recommended as a readily-available OTC remedy; however, persistent traveler's diarrhea is typically treated with a fluoroquinolone antibiotic. Chronic diarrhea in persons with radiation proctitis and short bowel syndrome may respond at least partially to use of psyllium fiber supplements to thicken the stool.

KEY POINT

Antimotility agents are not recommended for persons with infectious diarrhea, because the goal is to eliminate the causative organism from the body as rapidly as possible.

Probiotic Therapy

The use of probiotics has also received much attention in the research literature and has demonstrated some benefit in both the prevention and management of individuals with specific types of diarrhea. A meta-analysis of 33 studies involving more than 6,300 children suggests that probiotics, particularly *Lactobacillus rhamnosus* and *Saccharomyces boulardii,* can be beneficial in the prevention of antibiotic-associated diarrhea in otherwise healthy infants and children (Guo et al., 2019). Probiotics, particularly *Saccharomyces boulardii* and bifidobacterium, are also beneficial in reducing the duration of acute diarrhea (Yang et al., 2019). *Saccharomyces boulardii* CNCM1-745 was found to reduce the incidence of traveler's diarrhea (McFarland & Goh, 2019). Meta-analysis of studies testing the effects of probiotics in the prevention of *C. difficile*–associated diarrhea in adults also identified benefit, particularly among individuals with a higher risk of *C. difficile* (Goldenberg et al., 2017). A trial of a combination probiotic product containing *Lactobacillus acidophilus* and *Bifidobacterium longum* reduced daily number of stools, severity of diarrhea, and abdominal pain (Demers et al., 2014) in persons with diarrhea following pelvic radiation. A double-blind, randomized controlled trial of *Lactobacillus casei* in children with acute diarrhea resulted in significantly shorter duration of diarrhea, decreased abdominal distention, and lower markers of inflammation (Lai et al., 2019). Further research is needed to determine the specific agents, dosages, and indications for probiotic use in prevention and management of diarrhea.

KEY POINT

Early research suggests that probiotics may be of benefit in prevention and management of acute diarrheal syndromes; however, further study is needed to determine best agents and dosages.

Although research suggests benefit from probiotics in preventing and treating diarrhea due to acute problems, current meta-analytic results do not suggest a benefit for the induction or maintenance of remission in chronic diarrhea caused Crohn disease (Derwa et al., 2017; Ganji-Arjenaki & Rafieian-Kopaei, 2018). Probiotics may be beneficial for inducing and maintaining remission in ulcerative colitis (Derwa et al., 2017; Ganji-Arjenaki & Rafieian-Kopaei, 2018).

Stool Containment
Containment of stool typically involves disposable absorbent body worn absorbent products (BWAPs); other products include reusable continence products (see Chapter 16), fecal external pouches, or internal fecal management systems. In the United States, the most common method of containment is disposable absorbent pads, pull-ons, briefs (Gray et al., 2018) in adults, or diapers in children, which, in the case of infants and young children, raises infection control concerns in facilities such as daycare centers. Containment of stool is also a concern when adults suffering from diarrhea are unable to toilet independently and incontinent of stool. Diligent hygiene and skin care are critical, with regular checking of pads to reduce risk of skin erosion from fecal enzymes. Contaminated disposable products used at home pose an additional economic burden related to both the initial purchase and safe disposal of the products. An in vitro study of briefs and pads for urinary incontinence (not fecal incontinence) suggested that briefs may be more cost-effective than pads (Yamasato et al., 2014). Further research is required to determine the best products for individuals with fecal incontinence. An in vitro study comparing internal stool management systems demonstrated differences in the ability to contain infectious material such as *C. difficile* (Gray et al., 2014). Further study is needed to determine the ability of perianal pouches and/or internal bowel management systems to reduce the risk of transmission by effectively containing the stool.

External stool containment pouches (perianal pouches) have been available for many years and are sometimes considered the "first-line" approach to stool containment, so long as the perianal skin is intact. These pouches are attached to a flexible pectin-based adhesive skin barrier designed to adhere to the perianal skin and inner buttocks of the individual. Their use is limited because they do not adhere well to moist skin and are therefore ineffective when skin damage has already occurred. In addition, female clients may have inadequate tissue in the perineal bridge between the anal and vaginal openings for pouch adherence.

KEY POINT

Perianal pouches are considered the "first-line approach" to stool containment so long as the perianal skin is intact.

The use of a nasopharyngeal airway (rectal trumpet [RT]) for containment of stool has been implemented for the management of incontinent liquid stool, particularly in critically ill adults. More study is needed before definitive recommendations can be made (Beeckman et al., 2016; Beeson et al., 2017). A recent study in one transplant intensive care unit of 400 patients found three possible and nine probable cases of RT-associated hemorrhage (Glass et al., 2018).

Fecal containment systems (or internal bowel management catheters) are devices that are inserted rectally and maintained in place by inflation of an internal balloon; they are most appropriate for patients who are bedbound with high-volume liquid stool. Because these devices involve insertion of tubing into the rectum and through the sphincter, they do not provide perfect containment. Clinicians, patients, and families must be instructed to expect small amounts of leakage and resulting odor. In vitro research indicates that fecal containment systems may be effective in reducing the spread of *C. difficile*, but this has not yet been demonstrated in clinical practice (Gray et al., 2014) (**Fig. 21-1**). Chapter 22 discusses further stool containment options.

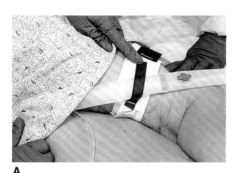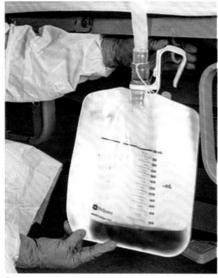

A **B**

FIGURE 21-1. Internal Fecal Containment Device. **A.** Tubing secured to leg by stabilization device. **B.** Drainage bag for fecal containment system.

Hygiene and Skin Care

Cleansing of skin wet with feces and/or urine should be provided using both a no-rinse perineal cleanser and soft disposable washcloth, or a disposable wipe impregnated with surfactants and moisturizers. The goal is effective cleansing with avoidance of trauma to the perineal and perianal skin. In some cases, a perineal bottle can be used to gently flush away the stool. The skin should be dried by gently rubbing with a soft absorbent cloth. ("Patting" the skin dry is not recommended; research on transepidermal water loss [TEWL] on the volar surface of the arm in healthy adults suggests that patting leaves the skin significantly wetter and at greater risk of frictional damage than gentle rubbing (Voegeli, 2008).) When the skin is dry, moisture barrier films, ointments, or pastes should be applied to protect the skin from the moisture and enzymes in the stool. If the skin is denuded, a product designed specifically for wet, weepy skin should be applied, such as a pectin-based powder followed by a clear acrylate liquid barrier, or a zinc oxide–based ointment.

All caregivers must be taught the critical importance of correct application and removal of the zinc oxide–based product; a no-rinse perineal cleanser and soft cloth should be used to gently remove the soiled layers of zinc oxide without causing trauma. Additional ointment can then be applied. Chapter 17 provides more detailed discussion on skin care and incontinence-associated dermatitis.

CONSTIPATION

DEFINITION

Constipation can be defined as difficult defecation characterized by one or more of the following: (1) hard or dry stools, (2) decreased frequency of stooling, (3) a sensation of incomplete rectal evacuation following a bowel movement, and (4) pain or straining associated with stool elimination. Initial identification of constipation is usually based on a reduction in the frequency of stooling in comparison to an individual's normal bowel pattern. The National Digestive Diseases Information Clearinghouse (NIDDIC) uses the criterion of fewer than 3 bowel movements per week in its patient education materials (National Digestive Diseases Information Clearinghouse, 2018), a definition accepted by many clinicians. However, there is considerable variation among individuals in regard to the frequency of bowel movements, and the American Gastroenterology Society (AGS) recommends a focus on the signs and symptoms rather than fixed criteria related to frequency of bowel movements (Bharucha et al., 2013a).

The NANDA International, Inc. and the American Gastroenterological Association (AGA) (Bharucha et al., 2013a) identify constipation and perceived constipation as two separate conditions; constipation represents a genuine problem with stool elimination, whereas perceived constipation represents the perception that there is a problem when in fact bowel function is normal. Perceived constipation is actually a common problem, due to the widespread misconception that normal bowel function is defined by a bowel movement that occurs at the same time every day. Nurses can help to address this problem by providing accurate information regarding the characteristics and variations in normal bowel elimination patterns. In addition to constipation and perceived constipation, NANDA also recognizes the nursing diagnosis "risk for constipation" and "risk for chronic functional constipation." Many of the interventions for persons at risk for constipation can be initiated by nurses independently, and early identification of at-risk individuals followed by implementation of a bowel management program can frequently prevent constipation, especially among hospitalized or institutionalized patients (e.g., individuals in long-term or rehabilitative care settings). **Table 21-3** summarizes the differences between the four main NANDA diagnostic categories related to constipation: constipation, perceived constipation, risk for constipation, and risk for chronic functional constipation (Ackley et al., 2020).

KEY POINT

NANDA recognizes four nursing diagnoses related to constipation: constipation, perceived constipation, risk for constipation, and risk for chronic functional constipation.

EPIDEMIOLOGY

In contrast to transient constipation, persistent constipation is a much more significant problem and the focus of most epidemiologic investigations. Based on analyses of the 2009–2010 National Health and Nutrition Examination Survey (NHANES) dataset that included the Bowel Health Questionnaire, the prevalence of chronic constipation was 11.2% in adults. Female gender, older age, depression, and frequent milk consumption were positively associated with chronic constipation in this population-based survey. The prevalence rates of chronic constipation vary by country and settings (ambulatory care, specialty care, hospital, long-term care). In ambulatory care constipation, symptoms were responsible for 3.0 million visits (Peery et al., 2019).

Chronic Constipation

Prevalence of constipation reported in the literature varies among different populations and geographical locations (Camilleri et al., 2017; Suares & Ford, 2011). Not surprisingly, the rate of constipation among hospitalized and disabled individuals is higher. In a Danish study, the incidence of constipation among hospitalized individuals was 143 cases per 1,000 patient days, and in new admissions was 39% (Noiesen et al., 2014). Among children with disability due to cerebral palsy, 57% had constipation and 55% used laxatives regularly (Noiesen et al., 2014). A meta-analysis

---

TABLE 21-3 NANDA DEFINITIONS AND CHARACTERISTICS FOR CONSTIPATION, PERCEIVED CONSTIPATION, RISK FOR CONSTIPATION, AND RISK FOR FUNCTIONAL CONSTIPATION

DIAGNOSTIC CATEGORY	KEY ELEMENTS OF DEFINITION	CHARACTERISTICS

Constipation	Decreased stool frequency
	Difficult passage of stools
	Incomplete stool passage
	Excessively dry, hard stool
		Subjective:
		  Rectal fullness
		  Rectal pressure
		  Abdominal pain
		  Abdominal tenderness
		  Fatigue
		Objective:
		  Decreased stool volume
		  Abdominal distention
		  Hard, formed stools
		  Hyperactive/hypoactive bowel sounds
		  Abdominal distention
		  Liquid stool

Perceived constipation	Self-diagnosed
	Laxative, enema, or suppository abuse
		Subjective:
		  Expectation of daily bowel movement
		  History of OTC medications to stimulate daily bowel movements
		Objective:
		  Absence of clinical signs of constipation

Risk for constipation	At risk for:
	  Difficult defecation
	  Passage of hard, dry stools
	  Incomplete stool passage
		Not applicable

Adapted from Ackley, B. J., et al. (2020). *Nursing diagnosis handbook: An evidenced-based guide to planning care* (12th ed.). St. Louis, MO: Elsevier.

of GI problems in children with autism spectrum disorder revealed more frequent complaints of constipation in these children as compared to children without autism spectrum disorder (McElhanon et al., 2014).

Clients with chronic constipation often report psychological distress (anxiety, depression) and reductions in quality of life. Chronic constipation can hinder work, school, and social life. Among children with chronic constipation, behavioral problems are much more common than among their peers without constipation (Joinson et al., 2019). Constipation is also associated with a significant reduction in both physical and mental quality of life (Albiani et al., 2013; Wald et al., 2007), which may be due in part to the complex interaction between the brain and gut. In an international survey of individuals with reported constipation according to Rome II or III criteria and a matched nonconstipated cohort, those with constipation reported lower health-related quality of life (HRQOL) than in nonconstipated controls, as measured by the SF-36 and interview scores. The results were similar to those reported in other studies involving participants with chronic diseases such as reflux, chronic obstructive lung disease, diabetes, or hypertension (Wald et al., 2007). Whether treatment of constipation would have a direct effect on improved HRQOL is unclear because of the multifactorial nature of chronic constipation.

KEY POINT

Chronic constipation is associated with a significant reduction in both physical and mental quality of life.

ASSESSMENT

A comprehensive history and physical examination are necessary for proper diagnosis and for development of an individualized treatment plan.

History

In addition to questions about medical and surgical history, focused questions should address the following:

- An individual's description of constipation symptoms and opinion regarding cause
- Stool frequency, usual stool form/consistency, and presence/absence of blood in the stool
- Any straining or pain associated with bowel movements
- Previously and currently used measures to manage constipation and found to be successful, including use of laxatives, suppositories, enemas, manual maneuvers to facilitate stool elimination, and digital removal of stool
- "Red flag" signs and symptoms associated with colorectal cancer (**Box 21-1**). If present, these mandate referral for further workup (including colonoscopy)
- Previous investigations of the problem and outcomes

BOX 21-1   RED FLAG BOWEL SYMPTOMS REQUIRING COLONOSCOPY

Recent onset of constipation
Onset of symptoms occurring after age 50
Age ≥50 years with no previous screening for colorectal cancer; African Americans screening at age ≥45 years
Visible or occult blood in stools
Symptoms of bowel obstruction
Family history of colorectal cancer in a first-degree relative
Unintentional weight loss
Narrowing of stool diameter
Rectal prolapse

Data from Rex, D. K., Boland, C. R., Dominitz, J. A., et al. (2017). Colorectal cancer screening: Recommendations for physicians and patients from the U.S. Multi-Society Task Force on Colorectal Cancer. *American Journal of Gastroenterology, 112*(7), 1016–1030. doi: 10.1038/ajg.2017.174.

Use of a standardized instrument such as the Bristol Stool Scale (see Fig. 6-7, in Chapter 6) aids in the differentiation between true and perceived constipation and also provides a less subjective baseline measure for monitoring response to treatment. The Bristol Stool Scale correlates positively with stool transit time and has demonstrated acceptable sensitivity and specificity for predicting both colonic and whole gut transit time (Saad et al., 2010).

KEY POINT

Assessment of the individual with chronic constipation must include screening for alarm symptoms (blood in the stool, unintentional weight loss, change in stool caliber, family history of colorectal cancer, etc.); these symptoms require referral for workup.

In neonates and children, a history of progressively worsening constipation is commonly associated with congenital absence of bowel ganglia (Hirschsprung disease), which results in a functional bowel obstruction. Neurogenic bowel dysfunction is a common cause of constipation in individuals with a history of neurologic lesions such as spina bifida, spinal cord injury, or back injury/surgery. Central nervous system diseases such as multiple sclerosis, Parkinson disease, and Alzheimer dementia are also associated with constipation, due in part to progressive loss of functional mobility as well as reduced dietary and fluid intake. Metabolic disorders, such as hypothyroidism, hypercalcemia (Black & Ford, 2018), and diabetic neuropathy, may also contribute to constipation, as can various medications (e.g., opioids and anticholinergics).

Further history should include questions about lifestyle such as exercise/activity and dietary and fluid intake. In many situations, it is lifestyle (and/or medications) that are the primary contributing factors to constipation. Correction of lifestyle factors is the first step in improvement of constipation. It is helpful to have the client describe a "usual day" and conduct a 24-hour recall of food and fluid intake (or to have the client complete a food and fluid intake diary). In asking the client about lifestyle factors, the nurse can begin the process of education about normal bowel function and the factors contributing to constipation. The nurse should also be alert to indicators of anxiety or depression as there may be a relationship between HRQOL and constipation.

It is imperative for nurses to recognize those at high risk for constipation and to initiate preventive measures. High-risk populations include individuals with decreased physical activity due to illness, injury, or surgery and those who require opioid analgesics for pain management, especially those with advanced cancer and hospice patients. Opioid-induced constipation is constipation that is due to opioid therapy (Crockett et al., 2019). The American Gastroenterology Association recommends the use of laxatives as first-line treatment for individuals with opioid-induced constipation (Crockett et al., 2019). Constipation among cancer patients is a common complication (Candy et al., 2018). Anticipatory education regarding fiber and fluid intake and judicious use of stool softeners and laxatives are essential to prevent severe constipation and possible fecal impaction.

Physical Examination

The focused physical examination should include an abdominal and anorectal examination and a perineal skin inspection. In women, a pelvic examination may be indicated to rule out enterocele and rectocele. The abdominal examination should include inspection for obvious distention or masses, palpation, and percussion; the nurse should percuss along the length of the colon to determine abnormal colon "loading" with stool (evidenced by a dull percussion note along the length of the colon, as opposed to the normal tympanic percussion note) and should palpate the abdomen to detect any masses, including evidence of retained stool in the sigmoid colon. Anorectal examination is done to assess sensation, determine presence of retained stool in the rectum, and assess the individual's ability to voluntarily contract and relax the sphincter on command. The perineal skin is inspected for dermatitis or ulceration.

TYPES OF CONSTIPATION

There are different types of constipation based on the underlying etiology and reflected in clinical presentation and symptom severity. **Table 21-4** provides a summary of the types of constipation, the underlying pathophysiologic process, and the signs and symptoms common to each type. Constipation may occur in isolation or due to an underlying pathology. The term "functional

TABLE 21-4 TYPES OF CONSTIPATION WITH UNDERLYING CAUSES AND TYPICAL DATA PRESENTATION

TYPE OF CONSTIPATION	UNDERLYING CAUSE(S)	SIGNS AND SYMPTOMS
Transient	Dietary changes	Subjective: 　Straining during defecation 　Decreased stool frequency from baseline Objective: 　Colonic tenderness on palpation 　Palpable fecal mass in sigmoid colon
	Environmental and daily habit changes	Subjective: 　Abdominal discomfort 　Recent history of travel 　Immobility 　History of toilet training (children) 　Decreased access to toilet facilities which are comfortable 　Inability to achieve physiologic position for defecation Objective: 　Abdominal distension 　Irritability 　Anorexia 　Fecal soiling
	Pregnancy due to increase in progesterone (smooth muscle relaxant) and iron supplementation	Subjective: 　Straining during defecation 　Decreased stool frequency from baseline 　Hard, dry stools Objective: 　Dry, pellet-like stools 　Hemorrhoids

TABLE 21-4 TYPES OF CONSTIPATION WITH UNDERLYING CAUSES AND TYPICAL DATA PRESENTATION (*Continued*)

TYPE OF CONSTIPATION	UNDERLYING CAUSE(S)	SIGNS AND SYMPTOMS

	Pharmacologic side effects
	   Iron supplements
	   Calcium supplements
	   Opioid analgesics
	   Antacids
	   NSAIDs
	   Chronic laxative use
	   Calcium channel blockers
	   Antihistamines
	   Antipsychotics
		Subjective:
		   Medication history
		Objective:
		   Symptom improvement with medication discontinuation

	Painful anorectal condition with deliberate defecation delay
	   Hemorrhoids
	   Anal fissure
		Subjective:
		   Painful defecation
		   Hard, dry stools
		   Anal itching or pain
		Objective:
		   Blood on stools or toilet tissue with bowel movement
		   Visible fissure or hemorrhoid
		   Pain with DRE

Functional: normal-transit	Persistent lifestyle deficits (fiber, fluids, and exercise)	Subjective:
		   Hard, dry stools
		   Straining at defecation
		   Sensation of incomplete evacuation or obstruction
		   <3 stools per week
		   Inadequate fluid or fiber intake
		   Limited exercise
		Objective:
		   Normal bowel sounds
		   Abdominal distention
		   Responds to laxative use
		   Responds to lifestyle changes (diet, fluids, exercise)

Functional: slow-transit	Medical conditions
	   Diabetes mellitus
	   Depression
	   Hypothyroidism
	   Multiple sclerosis
	   Spinal cord injury
	   Parkinson disease
		Subjective:
		   Massive, very infrequent stools
		   History of disease or condition affecting motility
		   Failed self-treatment with fiber, fluids, exercise, or stimulant laxatives
		Objective:
		   Reduced transit time confirmed with diagnostic studies
		   Lack of anal wink (sacral nerve involvement)
		   Elevated TSH (hypothyroidism)

Dysfunctional defecation	Tumors	Subjective:
		   Thinning of stool diameter
		   Rectal discomfort
		   Blood in stool
		   Failed self-treatment with laxatives
		   History of unexplained weight loss
		   Bowel urgency
		Objective:
		   Abdominal distension
		   Positive fecal occult blood test
		   Palpable mass on DRE
		   Abnormal barium enema
		   Abnormal colonic biopsy
		   Rectal prolapse
		   Low hemoglobin

(*Continued*)

TABLE 21-4 TYPES OF CONSTIPATION WITH UNDERLYING CAUSES AND TYPICAL DATA PRESENTATION (*Continued*)

TYPE OF CONSTIPATION	UNDERLYING CAUSE(S)	SIGNS AND SYMPTOMS
	Dyssynergia between pelvic floor and anal sphincter muscles	Subjective: 　Difficulty passing even soft stools 　Straining 　Prolonged toileting 　Sensation of incomplete evacuation 　Rectal pain Objective: 　Normal-transit time studies 　Difficulty relaxing anal sphincter when bearing down 　Abnormal pelvic muscle floor diagnostic testing
	Pelvic organ prolapse	Subjective: 　Difficulty passing even soft stools 　Straining 　Prolonged toileting 　Use of manual maneuvers to evacuate stool 　Urinary incontinence Objective: 　Rectal bleeding 　Visible protraction of organs 　Palpable protrusion of organs 　Weak anal sphincter contraction

constipation" refers to symptoms of difficult, infrequent, or incomplete defecation that are present in the absence of disease or pathology (Bharucha et al., 2013b). The Rome IV diagnostic criteria for functional constipation include presence on ≥3 days per month during the preceding 3 months and onset of symptoms ≥6 months prior to seeking treatment. The Rome IV criteria for constipation differ by age group and are listed in **Table 21-5**.

Normal-Transit Constipation

Normal-transit constipation occurs in individuals who have a normal peristaltic response to stimuli such as colonic distention, but who do not have enough stimuli to activate the peristalsis. It is the most common type of constipation (Black & Ford, 2018). The problem is most commonly caused by inadequate fiber and fluid intake leading to small-caliber stools that do not stimulate the bowel wall. Individuals with normal-transit constipation typically describe their stools as hard and pellet-like and may also describe associated complaints, such as straining to pass stool, abdominal pain, gas, and bloating. Normal-transit constipation typically responds well to lifestyle changes designed to produce soft formed stool, because peristaltic activity is normal. Normal transit constipation is a transient problem, most often due to dietary or environmental issues (Bharucha et al., 2013b). It is a common complaint among the elderly, pregnant women, or individuals whose normal routine has been disrupted by factors such as travel or even the use of public

restrooms, where relaxation may be difficult. A low-fiber, "junk food" diet rich in simple carbohydrates is a common cause. A lack of exercise, such as the immobility associated with hospitalization, and inadequate fluid intake can exacerbate the problem by further reducing peristaltic stimuli. In children, constipation may be triggered by toilet training, changes in school, or use of unfamiliar toilet facilities. Depending on precipitating factors, normal-transit constipation occurs sporadically or more frequently if associated with IBS.

Slow-Transit Constipation

Slow-transit constipation, in contrast, involves decreased frequency of both segmental and mass movements within the gut. Due to the marked reduction in peristaltic activity, the stool mass sits in the colon for prolonged periods, reabsorbing water and increasing in size. Defecation may not occur until the entire colon is filled with stool, at which point the colonic and rectal pressures exceed anal canal pressures and the stool is forced out. Many individuals with slow-transit constipation report very infrequent (and very large) bowel movements (1 to 4/month), with significant bloating. Slow-transit constipation does not respond well to fiber therapy, because the added fiber simply increases the size of the fecal mass but does not stimulate peristalsis. Response to stimulant laxatives is also poor, because those agents are designed to stimulate peristalsis. Stool softeners and osmotic agents may be more effective because they keep the

TABLE 21-5 ROME IV CRITERIA FOR DIAGNOSIS OF FUNCTIONAL CONSTIPATION BY AGE GROUPS FOR INDIVIDUALS NOT MEETING CRITERIA FOR IRRITABLE BOWEL SYNDROME (IBS)

ADULT	INFANT TO 4 YEARS OF AGE	DEVELOPMENTAL AGE >4 YEARS THROUGH ADOLESCENT

Two or more of the following present:
1. Symptoms present ≥25% of defecations
  • Straining
  • Hard or lumpy stools
  • Sensation of incomplete evacuation
  • Sensation of anorectal obstruction/blockage
  • Manual maneuvers (e.g., digital evacuation) to facilitate stool passage
2. Loose stools are rarely present without use of laxatives
3. Insufficient criteria for IBS
	At least two of the following present for at least 1 month:
	  • Two or fewer defecations per week
	  • History of excessive stool retention
	  • History of painful or hard bowel movements
	  • History of large-diameter stools
	  • Presence of a large fecal mass
	In toilet-trained children, the following additional criteria may be used:
	  • At least one episode/week of incontinence after the acquisition of toileting skills
	  • History of large-diameter stools that may obstruct the toilet
		Two or more of the following present:
		  • Two or fewer defecations in the toilet per week
		  • At least one episode of fecal incontinence per week
		  • History of retentive posturing or excessive volitional stool retention
		  • History of painful or hard bowel movements
		  • Presence of a large fecal mass in the rectum
		  • History of large diameter stools which may obstruct the toilet
		  • After evaluation symptoms cannot be fully explained by another medical condition

Symptoms must be present for past 3 months with onset ≥6 months	Symptoms must be present for at least 1 month	Symptoms must be present for at least 1 month

Source: Drossman, D., Chang, L., Chey, W. D., et al. (2016). *Rome IV functional gastrointestinal disorders: Disorders of gut-brain interaction* (4th ed.). Raleigh, NC: The Rome Foundation.

stool soft and facilitate elimination. Slow-transit constipation is a very challenging disorder, and more research is desperately needed to guide treatment.

KEY POINT

In normal-transit constipation, peristaltic function is normal; these individuals respond well to lifestyle changes that produce soft formed stool. Slow-transit constipation is associated with significant reduction in peristaltic activity and does not respond well to simple measures such as fiber therapy.

Transit time is the diagnostic tool used to objectively diagnose normal-transit constipation versus slow-transit constipation and can be measured with various different procedures. One approach is ingestion of a radiation-free wireless motility capsule (WMC) (Aburub et al., 2018) that measures pressure, pH, and transit (Saad, 2016). Due to the size of the capsule, this is infrequently performed in children (Vriesman et al., 2019). Video capsule endoscopy allows direct visualization of the bowel lumen as the capsule passes from stomach to small bowel to colon and rectum and evacuation (Rao et al., 2011). Orally ingested radio-opaque markers (Sitz markers) can be used in combination with serial radiographic examinations to determine the time for markers to reach various segments of the bowel. Scintigraphy studies involve ingestion of either a radioactive meal or nonabsorbable charcoal that has been marked with radioisotopes.

Transit time studies are usually initiated in a physician's office or outpatient facility. Nursing education involves bowel preparation for capsule endoscopy and the need to continuously wear a transmitter for 3 to 5 days (or until the capsule is expelled) with wireless remote procedures. Radio-opaque marker studies require frequent returns for x-rays and possible abdominal ultrasound procedures, and the patient may be asked to avoid use of any laxative agents until the study is complete. Neither wireless remote nor radiopaque marker studies require any type of bowel preparation.

KEY POINT

Transit time studies are used to differentiate between types of functional constipation (normal-transit, slow-transit, and defecation disorder).

Defecation Disorder

Defecation disorder constipation is the result of pelvic floor dysfunction, specifically the inability to coordinate pelvic floor and sphincter relaxation with abdominal muscle contraction; the individual strains to pass the stool but is unable to empty the rectum effectively due to the functional obstruction created by persistent contraction of the anal sphincter (dyssynergia). Dysfunctional defecation may occur in people with normal stool consistency as well as those who have severe constipation.

Dyssynergic defecation can also occur due to mechanical causes such as rectal tumors, strictures following anal trauma, and rectoanal intussusception. Enterocele (herniation of the small bowel into the vagina) and rectocele (prolapse of the rectum into the vagina) making defecation extremely painful and difficult, and the patient may, if asked, acknowledge that she has to insert 1 to 2 fingers into the vagina to enable defecation, this is called "splinting" (Grossi et al., 2017). Women with enterocele or rectocele may have coexisting symptoms including rectal bleeding and urinary incontinence (Grossi et al., 2017). Pelvic organ prolapse may result in obstructed defecation, requiring the woman to manually support the perineum to facilitate defecation (splinting). In obtaining the history of a patient with suspected obstructed defecation, it is essential to ask about manual maneuvers used to evacuate stool, because patients may not volunteer this information due to embarrassment.

Some of the conditions resulting in dyssynergic defecation are evident either on visual inspection or on anorectal examination (e.g., tumors and strictures). A preliminary assessment of pelvic floor dyssynergia can be made during anorectal examination by asking the patient to relax the sphincter and bear down as if trying to pass stool or gas. A normal response is visible relaxation of the anal sphincter accompanied by a downward push. The individual with pelvic floor dyssynergia will bear down but will be unable to relax the sphincter. However, some conditions can be identified only with defecography, a radiographic visualization of rectoanal function during attempted evacuation of contrast thickened to the consistency of stool. In the absence of symptoms, "red flags" or history suggesting risk of bowel cancer, colonoscopy is seldom indicated in the assessment of constipation.

Symptoms of a defecation disorder include prolonged toileting time, rectal pain, excessive straining followed by a sensation of incomplete emptying, and difficulty passing even soft stools (Camilleri et al., 2017). Transit time through the colon is usually normal, as the pathology involves the pelvic floor and anorectal junction. Prolonged defecatory dysfunction leads to complications including chronic rectal distention (megarectum), pelvic floor muscle spasticity, weakening of the perineal musculature, and rectal ulcerations. Various diagnostic tests can be used to confirm dyssynergic defecation: balloon expulsion, electromyography, water-perfused or high-resolution anorectal manometry, colonic manometry, contrast enema, and defecography, alone or in combination (Palmer et al., 2019). High-resolution anorectal manometry which provide greater detail on colon contractile activity is currently used in research settings (Prichard & Bharucha, 2018).

KEY POINT

Dyssynergic defecation disorder is the result of pelvic floor dysfunction (inability to coordinate pelvic floor and sphincter relaxation with abdominal muscle contraction) or a mechanical obstruction due to rectocele, enterocele in women or rectal prolapse, tumor, stricture, etc.

TREATMENT

Treatment of constipation is based on the underlying cause. Although the initial care for constipation may be initiated independently either by the generalist or by the continence nurse, other types of constipation require interdisciplinary care that involves gastroenterologists, colorectal and general surgeons, diagnostic imaging professionals, physical therapists, and advanced practice nurses. In addition to conventional medical and surgical care, clients may benefit from complementary therapy such as biofeedback therapy.

KEY POINT

Treatment of constipation is based on the specific type and underlying cause but typically involves lifestyle modifications to assure appropriate stool consistency and normal posture for defecation and selective use of laxatives and enemas.

Lifestyle Modifications

Lifestyle modifications can be taught to both adult clients and parents of children with simple constipation. The critical components of lifestyle modification include increased intake of fiber and fluid, increased activity, and elimination or reduction of constipating medications. Increased dietary fiber is recommended but must be accompanied by an increase in fluid intake to prevent further constipation. The current recommendation for fiber intake in adults is about 14 g/1,000 calories. For females between 21 and 50, this is 25 g/day and for adult males, 38 g/day, balanced with sufficient fluid intake (approximately 1,500 to 2,500 mL/day). For women over age 50, 21 g/day is recommended. Fiber affects bowel function in several ways, including (1) increased moisture content and softening of stool, (2) increased stool bulk, (3) decreased colonic transit time, and (4) promotion of normal microbial balance through its role as a prebiotic; the normal flora add further bulk to the stool. Chapter 6 discusses lifestyle modification in further detail.

KEY POINT

The current recommendation for fiber intake in adults is 14 g/1,000 calories; fiber acts to soften the stool, increase stool bulk, reduce colonic transit time, and promote normal microbial balance.

Dietary fibers differ in their solubility in water, as well as their fermentability within the colon. These differences result in different clinical effects. *Soluble, highly fermentable fiber* substances do not reduce fecal transit time and primarily "work" through a mild laxative effect and by adding water and bulk to the stool. Included in this group are fructo-oligosaccharides (FOS), pectin, guar gum, and inulin. OTC fiber supplements in this category include Fiber Choice and Benefiber. *Soluble fiber with reduced fermentation properties* is found in psyllium and β-glucans, such as oat bran. This type of fiber provides a much better laxative effect because it reduces transit time in addition to increasing stool bulk and retaining water to keep stool soft (Okawa et al., 2019). Various psyllium fiber supplements are available and include brand names such as Metamucil, Konsyl, Serutan, and Fiberall. *Insoluble, partially fermentable fiber* includes sources such as wheat bran, flax seed, whole grain cereals, quinoa, and vegetables. This type of fiber reduces fecal transit time and is therefore an effective laxative. Like soluble fibers that are only partially fermented in the colon, insoluble partially fermentable fibers provide an overall increase in bacterial species (Okawa et al., 2019). *Insoluble, nonfermentable fiber* is found in nuts, seeds, fruit, and vegetable peels, and the food additive cellulose; these substances reduce transit time significantly and provide a strong laxative effect. Citrucel is an OTC supplement containing cellulose. High-fiber foods and supplements that are fermentable cause increased flatulence; thus, individuals are usually advised to begin with low-dose supplementation and to gradually increase the daily dose until the desired stool consistency is obtained. Increased activity is also recommended, because activity stimulates peristalsis and decreases transit time (time required for stool to pass through the bowel), resulting in softer stool. Finally, the nurse should collaborate with the patient and prescribing provider to reduce or eliminate constipating medications, such as those with anticholinergic effects.

KEY POINT

Lifestyle modification is first-line treatment for normal transit constipation which includes fluid, fiber, and exercise. However, fiber supplements are not recommended in people who suffer slow-transit constipation.

Laxatives and Enemas
Although initial management of functional constipation usually includes lifestyle modifications (Camilleri et al., 2017), these measures may be insufficient in and of themselves. This is particularly true for patients with slow-transit constipation, for whom increased fiber intake may actually be contraindicated. Laxatives are usually a second line of treatment for both normal-transit and slow-transit constipation. Laxatives produce bowel movements through various physiologic mechanisms, including stool bulking, osmosis, and direct stimulation of peristalsis. **Table 21-6** provides information regarding the mechanism of action for different laxative categories and key nursing administration issues. The only type of laxatives routinely recommended on a long-term basis are high-fiber foods or fiber supplements, such as psyllium.

KEY POINT

Laxatives are considered second-line interventions for normal and slow-transit constipation.

Use of osmotic and stimulant agents for periods longer than 2 weeks should be supervised by an advanced practice nurse or physician. The continence nurse should realize that osmotic agents work by distending the bowel and *can* safely be used on a repetitive basis when needed, whereas stimulant laxatives activate the nerve cells within the bowel wall and are recommended for intermittent use only. Whenever any laxative is used, observation and documentation of stool frequency, form, color, and the ease or difficulty of stool elimination are important nursing assessments. Abdominal pain, nausea and/or vomiting, and fever all indicate possible peritoneal inflammation and are strict contraindications to laxative use.

KEY POINT

Osmotic agents work by distending the bowel and can safely be used on a repetitive basis when needed, whereas stimulant laxatives activate nerve cells within the bowel wall and are recommended for intermittent use only.

Laxatives are most commonly used on an "as-needed" basis for treatment of simple constipation, or in combination with lifestyle changes for those with functional normal-transit constipation. For some individuals with functional slow-transit constipation, laxatives may be required on a routine basis. For on-going use, osmotic agents are generally considered the agent of choice, for two reasons: (1) these agents "work" by distending the bowel and softening the stool and may be more effective than stimulant agents in patients with reduced peristalsis and (2) there are concerns that routine use of stimulant agents may adversely affect motility over the long term.

The continence nurse frequently needs to provide patient education regarding the safety of appropriately used laxative agents, because many people have been taught that long-term or routine use of *any* laxative is dangerous. While routine use of laxatives should not be used as a substitute for healthy lifestyle modifications, appropriate use of laxatives is an essential element of management for most individuals with slow-transit constipation, and patients should be counseled appropriately. A cross-sectional survey identified improved stool frequency and consistency with appropriate use of laxatives (Fosnes et al., 2011). Routine use of laxatives is also appropriate for management of constipation secondary to medication usage when the medication cannot be discontinued, such as the patient who requires opioid analgesics.

KEY POINT

Appropriate use of laxatives is an essential element of management for most individuals with slow-transit constipation, and patients should be counseled appropriately.

TABLE 21-6 COMMONLY PRESCRIBED LAXATIVES

GENERIC NAME BRAND NAME(S)	ACTION	NURSING ACTIONS
FIBER SUPPLEMENT		
Psyllium Metamucil Konsyl Fiberall	Absorb water to add bulk to the stool, which promotes peristalsis	Encourage fluid intake 1,500–2,000 mL/day Assess regularly for bloating, distention, bowel sounds Withhold for constipation accompanied by abdominal pain, nausea, vomiting, especially if accompanied by fever
OSMOTIC AGENTS		
Lactulose Polyethylene glycol (PEG) Miralax PEG with electrolytes Colyte Golytely	Draw water into the bowel lumen to increase water content of stool	Assess regularly for bloating, distention, bowel sounds Monitor for belching, flatulence, abdominal cramping Lactulose may increase glucose in diabetics PEG and lactulose not for use >2 weeks PEG with electrolytes used only for bowel preparation; extreme caution with persons who do not have gag reflex
HYPERTONIC AGENTS		
Phosphate/biphosphate Fleet enema Visicol OsmoPrep	Inhibit water and electrolyte reabsorption in small intestine, causing water retention and increasing peristalsis	Assess regularly for bloating, distention, bowel sounds Often used as bowel preparation for procedures Caution with renal or cardiac disease due to electrolyte changes Administer early in day to avoid sleep pattern disturbance
Magnesium salts Milk of magnesia Citrate of magnesia Slow-Mag	Draw water into bowel lumen via osmosis	Assess regularly for bloating, distention, bowel sounds Caution in persons with renal insufficiency
STIMULANTS		
Bisacodyl Dulcolax Carter's Little Pills Feen-A-Mint Sennosides Ex-Lax Senokot Fletcher's Castoria	Stimulation of peristalsis through direct action on the colon to produce fluid accumulation	Assess regularly for bloating, distention, bowel sounds May decrease absorption of other oral medications Assess regularly for bloating, distention, bowel sounds May change urine color
STOOL SOFTENERS		
Docusate sodium Colace Docusate calcium Surfak	Softens feces by absorption of water into stool	Assess regularly for bloating, distention, bowel sounds Administer with full glass of water or juice Do not administer within 2 hours of other laxative, especially mineral oil due to risk of increased absorption

Data from Deglin, J. H., Vallerand, A. H., & Sanoski, C. (2013). *Davis's drug guide for nurses* (13th ed.). Philadelphia, PA: F.A. Davis.

Persons with neurogenic bowel due to spinal cord injury, multiple sclerosis, or a progressive neurologic disease often require regular use of stool softeners combined with stimulant laxatives or suppositories. To prevent severe constipation, fecal impaction, and stool leakage, establishment of a regularly scheduled time of day for bowel evacuation and use of digital stimulation and/or a suppository is needed. A Cochrane review revealed very little high-quality evidence to support any specific laxative or bowel management protocol for individuals with neurogenic bowel due to central nervous system disease or injury (Coggrave & Norton, 2013). See Chapter 22 for further discussion of neurogenic bowel management.

Enemas are often administered for treatment of short-term constipation. Small-volume prepackaged hypertonic enemas are designed to stimulate rapid evacuation, but they may cause electrolyte disturbances and must therefore be used with caution in older (>70) patients as well as those with renal insufficiency and cardiac disease. Large-volume enemas are typically used for bowel cleansing, usually in preparation for a surgical or diagnostic procedure.

Management of Fecal Impaction

Fecal impaction is a potential complication of severe constipation and causes significant morbidity and patient distress; thus, the goal is prompt (and ideally painless) elimination of the obstructing fecal mass and measures to prevent recurrence. Whenever possible, the fecal mass is gently broken up by digital manipulation, and a cleansing enema is then administered to eliminate the retained stool. If the fecal mass is very hard, it may be necessary to first administer an oil-retention enema or a milk and molasses enema to soften the mass so that it can be broken up digitally. Once the mass has been broken up, a cleansing enema can be administered. (See Chapter 22 for further information on oil-retention and milk and molasses enemas.) An oral laxative may be given as well to assure effective colonic cleansing.

Digital Removal of Feces

Digital removal of feces is a procedure commonly included in fundamental nursing textbooks. However, the procedure is not without risks, and there is little research evidence to guide the practice (Mitchell, 2019). Although routine digital stimulation and/or evacuation are frequently required for individuals with neurogenic bowel conditions, the procedure should be considered a last resort for individuals with normal peristaltic function. Pain, bleeding, anal or rectal tears, and bradycardia due to vagal nerve stimulation are all potential complications of digital evacuation of stool (Falcon et al., 2016). In the spinal cord–injured individual with a lesion at thoracic vertebra 6 or higher, autonomic dysreflexia is an additional risk. Thus, the priority in nursing management should be prompt identification of patients at risk for constipation and aggressive intervention to prevent severe constipation and fecal impaction. When manual disimpaction is required, the procedure should be carried out with extreme caution and only after a complete bowel assessment has been performed (Mitchell, 2019). The continence nurse should always advocate for client safety during digital removal of feces.

> ### KEY POINT
>
> Although routine digital stimulation and/or evacuation are frequently required for individuals with neurogenic bowel conditions, the procedure should be considered a last resort for individuals with normal peristaltic function.

Alternative Therapies

Various complementary and alternative therapies are described in the literature for treatment of constipation. Although some may be useful, there is a lack of high-quality research to recommend these therapies for wide adoption in practice. Two separate studies identified a desire for symptom relief and symptom distress as major reasons for the use of alternative medicine (Stake-Nilsson et al., 2012; van Tilburg et al., 2008).

Chinese herbal medicine has received a great deal of research, disseminated primarily in Chinese journals. Unfortunately, many of the studies have methodological issues such as insufficient information on product quality, no or inappropriate comparison group, and small sample sizes. There is also limited information on potential for herb–drug interactions (Zhong et al., 2016). A systematic review of the effectiveness of abdominal massage revealed a similar problem with methodological rigor (Ernst, 1999). While complementary and alternative therapy may provide new directions for treatment of chronic constipation, more research, particularly well-designed clinical trials, must be conducted to measure their effectiveness.

Biofeedback

Biofeedback has been evaluated as a treatment for encopresis in children and dyssynergic defecation in both children and adults. Slow-transit constipation is less responsive to biofeedback than defecatory disorder. Approximately 60% of patients with defecatory dyssynergia experience long-term relief of symptoms (Narayanan & Bharucha, 2019). Many patients may not have access to treatment centers. A systematic review of 17 RCTs comparing biofeedback to other methods of treatment for constipation or encopresis did not find a significant difference between groups and concluded that there is insufficient evidence to recommend biofeedback as a treatment modality for these individuals (Woodward et al., 2014). Evidence regarding biofeedback suffers from the same methodologic deficiencies as those affecting studies of complementary and alternative therapy. However, given the paucity of treatment options and the fact that the modality is safe and provides at least modest benefit for some patients, it is an option to be considered when other strategies have failed, especially for treatment of defecation dyssynergia.

Sacral Neuromodulation

Sacral neuromodulation is a procedure done for persons who are not candidates for biofeedback or other strategies. Sacral neuromodulation is a long-term treatment approach that uses implantable electrodes and a stimulation device to modulate colonic function. Candidates are screened for response to sacral neuromodulation before permanent implantation. Specifically, temporary leads are placed percutaneously and attached to an external stimulator; subjects then maintain a bowel diary for an average of 2 weeks. If there is a significant improvement in bowel function, the individual undergoes surgery to implant the electrodes and stimulation device. One prospective study demonstrated improvement in bowel function that was sustained at 60 months in 23% of persons with constipation refectory to medical and behavioral treatment

(Maeda et al., 2017). Furthermore, 61% of individuals had device-related adverse events including abdominal pain, constipation, device dislocation, or implant site pain. Further study is needed to determine the role of sacral neuromodulation in addressing constipation.

Surgical Treatment

Surgical approaches to the treatment of chronic constipation include procedures designed to address specific anatomic problems (such as resection of an acontractile section of bowel) and procedures that enhance management of the underlying functional issue.

For women with obstructed defecation due to pelvic organ prolapse, rectocele or enterocele, surgical intervention involves correction of the underlying problem. For persons with slow-transit constipation, surgical options include total colectomy with ileoanal anastomosis, low anterior resection, and anterior resection (Kumar et al., 2013). For children with Hirschsprung disease, surgical treatment involves removal of aganglionic bowel, pulling the healthy bowel down, and connecting it to the anal opening (Kumar et al., 2013).

In contrast, the Malone antegrade continence enema (MACE procedure) is designed to enhance management of slow-transit constipation. Surgery involves creation of a small stoma connecting the abdominal wall to the proximal colon; to empty the bowel, the individual inserts a small catheter into the stoma and performs antegrade (to distal) "washouts" every day or every other day. (See Fig. 23-5, in Chapter 23.) The MACE has been used widely for children with chronic constipation and neurogenic bowel and is also now used for adults. Long-term results indicate positive patient satisfaction, though some individuals require revision due to stomal complications (Ellison et al., 2013), and others require additional surgical procedures such as partial colectomy, total colectomy with ileal–anal anastomosis, or total colectomy with Brooke ileostomy (Meurette et al., 2010). One pediatric surgical unit reported reversing 27.5% of procedures, with the majority of reversals due to the return of spontaneous, regular bowel movements (Peeraully et al., 2014).

KEY POINT

The Malone Antegrade Continence Enema permits "top-down" irrigations for individuals with chronic constipation and/or compromised bowel control.

IRRITABLE BOWEL SYNDROME

Functional GI disorders, including IBS, are among the most common and costly health care problems in the United States (Peery et al., 2019). Approximately 10% to 20% of adults experience chronic abdominal pain/discomfort and associated bowel changes (constipation and/or diarrhea) compatible with a diagnosis of IBS

(Drossman et al., 2016). In 2014, IBS accounted for over 585,061 outpatient visits and nearly 19 thousand emergency department visits. The public health impact is enormous with direct and indirect costs totaling approximately $3.1 billion/year (Peery et al., 2019); in addition, the symptom burden has a negative impact on quality of life (Heitkemper et al., 2011). In the United States as well as other Western countries, women seek health care services disproportionately more than men (Drossman et al., 2016).

IBS is typified by the presence of abdominal pain or discomfort associated with bowel pattern changes and/or relieved by bowel movements, with patients usually suffering from diarrhea, constipation, or mixed diarrhea and constipation. Effective, targeted therapies are limited in part by the fact that there is tremendous variability in bowel symptoms ranging from diarrhea, constipation, or mixed defecation patterns, and symptom severity ranges from mild to severe, or even disabling. **Box 21-2** lists the current diagnostic criteria for IBS.

KEY POINT

IBS is typified by the presence of abdominal pain or discomfort associated with bowel pattern changes and/or relieved by bowel movements, with patients usually suffering from diarrhea, constipation, or mixed diarrhea and constipation.

PATHOPHYSIOLOGY

The underlying pathophysiologic mechanisms of IBS likely involve an interplay among multiple factors, for example, visceral hypersensitivity, low-grade inflammation, increased GI permeability ("leaky gut"), abnormalities in the composition of the GI microbiota (bacteria, their genomes, metabolites, and interaction with the host), altered immune responses, autonomic nervous system dysfunction, altered bile acid metabolism, and psychological distress (Camilleri, 2018). Early life exposure to stress as well as ongoing psychologic distress may be significant factors in both the initiation and perpetuation of symptoms for some people with IBS. Recent studies of prognostic markers suggest that IBS can

---

BOX 21-2	DIAGNOSTIC CRITERIA FOR IRRITABLE BOWEL SYNDROME*

Irritable bowel syndrome is diagnosed by recurrent abdominal pain on average at least 1 day per week in the last 3 months, associated with two or more of the following:
- Related to defecation
- Associated with a change in frequency of stool
- Associated with a change in form (appearance) of stool

*Criteria fulfilled for the past 3 months with symptom onset at least 6 months prior to diagnosis.

develop from one or more of the following factors: adverse events and stress occurring early in life, significant life events producing moderate stress in adults, and/or luminal factors (e.g., infection or alterations in the GI microbiota that trigger immune activation) (Creed, 2019). IBS is a complex and not well-understood disease. It remains unclear whether stress is a primary causative factor or a risk factor. In a survey of young adults who were diagnosed with functional abdominal pain as children, 41% met the Rome III criteria for IBS (Horst et al., 2014). The presence of extraintestinal somatic conditions and depressive symptoms at the time of initial pediatric diagnosis was most predictive of adulthood IBS.

KEY POINT

The underlying pathophysiologic mechanisms of IBS likely involve an interplay among multiple factors, for example, visceral hypersensitivity, low grade inflammation, increased GI permeability ("leaky gut"), abnormalities in the composition of the GI microbiota (bacteria, their genomes, and interaction with the host), altered immune responses, autonomic nervous system dysfunction, altered bile acid metabolism, and psychological distress

Visceral hypersensitivity

Visceral hypersensitivity refers to increased sensitivity to luminal stimuli including gas and fecal material. Several studies have demonstrated that individuals with IBS are hypersensitive to colonic stimuli (Fuentes & Christianson, 2018). It has been suggested that hyperresponsiveness to visceral stimuli might explain the overlap of IBS with other conditions such as chronic pelvic pain, vulvodynia, and dysmenorrhea in women with IBS. The increased sensitivity may be due to peripheral factors including microbiome metabolites, inflammation, or abnormal central processing of afferent input.

Abnormalities in Gut Microflora

The largest microbial mass in the body is found in the GI tract, with estimates of >10^{13} organisms present. Recent studies have identified novel associations between the gut microbiota and diverse diseases such as obesity, diabetes, rheumatoid arthritis, colorectal cancer, IBD, Parkinson's, mental health disorders, and IBS (Hills et al., 2019). The microbiota affects immune and inflammatory responses within the GI tract itself, and research evidence suggests that the bacterial mix may also influence systemic inflammatory responses. For example, abnormal proportions of *Firmicutes* and *Bacteroides* have been identified in patients with type II diabetes (Dinan & Cryan, 2017; Grigorescu & Dumitrascu, 2016). These changes in the bacterial composition may induce a proinflammatory state as evidenced by elevated proinflammatory cytokine levels (Dinan & Cryan, 2017). A current hypothesis is that abnormalities in the bacterial mixture

activate mucosal immune responses that increase epithelial barrier permeability, activate nociceptive (pain) pathways, and cause dysfunction of the enteric nervous system, thus adversely affecting normal peristaltic activity (Dinan & Cryan, 2017; van Thiel et al., 2020).

Diet

Although dietary intake and IBS symptoms have long been linked, there are currently no data to prove a causal relationship between the two. While adults and children with IBS complain of subjective food intolerance more commonly than people without IBS (Chumpitazi et al., 2016), patients with IBS typically report dietary intake that is similar to their healthy counterparts. By convention, a patient with confirmed diet-related symptoms (e.g., celiac disease) is no longer considered to have IBS. Despite this, not only do the symptoms of IBS and celiac disease overlap but there is evidence that the prevalence of positive celiac serology as well as biopsy determined celiac disease is higher in individuals with IBS symptoms (Irvine et al., 2017).

An additional link between diet and IBS symptoms is the relationship between diet and the microbiome. Intake of poorly digested (fermentable) carbohydrates (i.e., oligo-, di-, and monosaccharides and polyols [FODMAPs]) alters the bacterial composition and activity resulting in increased gas production and abdominal pain/discomfort. The low-FODMAP diet has been shown to be effective in improving IBS symptoms in some patients (Muir & Gibson, 2013). Despite the improvement in symptoms, it may be challenging for adult patients to maintain a low FODMAP diet (Weynants et al., 2019). An interdisciplinary team approach involving dietitians in patient education regarding dietary changes is important (Rej et al., 2019).

Pharmacologic Influences

Various antibiotics alter bacterial balance by reducing bacterial diversity and creating a shift in bacteria taxa; these changes occur within the first few days of therapy. One week after a course of antibiotics either the prior stable state (norm) is reestablished or an altered stable state may become the "new" norm. The recovery of the gut microbiome even after a single dose of antibiotic is highly individualized (Koo et al., 2019). When the usual stable state and bacterial balance are altered, it can trigger changes in the immune response. For example, amoxicillin eradicates GI *Lactobacillus* spp. and alters levels of other aerobic and anaerobic bacteria; this can lead to increased mast cell protease expression and reduced immune response to specific antigens in the intestinal lumen. These changes in the bacterial balance and the immune response of the intestinal mucosa can increase the risk of GI infections such as *Clostridium difficile*. Proton pump inhibitors (PPIs) are another type of medication that may adversely affect the bacterial diversity and increase risk of inflammation (Takagi et al., 2018).

Genetic Predisposition

Family and twin studies have demonstrated that genetic predisposition may play a role in IBS development (Gazouli et al., 2016). Despite epidemiologic studies supporting a heritability contribution to the pathophysiology of IBS, a specific genetic cause has not been established. Candidate gene studies have examined specific variants in genes involved in mood, pain sensitivity, inflammation, immune function, and intestinal barrier proteins (Gazouli et al., 2016). Given the links between early childhood adversity, diet, microbiota, and IBS symptoms, the role of gene-environment interactions in IBS pathophysiology remains to be fully appreciated. Such study will require well-phenotyped 21 populations and use of standardized diagnosis and data collection protocols. Machine learning approaches using host and microbiota data may be needed to elucidate genetic and molecular factors contributing to symptoms.

ASSESSMENT AND DIAGNOSIS

There is no widely accepted biomarker for diagnosis of IBS or assessment of disease activity nor is there an accepted single causative factor (Drossman et al., 2016). The diagnosis and categorization of IBS are based on symptom-based Rome IV criteria (Drossman et al., 2016). Although these criteria are accepted and used by most clinicians, they do not capture all of the pathology associated with IBS that may impact the individual's response to therapy (e.g., pain severity and level of psychological distress). The Rome Committee developed the multidimensional clinical profile (MDCP) to characterize patients with IBS (Lin & Chang, 2018). Such an approach which takes into account clinical modifiers can serve as guide for clinicians to personalize therapy.

Diagnostic Criteria

At present, the diagnosis of IBS is based on the Rome IV criteria, coupled with the exclusion of organic disease via a careful history and physical examination and, when indicated, diagnostic procedures such as CT scan and endoscopy. The clinician should, however, be aware that many people with IBS experience symptoms other than those outlined in the Rome IV criteria and should conduct a comprehensive interview designed to capture all factors contributing to the individual's distress; for example, many individuals report increased intestinal gas and fecal urgency. Patients should be encouraged to keep a symptom diary, and it is helpful to use a validated tool such as the Bristol Stool Chart to accurately determine usual stool consistency. (See Fig. 6-7 in Chapter 6.) As noted in the diagnostic criteria, alterations in bowel patterns range from diarrhea to constipation and can be mixed or alternating. Because of the variability in patterns, specific subtypes were designated by the Rome IV criteria (Drossman et al., 2016) and are listed in **Box 21-3**.

BOX 21-3	SUBTYPING IRRITABLE BOWEL SYNDROME BY PREDOMINANT STOOL PATTERN

To subtype patients according to their bowel habit for research or clinical trials, the following subclassification may be used. The validity and stability of such subtypes over time are unknown and should be the subject of future research.

IBS with predominant diarrhea (IBS-D)
>25% of bowel movements with Bristol stool types 6 or 7* and <25% of bowel movement with Bristol stool types 1 or 2.†

IBS with predominant constipation (IBS-C)
>25% of bowel movements with Bristol stool types 1 or 2* and <25% of bowel movement with Bristol stool types 6 or 7.†

IBS with mixed bowel habit (IBS-M)
>25% of bowel movements with Bristol stool types 1 or 2* and >25% of bowel movement with Bristol stool types 6 or 7.†.

IBS Unclassified (IBS-U)
Patients who meet diagnostic criteria for IBS but whose bowel habits cannot be accurately categorized into 1 of the 3 groups (IBS-D, IBS-C, or IBS-M) should be categorized as having IBS-U

IBS subtype determination should be determined when the patient is evaluated off medications used to treat bowel pattern abnormalities.

*Bristol Stool Form Scale 6 to 7 (fluffy pieces with ragged edges, a mushy stool or watery, no solid pieces, entirely liquid).
†Bristol Stool Form Scale 1 to 2 (separate hard lumps like nuts "difficult to pass" or sausage shaped but lumpy).

KEY POINT

Diagnosis of IBS is based on the Rome IV criteria, coupled with the exclusion of organic disease via a careful history and physical examination and, when indicated, diagnostic procedures such as CT scan and endoscopy.

History and Physical Examination

IBS can usually be diagnosed by a thorough history and physical examination, with a focus on the types of symptoms, symptom severity, and presence of any "alarm" signs and symptoms. In addition to abdominal pain and discomfort associated with altered bowel function, patients with IBS often report various comorbid conditions, including headache with aura, chronic pelvic pain, temporomandibular joint syndrome, fibromyalgia, chronic fatigue, and, for women, menstrual discomfort. The clinician should be alert to any signs and symptoms that would suggest specific pathology and warrant further investigation; "alarm" signs and symptoms include fever, blood in the stool, anemia, unintentional weight loss, rectal bleeding, and increased levels of inflammatory markers.

The history should include queries as to the onset of symptoms, travel history (especially travel to areas where exposure to infectious enteric disease is likely), medication history to include OTC medications (with particular attention to recent intake of antibiotics), diet, and current and past stressors. Symptoms may begin in childhood or may be linked to a moderate-to-severe episode of enteritis or stress. The individual should be queried about any observed relationship between IBS symptoms and intake of foods containing gluten or complex fermentable carbohydrates (FODMAPs). Although the incidence of objectively proven celiac disease in the general population is quite low, some patients report that their symptoms improve with a gluten-free diet, and many report improved symptomatology with reduced intake of complex fermentable carbohydrates.

Diagnostic Tests

Diagnostic testing, in the absence of alarm symptoms, is usually limited to fecal occult blood testing and serum tests to rule out anemia and elevated levels of inflammatory markers such as C-reactive protein or fecal calprotectin (Chey et al., 2015). Screening for celiac disease is recommended for patients with IBS-D (IBS with diarrhea) and involves measurement of serum IgA antibody to tissue transglutaminase. Food allergy testing is rarely indicated in the diagnostic workup for IBS. Scanning and endoscopy are indicated only for patients with "alarm" symptoms.

MANAGEMENT

Management of IBS is symptom-based and includes individualized patient education, dietary modifications, routine exercise and stress management, and medications. A suggested algorithm is presented in **Figure 21-2**.

Patient Education

The first step in management of IBS, regardless of the predominant bowel pattern, is education. Individuals often have had symptoms for some time and may have consulted with other health care providers; many are very concerned that they have cancer or some other serious underlying condition. Developing a trusting relationship by actively listening to the history and concerns is foundational to effective management. Initial education should address the following points:

1. IBS is a common disorder that causes significant physical and emotional distress, but it is not life threatening and does not increase the risk for cancer.
2. At present, there is no known "cure" for IBS, but there are various treatment strategies that can significantly reduce symptoms and improve quality of life.
3. Determining the best treatment plan involves some trial and error and is unique for each individual.

As noted, there is currently no "cure" for IBS; thus, it is imperative for the clinician to work with the patient to establish realistic goals and strategies for self-management. A

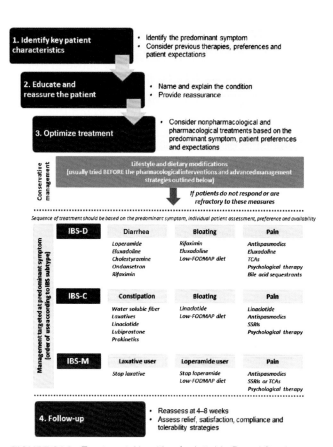

FIGURE 21-2. Treatment Algorithm for Irritable Bowel Syndrome. (From Moayyedi, P., Mearin, F., Azpiroz, F., et al. (2017). Irritable bowel syndrome diagnosis and management: A simplified algorithm for clinical practice. *United European Gastroenterology Journal, 5*(6), 773–788. doi: 10.1177/2050640617731968. Reprinted with permission from Fairview General Hospital, Cleveland, OH.)

very helpful initial strategy is to have the patient maintain a 2-week symptom diary that includes a Bristol Stool Form chart, in which the patient can simultaneously track their bowel symptoms and stool elimination patterns. This information can then be reviewed by the care provider and individual at follow-up visits and used as a baseline for assessment in improvement.

KEY POINT

Management of IBS is symptom based and individualized; it includes patient education, dietary modifications, routine exercise and stress management, and medications.

Dietary Modifications

Modification in diet is typically the first step in self-management of IBS. Foods known to create gas and the sensation of bloating are a logical focus for trial elimination and include beans, onions, celery, carrots, raisins, bananas, apricots, prunes, and Brussels sprouts. Elimination or reduction of FODMAPs and lactose-containing foods has been shown to be effective for some patients with IBS (Algera et al., 2019). A 2-week trial of dietary elimination is often recommended and should be enough to provide insight into any link between dietary intake and symptom severity. Identification of any foods that cause exacerbation of symptoms allows the patient to make his or her own decisions as to reduction, timing, or elimination; some individuals find long-term adherence to elimination of particular foods to be difficult and may elect selected intake as opposed to complete elimination.

Exercise/Activity and Stress Management

Physical activity may also help reduce symptoms. Limited research indicates that patients enrolled in an intervention trial experienced a reduction in symptoms following a 12-week exercise intervention program (Camilleri, 2018). Routine exercise may also help to reduce stress, which is known to be a trigger for symptom flares. Other stress management therapies may also be beneficial. For example, cognitively focused therapies such as cognitive-behavior therapy (CBT) may be helpful and can be delivered over the phone, Web site, or in person by a trained provider (Cangemi & Lacy, 2019; Lackner et al., 2018). However, the minimum number of sessions to deliver content related to relaxation and cognitive restructuring remains to be determined, and it can be challenging for patients to find providers who can provide this type of intervention.

Sleep disturbance can be regarded as one of the most important extraintestinal symptoms of IBS, which markedly affects quality of life and psychosocial well-being (Tu et al., 2017). Mind-body therapy such as hypnosis and sleep hygiene may help decrease symptoms (Ballou & Keefer, 2017; Thakur et al., 2018).

Pharmacologic Therapy

The choice of medication(s) is based on the predominant bowel syndrome (Ford et al., 2018; Moayyedi et al., 2019). For some patients, particularly those with IBS-C (IBS with constipation), the addition of psyllium/ispaghula improves stool bulk and intestinal transit time and reduces constipation (El-Salhy et al., 2017). Soluble fiber, osmotic laxatives, and newer agents including tenapanor (sodium/hydrogen exchanger 3 [NHE3] inhibitor), plecanatide, lubiprostone, and linaclotide may also be recommended for individuals with IBS-C resistant to lifestyle modification and OTC medications (Brenner et al., 2018; Chey et al., 2020; Ford et al., 2018; Hayat et al., 2019; Prichard & Bharucha, 2018). Osmotic laxatives, for example PEG, are commonly prescribed when the addition of soluble fiber is insufficient to normalize stool consistency and elimination. While laxatives frequently correct the constipation, they do not decrease the abdominal pain/discomfort and are used only as needed for constipation management. For patients who fail to respond to psyllium and PEG, lubiprostone or linaclotide may be prescribed. Lubiprostone

acts directly on the chloride channel activator to increase intestinal secretion and ultimately speed stool expulsion. Linaclotide is a guanylate cyclase agonist that stimulates intestinal secretion and peristalsis.

Several preliminary results indicate that serotonin norepinephrine reuptake inhibitors (SNRI) have efficacy in reducing pain as well as comorbid depression and anxiety (Camilleri, 2018). There is less evidence about selective serotonin reuptake inhibitors (SSRI) and tricyclic antidepressants in the management of IBS (Camilleri, 2018).

People with IBS-D may be prescribed antidiarrheal agents for short-term use such as loperamide. While effective in reducing IBS diarrhea, it does not reduce the abdominal pain/discomfort, which is a limiting factor in its use. Another agent that may be tried when bile acid malabsorption is suspected is a bile acid sequestrant (e.g., cholestyramine). For women only with severe diarrhea for whom other treatments are not effective after a 6-month period, the $5-HT_3$ receptor antagonist alosetron (Lotronex) may be trialed. Of note, health care providers (e.g., doctors) who prescribe alosetron must be specially certified to prescribe due to risk of ischemic colitis (Rising Pharmaceuticals, 2018). Other pharmacologic options include rifaximin, an antibiotic that reduces bacterial overgrowth in the small intestine, has been shown to reduce IBS-D symptoms especially bloating when used as a short course agent, that is 2-week, but retreatment often is needed (Levio & Cash, 2017; Li et al., 2016; Saadi & McCallum, 2013). Eluxadoline, a mu- and kappa-opioid receptor agonist and a delta-opioid receptor antagonist, was recently approved by the FDA due to its ability to effectively slow gut transit time (Cash et al., 2016; Ford et al., 2018; Fragkos, 2017; Moayyedi et al., 2019) although contraindicated in individuals without a gallbladder due to the risk of pancreatitis and sphincter of Oddi spasms (Levio & Cash, 2017). Rifaximin and eluxadoline should be considered first-line therapy for IBS-D if lifestyle modification and OTC medications proved to be ineffectual (Levio & Cash, 2017). Alosetron should only be initiated in women if all other therapies are exhausted due to the black box warning and risk for severe constipation and ischemic colitis (Friedel et al., 2001; Levio & Cash, 2017).

Antispasmodic agents may be prescribed on an as-needed basis for relief of cramping abdominal pain; the most commonly used agents are dicyclomine and hyoscyamine, which are direct-acting GI smooth muscle relaxants. For patients with IBS-D or IBS-M (IBS with mixed symptoms of constipation and diarrhea) in whom infectious enteritis is suspected, a trial of the nonabsorbable antibiotic rifaximin may be indicated as previously described. Antidepressants, in particular tricyclic agents, have been shown in randomized clinical trials to decrease symptoms such as abdominal pain and diarrhea in patients with IBS-D; in addition, they are associated with an improved sense of well-being. There is less evidence about SSRIs and SNRIs in the management of IBS.

Probiotics may be helpful for some patients with IBS (Moayyedi et al., 2019). Probiotics are believed to suppress the growth and luminal binding of pathogenic bacteria and thereby to improve epithelial barrier function and reduce inflammation. However, clinical studies are needed to evaluate safety, dosing, and concentrations of the various probiotics and to determine optimal duration of treatment (Moayyedi et al., 2019).

KEY POINT

Probiotics may be helpful for some patients with IBS; however, clinical studies are needed to evaluate the dose and concentration of various agents as well as the optimal duration of treatment.

 ## CONCLUSION

Functional bowel disorders such as constipation, diarrhea, and IBS are extremely common and exert a significant toll in terms of health care expenditures and quality of life. Effective management begins with a thorough history and focused physical examination to rule out "alarm symptoms" and to determine the specific disorder, associated symptomatology, and impact. Individuals with alarm symptoms must be promptly referred for further workup; individuals with no alarm symptoms can be managed symptomatically, with a focus on patient education, lifestyle modifications (e.g., fiber and fluid intake, dietary modifications, and exercise), and judicious use of pharmacologic agents (e.g., laxatives, antidiarrheals, and antispasmodic agents). A trusting patient/provider relationship is essential to effective management in all situations. Individuals with persistent diarrhea, slow-transit constipation, or dyssynergic defecation may require further workup and additional medical–surgical therapies.

REFERENCES

Aburub, A., Fischer, M., Camilleri, M., et al. (2018). Comparison of pH and motility of the small intestine of healthy subjects and patients with symptomatic constipation using the wireless motility capsule. *International Journal of Pharmaceutics, 544*(1), 158–164. doi: 10.1016/j.ijpharm.2018.04.031.

Ackley, B. J., Ladwig, G. B., Makic, M. B. F., et al. (2020). *Nursing diagnosis handbook: An evidenced-based guide to planning care* (12th ed.). St. Louis, MO: Elsevier.

Albiani, J. J., Hart, S. L., Katz, L., et al. (2013). Impact of depression and anxiety on the quality of life of constipated patients. *Journal of Clinical Psychology in Medical Settings, 20*(1), 123–132. doi: 10.1007/s10880-012-9306-3.

Algera, J., Colomier, E., & Simrén, M. (2019). The dietary management of patients with irritable bowel syndrome: A narrative review of the existing and emerging evidence. *Nutrients, 11*(9), 2162. doi: 10.3390/nu11092162.

Arnold, B. F., Barreto, M. L., Boisson, S., et al. (2011). Epidemiological methods in diarrhoea studies—An update. *International Journal of Epidemiology, 40*, 1678–1692. doi: 10.1093/ije/dyr152.

Ballou, S., & Keefer, L. (2017). Psychological interventions for irritable bowel syndrome and inflammatory bowel disease. *Clinical and Translational Gastroenterology, 8*(1), e214. doi: 10.1038/ctg.2016.69.

Barr, W., & Smith, A. (2014). Acute diarrhea. *American Family Physician, 89*(5), 180–189.

Beeckman, D., Van Damme, N., Schoonhoven, L., et al. (2016). Interventions for preventing and treating incontinence-associated dermatitis in adults. *The Cochrane Database of Systematic Reviews, 11*(11), CD011627. doi: 10.1002/14651858.CD011627.pub2.

Beeson, T., Eifrid, B., Pike, C. A., et al. (2017). Do intra-anal bowel management devices reduce incontinence-associated dermatitis and/or pressure injuries? *Journal of Wound Ostomy Continence Nursing, 44*(6), 583–588. doi: 10.1097/WON.0000000000000381.

Bharucha, A. E., Dorn, S. D., Lembo, A., et al. (2013a). American Gastroenterological Association medical position statement on constipation. *Gastroenterology, 144*(1), 211–217. doi: 10.1053/j.gastro.2012.10.029.

Bharucha, A. E., Pemberton, J. H., & Locke, G. R., III. (2013b). American Gastroenterological Association technical review on constipation. *Gastroenterology, 144*(1), 218–238.

Black, C. J., & Ford, A. C. (2018). Chronic idiopathic constipation in adults: Epidemiology, pathophysiology, diagnosis and clinical management. *Medical Journal of Australia, 16*(2), 86–91.

Brenner, D. M., Fogel, R., Dorn, S. D., et al. (2018). Efficacy, safety, and tolerability of plecanatide in patients with irritable bowel syndrome with constipation: Results of two phase 3 randomized clinical trials. *The American Journal of Gastroenterology, 113*(5), 735–745. doi: 10.1038/s41395-018-0026-7.

Cash, B. D., Lacy, B. E., Rao, T., et al. (2016). Rifaximin and eluxadoline—Newly approved treatments for diarrhea-predominant irritable bowel syndrome: What is their role in clinical practice alongside alosetron? *Expert Opinion on Pharmacotherapy, 17*(3), 311–322. doi: 10.1517/14656566.2016.1118052.

Camilleri, M. (2018). Management options for irritable bowel syndrome. *Mayo Clinic Proceedings, 93*(12), 1858–1872. doi: 10.1016/j.mayocp.2018.04.032.

Camilleri, M., Ford, A. C., Mawe, G. M., et al. (2017). Chronic constipation. *Nature Reviews Disease Primers, 14*(3), 17095. doi: 10.1038/nrdp.2017.95.

Candy, B., Jones, L., Vickerstaff, V., et al. (2018). Mu-opioid antagonists for opioid-induced bowel dysfunction in people with cancer and people receiving palliative care. *Cochrane Database of Systematic Reviews, 6*(6), CD006332. doi: 10.1002/14651858.CD006332.pub3.

Cangemi, D. J., & Lacy, B. E. (2019). Management of irritable bowel syndrome with diarrhea: A review of nonpharmacological and pharmacological interventions. *Therapeutic Advances in Gastroenterology, 12*, 1756284819878950. doi: 10.1177/1756284819878950.

Centers for Disease Control and Prevention. (2019). Surveillance for foodborne disease outbreaks United States, 2017: Annual report. Retrieved from https://www.cdc.gov/fdoss/pdf/2017_FoodBorne-Outbreaks_508.pdf

Chen, L. H., Leder, K., Barbre, K. A., et al. (2018). Business travel-associated illness: A GeoSentinel analysis. *Journal of Travel Medicine, 25*(1), 10. doi: 10.1093/jtm/tax097.

Chey, W. D., Kurlander, J., & Eswaran, S. (2015). Irritable bowel syndrome: A clinical review. *JAMA, 313*(9), 949–958. doi: 10.1001/jama.2015.0954.

Chey, W. D., Lembo, A. J., & Rosenbaum, D. P. (2020). Efficacy of tenapanor in treating patients with irritable bowel syndrome with constipation: A 12-week, placebo-controlled phase 3 trial (T3MPO-1). *The American Journal of Gastroenterology, 115*(2), 281–293. doi: 10.14309/ajg.0000000000000516.

Chumpitazi, B. P., Weidler, E. M., Lu, D. Y., et al. (2016). Self-perceived food intolerances are common and associated with clinical severity in childhood irritable bowel syndrome. *Journal of the Academy of Nutrition and Dietetics, 116*(9), 1458–1464. doi: 10.1016/j.jand.2016.04.017.

Coggrave, M., & Norton, C. (2013). Management of faecal incontinence and constipation in adults with central neurological diseases. *Cochrane Database of Systematic Reviews, 12*, CD002115. doi: 10.1002/14651858.CD002115.pub4.

Creed, F. (2019). Review article: The incidence and risk factors for irritable bowel syndrome in population-based studies. *Alimentary Pharmacology & Therapeutics, 50*(5), 507–516. doi: 10.1111/apt.15396.

Crockett, S. D., Greer, K. B., Heidelbaugh, J. J., et al. (2019). American Gastroenterological Association institute guideline on the medical management of opioid-induced constipation. *Gastroenterology, 156*(1), 218–226.

Dayananda, P., & Wilcox, M. H. (2019). A review of mixed strain *Clostridium difficile* colonization and infection. *Frontiers in Microbiology, 10*, 692. doi: 10.3389/fmicb.2019.00692.

Demers, M., Dagnault, A., & Desjardins, J. (2014). A randomized double-blind controlled trial: Impact of probiotics on diarrhea in patients treated with pelvic radiation. *Clinical Nutrition, 33*(5), 761–767. doi: 10.1016/j.clnu.2013.10.015.

Derwa, Y., Gracie, D. J., Hamlin, P. J., et al. (2017). Systematic review with meta-analysis: The efficacy of probiotics in inflammatory bowel disease. *Alimentary Pharmacology & Therapeutics, 46*(4), 389–400. doi: 10.1111/apt.14203.

Dinan, T. G., & Cryan, J. F. (2017). The Microbiome-Gut-Brain axis in health and disease. *Gastroenterology Clinics of North America, 6*(1), 77–89. doi: 10.1016/j.gtc.2016.09.007.

Drossman, D., Chang, L., Chey, W. D., et al. (2016). *Rome IV: Functional gastrointestinal disorders* (4th ed.). Raleigh, NC: The Rome Foundation.

Ellison, J. S., Haraway, A. N., & Park, J. M. (2013). The distal left Malone antegrade continence enema—Is it better? *The Journal of Urology, 190*(4 Suppl), 1529–1533. doi: 10.1016/j.juro.2013.01.092.

El-Salhy, M., Ystad, S. O., Mazzawi, T., et al. (2017). Dietary fiber in irritable bowel syndrome (Review). *International Journal of Molecular Medicine, 40*(3), 607–613. doi: 10.3892/ijmm.2017.3072.

Ernst, E. (1999). Abdominal massage therapy for chronic constipation: A systematic review of controlled clinical trials. *Forschende Komplementärmedizin, 6*(3), 149–151.

Falcón, B. S., Barceló López, M., Mateos Muñoz, et al. (2016). Fecal impaction: A systematic review of its medical complications. *BMC Geriatrics, 16*, 4. doi: 10.1186/s12877-015-0162-5.

Friedel, D., Thomas, R., & Fisher, R. S. (2001). Ischemic colitis during treatment with alosetron. *Gastroenterology, 120*(2), 557–560. doi: 10/1053/gast.2001.21177.

Fragkos, K. C. (2017). Spotlight on eluxadoline for the treatment of patients with irritable bowel syndrome with diarrhea. *Clinical and Experimental Gastroenterology, 10*, 229–240. doi: 10.2147/CEG.S12362120.

Ford, A. C., Moayyedi, P., Chey, W. D., et al. (2018). American College of Gastroenterology monograph on management of irritable bowel syndrome. *American Journal of Gastroenterology, 113*, 1. doi: 10.1038/s41395-018-0084-x.

Fosnes, G. S., Lydersen, S., & Farup, P. G. (2011). Effectiveness of laxatives in elderly—A cross sectional study in nursing homes. *BMC Geriatrics, 11*, 76. doi: 10.1186/1471-2318-11-76.

Fuentes, I. M., & Christianson, J. A. (2018). The influence of early life experience on visceral pain. *Frontiers in Systems Neuroscience, 12*, 2. doi: 10.3389/fnsys.2018.00002.

Ganji-Arjenaki, M., & Rafieian-Kopaei, M. (2018). Probiotics are a good choice in remission of inflammatory bowel diseases: A meta-analysis and systematic review. *Journal of Cell Physiology, 233*(3), 2091–2103. doi: 10.1002/jcp.25911.

Gazouli, M., Wouters, M. M., Kapur-Pojskić, L., et al. (2016). Lessons learned—Resolving the enigma of genetic factors in IBS. *Nature Reviews Gastroenterology & Hepatology, 13*(2), 77–87. doi: 10.1038/nrgastro.2015.206.

GBD Diarrhoeal Disease Collaborators. (2017). Estimates of global, regional, and national morbidity, mortality, and aetiologies of diarrhoeal disease: A systematic analysis for the Global Burden of Diseases Study 2015. *The Lancet, 17*(9), 909–948. doi: 10.1016/S1473-3099(17)30276-1.

Glass, D., Huang, D. T., Dugum, M., et al. (2018). Rectal trumpet-associated hemorrhage in the intensive care unit: A quality improvement initiative. *Journal of Wound Ostomy Continence Nursing, 45*(6), 516–520. doi: 10.1097/WON.0000000000000479.

Goldenberg, J. Z., Yap, C., Lytvyn, L., et al. (2017). Probiotics for the prevention of *Clostridium difficile*-associated diarrhea in adults and children. *Cochrane Database of Systematic Reviews, 12*, CD006095. doi: 10.1002/14651858.CD006095.pub4.

Gray, M., Kent, D., Ermer-Seltun, J., et al. (2018). Assessment, selection, use, and evaluation of body-worn absorbent products for adults with incontinence. *Journal of Wound Ostomy Continence Nurse, 45*(3), 243–264.

Gray, M., Omar, A., & Buziak, B. (2014). Stool management systems for preventing environmental spread of *Clostridium difficile*: A comparative trial. *Journal of Wound, Ostomy, and Continence Nursing, 41*(5), 460–465.

Grigorescu, I., & Dumitrascu, D. L. (2016). Implication of gut microbiota in diabetes mellitus and obesity. *Acta Endocrinologica, 12*(2), 206–214. doi: 10.4183/aeb.2016.206.

Grossi, U., Horrocks, E. J., Mason, J., et al. (2017). Surgery for constipation: Systematic review and practice recommendations: Results IV: Recto-vaginal reinforcement procedures. *Colorectal Disease, 19*(Suppl 3), 73–91. doi: 10.1111/codi.13781.

Guo, Q., Goldenberg, J. Z., Humphrey, C., et al. (2019). Probiotics for the prevention of pediatric antibiotic-associated diarrhea. *Cochrane Database of Systematic Reviews, 4*, CD004827. doi: 10.1002/14651858.CD004827.pub5.

Hayat, M., Zia, H., & Nusrat, S. (2019). Lubiprostone in the treatment of chronic idiopathic constipation: An update on health-related quality of life and patient-reported outcomes. *Patient Related Outcome Measures, 10*, 43–47. doi: 10.2147/PROM.S157905.

Heitkemper, M., Cain, K. C., Shulman, R., et al. (2011). Subtypes of irritable bowel syndrome based on abdominal pain/discomfort severity and bowel pattern. *Digestive Diseases and Sciences, 56*(7), 2050–2058. doi: 10.1007/s10620-011-1567-4.

Hills, R. D., Jr., Pontefract, B. A., Mishcon, H. R., et al. (2019). Gut microbiome: Profound implications for diet and disease. *Nutrients, 11*(7), 1613. doi: 10.3390/nu11071613.

Horst, S., Shelby, G., Anderson, J., et al. (2014). Predicting persistence of functional abdominal pain from childhood into young adulthood. *Clinical Gastroenterology and Hepatology, 12*(12), 2026–2032. doi: 10.1016/j.cgh.2014.03.034.

Irvine, A. J., Chey, W. D., & Ford, A. C. (2017). Screening for celiac disease in irritable bowel syndrome: An updated systematic review and meta-analysis. *American Journal of Gastroenterology, 112*(1), 65–76. doi: 10.1038/ajg.2016.466.

Joinson, C., Grzeda, M. T., von Gontard, A., et al. (2019). Psychosocial risks for constipation and soiling in primary school children. *European Child & Adolescent Psychiatry, 28*(2), 203–210. doi: 10.1007/s00787-018-1162-8.

Kirk, M. D., Pires, S. M., Black, R. E., et al. (2015). World Health Organization estimates of the global and regional disease burden of 22 foodborne bacterial, protozoal, and viral diseases, 2010: A data synthesis. *PLoS Medicine, 12*(12), e1001921. doi: 10.1371/journal.pmed.1001921.

Koo, H., Hakim, J. A., Crossman, D. K., et al. (2019). Individualized recovery of gut microbial strains post antibiotics. *NPJ Biofilms Microbiomes, 5*, 30. doi: 10.1038/s41522-019-0103-8. eCollection 2019.

Kotloff, K. L., Nataro, J. P., Blackwelder, W. C., et al. (2013). Burden and aetiology of diarrhoeal disease in infants and young children in developing countries (the Global Enteric Multicenter Study, GEMS): A prospective, case–control study. *Lancet, 382*(9888), 209–222.

Kumar, A., Lokesh, H., & Ghoshal, U. C. (2013). Successful outcome of refractory chronic constipation by surgical treatment: A series of

34 patients. *Journal of Neurogastroenterology and Motility, 19*(1), 78–84. doi: 10.5056/jnm.2013.19.1.78.

Lackner, J. M., Jaccard, J., Keefer, L. et al. (2018). Improvement in gastrointestinal symptoms after cognitive behavior therapy for refractory irritable bowel syndrome. *Gastroenterology, 155*(1), 47–57.

Lacy, B. E., Mearin, F., Chang, L., et al. (2016). Bowel disorders. *Gastroenterology, 150*, 1393–1407. doi: 10.1053/j.gastro.2016.02.031.

Lai, H. H., Chiu, C. H., Kong, M. S., et al., (2019). Probiotic *Lactobacillus casei*: Effective for managing childhood diarrhea by altering gut microbiota and attenuating fecal inflammatory markers. *Nutrients, 11*(5), 1150. doi: 10.3390/nu11051150.

Levio, S., & Cash, B. D. (2017). The place of eluxadoline in the management of irritable bowel syndrome with diarrhea. *Therapeutic Advances in Gastroenterology, 10*(9), 715–725. doi: 10.1177/1756283X17721152.

Li, J., Zhu, W., Liu, W., et al. (2016). Rifaximin for irritable bowel syndrome: A meta-analysis of randomized placebo-controlled trials. *Medicine, 95*(4), 2–6. doi: 10.1097/MD.0000000000002534.

Lin, L. D., & Chang, L. (2018). Using the Rome IV criteria to help manage the complex IBS patient. *The American Journal of Gastroenterology, 113*(4), 453–456. doi: 10.1038/ajg.2017.477.

Maeda, Y., Kamm, M. A., Vaizey, C. J., et al. (2017). Long-term outcome of sacral neuromodulation for chronic refractory constipation. *Techniques in Coloproctology, 21*(4), 277–286. doi: 10.1007/s10151-017-1613-0.

Makic, M. B. F., & Ackley, B. J. (2017). Diarrhea. In B. J. Ackley, G. B. Ladwig, & M. B. F. Makic (Eds.), *Nursing diagnosis handbook: An evidence-based guide to planning care* (11th ed., p. 332). Oxford, UK: Wiley Blackwell.

McElhanon, B. O., McCracken, C., Karpen, S., et al. (2014). Gastrointestinal symptoms in autism spectrum disorder: A meta-analysis. *Pediatrics, 133*(5), 872–883.

McFarland, L. V., & Goh, S. (2019). Are probiotics and prebiotics effective in the prevention of travellers' diarrhea: A systematic review and meta-analysis. *Travel Medicine and Infectious Diseases, 27*, 11–19. doi: 10.1016/j.tmaid.2018.09.007.

Meurette, G., Lehur, P. A., Coron, E., et al. (2010). Long-term results of Malone's procedure with antegrade irrigation for severe chronic constipation. *Gastroentérologie Clinique Et Biologique, 34*(3), 209–212. doi: 10.1016/j.gcb.2009.12.009.

Midenfjord, I., Polster, A., Sjövall, H., et al. (2019). Anxiety and depression in irritable bowel syndrome: Exploring the interaction with other symptoms and pathophysiology using multivariate analyses. *Neurogastroenterolgy & Motility, 31*(8), e13619. doi: 10.1111/nmo.13619.

Mitchell, A. (2019). Rationale and procedure for performing digital removal of faeces. *British Journal of Nursing, 28*(7), 430–433.

Moayyedi, P., Mearin, F., Azpiroz, F., et al. (2017). Irritable bowel syndrome diagnosis and management: A simplified algorithm for clinical practice. *United European Gastroenterology Journal, 5*(6), 773–788. doi: 10.1177/2050640617731968.

Moayyedi, P., Andrews, C. N., MacQueen, G., et al. (2019). Canadian Association of Gastroenterology clinical practice guideline for the management of irritable bowel syndrome (IBS). *Journal of the Canadian Association of Gastroenterology, 2*(1), 6–29. doi: 10.1093/jcag/gwy071.

Muir, J. G., & Gibson, P. R. (2013).The low FODMAP diet for treatment of irritable bowel syndrome and other gastrointestinal disorders. *Gastroenterology & Hepatology, 9*(7), 450-452.

Narayanan, S. P., & Bharucha, A. E. (2019). A practical guide to biofeedback therapy for pelvic floor disorders. *Current Gastroenterology Reports, 21*(5), 21. doi: 10.1007/s11894-019-0688-3.

National Digestive Diseases Information Clearinghouse. (2018). Constipation. Retrieved from https://www.niddk.nih.gov/health-information/digestive-diseases/constipation/definition-facts

Noiesen, E., Trosborg, I., Bager, L., et al. (2014). Constipation—Prevalence and incidence among medical patients acutely admitted to hospital with a medical condition. *Journal of Clinical Nursing, 23*(15/16), 2295–2302. doi: 10.1111/jocn.12511.

Ochoa, B., & Surawicz, C. M. (2012). Diarrheal diseases—Acute and chronic. Retrieved from https://gi.org/topics/diarrhea-acute-and-chronic/

Okawa, Y., Fukudo, S., & Sanada, H. (2019). Specific foods can reduce symptoms of irritable bowel syndrome and functional constipation: A review. *BioPsychoSocial Medicine, 13*, 10. doi: 10.1186/s13030-019-0152-5.

Oxford English Dictionary. (2019). Oxford, UK: Oxford University Press. Retrieved from https://www.lexico.com/en/definition/diarrhea

Palmer, S. L., Lalwani, N., Bahrami, S., et al. (2019). Dynamic fluoroscopic defecography: Updates on rationale, technique, and interpretation from the Society of Abdominal Radiology Pelvic Floor Disease Focus Panel. *Abdominal Radiology (NY).* doi: 10.1007/s00261-019-02169-y.

Peeraully, M. R., Lopes, J., Wright, A., et al. (2014). Experience of the MACE procedure at a regional pediatric surgical unit: A 15-year retrospective review. *European Journal of Pediatric Surgery, 24*(1), 113–116. doi: 10.1055/s-0033-1357502.

Peery, A. F., Crockett, S. D., Murphy, C., et al. (2019). Burden and cost of gastrointestinal, liver, and pancreatic diseases in the United States: Update 2018. *Gastroenterology, 156*(1), 254–272.e11. doi: 10.1053/j.gastro.2018.08.063.

Pietroni, M. A. C. (2019). Case management of cholera. *Vaccine,* (Suppl 1), A105–A109. doi: 10.1016/j.vaccine.2019.09.098.

Prichard, D. O., & Bharucha, A. E. (2018). Recent advances in understanding and managing chronic constipation. *F1000Research, 7,* F1000. doi: 10.12688/f1000research.15900.1.

Rao, S. S. C., Camilleri, M., Hasler, W. E., et al. (2011). Evaluation of gastrointestinal transit in clinical practice: Position paper of the American and European Neurogastroenterolgy and Motility Societies. *Neurogastroenterology & Motility, 23*, 8–23. doi: 10.1111/j.1365-2982.2010.0162.x.

Rej, A., Aziz, I., Tornblom, H., et al. (2019). The role of diet in irritable bowel syndrome: Implications for dietary advice. *Journal of Internal Medicine, 286*(5), 490–502. doi: 10.1111/joim.12966.

Rex, D. K., Boland, C. R., Dominitz, J. A., et al. (2017). Colorectal cancer screening: Recommendations for physicians and patients from the U.S. Multi-Society Task Force on Colorectal Cancer. *American Journal of Gastroenterology, 112*(7), 1016–1030. doi: 10.1038/ajg.2017.174.

Rising Pharmaceuticals. (2018). Alosetron—FDA prescribing information, side effects and uses. Retrieved from https://www.drugs.com/pro/alosetron.html

Saad, R. J. (2016). The wireless motility capsule: A one-stop shop for the evaluation of GI motility disorders. *Current Gastroenterology Reports, 18*(3), 14. doi: 10.1007/s11894-016-0489-x.

Saad, R. J., Rao, S. S. C., Koch, K. L., et al. (2010). Do stool form and frequency correlate with whole-gut and colonic transit? *American Journal of Gastroenterology, 105*(2), 403–411.

Saadi, M., & McCallum, R. W. (2013). Rifaximin in irritable bowel syndrome: Rationale, evidence and clinical use. *Therapeutic Advances in Chronic Disease, 4*(2), 71–75. doi: 10.1177/2040622312472008.

Sell, J., & Dolan, B. (2018). Common gastrointestinal infections. *Primary Care, 45*(3), 519–532. doi: 10.1016/j.pop.2018.05.008.

Stake-Nilsson, K., Hultcrantz, R., Unge, P., et al. (2012). Complementary and alternative medicine used by persons with functional gastrointestinal disorders to alleviate symptom distress. *Journal of Clinical Nursing, 21*(5–6), 800–808. doi: 10.1111/j.1365-2702.2011.03985.x.

Suares, N. C., & Ford, A. C. (2011). Prevalence of, and risk factors for, chronic idiopathic constipation in the community: Systematic review and meta-analysis. *American Journal of Gastroenterology, 106*, 1582–1591.

Takagi, T., Naito, Y., Inoue, R., et al. (2018). The influence of long-term use of proton pump inhibitors on the gut microbiota: An age-sex-matched case–control study. *Journal of Clinical Biochemistry and Nutrition, 62*(1), 100–105. doi: 10.3164/jcbn.17-78.

Thakur, E. R., Shapiro, J., Chan, J., et al. (2018). A systematic review of the effectiveness of psychological treatments for IBS in gastroenterology settings: Promising but in need of further study. *Digestive Diseases and Sciences, 63*(9), 2189–2201. doi: 10.1007/s10620-018-5095-3.

Thorpe, D. M., Byar, K. L., Conley, S. (2017). Chemotherapy-induced diarrhea. Retrieved from https://www.ons.org/pep/chemotherapy-induced-diarrhea

Tu, Q., Heitkemper, M. M., Jarrett, M. E., et al. (2017). Sleep disturbances in irritable bowel syndrome: A systematic review. *Neurogastroenterology Motility, 29*(3). doi: 10.1111/nmo.12946

van Thiel, I. A. M., Botschuijver, S., de Jonge, W. J., et al. (2020). Painful interactions: Microbial compounds and visceral pain. *Biochimica et Biophysica Acta (BBA)—Molecular Basis of Disease, 1866*(1), 165534. doi: 10.1016/j.bbadis.2019.165534.

van Tilburg, M. A. L., Palsson, O. S., Levy, R. L., et al. (2008). Complementary and alternative medicine use and cost in functional bowel disorders: A six-month prospective study in a large HMO. *BMC Complementary and Alternative Medicine, 8*, 46. doi: 10.1186/1472-6882-8-46.

Voegeli, D. (2008). The effect of washing and drying practices on skin barrier function. *Journal of Wound, Ostomy, and Continence Nursing, 35*(1), 84–90. doi: 10.1097/01.WON.0000308623.68582.d7.

Vriesman, M. H., Rajindrajith, S., Koppen, I. J. N., et al. (2019). Quality of life in children with functional constipation: A systematic review and meta-analysis. *Journal of Pediatrics, 214*, 141–150. doi: 10.1016/j.jpeds.2019.06.059.

Wald, A., Scarpignato, C., Kamm, M. A., et al. (2007). The burden of constipation on quality of life: Results of a multinational survey. *Alimentary Pharmacology & Therapeutics, 26*(2), 227–236.

Weynants, A., Goossens, L., Genetello, M., et al. (2019). The long-term effect and adherence of a low fermentable oligosaccharides disaccharides monosaccharides and polyols (FODMAP) diet in patients with irritable bowel syndrome. *Journal of Human Nutrition Diet, 33*(2), 159–169. doi: 10.1111/jhn.12706.

Woodward, S., Norton, C., & Chiarelli, P. (2014). Biofeedback for treatment of chronic idiopathic constipation in adults. *Cochrane Database of Systematic Reviews,* (3), CD008486.

World Health Organization. (2017). Diarrhoeal disease, Fact sheet. Retrieved from https://www.who.int/news-room/fact-sheets/detail/diarrhoeal-disease

World Health Organization. (2019). Zinc supplementation in the management of diarrhea. *e-Library of Evidence for Nutrition Actions (eLENA).* Retrieved from https://www.who.int/elena/titles/zinc_diarrhoea/en/

Yamasato, K., Kaneshiro, B., & Oyama, I. A. (2014). A simulation comparing the cost-effectiveness of adult incontinence products. *Journal of Wound, Ostomy, and Continence Nursing, 41*(5), 467–472. doi: 10.1097/WON.0000000000000045.

Yang, B., Lu, P., Li, M.-X., et al., (2019). A meta-analysis of the effects of probiotics and synbiotics in children with acute diarrhea. *Medicine, 98*(37), e16618. doi: 10.1097/MD.0000000000016618.

Zhong, L., Zheng, G., Da Ge, L., et al. (2016). Chinese herbal medicine for constipation: Zheng-based associations among herbs, formulae, proprietary medicines, and herb-drug interactions. *Chinese Medicine, 11*, 28. doi: 10.1186/s13020-016-0099-4.

CASE STUDIES

CASE STUDY: PATIENTS WITH IBS-D

Common patient presentation: KS is a 25-year-old woman who was referred to a gastroenterologist for colonoscopy to evaluate a recent exacerbation of diarrhea with increased abdominal cramping. Currently, she is a graduate student at a large university. She describes her current life as stressful due to financial concerns. She reports a history of depression. Her abdominal symptoms started 2 years ago. She complains of lower abdominal pain, bloating, gas, and frequent, loose stools; she denies seeing any blood in the stool. Despite these symptoms, her weight has remained stable. For the last 6 months, her abdominal pain has been at least 3 days per month and is not associated with menstruation. The pain is reduced with defecation. In addition, she reports feeling anxious, tired, and sleep deprived.

Basic workup: Her physical examination, vital signs, and body weight are within normal limits. There is no family history of organic GI disease. Her primary care provider orders a panel of laboratory tests (CBC, ESR, electrolytes, LFTs) and more stool studies (e.g., ova). These are WNL. Rectal examination revealed no hemorrhoids. No mucosal lesions were identified on colonoscopic examination, and random biopsies were taken from the descending and sigmoid colon. All findings were normal.

Individual management plan: The provider works with KS to establish a treatment plan. She is educated regarding the pathophysiology and management of IBS and is reassured that the symptoms can be managed with lifestyle changes and medications if needed. KS is encouraged to keep a symptom and stool diary for 2 weeks. She is asked to reflect on her dietary intake and stress levels when she experiences symptoms and to make a note of these as well. The goal is to identify triggers that are associated with "flares" of symptoms. Nonpharmacological approaches such as relaxation, stress management, and sleep hygiene are initiated. In her diary, KS notes that on those days when she doesn't eat breakfast, her symptoms are more intense. The continence nurse provides education regarding the relationship of diet including the timing of meals and symptoms. Despite these nonpharmacological approaches, KS's symptoms persist, and she is having difficulty continuing to attend school. Antidiarrheal and antispasmodic medications are prescribed, and KS reports that these are very beneficial in managing symptoms and that she is feeling better able to control her IBS and to complete her school assignments.

CASE STUDIES

CASE STUDY: PATIENT WITH CONSTIPATION

An 87-year-old woman receiving in-home hospice care due to inoperable aortic stenosis complained of constipation. The client reported that she had managed her bowels with a daily dose of milk of magnesia for the past 7 years, a treatment that was no longer effective. She reported no bowel movement for the past 2 days, a sensation of rectal fullness, and inability to defecate. "The cardiologist told me I shouldn't strain because of my heart," she reported to the hospice nurse. The nurse noted that in addition to the cardiac problems, the client required fentanyl for management of chronic rheumatoid arthritis pain and was on fluid restriction for chronic renal insufficiency and heart failure. Although still ambulatory, the client was unable to tolerate prolonged exercise without severe fatigue.

Diet recall for the previous 24 hours included the following: packet of instant oatmeal with milk, cup of coffee, ½ sandwich with ham, and a "microwave dinner." When asked, the client admitted that she restricted her fluids much more than prescribed by her physicians so that she did not have to go to the bathroom so often.

Physical examination revealed abdominal distention, hypoactive bowel sounds, and left lower quadrant abdominal tenderness on palpation. After consultation with the cardiologist and obtaining permission from the client, a digital rectal examination (DRE) was performed. The DRE revealed an external hemorrhoid at the anal opening and presence of a large, firm fecal mass in the rectal vault.

Because the etiology of constipation was complex, various nursing care measures were required:

Independent continence nursing actions:

1. Instruct client regarding the need to discontinue use of the stimulant laxative.

2. Review a list of high-fiber foods with the client to determine which, if any, she might be willing and able to include in the diet.

3. Instruct the client in tracking fluid intake to achieve full daily fluid allowance.

4. Instruct the client in optimal toileting position and ensure availability of necessary assistive devices to achieve a physiologic defecation position.

5. Provide bowel diary and stool form chart and instruct the client in completion between home visits.

Dependent continence nursing actions:

1. Obtain prescription for daily stool softener.

2. Obtain prescription for oil retention enema now and prn.

3. Obtain prescription for prn PEG laxative.

Interdependent continence nursing actions:

1. Monitor stool form and frequency with bowel diary.

2. Assess for flatulence, abdominal discomfort, or other complications of fiber therapy.

Response: Following administration of the oil retention enema, the continence nurse was able to gently break up the fecal mass. The patient was instructed to take the PEG laxative and reported a normal bowel movement following this. The patient also increased her fluid and fiber intake and began taking the stool softener; 1 week following the initial visit, the patient reported soft formed stools every other day.

QUESTIONS

1. A continence nurse is assessing a patient diagnosed with acute-onset diarrhea. What is the usual cause of this condition?
   A. Malabsorption syndrome
   B. Infectious process
   C. Motility disorder
   D. Chronic inflammatory bowel condition

2. A continence nurse is assessing a patient diagnosed with "fatty diarrhea." What is one of the most common causes of this bowel alteration?

   A. *Clostridium difficile*
   B. Cancer
   C. Radiation proctitis
   D. Lactose intolerance

3. Which type of watery diarrhea is high volume and unaffected by oral intake?
   A. Osmotic
   B. Secretory
   C. Functional
   D. Dysfunctional

4. The continence nurse is monitoring an infant for dehydration related to chronic diarrhea. What sign should arouse the nurse's suspicion of this life-threatening complication?
   A. Skin tenting
   B. Increased urinary output
   C. Hypertension
   D. Bradycardia

5. For which patient would antimotility agents be considered first-line therapy?
   A. A patient with infectious diarrhea
   B. A patient with traveler's diarrhea
   C. A patient with diarrhea caused by chemotherapy
   D. A patient with osmotic diarrhea

6. A continence nurse is caring for a patient who is experiencing slow-transit constipation. What treatment measure is recommended?
   A. Fiber therapy
   B. Stimulant laxatives
   C. Osmotic laxatives
   D. Antibiotic therapy

7. A female patient explains to a continence nurse that she has to "insert her finger into her vagina to enable a bowel movement." What is the probable cause of this patient's bowel alteration?
   A. Rectal–anal intussusception
   B. Rectocele
   C. Rectal tumor
   D. Megarectum

8. How would the continence nurse explain the action of fiber in the diet to patients with bowel alterations?
   A. Fiber hardens the stool.
   B. Fiber decreases stool bulk.
   C. Fiber reduces colonic transit time.
   D. Fiber increases colonic transit time.

9. What is the current theory regarding probiotics mechanism of action in prevention or treatment of a bowel dysfunction?
   A. Guards against parasite invasion in immunocompromised people
   B. Reduces inflammation in individuals with Crohn disease
   C. Enhances epithelial barrier and reduces inflammation in the gut
   D. Normalizes blood glucose in people with prediabetes

10. The continence nurse is counseling a patient recently diagnosed with irritable bowel syndrome (IBS). What teaching point would the nurse include?
   A. "IBS is a life-threatening disease causing physical and emotional distress."
   B. "IBS increases the risk for cancer."
   C. "At present, there is no known cure for IBS."
   D. "Treatment plans for IBS are standardized according to age."

ANSWERS AND RATIONALES

1. B. Rationale: Acute diarrhea is most often caused by infectious disease via the fecal–oral route through contaminated food or water containing pathogens such as viruses, bacteria, and parasites.

2. D. Rationale: *Fatty diarrhea* occurs due to malabsorption as seen with lactose intolerance. Surgical procedures (short bowel syndrome, bowel resection, gastric bypass), pancreatic disease, some medications, and Giardia may be associated with malabsorption and fatty diarrhea.

3. B. Rationale: Secretory diarrhea is usually high volume and unaffected by reduced oral/enteral intake.

4. A. Rationale: Nursing care involves careful monitoring of intake and output and identifying signs of dehydration. Dry mouth, decreased urinary output, skin tenting, hypotension, lethargy, tachycardia, and elevated temperature should arouse suspicion of dehydration with the potential for shock, especially in the pediatric patient.

5. C. Rationale: For diarrhea caused by chemotherapy, antimotility agents such as loperamide are frequently considered first-line therapy with progression to octreotide for persistent diarrhea.

6. C. Rationale: Slow-transit constipation osmotic agents are generally considered the agent of choice because these agents "work" by distending the bowel and softening the stool and may be more effective than stimulant agents in patients with reduced peristalsis.

7. B. Rationale: Women who have symptomatic rectocele may report using their fingers vaginally to manually reduce the prolapse to assist in bowel evacuation.

8. C. Rationale: *Soluble fiber such as* psyllium or oat bran provides a laxative effect by reducing transit time in addition to increasing stool bulk and retaining water to keep stool soft.

9. A. Rationale: Probiotics are believed to suppress the growth and luminal binding of pathogenic bacteria and thereby improve epithelial barrier function and reduce inflammation.

10. C. Rationale: IBS is a complex and not well-understood disease with pathophysiologic mechanisms involving an interplay among multiple factors. Currently, there isn't any cure for IBS; treatment focus is adequate symptom management.

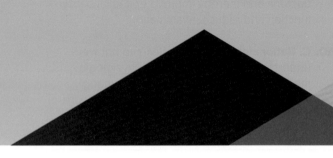

CHAPTER 22

FECAL INCONTINENCE: PATHOLOGY, ASSESSMENT, AND MANAGEMENT

Laurie Lonergan Callan and Kathleen Francis

OBJECTIVES

1. Discuss the impact of bowel dysfunction or fecal incontinence on lifestyle and quality of life and implications for psychosocial support and counseling.

2. Explain how each of the following contributes to normal bowel function and fecal continence: normal peristalsis; sensory awareness of rectal distention and ability to distinguish between solid, liquid, and gas; internal anal sphincter function; external anal sphincter function; and rectal capacity and compliance.

3. Relate the underlying pathology to management options for passive incontinence, urge incontinence, and seepage and soiling.

4. Describe data to be gathered during the interview and physical assessment that provide insight into peristaltic function, sensory awareness/sphincter function, and rectal capacity and compliance.

5. Synthesize data obtained during patient assessment to determine pattern of fecal incontinence and to develop an appropriate management program.

6. Explain indications and guidelines for a colonic cleanout program, sphincter exercises, instruction in urge inhibition, biofeedback, and stimulated defecation program.

7. Identify options for the patient with refractory fecal incontinence.

TOPIC OUTLINE

INTRODUCTION

Continence is a balance between the anal sphincter complex, stool consistency, rectal reservoir function, and neurological processes. Problems with any of these components can lead to fecal incontinence (Ruiz & Kaiser, 2017). Fecal incontinence (FI) is a serious problem associated with significant physical and psychological morbidity. Incontinence itself is not a definitive diagnosis and the initial focus in management is to determine the cause of the problem. Once etiologic factors have been identified, management is directed toward correction of the causative factors and restoration of continence. When continence cannot be fully achieved, even with advanced medical and surgical interventions, containment products are available to help manage the problem and diversion should be considered (Findlay & Maxwell-Armstrong, 2010).

While FI can affect an individual at any age, older men and women are more likely to develop this problem (Bharucha et al., 2017; Pretlove et al., 2006). The negative social stigma that surrounds this condition tends to leave sufferers and caretakers to cope quietly with their feelings of embarrassment, humiliation, and social isolation (Farage et al., 2008; Meyer & Richter, 2015); thus, sensitive and patient-focused nursing intervention is critical to positive outcomes and enhanced quality of life (QOL).

 OVERVIEW

Fecal continence is directly related to the individual's ability to sense rectal fullness and to control the urge to defecate or pass gas until an appropriate time and place (Halland & Talley, 2012; Van Koughnett & Wexner, 2013). It requires normal function of the gastrointestinal tract, intact sensory function and cognition, competence of the sphincters, and adequate rectal capacity and compliance and can be affected by various extrinsic and intrinsic factors, including comorbidities, medications, and diet.

KEY POINT

Fecal continence requires normal GI tract function, intact sensory function and cognition, competence of the sphincters, and adequate rectal capacity and compliance.

DEFINITIONS

The 2010 International Urogynecological Association (IUGA)/International Continence Society (ICS) Joint Report on the Terminology for Pelvic Floor Disorders defined FI simply as the involuntary loss of stool (Haylen, 2010). Others define FI as an affirmative response to the question: "In the past year, have you had any loss of control of your bowels, even a small amount that stained the underwear?" (Goode et al., 2005). *FI* has also been defined as the involuntary loss of mucus, liquid, or solid bowel contents; a lack of control over defecation; or the inability to control the evacuation of stool at a socially acceptable location and time (Bellicini et al., 2008; Doherty, 2004; Dunberger et al., 2011;

Findlay & Maxwell-Armstrong, 2010; Herbert, 2008; Mellgren, 2010; Meyer & Richter, 2015; Northwood, 2013; Ostaszkiewicz et al., 2008). Often part of the definition is a duration of 1 month or longer and an age of >4 years with previously achieved control (Paquette et al., 2015; Rao et al., 2017). The involuntary loss of flatus, without loss of mucus or stool, is defined as *anal incontinence* (AI) (Northwood, 2013).

Urge bowel incontinence involves a sudden urgent need to defecate that results in incontinence when the individual is unable to reach a toilet in time (Sharpe & Read, 2010). In contrast, *passive fecal incontinence* involves the passage of stool or gas without any awareness on the part of the individual. *Encopresis* is the term used to describe voluntary or involuntary fecal soiling; retentive encopresis refers to involuntary fecal soiling, usually in children who have already been toilet trained and usually in response to subconscious withholding of stool. Encopresis will be discussed in greater detail in Chapter 23. Among adults, the leakage of small amounts of stool into undergarments is commonly labeled as *partial fecal incontinence*, fecal leakage, anal leakage, *fecal soiling*, or *fecal seepage*; FI or bowel incontinence is the term used to denote larger accidents or complete loss of rectal contents (Bartolo & Paterson, 2009; Doughty, 2000).

KEY POINT

Urge bowel incontinence involves a sudden urgent need to defecate that results in incontinence when the individual is unable to reach a toilet promptly; in contrast, passive incontinence involves passage of stool or gas without any awareness on the part of the individual.

PREVALENCE AND INCIDENCE

Published FI incidence and prevalence rates vary and are generally believed to be inaccurate and low, based on evidence that FI is widely underreported or due to variance in the incontinence defining parameters (Rees & Sharpe, 2009). Throughout the literature, prevalence ranges from 7% to 25% in community-dwelling men and women, and tends to increase with age or with cognitive impairment (Bharucha et al., 2015; Forte et al., 2016; Meyer & Richter, 2015). Literature reports that FI affects <3% of young adults age 20 to 29 but more than 15% of adults age 70 and older (Forte et al., 2016; Rao et al., 2017). Women over the age of 40 tend to report more FI due to pelvic floor dysfunction or obstetrical injuries (Forte et al., 2016). It is hypothesized that the effects of the original obstetric injury may later be compounded by age-related issues: pelvic laxity, pudendal neuropathy, and menopause (Meyer & Richter, 2015).

There are limited data regarding the prevalence of FI in men, but the literature suggests that there may be a large number of symptomatic male patients who do not present to their medical practitioners despite the negative effect on QOL (Eva et al., 2003). Shamliyan et al. (2009) found cognitive impairment, poor general health, surgery, and radiation for prostate cancer were associated with FI in community-dwelling men.

Frailty (impaired physical activity, mobility, muscle strength, motor processing, cognition, nutrition, endurance, multiple comorbid chronic illnesses) is considered an independent risk factor for FI (Meyer & Richter, 2015). The prevalence rate of FI in nursing home residents has been reported as high as 47% to 50%; FI in these individuals is frequently associated with dementia and/or immobility (Forte et al., 2016a).

A higher incidence of FI is also found in patients with an acute illness and is often due to loose or liquid stools. In acute care settings, the incidence range has been reported as 17% to 33% (Hurnauth, 2011). Bliss and colleagues found that 33% of acutely ill patients suffered from FI and that hospitalized patients with liquid stools/diarrhea had higher rates of FI (43%) than did patients without diarrhea (27%) (Bliss et al., 2000).

KEY POINT

Acute illness is associated with a higher incidence of FI which is often due to loose or liquid stools.

IMPACT

FI causes considerable distress and can have a devastating effect on QOL for individuals and often for their family members. Based on QOL surveys, 6% of patients with mild FI symptoms, 35% with moderate FI, and 82% with severe FI report a moderate to severe impact on their QOL (Bharucha et al., 2005; Hussain et al., 2014). The unpredictability of FI disrupts a patient's daily routine and affects every aspect of life including diet, skin health, sexuality, marriage, friendships, employment opportunities, and the ability to exercise (Crowell et al., 2007; Roth, 2010). FI leads to social stigmatization and isolation and is a common cause for institutionalization of the elderly (Dunivan et al., 2010). FI is also a strong predictor of falls in the elderly.

Studies have found that people with FI are more apt to seek health care assistance if symptoms are more severe, if symptoms are perceived as dangerous, if there is loss of solid stool, or if having an established primary care provider to seek help from (Bharucha et al., 2015). Commonly reported psychological signs and symptoms related to FI include the following (Bharucha et al., 2017; Meyer & Richter, 2015; Roth, 2010):

- Reduced self-esteem and confidence; self-conscious about body image, loss of composure
- Reluctance to share information about the FI problem with others, including health care providers

- Increased risk of anxiety and depression disorders
- Higher risk scores on the Patient Health Questionnaire (PHQ), poor QOL scores
- Feelings of anger, grief, shame, embarrassment, fear, hopelessness, and frustration
- Lower sexual desire, satisfaction, and sexual functioning
- Poor self-perceived health
- More anxiety and planning needed to go out of the house or travel, or avoid leaving the house; dependence on others and isolation
- Having to "map out" public toilets
- Reduced work concentration, missed work, decreased productivity, or for some, forced retirement
- Anxiety about concealing the appearance of pads or adult briefs or hiding possible stains

Caregiver burden is also to be considered, as measured by hours of care, emotional distress, and/or having to arrange for home care or nursing home care for their family member with FI (Bharucha et al., 2015).

Studies report patients often shy away from discussing the sensitive subject of FI with their health care provider; therefore, health care providers should inquire if FI is a problem and how it affects their QOL. Researchers recommend using patient-preferred terminology to facilitate better communication and help to place your patient at ease; "accidental bowel leakage" is a preferred term for discussions with patients (Williams et al., 2018; Whitehead et al., 2016). Avoid phrases that might imply blaming the patient for stool leakage, belittling the impact of FI, or referring to incontinence as a "failure to control leakage" (Meyer & Richter, 2015).

Providers are generally more interested in frequency, amount of lost stool, and type of FI, whereas patients are more concerned with how the leakage affects personal hygiene and self-image. Questionnaires that combine severity scales and patient-reported QOL measures will help with this conversation. These scoring systems however, do not include physiologic components or objective test parameters for assessment of severity (Ruiz & Kaiser, 2017). Multiple assessment tools that have been developed for assessing FI. They can be classified based upon the parameters evaluated, that is, descriptive measures, severity measures, and impact measures (Hussain et al., 2014). The tools most commonly used in clinical practice are symptom severity questionnaires and health-related quality-of-life (HRQOL) impact scales (Bharucha et al., 2017). These tools can be very helpful to the clinician to more accurately assess the subjective impact of FI on the individual and family. However, not all assessment tools have been validated; thus, care must be taken if the tool is being used for research purposes (Bharucha et al., 2015). Some considerations when selecting a tool include ease of use by both the person and the practitioner, the parameters the tool is designed

to measure, the tool's ability to detect a change in the person's condition, and the population for which it was designed (Ruiz & Kaiser, 2017). See **Table 22-1** for a brief overview of currently available assessment tools specific to individuals with urinary and FI.

COSTS ASSOCIATED WITH FI

There are limited data available on the economic impact of FI. FI is associated with increased hospital stays and an increased nursing workload to maintain patients' hygiene (McKenna et al., 2001). Therefore, FI is costly to the patient and to society, with specific costs including the following (Goode et al., 2005; Meyer & Richter, 2015; Nix & Ermer-Seltun, 2004; Palmieri et al., 2005; Paterson et al., 2003): work absenteeism, impaired work performance, changes in job status and wages, nursing time (labor), skin care products, containment products and protective pads, laundry costs, consultations, medical and pharmacy services, and home and long-term care services. In addition, the potential economic impact of new medical and surgical treatment modalities (i.e., sacral nerve stimulation and perianal bulking agents) has been found to be quite expensive (Bharucha et al., 2015; Hurnauth, 2011).

Incontinence-associated costs in the United States are estimated at $22.5 to $19.5 billion, and 9% of that is attributed to costs for absorbent products (Fader et al., 2009). Farage et al. (2008) reported similar estimates of costs at $22.4 billion per year for incontinence-related care and $1.1 billion for disposable products.

⬤ TYPES AND PATHOLOGY OF FI

FI can be classified based on clinical presentation and on duration of the problem. Classification based on clinical presentation includes urge incontinence, passive incontinence, and flatus incontinence. Knowledge of normal defecation physiology (see Chapter 20) helps to understand the different pathophysiologies that lead to FI, with many patients having multifaceted anorectal dysfunctions (Bharucha et al., 2015)

PASSIVE INCONTINENCE

Passive incontinence involves the unrecognized leakage of mucus, fluid, or solid stool. FI that occurs with no awareness on the individual's part is often caused by cognitive impairment (dementia) or sensorimotor dysfunction (e.g., incontinence in the patient with a neurologic lesion such as spinal cord injury). Less commonly, this type of incontinence is caused by significant internal anal sphincter (IAS) dysfunction resulting in lower anal sphincter resting pressures. Passive incontinence can range from mild soiling of the underwear to total evacuation of the bowel without warning (Bartolo & Paterson, 2009; Ruiz and Kaiser, 2017; Stevens et al., 2003).

TABLE 22-1 TOOLS FOR ASSESSMENT OF FI: SEVERITY AND IMPACT ON QUALITY OF LIFE

ABBREVIATION	TOOL NAME	DESCRIPTION	AUTHOR(S)/ DEVELOPER(S)	REFERENCE CITATION
Wexner or CCIS	Cleveland Clinic Fecal Incontinence Score/Wexner Scale	Five questions to score symptoms related to FI in terms of severity (0–20), frequency (0–4), and quality of life (QOL) impact. Has undergone psychometric evaluation	Steven D. Wexner, Cleveland Clinic	Hussain et al. (2014), Rockwood (2004), Ruiz and Kaiser (2017), Sansoni et al. (2013), Thomas et al. (2006)
FISI	Fecal Incontinence Severity Index/ Rockwood	Tool developed by surgeons (with patient input) to assess severity of FI and AI independent of direct clinical assessment; scores range from 0 to 61; applies an external weighting system.	Todd Rockwood, James Church, James Fleshman, Robert Kane, Constantinos Mavrantonis, Alan Thorson, Steven Wexner, Donna Bliss, Ann Lowry, Univ of Minnesota, Dept of Colon and Rectal Surgery	Northwood (2013), Rockwood et al. (1999), Rockwood (2004)
BBUSQ-22	Birmingham Bowel and Urinary Symptom Questionnaire	22-item questionnaire covering a range of bowel and urinary symptoms in women; designed to evaluate the effects of pelvic surgery on FI and LUTS. Has undergone rigorous psychometric testing	L. Hiller, S. Radley, C. Mann, S. C. Radley, G. Begum, S. J. Pretlove, J. Salaman	Hiller et al. (2002), Northwood (2013)
FIQoLS	Fecal Incontinence QOL Scale	29-item questionnaire addressing specific QOL indicators; measures the effect of FI treatment on HRQOL in adults. Has undergone psychometric evaluation	Todd Rockwood, James Church, James Fleshman, Robert Kane, Constantinos Mavrantonis, Alan Thorson, Steven Wexner, Donna Bliss, Ann Lowry, Univ of Minnesota, Dept of Colon and Rectal Surgery	Hussain et al. (2014), Northwood (2013), Rockwood et al. (1999)
MHQ	Modified Manchester Health Questionnaire	31-item questionnaire that measures HRQOL in women with FI and AI. Has undergone psychometric evaluation	G. Bugg, E. Kiff, G. Hosker	Northwood (2013)
RFIS	Revised Fecal Incontinence Scale	Short, reliable, valid five-item scale designed to discriminate between different levels of incontinence severity. Has undergone psychometric testing		Sansoni et al. (2013)
SMIS	Vaizey/St. Mark's Incontinence Score	7-question questionnaire, with scores based on frequency (0–4) and severity (0–24) of symptoms; takes into consideration fecal urgency and management behaviors, along with QOL indicators. Has undergone psychometric evaluation	C. Vaizey, C. Carapeti, J. Cahill, M. Kamm	Rusavy et al. (2014), Sansoni et al. (2013)
ICIQ-B	International Consultation on Incontinence Questionnaire-Bowel Symptoms	QOL assessment tool that takes into account FI issues the patients identified as important. Proven validity, reliability, and responsiveness	Cotterill, Norton, Avery, Abrams, Donovan	Hussain et al. (2014)

CCIS, Cleveland Clinic Incontinence Score; QOL, quality of life; FISI, Fecal Incontinence Severity Index; FI, fecal incontinence; AI, anal incontinence; BBUSQ, Birmingham Bowel and Urinary Symptom Questionnaire; LUTS, lower urinary tract symptoms; FIQoLS, Fecal Incontinence QOL Scale; HRQOL, health-related quality of life; MHQ, Manchester Health Questionnaire; RFIS, Revised Fecal Incontinence Scale; SMIS, St. Mark's Incontinence Score; ICIQ-B, International Consultation on Incontinence Questionnaire-Bowels.

Passive incontinence can range from mild soiling to total evacuation of the bowel and is most commonly caused by cognitive impairment or sensorimotor dysfunction (neurogenic bowel).

URGE INCONTINENCE

Urge incontinence is characterized by a sudden need to defecate and the inability to reach the toilet before defecation occurs, resulting in involuntary passage of mucus, gas, liquid, or solid stool. Urge incontinence may be caused by external anal sphincter (EAS) dysfunction (with an intact internal sphincter, causing reduced squeeze pressures and/or squeeze duration), a colorectal motility disorder, or a reduced capacity and/or compliance of the rectal cavity (Bartolo & Paterson, 2009; Rao et al., 2017).

Urge incontinence may be caused by EAS dysfunction, a motility disorder, or diminished rectal capacity and compliance.

FLATUS INCONTINENCE

Flatus incontinence may be the first sign of FI. Fecal leakage, fecal soiling, and fecal seepage are minor degrees of FI and describe the incontinence of liquid stool, mucus, or very small amounts of solid stool. The leakage varies in severity, from staining, to soilage, to seepage, to small accidents in people who are continent and able to delay defecation the majority of the time (Bartolo & Paterson, 2009; Doughty, 2000). This pattern of incontinence may be caused by dysfunction of the IAS, which is normally responsible for preventing leakage of small volumes of stool or gas, or by sensory impairment that prevents prompt recognition of stool in the rectal vault (Rao et al., 2017).

Transient versus Chronic FI

Incontinence can also be classified based on duration; this classification includes transient and chronic FI. Transient FI refers to short-term (new-onset) incontinence caused by a change in stool consistency or sensory awareness; these individuals were continent until they became acutely ill, became severely confused, or developed severe diarrhea (Hurnauth, 2011). Management of these individuals is directed toward treatment of the underlying disease process, containment of the stool, and perianal skin protection. In contrast, chronic incontinence is a persistent or recurrent problem caused by chronic disease, injury to or denervation of the sphincter, cognitive impairment, or neurologic dysfunction (such as spinal cord injury). These individuals require a comprehensive management plan that is individualized

based on the specific type and cause of the FI (Doughty, 2000; Wishin et al., 2008).

Transient FI is usually caused by an acute diarrheal illness and/or alteration in mental status; management is focused on correction of the underlying disease process, containment of the stool, and perianal skin protection.

RISK FACTORS FOR FI

Continence is maintained by anatomical factors (endovascular cushions and the integrity of the anal sphincter and puborectalis), rectoanal sensation, rectal compliance, neuronal innervation, stool consistency, mobility, and psychological factors (Rao et al., 2017). There are multiple factors that predispose individuals to developing FI and multiple approaches to classifying those risk factors. Information about risk factors not only tells us which patients to screen but also guides treatment. In this text, we will categorize risk factors based on their impact on functional components of continence, because this approach provides the foundation for assessment and management of the individual with FI. Using this conceptual approach, the major risk factors can be grouped into the following categories: those related to gastrointestinal system function, bowel motility, and stool consistency; those related to neurologic control of defecation; those related to the integrity and innervation of the pelvic floor and anal sphincters; those affecting rectal capacity and compliance; and those affecting overall health status and mobility (**Table 22-2**). Other factors that have an impact on FI are age, gender, diet, and exercise (Bharucha et al., 2017; Forte et al., 2016; Mellgren, 2010; Meyer & Richter, 2015; Roth, 2010; Ruiz & Kaiser, 2017; Shamliyan et al., 2009).

CONDITIONS AFFECTING BOWEL MOTILITY AND STOOL CONSISTENCY

As explained in Chapter 20, one factor critical to continence is normal stool consistency; stool that is formed but soft is fairly easily retained even if the sphincter is somewhat weak, while high-volume liquid stool can overwhelm the strongest sphincter. Therefore, any condition producing liquid stool increases the risk of incontinence. The risk is further increased when the stool is high volume and/or in the individual with any degree of sphincter weakness.

Conditions resulting in diarrheal stool include bacterial and viral infections (e.g., *Clostridium difficile*), malabsorption syndromes (e.g., diet/gluten or lactose intolerance, fat malabsorption following cholecystectomy), hypersecretory tumors, constipation with paradoxical diarrhea,

TABLE 22-2 RISK FACTORS FOR FECAL INCONTINENCE

PREDISPOSING FACTORS	REFERENCE CITATION
1. Factors related to the integrity of the pelvic floor and anal sphincter(s)	
Obstetrical internal and/or external sphincter injury (due to forceps delivery, large head circumference, large birth weight, abnormal presentation at delivery)	Altman et al. (2007), Bartolo and Paterson (2009), Erekson et al. (2008), Groutz et al. (1999), Leung and Rao (2011), Mellgren (2010), Ruiz and Kaiser (2017)
Pelvic organ prolapse. rectal prolapse, rectocele, hemorrhoids, intussusception, fistula	Altman et al. (2007), Bartolo and Paterson (2009), Findlay and Maxwell-Armstrong (2010)
Vaginal parity	Erekson et al. (2008), Findlay and Maxwell-Armstrong (2010)
Trauma: Pelvic fractures, insertion of foreign bodies into anal canal, perineal lacerations. Sexual abuse. Anal intercourse	Roth (2010), Shamliyan et al. (2009)
Perianal surgery (sphincterotomy, hemorrhoidectomy, anal dilation)	Meyer & Richter, 2015
2. Factors related to overall health status	
Obesity (e.g., altered transit, change in flora, significant difference in stool consistency). Pelvic floor weakness in morbidly obese prior to bariatric surgery contributes to FI after surgery.	Altman et al. (2007), Bharucha (2010), Gallagher (2005), Halland and Talley (2012), Pares et al. (2012)
Medications: alpha-blockers, calcium channel blockers, nitric oxide donors, diabetes meds, anticholinergics, antipsychotics (see Table 22-3)	Doherty (2004), Farage et al. (2008), Gallagher (2005), Leung and Schnelle (2008)
Hysterectomy	Altman et al. (2007)
Diabetes	Altman et al. (2007), Bartolo and Paterson (2009)
Postreconstructive: low anterior resection, pouch surgery, radiation, hemorrhoidectomy, anorectal surgery	Bartolo and Paterson (2009), Doherty (2004), Erekson et al. (2008), Ruiz and Kaiser (2017)
Poor general health	Bellicini et al. (2008)
Prostate disease	Bellicini et al. (2008)
Enteral tube feedings	Bellicini et al. (2008)
Infectious: *Campylobacter*, *Salmonella*, *Shigellosis*, *Clostridium difficile/perfringens*, pseudomembranous colitis, perianal sepsis, human papillomavirus, cytomegalovirus, lymphogranuloma venereum, etc.	Farage et al. (2008), Findlay and Maxwell-Armstrong (2010), Sabol and Friedenburg (1997), Wishin et al. (2008)
Malignancy: Paget disease, Bowen disease, lichen sclerosus, anal intraepithelial neoplasia	Bartolo and Paterson (2009), Findlay and Maxwell-Armstrong (2010)
Increased severity of illness	Bliss et al. (2000)
3. Factors related to neurological integrity	
Dementia, alteration in cognitive function	Farage et al. (2008), Leung and Schnelle (2008), Mellgren (2010)
Neurological/muscular impairment: stroke, parkinsonism, spinal cord injury, cauda equina injury, multiple sclerosis, spina bifida, muscular dystrophies, myasthenia gravis, muscular weakness, amyloidosis, pudendal neuropathy	Bellicini et al. (2008), Coggrave (2007), Findlay and Maxwell-Armstrong (2010), Finne-Soveri et al. (2008), Formal et al. (1997), Mellgren (2010), Sharpe and Read (2010), Ruiz and Kaiser (2017)
4. Factors related to bowel pattern or function	
Accelerated colonic transit, bowel resection, conditions resulting in diarrhea. Loss of rectal wall compliance. Irritable or inflammatory bowel disease, fistula, radiation injury	Bharucha (2010), McKenna et al. (2001), Meyer & Richter (2015), Stevens et al. (2003)
Alteration in intestinal and colonic bacterial flora after bariatric surgery	Bharucha (2010), Roberson et al. (2010)
Diarrhea. Fecal impaction	Bharucha (2010), Bliss et al. (2000), Erekson et al. (2008), McKenna et al. (2001), Mellgren (2010)
Cholecystectomy and fat malabsorption	Bharucha (2010)
Constipation, fecal impaction	Leung and Schnelle (2008)
Congenital anorectal anomalies, atresia	Bellicini et al. (2008)
Colorectal disease, inflammatory bowel diseases, acute diverticulitis, superior mesenteric bowel disease, venous thrombosis, ischemic bowel disease	Bellicini et al. (2008), Doherty (2004), McKenna et al. (2001), Sabol and Friedenburg (1997), Ruiz and Kaiser (2017)
Anal sphincter dysfunction	Palmieri et al. (2005)

TABLE 22-2 RISK FACTORS FOR FECAL INCONTINENCE *(Continued)*

PREDISPOSING FACTORS	REFERENCE CITATION
5. Factors related to the living situation	
Use of restraints	Leung and Schnelle (2008)
Lack of timely toileting assistance	Leung and Schnelle (2008)
Inability to toilet themselves	Leung and Schnelle (2008)
6. Factors related to mobility	
Impaired mobility, physical disability	Bellicini et al. (2008), Finne-Soveri et al. (2008), Gallagher (2005), Leung and Schnelle (2008), Wishin et al. (2008)
Overuse/misuse of absorbent pads and undergarments	Leung and Schnelle (2008)
7. Other factors	
Older age	Bellicini et al. (2008), Bliss et al. (2000), Erekson et al. (2008), Farage et al. (2008)
Female gender	Bellicini et al. (2008)
Diet: lack of dietary fiber, high-fat diet	McKenna et al. (2001)
Lack of exercise	McKenna et al. (2001)
Smoking with chronic cough, increased intra-abdominal pressure	Halland and Talley (2012)

surgical procedures resulting in reduced bowel length (e.g., major small bowel resection or colectomy), inflammatory conditions affecting bowel motility (e.g., Crohn disease or ulcerative colitis), motility disorders (e.g., irritable bowel syndrome, diarrhea predominant), initiation of enteral feedings in a malnourished patient with flattening of the villi, and selected medications (e.g., antibiotics, prokinetic agents, magnesium-based antacids, sorbitol) (Hurnauth, 2011; Rao et al., 2017). Interestingly, severe constipation resulting in fecal impaction can also cause or contribute to FI, because a large bolus of stool in the rectum produces persistent relaxation of the IAS and permits leakage of liquid stool around the fecal bolus. (See Chapter 21 for an in-depth discussion of motility disorders.)

of the sphincter places the individual at high risk for recurrent episodes of FI (Ruiz & Kaiser, 2017). Congenital causes include spinal cord defects and anorectal malformations. Other conditions include spinal cord surgery and spinal cord lesions (e.g., spina bifida, spinal cord injury, lower back syndrome, multiple myelitis, or multiple sclerosis), and peripheral neuropathy (diabetes, effect of chemotherapy drugs). Altered mental status, cerebrocortical dysfunction, (psychiatric disorders, delirium, or dementia), or a central nervous system disorder (stroke, trauma, tumor, infection) can alter the individual's ability to appropriately process and respond to the signals of rectal distention. A spinal cord lesion can prevent transmission of signals from the rectum and sphincters to the brain and vice versa (Alavi et al., 2015).

KEY POINT

One factor critical to continence is normal stool consistency; stool that is formed is fairly easily retained even if the sphincter is somewhat weak, whereas high-volume liquid stool can overwhelm the strongest sphincter.

KEY POINT

Any condition that compromises the individual's ability to recognize the presence of stool in the rectum and to voluntarily contract the sphincter places the individual at high risk for recurrent episodes of incontinence.

CONDITIONS AFFECTING NEURAL CONTROL

The second group of risk factors includes conditions that affect neural control of defecation. As explained in Chapter 20, fecal continence is dependent on the individual's ability to recognize the presence of stool or gas in the rectum and to contract the external sphincter until he/she reaches a socially acceptable time and place to defecate. Thus, any condition that interferes with sensory recognition of rectal distention or with voluntary control

SPHINCTER DAMAGE OR DENERVATION

The third group of risk factors involves damage or denervation of the sphincters or pudendal neuropathy. There are three main muscles of the anal sphincter complex that maintain bowel continence: the EAS, the IAS and the puborectalis muscle. The sphincter provides squeeze pressure and the ability to retain stool in the rectum, and is especially needed when the stool is liquid and/or high volume. The puborectalis muscle and EAS are innervated by the pudendal nerve and contributes to 30% to 40% of the anal resting tone and provide the voluntary sphincter contraction. The IAS provides 50% to 55% of the resting tone of the anal canal and is associated with the fine-tuning of fecal control (Ruiz & Kaiser, 2017). Incontinence for solid stool suggests more severe sphincter weakness than does that for liquid stool alone. Conditions most commonly associated with sphincter defect or denervation include obstetric trauma with pudendal nerve injury (vaginal delivery, forceps delivery, occipitoposterior presentation, prolonged labor, episiotomies/perineum tear), diabetic neuropathy, anorectal malformations (imperforate anus, cloacal defect), surgical repairs (anorectal surgery for fistula, fissures, hemorrhoidectomy, sphincterotomy, anorectal carcinoma), coloanal or ileoanal reconstruction, and anorectal trauma (e.g., impalement injuries, anal intercourse) (Alavi et al., 2015; Paquette et al., 2015; Williams et al., 2018). A history of obstetrical injury may not present with FI symptoms for many years, symptoms are often associated with weight gain, aging, and onset of menopause. In addition, the degree of levator ani and puborectalis muscle atrophy or pelvic floor relaxation correlates closely with FI symptoms (Bharucha et al., 2015; Rao et al., 2017).

> **KEY POINT**
>
> Damage or denervation of the anal sphincter is a common cause of chronic FI and is usually caused by obstetric trauma, anorectal surgery, or anal trauma.

CONDITIONS AFFECTING RECTAL CAPACITY OR COMPLIANCE

The fourth group of risk factors includes conditions that alter rectal capacity or compliance. Normally, the sensation to defecate prompts voluntary contraction of the external sphincter and puborectalis muscle, then the sense of fullness and urgency decreases as the rectum adjusts to hold more stool (Rao et al., 2017). A fibrotic or inflamed rectum is unable to accommodate any volume of stool and is associated with severe urgency and urge incontinence. Conditions that increase rectal sensitivity are associated with reduced compliance and repetitive contractions during rectal distention. These include inflammatory conditions (e.g., infectious colitis, ulcerative colitis, Crohn's proctocolitis, or radiation proctitis) and rectal fibrosis caused by radiation or repetitive inflammation (Ruiz & Kaiser, 2017). In addition, patients undergoing low anterior resection (removal of the rectum) are at risk for incontinence due to loss of the rectal reservoir. These individuals typically experience intense fecal frequency and urgency until the segment of colon immediately proximal to the anal canal distends to form a pouch-like structure that acts as a "pseudo rectum." Individuals undergoing ileal pouch anal anastomosis procedures are at risk for incontinence until the pouch has adapted (distended) sufficiently to provide an adequate reservoir. Decreased rectal sensitivity can also contribute to fecal retention by decreasing the frequency and intensity of the urge to defecate; this allows stool to leak out before the EAS can contract (Rao et al., 2017).

Third-degree (involving the EAS) and fourth-degree anal lacerations (extending through the external and IASs) are strong risk factors for anal and FI (Rao et al., 2017). Pelvic organ descent and prolapse may result in a reduced reservoir and possibly more undesired or even ineffective evacuations (Ruiz & Kaiser, 2017). Rectal prolapse or intussusception also compromises sphincter function. In addition, any condition that causes severe debility or immobility can compromise the individual's ability to reach the toilet in a timely manner. Specific risk factors are listed in **Table 22-2**.

> **KEY POINT**
>
> A fibrotic or inflamed rectum is unable to accommodate and "store" any volume of stool and is associated with severe urgency and urge incontinence.

ASSESSMENT GUIDELINES

Accurate assessment of the patient with FI is critical to development of an appropriate individualized management plan. The novice practitioner will not be able to conduct the same level of expert assessment as an advanced practice continence nurse. However, the novice practitioner *can* use available tools and guidelines to conduct an effective baseline assessment including basic history and physical examination. For example, there are several tools available that assess the individual with FI in terms of symptom severity and impact on daily living and HRQOL. These questionnaires can be helpful to the affected individual as well as the nurse, because completion of the tool allows the person to articulate and quantify his or her symptoms, feelings, and experience (Alavi et al., 2015; Paquette et al., 2015). This is important because clinicians tend to underestimate symptom severity and impact on HRQOL. A table of available assessment tools was presented earlier in this chapter (see **Table 22-1**) and can be of tremendous assistance to the clinicians in determining the needs of their patients with FI.

> **KEY POINT**
>
> Use of structured tools to assess QOL is important, because clinicians tend to underestimate symptom severity and impact of FI on HRQOL.

PATIENT INTERVIEW

A comprehensive assessment of FI should include a thorough history, that includes identification of risk factors, patterns of incontinence (i.e., urge FI vs. passive FI vs. minor leakage), daytime versus nighttime FI, effect on skin, history of urinary tract infections (UTIs), symptom severity and impact on QOL (as discussed above), physical activity, food and fluid intake, all medications taken, and goals for treatment. The initial interview should include a basic focused history; additional data can be gathered over time as indicated.

Review of Systems

In addition to obtaining information about the onset of the problem, type and severity of incontinence, current management approaches, goals for treatment, and food/fluid/medications, the nurse should query the patient about past evaluations and treatments, comorbid conditions, and prior surgical procedures and should conduct a focused review of the following systems:

- Neurologic (i.e., history of stroke, spinal cord trauma or lesions, lower back problems or procedures, multiple sclerosis, cognitive status)
- Gastrointestinal (i.e., bowel resections, inflammatory bowel disease, irritable bowel syndrome, anorectal trauma, anorectal surgical procedures, hemorrhoids, anal intercourse)
- Obstetric/gynecologic (women) (number of vaginal deliveries, difficult deliveries, obstetric trauma, pelvic procedures, presence of pelvic organ prolapses, rectovaginal fistula)

As noted, a complete list of all medications should be obtained and should include over-the-counter and herbal agents as well as prescription medications that could affect bowel function (**Table 22-3**).

Essential Questions

The nurse could use the following questions and follow-up discussion to obtain insight into any derangements in bowel motility and stool consistency, sensory awareness and sphincter control, rectal capacity and compliance, and general ability to reach the bathroom in a timely manner (Kuoch et al., 2019; Whitehead et al., 2016):

1. How often do you have voluntary (controlled) bowel movements, and what is the consistency of the stool?
2. How often do you have involuntary leakage of stool, and what is the consistency of the stool?
3. Do you always know when there is stool or gas in your rectum? Can you differentiate between gas and liquid and solid?
4. If you get the urge to have a bowel movement, can you retain the stool long enough to get to the toilet without leakage?

5. Does bowel or stool leakage cause you to alter your lifestyle?
6. Would you like to receive treatment for accidental bowel leakage?

KEY POINT

The history should always include "key questions" related to stool frequency and consistency; sensory awareness; ability to differentiate between gas, liquid, and solid; and ability to delay defecation.

Contributing Factors

In conducting the interview and synthesizing the data, the continence nurse should be alert to the following potential contributing factors (Danielson, 2019; Doughty, 2000; Fader et al., 2010; Mellgren, 2010; Meyer & Richter, 2015; Roth, 2010; Ruiz & Kaiser, 2017):

- Reversible risk factors: intestinal infections, fecal impaction, foods and medications affecting bowel motility (**Tables 22-3 and 22-4**), and initiation of enteral feedings
- Functional ability: mobility, dexterity, visual and mental acuity, and any issues with the living environment
- Bowel incontinence pattern: incontinence of gas, liquid, and/or solid stool; frequency of stools—voluntary and involuntary; description of stool; and awareness of rectal distention and incontinent episodes.
- Obstetric history: episiotomies, forceps, multiparity, and hysterectomy
- Surgical history: bowel resections, rectal prolapse, hemorrhoids, fissures, anorectal surgery or trauma, and malignancy
- Sexual history: anal sex or sex appliances that might cause dilation of anal sphincter
- CNS disorders, neuropathy, back injury, and dementia
- Chronic diseases: diabetes, Crohn's, ulcerative colitis, irritable bowel, arthritis, Parkinson's, and MS
- Medications (**Table 22-3**)

FOCUSED PHYSICAL EXAMINATION

As is true of history taking, the physical examination can range from a basic examination to an extensive examination, depending on the individual's presenting symptoms and the examiner's level of expertise. A basic assessment should include an abdominal exam, an evaluation of anorectal anatomy, and a digital rectal examination to determine sphincter tone, presence of stool or masses, perineal sensation, presence or absence of the anocutaneous reflex (i.e., anal wink sign), and any pelvic organ prolapse such as cystocele, rectocele, enterocele, or uterine (Paquette et al., 2015).

Basic physical assessment includes abdominal and anorectal examinations.

TABLE 22-3 MEDICATIONS AFFECTING BOWEL MOTILITY

MEDICATION	PHARMACOLOGICAL EFFECT ON GASTRIC/ COLONIC MOTILITY	REFERENCE CITATION
ANTIDIARRHEAL MEDICATIONS		
Codeine	Opioid agonist: Binds to opioid receptors, inhibiting peristalsis	Epocrates (2019)
Diphenoxylate hydrochloride and atropine sulfate (Lomotil, Pfizer, New York, NY)	Difenoxin binds gut wall opioid receptors, inhibiting peristalsis	Epocrates (2019)
Difenoxin/atropine sulfate (Motofen, Valeant Pharmaceuticals, Quebec, Canada)	Difenoxin binds gut wall opioid receptors, inhibiting peristalsis	Epocrates (2019)
Loperamide (Imodium, Janssen Pharmaceutical, Titusville, NJ)	Binds gut wall opioid receptors, inhibits peristalsis, increases anal sphincter tone	Epocrates (2019)
Octreotide acetate (Sandostatin, Novartis Pharmaceuticals, Basel, Switzerland)	Synthetic analog of somatostatin; reduces volume of intestinal secretions	Epocrates (2019)
Bismuth subsalicylate (Maalox, Novartis, Basel, Switzerland; Pepto-Bismol, Procter & Gamble, Cincinnati, OH; Kaopectate, Chattem, Inc., Chattanooga, TN)	Reduces secretions, possesses antimicrobial effects	Epocrates (2019)
Cholestyramine (Questran, Bristol-Myers Squibb, NY; Prevalite, Upsher-Smith Laboratories, Minneapolis, MN)	Binds intestinal bile acids, which have a promotility effect in the colon	Epocrates (2019)
Crofelemer	Inhibits calcium activated chloride channels, normalizing water flow in gut, treatment of HI-associated diarrhea	Epocrates (2019)
Eluxadoline	Binds to opioid receptors to inhibit peristalsis, in IBS-D	Epocrates (2019)
MEDICATIONS TO TREAT CONSTIPATION		
Bulk-forming laxatives Psyllium (Metamucil, Procter & Gamble, Cincinnati, OH) Methyl cellulose (Citrucel, GlaxoSmithKline, Brentford, Middlesex, UK) Calcium polycarbophil (FiberCon, Pfizer, New York, NY)	Increase bulk, increase water absorption, may take several days to work, require adequate fluid intake	Epocrates (2019), Marples (2011), Woodward (2012)
Osmotic laxatives Sodium phosphate, magnesium hydroxide, magnesium citrate, polyethylene glycol, lactulose Lubiprostone (Amitiza, Takeda Pharmaceuticals, Deerfield, Il.)	Pull fluid into the lumen of the bowel via osmosis, thus softening the stool and promoting peristalsis; decrease intestinal permeability*	Epocrates (2019), Marples (2011), Woodward (2012)
Stimulant laxatives Bisacodyl Castor oil Sennosides, senna	Increase peristalsis, increase water absorption from large intestine, can cause electrolyte imbalance in frail elderly	Epocrates (2019), Marples (2011), Woodward (2012)
Stool softeners Docusate calcium, docusate sodium Mineral oil	Soften stool; facilitate mixture of stool, fat, and water; make stool easier to pass; little evidence to support use	Epocrates (2019), Marples (2011), Woodward (2012)
Probiotics	May improve stool consistency and bowel regularity by normalizing intestinal flora (more data needed regarding specific agents and dosages)	Marples (2011), Woodward (2012)
Guanylate cyclase-C agonist Linaclotide Plecanatide	Accelerates gut transit in healthy people and females with IBS-C Promotes luminal secretion through the CFTR receptor to treat chronic idiopathic constipation or constipation or IBS-C	Epocrates (2019)

TABLE 22-3 MEDICATIONS AFFECTING BOWEL MOTILITY (*Continued*)

MEDICATION	PHARMACOLOGICAL EFFECT ON GASTRIC/COLONIC MOTILITY	REFERENCE CITATION
Lubiprostone	Activates ClC-2 chloride channels, increasing intestinal fluid secretion and motility, reducing permeability	Epocrates (2019)
Methylnaltrexone	Antagonizes peripheral mu-opioid receptors, inhibiting opioid-induced constipation	Epocrates (2019)
MEDICATIONS THAT CONTRIBUTE TO FI		
Anticholinergics Antihistamines Antispasmodics Tricyclic antidepressants Antipsychotics	Can contribute to constipation, possess anticholinergic properties, prolong colonic transit time, have antiemetic and sedative effects	Bliss et al. (2006), Epocrates (2019), Wuong (2012)
Cardiovascular medications Calcium channel blockers Beta-adrenergic antagonists Diuretics Antiarrhythmics	Can contribute to constipation	Bliss et al. (2006), Epocrates (2019)
Central nervous system depressants Anticonvulsants Antiparkinsonian drugs	Can contribute to constipation	Bliss et al. (2006), Epocrates (2019)
Narcotic analgesics Opiates Barbiturates Opioid derivatives (methadone, morphine, oxycodone)	Opioid agonists; bind to opioid receptors, inhibiting peristalsis	Bliss et al. (2006), Epocrates (2019)
Antineoplastics Vinca alkaloids	Can cause constipation and/or diarrhea as a side effect	Bliss et al. (2006), Epocrates (2019)
Cholestyramine	Bile acid–binding agent; used in treatment of diarrhea	Bliss et al. (2006), Marples (2011)
Nonsteroidal anti-inflammatory drugs Ibuprofen Naproxen	May cause constipation	Bliss et al. (2006), Epocrates (2019)
Oxybutynin	Constipation is common side effect due to anticholinergic effects.	Bliss et al. (2006), Epocrates (2019)
MEDICATIONS THAT CAUSE LOOSE STOOLS/DIARRHEA		
Oral hypoglycemics	May cause diarrhea as a side effect, delay or decrease intestinal absorption of glucose	Bliss et al. (2006), Epocrates (2019)
Alzheimer disease medications Acetylcholinesterase inhibitors (donepezil)	Can cause diarrhea as a side effect; reversibly bind to and inactivate acetylcholinesterase, thus increasing levels of acetylcholine (which promotes peristalsis) (acetylcholinesterase inhibitor)	Bliss et al. (2006), Epocrates (2019)
Antibiotics Ampicillin Cefazolin, cephalexin, ceftriaxone, ceftazidime Ciprofloxacin Clindamycin, erythromycin	Alter intestinal mucosa and intestinal flora. Diarrhea is a common side effect.	Bliss et al. (2006), Epocrates (2019)

*Patient needs to have adequate fluid intake for these to be effective.

Abdominal Examination

Abdominal examination involves visual inspection for distention, percussion along the length of the bowel to assess for indicators of stool retention, and palpation of the lower quadrants to assess for evidence of stool reten-tion. (An advanced practice nurse should also conduct a thorough abdominal examination to detect any masses.) Indicators of chronic constipation/stool retention include dull note to percussion along most of the colon, pal-pable nodules of stool in the left lower quadrant, and

TABLE 22-4 FOODS AFFECTING BOWEL MOTILITY		
FOOD	EFFECT ON GASTRIC/COLONIC MOTILITY	REFERENCE CITATION
Caffeine	Stimulates gastrointestinal motility; can cause diarrhea and FI; if taken in excess may contribute to dehydration and constipation	Crosswell et al. (2010), Hansen et al. (2006)
Alcohol	Stimulates gastrointestinal motility, increases risk of FI	Crosswell et al. (2010), Hansen et al. (2006)
Lactose	Intolerance and malabsorption of lactose results in diarrhea. FI is secondary to diarrhea.	Crosswell et al. (2010), Hansen et al. (2006)
Spicy foods	Increase gastrointestinal motility, increase FI secondary to loose stools	Crosswell et al. (2010)
Nuts (high in insoluble fiber)	Increase gastrointestinal motility	Hansen et al. (2006)
Foods high in insoluble fibers: Unprocessed bran, bran cereals, whole wheat fiber, popcorn, nuts, cabbage, green beans, wax beans, eggplant, apples, carrots	Increase stool bulk, but do not absorb water; can move through the GI system basically intact. Increased stool bulk contributes to distention of colon wall, which triggers peristaltic activity.	Hunter et al. (2002), Wisten and Messner (2005)
Foods high in soluble fibers (fruit fiber/pectin): Oats, dried beans, squash, pectin, apples, citrus fruits, psyllium	Absorb water and have high water retention, thicken stool, reduce bowel transit time, slow digestion, have a lubricating effect on the intestinal mucosa	Wisten and Messner (2005)
Chocolate	Increases gastrointestinal motility and risk of FI	Crosswell et al. (2010), Hansen et al. (2006)
Foods with both soluble and insoluble fiber: Onions, cabbage, Brussels sprouts, cauliflower, apricots	Cause flatus	Crosswell et al. (2010)
Greasy/fatty foods: Fast food, pizza, bacon, gravy, fried foods	Increase gastrointestinal motility and risk of FI	Crosswell et al. (2010)
Fruits: Fresh fruit (raisins), fruit juice (orange, prune)	Increase gastrointestinal motility and risk of FI	Crosswell et al. (2010)
Cheeses, dairy products	Increase risk of FI if lactose intolerant, can cause constipation if eaten in large amounts (taking place of high-fiber foods)	Crosswell et al. (2010), Woodward (2012), Wuong (2012)

FI, fecal incontinence.

discomfort and resistance to palpation in the right lower quadrant. Normally, the percussion note over most of the air-filled colon is tympanic or resonant, there is no palpable stool in the left lower quadrant, and palpation of the right lower quadrant is met with no resistance and no symptoms of pain or discomfort.

Visual Anal Examination

A visual examination of the anus should be performed while the patient is at rest, during contraction, and while bearing down (Valsalva maneuver). The sphincter should be closed at rest; a patulous or gaping sphincter is indicative of a neurologic lesion causing denervation of the sphincter. The sphincter should visibly contract when the individual is instructed to "tighten as if you are trying not to pass stool or gas," and there should be no visible defects. Inability to voluntarily contract the sphincter is evidence of a neurological problem or muscle deficit. Observation during bearing down may reveal the presence of hemorrhoids, mucosal or rectal prolapse, or pelvic organ prolapse. If the sphincter remains tightly contracted when the individual is instructed to "bear down as if you are trying to eliminate stool or gas," it suggests compromised ability to coordinate pelvic floor and sphincter relaxation with abdominal muscle contraction (pelvic floor dyssynergia). The external perineum is assessed for any evidence of scarring, skin breakdown, perineal thinning, or fistula (Alavi et al., 2015).

KEY POINT

When doing the anorectal exam, the examiner should instruct the individual to contract the sphincter as if "trying not to pass stool or gas"; normal response is evidenced by 360 degrees of symmetrical tension that is felt as a strong squeeze and slight inward pull.

Digital Anorectal Examination

A digital anorectal examination should be done to assess for fecal impaction, fissure, fistula, hemorrhoids, enlarged or irregular prostate gland in males, masses, and the function of the pelvic floor musculature, including EAS and IAS tone and length (Paquette et al., 2015). Normal anal resting tone is a closed sphincter. During digital exam, sphincter tone may vary; however, when the individual is prompted to tighten the sphincter, normal function is evidenced by 360 degrees of symmetrical tension that is felt as a strong squeeze around the examining finger and a slight inward pull on the finger. Defects or gaps in the circumference of the external sphincter circumference can be palpated though it takes practice and experience to detect subtle abnormalities. During bearing down, a downward push should be felt, accompanied by sphincter relaxation; there should be no prolapse of the rectal vault (Doughty, 2000; Ruiz & Kaiser, 2017).

Neurologic Examination

A neurologic examination is indicated in situations where a neurologic deficit is suspected and should include anal reflex and perianal sensory testing. The anal reflex is elicited by gently stroking the perianal skin with a finger or q-tip; normally, this causes the anus to quickly contract, the so-called anal wink. No response may be indicative of neurological problems, though absence of the anal wink is not diagnostic in and of itself. Detection of any abnormalities during the physical examination warrants referral to the individual's primary care provider to consider anorectal physiologic testing, especially when there is additional evidence of denervation (Bartolo & Paterson, 2009; Doughty, 2000; Nix & Haugen, 2010).

BOWEL DIARY

Characterization of bowel habits is important, and the Bristol Stool Form Scale and bowel diaries can be useful. Bowel diaries provide objective information regarding the person's elimination patterns (Chapter 6, Fig. 6-8). Bowel diaries allow the clinician to understand the patient's symptoms over time in order to determine the severity of the FI and the effectiveness of therapeutic procedures (Doughty, 2000; Findlay & Maxwell-Armstrong, 2010). Studies show that a daily written report (bowel diary) is more reliable then verbal self-reporting based on recall. However, bowel diaries are limited by level of commitment and willingness to do them (Meyer & Richter, 2015). The health care provider can encourage the individual and emphasize the value of the information toward making a proper diagnosis and developing an effective treatment strategy. Examples of bowel diaries in the literature tend to evaluate both voluntary and involuntary stools for consistency, frequency of evacuation, volume and severity of incontinence, diet, discomfort, activity at time of incontinence, and/or presence of urgency. The Bristol Stool Scale (Chapter 6, Figs. 6-7 and 6-8) is often incorporated within the bowel diary to enhance stool consistency descriptions (see **Fig. 22-1**).

Date/time	Voluntary evacuation (amount and consistency)	Incontinent stool (amount and consistency)	Diet	Activity/ discomfort

FIGURE 22-1. Sample Bowel Diary. A bowel diary helps track changes in stool pattern over several days. Length of time depends, in part, on how often the individual has a bowel movement but should be recorded for at least a week. The bowel diary and Bristol Stool Chart should be used together to provide a complete record. Also see Chapter 6, Figure 6-8.

DIAGNOSTIC PROCEDURES

Additional diagnostic tests may be indicated for individuals with persistent diarrhea of unknown etiology, indicators of sphincter dysfunction, suspected prolapse, and suspected malignancy (Rao et al., 2017). Diagnostic procedures for the individual with persistent diarrhea include stool testing for ova and parasites; stool cultures for *Salmonella*, *Shigella*, *Campylobacter*, *Escherichia coli*, *Entamoeba histolytica*, and *C. difficile*; blood work (e.g., CBC, electrolytes, calcium, phosphorus, and albumin); and malabsorption studies (e.g., hydrogen breath test or stool acidity test) (Sabol & Friedenburg, 1997).

Anal sphincter imaging and physiologic function studies are typically indicated when there is a suspected sphincter defect, such as a gap in the circumferential contraction of the sphincter on examination, or evidence of diminished contractility. The clinician should implement measures to correct motility disorders and other reversible factors prior to conducting studies of sphincter structure and function (Bharucha et al., 2010; Dudding et al., 2010; Roberson et al., 2010; Ruiz & Kaiser, 2017). Specific studies are discussed below.

KEY POINT

Additional diagnostic tests may be indicated for selected individuals, including those with persistent diarrhea of unknown etiology, indicators of sphincter dysfunction, suspected prolapse, and suspected malignancy.

Endoanal Ultrasound

Ultrasonography uses a transducer emitting sound waves to create an image of organ structure; it is used to determine anal anatomic integrity and to identify any structural abnormalities of the internal and/or EAS. Endoanal ultrasound (EAUS) is the gold standard investigation for the structural assessment of the anal canal. It is considered to be a very sensitive tool for identifying sphincter defects. However, the presence of a sphincter defect may not necessarily correlate with severity of incontinence (Paquette et al., 2015; Rao et al., 2017).

Differentiating defects identified in the EAS from fatty tissue may be difficult and necessitate the use of newer high-resolution ultrasound probes to visualize defects clearer (Williams et al., 2018).

Anorectal Manometry

Anorectal manometry is used to assess sphincter function; it measures resting and squeeze pressures, high-pressure zone, rectal sensation, and the presence or absence of a rectoanal inhibitory reflex and provides assessment of rectal vault distensibility. High-resolution anorectal manometry (HRM) using an integrated probe allows for 3D-analysis and visualization of pressure profiles, providing data regarding rectal capacity and sensory awareness of rectal distention, which may improve assessment of defecation disorders (Ruiz & Kaiser, 2017; Wald, 2018). The response of the sphincters to rectal distention is evaluated simultaneously and should involve relaxation of the IAS and contraction of the EAS. Resting pressure reflects IAS function, and squeeze pressure reflects EAS function. Unfortunately, disturbances of anorectal structure and/or function do not always correlate well with reported symptom severity (Rao et al., 2017).

Electromyography

Electromyography is a neurologic examination of the pelvic floor muscles and the nerves that control the anal and rectal muscles, using either surface electrodes or needle electrodes. The patient is instructed to -contract the anal sphincter muscle and the electrodes measure the strength of the contraction. Needle electrodes provide more accurate data, but the individual may experience discomfort or pain with insertion. EMG provides data regarding sphincter innervation and contractility. While pudendal nerve terminal motor latency (PTNML) testing is used to identify neuropathy as a result of injury (obstetrical stretch, radiation, surgery) or systemic factors (diabetes, chemotherapy), it is not used that often in the evaluation of FI; (Paquette et al., 2015; Rao et al., 2017).

Defecography

Defecography is used to diagnose functional problems with rectal evacuation, such as rectal prolapse, rectocele, or rectoanal intussusception. The rectum is filled with a radiopaque paste, and imaging studies are obtained during rectal evacuation. It is a very difficult and embarrassing study for the patient and requires a skilled and empathetic examiner.

Proctosigmoidoscopy or Colonoscopy

Proctosigmoidoscopy or colonoscopy is indicated when there is any suspicion of malignancy (e.g., bleeding, change in bowel habits, and/or palpable rectal or abdominal mass). The examiner is able to directly visualize the intestinal mucosa and to obtain biopsies of any suspicious areas or lesions.

Magnetic Resonance Imaging

MRI uses radio waves and magnets to produce detailed pictures of internal organs and soft tissues without the use of x-rays. It may include the injection of contrast medium. It can provide detailed anatomic images of the IAS and EAS and is more accurate than ultrasound (US) in the diagnosis of sphincter defects and atrophy (Rao et al., 2017).

DATA SYNTHESIS

In summary, a thorough history and physical examination are required to identify the specific issues resulting in FI and to develop an appropriate management plan. All individuals require a basic history and physical examination; those with suspected sphincter defects, neurologic lesions, or persistent diarrhea may require additional studies. More advanced studies are also required for the patient who does not respond to basic management strategies.

In synthesizing the data and developing a management plan, the continence nurse should begin by answering the following questions.

- Is the incontinence transient or chronic? If the FI is new onset and due to either high-volume liquid stool or altered mental status, the focus should be on treatment of the underlying medical conditions, containment of the stool, and protection of the perianal skin. For individuals with chronic FI, the continence nurse should review the assessment data to determine the following:
- Is stool consistency normal (i.e., is stool soft and formed?)? Since stool consistency is a major determining factor for continence, the initial focus in management should be on correcting any abnormalities in stool consistency.
- Is the individual cognitively intact, or does he/she have incontinent stools with no apparent cognitive awareness? The individual with incontinence due to dementia will require a routine toileting program and may require regular stimulated defecation (anal washout) *or* management with absorptive products.
- Is sensory function intact, that is, does the individual always know when there is stool or gas in the rectum, and can the individual reliably discriminate between gas, liquid, and solid contents? If the individual usually senses stool in the rectum but sometimes leaks small volumes of stool without recognition, she/he should be referred for biofeedback to improve sensory function. If the individual never senses rectal distention due to a neurologic lesion or process, she/he will require a stimulated defecation program.
- Is sphincter function normal, or is there evidence of sphincter weakness or denervation? The individual with weak but contractile sphincter muscles will benefit from pelvic muscle exercises as initial management. The individual with total loss of sphincter contractility due to a neurologic lesion or process will require a stimulated defecation program.

- Is there evidence of inadequate rectal capacity and compliance (i.e., persistent intense urgency and ability to delay defecation for only a short period of time)? These individuals should be evaluated by a gastroenterologist and possibly colorectal surgeon for management of the underlying disease process.

MANAGEMENT OF FECAL INCONTINENCE

WOC nursing management of the patient with FI or AI will depend primarily on the underlying cause(s), the functional aspects of continence involved (as outlined in the section on data synthesis), and the specific care setting. Individualized and patient-focused management, protection of patient privacy, and maintenance of patient dignity are key nursing responsibilities in all settings. Initial treatment should focus on correcting the specific factors causing FI and on minimizing the physical and psychosocial impact (e.g., pain, skin damage, embarrassment) (Bharucha et al., 2015; Kelly, 2019; Stokes et al., 2016). Implementation of measures to contain stool and control odor is essential in situations in which bowel control cannot be immediately achieved. In addition, protocols that assure effective management of diarrhea and constipation should be developed in all care environments (Alavi et al., 2015; Bharucha et al., 2015; Wald, 2018).

MANAGEMENT OF TRANSIENT INCONTINENCE

Transient incontinence due to acute diarrhea and/or acute alteration in mental status is common among hospitalized patients (Bliss et al., 2017; Stokes, 2017). Typical causes include infectious or acute inflammatory processes (e.g., certain strains of flu, *C. difficile*, exacerbation of Crohn's or ulcerative colitis, antibiotic-associated diarrhea, medications with GI side effects, and radiation therapy or chemotherapy), heavy sedation, and/or delirium. Malnutrition or gluten sensitivity, protein deficiencies, and enteral feedings may also cause diarrhea (Bliss et al., 2017; Stokes, 2017). While restoration of normal stool consistency and

continence status is the ultimate goal for nursing management, stool containment and skin management may be the most immediate concerns, especially in critical care and acute care settings when there is high-volume liquid stool. An individualized program of management should be developed that includes skin cleansing with a mild agent and use of a pouching system or internal collection device to contain the effluent (Carr & Hunter, 2018; Park & Kim, 2014; Willson et al., 2014).

There are a variety of devices and products available for management of FI. These products can be divided into two major groups: (1) those designed to prevent fecal leakage onto the skin and (2) those designed to absorb the stool and protect the skin. Products that prevent leakage of stool onto the skin include fecal collection pouches, intra-anal devices, rectal tubes and trumpets, and internal bowel management systems. Absorbent pads and briefs are used for absorption and containment of the stool and must be used in conjunction with skin care products designed to prevent incontinence-associated dermatitis although available absorbent products are made to absorb fluid rather than contain stool (especially formed stool) and control odor (Gray et al., 2018; Park & Kim, 2014; Wald, 2018).

External Fecal Collection Pouches

External fecal pouches are products designed to collect and contain liquid fecal material in order to quantify the stool and protect the skin; they are recommended as the "first step" in management of large-volume liquid stool (see **Fig. 22-2**). An external pouching device adheres directly to the perianal skin and is replaced every 1 to 2 days and as needed for leakage. Benefits of external fecal pouches include the fact that they are noninvasive with no risk of damage to the sphincters or rectal tissue; they protect the perianal skin from breakdown; they are a closed system, which helps to prevent the spread of harmful organisms; they can be attached to ancillary drainage systems; they at least partially contain excrement and odor; and they help to reduce use of absorptive products and linens as well as nursing and caregiver time.

Disadvantages of fecal pouches include the following: their use is limited to nonambulatory patients who do not slide up and down in bed; it typically requires more than one caregiver to apply a rectal pouch (one to position the patient and one to apply the device); stool occasionally undermines the pouch and causes perianal skin breakdown if not changed in a timely manner; rectal exams cannot be performed; and rectal medication cannot be

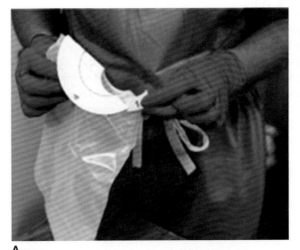

A

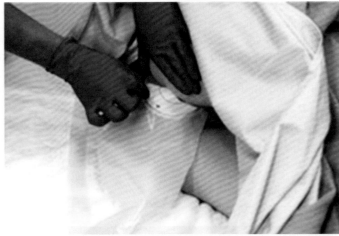

B

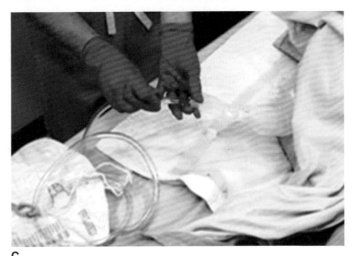

C

FIGURE 22-2. External Fecal Collection Device. The fecal incontinence pouch is used to protect the skin when the client is having frequent liquid stools. **A.** The paper backing is removed from the pouch's adhesive. **B.** The pouch is applied covering the anal opening. **C.** The tube from the pouch is attached to the tubing of the collection bag, which is positioned below the level of the client's buttocks. It is secured to the bed in the same manner as the urine collection bag.

administered with the pouch in place. A very significant disadvantage is the inability to use these devices effectively when there is perianal skin breakdown, because intact skin is required for a secure seal. In addition, removal from the patient with damaged skin carries the risk for additional skin breakdown (Carr & Hunter, 2018).

Internal Bowel Management Systems
Intended for use primarily in acute care settings, intra-anal bowel management systems (IBMS) are designed to divert liquid stool away from the perianal skin and into a collection device, thus providing for both quantification of fecal output and protection of the perianal skin. Indwelling devices should be used judiciously and in accordance with facility criteria and manufacturer's recommendations. Prior to placement of an intra-anal device, the nurse must carefully evaluate the patient to determine eligibility and to rule out contraindications (Whiteley et al., 2014; Carr & Hunter, 2018). See Box 22-1 for contraindications established by the manufacturers of these devices.

BOX 22-1	CONTRAINDICATIONS TO USE OF INTERNAL BOWEL MANAGEMENT SYSTEMS

Intra-anal devices should not be used in the following patients:

- Those known to be sensitive or allergic to any components within the system
- Those with clotting disorders
- Those who have had lower large bowel or rectal surgery in the last year
- Those with rectal or anal injury, severe rectal or anal stricture or stenosis (i.e., any patient if the distal rectum cannot accommodate the inflated cuff), confirmed rectal or anal tumor, severe hemorrhoids, or fecal impaction
- Those with suspected or confirmed rectal mucosa impairment (i.e., severe proctitis, ischemic proctitis, mucosal ulcerations)
- Those with indwelling rectal or anal devices in place, or who require enemas

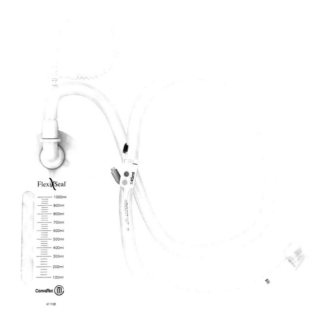

FIGURE 22-3. Example of a Fecal Management System: Internal Bowel Management. (Reprinted with permission from Hinkle, J. L., Cheever, K. H. (2017). *Brunner & Suddarth's textbook of medical-surgical nursing* (14th ed.). Philadelphia, PA: Wolters Kluwer Health.)

The device includes soft silicone tubing connected to a low-pressure intrarectal balloon on one end and to a collection device on the other end (**Fig. 22-3**). The retention balloon is placed into the rectum and then inflated with air, water, or saline. While the catheter and intrarectal balloon can be left inside the patient for an extended period (29 days), the stool collection bags are detached when full and disposed of appropriately. Some intra-anal devices allow for fecal sampling and for medication administration and irrigation; in addition, some are equipped with an indicator that signals maximum inflation of the intrarectal balloon and prevents further inflation (Carr & Hunter, 2018; Sammon et al., 2015).

Advantages of intra-anal devices include reduced risk of skin breakdown and discomfort; minimization of odor; enhanced patient dignity; protection of wounds, surgical sites, or burns from fecal contact; decreased exposure to infectious microorganisms; more accurate measurement of output (measurements on any plastic collection device are approximate as the print may slip and slide during stamping); reduced risk of catheter-associated UTIs; reduced soiling of linens; and reduced caregiver time required for hygienic care (Carr & Hunter, 2018; Gray et al., 2014).

Disadvantages related to use of intra-anal devices include risk of bleeding, especially among patients receiving anticoagulants or antiplatelet medications or those sustaining inadvertent traumatic balloon removal; damage to the rectal mucosa; anal erosions secondary to corrosive fecal enzymes or pressure from the indwelling device; blockage of the tubing; expulsion of the tube; and stool leakage around the device (Beeson et al., 2017;

Carr & Hunter, 2018; Mulhall & Jindal, 2013; Sammon et al., 2015). One researcher noted that the rate of anal mucosal injury increased over time from 1% at day 3 to 34% at day 14 (Sammon et al., 2015). It is recommended that the nurse monitor the number of days the IBMS is in place and reevaluate need for its use on daily basis with goal of discontinuation at the earliest possible date (Carr & Hunter, 2018; Sammon et al., 2015; Whiteley et al., 2014).

Intra-anal devices should not be used for chronic diarrhea as the devices are not intended for use for more than 29 consecutive days. It is essential for caregivers to be competent in placement and management of intra-anal devices. Frequent routine patient and device assessments should be performed to ensure the tubing is not beneath the patient and that there is no tension on the device; in addition, care must be taken with patient transfers to prevent traumatic removal of the device (Carr & Hunter, 2018; Sammon et al., 2015).

There are some direct costs associated with an intra-anal management device, with some cost variations between manufacturers. However, the costs may be offset by the savings from reduced use of linens, lower laundry costs, reduction in nursing time required for care, and reduced incidence of skin problems (Kowal-Vern et al., 2009). Use of the devices has been linked to improved nursing assessment and documentation and better patient outcomes.

KEY POINT

Prior to placement of an intra-anal device, the nurse must carefully evaluate the patient to determine eligibility and to rule out contraindications. Intra-anal devices should be used judiciously and in accordance with facility criteria and manufacturer's recommendations.

Rectal Trumpets

Thirty-two-French nasopharyngeal airways have been used off-label for management of FI; the "trumpet" (flared end of the airway) is inserted into the rectum and the straight end of the tube is connected to a gravity drainage system. This device should not be used in patients with leukopenia, perirectal abscess, or gastrointestinal bleeding. While very few studies have been done with these devices, outcomes have been mixed with one retrospective review reporting a three percent rate of rectal hemorrhages with its use (Glass et al., 2018). Since newer fecal management systems with safety data are available, rectal trumpet use is not generally recommended (Beitz, 2006; Carr & Hunter, 2018; Glass et al., 2018).

Rectal Tubes

Large lumen balloon-tipped indwelling catheters and rectal tubes have been used in the past for liquid stool diversion, for gas reduction, or to administer medications or enemas. Rectal tubes can divert stool away from the skin and can be attached to a closed system to prevent infectious contamination. They do not control odor. The balloons usually contain latex and can be inflated to over 500 cc. This overinflation can potentially cause ischemic injury to rectal wall or injury that can result in fistula formations (Carr & Hunter, 2018). The literature and expert opinions do not support the use of these devices especially since there are safer options available on the market today (Beitz, 2006; 2018; Carr & Hunter, 2018).

MANAGEMENT OF CHRONIC FECAL INCONTINENCE

As noted, chronic FI may be due to alterations in stool consistency, dementia, impaired sensory function, compromised sphincter function, neurologic lesions causing total loss of sensory function and sphincter control, changes in rectal capacity and compliance, or functional issues such as immobility or restraints (Pares et al., 2012). Restoration of normal controlled defecation is the goal for nursing management and begins with reversible factors, including elimination of any impacted stool and dietary, fluid, and medication modifications to normalize stool consistency; weight reduction, smoking cessation, and measures to improve mobility and functional status are also of benefit. Additional noninvasive interventions may include sphincter muscle exercises with or without biofeedback, bowel habit training, and stimulated defecation/transanal irrigation programs. Chapter 6 thoroughly explains lifestyle modification and behavioral measures to support optimal bowel health and elimination. For individuals who fail to respond to these noninvasive measures, surgical intervention should be considered. Currently available surgical options include sphincter repair, stimulated gracioplasty, artificial anal sphincter, sacral nerve modulation, magnetic anal sphincter implantation, injectable bulking agents, the antegrade continence enema (ACE) procedure, and diversion (colostomy) (Alavi et al., 2015; Bharucha et al., 2017; Forte et al., 2016; Ruiz & Kaiser, 2017; Wald, 2018; Whitehead et al., 2015).

The principles of bowel management and knowledge of treatment options should be used to develop an individualized program for prevention or management of FI. For example, evidence suggests that individuals undergoing bariatric surgery are at risk for FI and that measures to normalize stool consistency and to improve pelvic floor muscle strength prior to surgery can reduce the incidence of FI in these individuals (Richter et al., 2005; Roberson et al., 2010).

KEY POINT

Evidence suggests that individuals undergoing bariatric surgery are at risk for FI and that measures to normalize stool consistency and to improve pelvic floor muscle strength prior to surgery can reduce the incidence of FI in these individuals.

Management of Fecal Impaction

Fecal impaction most commonly occurs as an acute exacerbation of chronic constipation; risk factors include routine use of laxatives (possibly due to the underlying motility issue triggering the need for laxatives), immobility, neurologic lesions or disease states, and constipating medications (e.g., anticholinergic, antidiarrheal, and narcotic agents). Fecal impaction creates a mechanical obstruction that prevents the elimination of stool proximal to the impaction. Fecal impactions can increase the intraluminal pressure of the colon resulting in ischemic changes that could lead to ulcer formation or colonic perforations. The hard mass of stool also causes persistent relaxation of the internal sphincter; this allows liquid stool to pass around the fecal mass and causes fecal leakage (Falcon et al., 2016). Impactions most commonly occur at the level of the rectum but can also occur in the ascending or transverse colon (high impaction).

KEY POINT

Impactions most commonly occur at the level of the rectum but can also occur in the ascending or transverse colon; management is dependent on the level of impaction.

Rectal Impaction

When stool impaction is suspected, a digital rectal examination should be done; if there is a fecal mass in the rectum that is too hard and too large to evacuate, measures should be initiated to eliminate the fecal mass and to cleanse the proximal colon. Digital breakup should be attempted; if this is unsuccessful, lubricant and/or cathartic solutions should be administered rectally to soften the stool. Warm mineral oil enemas are frequently used to soften the stool and facilitate evacuation. They are typically given daily for 2 to 3 days, at which point the mass can usually be digitally broken up and removed. Anecdotal reports also support the use of a milk and molasses enema (typically a 1:1 mixture of molasses and milk, either powdered milk or cow's milk); the solution is warmed until it mixes thoroughly and then cooled for administration. Small volumes (60 to 90 mL) are instilled adjacent to the fecal mass, and the individual is asked to retain the mixture for about 30 minutes. Digital breakup is then attempted. This procedure is repeated until the fecal mass can be broken up and removed (Vilke et al., 2015).

Once the obstructing fecal mass has been removed, the proximal colon must be cleansed using suppositories, enemas, or laxatives. Oral polyethylene glycol or magnesium citrate solutions may be used to cleanse the proximal bowel so long as there are no contraindications (e.g., evidence of colonic distention or obstruction). Selection of a laxative must be made with any comorbidities in mind. For example, preparations containing magnesium, phosphate, or citrate should be avoided for individuals with heart failure or renal failure. Spontaneous evacuation of soft stool indicates that the bowel has been thoroughly cleansed (Mounsey et al., 2015; Minguez et al., 2016).

High Impaction

A high impaction occurs in the ascending or transverse colon and may be accompanied by nausea and vomiting, abdominal distention, and liquid stools. High impactions are treated with tap water or brand-name enemas to stimulate bowel movements. Some clinicians recommend use of oral mineral oil to lubricate the fecal mass prior to enema administration. MD Anderson Cancer Center utilizes a protocol involving powdered milk and molasses enemas, as follows: 6 ounces of hot water are mixed with 3 ounces of powdered milk (not cow's milk); 4.5 ounces of molasses are added and the mixture is stirred until the solution is uniform in color and at room temperature. The patient is positioned on his or her left side and the enema tube is inserted via the rectum about 12 inches (to reach the proximal descending and left transverse colon); the solution is instilled and then held for about 20 minutes. The procedure is repeated if needed with the patient in the left-side lying position and then with the patient in the right-side lying position. Once the fecal mass has been eliminated, oral laxatives are used to assure colonic cleansing, along with 2 L of fluid daily (Bisanz, 2011; Falcon et al., 2016).

Prevention of Recurrent Impaction

Once the impaction has been cleared, the continence nurse must institute measures to prevent recurrence. This usually includes increased fiber and fluid intake, increased mobility as tolerated, and avoidance of constipating drugs (if possible). Stool softeners may be needed if stools remain hard even after administration of adequate fiber and fluid. Osmotic laxatives can be given as needed, for example, whenever the individual has not had a bowel movement for 2 to 3 days despite use of fiber, fluids, and softeners. These agents "work" by pulling fluid into the lumen of the bowel, thus distending the bowel and promoting peristalsis. As a result, they can be used routinely if needed. In selecting an osmotic laxative, the nurse must always consider any contraindications to specific agents related to comorbid conditions.

Stimulant laxatives may be used when osmotic agents are ineffective; they work by stimulating the nerve cells within the bowel wall in addition to causing fluid secretion into the lumen of the bowel. Because they have direct effects on the nerve cells within the bowel wall, there are concerns that frequent repetitive use might have adverse effects on motility long term; thus, they are typically recommended for "PRN" use as opposed to routine use (Mounsey et al., 2015). For individuals with limited bowel control, enemas may be preferable to oral laxatives because the time frame for response is more predictable.

KEY POINT

Osmotic agents work by pulling fluid into the lumen of the bowel, thus distending the bowel and stimulating peristalsis; as a result, they can be used routinely if needed.

Measures to Normalize Stool Consistency and Bowel Function

Once any impacted stool has been removed, the continence nurse should focus on normalizing stool consistency and establishing a pattern for regular evacuation through dietary and fluid modifications to create soft formed stool and to reduce gas production, and use of medications as needed to assure normal stool consistency. Food intake patterns can also help to regulate bowel function. Bisanz (2011) suggests encouraging patients to take 64 ounces of fluids and ensuring the diet include 25 to 40 g of fiber daily. Three well-balanced meals and increased physical activity are also suggested. Individuals should be encouraged to eat at regular intervals every day and to avoid skipping meals (Bisanz, 2011; Mounsey et al., 2015). Patients should be advised to take advantage of the gastrocolic reflex and schedule toileting after meals. It is also suggested that patients use the correct seating position while toileting to straighten the anorectal junction; sit with feet on floor, knees higher than hips, lean forward slightly (Bisanz, 2011; Mounsey et al., 2015). See Figure 6-6 for the correct position for opening the bowels.

KEY POINT

Once any impacted stool has been removed, the continence nurse should focus on normalizing stool consistency and establishing a pattern for regular evacuation.

As explained previously, liquid stool may overwhelm the sphincters, and chronic constipation places the individual at risk for fecal impaction and subsequent leakage of liquid stool. Consequently, establishment of normal stool consistency is an essential element of management for most people with FI. Adequate hydration must be assured, watery to loose stools need to be thickened to decrease frequency and volume, and hard stools need to be softened. Both diarrhea and constipation may be positively affected by adequate fluid intake, dietary modifications, and use of fiber supplements. Medications may be recommended when these lifestyle measures provide insufficient effects or while waiting for advised fluid and dietary modifications to take effect (Bliss et al., 2014; Bharucha et al., 2017; Mounsey et al., 2015; Ribas and Munoz-Duyos, 2018).

Management of Diarrhea

This topic is addressed in Chapter 21, but the critical elements will be briefly highlighted here as well. All individuals with diarrhea should be counseled regarding the critical importance of fluid replacement, which should be initiated whenever there are frequent liquid stools. A simple and practical recommendation is to consume 8 ounces of liquid immediately following each loose stool in addition to their usual fluid intake. Good fluid choices include bouillon, broth-based soups, low-sugar sports drinks, herbal teas, gelatin (Jell-O), and water. Carbonated diet beverages, orange or prune juice, caffeinated beverages, alcoholic beverages, and chocolate should be avoided since they increase gastrointestinal motility and could worsen diarrhea. Liquids at room temperature may be better tolerated than those that are hot or cold. Milk should be limited or avoided altogether until diarrhea is no longer a problem, especially for those with known lactose intolerance. In contrast, yogurt with probiotics may help to restore normal colonic flora and thus, reduce diarrhea (Crosswell et al., 2010; Hansen et al., 2006; Shiller et al., 2017).

Dietary modifications may also help to reduce diarrheal episodes. For example, greasy, deep-fried, and fatty foods such as bacon and pizza, some fast foods, and rich sauces and gravy may worsen diarrhea and increase the risk of FI. Foods and fluids with high sugar content, those sweetened with sorbitol, very spicy foods such as chili, and nuts and fruits (figs, plums, prunes, and oranges) may also be bothersome as they increase gastrointestinal motility. Products containing gluten (pasta, wheat flour, baked goods) can cause or worsen diarrhea, specifically in individuals who are gluten sensitive (Hansen et al., 2006; Shiller et al., 2017). Finally, foods that form gas can also cause diarrhea. Some of these gas-forming foods include onions, beans, cabbage, peas, broccoli, cauliflower, whole grain breads and cereals, nuts, and popcorn (Crosswell et al., 2010; Shiller et al., 2017).

The BRAT diet is widely recommended for short-term relief of diarrhea: *B*ananas, *R*ice, *A*pples or *A*pplesauce, and *T*oast (low-fiber or white bread) or *T*apioca. Bananas may be more effective when they are green. See **Table 22-4** for foods that slow motility.

Bulk-forming fiber supplements can also be used to thicken the stool. A teaspoon of methyl cellulose (Citrucel) or 3.4 g of psyllium (Metamucil) mixed with 2 ounces of water and ingested immediately before or after a meal may help to thicken small bowel contents and to slow motility through the bowel. No additional liquid should be taken for about 1 hour (Bisanz, 2011; Bliss et al., 2014; Shiller et al., 2017).

Management of Constipation

As noted previously, correction of constipation requires provision of adequate fiber and fluid, measures to increase mobility, elimination of constipating medications when feasible, and judicious use of stool softeners and laxatives as well as prompt response to the urge to defecate. Recommended fluid intake for adults is usually about 1.5 to 2.5 L of fluids or 30 mL/kg body weight/day up to 2.5 L. Daily fiber intake of 25 to 38 g/day is recommended (Mounsey et al., 2015). Factors to consider in making recommendations for a specific individual include weight, activity level, atmospheric temperature, and any conditions requiring fluid restriction, such as congestive heart failure. Liquids typically include water, tea, coffee, and fresh fruit juices, as well as foods with high water content, such as Jell-O or popsicles. Potentially dehydrating fluids, such as alcohol or caffeine in high volumes, should be avoided or limited, as should fluids with high sugar content.

Individuals on fluid restriction may be at high risk for constipation because they are unable to consume adequate fiber and fluid. A review of the literature suggests that use of combination therapies, such as osmotic laxatives, stool softeners, and/or stimulant laxatives may be effective for this population (Forte et al., 2016; Mounsey et al., 2015; Wagg et al., 2017). As with all treatment plans, therapy should be individualized and individuals should be instructed to follow manufacturers' guidelines in regard to dosage of OTC products (Wilde et al., 2014).

Dietary measures to prevent constipation include reduced intake of high-fat and processed foods and increased intake of dietary fiber. High-fat foods slow motility and should be avoided or consumed in limited amounts; these include ice cream, cheese, whole milk, pizza, French fries, potato chips, and high-fat meats. Fast food should also be avoided or limited, because processing of fast food removes most of the beneficial dietary fiber; processed foods include all prepackaged foods, white or polished rice, refined sugars, refined white flour, doughnuts and pastries, and hot dog and hamburger buns.

Foods high in dietary fiber add bulk to the stool, thus promoting peristalsis and acting as natural stool-softening agents. Fresh fruits and raw vegetables are excellent choices of dietary fiber, as are high-fiber cereals and foods made with whole grains (Bisanz, 2011). Foods sweetened with sorbitol can help to relieve constipation because sorbitol is an osmotic laxative; licorice and green pumpkin seeds (pepitas) have also been reported to have natural laxative properties. **Table 22-4** lists foods that promote soft stool and help to prevent constipation.

Various fiber supplements are available for individuals who are unable or unwilling to ingest a high-fiber diet. Medicinal fiber supplements can be divided into two categories: soluble and bulk-forming. Soluble fiber dissolves in water, remains gelatinous in the bowel, and slows peristalsis so that nutrients can be absorbed. Bananas contain natural inulin fiber, which has a softening effect but does not add bulk to the stool. Benefiber, Fiber Choice, and ReCleanse Fiber Powder are manufactured products that also contain natural inulin. Bulk-forming fiber supplements work by absorbing water; with liquid stool, this results in thickening of the stool, and with hard stool, the fiber adds bulk to the stool, which attracts water and softens the stool. Examples of bulk-forming fiber supplements include psyllium and methyl cellulose (Bisanz, 2011; Bliss et al., 2014; Mounsey et al., 2015). Individuals using fiber supplements are generally encouraged to take them daily, to titrate the dose to obtain appropriate stool consistency, and to assure adequate fluid intake. Adequate fluid intake is particularly important with bulk-forming agents. Individuals beginning fiber supplements should be informed that increased production of gas is common during the first few weeks of fiber therapy.

KEY POINT

Dietary modifications and use of fiber supplements can be beneficial in management of both constipation and diarrhea.

Medications are a common contributing factor to constipation; thus, management of the individual with constipation involves a thorough review of all medications being taken (including over-the-counter and herbal agents) and consultation with the prescribing provider regarding possible substitutions or dose modifications for medications known to cause constipation. If the patient requires continued use of the medication, constipation should be prevented through a program that includes adequate fiber and fluid intake (unless contraindicated), stool softeners, and osmotic and stimulant laxatives. See **Table 22-3** for medications that commonly cause constipation.

KEY POINT

Medications are a common contributing factor to constipation; if the patient requires continued use of the medication (e.g., opioid analgesics), the patient should be placed on a program to prevent constipation (e.g., fiber supplements if tolerated, stool softeners, and laxatives as needed).

Various medications can be taken to promote peristalsis and relieve constipation, including suppositories, enemas, and oral laxatives. Enemas and suppositories should be avoided in individuals with low blood counts, due to the risk of bleeding or infection. Oral agents should be used only when there is no distal obstruction or impaction and should be selected based on any comorbid conditions, as noted earlier.

In general, fiber supplements and stool softeners are used to prevent constipation, and osmotic and stimulant laxatives are used to treat constipation. There are a wide variety of osmotic agents, including saline- and magnesium-based products, sorbitol, lactulose, and polyethylene glycol; all work by pulling fluid into the lumen of the bowel, which stimulates peristalsis and helps to soften the stool. The two stimulant laxatives widely used are senna and bisacodyl; both promote intestinal motility and increase fluid secretion into the bowel thereby increasing peristalsis through direct action on the nerves in the bowel wall. Softener–stimulant combinations have dual effects, as the classification suggests. Stimulant laxatives should be used with caution in the elderly and have some adverse effects with long-term use. These should only be considered after fiber and osmotic laxatives have been tried (Forte et al., 2016; Mounsey et al., 2015; Wagg et al., 2017).

KEY POINT

In general, fiber supplements and stool softeners are used to prevent constipation, and osmotic and stimulant laxatives are used to treat constipation.

Medications should be titrated to maintain soft formed stools on a regular basis. Stool softeners, stimulant laxatives, and combination products can be purchased at drug and grocery stores without a prescription. Store-brand stimulant laxative/stool softeners should work as well as brand names and may cost less. Liquid forms of these medications are also available and may be prescribed by a physician.

Healthy Bowel Habits

Patients need to be taught the fundamentals of normal bowel function and bowel hygiene, which includes prompt response to the "call to stool" (see Chapter 6). Prerequisites to an effective bowel habit training program include elimination of retained stool (via enemas or laxatives) and establishment of soft formed stool via fiber, fluid, activity, and softeners if needed. Any known personal stimuli for defecation should be used, such as warm tea or coffee, prune juice, or yogurt with probiotics. The individual must also be taught the best posture for bowel evacuation, which is sitting upright on the commode with feet apart and flat on the floor (see Chapter 6, Fig. 6-6). Some mild straining or abdominal muscle contraction might be necessary to increase intra-abdominal pressure.

KEY POINT

Healthy bowel habits include prompt response to the urge (call) to defecate, use of any personal stimuli to defecation (such as warm tea, coffee, or prune juice), and correct posture for defecation (sitting upright with feet flat on floor or step stool).

Management of Flatus Incontinence

Passing gas is a natural elimination process that occurs on a daily basis; however, there are extreme variations among individuals in terms of daily volume. Factors affecting the volume of gas production include the amount of high-fiber foods and cruciferous vegetables ingested (vegetables with peels, cabbage and related vegetables, grains, high-fiber breads, beans, cereals, nuts, and seeds) and, to a much lesser extent, the amount of air that is swallowed. Carbonated beverages, chewing gum, and drinking through straws increases the volume of swallowed air and may increase gas production in selected individuals; however, most swallowed air is absorbed prior to reaching the distal bowel. Individuals who report persistent high-volume gas production should be evaluated for an unrecognized malabsorption syndrome, such as lactose intolerance or gluten intolerance. Individuals who have flatus incontinence should be taught measures to reduce gas production and should also be taught sphincter strengthening exercises; if the flatus incontinence occurs without the individual's awareness of gaseous rectal distention, biofeedback may be indicated to improve sensory awareness. The most obvious strategy for reducing gas production is to reduce the intake of gas-producing foods. Additional measures include the use of simethicone and alpha-galactosidase. Simethicone breaks large gas bubbles into smaller bubbles so that it is more likely to be absorbed and less likely to cause distress. Alpha-galactosidase is an enzyme that helps to break down complex carbohydrates to prevent bacterial action and gas production. Both of these products are readily available over the counter (Bisanz, 2011; Mounsey et al., 2015).

KEY POINT

Management of flatus incontinence includes measures to reduce gas production and instruction in sphincter-strengthening exercises.

Noninvasive Therapeutic Techniques

A variety of noninvasive therapeutic techniques, such as pelvic floor muscle training (PFMT), biofeedback (BF), and electrical stimulation (ES) are available for the treatment of FI. These therapies can be used alone or in combination with each other and with conservative medical management (Bliss et al., 2017; Ruiz & Kaiser, 2017).

Pelvic Floor Muscle Exercises

PFMT is an established mode of therapy for urinary incontinence (UI). PFMT is currently recommended by the 6th International Consultation on Incontinence as an early intervention that can be used with other conservative management options (Bliss et al., 2017). The technique involves having the patient contract the pelvic floor muscles, including the EAS and the puborectalis, while keeping the abdominal muscles relaxed. The patient is instructed to do this multiple times a day to increase the strength of the pelvic floor muscles (Bliss et al., 2017;

Wald, 2018). PFMT is of potential benefit to individuals who recognize rectal distention but have difficulty retaining stool due to weak or damaged sphincter muscles. The techniques for teaching and performing pelvic muscle exercises are essentially the same whether the individual has urinary, fecal, or mixed incontinence. The goal of sphincter exercises is to condition the external sphincter in terms of duration and speed of contraction in order to prevent fecal leakage, and the retraining may be used in conjunction with other conservative measures to improve fecal continence in patients with intact sensation, cognition, and volitional contraction of the sphincter (Bates et al., 2017; Wilde et al., 2014).

KEY POINT

The techniques for teaching and performing pelvic muscle exercises for individuals with FI are essentially the same as those for individuals with UI; the individual must be able to isolate and voluntarily contract the pelvic floor muscles without recruiting the abdominal muscles. Pelvic floor muscle exercise is recommended as an early intervention that can be used with other conservative management interventions

---

Wilde et al. (2014) describe the following steps in teaching PFMT: (1) assist the cognitively aware and compliant patient to identify and isolate the pelvic floor muscles; (2) teach the individual to contract the pelvic floor muscles without additionally contracting the abdominal muscles; and (3) establish an exercise program that specifies number of contractions and goal for duration of contraction. Isolating the pelvic floor muscles may initially be difficult for the individual. Sitting straight up in a chair with feet flat on the floor and pretending to "hold back flatus" may help the patient to identify the specific muscles. The clinician or therapist may also insert a gloved finger into the vagina or rectum and have the patient squeeze around the examining finger. Some clinicians have suggested the patient stop the flow of urine midstream to check that he or she is contracting the appropriate muscle group; this should be done *only* to assess muscle strength and not on a routine basis.

Once the patient can consistently isolate and contract the muscle, she/he is placed on an individualized exercise program to improve the strength, muscle coordination, and endurance of the muscles. Usually, a 12-week program is initiated in which the patient begins with a series of 10 pelvic floor muscle contractions at three different times during the day. The ultimate goal is that each individual contraction would last 10 seconds. However, the person with very weak muscles who is unable to hold the contraction for even 4 seconds may become discouraged; thus, an individualized goal should be established, for example, 3- to 5-second contractions at first, with gradual increase in duration to the sustained 10-second contraction. Once the patient is able to sustain

10-second contractions, the number of contractions may be increased as negotiated with the therapist. Although the exercises may be done lying, sitting, or standing, patients who have trouble isolating the pelvic floor muscles (and keeping the abdominal muscles relaxed) may be more successful if they perform the exercises while bending forward with arms pressed against a table or chair back or leaning forward with arms pressed against a wall. Biofeedback may also be a useful adjunct to standard pelvic muscle exercise therapy for some individuals.

The patient needs to be reminded that strength and endurance are built gradually over time, as is true with any exercise program. In addition, maintenance "toning" exercises should be continued throughout life. Another strategy to promote patient adherence and confidence in her/his progress is to have the patient keep a bowel diary to track FI episodes; this provides objective evidence of progress (reduced episodes of incontinence) that may serve to encourage and motivate the individual (Wilde et al., 2014), (see Chapter 6 for PFMT details).

Biofeedback

Biofeedback is used in combination to PMFT to assist the patient to gain awareness of the pelvic floor muscles while they are performing PFMT exercises (Alavi et al., 2015; Bates et al., 2017; Ruiz & Kaiser, 2017; Wald, 2018). It can be used to improve sensory awareness, improve pelvic muscle strength and function, or improve coordination between abdominal and pelvic floor muscles. When coupled with pelvic floor exercises, biofeedback has been successful in improving continence for patients with FI refractory to lifestyle and medical treatment alone. Some sensation of rectal fullness and the ability to at least weakly contract the pelvic muscles must be present for biofeedback to be successful. Biofeedback may be used in conjunction with digital feedback, electrical stimulation, and manometric or US response monitoring (Alavi et al., 2015; Bates et al., 2017; Bliss et al., 2017). Several different regimens have been defined and utilized in various studies; at present, there are insufficient data to support any one regimen as being superior (Bliss et al., 2017; Ruiz & Kaiser, 2017; Wald, 2018). Biofeedback with adjunctive pelvic floor muscle exercises is suggested to be more effective than pelvic muscle exercises or biofeedback alone (Bates et al., 2017; Ruiz & Kaiser, 2017).

KEY POINT

Biofeedback can be used to improve sensory awareness, improve pelvic muscle strength and function, and/or improve coordination between abdominal and pelvic floor muscles.

Biofeedback can also be used to improve rectal sensation in individuals with blunted or delayed awareness of rectal filling. A balloon is placed into the rectum and gradually inflated to the point of awareness and then gradually deflated with the patient focusing on the sensation. Over time, the patient is "taught" to recognize lower levels of rectal distention and to immediately contract the sphincter in response to the sensation of fullness. As noted earlier, prompt recognition of stool in the rectum is an essential element of continence that prompts the individual to contract the EAS and to move to a toilet in a timely manner (Wald, 2018). Therapy requires motivation and a commitment between the therapist and patient for weeks, even months, to realize success. All candidates, especially the elderly, must be able to understand and comply with directions (Mounsey et al., 2015; Wald, 2018).

Biofeedback involves placement of a pressure-sensitive probe intravaginally or rectally. The probe detects and measures the strength and coordination of the sphincter and levator ani muscles at baseline and can be used to monitor improvement over time (Bates et al., 2017). The patient can actually see the monitor screen as he or she is performing the contractions, which provides visual feedback that he or she is recruiting the appropriate muscles and that contractions are becoming stronger (Bates et al., 2017) (**Fig. 22-4**). This visual feedback is helpful in supporting continued patient compliance with the treatment program. The frequency of in-clinic biofeedback therapy sessions is determined by the physical therapist and patient. Some biofeedback systems are portable and battery operated and can be used by the patients in their homes. The literature suggests that portable, at-home therapies may improve treatment outcomes when compared to clinic-based options (Bliss et al., 2017).

Electrical Stimulation

Electrical stimulation directly to the anal sphincter is another option for strengthening sphincter function and may be used in combination with biofeedback therapy.

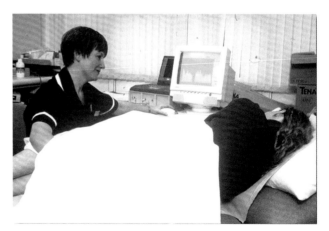

FIGURE 22-4. A Patient and Therapist during Biofeedback Treatment. (From Corman, M., Nicholls, R. J., Fazio, V. W., et al. (2012). *Corman's colon and rectal surgery*. Philadelphia, PA: Lippincott Williams & Wilkins.)

Sensors are placed intravaginally or intra-anally; alternatively, skin electrodes can be used with placement at specific points on the perineum. The stimulation device delivers a slight charge to the area, which causes the muscle to contract for the duration of the charge. The stimulation is said to feel like "pins and needles," similar to when your arm or foot "falls asleep." The charge is increased in strength and duration gradually over time. This therapy may be continued at home with a home unit; the individual should return to the clinic at regular intervals for evaluation of strength measurements and recalibration of the E-stim machine. At present, electrical stimulation is not widely recommended, due in part to the lack of substantial evidence regarding the technique and outcomes (Bliss et al., 2017). Better outcomes may be achieved among patients receiving E-stim as opposed to biofeedback; however, substantially more data are needed before E-stim can be widely recommended, and these data are also needed to obtain coverage by third-party payers. In addition, effective outcomes require a very skilled physical therapist as well as a compliant patient (Van Koughnett & Wexner, 2013).

As noted, third-party coverage for the cost of biofeedback and electrical stimulation is currently limited; however, this will probably improve once substantial data regarding efficacy can be provided. It should be noted that these advanced therapies are adjunctive to dietary and medication counseling and do not replace these basic interventions.

Neurogenic Bowel Management: Stimulated Defecation

By definition, neurogenic bowel involves loss of neural control of defecation; the individual with neurogenic bowel manifests changes in colon motility and/or loss of anorectal control, depending on the level of the injury. If the injury is above the level of the conus medullaris (L1–L2), the symptoms include increased bowel motility and poor anorectal sphincter relaxation. Rectal hypertonia and increased gastric transit time predisposes these patients to reflex defecation and incontinence (Cotterill et al., 2017; Dickinson et al., 2017; Stoffel et al., 2018). Injuries below the level of the conus medullaris (S1–S3), usually present with areflexic colon with loss of sphincter tone (Cotterill et al., 2017; Stoffel et al., 2018). Complete spinal cord lesions often result in slower colonic transit time (compared to incomplete injuries) and can predispose patient to constipation resulting in bloating, hard stools, and need for manual disimpaction (Dickinson et al., 2017; Stoffel et al., 2018). Conditions associated with neurogenic bowel include multiple sclerosis, spina bifida, cauda equina syndrome, stroke, spinal cord injury, cerebral palsy, and Parkinson disease (Dickinson et al., 2017).

Restoration of controlled defecation requires the individual to establish a schedule for elimination and to use peristaltic stimulants to initiate the evacuation process;

prior to beginning the program, any impacted stool must be removed and soft formed stool must be established through dietary and fluid management. The bowel must then be stimulated to empty daily or every other day to avoid passive incontinence, which has an extremely detrimental psychological effect on the lives of people with neurogenic bowel. An effective bowel management/stimulated defecation program typically requires 30 to 60 minutes a day devoted to thoroughly cleaning out the bowel and allows people to go on about their day without worrying about an accident (Cotterill et al., 2017; Stoffel et al., 2018).

> **KEY POINT**
>
> The individual with neurogenic bowel is unable to sense rectal distention and unable to voluntarily control the sphincter; restoration of controlled stool elimination requires establishment of a routine schedule for defecation and use of a peristaltic stimulus.

Dietary and fiber measures should be individualized to optimize stool consistency and bowel motility (Cotterill et al., 2017; Dickinson et al., 2017). As mentioned earlier in this chapter, dietary measures to prevent constipation include increased intake of dietary fiber. Although the effect of diet on symptoms in neurogenic bowel are not fully understood, researchers found diets high in fiber increased colonic transit time, thereby increasing rates of constipation. In addition, the literature suggests that a low-residue diet combined with adequate fluid intake and a bowel regimen improved colonic transit time and reduced constipation and abdominal pain (Cotterill et al., 2017; Stoffel et al., 2018).

Oral laxatives are not routinely used for individuals with neurogenic bowel, due to the unpredictability of their results; constipation in these individuals is usually better managed with suppositories and enemas as well as dietary and fluid modification. Occasionally, low-dose laxative agents or softener–stimulant combinations may be used in the evening followed by a stimulated defecation program in the morning; however, the dose and timing must be carefully titrated to prevent fecal accidents.

Once any retained stool has been eliminated and normal stool consistency has been established, the individual should establish a schedule for elimination; stimulated defecation should be scheduled for the same time of day every day (or every other day) when the individual has the time to devote to stimulating the bowel and waiting for defecation to occur. Some patients may choose to lie in bed to administer the agent, followed by transfer to the toilet or commode chair; others may elect to administer the stimulus while seated on the toilet or commode chair or while seated on the shower chair or bench to save time with showering and personal cleanup after evacuation. For instance, the individual may use digital stimulation, a suppository, or a mini-enema to promote peristalsis and to move the fecal mass into the rectum. Choice of the agent is individual and may change over time with aging or changes in physical condition. How quickly the stimulant works also varies from person to person.

Digital Stimulation

Digital stimulation is performed with a lubricated gloved finger inserted about an inch into the anal canal. Circular sweeps in the canal stimulate peristalsis as well as relaxation of the internal sphincter. Stimulation may need to be repeated for 5 to 10 minutes to initiate and prolong peristalsis. Usually, evacuation occurs in approximately 20 minutes. Performing digital stimulation depends on the person's ability to physically reach the anus and to maintain balance in a position to perform the finger movement. A wand-like device with a "finger" is commercially available. Some individuals rely on a caregiver to perform the procedure. This option is the most economical but does not necessarily provide effective results for everyone (Dickinson et al., 2017; Hammond & Burns, 2000). For patients with injury below conus medullaris, digital stimulation is not effective because the anal sphincter is denervated (Dickinson et al., 2017). Therefore, these patients may require manual evacuation of stool.

Suppository

Use of chemical stimulants, such as rectal suppositories or mini-enemas, can be effective in causing a reflex contraction of the rectum. It is suggested that the user confirm the presence of stool in rectum via digital exam prior to use (Apostolidis et al., 2017). Common choices include glycerin, bisacodyl, or carbon dioxide suppositories. Glycerin works by stimulating peristalsis and lubricating the rectum. Bisacodyl stimulates the nerves in the colon wall. Carbon dioxide produces carbon dioxide gas in the rectum, which expands the colon and stimulates peristalsis (Cotterill et al., 2017; Dickinson et al., 2017).

Suppositories can be readily purchased and are not expensive; "trial and error" is typically needed to determine the type that is most effective for a particular individual. Devices for suppository insertion are available if needed. Over time, the suppository used initially may become less effective and the individual may need to use another type.

Mini-enemas

The third option for bowel stimulation is the use of small enemas. Mineral oil enemas lubricate the intestine, and mini-enemas stimulate the rectal lining and keep the stool soft (Cotterill et al., 2017). Mini-enemas usually work in 15 to 20 minutes.

Tap Water Enemas or Transanal Irrigation

A fourth option for stimulating defecation is use of warm tap water enemas or transanal irrigations; these options work by distending the bowel, which stimulates peristalsis. This option is used only when the individual gets inadequate results with digital stimulation and/or suppositories or mini-enemas. The enema should be administered through a balloon-tipped catheter inserted into the rectum, in order to provide adequate retention of the enema solution. The catheter is inserted into the rectum and the balloon is inflated; the enema tubing is then connected to the catheter and the fluid is allowed to flow into the rectum and distal bowel. Once the fluid has been instilled, the balloon can be deflated and the catheter can be removed. This option works by distending the bowel and activating the enteric nervous system; it is therefore sometimes effective for individuals with sacral-level lesions and loss of autonomic innervation.

Transanal irrigation is seen as a safe, conservative, and effective neurogenic bowel management therapy that has gained popularity in the market over the last few years (Dickinson et al., 2017). Examples of anal irrigation systems include Peristeen Anal Irrigation System (Coloplast) and Qufora Irrisedo Balloon and mini (MacGregor Healthcare Ltd.) The purpose of the irrigation is to flush the stool out the rectum and colon using tepid tap water.

The kit includes a hydrophilic-coated rectal balloon, a clear plastic water reservoir, and a handheld unit that allows the individual to inflate the balloon and to control water instillation into the bowel; the unit requires minimal hand strength for manipulation. One major advantage to this system as opposed to a standard "enema" unit is the rectal balloon, which comes with the unit and is designed specifically for intrarectal use; the other advantage is the delivery system for the water, which propels the fluid proximally to provide more effective evacuation. For most individuals, the time frame required for evacuation is only 20 to 30 minutes. Manufacturer's instructions for use should be followed to maximize safety and efficacy. The risk of rectal perforation should be discussed with the patient prior to introducing this into the treatment plan (Dickinson et al., 2017). This is a prescription item, and the patient must be trained in its use by a nurse or physician.

Oral Laxatives

Oral pharmacological agents may be used in conjunction with the stimulated defecation program to maximize effectiveness, but dose and timing must be carefully titrated to prevent incontinent episodes. Whatever the specific stimulus to defecation used by a specific individual, bowel evacuation is thought to be complete if no more stool is ejected after two digital stimulations or if mucus without stool is expelled.

Neurogenic Bowel Management: MACE Procedure

The Malone antegrade continence enema (MACE) is a procedure growing in popularity that was originally (and effectively) used in children with spina bifida. The reversed appendix (or narrowed tubular section of bowel) is implanted into the colon and connected to the abdominal surface as a small skin-level stoma; this permits the individual to intubate the stoma with a narrow lumen catheter and to administer antegrade (top-down) enemas through the catheter to flush the distal bowel while sitting on the toilet (see Chapter 23, Fig. 23-6). In most situations, the appendix or tubular section of bowel is implanted into the cecum, ascending colon, or right transverse colon, though in some situations, it is implanted into the left transverse or descending colon. This procedure provides an alternative to stimulated defecation programs for individuals with neurogenic bowel and no voluntary control of defecation. In recent years, increasing numbers of spinal cord–injured individuals (especially women) are electing this procedure, both to regulate stool elimination and to eliminate chronic UTIs related to urethral contamination by stool. The daily or QOD enema usually involves tap water, though some individuals add small amounts of glycerin. The volume varies from individual to individual and is titrated to assure adequate colonic washout. Stoma complications, especially stenosis, are relatively common, and retrograde leakage can occur, especially if the colon becomes distended with stool (Dickinson et al., 2017; Ellison et al., 2013; Ruiz and Kaiser, 2017). This procedure is discussed in more detail in Chapter 23 and see Figure 23-6.

Effective management options for the individual with neurogenic bowel, such as the spinal cord–injured person, depend in part on whether the person has upper or lower motor neuron dysfunction. Lower motor neuron dysfunction is characterized by flaccid paralysis of the sphincter and frequent fecal leakage, whereas upper motor neuron dysfunction is characterized by increased sphincter tone. Stimulated defecation is more likely to be effective with individuals who have upper motor neuron dysfunction; the MACE procedure can be used with either type of dysfunction. The key elements of management for any patient with neurogenic bowel, as discussed above, are establishment of soft formed stool and a regular schedule for elimination. Elimination can then be managed either with stimulated defecation or with the MACE procedure, with the goal of producing daily or every other day bowel movements and no leakage in between movements (Dickinson et al., 2017; Ruiz & Kaiser, 2017).

Neurogenic Bowel Management: Colostomy

An end colostomy is another option for individuals with neurogenic bowel who do not respond to conservative management. An end colostomy may improve QOL for the person who is spending considerable time on a bowel management program with variable or unsatisfactory results (Bleier & Kann, 2013). The colostomy can be managed with an odor-proof pouch or through retrograde washouts (colostomy irrigation) performed daily or every other day.

KEY POINT

Surgical options for the individual with neurogenic bowel include the MACE procedure and fecal diversion (colostomy).

SURGICAL MANAGEMENT OPTIONS

Individuals who fail to respond to conservative measures should be referred for evaluation for possible surgical intervention. Surgical options currently available include sphincter repair, injection of bulking agents, neuromodulation (sacral nerve stimulation), MACE procedure, and fecal diversion. The MACE procedure and fecal diversion have already been described; the remaining options will be described briefly in terms of indications, contraindications, mechanism of action, and level of evidence to support use.

Sphincter Repair: Sphincteroplasty

Sphincteroplasty is the time-honored standard of care for management of FI for patients with EAS injury, but no neurologic deficit (O'Connell et al., 2017; Ruiz & Kaiser, 2017). The most common procedure is the anterior overlapping sphincteroplasty; this procedure is generally successful in management of obstetric trauma involving the EAS so long as the IAS remains intact (Ruiz & Kaiser, 2017; Van Koughnett & Wexner, 2013). With a curvilinear incision on the perineum, the EAS is isolated. The ends of the sphincter are overlapped and sewn together creating more bulk to the sphincter (O'Connell et al., 2017). Long-term follow-up studies for this procedure have been disappointing as the results appear to deteriorate over time (O'Connell et al., 2017; Wald, 2018). Consequentially, procedure is largely reserved for women with postpartum sphincter injury (Wald, 2018).

Artificial Anal Sphincter

Initially developed for UI, artificial sphincters (AS) have been revised and altered for use with FI. The AS was an approved treatment in the United States and was usually reserved for cases in which the only other alternative for extreme FI was a diverting colostomy. The procedure involved creating a perineal incision to implant the silicone sphincter, or "cuff," around the existing sphincter. Then a channel was created to support an attached reservoir and hydraulic pump system that would control inflation and deflation of the cuff, thereby simulating contraction and relaxation of the sphincter. The reservoir was then implanted in the groin, and the manually operated pump placed in the scrotum or the labia majora. The fluid from the reservoir was to be used to fill the cuff, which compresses the anal canal and provides continence. When the individual felt the need to defecate, she/he used the manually operated pump to transfer the fluid back into the reservoir, thereby deflating the cuff and opening the anal canal. Continence results were good, but studies reported high infection rates of >40%, and failure rates of >72%, requiring reimplantation (O'Connell et al., 2017; Wald, 2018). Currently this product is not commercially available (O'Connell et al., 2017; Ruiz & Kaiser, 2017).

Magnetic Artificial Sphincter

The magnetic artificial sphincter (MAS) is an alternative to the AS and involves surgical implantation of a ring of magnetic titanium beads into the anal sphincter; the magnets hold the anal canal closed until abdominal muscle contraction forces them open to permit defecation. The procedure for implantation of MAS is similar to the procedure used to implant AS except it takes around 45 minutes to implant and requires only an overnight stay. The MAS is immediately functional, and without the need for patient manipulation. In order to qualify for this procedure, the individual must fail conventional measures to manage the FI. Early results are positive, but more long-term and comparative studies are needed before definitive recommendations can be made (O'Connell et al., 2017; Ruiz & Kaiser, 2017).

Graciloplasty

Unstimulated muscle transposition or graciloplasty is another neosphincter procedure that involves transfer of the gracilis muscle or the gluteus maximus muscle; the muscle segment is then wrapped around the anal sphincter and sutured into place to support the anal sphincter. The gracilis and gluteal muscles are the muscles of choice because of their immediate location adjacent to the anal area as well as the nerve innervation, which will tolerate the change in anatomic location. Success rates following graciloplasty have been variable with deterioration reported by patients over 5-year follow-up. Patients were unable to consciously maintain contraction on the muscle (Ruiz & Kaiser, 2017) In addition, high donor site and perirectal complication rates were reported. As a result, the 2017 ICS recommendations state that "unstimulated graciloplasty should not be routinely offered."

Results have been improved with the implantation of a pulse generator device (O'Connell et al., 2017; Ruiz &

Kaiser, 2017). Nerve-stimulating leads are placed at the nerve origin and are then connected to a pacemaker-like generator. The pacemaker is placed in a surgically created subcutaneous pocket on the lower abdominal wall. The muscles that encircle the anal sphincter are held in a state of tonic contraction to prevent bowel evacuation. When the individual senses rectal distention and the urge to defecate, she/he passes a magnet over the pacemaker; this temporarily turns the generator off, which relaxes the sphincter and permits stool elimination. At present, the generator used in this procedure is not available in the United States, and because of the high morbidity rates associated with the procedure, its use has been limited in countries with access to the generator (O'Connell et al., 2017; Ruiz & Kaiser, 2017).

KEY POINT

Individuals with FI who fail to respond to behavioral strategies should be referred for surgical evaluation; surgical options at present include sphincter repair, anal bulking procedures, and sacral nerve stimulation (neuromodulation). Sacral neuromodulation is associated with the best overall outcomes.

Injectable Bulking Agents

Anal canal bulking agents have been developed based on some degree of success with urethral bulking agents for UI. In an outpatient setting, and without anesthesia, biomaterials are injected into the sphincter muscle or the submucosal tissues (Ruiz & Kaiser, 2017; Wald, 2018). Dextranomer/hyaluronic acid (NASHA Dx) is the only FDA-approved bulking agent for FI (Bharucha et al., 2017). Another bulking agent available in the United Kingdom is composed of a cross-linked porcine collagen (Permacol) (Wald, 2018). Bulking agents are intended to supplement the function of the intact IAS. Based on the limited data available at present, injectables appear to provide modest improvement in incontinence scores, with limited durability of results; many individuals require repeat injections. Some authors question the efficacy of bulk injections, with variable reported success rates between 6% and 50% for complete continence after 6 months (Bharucha et al., 2017; Wald, 2018). Thus, some authors suggest that this therapy may be most effectively used for individuals with seepage and soiling as opposed to those with frank FI (Bleier & Kann, 2013; Wald, 2018). Studies that characterize clinical significance using FIQOL scores as well as anorectal measurements are needed.

Sacral Nerve Stimulation

Sacral nerve stimulation was originally designed and tested for the management of UI but has been found to be very effective in the management of FI as well, with studies dating back to the mid-1990s (Bharucha & Rao, 2014). In May 2011, the FDA approved sacral nerve stimulation therapy for patients with FI who failed conservative therapy including dietary modifications, biofeedback, and medications (McNevin et al., 2014). Placement is a two-step process. Initially, an outpatient procedure is performed in which an electrode is passed through the foramina of S2–S4 and connected to an external temporary stimulator. The patient then undergoes a 2- to 3-week trial of pelvic nerve stimulation using the percutaneous wire electrodes and external stimulator; if there is significant improvement, a second procedure is performed in which the electrodes are permanently implanted and the permanent stimulator is implanted in the gluteal muscle area (O'Connell et al., 2017; Ruiz & Kaiser, 2017). The exact mechanism of action is not specifically understood (Halland & Talley, 2012) but is thought to involve altered muscle function, improved sensory function, and altered motility.

Unlike AS devices, sacral nerve stimulators do not have to be switched off (or deflated) to allow defecation. Sacral nerve stimulation appears to be effective for individuals with both external and internal sphincter injuries and is now often used as a first-line treatment when more conservative management has not been successful; 5-year success rates as high as 89% have been reported (Ruiz & Kaiser, 2017). This therapy has also been shown to improve QOL scores for individuals struggling with FI (Bharucha & Rao, 2014; O'Connell et al., 2017; Ruiz & Kaiser, 2017).

SKIN CARE AND CONTAINMENT

Skin care for the individual who is incontinent of stool should be individualized. Thorough cleansing after each episode of leakage is essential. The need for skin protectants in addition to cleansing depends on the frequency of leakage, the viscosity and amount of stool, and whether the stool contains corrosive enzymes. For occasional seepage of small amounts of stool, cleansing alone may be adequate; perineal skin cleansers should be used as opposed to soap and water. However, if the frequency and volume is high, cleansing should be followed by use of a moisturizing and moisture barrier product; acceptable barrier products include liquid film barriers that do not wash off with cleansing, and moisture barrier ointments containing petrolatum, zinc oxide, and/or dimethicone.

Skin exposure to high-volume liquid stool with irritating enzymes requires a more aggressive approach to skin protection. Gentle cleansing of the skin with a soft cloth and a no-rinse cleanser containing a surfactant to loosen the irritants should be followed by application of skin barrier ointment (Gray et al., 2012). Use of zinc oxide barriers is helpful, but the zinc oxide can be difficult to remove. Care should be taken not to forcefully scrub the fecal soiled areas; mineral oil or a perineal cleanser should be used to remove the soiled layers of the zinc oxide ointment, with the base layer left intact as long as it is not soiled (Beeckman et al., 2009, Gray et al., 2012). Chapter 17 discusses structured skin care program for individuals suffering from incontinence.

Fecal leakage has variable consistency and is not absorbed easily if at all by containment absorbent products. In fact, their use may contribute to further skin irritation and even breakdown because of more prolonged exposure to the irritants in the stool. For patients with light FI, absorbent pads designed to be placed between the cheeks of the buttocks over the anus can be effective in containing leakage on the perineal skin and is preferred by patients over other body-worn absorbent products (BWAPs) although not specifically designed for FI (Gray et al., 2018). In addition, absorptive products do not effectively conceal odor, so the product should be changed as soon as possible following soiling. If an individual needs a containment product, the nurse must consider stool frequency, volume, and viscosity and whether the individual suffers with UI as well. The trend in inpatient care settings is to avoid use of BWAPs unless the patient is ambulatory. The seal around the leg openings should be snug enough to provide security while ambulating; the seal is also snug enough to mask odor for at least a short period of time. Better absorbent product designs are needed for FI containment (Cottendon et al., 2017). Chapter 16 further examines BWAPs and other containment devices.

Some garments are made specifically for those with minor FI for purposes of swimming or pool therapy. Small disposable pads are available for placement between the buttocks to absorb scant fecal seepage. Costs vary from product to product, and there is no third-party reimbursement for most absorptive and containment products. When recommending absorptive and containment products, the nurse must consider the patient's ability to use the products properly, the patient's preferences, and any financial concerns and limitations. At present, no products have been developed that effectively deal with odor or the noise related to flatus, which may occur independently or in combination with fecal leakage (Fader et al., 2010; Willson et al., 2014).

KEY POINT

Currently, there is a lack of BWAPs designed to effectively contain stool and odor; products must be carefully selected based on stool volume and consistency, and skin care with routine use of moisture barrier products is essential.

ANAL PLUGS

The anal plug is an absorbent porous device that is positioned in the rectum to prevent accidental stool leakage; gas can pass through the device. It is a small white device similar to a tampon that is worn for up to 12 hours (Bates et al., 2017); when activated by moisture, the plug expands into a "tulip"-shaped structure. The string on the plug is positioned between the buttocks and is used for plug removal. After removal, the plug should be disposed of in the waste bin, not flushed in the toilet. Anal plugs are more appropriate for fecal seepage episodes versus large-volume FI. They are not recommended for patients at risk for autonomic dysreflexia, such as patients with SCI, and for those with an established bowel routine (Cottonden, 2017). The device requires a prescription and is available in varying sizes and designs (Willson et al., 2014). An empty rectal vault is required to allow full expansion of the plug.

The anal plug is one of the few continence devices an individual may use independently. Thus, it is critical for the nurse to carefully evaluate the individual's dexterity and ability to correctly use the plug. It is also critical to provide sufficient education to assure that the patient can use the plug correctly and with confidence. Although the plugs have been found to be helpful in preventing stool leakage in some patients, the plugs can be difficult to tolerate (Bates et al., 2017; Deutekom & Dobben, 2012). At this time, anal plugs are not available in the United States.

PATIENT EDUCATION

FI is not necessarily a sign of aging, though the risk increases with age, and is more prevalent than imagined. Cultural taboos and embarrassment keep affected individuals from bringing the problem to the attention of a knowledgeable care provider. FI is usually related to conditions that can be reversed or remedied, and ongoing attention and self-care is key to effective management, as is true with other chronic conditions (Peden-McAlpine et al., 2008). Individualized dietary modifications, adequate hydration, and compliance with prescribed medications and bowel habit routine are the conservative measures initially employed to address FI (Crosswell et al., 2010). Pelvic muscle exercises are recommended for individuals with compromised sphincter function, and stimulated defecation programs are the treatment of choice for those with neurogenic incontinence. In addition, there is a myriad of containment products in various sizes, absorbencies, and price ranges, although items specific for men are limited (Bliss et al., 2017; Gray et al., 2018). Qualified

continence nurses should be able to assist in the selection of appropriate garments and skin protection agents for individual patients and in patient/caregiver education regarding their use. When FI is not responsive to conservative treatments, surgical interventions may be considered; individuals must be educated regarding options, advantages and disadvantages, and requirements for lifelong management (Roth, 2010).

KEY POINT

Ongoing patient education and support are essential to positive outcomes for the individual with FI.

Individualized education and support are required to assist patients with both conservative and advanced management and are essential to positive outcomes. While the continence nurse is most commonly involved in patient education regarding dietary and fluid modifications, appropriate use of medications, and pelvic floor strengthening exercises, the continence nurse should also be able to inform patients about other therapy options and should be able to make appropriate referrals. The continence nurse should consistently communicate to the individual her/his commitment to helping the individual identify and master strategies that reduce incontinent episodes and improve QOL (Halland & Talley, 2012).

CONCLUSION

FI is a devastating condition in terms of QOL; due to the embarrassment and stigma, individuals are reluctant to report the problem, even to their health care providers. Effective management begins with careful assessment to determine the contributing problems; most commonly, causative factors include alterations in GI tract function and stool consistency, sphincter damage or denervation, compromised sensory awareness or cognition, and/or altered rectal capacity and compliance. Management is directed toward the specific problems affecting the individual and includes elimination of impacted stool, measures to correct stool consistency and to normalize bowel function, sphincter strengthening exercises, biofeedback to improve sensory awareness and sphincter strength, and stimulated defecation programs for those with sensorimotor loss resulting in neurogenic bowel. Surgical options are available for those who fail to respond to primary measures; those with the greatest success to date include the MACE procedure and sacral nerve stimulation.

REFERENCES

Alavi, K., Chan, S., Wise, P., et al. (2015). Fecal incontinence: Etiology, diagnosis, and management. *Journal of Gastrointestinal Surgery, 19*, 1910–1921.

Altman, D., Falconer, C., Rossner, S., et al. (2007). The risk of anal incontinence in obese women. *International Urogynecology Journal and Pelvic Floor Dysfunction, 18*(11), 1283–1289.

Andromanakos, N., Filippou, D., Pinis, S., et al. (2013). Anorectal incontinence: A challenge in diagnostic and therapeutic approach. *European Journal of Gastroenterology and Hepatology, 25*, 1247–1256.

Apostolidis, A., Drake, M., Emmanuel, A., et al. (2017). Neurological urinary and faecal incontinence. In P. Abrams, L. Cardozo, A. Waggs, et al. (Eds.), *Incontinence* (6th ed., Vol. 1, pp. 1178–1303). ICI-ICS. Bristol, UK: International Continence Society.

Bartolo, D., & Paterson, H. (2009). Anal incontinence. *Best Practice & Research Clinical Gastroenterology, 23*, 505–515.

Bates, F., Bliss, D. Z., Bardsely, A., et al. (2017). Management of fecal incontinence in community-living adults. In D. Z. Bliss (Ed.), *Management of fecal incontinence for the advanced practice nurse* (pp. 93–126). Cham, Switzerland: Springer International Publishing AG.

Beeckman, D., Schoonhoven, L., Verhaeghe, S., et al. (2009). Prevention and treatment of incontinence-associated dermatitis: Literature review. *Journal of Advanced Nursing, 65*(6), 1141–1154.

Beeson, T., Eifrid, B., Pike, C. A., et al. (2017). Do Intra-anal bowel management devices reduce incontinence-associated dermatitis and/or pressure injuries? *Journal of Wound, Ostomy and Continence Nursing, 44*(6), 583–588.

Beitz, J. (2006). Fecal incontinence in acutely and critically ill patients: Options in management. *Ostomy Wound Manage, 52*(12), 56–58, 60, 62–66.

Bellicini, N., Molloy, P., Caushaj, P., et al. (2008). Fecal incontinence: A review. *Digestive Diseases and Sciences, 53*(1), 41–46. doi: 10.1007/s10620-007-9819-z.

Belmonte-Montes, C., Hagerman, G., Vega-yepez, P., et al. (2001). Anal sphincter injury after vaginal delivery in primiparous females. *Diseases of the Colon and Rectum, 44*(9), 1244–1248. doi: 10.1007/BF02234778.

Bharucha, A., Zinsmeister, A., Locke, G., et al. (2005). Prevalence and burden of fecal incontinence: A population-based study in women. *Gastroenterology, 129*(1), 42–49. doi: 10.1053/j.gastro.2005.04.006.

Bharucha, A. (2010). Incontinence: An underappreciated problem in obesity and bariatric surgery. *Digestive Diseases and Sciences, 55*, 2428–2430. doi: 10.1007/s10620-010-1288-0.

Bharucha, A., & Rao, S. (2014). An update on anorectal disorders for gastroenterologists. *Gastroenterology, 146*(1), 37–45.

Bharucha, A. E., Dunivan, G., Goode, P. S., et al. (2015). Epidemiology, pathophysiology, and classification of fecal incontinence: State of the Science Summary for the National Institute of Diabetes and Digestive and Kidney Diseases (NIDDK) Workshop. *American Journal of Gastroenterology, 101*(1), 127–136.

Bharucha, A. E., Rao, S. S., & Shin, A. S. (2017). AGA CLINICAL PRACTICE UPDATE: Surgical interventions and the use of device-aided therapy for the treatment of fecal incontinence and defecatory disorders. *Clinical Gastroenterology and Hepatology, 15*, 1844–1854.

Bisanz, A. (2011). *Bowel management: A guide for patients.* Houston, TX: The University of Texas, MD Anderson Cancer Center.

Bleier, J., & Kann, B. (2013). Surgical management of fecal incontinence. *Gastroenterology Clinics of North America, 42*, 815–836.

Bliss, D. Z., Doughty, D. B., & Heitkemper, M. M. (2006). Pathology and management of bowel dysfunction. In D. B. Doughty (Ed.), *Urinary & fecal incontinence: current management concepts* (3rd ed., pp. 425–452). St. Louis, MO: Mosby-Elsevier.

Bliss, D., Johnson, S., Savik, K., et al. (2000). Fecal incontinence in hospitalized patients who are acutely ill. *Nursing Research, 49*(2), 101–108.

Bliss, D., Mimura, T., Berghmans, B., et al. (2017). Assessment and conservative management of faecal incontinence and quality of life in adults. In P. Abrams, L. Cardozo, A. Waggs, et al. (Eds.), *Incontinence* (6th ed., Vol. 2, pp. 1993–2085). Tokyo, Japan: ICS ICUD.

Bliss, D. Z., Savik, K., Jung, H. J., et al. (2014). Dietary fiber supplementation for fecal incontinence: a randomized clinical trial. *Research in Nursing & Health, 37*(5), 367–378. doi: 10.1002/nur.21616.

Carr, M., & Hunter, K. F. (2018). Management of fecal incontinence in acutely ill and critically ill hospitalized adults. In D. Z. Bliss (Ed.), *Management of fecal incontinence for the advanced practice nurse* (pp. 187–210). Cham, Switzerland: Springer International Publishing AG.

Coggrave, M. (2007). Transanal irrigation after spinal cord injury. *Nursing Times, 103*(26), 47, 49.

Colavita, K., & Andy, U. U. (2016). Role of diet in fecal incontinence: A systematic review of the literature. *International Urogynecology Journal, 27*, 1805–1810.

Cottenden, A., Fader, M., Beeckman, D., et al. (2017). Management using continence products. In P. Abrams, L. Cardozo, A. Waggs, et al. (Eds.), *Incontinence* (6th ed., Vol. 2, pp. 2303–2426). Tokyo, Japan: ICS ICUD.

Cotterill, N., Madersbacher, H., Wyndaele, J. J., et al. (2017). Neurogenic bowel dysfunction: Clinical management recommendations of the Neurologic Incontinence Committee of the Fifth International Consultation on Incontinence 2013. *Neurourology and Urodynamics, 37*, 46–53.

Crosswell, E. B., Bliss, D. Z., & Savik, K. (2010). Diet and eating pattern modifications used by community-living adults to manage their fecal incontinence. *Journal of Wound, Ostomy, and Continence Nursing, 37*(6), 677–682.

Crowell, M., Schettler, V., Lacy, B., et al. (2007). Impact of anal incontinence on psychosocial function and health-related quality of life. *Digestive Diseases and Sciences, 52*, 1627–1631.

Danielson, J. K. (2019). Persistent fecal incontinence into adulthood after repair of anorectal malformations. *International Journal of Colorectal Disease, 34*, 551–554.

Deutekom, M., & Dobben, A. (2012). Plugs for containing faecal incontinence. *Cochrane Database of Systematic Reviews, 4*, CD005086.

Dickinson, T., Eustice, S., & Cotterill, N. (2017). Management of fecal incontinence in adults with neurogenic bowel dysfunction. In D. Z. Bliss (Ed.), *Management of fecal incontinence for the advanced practice nurse* (pp. 171–185). Cham, Switzerland: Springer International Publishing AG.

Doherty, W. (2004). Managing faecal incontinence or leakage: The Peristeen anal plug. *British Journal of Nursing, 13*(21), 1293–1297.

Doughty, D. (2000). Chapter 13. Pathophysiology of bowel dysfunction and fecal incontinence, Chapter 14. Assessment and management of patients with bowel dysfunction and fecal incontinence. In D. Doughty (Ed.), *Urinary & fecal incontinence, nursing management* (2nd ed., pp. 325–383). St. Louis, MO: Mosby, Inc.

Dudding, T., Pares, D., Vaizey, C., et al. (2010). Sacral nerve stimulation for the treatment of faecal incontinence related to dysfunction of the internal anal sphincter. *International Journal of Colorectal Disease, 25*, 625–630. doi: 10.1007/s00384-010-0880-2.

Dunberger, G., Lind, H., Steineck, G., et al. (2011). Loose stools lead to fecal incontinence among gynecological cancer survivors. *Acta Oncologica, 50*(2), 233–242.

Dunivan, G., Heymen, S., Palsson, O., et al. (2010). Fecal incontinence in primary care: Prevalence, diagnosis, and health care utilization. *American Journal of Obstetrics and Gynecology, 202*(5), 493.e1–493.e6.

Echols, J., Friedman, B., Mullins, R., et al. (2007). Clinical utility and economic impact of introducing a bowel management system. *Journal of Wound, Ostomy and Continence Nursing, 34*(6), 664–670.

Ellison, J., Haraway, N., & Park, J. (2013). The distal left Malone antegrade continence enema—is it better? *Journal of Urology, 190*(4 Suppl), 1529–1533.

Epocrates. (2019). Drugs: Gastrointestinal. Retrieved October 28, 2019, from Epocrates online: https://online.epocrates.com.

Erekson, E., Sung, V., & Myers, D. (2008). Effect of body mass index on the risk of anal incontinence and defecatory dysfunction in women. *American Journal of Obstetrics and Gynecology, 198*(5), 596.e1–596.e4.

Eva, U., Gun, W., & Preben, K. (2003). Prevalence of urinary and fecal incontinence and symptoms of genital prolapse in women. *Acta Obstetricia et Gynecologica Scandinavica, 82*(3), 280–286.

Fader, M., Bliss, D., Cottenden, A., et al. (2010). Continence products: Research priorities to improve the lives of people living with urinary and/or fecal leakage. *Neurourology and Urodynamics: Official Journal of the International Continence Society, 29*(4), 640–644.

Fader, M., Cottenden, A., & Getliffe, K. (2009). Absorbent products for moderate-heavy urinary and/or faecal incontinence in women and men. *Cochrane Database of Systematic Reviews, 4,* CD007408. doi: 10.1002/14651858.CD007408.

Falcon, B. S., Lopez, M. B., Munoz, B. M., et al. (2016). Fecal impaction: A systematic review of its medical complications. *BMC Geriatrics, 22*(4), 1–8.

Farage, M., Miller, K., Berardesca, E., et al. (2008). Psychosocial and societal burden of incontinence in the aged population: A review. *Archives of Gynecology and Obstetrics, 277*(4), 285–290. doi: 10.1007/s00404-007-0505-3.

Findlay, J., & Maxwell-Armstrong, C. (2010). Current issues in the management of adult faecal incontinence. *British Journal of Hospital Medicine, 71*(6), 335–339.

Finne-Soveri, H., Sørbye, L., Jonsson, P., et al. (2008). Increased work-load associated with faecal incontinence among home care patients in 11 European countries. *European Journal of Public Health, 18*(3), 323–328.

Formal, C., Cawley, M., & Stiens, S. (1997). Spinal cord injury rehabilitation. 3. Functional outcomes. *Archives of Physical Medicine and Rehabilitation, 78*(3 Suppl), S59–S64.

Forootan, M., Bagheri, N., & Darvishi, M. (2018). Chronic constipation: A review of literature. *Medicine, 27*(20), 1–9.

Forte, M., Andrade, K., Butler, M., et al. (2016). *Treatments for fecal incontinence; comparative effectiveness review No. 165.* Minnesota Evidence-based Practice Center (EPC) No. 290-2012-00016-I, Agency for Healthcare Research and Quality. Rockville, MD: AHRQ Publication. Retrieved from www.effectivehealthcare.ahrq.gov/reports/final.cfm

Gallagher, S. (2005). Challenges of obesity and skin Integrity. *The Nursing Clinics of North America, 40,* 325–335.

Glass, D., Huang, D. T., Dugum, M., et al. (2018). Rectal trumpet-associated hemorrhage in the intensive care unit: A Quality improvement initiative. *Journal of Wound, Ostomy and Continence Nursing, 45*(6), 522–520.

Goode, P., Burgio, K., Halli, A., et al. (2005). Prevalence and correlates of fecal incontinence in community-dwelling older adults. *Journal of the American Geriatrics Society, 53*(4), 629–635.

Gordon, D., Groutz, A., Goldman, G., et al. (1999). Anal incontinence: Prevalence among female patients attending a urogynecologic clinic. *Neurourology and Urodynamics: Official Journal of the International Continence Society, 18*(3), 199–204.

Gray, M., Beeckman, D., Bliss, D. Z., et al. (2012). Incontinence-associated dermatitis: A comprehensive review and update. *Journal of Wound, Ostomy and Continence Nursing, 39*(1), 61–74. doi: 10.1097/WON.0b013e31823fe246.

Gray, M., Bliss, D. Z., & Trammel, S. H. (2017). Management of skin damage associated with fecal and dual incontinence. In D. Z. Bliss (Ed.), *Management of fecal incontinence for the advanced practice nurse* (pp. 257–289). Cham, Switzerland: Springer International Publishing AG.

Gray, M., Kent, D., Ermer-Seltun, J., et al. (2018). Assessment, selection, use, and evaluation of body-worn absorbent products for adults with incontinence. *Journal of Wound, Ostomy and Continence Nursing, 45*(3), 243–264.

Gray, M., Omar, A., & Buziak, B. (2014). Stool management systems for preventing environmental spread of *Clostridium difficile. Journal of Wound, Ostomy, and Continence Nursing, 41*(5), 460–465.

Groutz, A., Fait, G., Lessing, J., et al. (1999). Incidence and obstetric risk factors of postpartum anal incontinence. *Scandinavian Journal of Gastroenterology, 34*(3), 315–318.

Halland, M., & Talley, N. (2012). Fecal incontinence mechanisms and management. *Current Opinion in Gastroenterology, 28,* 57–62.

Hammond, M., & Burns, S. (2000). *Yes, you can! A guide to self-care for persons with spinal cord injury* (3rd ed.). Washington, DC: Paralyzed Veterans of America.

Hansen, J. L., Bliss, D. Z., & Peden-McAlpine, C. (2006). Diet strategies used by women to manage fecal incontinence. *Journal of Wound, Ostomy, and Continence Nursing, 33*(1), 52–61.

Haylen, B. D. (2010). An International Urogynecological Association (IUGA)/International Continence Society (ICS) joint report on the terminology for female pelvic floor dysfunction. *Neurourology and Urodynamics, 29,* 4–20. doi: 10.1002/nau.22922.

Herbert, J. (2008). Use of anal plugs in faecal incontinence management. *Nursing Times, 104*(13), 66–68.

Hiller, L., Radley, S., Mann, C., et al. (2002). Development and validation of a questionnaire for the assessment of bowel and lower urinary tract symptoms in women. *BJOG, 109*(4), 413–423.

Hunter, W., Jones, G. P., Devereux, H., et al. (2002). Constipation and diet in a community sample of older adults. *Nutrition and Dietetics, 59*(4), 253–259.

Hurnauth, C. (2011). Management of fecal incontinence in acutely ill patients. *Nursing Standard, 25*(22), 48–56.

Hussain, Z., Lim, M., & Stojkovic, F. (2014). The test-retest reliability of fecal incontinence severity and quality-of-life assessment tools. *Diseases of the Colon and Rectum, 57*(5), 638–644.

Kelly, A. M. (2019). Constipation in community-dwelling adults with intellectual disability. *British Journal of Community Nursing, 24*(8), 392–396.

Kelly, M. S., Dorgalli, C., McLorie, G., et al. (2017). Prospective evaluation of Peristeen transanal irrigation system with the validated neurogenic bowel dysfunction score sheet in the pediatric population. *Neurourology and Urodynamics, 36,* 632–635.

Kowal-Vern, A., Poulakidas, S., Barnett, B., et al. (2009). Fecal containment in bedridden patients: economic impact of 2 commercial bowel catheter systems. *American Journal of Critical Care, 18*(3 Suppl), S2–S15.

Kuoch, K., Hebbard, G., O'Connell, H., et al. (2019). Urinary and faecal incontinence: Psychological factors and management recommendations. *The New Zealand Medical Journal (Online), 132*(1503), 25–33.

Leung, F., & Rao, S. (2011). Approach to fecal incontinence and constipation in older hospitalized patients. *Hospital Practice, 39*(1), 97–104. doi: 10.3810/hp.2011.02.380.

Leung, F., & Schnelle, J., (2008). Urinary and fecal incontinence in nursing home residents. *Gastroenterology Clinics of North America, 37*(3), 697–707.

Markland, A. D., Burgio, K. L., Whitehead, W. E., et al. (2015). Loperamide versus psyllium fiber for treatment of fecal incontinence: The fecal incontinence prescription (Rx) management (FIRM) randomized clinical trial. *Diseases of the Colon and Rectum, 58*(10), 983–993.

Marples, G. (2011). Diagnosis and management of slow transit constipation in adults. *Nursing Standard, 26*(8), 41–48.

McKenna, S., Wallis, M., Brannelly, A., et al. (2001). The nursing management of diarrhoea and constipation before and after the implementation of a bowel management protocol. *Australian Critical Care, 14*(1), 10–16.

McNevin, M., Moore, M., & Bax, T. (2014). Outcomes associated with Interstim therapy for medically refractory fecal incontinence. *American Journal of Surgery, 207*(5), 735–737.

Mellgren, A. (2010). Fecal incontinence. *The Surgical Clinics of North America, 90*(1), 185–194.

Meyer, I., & Richter, H. (2015). Impact of fecal incontinence and its treatment on quality of life in women. *Women's Health, 11*(2), 225–238.

Minguez, M., Higueras, A. L., & Judez, J. (2016). Use of polyethylene glycol in functional constipation and fecal impaction. *Revista Espanola De Enfermedades Digestivas, 108*(12), 790–806.

Montenegro, M., Slongo, H., Juliato, C. R., et al. (2019). The impact of bariatric surgery on pelvic floor dysfunction: A systematic review. *Journal of Minimally Invasive Gynecology, 26*(5), 822–825.

Mounsey, A., Raleigh, M., & Wilson, A. (2015). Management of constipation in older adults. *American Family Physician, 92*(6), 500–504.

Mulhall, A. M., & Jindal, S. K. (2013). Massive gastrointestinal hemorrhage as a complication of the Flexi-Seal Fecal management system. *American Journal of Critical Care, 22*(6), 537–543.

Nix, D., & Ermer-Seltun, J. (2004). A review of perineal skin care protocols and skin barrier product use. *Ostomy/Wound Management, 50*(12), 59–67.

Nix, D., & Haugen, V. (2010). Prevention and management of incontinence-associated dermatitis. *Drugs & Aging, 27*(6), 491–496.

Northwood, M. (2013). Fecal incontinence severity and Quality-of-Life instruments. *Journal of Wound, Ostomy, and Continence Nursing, 40*(1), 20–23.

O'Connell, P., Knowles, C., Maeda, Y., et al. (2017). Surgery for faecal incontinence. In P. Abrams, L. Cardozo, A. Waggs, et al. (Eds.), *Incontinence* (6th ed., Vol. 2, pp. 2087–2142). ICI-ICS. Bristol, UK: International Continence Society.

Ostaszkiewicz, J., O'Connell, B., & Millar, L. (2008). Incontinence: Managed or mismanaged in hospital settings? *International Journal of Nursing Practice, 14*(6), 495–502. doi: 10.1111/j.1440-172X. 2008.00725.x.

Palmieri, B., Benuzzi, G., & Bellini, N. (2005). The anal bag: A modern approach to fecal incontinence management. *Ostomy/Wound Management, 12*, 44–52.

Paquette, I., Varma, M., Kaiser, A., et al. (2015). The American Society of Colon and Rectal Surgeons Clinical practice guideline for treatment of fecal incontinence. *Diseases of the Colon and Rectum, 58*(7), 623–636.

Pares, D., Vallverdu, H., Monroy, G., et al. (2012). Bowel habits and fecal incontinence in patients with obesity undergoing evaluation for weight loss: The importance of stool consistency. *Diseases of the Colon & Rectum, 55*(5), 599–604.

Park, K. H., & Kim, K. S. (2014). Effect of a structured skin care regimen on patients with fecal incontinence. *Journal of Wound, Ostomy and Continence Nursing, 41*(2), 221–227.

Paterson, J., Dunn, S., Kowanko, I., et al. (2003). Selection of continence products: Perspectives of people who have incontinence and their carers. *Disability and Rehabilitation, 25*(17), 955–963.

Peden-McAlpine, C., Bliss, D., & Hill, J. (2008). The experience of community-living women managing fecal incontinence. *Western Journal of Nursing Research, 30*(7), 817–835.

Pittman, J., Beeson, T., Terry, C., et al. (2012). Methods of bowel management in critical care: A Randomized controlled trial. *Journal of Wound, Ostomy and Continence Nursing, 39*(2), 633–639.

Pretlove, S., Radley, S., Toozs-Hobson, P., et al. (2006). Prevalence of anal incontinence according to age and gender: A systematic review and meta-regression analysis. *International Urogynecology Journal and Pelvic Floor Dysfunction, 17*(4), 407–417.

Rao, S. S., Bharucha, A. E., Chiarioni, G., et al. (2017). Anorectal disorders. *Gastroenterology, 150*(6), 1430–1442.e4.

Rees, J., & Sharpe, A. (2009). The use of bowel management systems in the high-dependency setting. *British Journal of Nursing, 18*(7), S19–S20, 22, 24.

Ribas, Y., & Munoz-Duyos, A. (2018). Conservative treatment for severe defecatory urgency and fecal incontinence: Minor strategies with major impact. *Techniques in Coloproctology, 22*, 673–682.

Richter, H., Burgio, K., Clements, R., et al. (2005). Urinary and fecal incontinence in morbidly obese women considering weight loss surgery. *Obstetrics & Gynecology, 106*(6), 1272–1277.

Roberson, E., Gould, J., & Wald, A. (2010). Urinary and fecal incontinence after bariatric surgery. *Digestive Diseases and Sciences, 55*(9), 2606–2613.

Rockwood, T. H. (2004). Incontinence severity and QOL scales for fecal incontinence. *Gastroenterology, 126*(1 Suppl 1), S106–S113.

Rockwood, T., Church, J., Fleshman, J., et al. (1999). Patient and surgeon ranking of the severity of symptoms associated with fecal incontinence. *Diseases of the Colon and Rectum, 42*(12), 1525–1531.

Rockwood, T., Church, J., Fleshman, J., et al. (2000). Fecal incontinence quality of life scale. *Diseases of the Colon and Rectum, 43*(1), 9–16.

Roth, L. (2010). Fecal incontinence. *Medicine and Health, Rhode Island, 93*(11), 356–358.

Ruiz, N. S., & Kaiser, A. M. (2017). Fecal incontinence—Challenges and solutions. *World Journal of Gastroenterology, 23*(1), 11–24

Rusavy, Z., Jansova, M., & Kalis, V. (2014). Anal incontinence severity assessment tools used worldwide. *International Journal of Gynaecology and Obstetrics, 126*, 146–150. doi: 10.1016/j.ijgo.2014.02.025.

Sabol, V., & Friedenburg, F. (1997). Diarrhea. *AACN Clinical Issues, 8*(3), 425–436.

Sammon, M. A., Montague, M., Frame, F., et al. (2015). Randomized controlled study of the effects of 2 fecal management systems on incidence of anal erosion. *Journal of Wound, Ostomy and Continence Nursing, 42*(3), 279–286.

Sansoni, J., Hawthorne, G., Fleming, G., et al. (2013). The revised faecal incontinence scale: A clinical validation of a new, short measure of assessment and outcomes evaluation. *Diseases of the Colon and Rectum, 56*(5), 652–659.

Shamliyan, T., Bliss, D., Du, J., et al. (2009). Prevalence and risk factors of fecal incontinence in community-dwelling men. *Reviews in Gastroenterological Disorders, 9*(4), E97–E110.

Sharpe, A., & Read A. (2010). Sacral nerve stimulation for the placement of faecal incontinence. *The British Journal of Nursing, 9*(7), 415–419.

Shiller, L. R., Pardi, D. S., & Sellin, J. H. (2017). Chronic diarrhea: Diagnosis and management. *Clinical Gastroenterology and Hepatology, 15*, 182–193.

Stevens, T., Soffer, E., & Palmer, R. (2003). Fecal incontinence in elderly patients: common, treatable, yet undiagnosed. *Cleveland Clinic Journal of Medicine, 70*(5), 441–448.

Stoffel, J., Van der Aa, F., Wittmann, D., et al. (February 22, 2018). Neurogenic bowel management for the adult spinal cord injury patient. *World Journal of Urology, 36*, 1587–1592.

Stokes, A. L., Crumley, C., Taylor-Thompson, K., et al. (2016). Prevalence of fecal incontinence in the acute care setting. *Journal of Wound, Ostomy and Continence Nursing, 43*(5), 517–522.

Thomas, S., Nay, R., Moore, K., et al. (2006). *Continence outcomes measurement suite project (Final Report).* Australian Government Department of Health and Ageing. Retrieved March 2013, from http://www.bladderbowel.gov.au/assets/doc/ncms/Phase1-2InformationAndEvidence/11DevelopementofOutcomeMeasurementSuiteforContinenceConditions.pdf

Van Koughnett, J. A., & Wexner, S. (2013). Current management of fecal incontinence: Choosing amongst treatment options to optimize outcomes. *World Journal of Gastroenterology, 19*(48), 9216–9230.

Vilke, G. M., DeMers, G., Patel, N., et al. (2015). Safety and efficacy of milk and molasses enemas in the emergency department. *The Journal of Emergency Medicine, 48*(6), 667–670.

Wagg, A., Chen, L. K., Johnson, T., et al. (2017). Incontinence in frail older persons. In P. Abrams, L. Cardozo, A. Waggs, et al. (Eds.), *Incontinence* (6th ed., Vol. 2, pp. 1311–1441). Tokyo, Japan: ICS ICUD.

Wald, A. (2018). Diagnosis and management of fecal incontinence. *Current Gastroenterology Reports, 20*(9), 9. doi: 10.1007/s11894-018-0614-0.

Wheeler, T. L., de Groat, W., Eisner, K., et al. (2018). Translating promising strategies for bowel and bladder management in spinal cord injury. *Experimental Neurology, 306*, 229–176.

Whitehead, W., Palsson, O., & Simren, M. (2016). Treating fecal incontinence: an unmet need in primary care medicine. *North Carolina Medical Journal, 77*(3), 211–215.

Whitehead, W., Rao, S., Lowry, A., et al. (2015). Treatment of fecal incontinence: State of the science summary for the National Institute of Diabetes and Digestive and Kidney Diseases workshop. *American Journal of Gastroenterology, 110*(1), 138–146.

Whiteley, I., Sinclair, G., Lyons, A. M., et al. (2014). A Retrospective review of outcomes using a fecal management system in acute care patients. *Ostomy Wound Management, 60*(12), 37–43.

Wilde, M., Bliss, D., Booth, J., et al. (2014). Self-management of urinary and fecal incontinence. *American Journal of Nursing, 114*(1), 38–45.

Williams, K., Shalom, D., & Winkler, H. (2018). Faecal incontinence: a narrative review of clinic-based management for the general gynaecologist. *Journal of Obstetrics and Gynaecology, 38*(1), 1–9.

Willson, M., Angyus, M., Beals, D., et al. (2014). Executive Summary: A quick reference guide for managing fecal incontinence. *Journal of Wound, Ostomy and Continence Nursing, 41*(1), 61–69.

Wishin, J., Gallagher, T., & McCann, E. (2008). Emerging options for the management of fecal incontinence in hospitalized patients. *Journal of Wound, Ostomy, and Continence Nursing, 35*(1), 104–110.

Wisten, A. M., & Messner, T. (2005). Fruit and fiber (Pajala porridge) in the prevention of constipation. *Scandinavian Journal of Caring Sciences, 19*(1), 71–76. doi: 10.1111/j.1471-6712.2004.00308.x.

Woodward, S. (2012). Assessment and management of constipation in older people. *Nursing Older People, 24*(5), 21–26.

Wuong, S. (2012). Literature review: Management of constipation in people with Parkinson's disease. *The Australian and New Zealand Continence Journal, 18*(4), 112–118.

Yeung, H. Y., Lyer, P., Pryor, J., et al. (2019). Dietary management of neurogenic bowel in adults with spinal cord injury: An integrative review of literature. *Disability and Rehabilitation, 14*, 1–12.

Zhou, X. L., He, Z., Chen, Y. H., et al. (2017). Effect of a 1-piece drainable pouch on incontinence-associated dermatitis in intensive care unit patients with fecal incontinence. *Journal of Wound, Ostomy and Continence Nursing, 44*(6), 568–571.

CASE STUDY

A 72-year-old female with a medical history of hypertension, diabetes, and high cholesterol lives in an assisted living center. She takes a beta-blocker, metformin, and a statin medication. She feels well and has no physical symptoms, but she mentions she sometimes has accidents of stool during the day. Her obstetrical history consists of three vaginal births without complications. She reports occasional constipation and takes a stool softener and it helps. She denies diarrhea or abdominal pain. She admits this problem has been going on for many years and is one of the reasons she lives in an assisted living center. She reports her accidents occur frequently enough that she is afraid to go out and it has made a big difference in her lifestyle. She usually has family and friends come to visit her, and she avoids going anyplace where a bathroom is not readily available. She reports some sensation of urgency before the incontinence occurs but not always. She wears adult briefs all the time now. Her perineal area is slightly erythematous and tender; she states she uses diaper rash cream to try to protect her skin.

What predisposing factors does this patient have for FI? Vaginal births, age, possible mobility issues, diabetes, side effects of medications—beta-blocker and metformin and possibly statin. Possibly diet and fluid intake.

What other history is needed to help determine contributing factors? Usual frequency of defecation, accurate history of FI (frequency, consistency and volume of stool, any triggering events), usual consistency of stool with voluntary defecation, current management of constipation (to include use of stool softeners and laxatives), obstetric history to include episiotomy or change in continence after births, any other abdominal/intestinal/anorectal surgeries, history of any bowel disorders, and ability to sense rectal distention and to accurately differentiate between gas, liquid, and solid.

What would you ask about her diet and fluid intake? Usual daily fluid intake; any dehydrating fluids; usual caffeine intake; dietary fiber intake; any foods that cause increased flatus, dyspepsia, diarrhea, constipation, or GI irritability; foods usually eaten; and any food allergies.

How do her medications contribute? May contribute to altered stool consistency (diarrhea or constipation).

What physical assessments should be performed to help determine underlying cause? Digital examination to assess sphincter tone and strength/endurance and assessment for retained stool in rectal vault, rectal masses, hemorrhoids, and perineal scars. Abdominal exam: inspection, percussion, and palpation to rule out retained stool. Functional status exam: mobility and cognitive status, ability to perform toileting on own, and dressing ability.

What interventions have already been tried? Stool softener, adult briefs, skin barrier creams, dietary changes, moved into assisted living, and restricts her travel.

What interventions can the nurse offer? Measures to normalize stool consistency (dietary modifications, fiber and fluid intake, medications as indicated); instruction in bowel hygiene (prompt response to "urge to go," correct posture, establishment routine time for attempted defecation); sphincter strengthening exercises; skin care; education regarding effects of chronic disease on bowel, effects of meds on bowel function, effects of diet and fluid choices on bowel function, and prevention and management of constipation; discussion about QOL issues and strategies to help her regain her ability to go out without fears; and education on containment products.

QUESTIONS

1. A 75-year-old female patient confides to the continence nurse that she "frequently gets a sudden urge to move her bowels and sometimes has trouble getting to a bathroom in time." What is the label for this type of incontinence?
   A. Passive fecal incontinence
   B. Urge bowel incontinence
   C. Encopresis
   D. Fecal seepage

2. Which patient would the continence nurse place at higher risk for fecal incontinence related to sphincter denervation? A patient:
   A. with irritable bowel syndrome
   B. experiencing cerebrocortical dysfunction
   C. with a malabsorption syndrome
   D. who is post-anorectal surgery

3. Which technique would the continence nurse perform when conducting an abdominal examination on a person who reports fecal incontinence?
   A. Visual inspection for tumors
   B. Percussion to detect distention
   C. Palpation of the lower quadrants to assess for stool retention
   D. Auscultation for stool in the left lower quadrant

4. The continence nurse asks a patient to "bear down" during a *visual* examination of the anus. What bowel alteration might be assessed using this technique?
   A. Neurologic lesion
   B. Rectal prolapse
   C. Pelvic floor dyssynergia
   D. Rectal polyps

5. During an anorectal examination, the examiner elicits the "anal wink." No response to this test may be indicative of:
   A. Neurological problems
   B. Colon cancer
   C. Anal fissures
   D. Infection

6. The continence nurse is caring for a patient with a fecal pouch. Which statement accurately describes an advantage/disadvantage associated with this device?
   A. It only takes one caregiver to apply the rectal pouch.
   B. Use of a fecal pouch is limited to nonambulatory patients.
   C. Rectal exams can be performed when using a fecal pouch.
   D. Fecal pouches are effective when there is perianal skin breakdown.

7. The continence nurse is providing teaching to a patient who is undergoing bariatric surgery. What intervention would the nurse recommend?
   A. Bowel habit training
   B. Stimulated defecation program
   C. Sphincter muscle exercises with biofeedback
   D. Pelvic floor strengthening exercises

8. The continence nurse is caring for a patient who has a high impaction. What initial intervention is recommended?
   A. Administer a tap water enema.
   B. Administer oral laxatives.
   C. Perform digital breakup.
   D. Encourage fluid, fiber, and activity.

9. Which beverage would the continence nurse recommend to replace fluid for a patient experiencing diarrhea?
   A. Hot chocolate
   B. Orange juice
   C. Broth-based soups
   D. Ginger ale

10. What initial intervention would the continence nurse recommend for a patient who is experiencing acute constipation?
    A. Fiber supplements
    B. Osmotic laxative
    C. Stool softener
    D. Mineral oil enema

ANSWERS AND RATIONALES

1. B. Rationale: Urge bowel incontinence involves a sudden urgent need to defecate that results in incontinence when the individual is unable to reach a toilet promptly.

2. D. Rationale: Damage or denervation of the anal sphincter is a common cause of chronic FI and is usually caused by obstetric trauma, anorectal surgery, or anal trauma.

3. C. Rationale: Abdominal examination involves visual inspection for distention, percussion along the length of the bowel to assess for indicators of stool retention, and palpation of the lower quadrants to assess for evidence of stool retention.

4. B. Rationale: Observation during "bearing down" may reveal the presence of hemorrhoids, mucosal or rectal prolapse, or pelvic organ prolapse.

5. A. Rationale: Neurologic examination is indicated in situations where a neurologic deficit is suspected and should include anal reflex and perianal sensory testing. The "anal wink" tests the function of the pudendal nerve, which innervates the external anus sphincter.

6. B. Rationale: Disadvantages of external fecal pouches include being limited to nonambulatory patients who do not slide up and down in bed and it typically requires more than one caregiver to apply a rectal pouch. Perianal skin must be intact for it to adhere well.

7. D. Rationale: Evidence suggests that individuals undergoing bariatric surgery are at risk for FI and that measures to normalize stool consistency and to improve pelvic floor muscle strength prior to surgery can reduce the incidence of FI in these individuals.

8. A. Rationale: High impactions are treated with tap water or brand-name enemas to stimulate bowel movements; some clinicians recommend use of oral mineral oil to lubricate the fecal mass prior to enema administration.

9. C. Rationale: A simple and practical recommendation is to consume 8 ounces of liquid immediately following each loose stool in addition to their usual fluid intake; good choices include bouillon, *broth-based soups*, low-sugar sports drinks, herbal teas, gelatin (Jell-O), and water.

10. B. Rationale: Osmotic laxatives are a good choice for acute constipation; they work by pulling fluid into the lumen of the bowel, which stimulates peristalsis and helps to soften the stool. Stimulants activate the enteric nervous system to promote peristalsis and can lead to abrupt evacuations and electrolyte imbalance especially in the elderly.

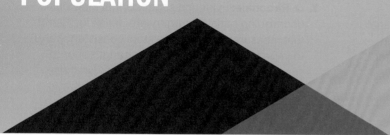

OBJECTIVES

1. Describe the pathology, clinical presentation, assessment, and management options for each of the following: retentive encopresis, nonretentive encopresis, and neurogenic bowel.

2. Explain how each of the following affects bowel function and continence: anal rectal malformations/imperforate anus, high and low lesions;

Hirschsprung disease; and neurogenic bowel conditions such as myelomeningocele.

3. Discuss the impact of developmental stage on management of bowel dysfunction and/or fecal incontinence.

4. Identify key concepts to be considered in management of the child or adolescent with bowel dysfunction or fecal incontinence.

TOPIC OUTLINE

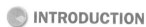
INTRODUCTION

The physiology of normal defecation and fecal continence has been covered in Chapter 20, and motility disorders and fecal incontinence (FI) in the adult population have been discussed in Chapters 21 and 22. This chapter focuses on types of bowel dysfunction and FI unique to the pediatric population and the impact of developmental stage on management approaches.

FETAL DEVELOPMENT OF THE GASTROINTESTINAL SYSTEM

Normal bowel function in the infant and child is dependent partly on normal fetal development of the gastrointestinal (GI) system. Although a detailed description of fetal GI tract development is beyond the scope of this text, a brief review of the critical aspects that are most likely to be involved in congenital anomalies is provided.

DEVELOPMENT OF PRIMITIVE GUT

Development of the GI tract begins during the 4th week of fetal life, when the primitive gut arises from the dorsal part of the yolk sac. The primitive gut can be divided into three segments: the foregut, the midgut, and the hindgut. The foregut develops into the pharynx, lower respiratory system, esophagus, stomach, upper portion of the duodenum, liver, pancreas, and biliary system. The vascular supply for these bowel segments is provided by the forerunner to the celiac artery. The midgut evolves into the small bowel distal to the orifice of the bile duct, the cecum, appendix, ascending colon, and most of the transverse colon. The blood supply for the midgut is provided by the superior mesenteric artery, and these segments of bowel are attached to the posterior abdominal wall by the dorsal mesentery. The hindgut forms the left transverse colon, descending colon, sigmoid colon, rectum, and proximal portion of the anal canal. The inferior mesenteric artery provides the blood supply for the bowel segments arising from the hindgut (Mazier et al., 1995).

KEY POINT

Development of the gastrointestinal tract begins during the 4th week of fetal life.

MIDGUT DEVELOPMENT/ROTATIONAL ANOMALIES

The midgut undergoes an interesting sequence of events during its development, and any defect in the normal sequence can produce congenital complications involving the small bowel and proximal colon. As the midgut lengthens and enlarges, it becomes too large for the developing fetal abdomen; as a result, the midgut herniates into the umbilical cord. When the fetal abdomen enlarges sufficiently to accommodate the midgut, these segments of bowel "return" to the abdominal cavity; however, they rotate in a counterclockwise position during their return. The small bowel segment of the midgut is the first to return, and it passes into the abdominal cavity in a position that is posterior to the superior mesenteric artery. The ascending and transverse colon segments then return and assume a position anterior to the superior mesenteric artery. The mesentery for the midgut attaches to the posterior abdominal wall close to the duodenum and ascending colon, which causes these segments of the bowel to assume a retroperitoneal position. Abnormalities in rotation may produce obstructive syndromes in the neonatal period (Mazier et al., 1995).

DEVELOPMENT OF PATENT LUMEN

Another aspect of fetal development that is critical to normal GI function after birth is the establishment of a patent lumen. Normal development of the GI "tube" involves endodermal proliferation, which temporarily occludes the lumen of the gut. However, this period of occlusion is normally followed by recanalization. Failure to recanalize the lumen may result in atresia (complete obstruction of the lumen), stenosis, cysts, or intestinal duplication (Mazier et al., 1995; Walker et al., 1990).

SEPARATION BETWEEN GASTROINTESTINAL AND GENITOURINARY SYSTEMS

A final aspect of GI development that is critical to normal function is the separation between the GI and the genitourinary systems. In very early stages of fetal development, the rudimentary reproductive, urinary, and intestinal ducts terminate in a common hollow cavity known as the "cloaca." At about week 4, the urorectal septum begins to form. This sheet of connective tissue divides the cloacal cavity into two separate compartments: the anterior compartment develops into the lower genitourinary tract and the posterior compartment develops into the rectum and anal canal. Congenital anorectal defects such as imperforate anus occur when this developmental sequence is interrupted or altered (Mazier et al., 1995).

FECAL ELIMINATION IN CHILDREN

Bowel function may be described in terms of stool frequency, stool consistency, and stool size (caliber). Unfortunately, it is difficult to define "normal" bowel habits among a healthy population because of the many variables that influence the frequency and consistency of fecal elimination. This variability is well documented among adult populations and is thought to be attributable in large part to differences in dietary intake; for example, studies among adults in Western societies reveal a variability in bowel movement frequency ranging from three times daily to three times weekly—bowel movement frequency fell within this range for 94% to 99% of the study population (Walker et al., 1990).

In infancy, normal stool frequency is much higher than among children and adults. During the infant's first week of life, an infant averages three to four stools a day, which usually decreases to two stools a day later in infancy and as a toddler. After the preschool years, the child may stool daily or every other day. Normal, healthy breastfed infants may go several days or longer without a bowel movement. Beyond the neonatal period, childhood constipation is usually not related to an organic condition (Nurko & Zimmerman, 2014). There are reported differences between breast-fed and formula-fed infants. Breast-fed infants have fewer stools during the first week of life but a significantly higher number of stools thereafter as compared to formula-fed infants (Walker et al., 1990). These differences in stool frequency gradually diminish after 8 weeks; by 16 weeks of age, when many infants have been introduced to solid foods, there is no difference in stool frequency between the two groups (Walker et al., 1990).

Stool frequency among preschool children is reported to be comparable to stool frequency among adults, with significant variation reported among various populations. Individuals following high-fiber and vegetarian diets typically have a greater number of bowel movements than individuals following a meat-based, low-fiber diet.

ACQUISITION OF FECAL CONTINENCE

Total control over bowel elimination is generally achieved by 4 years of age (O'Rorke, 1995), and most children achieve bowel and bladder control during *waking* hours by age 3. In order to achieve continence, the child must have functioning sphincters, normal rectal sensation, and normal rectosigmoid motility. In addition, the child must demonstrate both physiologic and developmental "readiness"; most children demonstrate "readiness" between 18 and 30 months of age (Christophersen, 1991). The two physiologic "readiness criteria" include *reflex sphincter control*, which can be demonstrated as early as 9 months of age, and *myelinization of the pyramidal tracts*, which is complete between 12 and 18 months of age. Some authors suggest that bladder control should be added to the list of readiness criteria; they define bladder control as the ability to empty the bladder completely with voiding and to stay dry for several hours (Christophersen, 1991). Psychological and cognitive "readiness" is equally critical but less predictable in terms of time frames for accomplishment.

Developmental criteria include motor skills such as walking to the bathroom, sitting on the toilet, clothing manipulation (such as pulling pants up and down), and flushing the toilet. Cognitive readiness is indicated by the child's ability to communicate impending urination or defecation, either through facial expressions or posturing, and instructional readiness. Instructional readiness includes both receptive language (such as words to describe voiding or defecation) and the ability to follow one-step or two-step commands. Some authors suggest that the most appropriate time frame for initiating toilet training for most children is between 24 and 30 months of age (Christophersen, 1991). O'Rorke summarizes a comprehensive approach that has been proven successful but notes that one approach may not be feasible for all parents (O'Rorke, 1995).

BOWEL DYSFUNCTION AND FECAL INCONTINENCE

CHILDHOOD CONSTIPATION

In pediatrics, a major cause of bowel dysfunction is "constipation." Constipation is common world-wide problem in childhood with reported cases ranging from 0.7% to 29.6%, accounting for 3% to 5% of pediatric primary care visit and 20% to 25% of visits to gastroenterology practices. Constipation is defined as infrequent defecation, painful defecation, or both. The definition of constipation developed by the North American Society of Gastroenterology, Hepatology, and Nutrition (NASPGHAN) is "a delay or difficulty in defecation, present for 2 weeks or more, and sufficient to cause significant distress to the patient." Internationally, the Paris Consensus on Childhood Constipation Terminology (PACCT) defines constipation as "a period of 8 weeks with at least 2 of the following symptoms: defecation frequency less than three times per week, FI frequency greater than once per week, passage of large stools that clog the toilet, palpable abdominal or rectal fecal mass, stool withholding behavior, or painful defecation" (Borowitz & Curffari, 2018). Constipation occurs in all age groups in pediatrics. Childhood constipation develops during 3 stages: infants during weaning; toddlers during toilet training, and in school-aged children. Several studies have reported that about half of childhood constipation occurs during the first year of life. Before puberty, it is equally common between genders. After puberty and into young adulthood, females are more likely to develop constipation than males (Borowitz & Curffari, 2018).

KEY POINT

Constipation is defined as infrequent defecation, painful defecation, or both. It occurs in all pediatric age groups and generally develops during three developmental milestones: infants during weaning; toddlers during toilet training, and in school-aged children.

Constipation which is a "symptom" not a disease becomes challenging in pediatrics, as the infant/child/adolescent unlike the adult is developing physically, cognitively, and emotionally. There are so many milestones they need to achieve such as transitioning from breastfeeding/formula to solids; toilet training, learning to communicate; physical growth; the stresses of adjusting to new environment (preschool, different schools, teachers, activities); and learning roles and responsibilities, social expectations such as family life or developing friendships, etc. It is not surprising that a child can physically internalize their stress, which can affect their appetite, urinary or bowel function which can lead to withholding behaviors, constipation, bowel dysfunction, and/or incontinence. In working with this age group, health care providers are working with the child/patient as well as the parents/caregivers, so treatment and explanations need to be tailored to the child's abilities and developmental level as well as the needs/abilities of the adult caregiver.

The majority of childhood constipation is "functional" with only 5% to 10% due to an organic cause. *Functional constipation* is a term that encompasses a group of disorders associated with persistent, difficult, infrequent, or incomplete defecation without an anatomical or biochemical etiology (Sood et al., 2019). Functional consti-

pation has no organic cause, and its etiology is felt to be multifactorial. The most frequent cause is painful defecation associated with hard stool. This discomfort then leads to stool withholding behavior evidenced by arching the back, stiffening the legs among infants, and crossing of legs or other postures in older children. Toilet training is the second most reported cause as 1 out of 5 children display toileting refusal by stool withholding behavior and incontinence (Philichi, 2018; Tobias et al., 2008).

KEY POINT

Functional constipation is a term that encompasses a group of disorders associated with persistent, difficult, infrequent, or incomplete defecation without an anatomical or biochemical etiology. The cause is multifactorial with an experience of passing a painful, hard stool as the main trigger that results in a stool withholding behavior.

A joint evidence-based guideline for the evaluation and treatment of functional constipation was developed in 2014 by the American Society for Pediatric Gastroenterology, Hepatology, and Nutrition and the European Society for Paediatric Gastroenterology, Hepatology and Nutrition. The Guidelines included definitions for intractable constipation and fecal impaction. Intractable constipation is constipation not responding to optimal conventional treatment for at least 3 months. Fecal impaction is defined as a hard mass in the lower abdomen indentified on physical examination or excessive stool in the distal colon on abdominal radiography (Tabbers et al., 2014). The guideline recommended the use of Rome III definition to diagnose functional constipation. The Rome III was subsequently updated in 2016, and presently, the Rome IV is utilized in defining functional constipation (see **Fig. 23-1**). Significant changes of Rome IV included the following:

- For younger children (0 to 4 mental age in years), "large diameter stools that may obstruct a toilet" was eliminated.
- "Fecal incontinence with at least one episode a week" was eliminated as criteria for young children who are not toilet trained.
- The duration of symptoms for all children was shortened from 2 months to 1 month for the age group 4 years to adolescence (Levy et al., 2017; Russo et al., 2019).

In addition to developmental milestones that increase the risk of functional constipation, stressful life events such as sexual abuse or a sudden loss of a parent may cause the child to develop other elimination dysfunctions such as FI with or without constipation or FI combined with urinary incontinence (UI). According to Koppen et al. (2016), 20% of children who exhibit symptoms of FI without constipation or any other underlying etiology

ROME IV CRITERIA IN PEDIATRICS
FUNCTIONAL CONSTIPATION

INFANTS AND TODDLERS UP TO 4 YEARS OLD

At least two of the following present for at least one month:
- Two or fewer defecations per week
- History of excessive stool retention
- History of painful or hard bowel movements
- History of large-diameter stools
- Presence of a large fecal mass

In toilet-trained children, the following additional criteria may be used:
- At least one episode/week of incontinence after the acquisition of toileting skills
- History of large-diameter stools that may obstruct the toilet

CHILDREN WITH DEVELOPMENTAL AGE OF AT LEAST 4 YEARS

At least two of the following present at least once/week for at least one month:
- Two or fewer defecations in the toilet
- At least one episode of fecal incontinence per week
- History of retentive posturing or excessive volitional stool retention
- History of painful or hard bowel movement
- Presence of large fecal mass in the rectum
- History of large-diameter stools that may obstruct the toilet
- The symptom cannot be fully explained by another medical condition

FIGURE 23-1. Rome IV Criteria for the Diagnosis of Functional Constipation in Children.

are diagnosed with functional nonretentive fecal incontinence (FNRFI), also known as primary nonretentive encopresis, which will be discussed later in the chapter.

Based on the previously cited time frames for "usual" acquisition of continence, one may consider a child who has not acquired bowel control by 4 years of age to be "fecally incontinent." There are several terms that are used to refer to bowel control problems among children, and these terms are defined as follows (Seth & Heyman, 1994):

- *Fecal incontinence:* Recurrent uncontrolled passage of fecal material for at least 1 month in an individual with a developmental age of at least 4 years.
- *Fecal soiling.* Any amount of stool deposited in the underwear, regardless of the cause.
- *Encopresis.* Fecal soiling usually associated with functional constipation; also used to refer to FI not caused by an organic or anatomic lesion.
- *Functional constipation.* Constipation not caused by organic or anatomic abnormalities *or* the requirement for medication to regulate bowel function after 4 years of age.

KEY POINT

Encopresis is fecal soiling associated with functional constipation (constipation not caused by organic or anatomic abnormalities); functional constipation is constipation not caused by organic or anatomic abnormalities.

Children with FI fall into four main groups: (1) children with functional fecal retention and overflow soiling (retentive encopresis), that is, fecal soiling caused by stool withholding behavior; (2) children with functional nonretentive fecal soiling (nonretentive encopresis), that is, fecal soiling without stool-withholding behavior; (3) children with anorectal malformations (ARM); and (4) children with neurologic lesions such as spina bifida. The pathophysiology of the dysfunction differs in each of these groups, and different management programs are required based on the underlying pathophysiology. Therefore, each of these groups will be addressed separately in terms of assessment/evaluation of each condition and treatment options.

ENCOPRESIS

Olaru et al. (2016) in their review of the literature define **encopresis** as a disorder characterized by repeated stool evacuation in inappropriate places in children over the age of four. The behavior can be either involuntary or intentional and have been present for a minimum of 3 months and presented at least once a month and is not the direct effect of a substance or medical condition. The etiology of this condition can be related to biological and developmental mechanisms as well as psychosocial and environmental factors.

Encopresis accounts for 3% to 5% of visits to a general pediatric outpatient clinic and up to 25% of visits to pediatric gastroenterologists (Yousseff & Lorenzo, 2001). Encopresis is reportedly three to six times more common among males than females and is noted in 3% of 4-year-olds and 1.6% of 10-year-olds. Encopresis presents predominantly in children between 3 and 7 years of age; in one study, 35% of children with encopresis had experienced hard stools within the first 6 months of life, 40% had experienced delays in toilet training, and 60% had reported painful defecation during the first 3 years of life (Abi-Hanna & Lake, 1998).

Causative factors remain unclear; however, socioeconomic status, family size, ordinal position of the child within the family, and age of parents have not been found to correlate positively with incidence of encopresis. There is a correlation between enuresis (urinary incontinence) and encopresis; 25% of children with encopresis also have enuresis. This is thought to be due to the close proximity of the rectum and bladder; an overly full rectum can partially obstruct the bladder neck and urethra, resulting in incomplete emptying of the bladder and subsequent leakage. In addition, the nerves that supply the bladder and bowel originate from the same (sacral) area. If there are problems with innervation and coordination of the anal sphincter, there may be coexisting problems with innervation and coordination of the urethral sphincter, leading to dual bowel and urinary incontinence.

Classifications

Encopresis is sometimes classified as "primary" or "secondary" and as "retentive" or "nonretentive." Primary encopresis refers to the condition in a child who has reached 4 years of age and has never achieved sustained bowel control (i.e., fecal continence lasting for at least 1 year), whereas secondary encopresis is used to indicate the condition in a child who has been successfully toilet-trained and has maintained continence for at least 1 year and then "relapsed" in response to some secondary disorder (Steinberg, 2008; Stern et al., 1988). Approximately 50% to 60% of all encopretic children have secondary encopresis.

Retentive encopresis is the term used to refer to FI clearly associated with constipation; these children retain stool and may even develop a megacolon. *Nonretentive encopresis* is defined as FI in a child who has no evidence of constipation; it is usually additionally classified as primary nonretentive encopresis (incontinence in a child who has never acquired bowel control) and secondary nonretentive encopresis (incontinence in a child who successfully completes toilet training but later regresses) (Boon & Singh, 1991). It is generally thought that primary nonretentive encopresis or FNRFI may be caused either by an organic problem or by emotional stressors, whereas secondary nonretentive encopresis is almost always caused by psychological issues (Boon & Singh, 1991). Encopresis can also be classified as diurnal or nocturnal, but this classification is rarely used because nocturnal encopresis is quite uncommon.

KEY POINT

Fifty to sixty percent of children with encopresis have secondary encopresis, meaning that the child had attained continence and then "relapsed," usually as a result of psychological stress.

Etiology

Although the cause of encopresis is not well understood, Levine (1982) postulated that in many children, encopresis represents a functional bowel disorder that can be at least partly explained from a developmental perspective. He hypothesized that as children pass through critical developmental stages, the environment, people in their lives, or critical life events may contribute to a functional bowel disorder. This hypothesis is supported by evidence that the history of many children with encopresis is positive for several of these "risk" factors (Levine, 1982). Levine outlined the developmental stages and issues as follows:

Stage I: early experience and predisposition (infancy and toddler years). Children with a tendency toward constipation during this period, due either to genetics or to dietary factors, are at greater risk for the development of encopresis when they are older. The major risk factor during this stage is functional constipation, which may develop as a result of immature bowel function, surgical correction of congenital anomalies (such as imperforate anus), parental overreaction to toileting, or aggressive bowel management. These factors may lead to voluntary withholding of stool, in which defecation is perceived as a negative experience.

Stage II: training and autonomy (2 to 5 years of age). During this stage, the child is beginning to develop autonomy and independence, and potentiating factors for bowel dysfunction include psychosocial stressors (birth of sibling/sibling rivalry, mother returning to work, parental discord) during toilet training, coercive or extremely permissive toilet training, fears of toileting (such as monsters that bite when one sits down on the toilet), and painful or difficult defecation.

Stage III: extramural function (early school years). Extramural function refers to the time frame during which the child enters school. These children are faced with a new routine, which includes using the school bathroom or withholding stool until they return home. Dietary habits, such as excessive ingestion of milk and decreased intake of fruits, vegetables, and fiber, may contribute to constipation. Additional potential risk factors include frenetic lifestyles, psychosocial stressors that evolve with school relationships, and illness or injury that results in prolonged inactivity with a resulting change in bowel function.

Psychosocial stressors at any stage can cause enough distraction to prevent a child's full attention to the urge to defecate. There are also reports of children with the diagnosis of autism spectrum disorder and attention deficit/hyperactivity disorder (ADHD) having FI (Beaudry-Bellefeuille, 2017; Niemczyk et al., 2015). Children with ADHD may be at greater risk due to their distractibility, difficulty linking actions to consequences, and inability to focus and sit still to finish a task. Improving their ability to attend is an essential first step in managing these children. Cohen (2007) also suggested the possibility of a link between autism and changes in bowel function, as children with this condition seem to have more bowel symptoms than other children. For example, constipation, diarrhea, and gastroesophageal reflux are commonly seen among children with autism. From a developmental perspective, children with autism may have more problems related to food and feeding; selective eating is quite common among these children, which makes it difficult to ensure a healthy diet. As a result, these children may have harder stools, which causes discomfort during evacuation and can lead to stool withholding. Autistic children and other children with special needs may also require more patience with toilet training; however, Cohen emphasizes that stool withholding and toilet training are often two separate issues in the special needs population. In some cases, the health care provider is only able to successfully treat stool withholding and is not able to address toilet training issues; however, successful treatment of stool withholding will in and of itself have a great impact on the child's life. Health care providers have to also be alert to children and adolescents who have been physically or sexually abused as they may have developed a stool withholding pattern that can result in fecal soiling; in these cases, the emotional effects of the abuse are more often the cause of the soiling than the physical effects. Recent studies continue to verify children with autism spectrum disorders experience an increased incidence of stooling issues (Beaudry-Bellefeuille, 2017).

It is clear that the risk factors for each individual child are likely to be somewhat different. It is therefore critical to perform a comprehensive assessment as a basis for an individualized treatment plan (Levine, 1982).

KEY POINT

The risk/etiologic factors for each child with encopresis are likely to be somewhat different; therefore, a comprehensive assessment is required as the basis for an individualized management program.

Clinical Presentation

There seem to be three major clinical patterns among children with encopresis. In more than 95% of cases,

encopresis is due to functional constipation. In this condition, retention of stool causes rectal distention, with resultant leakage of stool around the retained bolus. Because the rectum is chronically distended, the stretch receptors fail to signal the child that defecation is imminent. As a result, these children commonly have several fecal accidents per day as they are not capable of sensing rectal distention and the need to go to the bathroom. The stool size is usually small and the consistency of the stool is generally loose. These children are sometimes misdiagnosed as having diarrhea based on parental reports of odorous, thin, ribbon-like, or diarrheal stools.

KEY POINT

Ninety-five percent of children with encopresis have functional constipation, characterized by chronic stool retention and rectal distention; this causes loss of sensory awareness of the need to defecate and chronic relaxation of the internal anal sphincter, which permits leakage of stool around the fecal mass and resultant incontinence.

A much less common pattern of encopresis is the nonretentive pattern; children with this condition may experience stress-related diarrhea, which appears to be related to the disorder known as "irritable bowel syndrome" among adults, or may experience daily incontinence of stool that is of normal size and consistency.

The third and least common pattern is manipulative soiling, in which the child uses incontinent episodes to manipulate the environment (e.g., to avoid school or to passively display anger toward family members).

Almost all children with encopresis retain stool at least intermittently. Typically, the retention develops gradually over time. Some children with encopresis actually defecate daily but fail to effectively empty the lower bowel; because of this failure to empty, stool gradually amasses in the rectum and colon. The child may be asymptomatic or may complain of recurrent abdominal pain. Retained stool may be palpable on abdominal examination (if the child has significant colonic retention) or may be evident only on rectal examination (if the retained stool is confined to the rectum).

As rectal and colonic distention progress, sensory feedback from the bowel becomes impaired; that is, rectal distention no longer causes sensory awareness of the need to defecate. In addition, distention of the rectal wall overstretches the muscle fibers, which reduces contractile force. There is no awareness of the need to defecate and no propulsive force to eliminate the stool. As a result, stool continues to accumulate in the rectum, where continued water absorption creates a hard fecal mass. As the fecal mass becomes larger and harder, elimination becomes progressively more difficult and more painful; defecation may result in fissures or hemorrhoids. Painful defecation further contributes to the vicious cycle of stool retention.

Soiling occurs in the presence of retained stool because the retained stool causes sphincter dysfunction. The constant distention of the rectum causes persistent relaxation of the internal sphincter, mediated by the rectoanal inhibitory reflex (RAIR). Relaxation of the internal sphincter permits liquid stool and mucus to seep around the impaction and into the anal canal. Continence past that point is dependent on external sphincter contraction; however, the child with chronic retention usually fails to sense rectal distention and fecal seepage into the anal canal and therefore does not voluntarily contract the external sphincter. Even if the child does recognize the leakage, he or she is able to contract the sphincter for only a short period of time. When the external sphincter returns to resting tone, the anal canal pressures are insufficient to prevent leakage, and soiling occurs. In addition, prolonged rectal distention and high intrarectal pressures can produce a "paradoxical" response of the sphincter; that is, increased rectal volume causes reduced sphincter muscle tone and increased risk of soiling, as compared to the normal response of increased sphincter tone.

KEY POINT

Soiling occurs in the presence of retained stool because the retained stool causes persistent relaxation of the internal sphincter, mediated by the rectoanal inhibitory reflex. Relaxation of the internal sphincter permits liquid stool and mucus to seep around the impaction and into the anal canal. The child will often fail to respond to rectal distention and if prolonged, the external anal sphincter looses tone furthering the risk of fecal soiling.

Children with encopresis present with a wide range of associated symptoms. Children with recent onset of retention and incontinence typically complain of abdominal pain; in contrast, children with long-standing encopresis seldom complain of pain because they generally have developed tolerance to colonic distention. The presence of associated enuresis is also variable. In children who do present with enuresis, effective treatment of the stool retention may alleviate the child's problems with bladder control. Encopresis at night is relatively rare and seems to be associated with a poor prognosis (Levine, 1982).

Encopresis has a major effect on lifestyle and on self-esteem. The inability to control defecation is extremely humiliating to these children, who live in constant fear of discovery, exposure, ruthless teasing, bullying, and ridicule. In addition, these children are often punished and told that their problem with incontinence is an attention-

getting act or a result of their own laziness. They may be told that they are negligent when they fail to change foul-smelling undergarments after an accident. Parents fail to realize that the sense of smell in these children (as in all people) accommodates to their own odors and that the child is frequently genuinely unaware of the accident and the offensive odor. Despite the fact that these children live with daily emotional trauma, acting-out behavior is not common; instead, these children are likely to isolate themselves to varying degrees and to show excessive dependence.

KEY POINT

Encopresis has a major negative effect on lifestyle and self-esteem and on family and social relationships. Thus, psychosocial factors should be an area of major concern when one is assessing and managing the child with encopresis.

Encopresis also has a tremendous influence on the other family members. Parents generally feel frustrated and possibly angry or guilty regarding their child's "failure to acquire continence." In addition, the fear of "accidents" may profoundly affect family activities; car trips, visits to friends, and even restaurants may be avoided because of the fear of embarrassment. Siblings may hesitate or refuse to invite friends over because of fecal odor or fear that the child could have an embarrassing accident. The stress generated by these limitations and adaptations may increase tension and conflict among family members and between various family members and the encopretic child. Thus, psychosocial factors should be an area of major concern when one is assessing and managing the child with encopresis.

Assessment

The assessment of a child with a bowel dysfunction requires a thorough history (**Boxes 23-1 and 23-2**), a focused physical examination (**Table 23-1**), and possibly radiographic studies or anorectal physiology testing (**Table 23-2**) (Stadtler, 1989). The initial comprehensive assessment of a child with a bowel dysfunction requires a thorough medical and developmental history and psychosocial assessment with focused questions regarding the specific bowel symptoms experienced especially stooling pattern, stool characteristics, and leakage pattern if present (see Bristol Stool Scale in Chapter 6, Figs. 6-7 and 6-8). In pediatrics, most children do not usually experience chronic conditions as seen in adults, so the "review of systems" is abbreviated. However, there needs to be an extensive review of the child's bowel history that can provide the clinician enough information regarding the type of bowel dysfunction to determine therapeutic treatment options.

BOX 23-1 GENERAL PEDIATRIC HISTORY-TAKING GUIDELINES

History taking is vital when assessing a child with a bowel condition. There are differences in history taking from an adult as outlined below:

1. Chief Complaint: a statement of the primary problem
2. History of Present Illness: a statement identifying the historian that person's relationship to the patient and their reliability who provides a concise, chronological account of the illness which includes any previous treatment with full description of symptoms (pertinent positives) and pertinent negatives. It relates to the differential diagnosis for the chief complain
3. Past Medical History:
   a. Major medical illnesses
   b. Major surgical illnesses—operations/dates
   c. Trauma: for example, fractures, lacerations
   d. Previous hospital admissions with dates and reason for admissions
   e. Current medications
   f. Allergies
   g. Immunization status
4. Pregnancy and Birth History
   a. Maternal healthy during pregnancy: infectious illnesses, trauma, hypertension, gestational diabetes, drugs, alcohol, smoking
   b. Gestational age at delivery
   c. Labor and delivery—length of labor, fetal distress, types of delivery, abnormalities during delivery
   d. Neonatal history: birth measurements (weight and length), APGAR scores, respiratory status at birth, hyperbilirubinemia, birth injuries, feeding (breastfed or bottle), stooling consistency and frequency, and length of stay
5. Developmental History:
   a. Developmental milestones achieved (smiling, rolling, sitting, crawling, walking, language acquisition, etc.)
   b. School: present grade, problems interactions
   c. Behavior, enuresis, habits, teasing about accidents, withdrawn, attention deficit hyperactivity disorder (note: there is an association between ADHD and withholding behavior or incomplete bladder emptying and constipation)
   d. Toilet training: age of introduction, problems with achieving continence, bedwetting/enuresis
6. Feeding History
   a. Breast of bottle fed—type of formula, frequency and amounts, reasons for formula changes; duration of breastfeeding/formula use
   b. Solids: start date, tolerance to consistency of the solids, transition to table foods
   c. Current diet: (overall appetite)
      i. Intake of foods at different meals (breakfast/lunch/dinner/snacks)—amount eaten, frequency
      ii. Specifically foods higher in fiber (vegetables/fruits/etc.)
      iii. Known foods that constipate child and those that cause looser stools

      iv. Fluid intake (types/amount/frequency/total liquid intake in 24 hours). Note: excessive intake of milk can lead to constipation
      v. If on enteral feedings note type of formula, amount, frequency, and water flushes with feedings and medications, bolus or continuous feedings, and rate administered
7. Review of Systems: (very abbreviated for infants and younger children)
   a. Weight—recent changes/ability to gain/challenges with weight
   b. HEENT: unusual shape or size of head; visual or hearing problems, dysphasia; dentition/caries/excessive drooling
   c. Cardiac: heart murmurs, chest pain, palpitations, cyanosis, and dyspnea
   d. Respiratory: cystic fibrosis, wheezing, pneumonia, bronchitis, chronic cough, TB
   e. GI: stool color and character (use of Bristol chart); constipation, diarrhea, and vomiting; abdominal pain, colic, presence of GERD, Hirschsprung disease, and anorectal malformation; short gut/absorption disorder; prune belly, gastroschisis, pseudoobstruction, and use of feeding tubes/devices
   f. GU: frequency (approximate volume, color of urine) dysuria, bladder distention, hematuria, discharge, and quality of the urinary stream; catheterization (amount, frequency, and type of catheter used); renal anomaly (e.g., fused or absent kidney, anomalies of the ureters/bladder, urethra, penis, and scrotum), bladder or kidney infections or kidney stones
   g. Neurological: presence of seizures, headaches, neuropathy, hypotonia, sacral teratoma, sacral agenesis, Pilonidal dimple covered by a tuft of hair, and Down syndrome
   h. Musculoskeletal: joint pains, scoliosis, gluteal cleft deviation weakness, fractures, ambulatory or not, gait discrepancy, abnormal abdominal musculature, spasticity of muscles, and use of orthotics/walkers/wheelchair
   i. Endocrine: celiac disease, hypothyroidism
   j. Pubertal: secondary sexual characteristics, menses and affect on GI or GU system, sexually active. Note: withholding behavior is associated with sexual abuse
   k. Skin and lymph: rashes, eczema, lumps, infections, bruising and bleeding, abnormal pigmentation
8. Family History:
   a. Illnesses: cardiac disease, diabetes, inflammatory bowel disorders, constipation, asthma, allergies, congenital neurological conditions (muscular dystrophy; spina bifida; microcephaly)
   b. Developmental delays: mental retardation; congenital anomalies, chromosomal problems, consanguinity; growth problems
9. Social
   a. Living situation—homelessness, multiple families in a single dwelling
   b. Multiple caregivers

BOX 23-2   SPECIFIC HISTORY-TAKING GUIDELINES FOR A CHILD WITH A BOWEL CONDITION

- *Size and consistency of stools:* that is, "pellets," "balls," "logs," "ribbon-like" (obtain approximate length and diameter of stools if possible); liquid, mushy, soft, formed, hard, or variable consistency. (It is helpful to use the Bristol chart to identify the type of stool.) See Chapter 6, **Figures 6-7 and 6-8**.
- *Frequency and consistency of voluntary bowel movements (if applicable)*: Determine the age of the child when constipated stools were seen.
- *Pain:* Does the child experience any pain or bleeding when passing stools? Does the child have any abdominal discomfort while defecating and does it subside with defecation?
- *Other physical symptoms:* Does child experience any fever, nausea, vomiting, weight loss, or decreased appetite?
- *Detailed description of stooling "accidents":* frequency (daily, multiple times weekly, etc.), any associated or precipitating events, volume of incontinent stools (smear, teaspoon, tablespoon, ½ cup, "diarrhea," etc.), do accidents contain formed stool or if consistently liquid, this may be indication of impaction, number of underwear (or liners) soiled in 1 day, current management. (Is child aware that an accident has occurred? Is child able to clean himself or herself up after an accident? Does school or day care staff assist with management?)
- *Sensory awareness of rectal filling and defecation:* Can child sense rectal distention? Is child able to differentiate between gas, liquid, and solid? Is sensory awareness consistent or variable, and, if variable, how often is child able to recognize rectal distention? (It is helpful to ask the child to point to where he or she feels the urge to have a bowel movement; many children with diminished or absent rectal sensation point to the left abdomen, indicating that their sensory awareness is related to peristaltic activity as opposed to rectal distention.)
- *Current bowel management program:* Has a bowel program been established? If so, what does it involve—digital stimulation? suppositories? enemas? regular toileting? medications? (If medications taken, determine strength, dose, and frequency.) Is child independent in bowel program and medication administration, or is assistance needed—if assistance is needed, how much assistance and who is providing it at present? What is the frequency of the current program; that is, how often are medications taken? Stimulants used to initiate defecation? Routine toileting performed? Is the currently established bowel program effective? If not, what problems are associated with the current program?
- *Specific toileting behaviors:* What position does the child assume while toileting, that is, are his or her feet firmly positioned on the floor or in the air? Does the child have enough trunk stability to sit without having to support himself or herself? Is the child able to effectively do a Valsalva maneuver to "push the stool out"? (It may help to have the child demonstrate how he or she "pushes stool out.") How long does the child take to defecate? If current bowel program includes routine toileting, how much encouragement does the child require to adhere to the program? Does the young child exhibit any "withholding behaviors" for example, squatting; crossing ankles; stiffening body; holding onto furniture or mother; flushing, sweating, and crying; or hiding during defecation?

- *Dietary status:* Have any dietary modifications been made to address the problems with bowel function? If yes, what are they and what effect have they had? What types of high-fiber foods does the child eat and in what volume? What is the child's usual volume of liquid intake? Does the child have access to liquids in the school or day care setting? Is the child receiving any fiber supplementation, and, if so, what formula and in what volume? Is the child's dental status satisfactory, or are there dental problems contributing to inadequate fiber intake?
- *Environmental/social changes:* Determine if the child has had any recent stress, change in routine (e.g., started preschool or change in classroom), diet changes such as introduction of solids or cow's milk, illness or new home/school? Does the caregiver notice that the child consistently has difficulty stopping any activity to go to the bathroom or is in a hurry with defecation, not spending enough time to completely empty the rectum of stool? Has there been changes within the family (e.g., birth of another child, death, divorce, or major illness with a family member)?
- *Urological status:* Is the child continent of urine but incontinent of stool? How often does the child void during the day? Does the child complain of discomfort with urination? If the child is emptying his or her bladder with clean intermittent catheterization (CIC), at what frequency does the child catheterize? Has the child had any urinary tract infection (UTI)? Does the child exhibit withholding behavior with urine? Does the child have any urinary accidents? Does the child have problems with enuresis/bedwetting at night?
- *Goals and motivation:* What is the child's perception of the problem with FI? What are the child's and parents' goals for management? How much assistance does the child require, and how much assistance and support are the parents able and willing to provide?

Developmental Status

- *Time frame for achievement of developmental milestones:* Age at which toileting introduced and response to toileting. (The clinician should be aware that parents of children with congenital conditions sometimes tend to "excuse" the child from learning normal toileting behavior. The clinician should counsel the parents re: the importance of normalizing their child's life as much as possible and should explain that the child should be exposed to normal toileting by 3 years of age unless the child is cognitively impaired.)
- *Current continence status:* If child is in school, how much distance is there between the classrooms and the bathroom facilities? Do the bathroom facilities provide privacy? Does the child have accidents at school? If so, how often and how are these handled?
- *Current academic status:* Has the child been diagnosed with a specific disorder such as attention deficit disorder or developmental delay? Is the child in a regular classroom or a special education program? (If the child is in a special education program, ask about the services provided. Some special education programs provide toileting assistance.) How is the child's attendance record in school?

(Continued)

BOX 23-2 SPECIFIC HISTORY-TAKING GUIDELINES FOR A CHILD WITH A BOWEL CONDITION (*Continued*)

Psychosocial Status

- *Behavioral issues:* Is the child seeing a therapist for any behavioral or emotional problems? Has there been any abuse or neglect (sexual/physical/emotional)?
- *Peer relationships:* What is the child's peer group like? Are the child's friends aware of the problem, and, if so, what is their response? Are the child's peers able to detect any odor or problem with stool elimination? Is the child having any problems at school?
- *Extracurricular activities:* Does the child participate in school or extracurricular events? Does the child attend sleepovers or camps? Does the child participate in sports? How is the problem with bowel function handled in these settings?
- *School and teacher support:* Are the school staff and the teacher aware of the child's medical needs and problems? Are they sensitive and supportive regarding the child's toileting needs? Is the child in a "regular" classroom setting or receiving "special-educational" support?
- *Incentive program:* What type of incentive program is best suited for this child if a bowel program is implemented?

MacLeod, J. (1998). Fecal incontinence: A practical program of management. *Endoscopy Review, 5*, 45–56.

Walker, W. A., Durie, P. R., Hamilton, J. R., et al. (1996). *Pediatric gastrointestinal disease* (Vol. 2, 2nd ed., pp. 2077–2091). St. Louis, MO: Mosby.

From Nurko, S., & Zimmerman, L. A. (2014). Evaluation and treatment of constipation in children and adolescents. *American Family Physician, 90*(2), 82–90; Dos Santos, J., Lopes, R. I., & Koyle, M. A. (2017). Bladder & bowel dysfunction in children: An update on the diagnosis and treatment of a common, but underdiagnosed pediatric problem. *Canadian Urological Association Journal, 11*(1-2 Suppl 1), S64–S72. doi: 10.5489/cuaj.4411.

TABLE 23-1 PHYSICAL EXAMINATION OF A CHILD WITH A BOWEL CONDITION

EXAMINATION	NORMAL FINDING	ABNORMAL FINDING	REFERRAL AND WHY
General	Happy, interactive, cooperative	Altered consciousness, distressed, dehydrated	Check with caregivers as the abnormal findings may be "normal" for this child and the child is receiving care
Head	Normal size and shape; fontanelle flat	Cranial sutures overriding, enlarged head or microcephalic	Check with caregivers as the abnormal findings may be "normal" for this child and the child is receiving care
Eyes	EOM, able to track objects; PERL	Strabismus, blindness	Check with caregivers as the abnormal findings may be "normal" for this child and the child is receiving care
Ears	Equal position of ears; able to hear	Position of ear altered, unable to hear, drainage from ear	Check with caregivers as the abnormal findings may be "normal" for this child and is receiving care
Nose	Nasal septum present; no discharge	Bleeding; purulent discharge	Check with caregivers as the abnormal findings may require a referral to an ENT or ED
Mouth and Throat	Lips pink, oral mucosa moist and pink; number teeth; no caries or plaque; if visible normal palate	Lips cyanotic; oral mucosa dry; teeth with caries, discolored, plaque; upper palate with high arch; gag reflex absent	Check with caregivers as the abnormal findings may be "normal" for this child and the child is receiving care. This may require a referral to the ED
Lungs	Abdominal breathing is normal in infants and older child with even expansion of the chest wall; lungs clear to auscultation	Abnormal breathing or increased respiratory rate; use of accessory muscles, chest retraction; rales; wheezing and rhonchi	Check with caregivers as the abnormal findings may be "normal" for this child and the child is receiving care. If not may need to send the child to the ED
Cardiovascular	HR within normal limits; NSR; good pulses	Increased heart rate; murmurs; poor pulses—extremities cool, clamy, cyanosis	Check with care-givers as the abnormal findings may be "normal" for this child and the child is receiving care. If not may need to refer the child to the ED
Abdomen	Usually infants with protuberant abdomen flatter as they get older; bowel sounds present and abdomen soft	Infants with overly protuberant abdomen, distended; hypoactive bowel sounds; tenderness with palpation; hernias visible	Check with caregivers as the abnormal findings may be "normal" for this child and the child is receiving care. If abdomen is very distended and painful, refer to the ED3.

TABLE 23-1 PHYSICAL EXAMINATION OF A CHILD WITH A BOWEL CONDITION (*Continued*)

EXAMINATION	NORMAL FINDING	ABNORMAL FINDING	REFERRAL AND WHY
Musculoskeletal	Spine is straight; has full range of motion of all extremities; good muscle strength for age; no deformities; extremities are symmetrical; ambulates straight	Spine: kyphosis, lordosis, or scoliosis. Sacral dimple with or without tuft of hair—near the perineum; masses over the spine extremities limited range of motion; spastic; gluteal cleft deviation; deformities; in-toeing, out-toeing, bow legs; limp; hips (+) for Ortolani and Barlow signs. Abdominal musculature is abnormal	Check with caregivers as the abnormal findings may be "normal" for this child and the child is receiving care • May require a referral to neurologist or orthopedic specialist
Neurological	Good muscle tone and strength and reflexes	Hyper or hypotonia; spasticity of extremities; poor reflexes; presence of seizures. Gait abnormality. Absent anal and cremasteric reflex. Abnormal deep tendon reflexes of lower extremities	Check with caregivers as the abnormal findings may be "normal" for this child. • May require a referral to neurologist
Genital-Urinary	Normal genitalia—boys circumcised or not; with testes bilaterally. Labial development in adolescent girls. Anus is closed with anal wink. If a teen note Tanner stage of development.	Hypospadias; presence of hernias; absence of testes; anus displaced or laxed. Rectal prolapse may be visible. Bladder is distended.	Check with caregivers as the abnormal findings may be "normal" for this child and surgical correction may be considered with a urologist and/or pediatric surgeon
Skin	Good turgor, skin intact. Normal birthmarks: nevi, Mongolian spots, small hemangioma	Multiple or large hemangiomas, scars, bruises, especially in patterns suggestive of abuse, rash, poor skin turgor—possible dehydration	Large hemangiomas may require a surgical/vascular referral. Possible abuse is a referral to a Child Protective Agency
Rectal/Anal Area	Anus is approximately halfway between the base of the scrotum/labia minora and the tip of the coccyx. • Anus is contracted, slightly puckered and able to elicit an anal wink • Rectal examination if done, rectum should be empty, if stool present, should be soft	Assess for sacral dimples or pits; if anus is positioned anteriorly there is an increased risk for constipation or may result in abnormal defecation dynamics which some pediatric surgeons believe is a form of an imperforate anus with perineal fistula • If rectal examination done: a child with Hirschsprung disease is small and empty of stool, after the finger is removed there may be a gush of liquid stool as obstruction has been partially relieved. Rectum of a child with functional constipation is enlarged and stool is present just beyond the anal verge. • Anal fissures, fistulae, or hemorrhoids may be present	

Sources: MacLeod, J. (1998). Fecal incontinence: A practical program of management. *Endoscopy Review, 5*, 45–56; Walker, W. A., Durie, P. R., Hamilton, J. R., et al. (1996). *Pediatric gastrointestinal disease* (Vol. 2, 2nd ed., pp. 2077–2091). St. Louis, MO: Mosby. Borowitz, S. M., & Cuffari, C. (December 14, 2018). Pediatric Constipation. Retrieved from https://Emedicine.medscape.com/article/928185-print

Box 23-1 provides a sample in gathering a general pediatric history, while **Box 23-2** outlines the medical and developmental history, and psychosocial assessment in any child with a bowel condition. **Table 23-1** provides a guide in performing a focus physical examination regarding any child with a bowel dysfunction. **Table 23-2** outlines differential diagnosis of common pediatric bowel dysfunctions and applicable diagnostics if warranted.

KEY POINT

The initial assessment of a child with a bowel dysfunction requires a thorough medical and developmental history and psychosocial assessment with focused questions regarding the specific bowel symptoms experienced especially stooling pattern, stool characteristics, and leakage pattern if present. Bristol Stool Scale chart is a valuable tool to obtain more objective findings regarding stool characteristics along with a bowel diary.

TABLE 23-2 DIFFERENTIAL DIAGNOSIS AND RECOMMENDED DIAGNOSTIC EVALUATION

BOWEL DYSFUNCTION	RECOMMENDED DIAGNOSTIC EVALUATION
Functional Constipation	History and physical examination, no testing
	A plain abdominal radiography may be used if fecal impaction is suspected but the physical examination is unreliable/not possible or the history is vague
Anatomic Malformation of the Colon and Rectum	
Imperforate anus, anal or colonic stenosis, anteriorly displaced anus	Physical examination, barium enema
Spinal cord abnormalities	
Meningomyelocele, spinal cord tumor	Spinal computed tomography scan, magnetic resonance imaging, anorectal manometry, urodynamics. Defecography, electromyography, colonic transit study
Metabolic Conditions	
Hypothyroidism	Thyroid studies
Hypercalcemia, hyperkalemia	Serum calcium and potassium levels

Used with permission from AAFP. Copyright © 2014 by the American Academy of Family Physicians. Nurko, S., & Zimmerman, L. A. (2014). Evaluation and treatment of constipation in children and adolescents. *American Family Physician, 90*(2), 82–90. Retrieved from https://www.aafp.org/afp/2014/0715/p82.html

In the evaluation of children with encopresis if medical conditions such as Hirschsprung's, cystic fibrosis, or hypothyroidism have been ruled out, laboratory tests are generally not beneficial. An abdominal radiograph may be useful when the history is vague or the child is not cooperative with the examination (Beinvogl et al., 2017). The North American Society for Pediatric Gastroenterology, Hepatology and Nutrition (NASPGHAN) and the European Society for Pediatric Gastroenterology, Hepatology and Nutrition (ESPGHAN) as well as the Rome IV criteria do not support routine use of abdominal x-rays for functional constipation (Beinvogl et al., 2017). The recommended instances for use of an abdominal x-ray include an unreliable patient history, psychological factors that make a digital rectal examination inappropriate, obesity, or patients with a suspicion of sexual abuse history. A barium enema may be considered when looking for medical causes of constipation such as Hirschsprung's. Abdominal and pelvic ultrasound studies can show if the child has stool retention or if other abnormalities exist. The ultrasound can also show whether a child empties their bladder; this is important because severe constipation and rectal distention can partially obstruct the bladder neck and urethra, resulting in incomplete emptying. It is not uncommon for children with severe constipation to report coexisting problems with UI or urinary tract infections resulting in a disorder defined as bowel and bladder dysfunction (BBD) (Dos Santos et al., 2017).

Lumbosacral spine films or magnetic resonance imaging may be needed if examination of the lower extremities indicates an abnormality or if there are any sacral abnormalities noted. However, the history and physical examination are usually the only diagnostic tools necessary to identify retentive encopresis and to rule out organic factors. Few cases of retentive encopresis and even fewer cases of nonretentive encopresis have an organic etiology.

Management: General Principles

Some years ago, Mikkelsen (2001) conducted a literature review and stated that there had been less progress in understanding the etiology and treatment of encopresis than enuresis. More recently, Reid and Bahar (2006) reviewed the literature on the management of encopresis; they noted a major emphasis on careful history taking, especially in regard to the psychoemotional aspects of the child's environment and on educating children and families about the condition. Frequently, constipation and subsequent hard stools lead to fecal retention due to the painful evacuation; thus, treatment must include measures to correct constipation, such as dietary modifications, that is, increased fiber and fluid intake. (See **Table 23-3** for high-fiber diet and **Fig. 23-2A and B** for algorithm for the treatment of functional constipation). Loening-Baucke et al. (2004) reexamined the benefits of adding fiber to the diet and determined that fiber is of benefit in the treatment of constipation with or without encopresis. ESPGHAN and NASPGHAN, in their evidence-based review, recommend that there be "normal fiber and fluid intake." The evidence also demonstrated that polyethylene glycol (PEG) and enemas are equally effective for fecal disimpaction (Tabbers et al., 2014). The use of laxatives is also a critical part of the treatment plan for these children (Hyams et al., 2016). Several centers currently recommend avoiding the use of enemas and/or suppositories as administering medication via the rectum can increase a child's aversion to defecation and can therefore increase their constipation problem. There have also been reports suggesting that repeated enemas can induce secondary anger, complicating the original cause of encopresis. Currently, the majority of treatment programs emphasize dietary modifications with increased fiber and water, regular daily toileting, and a reward system.

TABLE 23-3 HIGH-FIBER DIET

General Guidelines

Dietary fiber is beneficial in that it adds bulk to the stool, reduces stool transit time, reduces intestinal intraluminal pressures, and slows gastric emptying.

Adequate fluid intake is essential when fiber is added to the diet. Fiber intake should be increased gradually to avoid unpleasant side effects.

A good approach is to use the following chart to identify high-fiber foods and to replace low-fiber foods in the diet with high-fiber foods until the desired "fiber intake goal" is reached.

FOOD	SERVING SIZE	FIBER IN GRAMS
Breads		
Cracked wheat	1 slice	2.1
Raisin	1 slice	0.4
Rye	1 slice	1.2
White	1 slice	0.8
Whole wheat	1 slice	2.1
Hamburger roll or bun	1 at 3½ inch diameter, 1½ inch height	1.2
Bagel, 100% whole wheat	1	5.4
Bagel, oat bran	1	7.7
Bran muffins made with Kellogg's All-Bran or Bran Buds cereal	1	3.2
Bran muffin made with Kellogg's 40% Bran Flakes cereal	1	1.3
Pancakes	1 at 4 inches diameter	0.5
Taco shell (tortilla)	1	0
Cereals		
Kellogg's All-Bran	⅓ cup (1 ounce)	9.0
Kellogg's Bran Buds	⅓ cup (1 ounce)	8.0
Kellogg's Cracklin' Bran	⅓ cup (1 ounce)	4.0
Kellogg's Most	¾ cup (1 ounce)	4.0
Bran flakes	1 cup	5.0–9.2
Fiber One	1 cup	27.5
Granola	1 cup	5.8–6.0
Grape Nuts	½ cup	5.4
Raisin Bran	1 cup	6–7.9
Oat bran, cooked	1 cup	6.4
Wheat germ toasted	½ cup	8.0
Macaroni, vegetable, tricolored	1 cup	5.8
Vegetables		
Avocado	Half	2.2
Asparagus (boiled, cut)	½ cup	1.1
Beans:		
Azuki bean, cooked	½ cup	5.8
Black, cooked	½ cup	7.5

TABLE 23-3 HIGH-FIBER DIET (*Continued*)

FOOD	SERVING SIZE	FIBER IN GRAMS
Garbanzo, canned	1 cup	9.1
Kidney, canned	½ cup	5.9
Mung, boiled	½ cup	5.8
Pinto, cooked	½ cup	7.3
Bean sprouts	½ cup	1.6
Broccoli, steamed or stir fried	1 cup	5.0
Brussels sprouts (boiled)	1 cup	7.2
Cabbage, shredded, boiled	½ cup	2.3
Carrots, drained, boiled	½ cup	2.3
Cauliflower, boiled	½ cup	1.1
Cucumber, raw	1 ounce	0.1
Eggplant, peeled, drained	½ cup	2.5
Green beans, cut, boiled	½ cup	2.0
Green pepper	1 medium	0.8
Lentils, dry, boiled	1 cup	9.0
Lettuce	6 medium leaves	1.4
Mushrooms, raw	½ cup	0.9
Okra	½ cup	2.6
Peas, boiled, drained	½ cup	4.2
Radishes	10 medium	0.5
Spinach, boiled	½ cup	5.7
Squash, acorn, baked or mashed	½ cup	5.3
Tomato, raw	1 medium	2.0
Tomato, paste, canned	½ cup	5.4
Taro, sliced, cooked	1 cup	6.7
Turnips, boiled, mashed	½ cup	3.2
Fruits		
Apple with peel	1 medium	3.3
Apple, dried, rings	10 each	5.8
Applesauce, canned	½ cup	2.6
Apricots	2 medium	1.6
Apricots, dried halves	½ cup	5.0
Banana	½ small	1.6
Cantaloupe	¼ whole	1.6
Cherries, sweet	10 large	1.2
Dates, dried	5	3.1
Figs, dried	5	8.7
Grapefruit, fresh	½ whole	0.6
Grapes, seedless	12	0.3
Guava	2	9.7
Lemon, fresh	1 slice	0.3
Mango	1 cup	5.0
Nectarines	1 medium	3.0
Oranges	1 small	2.4
Peach, fresh	1 medium	1.4
Peach, dried halves	10	12.2
Pear, dried, halves	10	13.1

(*Continued*)

TABLE 23-3 HIGH-FIBER DIET (Continued)		
FOOD	SERVING SIZE	FIBER IN GRAMS
Fruits (Continued)		
Pineapple, fresh	½ cup	0.9
Plums, fresh	2 medium	0.4
Pomegranate	1	5.5
Prunes, dried	10	7.8
Prunes, stewed	½ cup	7.0
Raisins	2 tablespoons	1.2
Strawberries	½ cup	1.7
Nuts and Seeds		
Almonds, dry roasted	½ cup	6.8
Coconut, fresh grated	1 cup	7.5
Coconut cream, canned	1 cup	6.5
Coconut cream, raw	1 cup	5.3
Coconut milk, fresh, frozen	1 cup	5.3
Coconut milk, raw	1 cup	5.3
Macadamia, chopped	½ cup	5.1
Mixed, dry roasted with peanuts	½ cup	6.2
Peanuts, boiled without shell	1 cup	5.5
Peanuts, dry roasted	½ cup	5.0
Pistachio, dry roasted	½ cup	5.0

From Seth, R., & Heyman, M. (1994). Management of constipation and encopresis in infants and children. *Gastroenterology Clinics of North America, 23*(4), 621–636, and Hawaii Academy of Nutrition and Dietetics. (2018). *Hawaii Diet Manual* (9th ed.). Honolulu, Hawaii: Hawaii Academy of Nutrition and Dietetics.

Some centers have incorporated "treatment sessions" for the parent(s) and child and have documented cessation of soiling in 85% of those children who had been refractory to medical management alone. Reid and Bahar (2006) described a program involving intensive psychoanalytical therapy over a 3-year period for both the parent and child. These behavioral sessions addressed three themes that have been shown to result in anger or resentment: (1) parental conflict, (2) a newborn baby, and (3) tormenting older sibling(s). The children in this study were encouraged to play with a variety of age-appropriate toys. This facilitated the child's expression of feelings regarding the stressful situation(s) that had occurred in his or her family. Identification of the issue(s) of concern enabled the therapists to assist the parents in resolving the problems, which resulted in resolution or improved control of the bowel problem. In reviewing the evidence, ESPGHAN and NASPGHAN did not recommend routine use of intensive behavioral psychoanalytical therapy program in addition to conventional treatment. They recommended demystification, explanation, and guidance for toilet training if the child has a developmental age of at least 4 years. They did feel, however, that it would be beneficial to refer children with constipation and behavioral abnormalities to a mental health provider (Tabbers et al., 2014).

Newer treatment options being utilized include reflexotherapy for soiling, encopresis, and constipation. Bishop et al. (2003) provided six 30-minute sessions of reflexology to the child's feet with improvement in symptoms. Specifically, they reported that six sessions of reflexology resulted in reduced incidence of soiling and increased frequency of bowel movement. However, this was a small study ($n = 50$), and the authors concluded that further study is needed before recommendations can be made. Chase and Shields (2011) conducted a review of the literature and concluded that the evidence for efficacy of nonpharmacological, nonsurgical, and nonbehavioral treatments of functional constipation is poor. The efficacy of chiropractic treatment, reflexology, acupuncture, and/or transcutaneous electrical stimulation (TENS) has not been established, although preliminary findings support further study. Acupuncture and TENS were the two more promising treatment options. At this point in time, ESPGHAN and NASPGHAN felt that the evidence does not support the use of transcutaneous nerve stimulation in children with intractable constipation. In one study, TENS deceased transit time in treated patients but not in stool pattern and frequency (Tabbers et al., 2014).

Biofeedback training has been used in conjunction with other behavioral measures. Biofeedback is based on reinforcement and is derived from psychological learning theory. It uses instrument-assisted exercises to improve physiologic control. Biofeedback has been used with children with constipation and/or encopresis to improve rectal sensation, strengthen and improve control of the external sphincter, and coordinate muscle contraction and relaxation to achieve continence. In more than half of the children with constipation/encopresis, the anal sphincter contracts instead of relaxing during defecation (DiLorenzo & Benninga, 2004). The quality of evidence regarding the use of biofeedback in the treatment of FI is low, and more studies are needed. ESPGHAN and NASPGHAN did recommend the use of biofeedback (Tabbers et al., 2014).

Management of the child with encopresis is variable, depending on the specific form of the encopresis (retentive vs. nonretentive) and on the unique characteristics of the individual patient and his or her family. Management of retentive and nonretentive encopresis is therefore discussed separately.

Management of Retentive Encopresis

Effective management of retentive encopresis requires a very comprehensive approach. A number of clinicians recommend beginning treatment with intensive psychoeducation to demystify the shame and blame around the stool accidents. They emphasize the importance of reassuring the child and the parents that this is a common childhood problem and that it is no one's "fault" (Levine,

1982; Schonwald & Rappaport, 2004). The clinician should review the pathologic sequence of events leading to the current condition of a "stretched-out bowel," reduced sensory awareness of rectal filling, and reduced contractility of the colonic and rectal musculature. The overall principles of treatment are explained, and a specific treatment plan is developed with the child and parents. The importance of long-term follow-up care should also be addressed in this initial discussion regarding management (see **Table 23-1**).

The next phase of treatment is the cleaning-out phase, the objective of which is to eliminate all retained stool from the colon and rectum. This may be accomplished by PEG enemas, suppositories, laxatives, or combination therapy. A review of the current literature recommended the use of PEG with or without electrolyte for 3 to 6 days as first-line treatment for children presenting with fecal impaction. If PEG is not available, a daily enema for 3 to 6 days is recommended to clear the impaction (Tabbers et al., 2014). In selecting a cleansing protocol, it is important to assess for impaction, since the use of laxatives and suppositories may be contraindicated in these children. Laxatives cannot eliminate a true impaction, and the increased peristaltic activity can cause severe cramping pain, which may lead to an emergency room visit. Suppositories are contraindicated because they are unable to break up the impaction or to facilitate elimination of a large fecal mass; in fact, they generally become imbedded in and contribute to the fecal mass and fail to aid in the cleansing objective (Schmitt & Mauro, 1992).

KEY POINT

Management of retentive encopresis begins with education and reassurance for the child and parents, followed by "cleanout" (i.e., measures to eliminate all retained stool from the colon and rectum).

Several protocols have been recommended for the cleanout phase of treatment. Bigg and Dery (2006) found that a common protocol for children 2 years or older is to administer a mineral oil enema followed by a phosphate enema. They noted although enemas provide rapid rectal disimpaction, this approach is invasive and possibly traumatic for a child. Likewise, other clinicians support avoidance of enemas and suppositories if possible, and randomized studies have found varying doses of PEG to be effective for disimpacting children, with reasonable acceptance by parents and children. Other oral medications utilized include mineral oil, senna, and magnesium citrate. Nurko et al. (2008) conducted a prospective, randomized, multicenter double-blinded, placebo-controlled study to determine dose ranges for PEG 3350 for children with functional constipation. The study

confirmed the efficacy and safety of PEG 3350 for short-term treatment of children with functional constipation, with a recommended starting dose of 0.4 g/kg/d. An earlier study by Pashankar et al. (2003) found that long-term PEG therapy was effective for the treatment of chronic constipation with and without encopresis in children.

Other clinicians have tried variations of Levine's protocol. Levine recommended as many as four 3-day cycles of day 1, two adult-sized fleets enemas; day 2, bisacodyl suppository; and day 3, bisacodyl tablet (Doughty, 2006). For example, Sprague-McRae (1990) reported success with the following adaptation: day 1, Fleet enema morning and evening; day 2, bisacodyl suppository morning and evening and Fleet enema in evening; and day 3, bisacodyl tablet taken orally in evening. This team recommends a pediatric-sized Fleet enema for children between 4 and 7 years of age or <50 pounds and an adult-sized Fleet enema for children >7 years of age or >50 pounds (Ingebo & Heyman, 1988). In 1994, Seth and Heyman reported successful cleansing without the use of enemas. Their approach was to use mineral oil at a dose of 15 to 30 mL/kg/d, not to exceed 240 mL/d; this was used only for children >1 year of age. They documented initial cleansing within 3 or 4 days, with a 98% success rate and minimal side effects (one patient complained of abdominal cramps). Administration of mineral oil is facilitated by keeping it cold and mixing it in a 1:1 ratio with a fat-based substance such as pudding, yogurt, or chocolate syrup.

Other clinicians have also reported beneficial results with mineral oil; for example, Abrahamian and Lloyd-Still found that 47% of their pediatric population became completely asymptomatic after treatment with laxatives and mineral oil and an additional 36% were effectively controlled with laxatives after the original cleansing treatment (Howe & Walker, 1992). Clinicians selecting mineral oil for initial cleansing are cautioned to avoid its use in very young children and in children with gastroesophageal reflux or vomiting because of the potential for and danger of aspiration. In addition, it is generally recommended that the mineral oil be given 2 or 3 hours after meals or that a multivitamin tablet be given as part of the treatment because mineral oil inhibits absorption of fat-soluble vitamins (Howe & Walker, 1992).

Children with severe impactions usually require hospitalization and oral or nasogastric administration of a PEG-electrolyte solution; this approach may also be required for children who are unresponsive to outpatient management or who cannot cooperate with the cathartic procedure (Boon & Singh, 1991; Gunn & Nechyba, 2002).

After successful colonic cleansing, a program is initiated to establish regular evacuation of soft formed stool and to eliminate withholding of stool and the evacuation of large stools. Components of the bowel retraining maintenance phase include medications and behavioral interventions. In the review by ESPGHAN and NASP-GHAN, PEG with or without electrolytes is recommended as the first-line maintenance treatment. The starting dose will vary according to the age of the child. The dose should be adjusted according to the clinical response. Lactulose is recommended as the first-line maintenance treatment *if* PEG is not available. Base on expert opinion, the use of milk of magnesia, mineral oil, and stimulant laxatives may be considered as an additional or second-line treatment. Maintenance treatment should continue for at least 2 months. All symptoms of constipation should be resolved for at least 1 month before discontinuation of treatment. Treatment should be decreased gradually. If the child is in the developmental stage of toilet training, medication should only be stopped once toilet training is achieved (Tabbers et al., 2014).

KEY POINT

PEG with or without electrolytes is recommended as the first-line maintenance treatment. Lactulose is recommended as the first-line maintenance treatment if PEG is not available. Based on expert opinion, the use of milk of magnesia, mineral oil, and stimulant laxatives may be considered as an additional or second-line treatment.

Additional medications that may be used include lactulose, malt soup extract (Maltsupex), milk of magnesia, Haley's M-O, senna (Fletcher's Castoria), and bisacodyl (Dulcolax). Suppositories and enemas may be used to stimulate defecation on an as-needed basis. **Table 23-4** provides dosage guidelines for each of the commonly used softener or stimulant agents based on the child's age and size.

Medications are generally used for at least 2 months and may be used for as long as 6 months. The goal is to prevent recurrent stool retention and to gradually restore the colon and rectum to normal size and function. Parents generally need to be reassured that laxatives are safe and not habit forming and that their child will have the laxatives tapered off once normal bowel function has been reestablished. Parents are also taught how to appropriately titrate the doses of PEG or mineral oil and any other medications and how to intervene if the child fails to have a bowel movement for 2 consecutive days.

KEY POINT

Parents of encopretic children need to be reassured that laxatives are safe and not habit forming and that they will be discontinued once normal bowel function has been reestablished.

In addition to using stool softeners and stimulants to normalize fecal elimination, the child's diet should be modified to eliminate constipating foods and fluids (such as excessive intake of milk and other dairy products) and to increase the intake of fiber if inadequate. Constipation may be precipitated by ingestion of cow-milk proteins. In a study of 27 Italian children aged 5 to 36 months who had chronic constipation, the constipation resolved in 78% of the children when soy milk was substituted for cow milk. In the majority of this population, constipation recurred when cow milk was reintroduced (Borowitz & Curffari, 2018). In infants and the young child, removing cow-milk protein from the diet for a period of time can be considered to determine if this relieves constipation. A dietary consultation may be helpful to the parents and child in determining ways to add fiber to the child's diet. The family should be provided with a list of fiber-containing foods (**Table 23-3**), and the child should be included in discussing ways by which to add fiber to the diet. It may be helpful to develop a sample meal plan so that the parents can see how to incorporate fiber-containing foods into daily menus.

In determining the fiber-intake goal for a particular child, the clinician should be aware that the American Academy of Pediatrics has recommended 0.5 g of fiber per kilogram of body weight up to a maximum of 35 g daily. Another formula for estimating fiber intake needs in children at least 3 years of age is as follows: "Child's age in years + 5 = desirable grams of fiber per day" (e.g., a 3-year-old child should receive 3 + 5 g, or 8 g, of fiber daily). The clinician also needs to remember that high-fiber foods are more filling and lower in calories than low-fiber foods. Given a child's small stomach, there is the potential for inadequate ingestion of calories when a high-fiber diet is begun. In addition, high-fiber foods can impede the absorption of minerals such as calcium, iron, copper, magnesium, phosphorus, and zinc; therefore, the child's weight should be monitored, and it is usually helpful to recommend a multivitamin–mineral compound daily.

In addition to measures to establish soft formed stool, the management program must include a toileting routine. It is not sufficient to teach the child to respond promptly to the urge to defecate, because the urge to defecate may not develop for 6 to 9 months following the initiation of treatment. Thus, it is essential to establish a regular schedule for sitting on the toilet and attempting defecation; this promotes appropriate elimination of stool into the toilet and helps to eliminate soiling. Having the child sit on the toilet for 5 to 10 minutes after breakfast and dinner will take advantage of the natural gastrocolic reflex, which increases the chance of successful defecation. In addition to encouraging the child to adhere to an established toileting routine, the entire family should be assisted to work on eliminating any negative issues regarding toileting that may have developed over time.

TABLE 23-4 DOSAGE GUIDELINES FOR STOOL SOFTENERS AND STIMULANTS

TYPE OF AGENT	GUIDELINE
Stool Softeners	
>**Mineral oil***	Age <1 year old: not recommended as well as neurologically impaired children and those high risk for GERD >1 year: 6 mL/kg once to twice/day
	2–11 years: 30–60 mL daily
	>11 years: 60–150 mL daily
	Disimpaction: 15–30 mL/year of age, up to 240 mL daily
	Maintenance: 1–3 mL/kg/d
Lactulose or sorbitol	First choice for clean-out if PEG not available: 1–2 g/kg one to two times/day or 1.5–3 mL/kg/d
	Maintenance: 1–2 g/kg one to two times/day or 1.5–3 mL/kg/d
Lavage	
Polyethylene glycol (PEG)—with or without electrolyte solution	For disimpaction:
	First choice—outpatient: 1–1.5 g/kg/d orally for 3–6 days with maximum dose 100 g/day
	If hospitalized: 25 mL/kg/h (to 1,000 mL/h) by nasogastric tube until clear
	or
	20 mL/kg/h for 4 hours/day
	For maintenance—outpatient: (children): 0.2–0.8 g/kg
Laxatives**	
Barley Malt extract (Maltsupex) liquid or powder	2–10 mL/240 mL of milk or juice (suitable for infants drinking from a bottle)
Magnesium hydroxide (Phillips' milk of magnesia or Haley's M-O)	2–5 years: 0.4–1.2 g/day, once or divided
	6–11 years: 1.2–2.4 g/day, once or divided
Magnesium citrate	12–18 years: 2.4–4.8 g/day, once or divided
Senna preparation (Senokot)	2–6 years old: −2.5 to 5 mg once or twice a day
	6–12 years old: 7.5–10 mg/day
	>12 years: 15–20 mg/day
Bisacodyl (Dulcolax)	3–10 years: 5 mg/day
	>10 years: 5–10 mg/day
Sodium Picosulfate	1 month to 4 years: 2.5–10 mg daily
	418 years: 2.5–20 mg daily
Rectal Suppositories	
Glycerin suppository	Use PRN (as needed) to stimulate defecation
	Children: 1 infant suppository 1–2 times per day
	Children >6 years: 1 adult suppository 1–2 times per day
Bisacodyl (Dulcolax) suppository	2–10 years: 5 mg suppository daily
	>10 years: 5–10 mg suppository daily
Enemas	
Docusate sodium (Enemeez—minienema)‡	One unit rectally—to be used as an enema and not a suppository (available in containers of 30 single-use, 5-mL tubes)
	Sodium docusate enema: <6 years: 60 mL and >6 years: 120 mL
	Glycerin enema: 5–10 mL of glycerin in 500 mL normal saline solution
Mineral oil enema	2–11 years: 30–60 mL as a single dose
	Adolescents: as a retention enema, contents of one enema (range 60–150 mL/d) as a single dose
Sodium phosphate (Fleet) enema	<1 year old: to be avoided
	1–18 years: 2.5 mL/kg, max 133 mL/dose
Miscellaneous	
Pre or Probiotics	Routine use of probiotics is not recommended as evidence does not support the use of pre- or probiotics in the treatment of childhood constipation

*If mineral oil preparation is used, multivitamin supplementation recommended because of potential for reduced absorption of fat-soluble vitamins.
**Lubiprostone (Amitiza)—safety and effectiveness has not been established for <6 years and effectiveness has not been established in patients >6 years.
Linaclotide (Linzess)—only 6 to 17 years: safety and efficacy not established, contraindicated for children <6 years.
Prucalopride (Motegrity)—safety and efficacy not established.
‡Enemeez was the only medication not listed in the position statement.
Source: Baker, S., et al. (1999). Constipation in infants and children: Evaluation and treatment of the North American Society for Pediatric Gastroenterology and Nutrition. *Journal of Pediatric Gastroenterology and Nutrition, 29,* 612–626.

It is recommended that small rewards be used for positive reinforcement (e.g., stickers or special toys in the bathroom for preschoolers; stickers or handheld computer games for school-age children; and magazines and the assurance of privacy for adolescents). The "reward" should not be costly, and special age-appropriate rewards should be earned only by more advanced achievement, such as a certain number of days without soiling. The goal is to help the child accept responsibility for his or her actions and needs but to avoid any sense of punishment for an accident.

In establishing the medication and toileting schedule for any individual child, it is important to be flexible and creative and to assist the child and family to incorporate the care routine into their daily schedule with minimal disruption. It is also important to monitor the child response and to taper the medications as the increased fiber and attention to toileting produce softer, more frequent stools. The goal of therapy is passage of soft, normal caliber stools every 1 to 2 days without FI. Sood et al. (2019) indicated that laxatives need to be taken for months and sometimes years to achieve daily soft stool. They felt once the child has achieved regular bowel habits (using the toilet independently), the frequency of mandatory toileting and the use of laxatives can be reduced gradually to prevent soiling and maintain one to two bowel movements per day. Sood et al. recommend waiting at least 6 months until optimal bowel habits are achieved and stable, before instituting medication modifications. In addition, parents need to be counseled on not stopping medications without consulting the child's clinician. Follow-up is critical to insure improvement. Recovery rates were reported to be approximately 30% to 50% within 1 year and 48% to 75% after 5 years (Sood et al., 2019). Most children with functional constipation will have good clinical outcomes in adulthood if they are treated adequately during childhood. Philichi (2018) reported at least one relapse will occur in 50% of children within the first 5 years after treatment. As many as 25% to 50% of children will remain constipated into early adulthood. An optimal prognosis is anticipated if vigorous treatment is not delayed and close monitoring is provided (Philichi, 2018). See **Figure 23-2A and B** for treatment algorithm of functional constipation and encopresis in the infant <6 months and children.

Management of Nonretentive Encopresis

As noted earlier, nonretentive encopresis is most commonly caused by psychological issues, though primary nonretentive encopresis may also be caused by organic problems. Therefore, it is essential to explore psychological issues when assessing the child and establishing a management plan.

The assessment of a child with *primary nonretentive encopresis* may reveal an organic cause of the encopresis but more commonly will reveal a history of coercive toilet training and the failure to achieve complete fecal continence. The parents may have been punitive in their approach to toilet training, and the child may have begun to use soiling as a way of getting back at them. Alternatively, the parents may have been controlling and intrusive though not punitive; in this case, the child may have reacted with anger and resentment. If the assessment reveals either a punitive or a controlling approach to toilet training and bowel management, the clinician should instruct the parents to stop trying to toilet train the child and to seek counseling and family therapy. The emphasis during counseling should be on development of positive parent–child relationships with appropriate use of positive reinforcement.

The history of a child with *secondary nonretentive encopresis* usually reveals psychosocial stressors in the home or the school environment that have caused the child to regress to an earlier developmental stage. Since the cause of the incontinence is psychological, the focus during treatment is on encouraging the child to identify and talk about the stressful situation that precipitated the regression. The child is reassured that he or she is not at fault for soiling and that there has been no change in the parents' unconditional love. This reassurance can help to eliminate or reduce guilt and blame. In planning and implementing treatment for a child with secondary nonretentive encopresis, it is important to provide the child with time to develop some control over the psychological crisis before introducing him or her to a bowel retraining program for correction of the FI.

As noted above, the primary focus in treatment of the child with nonretentive encopresis is on resolution of the psychological issues that triggered the bowel dysfunction. Secondary management usually involves implementation of a comprehensive bowel management program, which typically includes many of the elements already described under management of retentive encopresis: medications when indicated, establishment of a routine toileting program, encouragement to respond promptly to defecatory urges, periodic underwear checks, and positive reinforcement for appropriate toileting. The child or family may also be under the care of a psychologist or psychiatrist, or the clinician may observe signs and symptoms that prompt a follow-up psychiatric/psychological consultation (such as conduct disorder, depression, or learning disabilities). Whenever the patient

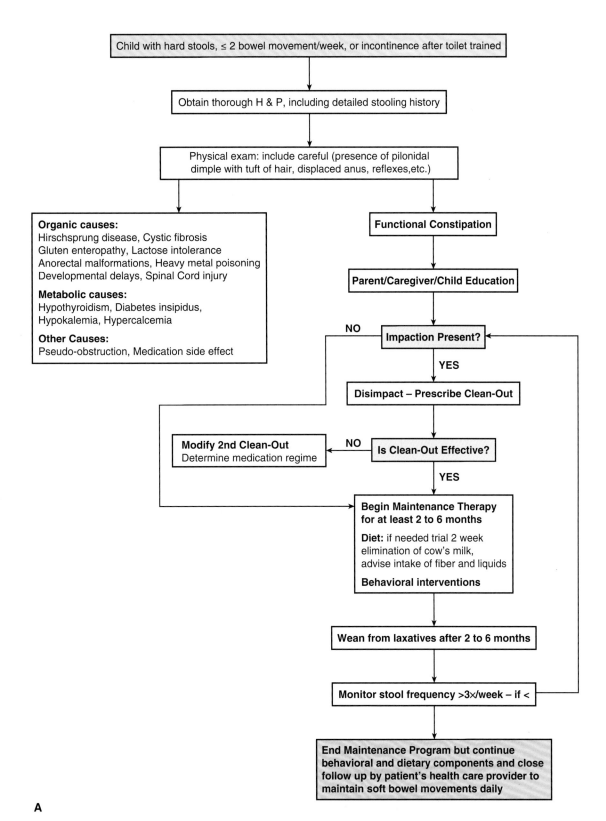

A

FIGURE 23-2. **A.** Treatment of functional constipation or encopresis in pediatrics.

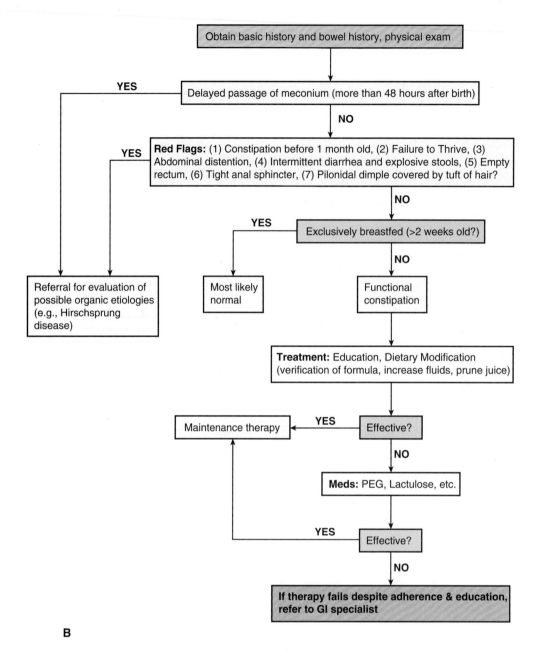

B

FIGURE 23-2   (*Continued*) **B.** Treatment of functional constipation in infants younger than 6 months.

and family are under psychiatric or psychological care, it is critical for the continence nurse clinician to work in collaboration with the mental health professional. It may also be of tremendous benefit to enlist the cooperation of the staff at the child's school, preschool, or daycare setting.

Carefully monitored long-term follow-up care is critical for any child with encopresis. As explained, the initial goal

is to establish regular voluntary elimination of soft formed stool and to eliminate withholding of stool and large fecal masses. Once an acceptable bowel elimination pattern has been in place for 4 to 6 months (such as two or three bowel movements per day), the child is gradually weaned off stool softeners. Data indicate that such a program results in complete and long-lasting remission in approximately 65% of the children, with an additional 30% reporting substantial improvement (Nolan & Oberklaid, 1993).

Children who continue to soil should have follow-up evaluation to determine the cause of the persistent problem; in some of these children, the problem may be paradoxical contraction of the external sphincter during attempted defecation (Nolan & Oberklaid, 1993). Benninga et al. evaluated the effectiveness of biofeedback retraining in 29 patients with chronic constipation and encopresis ranging in age from 5 to 16 years. Sixteen of these children exhibited inappropriate contraction of their external sphincters, and eight evidenced diminished rectal sensation. Biofeedback training was effective in teaching 26 of the children how to correctly relax the external anal sphincter and in normalizing rectal sensation in 18 (Seth & Heyman, 1994). Although research is limited, biofeedback should be considered for children with intact nerve pathways but attenuated rectal sensation or compromised ability to correctly contract and relax the pelvic floor and sphincter muscles or a lack response to other treatment modalities.

The ultimate goal in treating encopresis is to restore the child to normal bowel function and a normal lifestyle and to prevent long-lasting psychological and emotional problems that may develop secondary to chronic FI. Parents frequently report an overall improvement in the child's demeanor, appetite, and level of activity after successful treatment. The success of the treatment program is highly dependent on the child's willingness to address his or her problem with encopresis and on the parents' willingness to assist the child to remain compliant with the treatment program. As outlined, the treatment program is usually multifaceted and long term and must be carried out by the family members themselves, who are frequently juggling multiple other responsibilities and complex schedules. It is therefore essential for the health care clinician to establish rapport with the child and family and to work collaboratively with them to establish a workable treatment plan that incorporates the key elements of education, counseling, pharmacotherapy, and behavioral modification.

KEY POINT

The ultimate goal in treating encopresis is to restore the child to normal bowel function and a normal lifestyle and to prevent long-lasting psychological and emotional problems that may develop secondary to chronic fecal incontinence.

NEUROGENIC BOWEL

FI is defined as the involuntary loss of stool (or rectal contents) at any time of life after toilet training. The term FI is used to indicate the involuntary passage of either solid or liquid stool at least once during the preceding 3 months; the term anal incontinence also includes the involuntary passage of flatus (Thomas & Chandler, 2007). Neurogenic bowel is described as a colonic dysfunction caused by neurologic dysfunction or damage; it is manifest by problems with storage and evacuation that result clinically in constipation and/or incontinence (Thomas & Chandler, 2007). Neurogenic bowel and FI can be due to an organic or anatomic lesion, such as anorectal malformation, anal surgery, or trauma, or associated

conditions such as meningomyelocele and other neuromuscular conditions. In pediatrics, there are several congenital conditions that can lead to FI. The most common of these conditions include the following: short gut syndrome; imperforate anus; Hirschsprung disease; meningomyelocele; and neuromuscular disorders, such as cerebral palsy, muscular dystrophy, and the various forms of hypotonia (Thomas & Chandler, 2007). Each of these conditions will be briefly described, as a basis for understanding treatment options.

KEY POINT

Neurogenic bowel denotes colonic dysfunction caused by neurologic damage or dysfunction; it is manifest by problems with both storage and evacuation and results clinically in constipation and/or incontinence.

Imperforate Anus/Anorectal Malformation

This condition includes several congenital ARM resulting from abnormal embryological development of the hindgut. The incidence rate is about 1 in 5,000 births in the United States. This anorectal anomaly may occur in isolation or as part of other conditions or syndromes such as VACTERL (vertebral, anorectal, cardiovascular, tracheoesophageal, renal, and limb) syndrome. Imperforate anal lesions are divided into "high" or "low" lesions, depending on whether the distal end of the bowel terminates above or below the puborectal component of the levator ani complex (Jinbo, 2004). (See **Table 23-5** for the Wing Spread Classification and **Fig. 23-3** for illustration of imperforate anus.)

"Low defects" are characterized by complete formation of the distal bowel, including the anal canal, and descent of the anorectal junction and anal canal through the levator mechanism and the striated muscle complex; "low" defects involve anal stenosis or a "mismatch" between the anus and the perineal opening. Generally, low defects can be treated through simple dilatation or a minor perineal operation, and these children usually achieve normal continence (Jinbo, 2004).

With "intermediate-level defects," the distal bowel (rectum and anorectal junction) extends partially through the levator ani muscle but the anal canal and anus are missing; typically, a fistulous tract is present between the bowel and vagina in girls or between the distal bowel and rectobulbar urethra in boys. Surgery is typically required to establish communication between the distal bowel and the perineum. Because the internal and external anal sphincters are intact these children typically acquire continence with limited if any difficulty (Mazier et al., 1995).

In contrast, with "high defects," the distal bowel ends above the level of the levator ani muscle and the internal anal sphincter is usually absent, although there may be a slight thickening of the distal circular muscle at the end of the bowel. The external sphincter is almost always

TABLE 23-5 WINGSPREAD CLASSIFICATION FOR ANORECTAL ANOMALIES

FEMALE	MALE
High Lesions	**High Lesions**
Anorectal agenesis	Anorectal agenesis
With rectovaginal fistula	With rectoprostatic urethral fistula
Without fistula	Without fistula
Rectal atresia	Rectal atresia
Intermediate Lesions	**Intermediate Lesions**
Anal agenesis with rectovestibular fistula	Anal agenesis with rectobulbar urethral fistula
Anal agenesis with rectovaginal fistula	Anal agenesis without fistula
Anal agenesis without fistula	
Low Lesions	**Low Lesions**
Anovestibular fistula	Anocutaneous fistula
Anocutaneous fistula	Anal stenosis
Anal stenosis	
Cloacal Malformations	**Cloacal Malformations**
Rare Malformations	**Rare Malformations**

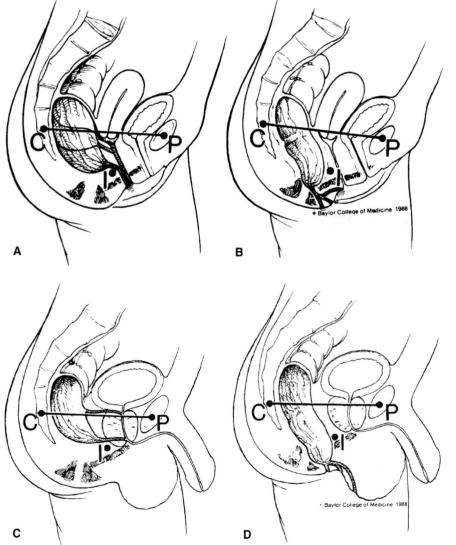

FIGURE 23-3. Imperforate Anus in the Female and Male. **A.** High lesion with fistula to vagina. **B.** Low lesion with fistula to vestibule or perineum. **C.** High lesion with fistula to urethra. **D.** Low lesion with fistula to perineum or median raphe. (Used with permission from Crocetti, M., & Barone, M. A. (2004). *Oski's essential pediatrics*. Philadelphia, PA: Lippincott Williams & Wilkins.)

present—at least in part; in addition, the levator ani and puborectalis muscles are almost always present, although in these lesions, the puborectal muscle is quite small and tightly adherent to the urethra or vagina. Most of the higher lesions end with a fistula from the bowel to the bladder, urethra, or vagina. Often, there are associated anomalies in the genitourinary tract, spine, and/or heart. The high lesions are more common in boys, but there are no other known genetic factors (Walker et al., 1996). In girls, high lesions are usually associated with a high rectovaginal fistula. High defects require a temporary diverting colostomy and reconstructive surgery, known as a pull-through procedure, which is usually done between birth and 6 months of age. Once the anastomosis and anoplasty are healed and necessary dilatations have been completed, the colostomy is closed (Walker et al., 1996).

KEY POINT

Imperforate anus refers to a spectrum of disorders involving fetal development of the distal bowel, anal canal, and sphincters; these abnormalities are usually classified as either "low" or "high" lesions, depending on whether the distal end of the bowel ends below or above the levator ani muscle complex.

Potential complications following the pull-through procedure include stricture of the anocutaneous anastomosis, recurrent rectourinary fistula, mucosal prolapse, anterior anal malposition, constipation, and incontinence. FI is by far the most troublesome. The most important determinant of continence is the level of the initial lesion, and only a small number of those with high lesions achieve normal continence before school age. Most children continue to improve to the point of social continence by adolescence.

KEY POINT

The continence prognosis for children with "low" imperforate anus lesions is good, because the sphincters are intact. In contrast, the continence prognosis for children with "high" lesions is variable, because the internal anal sphincter is missing and the external sphincter may be incomplete.

Hirschsprung Disease

Hirschsprung disease is a congenital condition representing a failure of the cephalocaudal migration of neural crest cells into the hindgut, with subsequent lack of development of the autonomic ganglion cells in Meissner and Auerbach plexuses. The resultant loss of peristalsis causes a functional obstruction, followed by dilation of the proximal segment (**Fig. 23-4**). The proximal border of the defect is most often within the rectum or sigmoid colon (short-segment disease). In a smaller percentage of cases, longer segments of colon are involved (long-segment disease); in rare instances, the entire

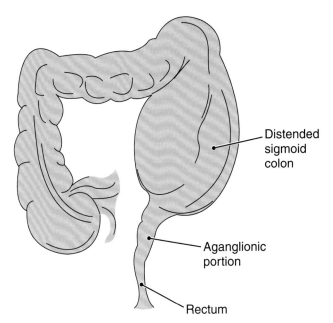

FIGURE 23-4. Hirschsprung Disease. Distal (aganglionic) bowel collapses due to absence of innervation and peristalsis; proximal (ganglionic) bowel becomes severely dilated. (Used with permission from Pillitteri, A. (2003). *Maternal and child nursing* (4th ed.). Philadelphia, PA: Lippincott Williams & Wilkins.)

colon is aganglionic. Hirschsprung disease accounts for a major proportion of cases of neonatal obstruction. Forty-six percent of all patients with Hirschsprung disease are diagnosed in the neonatal period (Mazier et al., 1995).

Hirschsprung disease involves absence of ganglion (nerve) cells in the distal bowel; the affected bowel is unable to contract to propel stool distally, which creates a functional obstruction. Most children present with "short-segment disease," which means that the dysfunctional segments are the internal sphincter, rectum, and possibly part of the sigmoid colon.

In a recent review of Hirschsprung disease, Amiel et al. (2008) reported the incidence of Hirschsprung disease as one in 5,000 live births; the male:female ratio is 4:1. The male:female ratio is higher for short-segment Hirschsprung disease compared with long-segment Hirschsprung disease. The incidence varies among ethnic groups, with rates of 1.0, 1.5, 2.1, and 2.8 per 10,000 live births in Hispanics, Caucasian Americans, African Americans, and Asians, respectively (Amiel et al., 2008). This disease occurs as an isolated trait in 70% of cases; a chromosomal abnormality is associated in 12% of cases and associated congenital anomalies in 18% (Amiel et al., 2008). There is also a genetic predisposition to Hirschsprung disease.

Infants with short-segment disease may initially be diagnosed as "constipated"; if the diagnosis of Hirschsprung disease is delayed, the affected child suffers from persistent constipation, with development of malodorous, ribbon-like stools, and an enlarged abdomen with palpable fecal masses. The infant may present with intermittent bouts of intestinal obstruction from fecal impaction, hypochromic anemia, hypoproteinemia, and failure to thrive (Jinbo, 2004).

Assessment of the child with suspected Hirschsprung disease involves a rectal examination, which typically reveals an absence of fecal material in the rectum and a narrow or snug rectum and anorectal junction during digital examination. A rectal biopsy is the most reliable method of diagnosis; histologic examination reveals an absence of ganglion cells. Manometric studies or pressure readings reveal failure of sphincter relaxation and absence of the RAIR, that is, failure of the internal sphincter to relax in response to rectal distention (Jinbo, 2004).

When the condition is diagnosed at birth, the functional (ganglionic) colon is anastomosed to the anal canal, and diversion may not be required. In contrast, when there is a delay in diagnosis, the functional obstruction results in significant dilation of the proximal bowel, and a temporary colostomy is required to decompress the dilated colon; the stoma is created in the dilated (functional) section of the colon (the distal point of bowel found to have ganglion cells on frozen section). Once the distended colon has been decompressed, the functional bowel is anastomosed to the anal canal, and the colostomy is closed (Doughty, 2006).

KEY POINT

Infants with short-segment Hirschsprung disease may not be diagnosed in the early neonatal period, because the functional bowel is initially able to compensate and push stool through the dysfunctional segment. By the time these children are diagnosed, the proximal bowel is typically very dilated; therefore, a temporary colostomy is required to decompress the bowel, and the stoma is usually very large.

Potential postoperative complications include incomplete removal of the aganglionic section and abnormal spasticity of the internal sphincter, which can be corrected by performing a posterior sphincterotomy. In addition, postoperative incontinence may be a problem, and enterocolitis before or after surgery is an ominous complication that accounts for 30% of deaths in young infants (Roy et al., 1995).

KEY POINT

Definitive management of Hirschsprung disease requires a "pull-through" procedure, in which the functional (ganglionic) bowel is anastomosed to the anal canal.

Spina Bifida

Spina bifida is a syndrome caused by abnormal embryonic development of the neural tube and its surrounding structures (Molnar, 1985). The incidence of neural tube defects in the United States is about one in 1,000 live births. It is one of the leading causes of disability in

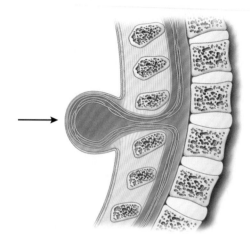

FIGURE 23-5. Spina Bifida with Myelomeningocele. (Used with permission from Werner, R. (2012). *Massage therapist's guide to pathology.* Philadelphia, PA: Lippincott Williams & Wilkins.)

children. There are higher incidence rates in some geographic areas, especially in the British Isles, where the incidence rate is 4.5 per 1,000 live births. With subsequent births, the incidence rate is 5% higher, rising to 10% after two affected siblings (Molnar, 1985).

One of the possible etiologies for this condition is low folic acid levels during the preconception period, which may cause failure of the neural tube to close completely; this closure normally occurs at 28 days of embryonic development. There are varying degrees of severity for this neural tube defect; the types of defects are as follows:

1. *Spina bifida occulta*—There is complete closure of the spinal column and no visible protrusion of the spinal cord or meninges; BBD are rare.
2. *Meningocele*—There is a visible opening of the spinal column, with a visible sac that contains spinal fluid and meninges. The spinal cord is normal and is not in the sac. If repairs go well, bowel and bladder function may be normal.
3. *Myelomeningocele*—This is the most common of neural tube defects, where there is a visible opening of the spinal column with a sac that contains spinal fluid, meninges, and the spinal cord; the cord typically is damaged due to compression. BBD are common especially if the lesions are above the sacral area (Smith, 1991) (**Fig. 23-5**).

Thomas and Chandler (2007) reported that 78% of children with spina bifida have abnormal bowel function and 40% use digital stimulation to facilitate fecal evacuation.

KEY POINT

Spina bifida with myelomeningocele can be conceptualized as a "congenital spinal cord injury"; the majority of these children have abnormal bowel function (neurogenic bowel).

Neuromuscular Disorders

The list of locations and the neuromuscular conditions that could result in neurogenic bowel and bladder includes the following:

1. Cerebral cortex: cerebral palsy, degenerative CNS lesions, infections (meningitis)
2. Spinal cord: spinal muscular atrophies; infantile poliomyelitis, spinal cord injuries, tumors, or malformations; spina bifida with meningomyelocele
3. Neuromuscular junction: myasthenia gravis; botulism
4. Muscle diseases (dystrophy): Duchenne's muscular dystrophy; myotonic dystrophy

Collectively, children who require imperforate anus repairs or pull-through procedures for Hirschsprung disease and children with meningomyelocele or spinal cord disorders who have bowel incontinence can be viewed as having some level of neurologic bowel impairment. Assessment and treatment of these children follow similar pathways, except for specific differences, which are emphasized among the various conditions.

KEY POINT

Collectively, children who require imperforate anus repairs or pull-through procedures for Hirschsprung disease and children with spinal cord disorders such as myelomeningocele can be viewed as having some degree of neurogenic bowel.

ASSESSMENT OF THE CHILD WITH A NEUROGENIC BOWEL

Children with neurogenic bowel conditions should have a comprehensive evaluation during each health care visit. Questions regarding health history and current care should be directed to the child with input from their parents/caregivers as needed. The initial encounter involves a thorough assessment including past medical history, developmental and psychosocial history, bowel management programs previously utilized, toileting behaviors, stooling patterns, diet, family lifestyle, and determination of the child's goals. With this in-depth assessment, the provider is equipped to monitor and alter plans based on the child's unique needs. **Box 23-3** provides guidelines for obtaining a comprehensive history from the child or adolescent with neurogenic bowel and fecal incontinence.

KEY POINT

Assessment of the child/adolescent with neurogenic bowel must include attention to developmental and psychosocial issues as well as a comprehensive assessment of bowel function and previous and current strategies for management.

PHYSICAL EXAMINATION

The physical assessment is critical in determining the extent of stool retention and determining potential causes of lower bowel dysfunction, especially disorders affecting the lumbar sacral area. Provision of privacy is of utmost importance while examining an older child or adolescent.

Visual Inspection of Sacral Area

General inspection should include assessment of the sacral area for abnormalities, which would be indicative of potential neurologic lesions affecting the perianal, gluteal, and lower extremity regions. Physical signs of underlying disorders include flat buttocks (commonly seen in sacral agenesis) and a pilonidal dimple or tuft of hair, commonly seen in the individual with spina bifida occulta or an associated tethered cord. Motor and sensory function in the lower limbs and spinal area should also be assessed (Currie, 2000).

Abdominal Examination

During the physical examination, abdominal inspection, percussion, and palpation are done to assess for fecal retention as well as scars from prior surgeries. The presence and location of any type of urinary or bowel diversion and the stomal openings are also assessed. It may also be helpful to evaluate sexual maturity and to note any indicators of *precocious puberty;* it is not uncommon for children with meningomyelocele or hormonal imbalance to begin sexual development at a much younger age—commonly, <8 years of age (Steinberg, 2008).

Anal Inspection

Inspection of the anus should include anal placement, any visible indicators of sphincter muscle laxity (e.g., gaping or "patulous" anus), rectal prolapse, and perianal skin integrity (e.g., perianal fissures, rash, or incontinence-associated dermatitis). An anteriorly displaced anus (anterior ectopic anus) may cause constipation and straining with defecation in some individuals, although it is considered a normal finding in many patients. External examination of the anus should also include assessment for the anal wink and/or bulbocavernosus reflex (anal contraction in response to stroking of the perianal skin or to light compression of the glans penis or stroking of the clitoris); the presence of the anal wink and/or bulbocavernosus reflex indicates intact nerve pathways between the sacral cord and the perineum. It may also be helpful, especially in a child with a history of imperforate anus or spinal cord disorder, to assess sensation circumferentially around the anus; injury or denervation may cause loss of sensation. If no reflexes are elicited and the anus exhibits no tone, EMG studies can validate sphincter denervation and absence of sphincter contractility (Currie, 2000).

Rectal Examination

The rectal examination may be deferred until there is a trusting relationship established between the child and

BOX 23-3 SPECIFIC HISTORY-TAKING GUIDELINES FOR A CHILD WITH A NEUROGENIC BOWEL CONDITION

Medical History

The questions in this section are specific to the underlying cause of the neurogenic bowel dysfunction and are therefore grouped accordingly:

Imperforate Anus

- *Level of anomaly, if known*: Was a "high" or a "low" defect, and what prognosis was given at the time of repair? Were any tests done to evaluate the potential for continence?
- *Sacral anomalies*: Was sacrum intact, or were abnormalities noted? (This is significant because children with imperforate anus combined with sacral anomalies are at greater risk for incontinence.)
- *Urologic problems*: Were any urologic defects or problems noted? Were any tests completed to evaluate the urologic system?
- *Corrective surgeries*: Number of corrective surgeries performed and any available data regarding the specific procedures
- *Medical–surgical follow-up study after repair*: Last checkup by surgeon? Problems with constipation and overflow stooling? Any studies done to rule out retained stool and dilatation of rectosigmoid colon?

Hirschsprung Disease

- *Extent of colonic involvement and type of surgery done to correct the problem (if known)*: Any anal dilatations required postoperatively? If yes, when was last procedure done? It is important to carefully question the child or parents re: the caliber of stools; ribbon-like or pencil-thin stools may be indicative of anal stenosis, which is a common complication after surgical repair of Hirschsprung disease.

- *History of constipation after repair*: Current frequency and consistency of stools? Any use of softeners, stimulants, enemas, or suppositories? (These children are at significant risk for constipation caused by anal stenosis, dilatations causing an aversion to defecation, incomplete removal of the aganglionic bowel, or recurrent aganglionosis.)
- *History of enterocolitis (fever, abdominal pain, and diarrhea)*: Treatment required.

Myelomeningocele or Spinal Disorder

- *Level of lesion*: Children with lesions at or above the sacral cord usually present with a neurogenic bowel and bladder though some children have incomplete lesions with sparing of some of the sacral pathways (these children may retain some degree of bowel control).
- *Any additional neurologic or spinal cord problems, such as tethered cord?* If yes, effect on bowel and bladder function?
- *Mobility and independence in ADLs to include toileting:* Is child able to ambulate with or without assistive devices? Is child able to self-toilet and to carry out own bowel program? If not, how much assistance is required, and who is available to provide the assistance needed to implement the program? Are assistive devices needed to facilitate the patient's transfer to the toilet and ability to maintain balance while on the toilet?
- *Urologic status:* Current bladder management (that is, spontaneous voiding vs. Credé's maneuver vs. clean intermittent catheterization); history of chronic UTIs; and usual frequency of antibiotic therapy (there is a potential for antibiotic therapy to cause diarrhea and disrupt bowel program).

Data from MacLeod, J. (1998). Fecal incontinence: A practical program of management. *Endoscopy Review, 5*, 45–56.
Data from Walker, W. A., Durie, P. R., Hamilton, J. R., et al. (1996). *Pediatric gastrointestinal disease* (Vol. 2, 2nd ed., pp. 2077–2091). St. Louis, MO: Mosby.

---

health care provider. Creating a trusting relationship is crucial, especially if the health care provider will be involved in providing biofeedback or in working with the child to establish compliance with a bowel management program. It may be helpful to ask the primary physician about the results of his/her rectal examination, to avoid repeated uncomfortable examinations (Jinbo, 2004).

If a rectal examination is performed, it is important to obtain the child's consent and cooperation and to perform the examination as gently as possible. During the examination, the nurse should note sphincter tone and any internal hemorrhoids, anal fissures, strictures, tenderness, or irregularities in the rectal vault. The nurse should note the amount and consistency of stool in the rectal ampulla and the size of the rectum and should then ask the child to contract the anal sphincter as if trying not to pass gas or stool and finally to "bear down" as if trying to expel stool.

These maneuvers allow the nurse to assess sphincter tone and contractility, as well as the child's ability to

voluntarily control the sphincter, and to coordinate sphincter relaxation and abdominal muscle contraction (Currie, 2000). It also allows the nurse to assess for rectal prolapse, which sometimes is found in children or adolescents who have undergone anoplasty and in those with spinal disorders such as meningomyelocele. If rectal prolapse is present, the nurse should further assess for bleeding and tenderness and should refer any child or adolescent with significant prolapse for surgical evaluation (Currie, 2000).

KEY POINT

Once rapport has been established and the child/adolescent has given permission, a rectal examination should be performed; this examination permits the nurse to assess for retained stool, baseline sphincter tone, perineal hygiene, and the individual's ability to voluntarily contract the sphincter and to coordinate sphincter relaxation and abdominal muscle contraction.

During the rectal examination, it is also important to assess perineal hygiene. If the underwear is soiled or there is fecal material present due to inadequate cleansing, the nurse should determine the patient's awareness of the soiling and should specifically query the individual as to sensory awareness of rectal distention and of stool passage. The nurse should also be alert to the presence of rash or erythema and should discuss with the patient his or her hygiene and skin care routines (Currie, 2000).

DIAGNOSTIC TESTS

Several tests play a valuable role in further assessing the pathophysiology of FI and neurogenic bowel. Anorectal manometry, defecography, rectal compliance, and electromyography can all be helpful in the evaluation of rectal and sphincter function. A child with a spinal cord lesion such as myelomeningocele may benefit from anorectal manometry or defecography studies to assess their rectal sensation and ability to voluntarily control the sphincter (Currie, 2000). These children may also have problems with colonic motility, due to loss of autonomic innervation; if the individual reports persistent constipation, transit studies should be considered.

An abdominal x-ray may be helpful in assessing the amount of stool present in the colon, especially if there is a history of constipation. The presence of stool in various segments of the colon provides insight as to peristaltic activity and high versus low impaction (Jinbo, 2004).

An infant born with Hirschsprung disease usually had a rectal biopsy and/or barium enema done at the time of diagnosis. If the child continues to have problems with defecation following the pull-through procedure, additional studies may be indicated and may include anorectal manometry, colonic transit studies, or colonic manometry in addition to possible repeat biopsy and barium enema (Jinbo, 2004).

If any individual with a neurogenic bowel exhibits signs and symptoms of neurological decompensation (e.g., increase in incontinence episodes, increased problems with gait or mobility, or back pain/discomfort), CT scans or MRI studies are usually indicated to evaluate the spinal cord. During growth spurts or periods of weight gain, these children and adolescents are at risk for developing a tethered cord and need to be monitored accordingly. In some instances, deterioration in bowel or bladder function is the first indication of a tethered cord or spinal problem. CT scans or MRI studies may also be ordered to evaluate the status of imperforate anus or Hirschsprung disease repairs (Jinbo, 2004).

TREATMENT AND MANAGEMENT OF A CHILD WITH A NEUROGENIC BOWEL

Due to the marked variations in the degree of neurological involvement, there is not one single treatment protocol for neurogenic bowel; rather, there are a variety of management options.

BEHAVIORAL MEASURES

Initially, as noted, the patient should be evaluated for evidence of stool retention If the colon is filled with stool, a bowel cleanout is necessary to prevent overflow incontinence. The child will need to be given stool softeners and laxatives for cleanout and until bowel regularity is achieved (**Table 23-3**). If the child is unable (or unwilling) to take in enough dietary fiber, then fiber supplements should be offered, with the goal of establishing stool that is soft but formed and therefore both easily be retained by a weak sphincter and also effectively eliminated with minimal straining. Behavioral therapy should include sitting on the toilet and attempting defecation two to three times a day (after meals) until a predictable pattern of elimination has been established. Careful observation is needed to ensure that the child is maintaining the optimal position for defecation and is allowing sufficient time for the stool to pass. The child's feet should be supported with a stool to ensure relaxation of the pelvic floor.

BIOFEEDBACK

It is inconclusive as to whether biofeedback is beneficial for these individuals; however, the incorporation of biofeedback into the program may help to improve sensory awareness and coordination of sphincter relaxation and abdominal muscle contraction. If the child has some external sphincter tone, biofeedback may optimize the degree of strength of the external sphincter.

Heymen et al. (2001) identified the following potential benefits of biofeedback: improved strength of the pelvic floor muscles in response to rectal filling, increase in the patient's ability to perceive distention of the rectum, or both. Thus, biofeedback treatment protocols can be designed to accomplish any of the following goals: (1) improve coordination of pelvic floor muscle contraction in response to rectal distention, (2) improve sensory awareness of rectal distention without strengthening pelvic floor muscles, or (3) strengthen the pelvic floor muscles without increasing sensory awareness of rectal distention (Heymen et al., 2001).

The data regarding use of biofeedback for treating children with imperforate anus are limited; however, Rao et al. (1996) and Leung et al. (2006) concluded that biofeedback training is an effective treatment for these children. Specifically, these investigators found that biofeedback helped children and adolescents to improve their squeeze pressure (external sphincter contractility) and their ability to maintain the sphincter contraction. Clinically, this enabled the participants to more effectively retain liquid in the rectum. They also found improved rectoanal coordination with a reduction in rectal pressure and an increase in the continence index. Used in combination with behavior modification, biofeedback has been found to be a clearly superior mode of treatment (Heymen et al., 2001). This author has also found, in treating this population of children, that several have developed paradoxical contractions; that is, when they Valsalva to defecate, there is an increase in external sphincter tone (as opposed to relaxation), which causes inadequate emptying of the rectal vault. Biofeedback has been helpful in teaching these children to relax the external sphincter muscle, which improves emptying of the rectal vault and decreases stooling accidents. Wald (1981) reported in children with myelomeningocele who suffered from fecal soiling and underwent biofeedback therapy to reduce FI had a good clinical response. Four out of the eight children (ages ranging from 5 to 17 years) had complete resolution of fecal soiling or a 75% reduction in FI episodes. It was noted that those who had a therapeutic response also had intact anal sensation (demonstrated on anal manometry prior to biofeedback) and an ability to contract external anal sphincter or gluteal muscles following clinician instruction. Additional research is needed examining the benefits of biofeedback in this population.

PERISTALTIC STIMULI (STIMULATED DEFECATION)

If the child/adolescent cannot initiate a bowel movement, either with routine toileting or in response to some sensory awareness of the urge to defecate, use of a suppository or mini-enema can be helpful in stimulating peristalsis and evacuation. If the child does not respond to these stimuli, further studies are indicated to assess for a megarectosigmoid colon, and if present, referral for surgical evaluation is indicated.

MANAGEMENT OF OBSTRUCTION

All children and adolescents who have undergone pull-through procedures need to be carefully monitored for obstructive symptoms. If obstructive symptoms occur, it is important to determine the cause of the obstruction through diagnostic testing. Management is then dependent on the specific causative factor. If anatomical problems, such as anal stenosis or strictures, are causing the obstruction, further dilatation or surgery may be indicated. If biopsy reveals recurrent aganglionosis in the child with Hirschsprung disease, further surgery is required. If dysmotility is a problem, medications can be initiated to reduce transit time. If outlet problems are due to a hypertonic sphincter, a rectal myectomy may be necessary. This author has also utilized biofeedback with a small number of children with Hirschsprung disease to teach relaxation of the pelvic floor musculature, which reduces sphincter tone and improves evacuation.

If dietary modifications (increased fiber and fluid intake), medications, and behavioral measures are insufficient in children with outlet dysfunction with refractory chronic constipation, a rectal myectomy may be required (Redkar et al., 2012) as previously noted. If the child and caregiver are comfortable with digital stimulation, this can be introduced along with behavior management to enable them to defecate at a given time daily. Digital stimulation is an inexpensive way of eliciting rectal emptying but works only if the reflex arc is intact. In addition, children and adolescents with outlet dysfunction need to be monitored for enterocolitis (inflammation of the gut) and require referral and aggressive management to eliminate the obstruction. Symptoms of enterocolitis may include fever, pain, bleeding or mucous-like discharge from the rectum, diarrhea, abdominal cramps and pain, nausea and vomiting, as well as loss of appetite and necessitate a prompt referral since enterocolitis can progress rapidly even leading to death (International Foundations for Gastrointestinal Disorders, n.d.).

ANAL IRRIGATION

Children with weak sphincters may find the use of enemas (anal irrigations or rectal "washouts") helpful in attaining continence. Utilizing a balloon-tipped catheter or bowel management tube allows the enema solution to be retained in a child with a weak anal sphincter. The bowel management tube is a silastic catheter with a balloon (30 to 50 mL) that is inflated to facilitate retention of the enema fluid; due to the possibility of latex allergies, especially in the spina bifida or meningomyelocele population, latex exposure should be minimized and silicone or silastic catheters should be used. Since proper volume and retention are difficult due to poor sphincter control, the balloon helps to "seal" the lower rectum as the enema solution is administered. "Cone enema" or a colostomy irrigation kit can also be utilized as a continence enema (Smith, 1991), or an anal irrigation system can be used, as described in Chapter 22. The child can then transfer to the toilet with the seal in place and expel the contents of the colon when the balloon or cone is released. While this is usually an effective approach to controlled evacuation, children or adolescents with concomitant colonic dysmotility may prematurely expel the balloon or may experience incomplete evacuation despite administration of high-volume enemas; these individuals may experience increased incontinent episodes as the enema solution and stool is expelled slowly over a prolonged period of time. If this is a persistent problem, the enema/washout should be discontinued and another therapy approach should be explored.

> **KEY POINT**
>
> Management of the child/adolescent with neurogenic bowel must be individualized and includes strategies such as dietary modification and medications to establish soft formed stool, routine toileting, biofeedback, stimulated defecation programs, anal irrigations, and surgical intervention.

The balloon-tipped catheter can also be used as a biofeedback device, to help the child or adolescent learn to sense rectal filling. However, this is effective and appropriate only in children and adolescents who have normal cognitive function and some degree of innervation/sensory awareness.

SURGICAL INTERVENTION (MACE OR ACE PROCEDURE)

In many instances when the anal sphincter is weak or denervated, successful administration of retrograde enemas is difficult. In addition, this approach to bowel regulation frequently limits the child or adolescent in achieving independence with care. If diet regulation, medication, enemas, and/or biofeedback fail to produce a positive response, other surgical interventions (e.g., a Malone antegrade continence enema [MACE] or antegrade continence enema [ACE] procedure or creation of a colostomy) may be indicated (Jinbo, 2004). In the late 1980s, the "MACE" or Malone antegrade continence enema was introduced (Malone et al., 1990). This new operative technique involved reimplanting the appendix in a nonrefluxing manner into the cecum with the other end brought out on the abdominal wall as a continent stoma (Churchill et al., 2001) (**Fig. 23-6**). (The stoma is normally continent of both stool and gas.) The "cecostomy button" technique is a variation of this procedure; a low profile device is placed into the tract between the abdominal wall and the bowel and is accessed daily for administration of the solution (Duel & Gonzalez, 1999; Lee et al., 2002). With each of these procedures, antegrade

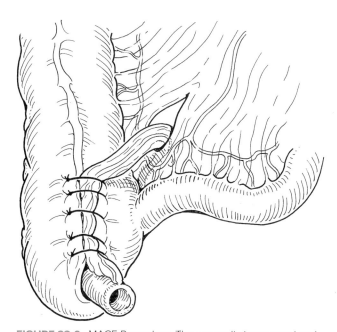

FIGURE 23-6. MACE Procedure. The appendix is removed and reimplanted into the cecum (or transverse or descending colon); other end of appendix brought to abdominal wall as stoma. This permits antegrade "washouts" through the stoma. (Used with permission from Keighley, M. R. B., & Williams, N. S. (2008). *Surgery of the anus, rectum, and colon* (3rd ed.). Philadelphia, PA: W.B. Saunders).

washouts are administered through the catheterizable channel or low profile device to produce colonic emptying. Many children and adolescents with neurogenic bowel, especially those with myelomeningocele, have benefited from this procedure and have found routine irrigations less invasive than having a colostomy or doing retrograde enemas.

In the past decade, there have been several modifications to the ACE procedure. When the appendix is not available or is unsuitable, a neoappendix can be created using the Monti technique. A segment of ileum or colon is detached from the GI tract, while its blood supply is preserved. This segment of bowel is opened to form a rectangle and then reconfigured into a tube-like structure that is tunneled in an antireflux fashion into the bowel wall; it provides a continent, catheterizable conduit through which daily antegrade enemas can be administered (Jinbo, 2004).

Mitrofanoff has placed these ACE conduits (and stomas) in the splenic flexure because the formed stool that needs to be expelled is stored in the left side of the colon (primarily left transverse and descending colon). There have even been modifications to this procedure where a Monti tube is created from the large bowel and placed at the splenic flexure (Heymen et al., 2001). The ACE procedure is also being done laparoscopically (Lynch et al., 1999).

The amount, frequency, and type of solutions vary and include normal saline, hypertonic phosphate, PEG 3,350 (Miralax), and tap water. Yerkes et al. (2001) studied the routine use of tap water as an irrigant, as there have been reported cases of hypernatremia with saline irrigations and electrolyte abnormalities with the use of hypertonic phosphate solutions. They found no significant hyponatremia or hypochloremia in any patient who used tap water for continence irrigations. However, although rare, electrolyte abnormalities with potential morbidity are a possible complication of tap water irrigation, and patients should therefore be monitored closely for any signs of electrolyte disturbances (Yerkes et al. 2001).

Kokoska et al. (2001) described their experience with irrigants and reported best results with normal saline and PEG 3,350; their third choice was a one-to-one solution of glycerin and saline. Due to the potential for electrolyte imbalance with the various solutions, it is recommended that serum electrolyte studies be done to assess the child's tolerance to a solution (Kokoska et al., 2001; Yerkes et al., 2001). Graf et al. (1998) reviewed the literature on types and amounts of solutions utilized for irrigation. They found that the volume used varied from 80 mL to 1 L administered over 5 to 60 minutes. In the majority of patients, colonic evacuation occurred within 1 hour of enema administration. Enemas were given daily to once a week. They concluded that the type of solution, volume, and frequency must be individualized for each patient (Thies & McAllister, 2001).

Siddiqui et al. (2011) did a retrospective review of 117 patients who underwent the ACE procedure. These patients were started on normal saline irrigations and transitioned to GoLytely (PEG-3350 and electrolyte solution) if irrigations were unsuccessful. Other additives were used in 34% of the patients and included bisacodyl (28%), glycerin (5%), phospho-soda (1%), and magnesium citrate (1%). Eighty percent of patients on these alternative additives were managed successfully. The mean age of the placement ACE was 11 years, and the mean irrigation dose was 847 ± 55 mL.

KEY POINT

The MACE/ACE procedures permit antegrade washouts of the distal colon, and in general, children/adolescents and their families have been very satisfied with the results. However, the clinician must work with the individual child/adolescent to determine the optimal frequency of irrigation and the best volume and type of irrigant solution.

The MACE procedure and its variants have been performed for over a decade, and in general, children and adolescents (and their families) have been very satisfied with the results. However, clinicians and patients must always be aware that there are potential complications, which include appendiceal and stomal necrosis; stomal stenosis; stomal leakage; difficulty catheterizing the stoma; pain with enema administration; wound infection; adhesions resulting in bowel obstruction; hypertrophic granulation tissue at the stoma site; mucus discharge and dermatitis around the stoma; cecal volvulus; nausea and dizziness during phosphate enema usage; and hyperphosphatemia with the use of phosphate solutions (Thies & McAllister, 2001). Positive outcomes with this procedure are dependent on patient/family motivation and on compliance with the enema regimen. Some centers believe that this procedure is more successful in children over 5 years of age as they are more motivated and have a better understanding of the care required (Graf et al., 1998; Thies & McAllister, 2001).

If all options for bowel management have been attempted without success, the child and their family should be given the option of having a colostomy created. Although this sounds like a dramatic option, the child with intractable FI may find this quite rewarding, as they will actually regain "control" of defecation.

KEY POINT

If all options for management of neurogenic bowel have been trialed without success, the patient should be offered construction of a colostomy; while this may seem dramatic, it can provide significant improvement in quality of life.

The algorithm shown in **Figure 23-7** depicts a common approach to managing a child with a neurogenic bowel. Treatments are, however, always individualized according to the child and his or her individual symptoms.

KEY CONCEPTS IN THE MANAGEMENT OF THE INDIVIDUAL WITH A NEUROGENIC BOWEL

Ideally, it is hoped that adolescents with a neurogenic bowel have had ongoing monitoring and treatment for incontinence following the initial diagnosis. However, if an adolescent has had no prior treatment, there are several key concepts in working with a child and their caregiver.

Development of Rapport

The first concept for effective management of any adolescent with a chronic illness is the importance of a good rapport between the adolescent and health care provider. Due to the number of tests and examinations, many adolescents are suspicious of health care providers. It is especially important that trust be established if the health care provider needs to provide any type of therapy, such as biofeedback or electrical stimulation. These procedures can be seen as "invasive" or intimidating since leads or sensors are placed in or on the perineum. A good relationship also enables the adolescent to feel comfortable in discussing their feelings or reporting incontinence events. Caregivers need to be counseled regarding avoidance of punishment or blame for bowel incontinence and should be encouraged to assist with a positive reinforcement program, such as incentives for positive behaviors (Jinbo, 2004; Michaud et al., 2007).

Interdisciplinary Approach

A second key concept is an interdisciplinary team approach to management and care. An adolescent with FI experiences many stressful emotional situations and would benefit from the counseling of a mental health professional (i.e., psychologist, psychiatrist, or counselor). The counselor or therapist can reinforce the treatment plan during therapy sessions with the adolescent and caregiver. It is a good proactive measure to routinely refer adolescents with multiple congenital problems and with long-standing incontinence for counseling, since many of these children are "suffering silently" and would benefit from ongoing counseling to help them deal with this problem as well as their disability (Jinbo, 2004). In school, a referral to the school health nurse is helpful so that the adolescent can be assisted in maintaining his or her bowel program, such as reminders to go to the toilet or access to private bathrooms. School nurses are also encouraged to incorporate activities of daily living (ADL) skills into

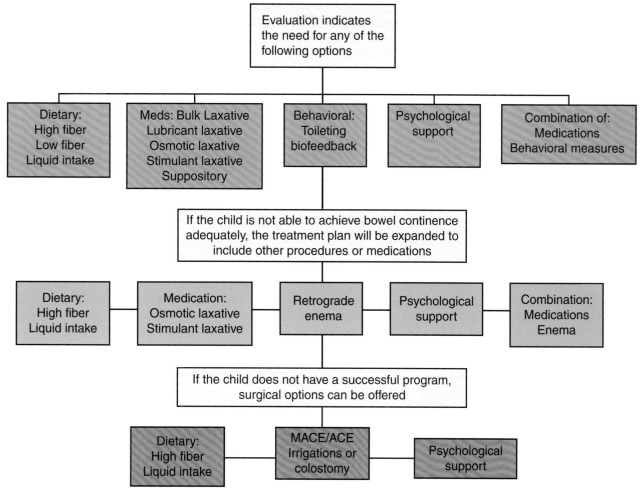

FIGURE 23-7. Algorithm for Management of Neurogenic Bowel.

the adolescent's Individualized Educational Plan (IEP) if there is a need to do procedures (such as catheterizations or behavior interventions) in the school setting (Michaud et al., 2007).

Patient and Caregiver Education

Education of the caregiver and adolescent is crucial, including a review of normal bowel function and a discussion of the causes of neurogenic bowel; it is also important to explain the options for management and to assure that the patient and family understand the treatment plan. This helps to promote cooperation and compliance. Information must be presented in a manner that is consistent with the adolescent's cognitive ability to understand the material. For example, instead of encouraging an adolescent with FI to eat more fiber because these foods are healthier, it would be best to introduce the use of fiber to help bulk the stool and decrease weight and accidents (Michaud et al., 2007) (**Tables 23-6 and 23-7**).

TABLE 23-6 CLINICAL KEY POINTS IN EDUCATING CHILDREN AND FAMILIES FOR ANY BOWEL CONDITION

Clinician Key Points

Education of the patient and family are key to success and adherence to a bowel management plan.

Education of caregivers should remove the negative connotations that can arise between the child and the caregiver.

- For example, if soiling is due to "overflow incontinence," this does not equate to a child exhibiting this behavior willfully or defiantly, but there is a physiological loss of bowel continence. Therefore, the child should not be punished or disciplined for the accident.

Review educational plan with all children/families seeking assistance with their bowel problems.

- If the child is old enough, he or she should be included in the educational process.

Explanations should be simple yet informative/factual and tailored to the type of bowel condition that is being addressed.

- Use of medical terminology needs to be minimal and/or defined whenever utilized.

TABLE 23-7 EDUCATIONAL KEY POINTS WHEN EDUCATING CHILDREN/PARENTS REGARDING BOWEL CONDITIONS

Educational Components and Tips in Delivery

1. Use a diagram to explain the different parts of the GI tract beginning with the mouth and ending with the anus. Naming each segment and explaining its basic function provides the child/family an overview of the digestive process.
   - Example the mouth is the beginning of the GI tract where the food is mechanically (by the teeth) broken down and swallowed.
2. The colon, rectum, and anus play an important role in the development of constipation or diarrhea additional information, for example, the gastric colic reflex, colonic motility, colonic/rectal distention stretch to accommodate the buildup of stool and the role of the anal sphincter.
   - With the younger child, their body size, especially in the lower abdominal/pelvis area, is smaller such that the distention of the rectum can push/extend toward the bladder, urethra, ureters, and affect the flow of urine. This can result in bladder infections, leakage of urine, or the sensation of incomplete bladder emptying.
3. Review the process of defecation to include the movement of stool into the rectum, causing rectal distention which triggers a message to the brain via the spinal cord to enable the individual to find a toilet. When ready to defecate, contraction of the rectum simultaneously relaxes the sphincter and defecation occurs with the release of stool.
4. The development of a bowel management plan should be reviewed. This plan provides individual instructions on how to manage fecal incontinence or constipation. (The plan can be as simple as sitting on the toilet after meals or more involved needing to do a daily enema). The child and family should be advised that this plan will need to be adjusted and tailored to the unique characteristics of the child/patient.
5. *Medication:* Assure families using laxatives continuously for months may be indicated and reassure caregivers as to the safety of long-term laxative use and the importance of continuous treatment with these medications. Encourage to call if needed!
6. Address common misconceptions about laxative dependency and the increased risk of colon cancer due to long-term use of laxatives (Borowitz & Cuffari, 2018, p. 3).
7. If a cleanout is needed this should be done before the implementation of a bowel management program.
8. Timing of taking medication, initiating a bowel movement should be based on the individual's cycle of having a bowel movement. For example, if the patient historically moves their bowel after breakfast, the bowel program should revolve around having bowel movements occur "after breakfast"—so giving a suppository or enema should occur after breakfast.
9. If medication is required, the effectiveness of the medication should be timed. For example, the medication is given/taken to enable the individual to defecate whenever he or she would have normally defecated, for example, after breakfast or after dinner.
10. Child and family need to be advised that consistency in administering medication or procedures to stimulate defecation should be maintained as close to the time as possible as the body can be "trained" to pass stools at that given time. They are also reminded that the bowel management plan "does not stop while on vacation" as the flow of stool should not be interrupted as this can result with the child regressing to their original stooling problems.
11. Older children should be encouraged to participate in their own care, so if the child's bowel program is based on medication, parents can fill medicine containers and the child is instructed to take his or her medication at the prescribed time. The parent can monitor the child by checking the container daily to be sure the medication is taken as well as reminders to take the medication.
12. *Nutrition:* Based on the child's nutritional status/needs, discuss the balance between obtaining enough fiber and fluid intake. If more fiber is needed direct them to lists of high fiber foods. A quick method to determine the amount of fiber needed is (child's age + 5 = the daily grams of fiber needed). The avoidance of sweetened drinks such as sodas and juices and encouraging water should be recommended. The balance of adequate milk or milk products for calcium—excessive intake of milk can lead to constipation. Encourage drinking water and packing a water bottle/flask to take to school.
13. *Behavioral Interventions:* If the child has no obvious stooling pattern, the parents/caregiver may consider designating a timeframe based on "their" schedule. Since children may attend preschool or regular school, it may be too hectic for the parent to wake up the child early to have a bowel movement before leaving for school/work. Subsequently, the parents can target the bowel management program for the late afternoon or early evening.
14. Parents/caregivers with younger children going to baby sitters or preschool, should be encouraged to establish the child's stooling pattern to occur in the late afternoon/early evening, such that the child is able to defecate in a more relaxed environment. This timing can be maintained as the child transitions to a regular school environment.
15. If the child is in a preschool or school, advise the family to speak to the school counselor/teacher and advise them of the child's condition and arrangements should be made to request their assistance with the bowel management program. Example: allowing the child to access the bathroom whenever needed and/or request reminders for the child to toilet after meals.
16. Toileting practice should be reviewed: a child should sit on the potty or toilet with both feet supported on a stool/box/etc. Their knees should be elevated, their feet supported, and they are leaning slightly forward (35 degrees angle), enabling the pelvic floor to more relaxed and better flow of stool. See **Figure 23-8**. Optimal Position for Pooping.
17. The child needs to be encouraged to sit on the toilet (if possible) for 5–10 minutes. They can be provided books, small games to play while sitting, singing, etc. A timer can be used to monitor their sitting time. Small rewards can be given as they achieve their toileting time or defecate.
18. Using the effect of the gastrocolic reflex (a physiological reflex that controls the motility within the colon—the colon has increased motility in response to the stretch of the stomach/ingestion of food) the bowel program should incorporate toileting after meals.

TABLE 23-7 EDUCATIONAL KEY POINTS WHEN EDUCATING CHILDREN/PARENTS REGARDING BOWEL CONDITIONS (*Continued*)

19. If the child has not been toilet trained, discussion with the parents/caregivers may require that toilet training be delayed until the child is able to have more regular bowel movements and/or passing stools of softer consistency. If toilet training was attempted and the child was resistant or fearful, toileting should be delayed. Once the child is stooling regularly and shows signs of readiness to begin toilet training (e.g., rectal awareness), the parents/family can try to introduce toilet training, but need to postpone if there are signs of regression by the child.

20. As noted above, it may be helpful to have a reward system developed with the parent/family, which can be simple praising of the child, stickers on a chart, reading their favorite story, or going to a park to play.

21. It is helpful to monitor the child's response to the bowel program closely especially if on medication—close communication with the continence nurse (e.g., every 2–3 days) helps to insure that adjustments can be made in a timely way to avoid stools that are too loose or infrequent; avoiding abdominal discomfort; or addressing concerns or questions that may arise.

22. If the child has emotional needs, a referral for counseling should be encouraged to deal with their possible anxieties, bullying, etc.

Sources: Levy, E. I., Lemmens, R., Vandenplas, Y., et al. (2017). Functional constipation in children: Challenges and solutions. *Pediatric Health, Medicine and Therapeutics, 8*, 19–27. doi: 10.2147/PHMT.S110940; Philichi, L. (2018). Management of childhood functional constipation. *Journal of Pediatric Health Care, 32*(1), 108–111. doi: 10.1016/j.pedhc.2017.08.008; Sood, M. R., Li, B. U. K., & Hoppin, A. G. (2019). Chronic functional constipation and fecal incontinence in infants, children, and adolescents: Treatment. *UpToDate*. Retrieved from https://www.uptodate.com/contents/chronic-functional-constipation-and-fecal-incontinence-in-infants-children-and-adolescents-treatment/; and Tabbers, M. M., DiLorenzo, C., Berger, M. Y., et al. (2014). Evaluation and treatment of functional constipation in infants and children: Evidence-based recommendations from ESPGHAN and NASPGHAN. *Journal of Pediatric Gastroenterology and Nutrition, 58*(2), 258–274. doi: 10.1097/MPG.0000000000000266.

Developing a treatment plan in collaboration with the child and caregiver is helpful, as both parties can take ownership and responsibility for the various treatment options. Listening carefully to the adolescent is important in assuring adherence with the treatment plan. In many instances, the adolescent has experienced the use of various medications or treatments and may have preconceived ideas of how these treatments affect their bodies. The adolescent may also have employment or extracurricular activities that should be incorporated into the treatment plan. For example, if the adolescent has difficulty getting up in the morning, doing enemas in the morning may not be the optimal time for him or her. Trying to accommodate an adolescent's schedule into the treatment plan may necessitate administering an enema in the evening when the schedule is not as hectic. In middle adolescence, when there is a lot of effort at establishing identity, it is not uncommon for adolescents to have periods of rebellion when they feel that their lives are too tightly controlled; during this period, health care providers may need to compromise on different aspects of the adolescent's treatment plan. During late adolescence, there is more acceptance of their condition, and there may be more instances where adolescents exhibit more control over their condition (Currie, 2000).

Correct position for opening your bowels

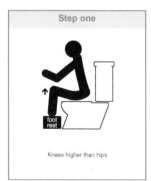

Step one

Knees higher than hips

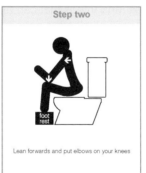

Step two

Lean forwards and put elbows on your knees

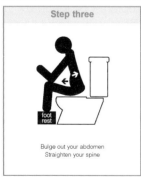

Step three

Bulge out your abdomen
Straighten your spine

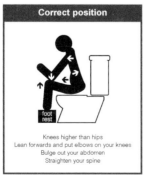

Correct position

Knees higher than hips
Lean forwards and put elbows on your knees
Bulge out your abdomen
Straighten your spine

FIGURE 23-8. Correct Position for Opening the Bowels. (Reproduced by the kind permission of Ray Addison, Nurse Consultant in Bladder and Bowel Dysfunction. Wendy Ness, Colorectal Nurse Specialist. Produced as a service to the medical profession by Norgine Ltd.)

> **KEY POINT**
>
> Key concepts in effective management of the pediatric population include development of rapport, an interdisciplinary approach, patient and family education, and ongoing follow-up.

Follow-Up

Close follow-up with the adolescent and his or her family is essential during establishment and maintenance of a bowel management program. If the adolescent and their family/caregiver(s) are not able to return for follow-up appointments within the first week or two, a telephone follow-up should be done. The adolescent and family/

caregiver(s) should be advised that each bowel management program is tailored individually to each child and that ongoing communication is essential in obtaining success. It is also helpful to emphasize that bowel control does not occur "overnight" and that finding the "right" treatment plan may take time. In addition, bowel management programs need to be maintained even when on vacation or admitted to a hospital, and the adolescent needs to understand that his or her bowel control will be affected by dietary changes as well as medications and illnesses. Keeping the adolescent focused and motivated during the process can be challenging; incentives can be utilized as a means of reinforcing positive behaviors and compliance with the bowel program. Sending reports and consultation notes to the primary physician, who may have referred the adolescent, is helpful in keeping all health care providers apprised of the situation and helping them be supportive of the interventions offered (Jinbo, 2004).

Figure 23-7 depicts the flow of patient management in neurogenic bowel, based on assessment findings and response to treatment. Although treatment regimens differ based on the needs of the specific child, three typical cases are provided at the end of the chapter that illustrate management based on the underlying condition and severity of incontinence.

 DIARRHEA

As noted earlier, chronic constipation is a common contributor to incontinence in children. Diarrhea can also cause incontinence; it most frequently occurs as a response to an acute infectious process or as the result of a chronic condition or disease state.

ACUTE DIARRHEA

"Acute diarrhea" is an increase in the number of stools and an alteration in stool consistency, as compared to the patient's normal stooling pattern. It is usually caused by viral, bacterial, or protozoal agents. In children, rotavirus and Norwalk-like virus are responsible for up to 50% of acute diarrheal cases during winter months (Jackson & Vessey, 2000). History will usually reveal a sudden onset of illness, and there may be other systemic symptoms, such as fever, cough, rash, or decreased activity level. With resolution of the infectious process, the diarrhea subsides as do the incontinent episodes.

CHRONIC DIARRHEA

Chronic diarrhea is an increase in the frequency, fluidity, or volume of stool, compared to the child's normal pattern, for longer than 14 to 21 days. Stool output in excess of 10 g/kg/d in infants and >200 g/d in children is considered indicative of diarrhea (Jackson & Vessey, 2000). Disease states that commonly lead to diarrhea include short gut syndrome, irritable bowel syndrome, Crohn disease or ulcerative colitis, celiac disease, and cystic fibrosis. Children with peritoneal shunt infections commonly exhibit nausea, vomiting, and diarrhea as well as fever and abdominal pain. Children with congenital heart disease must be monitored closely during any episode of diarrhea, as it can be indicative of digoxin toxicity or worsening congestive heart failure (vs. an episode of acute gastroenteritis). Oncology patients may develop chemotherapy-induced diarrhea. Children with cerebral palsy who have limited mobility are frequently plagued with impactions that exhibit as constant diarrhea (because the liquid stool seeps around the impacted stool in the presence of persistent internal sphincter relaxation); it is critical to carefully balance fiber, liquid, and stool softeners in these children and to assess for impaction before treating episodes of "diarrhea." Any child with diarrhea requires careful assessment, since diarrhea in children is typically symptomatic of another condition that needs to be addressed. Once the underlying problem is corrected, the diarrhea and incontinence typically resolve.

 CONCLUSION

Bowel management in the pediatric population is both challenging and rewarding. Fortunately, our society is moving toward a little more openness in discussion of elimination. There are more books for children and parents that explain problems with control of "poop" and "gas" and things that can be done to normalize and control their elimination patterns. Common problems include chronic constipation and encopresis; these problems are very responsive to management strategies including cleanout regimens, establishment of soft formed stool via increased fiber and fluid intake, and routine toileting. Neurogenic bowel is a less common but very difficult problem that is characterized by compromised sensory function and sphincter function. Management of these children requires in-depth assessment and individualized therapy; treatment strategies include correction of stool consistency, toileting programs, biofeedback, use of medications, use of peristaltic stimuli to regulate evacuation, and surgical options including ACE procedures and colostomy formation.

Fundamental principles in working with children and adolescents include establishment of rapport, a multidisciplinary approach, ongoing education of the child and caregivers, and positive reinforcement. Ultimately, the goal is not only to normalize bowel function and provide continence but also to promote positive self-esteem; thus, the clinician must always remember:

The young child is dependent on adults for many things, but the most important is a sense of being cared for ...
—*Mally, T. (1974). Montessori and your child. New York,*
NY: Schocken Books.

CASE STUDY: MILD INCONTINENCE

Jasmine is a 13-year-old patient who just arrived in Hawaii from the Pacific Basin. Jasmine was born with an imperforate anus, and repair was done shortly after birth. According to her mother, Jasmine has been constipated several times a year and occasionally has been to the emergency room because of severe constipation. Jasmine is usually given an enema with good results and then discharged home.

Jasmine's mother states Jasmine is now having problems with very watery stools similar to diarrhea. Her mother also reports that Jasmine had a small amount of stool about 5 days ago. Jasmine stated it was five small balls of stool and added that she has not felt very hungry for the past 5 days.

PHYSICAL EXAMINATION

Constitutional: Jasmine is a well-developed, 13-year-old, ambulatory teen who is very alert and in no acute distress.

Weight: Jasmine weighs 104 pounds.

Abdomen: She has a distended abdomen, with palpable nodules of stool in the left lower quadrant, as well as along the transverse colon. No discomfort noted during palpation.

Perineum: Jasmine's anus had no signs of fissures, and her rectal vault was filled with small balls of stool. Sphincter tone was within a normal range. Perianal area was intact with no signs of any skin breakdown. Fecal staining noted on underwear.

X-ray: An abdominal x-ray revealed that Jasmine was impacted with stool throughout her colon.

Impression: Jasmine has a history of constipation and was currently impacted.

PLAN

1. Cleanout with a full capful of Miralax in 8 ounces of fluid twice a day in addition to Senokot 2 tabs. Recommend a clear liquid diet during the cleanout.

2. Maintenance dose after cleanout: administer Senokot 1 tab daily with one capful of Miralax in 8 ounces of fluid and titrate to keep stools soft and not loose. Resume diet for her current age after cleanout is complete.

3. Follow-up in 1 week.

CASE STUDY: MODERATE INCONTINENCE

Sarah is a 12-year-old girl who was involved in a motor vehicle accident (MVA) that left her paralyzed from the waist down due to a partially severed spinal cord. She does have occasional sensations of rectal filling but is not able to consistently initiate a bowel movement. She has had a moderate amount of slightly firm stool over the past 2 days.

PHYSICAL EXAMINATION

Constitutional: Sarah is a 12-year-old, thin but well-developed paraplegic, who sits in her wheelchair in no acute distress.

Chest: Sarah is developing breast buds.

Abdomen: Sarah's abdomen is flat, but she has palpable stool along the left lower quadrant.

Perineum: Her anus is closed, and she has a fairly high sphincter tone. Her rectal vault was full of stool.

Impression: She is status post-MVA with paraplegia and a neurogenic bowel.

PLAN

1. Recommend use of Fleet enema × 1.

2. Start Miralax ½ capful daily in 4 ounces of fluid, increase or decrease to keep stools soft and formed.

3. Recommend toileting after meals and utilize a glycerin suppository if no bowel movement × 1 day.

4. Will continue to monitor and if Sarah continues to have inadequate emptying, will recommend use of Bisacodyl suppository or weekly Fleets enema.

CASE STUDY: SEVERE INCONTINENCE

John is an 11-year-old who was born with S1–S2 spina bifida. Over the years, he, with the support of his parents, has tried a variety of oral medications, suppositories, and enemas with no success at achieving continence. John and his parents decided that he would do the ACE procedure in hopes of becoming continent. He is 6 weeks post-ACE procedure and has arrived with his parents for his second follow-up visit. Immediately post-op, John was doing well on daily 500 to 600 mL normal saline irrigations, evacuating his stool within 30 to 45 minutes. However, he and his mother noticed that after irrigating, he needs to sit on the toilet for 1.5 to 2 hours. He administers the irrigations shortly after dinner over a 5- to 10-minute period. Often, he will have a large accident 2 to 3 hours later. He is otherwise accident free. John is learning to catheterize and irrigate his stoma using a 10-French Coudé catheter.

PHYSICAL EXAMINATION

Constitutional: John is a well-developed child who is ambulatory with braces.

Weight: 70 pounds

Abdomen: John's abdomen is fairly flat and soft with active bowel sounds. He has a flush stoma that is barely visible in his umbilicus. His peristomal skin is intact.

Perineum: He has a lax anal sphincter; however, perianal skin is clean; no rash noted.

Extremities: John wears braces on bilateral lower extremities.

Impression: John has a prolonged evacuation of ACE irrigation solution.

PLAN

1. Discussed with John and his mother about increasing the volume of the saline solution to 700 to 800 mL of normal saline versus the use of one capful of Miralax in 500 mL of water. They decided to see if the increased volume of saline would expedite evacuation. If they continue to have a prolonged evacuation time, they will switch to the Miralax mixture.

2. They will follow up in the next 3 to 4 weeks.

REFERENCES

Abi-Hanna, A., & Lake, A. M. (1998). Constipation and encopresis in childhood. *Pediatrics in Review, 19*, 23–30.

Amiel, J., Sproat-Emison, E., Garcia-Barcelo, M., et al.; for the Hirschsprung Disease Consortium. (2008). Hirschsprung disease, associated syndromes and genetics: A review. *Journal of Medical Genetics, 45*, 1–4.

Beaudry-Bellefeuille, I. (2017). Defecation-specific behavior in children with functional defecation issues: A systematic review. *The Permanente Journal, 21*, 17–47. doi: 10.7812/TPP/17-047.

Beinvogl, B., Sabharwal, S., McSweeney, M., et al. (2017). Are we using abdominal radiographs appropriately in the management of pediatric constipation? *The Journal of Pediatrics, 191*, 179–83. doi: 10.1016/T.jpeds.2017.08.075.

Biggs, W. S., & Dery, W. H. (2006). Evaluation and treatment of constipation in infants and children. *American Family Physician, 73*(3), 469–477.

Bishop, E., McKinnon E., Weir, E., et al. (2003). Reflexology in the management of encopresis and chronic constipation. *Pediatric Nursing, 15*(3), 20–21.

Boon, R. F., & Singh, N. (1991). A model for the treatment of encopresis. *Behavior Modification, 15*(3), 355–371.

Borowitz, S. M., & Curffari, C. (December 14, 2018). Pediatric constipation. *Medscape.* Retrieved from https://emedicine.medscape.com/article/928185

Chase, J., & Shields, N. (2011). A systematic review of the efficacy of non-pharmacological, non-surgical and non-behavioural treatments of functional chronic constipation in children. *The Australian and New Zealand Continence Journal, 17*(2), 40–50.

Christophersen, E. (1991). Toileting problems in children. *Pediatric Annals, 5*(20), 240–244.

Churchill, B. M., Abramson, R. P., & Wahl, E. F. (2001). Dysfunction of the lower urinary and distal gastrointestinal tracts in pediatric patients with known spinal cord problems. *Pediatric Clinics of North America, 48*(6), 2–51.

Cohen, A. (2007). *Constipation, withholding and your child.* Philadelphia, PA: Jessica Kingsley Publishers.

Currie, D. M. (2000). Bowel management in children with fecal incontinence. *Physical Medicine and Rehabilitation: State of the Art Reviews, 14*(2), 311–322.

DiLorenzo, C., & Benninga, M. A. (2004). Pathophysiology of pediatric fecal incontinence. *Gastroenterology, 126*, S33–S40.

Dos Santos, J., Lopes, R. I., & Koyle, M. A. (2017). Bladder and bowel dysfunction in children: An update on the diagnosis and treatment of a common, but underdiagnosed pediatric problem. *Canadian Urological Association Journal, 11*(1-2 Suppl 1), S64–S72. doi: 10.5489/cuaj.4411.

Doughty, D. B. (2006). *Urinary and fecal incontinence: Nursing management* (3rd ed.). St. Louis, MO: Mosby, Inc.

Duel, B. P., & Gonzalez, R. (1999). The button cecostomy for management of fecal incontinence. *Pediatric Surgery International, 15*, 559–561.

Graf, J. L., Strear, C., Bratton, B., et al. (1998). The antegrade continence enema procedure: A review of the literature. *Journal of Pediatric Surgery, 33*, 1294–1296.

Gunn, V., & Nechyba, C. (2002). *The Harriet Lane handbook—Current pediatrics* (16th ed.). St. Louis, MO: Mosby, Inc.

Hawaii Academy of Nutrition and Dietetics. (2018). *Hawaii Diet Manual* (9th ed.). Honolulu, Hawaii: Hawaii Academy of Nutrition and Dietetics.

Heymen, S., Jones, K. R., Ringel, Y., et al. (2001). Biofeedback treatment of rectal incontinence. *Diseases of the Colon and Rectum, 44*(5), 728–736.

Howe, A. C., & Walker, C. E. (1992). Behavioral management of toilet training, enuresis, and encopresis. *Pediatric Clinics of North America, 39*, 413–432.

Hyams, J. S., Lorenzo, C. D., Saps, M., et al. (2016). Functional disorders: Children and adolescents, *Gastroenterology, 150*, 1456–1468.

Ingebo, K., & Heyman, M. (1988). Polyethylene glycol—electrolyte solution for intestinal clearance in children with refractory encopresis. *American Journal of Diseases of Children, 142*, 340–342.

International Foundation for Gastrointestinal Disorders (IFFGD). (n.d.). Retrieved form https://www.aboutkidsgi.org/hirschsprung-s-disease/enterocolitis-after-treatment-for-hirschsprung-s-disease.html

Jackson, P. L., & Vessey, J. (2000). *Primary care of the child with a chronic condition*. St. Louis, MO: Mosby.

Jinbo, A. K. (2004). The challenge of obtaining continence in a child with a neurogenic bowel disorder. *Journal of Wound, Ostomy, and Continence Nursing, 31*(6), 336–350.

Kokoska, E. R., Keller, M. S., & Weber, T. (2001). Outcome of the antegrade colonic enema procedure in children with chronic constipation. *American Journal of Surgery, 182*(6), 625–629.

Koppen, I. J. N., von Gontard, A., Chase, J., et al. (2016). Management of functional nonretentive fecal incontinence in children: Recommendations from the International Children's Continence Society. *Journal of Pediatric Urology, 12*(1), 56–64.

Lee, S. L., DuBois, J. J., Montes-Garces, R. G., et al. (2002). Surgical management of chronic unremitting constipation and fecal incontinence associated with megarectum: A preliminary report. *Journal of Pediatric Surgery, 37*(1), 76–79.

Levine, M. (1982). Encopresis: Its potential, evaluation, and alleviation. *Pediatric Clinics of North America, 29*(2), 315–329.

Leung, M. W. Y., Wong, B. P. Y., Leung, A. K. P., et al. (2006). Electrical stimulation and biofeedback exercise of pelvic floor muscle for children with fecal incontinence after surgery for anorectal malformation. *Pediatric Surgery International, 22*, 975–978.

Levy, E. I., Lemmens, R., Vandenplas, Y., et al. (2017). Functional constipation in children: Challenges and solutions. *Pediatric Health, Medicine and Therapeutics, 8*, 19–27. doi: 10.2147/PHMT.S110940.

Loening-Baucke, V., Miele, E., & Staiano, A. (2004). Fiber (Glucomannan) is beneficial in the treatment of childhood constipation. *Pediatrics, 113*(3), e259–e264.

Lynch, A. C., Beasley, S. W., Robertson, R. W., et al. (1999). Comparison of results of laparoscopic and open antegrade continence enema procedures. *Pediatric Clinics of North America, 15*, 343–346.

MacLeod, J. (1998). Fecal incontinence: A practical program of management. *Endoscopy Review, 5*, 45–56.

Malone, P., Ransley, P., & Kiely, E. (1990). Preliminary report: The antegrade continence enema. *Lancet, 336*, 1217–1218.

Mazier, W., Levien, D., Luchtefeld, M., et al. (1995). *Surgery of the colon, rectum, and anus*. Philadelphia, PA: WB Saunders.

Michaud, P. A., Suris, J. C., & Viner, R. (2007). *The adolescent with a chronic condition*. (Discussion Paper.). Geneva, Switzerland: World Health Organization.

Mikkelsen, E. J. (2001). Enuresis and encopresis: Ten years of progress. *Journal of the American Academy of Child and Adolescent Psychiatry, 40*, 1146–1158.

Molnar, G. (1985). *Pediatric rehabilitation*. Baltimore, MD: Lippincott Williams & Wilkins.

Niemczyk, J., Equit, M., Hoffman, L., et al. (2015). Incontinence in children with treated attention-deficit/hyperactivity disorder. *Journal of Pediatric Urology, 11*(3), 141e1–141e6. doi: https://doi.org/10.1016/j.jpurol.2015.02.009.

Nolan, T., & Oberklaid, F. (1993). New concepts in the management of encopresis. *Pediatrics in Review, 14*(11), 447–451.

Nurko, S., Youssef, N. N., Sabri, M., et al. (2008). PEG3350 in the treatment of childhood constipation: A multicenter, double-blinded, placebo-controlled trial. *The Journal of Pediatrics, 153*, 254–261.

Nurko, S., & Zimmerman, L. A. (2014). Evaluation and treatment of constipation in children and adolescents. *American Family Physician, 90*(2), 82–90. Retrieved from https://www.aafp.org/af/2014/0715/p82.html

Olaru, C., Diaconescu, S., Trandafir, L., et al. (2016). Chronic functional constipation and encopresis in children in relationship with the psychosocial environment. *Gastroenterology Research and Practice, 2016*. doi: 10.1155/2016/7828576.

O'Rorke, C. (1995). Helping children overcome fecal incontinence. *American Journal of Nursing, 95*, 16.

Pashankar, D. S., Bishop, W. P., & Loening-Baucke, V. (2003). Long-term efficacy of polyethylene glycol 3350 for the treatment of chronic constipation in children with and without encopresis. *Clinical Pediatrics, 42*, 815–819.

Philichi, L. (2018). Management of childhood functional constipation. *Journal of Pediatric Health Care, 32*(1). doi: 10.1016/j.pedhc.2017.08.008.

Rao, S. S. C., Welcher, K. D., & Happel, J. (1996). Can biofeedback therapy improve anorectal function in fecal incontinence? *The American Journal of Gastroenterology, 91*(11), 2360–2365.

Redkar, R. G., Mishra, P. K., Thampi, C., et al. (2012). Role of rectal myomectomy in refractory chronic constipation. *African Journal of Paediatric Surgery, 9*, 202–205. Retrieved from http://www.afrjpaedsurg.org/text.asp?2012/9/3/202/104720

Reid, H., & Bahar, R. J. (2006). Treatment of encopresis and chronic constipation in young children: Clinical results from interactive parent–child guidance. *Clinical Pediatrics, 45*, 157–164.

Roy, C., Silverman, A., & Alagille, D. (1995). *Pediatric clinical gastroenterology*. St. Louis, MO: Mosby.

Russo, M., Strisciuglio, C., Scarpato, E., et al. (January, 2019). Functional chronic constipation: Rome III Criteria versus Rome IV Criteria. *Journal of Neurogastroenterology Motility, 25*(1), 123–128. Retrieved from https://www.ncbi.nim.nih.gove/pmc/articlesPMC6326211/

Schmitt, B. D., & Mauro, R. (1992). 20 common errors in treating encopresis. *Contemporary Pediatrics, May*, 47–65.

Schonwald, A., & Rappaport, L. (2004). Encopresis: Assessment and management. *Pediatrics in Review, 25*(8), 278–283.

Seth, R., & Heyman, M. (1994). Management of constipation and encopresis in infants and children. *Gastroenterology Clinics of North America, 23*(4), 621–636.

Siddiqui, A. A., Fishman, S. J., Bauer, S. B., et al. (2011). Long-term follow-up of patients after antegrade continence enema procedure. *Journal of Pediatric Gastroenterology & Nutrition, 52*(5), 1–21. doi: 10.1097/MPG.0b013e3181ff6042.

Smith, K. (1991). Myelomeningocele: Managing bowel and bladder dysfunction in the school-aged child. *Progressions, 3*(2), 3–11.

Sood, M. R., Li, B. U. K., & Hoppin, A. G. (2019). Chronic functional constipation and fecal incontinence in infants, children, and adolescents: Treatment. *UpToDate*. Retrieved from https://www.uptodate.com/contents/chronic-functional-constipation-and-fecal-incontinence-in-infants-children-and-adolescents-treatment/

Sprague-McRae, J. M. (1990). Encopresis: Developmental, behavioral, and physiological considerations for treatment. *The Nurse Practitioner, 15*(6), 8–24.

Stadtler, A. (1989). Preventing encopresis. *Pediatric Nursing, 15*(3), 282–284.

Steinberg, L. (2008). *Adolescence* (8th ed.). New York, NY: McGraw-Hill.

Stern, P., Lowitz, G., Prince, M., et al. (1988). The incidence of cognitive dysfunction in an encopretic population in children. *Neurotoxicology, 9*(3), 351–358.

Tabbers, M. M., DiLorenzo, C., Berger, M. Y., et al.; European Society for Pediatric Gastroenterology, Hepatology, and Nutrition, & North American Society for Pediatric Gastroenterology. (2014). Evaluation and treatment of functional constipation in infants and children: evidence-based recommendations from ESPGHAN and NASPGHAN. *Journal of pediatric gastroenterology and nutrition, 58*(2), 258–274. doi: 10.1097/MPG.0000000000000266.

Thies, K. M., & McAllister, J. W. (2001). The health and education leadership project: A school initiative for children and adolescents with chronic health conditions. *The Journal of School Health, 71*(5), 167–172.

Thomas, R., & Chandler, B. (2007). Management of bowel dysfunction in neurological rehabilitation—A review. *Critical Review in Physical and Rehabilitation Medicine, 19*(4), 251–274.

Tobias, N., Mason, D., Lutkenhoff, M., et al. (2008). Management principles of organic causes of childhood constipation. *Journal of Pediatric Health Care, 22*(1), 12–23. doi: 10.1016/j.pedhc.2007.01.001.

Wald, A. (1981). Use of biofeedback in treatment of fecal incontinence in patients with meningomyelocele. *Pediatrics, 68*(1), 45–49.

Walker, W. A., Durie, P. R., Hamilton, J. R., et al. (1990). *Pediatric gastrointestinal disease* (Vol. 2, 2nd ed.). St. Louis, MO: Mosby.

Walker, W. A., Durie, P. R., Hamilton, J. R., et al. (1996). *Pediatric gastrointestinal disease* (Vol. 2, 2nd ed.). St. Louis, MO: Mosby.

Yerkes, E. B., Rink, R. C., King, S., et al. (2001). Tap water and the Malone Antegrade Continence enema: A safe combination? *The Journal of Urology, 166*, 1476–1147.

Youssef, N. N., & Di Lorenzo, C. (2001). Childhood constipation evaluation and treatment. *Journal of Clinical Gastroenterology, 33*, 199–205.

QUESTIONS

1. A continence nurse is assessing an 8-year-old child who is diagnosed with encopresis. Which of the following are important components of the assessment in determining treatment plan?
A. Developmental milestones
B. Present stooling consistency, stooling pattern, and accidents
C. Name of the schools attended
D. Child's usually temperament and behavior at home

2. The continence nurse is counseling the parents of a 5-year-old male who has fecal incontinence not caused by an organic or anatomic lesion. What is the term for this condition?
A. Chronic diarrhea
B. Fecal soiling
C. Encopresis
D. Functional constipation

3. What is the primary goal for initial management of retentive encopresis?
A. Finding the underlying cause
B. Establishing a reward/punishment system
C. Choosing a medication regimen
D. Education followed by "cleanout"

4. The continence nurse is teaching the parents of a 6-year-old encopretic child how many grams of fiber the child should consume each day. What amount is recommended?
A. 11 g
B. 12 g
C. 14 g
D. 15 g

5. What is the primary focus when treating secondary nonretentive encopresis?
A. Finding the organic problem causing the encopresis
B. Adding fiber to the diet
C. Resolving psychological issues that triggered encopresis
D. Choosing a laxative that is effective

6. Which GI disorder results in loss of peristalsis causing a functional obstruction and dilation of the proximal segment?
A. Hirschsprung disease
B. Imperforate anus
C. Spina bifida
D. Cerebral palsy

7. The continence nurse is assessing an adolescent with neurogenic bowel and he reported that he has been having UTIs every other month. What should the nurse be concerned about?
A. Cause of their neurogenic bowel
B. Has the adolescent been examined by a urologist
C. Possible impaction contributing to incomplete bladder emptying
D. The adolescent has poor intake of fiber and liquid

8. The continence nurse documents "patulous" anus upon assessment of an adolescent with neurogenic bowel. What bowel disorder does this condition indicate?
A. Perianal fissure
B. Incontinence-associated dermatitis
C. Internal hemorrhoids
D. Sphincter muscle laxity

9. What test is usually performed at the time of diagnosis for Hirschsprung disease in an infant?
A. CT scans
B. MRI studies
C. Defecography
D. Rectal biopsy

10. An adolescent with a neurogenic bowel is scheduled for surgery to place a low-profile device into the tract between the abdominal wall and the bowel to administer antegrade washouts and produce colonic emptying. What is the name of this surgical technique?
A. Pull-through procedure
B. Bowel resection
C. Cecostomy button
D. Colostomy

ANSWERS AND RATIONALES

1. B. Rationale: The initial comprehensive assessment of a child with a bowel dysfunction requires a thorough medical and developmental history and psychosocial assessment with focus questions regarding the specific bowel symptoms experienced especially stooling pattern, stool consistency, and leakage pattern if present.

2. C. Rationale: Encopresis is fecal soiling associated with functional constipation (constipation not caused by organic or anatomic abnormalities); functional constipation is constipation not caused by organic or anatomic abnormalities.

3. D. Rationale: Management of retentive encopresis begins with education and reassurance for the child and parents, followed by "cleanout" (i.e., measures to eliminate all retained stool from the colon and rectum).

The next phase of treatment is the cleaning-out phase, the objective of which is to eliminate all retained stool from the colon and rectum.

4. A. Rationale: A formula to determine the grams of fiber per day for a child 3 years or older is age + 5 = grams of fiber per day, in this case scenario, age 6 + 5 = 11 g of fiber per day.

5. C. Rationale: The history of a child with *secondary nonretentive encopresis* usually reveals psychosocial stressors in the home or the school environment that have caused the child to

regress to an earlier developmental stage. Since the cause of the incontinence is psychological, the focus during treatment is on encouraging the child to identify and talk about the stressful situation that precipitated the regression.

6. A. Rationale: Hirschsprung disease involves absence of ganglion (nerve) cells in the distal bowel; the affected bowel is unable to contract to propel stool distally, which creates a functional obstruction.

7. C. Rationale: The distention of the rectum with an impaction can push/extend toward the bladder, urethra, ureters and affect the flow of urine. This can result in bladder infections, leakage of urine, or the inability to effectively empty the bladder.

8. D. Rationale: Patulous anus represents laxity or gapping of the external anal sphincter usually due to pudendal nerve damage.

9. D. Rationale: A rectal biopsy is the most reliable method of diagnosis of Hirschsprung disease; histologic examination reveals an absence of ganglion cells.

10. C. Rationale: The "cecostomy button" technique is a variation of the MACE procedure; a low profile device is placed into the tract between the abdominal wall and the bowel and is accessed daily for administration of the solution to produce colonic emptying.

Abdominal leak point pressure: level of intra-abdominal pressure required to push urine through a partially closed sphincter; measurement obtained during filling cystometry by having patient perform various coughing or straining measures to determine abdominal pressure at which leakage occurs

Ablative techniques: used for BPH and involve the use of lasers to vaporize prostatic tissue

Absorbent product capacity: measures of ability of absorbent products to hold urine; three commonly used tests are as follows: retain moisture under pressure; the *absorptive capacity test* measures how quickly an absorbent product acquires a given amount of fluid: and the *total absorbent capacity test* measures how much fluid a product can absorb

Acetylcholine: major parasympathetic neurotransmitter; mediates detrusor muscle contraction

Active surveillance: conservative approach to management of localized prostate cancer in which active treatment is deferred and the patient undergoes routine monitoring for any evidence of disease progression, at which time treatment can be initiated (just in time treatment)

Acute diarrhea: diarrheal episodes lasting <14 days

Adiposity-based chronic disease (ABCD): new term for the condition of obesity that better reflects several adverse health consequences caused by excess adipose tissue or adiposity

Acute/transient urinary incontinence: newly occurring urinary incontinence of relatively sudden onset; typically <6 months in duration; caused by reversible factors

Acute urinary retention (AUR): sudden inability to pass urine; causes a painful, palpable, or percussible bladder

- *precipitated AUR*: results from a definable trigger even, for example, surgical procedure, medications
- *spontaneous AUR*: acute urinary retention in the absence of an identifiable trigger event

Alpha-adrenergic agonists: medications that increase tone in bladder neck and proximal urethra, thereby increasing bladder outlet resistance

Alpha-adrenergic antagonists: medications that reduce tone in the bladder neck and proximal urethra, thus reducing bladder outlet resistance

American Spinal Injury Association (ASIA): a system to classify the severity of the impairment associated with SCI; ASIA A SCI is a "complete injury" with no sensory or motor function below the level of the SCI; ASIA B SCI is defined as "sensory incomplete" with preservation of sensory but no motor function below the level of the injury

Anal bulking agents: biomaterials that can be injected into the sphincter muscle or submucosal tissue to supplement internal anal sphincter (IAS) function

Anal incontinence: involuntary loss of flatus without loss of mucus or stool

Anal verge: dividing line between squamous epithelium of anal canal (anoderm) and perianal skin

Anal wink (anocutaneous reflex): reflex contraction of external anal sphincter (EAS) in response to stroking of perianal skin at 3 o'clock and 9 o'clock; indicates intact pudendal nerve pathways

Anorectal angle: 90-degree angle between rectum and anal canal that is created by the "sling-like" effect of the puborectalis muscle and that promotes fecal continence; with straining, angle is increased to 135 degrees, which promotes stool elimination

Anorectal manometry: diagnostic test that measures resting and squeeze pressures in anal canal as well as assessment of rectal capacity and distensibility

Antegrade continence enema (ACE) procedure (also known as Malone antegrade continence enema, or MACE procedure): surgical procedure in which small stoma is created between the abdominal wall and proximal colon; permits antegrade "washouts" that can be used to manage chronic refractory constipation or fecal incontinence due to neurogenic bowel

Anticholinergic/antimuscarinic: medications that reduce urinary urgency and increase bladder storage capacity by blocking the activation of cholinergic/muscarinic receptors in the urothelium and detrusor

Artificial anal sphincter: surgical placement of inflatable cuff around the anal sphincter; cuff connected to reservoir implanted in groin and manually operated pump placed in scrotum or labia. When cuff is inflated, anal canal is closed; when defecation is desired, the fluid is transferred to the reservoir via manual activation of the pump, which opens the anal canal

Asymptomatic bacteriuria (ASB): the presence of bacteria in the urine *without* signs and symptoms of infection. All individuals with catheters will develop significant microbial colonization within a few days; ASB does not require treatment

Atresia: complete obstruction of bowel lumen

Atrophic urethritis/vaginitis (see genitourinary syndrome of menopause): thinning and drying of urethral and vaginal epithelium due to estrogen deficiency

AUA symptom score: (see IPSS)

Augmentation enterocystoplasty: a reconstructive surgical procedure using an intestinal segment to enlarge bladder capacity, improve bladder wall compliance, and reduce or abolish neurogenic detrusor overactivity

Augmentation cystoplasty: surgical procedure that uses segment of small bowel to enlarge bladder and increase bladder capacity

Autonomic dysreflexia (AD): a dangerous complication of urinary retention caused from overstimulation of the sympathetic nervous system in patients with SCI at or above T6. It is characterized by uncontrolled hypertension and bradycardia, pounding headache and the individual appears flushed and diaphoretic

Balanced bladder: one that empties completely and is not associated with recurring UTI or upper urinary tract distress; an imbalanced bladder does not empty completely and is associated with recurring UTI and/or upper urinary tract distress

Benign prostatic hyperplasia (BPH): nonmalignant enlargement of the prostate gland

Beta$_3$-adrenergic agonists: class of medication that enhances bladder relaxation by binding to the beta$_3$-adrenergic receptors in the bladder; use in individuals suffering from overactive bladder

Beta$_3$-adrenergic antagonist: class of medications that blocks beta$_3$-adrenergic receptors from relaxing, thereby promoting bladder contractility, in theory

Biofeedback: use of visual or auditory feedback to improve awareness of physiologic activities; may be used in conjunction with pelvic muscle exercise program to improve sensory awareness, pelvic muscle strength and function, and/or coordination between abdominal and pelvic floor muscles

Biofilm: a polysaccharide matrix in which organisms attach, live, and multiply on surfaces (urinary epithelium, external and internal catheter) to promote antibiotic resistance and spread of the biofilm to other surfaces

Bladder diary: record of voiding and leakage episodes and associated symptoms; some diaries include record of fluid intake (type and amount)

Bladder outlet obstruction (BOO): blockage that occurs at the bladder base or bladder neck that reduces or stops the flow of urine into the urethra; it can be caused by a functional (detrusor sphincter dysfunctions) or mechanical (prostatic enlargement, stricture) blockage

Bladder pain syndrome (BPS) or interstitial cystitis: defined by International Continence Society (ICS) as the complaint of suprapubic pain related to bladder filling, accompanied by other symptoms such as increased daytime and night-time frequency, in the absence of proven urinary infection or other obvious pathology

Bladder training program (Bladder drill): behavioral therapy that involves gradual lengthening of voiding interval with the use of behavioral strategies to control urgency

Bladder–sphincter coordination: sphincter relaxation prior to detrusor contraction; controlled by central nervous system and pontine micturition center

Bladder–sphincter dyssynergia (DSD): failure of the bladder neck muscle fibers (internal sphincter) to relax during voiding

Bladder wall compliance: the relationship between bladder volume and intravesical pressure during bladder filling/storage; normal function is characterized by a distensible bladder that fills with minimal increase in intravesical pressure

Blue pads: disposable underpads used as temporary protection for chairs and beds during clinical procedures; they are not to be used as incontinence pads; lack an absorbent filling and can allow pooling of urine on the thin plastic surface, placing the individual at risk of skin wetness and skin breakdown

Body worn absorbent products (BWAPs): disposable or washable body worn products used to contain urinary and/or fecal incontinence; products include pull-ons, briefs, pads/liners/leaf/shields/guards, and penile wraps

Bowel diary: record of stool elimination that documents time, volume, and consistency of voluntary and involuntary stools, as well as associated symptoms (and possibly diet and fluid intake)

Bristol stool scale: a tool commonly used to categorize stool consistency

Bulbocavernosus reflex (BCR): anal contraction in response to tapping of the clitoris or squeezing of the glans penis; one indication of intact neurologic pathways between the sacral cord and pelvic floor

Catheter-associated urinary tract infection (CAUTI): UTI in an individual with an indwelling catheter at least

48 hours in place prior to the UTI or day after the catheter was removed. It is considered a "complicated" UTI and is the most severe and common catheter-associated complication because it may lead to urosepsis and septicemia

Catheter bypassing: bladder forcing urine leakage around the catheter; often caused by bladder spasms and blockages (kinked tubing, stool impaction, clots, encrustations)

Catheter coating: consists of a hydrogel to reduce friction with insertion or antimicrobial such as an antibiotic or silver coating to reduce bacteriuria or catheter-associated urinary tract infection (CAUTI)

Catheter construction: is the type of material used in creating the catheter and has significant implications for clinical use:

- *latex impregnated with polytef particles* reduce fluid absorption into the catheter surface and aid in a smooth insertion; uncoated latex is not used for urethral catheters as there is a high contact sensitivity to the material
- *hydrogel-coated latex catheters* hydrophilic (water-loving) polymers, a gel-like substance made mostly of water covering a catheter to reduce fluid absorption into the catheter surface and friction to aid in a smooth insertion
- *silicone (pure) catheters* pure silicone catheters contain no latex and provide the advantage of a thinner wall and wider lumen as compared to latex-based catheters
- *silastic catheters* silicone-coated catheter but latex based

Catheter obstruction: anything that inhibits or completely stops the drainage of urine from the bladder through the catheter tube, that is, blood clots, encrustations, kinks in catheter

Catheter valve: tap-like device applied to the end of an indwelling catheter to promote normal bladder function, capacity, and tone by allowing urine to be stored in the bladder and then emptied into the toilet or other receptacle (leg or drainage bag) at regular intervals during the day

Celiac disease: autoimmune disorder where the ingestion of gluten triggers an individual's white blood cells to attack the villi in the small intestine leading to altered digestion and absorption of nutrients. Ongoing damage to the intestine may cause diarrhea, fatigue, weight loss, bloating, gas, osteoporosis, itchy skin rashes, joint pain, and anemia

Central obesity: excess fatty tissue in the abdominal area

C-fibers: nerve fibers present in bladder wall that transmit signals of severe discomfort or pain; activated by extreme distention, inflammation of bladder wall, or noxious substances in urine

Chronic diarrhea: diarrhea persisting >30 days

Chronic pelvic pain (CPP): American College of Obstetricians and Gynecologists (ACOG) defines CPP as noncyclic pain of 6 or more months' duration that is localized to the pelvis, anterior abdominal wall at or below the umbilicus, the lumbosacral back, or the buttocks and is of such severity that it may cause functional disability or lead one to seek treatment

Chronic urinary incontinence (CUR): urinary incontinence that lasts >6 months despite correction of reversible factors

- *high-pressure CUR*: chronic urinary retention in the presence of high bladder pressure; often leads to hydronephrosis
- *low-pressure CUR*: chronic urinary retention is the presence of low bladder pressure (a very compliant bladder)

Chronic urinary retention: nonpainful bladder that remains palpable or percussible after the patient has passed urine

CI (confidence interval): studies typically report the 95% CI associated with an OR or RR. It defines a range of values that you can be 95% certain contains the population or sample mean

Closing reflex: brief increase in external anal sphincter (EAS) activity that occurs following stool evacuation; triggers anal canal closure

CMS (Centers for Medicare & Medicaid Services): federal agency that administers the nation's major health care programs including Medicare, Medicaid, and Children's Health Insurance Program as well as collects and analyzes data, produces research reports, and works to eliminate instances of fraud and abuse within the health care system. See Medicare Part A, B, C, and D

Colonic transit time: time required for stool to pass through the colon and to be evacuated per the anus

Comorbid conditions: refers to one or more diseases or chronic *conditions* that occur along with another *condition such as bowel or bladder dysfunction* in the same person at the same time

Complex cystometrogram (CMG): measurement of both intravesical and intra-abdominal pressures; the pressure-sensitive catheter equipped with a transducer placed in the bladder measures bladder pressures (Pves), and a similar catheter placed into the rectum measures abdominal pressures (Pabd)

Compliance: ability of bladder (or rectum) to distend with urine or stool while maintaining low intravesical (or intrarectal) pressures

Constipation: difficult defecation characterized by one or more of the following: hard or dry stools; reduced frequency of stool elimination; sensation of incomplete evacuation following a bowel movement; or pain or straining associated with stool elimination

Continence care nurse: a nurse who specializes in the care of individuals who suffer from bowel and bladder dysfunction and incontinence

Continent catheterizable stoma: usually constructed from appendix or colon segment to create a catheterizable channel to empty the bowel or bladder when conventional elimination is not possible

Coudé-tipped catheters: have an angled tip and are useful for men with prostatic hypertrophy and mild obstruction as they slip around the prostatic curve more readily than a straight catheter

Cyanoacrylates: film-forming liquid skin protectants that adhere to weeping skin and resists washing off when cleansing perigenital skin following an incontinent episode

Cystometrogram (CMG): provides data regarding bladder capacity, sensory awareness of bladder filling, detrusor stability, and bladder wall compliance. CMG can be simple or complex measurements; see Simple CMG and Complex CMG

Cystoscopy: lighted scope place through the urethra and into the bladder to visualize bladder mucosa for malignancy, stones, or foreign bodies, bladder wall thickening (trabeculation), bladder neck abnormalities, and presence or absence of bladder diverticulum

Defecography: simulation of defecation using radiopaque stool substitute and fluoroscopic imaging

Delirium: transient (reversible) alteration in mental status/cognition

Dementia: irreversible decline in cognitive function

Dentate line: midpoint of anal canal; above this point, anal canal is lined with columnar epithelium, and distal to this point, it is lined with squamous epithelium, which is richly innervated with sensory receptors (anoderm)

Detrusor: smooth muscle of bladder

Detrusor overactivity: involuntary contractions of detrusor muscle that occur during filling phase of urodynamic study

Detrusor sphincter dyssynergia: failure of sphincter relaxation in response to detrusor contraction; creates significant risk for upper tract dysfunction

Detrusor underactivity: weak and/or poorly sustained bladder muscle contraction resulting in prolonged flow of urine and possibly incomplete bladder emptying

Diarrhea: alteration in bowel elimination characterized by increase in both frequency and volume of stools and reduced consistency of stool, as compared to individual's normal bowel elimination patterns

DIPPERS: a mnemonic often used to help guide assessment of reversible factors contributing to urinary incontinence: delirium, infection, pharmaceuticals, psychological, excess urine output, mobility, stool impaction

Dysfunctional voiding: abnormal voiding pattern characterized by intermittent flow pattern, intermittent detrusor contractions, and increased pelvic floor/sphincter activity during voiding in neurologically intact individual

Dysfunctional voiding symptoms score: an assessment tool used to assess the impact of dysfunctional voiding on the individual's quality of life and to track progress with treatment

Dyssynergic defecation: result of pelvic floor dysfunction (inability to relax the external anal sphincter during defecation) creating a functional obstruction *or* a mechanical obstruction such as a rectal prolapse, pelvic organ prolapse, tumor, etc.

Electromyography: neurologic examination of pelvic floor nerve/muscle function using either surface electrodes or needle electrodes

Encopresis: fecal soiling usually associated with functional constipation; fecal incontinence in children not caused by an organic or anatomic lesion. May be classified as

"primary" (child >4 years of age who has never achieved bowel control) or "secondary" (child who was continent of stool for at least 1 year and has relapsed due to some secondary condition). Also classified as retentive and nonretentive

Encopresis is a voluntary or involuntary fecal soiling; retentive encopresis refers to involuntary fecal soiling, usually in children who have already been toilet trained and usually in response to subconscious withholding of stool

Encrustations: gravel-like substance created by urease producing bacteria that splits urea in urine into ammonia, thereby elevating urine pH and causing precipitation of urine mineral ions into calcium and magnesium phosphate crystals that can lead to catheter blockage

Endoanal ultrasound: use of transducer emitting sound waves to create image of anal sphincters and to identify any structural abnormalities

Endometriosis: syndrome is characterized by growth of endometrial tissue outside the endometrium of the uterus

Endopelvic fascia: layer of pelvic floor comprised of collagen, elastin, and smooth muscle that connects pelvic organs to bony pelvis

Enteric nervous system (ENS): intraintestinal nervous system that consists of sensory receptors, motor neurons, and interneurons located in Meissner and myenteric (Auerbach) plexuses; mediates peristaltic activity in response to stretch and tension in bowel wall and intraluminal substances/irritants

Enterostomal therapy (ET): historically, enterostomal therapy evolved out of a need to educate people with a urinary or fecal ostomy by those who also had an ostomy. Later it evolved into a nursing specialty and expanded the scope of practice to include skin and wound care as well the care of the individual with urinary and bowel dysfunction. Currently, the nurse specialist is known as a Wound Ostomy and Continence (WOC) nurse

Enuresis: International Continence Society defines as a complaint of intermittent incontinence that occurs during periods of sleep also known as nocturnal enuresis or "bed wetting." It is further divided into monosymptomatic and nonmonosymptomatic enuresis:

- *monosymptomatic enuresis:* enuresis in children who have not history of bladder dysfunction; can be primary, occurring in a child who had never achieved at least 6 months of nighttime dryness, or secondary, developing after at least 6 months of nighttime dryness
- *nonmonosymptomatic enuresis:* enuresis accompanied by any other LUT symptoms such as increased/decreased voiding frequency, daytime incontinence, urgency, hesitancy, straining, a weak stream, intermittency, holding maneuvers, a feeling of incomplete emptying, postmicturition dribble, and genital or LUT pain

External anal sphincter (EAS): sphincter composed of both striated and smooth muscles that overlap internal anal sphincter and terminate at anus; striated muscle component under voluntary control and permits individual to delay defecation; smooth muscle component controlled by enteric and autonomic nervous systems

External collection devices (ECDs): devices that adhere to the external genitalia or pubic area and collect urinary output; they are further divided into the following categories: condom catheters, reusable body worn urinals, nonsheath glans adherent, and female suction devices

External fecal pouches: external containment device attached to a flexible pectin-based adhesive skin barrier designed to adhere to the perianal skin and inner buttocks of an individual to collect incontinent liquid stool; it resembles a one-piece ostomy pouch

External urethral sphincter (rhabdosphincter): striated muscle located at midurethra in women and just distal to prostate gland in men innervated by branches of pudendal nerve and under voluntary control

Extraurethral incontinence: urinary leakage through channels other than the urethra, usually due to a fistula or ectopic ureter

Fast-twitch muscle fibers: muscle fibers that provide rapid strong contractions; comprise 1/3 of pelvic floor muscle fibers

Fatty diarrhea: diarrhea caused by malabsorption syndrome (e.g., lactose intolerance), surgical procedure resulting in malabsorption (e.g., gastric bypass), medications causing malabsorption, or specific parasitic infections (e.g., Giardia)

Fecal continence: ability to control stool elimination; defecation that occurs at socially appropriate place and time

Fecal incontinence: accidental (involuntary) passage of stool or gas at undesirable time or place; inability to control evacuation of stool at socially appropriate place and time; can be classified as

- *urge fecal incontinence*—sudden urgent need to defecate that results in incontinence when the individual is unable to reach a toilet in time; usually due to incompetent external anal sphincter (EAS)
- *passive fecal incontinence*—passage of stool or gas without any awareness on the part of the individual; usually caused by cognitive impairment or sensorimotor dysfunction and ranges in severity from mild soiling to total evacuation of rectal contents
- *flatus incontinence*—fecal leakage, soiling, or seepage of minor degrees including liquid stool, mucus, or very small amounts of solid stool.

Fiber (dietary fiber and fiber supplements): foods and supplements that promote normal microbial balance in colon, add water and bulk to stool, and may reduce transit time. Classified as soluble (fiber that dissolves in water) versus insoluble (fiber that does not dissolve in water) and fermentable (fiber that is broken down by bacteria and produces gas) versus nonfermentable (fiber that is not broken down by bacteria and does not produce gas)

Filling cystometry: test that evaluates filling phase of micturition cycle and provides information re bladder capacity, sensory awareness, bladder wall compliance, and presence/absence of overactive bladder contractions. Involves placement of pressure-sensitive catheter into the bladder, followed by retrograde filling of the bladder

FODMAPs (Fermentable Oligo-, Di-, Monosaccharides, And Polyols): group of short chain carbohydrates that are poorly absorbed (onions, garlic, dried fruits, beans, lentils, wheat and rye bread, dairy, nuts, sweeteners, etc.) that can produce bloating, gas, abdominal pain, constipation, and/or diarrhea in some people with functional bowel disorders

Frailty: a medical syndrome with multiple causes and contributors that is characterized by diminished strength, endurance, and physiologic function and increases an individual's vulnerability for developing increased dependency and/or death

F-Tag 690: represents federally mandated guidelines to promote continence restoration (bowel and bladder)

of residents in long-term care and proper utilization of indwelling catheters

Functional bowel disorders: umbrella term that describes disorders of bowel motility in which there is no structural or tissue abnormality to explain the symptoms; includes diarrhea, constipation, and irritable bowel syndrome; often referred as a "gut–brain" disorder

Functional constipation: chronic constipation not caused by organic or anatomic abnormalities

Functional diarrhea: diarrhea caused by motility disorder

Functional intervention training: program in which caregivers incorporate musculoskeletal strengthening exercises into toileting routines

Functional urinary incontinence: urinary leakage caused by factors outside the urinary tract that compromise the individual's ability to respond appropriately to signals of bladder filling (e.g., impaired mobility or cognitive impairment)

Gastrocolic reflex: increase in peristaltic activity in response to food intake

Genitourinary syndrome of menopause (GSM): previously known as atrophic vaginitis or vulvovaginal atrophy; a relatively new term used to describe symptomatic vulvovaginal atrophy as well as lower urinary tract symptoms related to a decrease in estrogen and other sex hormones

Giggle incontinence: a unique condition seen in girls where laughter triggers complete incontinence of urine

Guarding reflex: progressive "reflex" increase in outlet resistance in response to bladder filling

Habit training: see Toileting programs

Hirschsprung disease (aganglionic megacolon): congenital absence of ganglion cells in bowel wall resulting in functional bowel obstruction due to absence of peristaltic activity in aganglionic section. Most cases are "short segment" (aganglionic segment limited to rectum or rectum and sigmoid); a small percentage involve greater lengths of the colon or, occasionally, the entire colon

Hostile bladder: bladder outlet obstruction and risk to upper urinary tracts from elevated detrusor pressures and/or low bladder wall compliance in individuals with neurogenic bladder dysfunction

Hydronephrosis: distention of the kidneys; can result from back pressure from increases in bladder pressure due to urinary retention particularly when bladder compliance is low

Ileocecal valve: one-way valve located at the junction of the ileum and cecum that controls passage of stool from small bowel into colon and prevents retrograde flow of stool from colon into small intestine

Imperforate anus: congenital anomaly involving distal colon/rectum and anal canal/sphincters; further classified as "high" or "low" lesion, depending on whether the distal end of the bowel terminates above or below the levator ani complex

Incidence: refers to the number of individuals who develop a specific disease or experience a specific health-related event during a particular time period

"Incident to" billing: mechanism for Medicare that allows services provided in an outpatient setting to be delivered by auxiliary personnel and billed under the provider's national provider identification (NPI)

Incontinence-associated dermatitis (IAD): skin damage caused by exposure to stool or urine

Infectious diarrhea: diarrhea caused by pathogenic organisms (viruses, bacteria, parasites)

Intermittent catheterization (IC): the act of inserting and then removing the catheter once urine has drained via the urethra or other catheterizable channel such as a Mitrofanoff continent urinary diversion

Internal anal sphincter: thick band of smooth muscle that is an extension of the circular muscle of the rectum; primary contributor to continence at rest; composed of slow-twitch muscle fibers innervated by enteric nervous system and autonomic nervous system; not under voluntary control

Internal bowel management system: system designed to divert liquid stool away from perianal skin and into collection device; comprised of low-pressure intrarectal balloon, soft silicone tubing, and collection device

Internal urethral sphincter: smooth muscle fibers within bladder neck that contribute to continence at rest; innervated by autonomic nervous system and not under voluntary control

International Prostate Symptom Score (IPSS): also known as the American Urologic Association score and one of the most common tools employed to assess LUTS in men

Interstitial cystitis: bladder pain syndrome of poorly understood etiology

Intertriginous dermatitis (ITD): a form of moisture-associated skin dermatitis (MASD) characterized by inflammation of the skin caused by moisture, bacteria, and fungi where opposing skin surfaces touch and may rub, such as the groin, gluteal cleft, under the pannus, etc.

Irritable bowel syndrome (IBS): functional bowel disorder typified by abdominal pain or discomfort associated with alterations in bowel elimination and relieved by bowel movements; further classified as

- *IBS-C* (IBS associated with constipation)
- *IBS-D* (IBS associated with diarrhea)
- *IBS-M* (IBS associated with alternating diarrhea and constipation)

KNACK maneuver: voluntary contraction of pelvic floor muscles during activities that increase intra-abdominal pressure and cause stress urinary incontinence, for example, sneezing, lifting

Lamina propria: suburothelial layer of bladder wall, located between urothelium and detrusor muscle; composed of interstitial cells, fibroblasts, blood vessels, and afferent/efferent nerves

Lapides classification system: classification system for neurogenic bladder dysfunction based on clinical and cystometric manifestations

Latchkey urgency (key in the lock or key in the door): an overwhelming need to urinate when reaching home

Laxative: agent that promotes bowel movements through several physiologic mechanisms: stool bulking, osmosis, and direct stimulation of peristalsis. Further classified as osmotic and stimulant laxatives

Levator ani: primary muscle group of pelvic floor; composed of three connected muscles (pubococcygeus, puborectalis, and iliococcygeus)

Lifestyle interventions: weight loss, smoking cessation, bowel management, exercise, appropriate fluid intake, and reduced caffeine consumption to reduce bladder or bowel dysfunction symptoms

Lower motor neuron neurogenic bladder: a noncontracting (acontractile or areflexic) detrusor due to sacral cord injury or lesion

Lower urinary tract (LUT): ureters, bladder, and urethra

Lower urinary tract symptoms (LUTS): subjective indicators of lower urinary tract dysfunction. Divided into three categories:

- *storage LUTS*: frequency, urgency, dysuria, nocturnal polyuria, and leakage
- *voiding LUTS*: hesitancy, poor or intermittent stream, straining to void, and terminal dribble
- *postvoid LUTS*: postvoid dribbling and sensation of incomplete emptying

Magnetic artificial sphincter: implantation of ring of magnetic titanium beads into anal sphincter, which holds walls of anal canal together in closed position until abdominal muscle contraction overrides the resistance and opens the anal canal

Mass movements: series of peristaltic contractions that rapidly propel stool from transverse colon to rectum

Medical adhesive–related skin injury (MARSI): skin damage resulting from the use of medical adhesives including contact dermatitis, allergic dermatitis, maceration, folliculitis, and mechanical skin damage, that is, epidermal stripping, friction blisters, and skin tears

Medicare: Federal government insurance program that covers people 65 or older and those with disabilities or end-stage renal disease. Coverage is determined by the location and types of services:

- *Medicare Part A*—covers hospital and hospice visits, stays in skilled nursing facilities, and home health
- *Medicare Part B*—covers 80% of expenses incurred with outpatient visits/care, some home health and durable medical equipment
- *Medicare Part C*—insurance coverage by private-run insurance companies
- *Medicare Part D*—helps cover the cost of prescriptions

Meissner plexus: nerve plexus located in submucosal layer of bowel wall; primary functions are to detect intraluminal substances, control GI blood flow, and regulate epithelial cell function

Microbiome: combined genetic material of the microorganisms in a particular environment such as the gut that protects individuals against germs, aides in digestion, metabolism and possible resistance to diseases or unhealthy conditions

Micturition reflex (voiding reflex): involuntary process of bladder emptying, or micturition controlled by the autonomic nervous system. If appropriate time to urinate, the pontine micturition center (PMC) is activated by a midbrain structure (PAG) to initiate the micturition reflex, the PMC sends input to the spinal cord that inhibits sympathetic stimulation of the bladder neck and innervation of the external sphincter via Onuf nucleus (thus causing both internal and external sphincter relaxation) and activates the parasympathetic pathways causing detrusor contraction to emptying the bladder

Mixed urinary incontinence (UI): mixed stress/urge UI; leakage of urine associated with activities that cause increase in intra-abdominal pressure in combination with leakage associated with urgency

Moisture-associated skin damage (MASD): an umbrella term to describe skin that is damaged from repeated exposure to different sources of moisture such as water, urine, or stool, perspiration, mucus, or saliva

Myenteric (Auerbach) plexus: nerve plexus located between longitudinal and circular muscle layers of bowel wall; plays primary role in regulating colonic motility

Neurogenic bowel: loss of neural control of defecation; characterized by absent or markedly reduced ability to sense rectal distention and to voluntarily contract the external anal sphincter (EAS)

Neurogenic incontinence (reflex incontinence): urinary incontinence caused by a neurologic lesion (such as a spinal cord injury or multiple sclerosis) that disrupts the neurologic pathways that provide voluntary control of voiding

Neurogenic lower urinary tract dysfunction (NLUTD): lower urinary tract dysfunction caused by disturbance of neurologic control mechanisms (most commonly a lesion between the sacral cord and brain)

Neuromodulation: therapeutic modality that uses electrical signals to alter involuntary reflexes of lower urinary tract, thus reducing involuntary detrusor contractions

Neurotransmitters: chemical messengers that regulate detrusor relaxation and contraction and act at specific receptor sites on the smooth muscle

Nicotinic receptors: receptors that react to the neurotransmitter acetylcholine, resulting in contraction of the periurethral and rhabdosphincter muscles and closure of the sphincter mechanism

Nocturia: waking at night one or more times to void

Nocturnal enuresis: (see enuresis)

Nocturnal polyuria: a condition in which the day/night ratio of urine production is reversed

Nonretentive encopresis: fecal soiling not associated with stool-withholding behavior

Norepinephrine: major sympathetic neurotransmitter; mediates sphincter contraction

Normal transit constipation: constipation in individual with normal peristaltic response to stimuli such as colonic distention; caused by dietary/environmental factors leading to reduced peristaltic stimuli (e.g., small-caliber stools)

Obstructed defecation: difficult elimination of stool caused by pathology involving the pelvic floor and anorectal junction

OLDCART: acronym to help provide a systematic approach to interviewing a patient about a presenting symptom such as urinary incontinence: O-onset, L-location, D-duration, C-character, C-consistency, A-aggravating factors, R-relieving factors

OnabotulinumtoxinA: a pharmacologic agent to treat neurogenic detrusor overactivity; the neurotoxin is injected directly into the detrusor wall during a cystoscopic procedure

Onuf nucleus: collection of cells in sacral cord that receive input from pontine storage center and mediate contraction of striated sphincter via pudendal nerve

OR (odds ratio): compares the likelihood (odds) of an outcome in individuals with a characteristic (risk factor) of interest (e.g., a breech delivery) to the likelihood in the group without the risk factor (those who did not have a breech delivery). An OR of 1 means that the outcome is equally likely in those with and without the characteristic being examined

Osmotic diarrhea: diarrhea caused by presence of high osmolar substances within the lumen of the bowel that pull fluid into gut

Osmotic laxative: agent that "works" by pulling fluid into the lumen of the bowel, thus softening the stool and causing colonic distention and peristalsis

Overactive bladder: symptom complex comprised of urinary urgency, with or without urgency incontinence, usually with increased daytime frequency and nocturia, in the absence of UTI or other obvious pathologies

Oxford grading system: internationally accepted muscle grading system used to score pelvic muscle tone, accessory muscle use, and muscle hypertonus during digital vaginal examination

Pabd: urodynamic measurement of intra-abdominal pressure obtained by pressure-sensitive catheter placed in the rectum

Parasympathetic nervous system: branch of autonomic nervous system; mediates detrusor muscle contraction and promotes intestinal peristaltic activity

Paruresis: inability to urinate in presence of others; also called shy bladder syndrome

Passive fecal incontinence: see Fecal incontinence

Pdet: urodynamic measurement of pressures created by bladder wall stiffness and detrusor muscle contractions; obtained by computer subtraction of Pabd from Pves

Pediatric urinary incontinence quality of life score (PIN-Q): a questionnaire used to assess the impact the symptoms have on the child's quality of life and to track treatment progress

Pelvic floor: network of fascia, ligaments, and muscles that support pelvic organs and oppose downward displacement

Pelvic floor dyssynergia: inability to coordinate pelvic floor and sphincter relaxation and abdominal muscle contraction; persistent contraction of anal sphincter and pelvic floor leading to obstructed defecation

Pelvic floor muscle training/exercises (PFMT): program involving routine repetitive contractions of pelvic floor muscles with goal of increasing pelvic floor muscle strength (contractility) and endurance. Patient must learn to isolate and voluntarily contract the pelvic floor muscles while (ideally) keeping the abdominal and gluteal muscles relaxed

Pelvic floor myofascial pain (PFMF): pain in the pelvic floor muscles characterized by the development of trigger points (TrP)

Pelvic organ prolapse (POP): the herniation of a pelvic organ toward and through the vaginal introitus

Penile compression device (penile clamps): mechanical devices designed to prevent urine leakage by compressing the penis

Perceived constipation: perception of problem with stool elimination when bowel function/stool elimination is actually normal

Percutaneous tibial nerve stimulation (PTNS): also referred to as posterior tibial nerve stimulation. Form of neuromodulation used to treat overactive bladder (OAB); thought to diminish abnormal reflex arcs associated with overactive bladder by modulating afferent signals from the bladder to the spinal cord; a fine needle electrode is inserted into the lower, inner aspect of the leg, slightly cephalad to the medial malleolus near but not on the tibial nerve

Periaqueductal gray (PAG): section of midbrain that integrates and forwards signals regarding bladder filling to prefrontal cortex. Under inhibitory control by prefrontal cortex; when inhibitory control released, PAG directs pontine micturition center to mediate coordinated voiding (micturition reflex)

Perigenital: skin located in area that is exposed to urinary or fecal incontinence: vulva, inner groin, thighs, gluteal cleft, buttocks, scrotum

Perineal body: fibrous muscular structure that is centrally located between the urogenital and anal triangles; frequently called the "central tendon" due to multiple attachments and playing a major role in pelvic floor strength

Perineal membrane: triangular fibrous structure that spans anterior pelvis and limits descent of pelvic organs

Pessary: vaginal device to stabilize and support the bladder neck and to compress the urethra to prevent urine leakage during increased intra-abdominal pressure

Phasic detrusor contractions: involuntary detrusor contractions that occur during filling phase of urodynamic study and may or may not result in urinary leakage

Phytotherapeutic agents: (see Plant Extracts)

PICOT: acronym use when searching for evidence representing the following **P**atient population of interest; **I**ntervention of interest; **C**omparison of interest; **O**utcome of interest; **T**ime

Plant extracts: (phytotherapeutic agents) are commonly used by men with LUTS related to BPH: saw palmetto (*Serenoa repens*), stinging nettle (*Urtica dioica*), extracts of the African plum tree (*Pygeum africanum*), pumpkin seed (*Cucurbita pepo*), South African star grass (*Hypoxis rooperi*), and rye pollen (*Secale cereale*)

Polyuria: defined by International Continence Society (ICS) as excessive production of urine

- *global polyuria*—urine production >40 mL urine/kg body weight for 24 hours or 2.8 L (70 kg individual) causing daytime urinary frequency and nocturia even in the face of normal bladder capacity
- *nocturnal polyuria*—nocturnal output >20% of the daily total in younger adults and >33% of the daily total in older adults

Pontine micturition center (PMC) or Barrington nucleus: midbrain structure responsible for assuring that bladder neck and rhabdosphincter are relaxed before the bladder contracts

Pontine storage center (PSC) or M center: midbrain structure responsible for maintaining contraction of striated sphincter during storage phase

Postobstructive diuresis: marked polyuria (>4 to 5 L/day) after bladder drainage in patients with urinary retention

Postoperative urinary retention (POUR): inability to urinate following anesthesia possible due to analgesic drugs or procedure near the urogenital tract disrupting neural control of micturition

Postvoid residual urine (PVR): amount of urine remaining in the bladder after voiding; may be measured by ultrasound or by catheterization

Postvoid symptoms: symptoms, including incomplete emptying, re-voiding ("encore" or "double voiding"), incontinence (dribbling), and postmicturition urgency experiences after cessation of voiding

Prebiotic: nondigestible food ingredient such as dietary fiber that promotes the growth of beneficial microorganisms (probiotics) in the intestine

Prefrontal cortex: area of cortex that controls decision-making regarding when and where to void

Pressure flow study: voiding phase of urodynamic study; patient voids into uroflow commode while pressure-sensitive catheter remains in place in the bladder. Provides simultaneous measurement of urine flow and pressures generated by detrusor muscle contraction

Prevalence: National Health Institute (NIH) defines as the proportion of a population who have a specific characteristic in a given time period

Probiotic: live microorganisms that are beneficial to gut health; often taken as a supplement to prevent antibiotic-induced diarrhea

Prompted voiding: see Toileting programs

Prostatitis: inflammation of the prostate gland that can be chronic, bacterial (acute or chronic), or asymptomatic

PSA velocity: rise in PSA value over 1 year; an increase of more than 0.75 ng/mL usually triggers the need for a biopsy

Puborectalis muscle: component of levator ani muscle that creates a U-shaped sling around the anorectal junction and the anorectal angle that supports fecal continence

Pudendal neuralgia: pelvic pain syndrome thought to be caused by injury to the pudendal nerve

p-value: indicates whether the results of a study are statistically significant, that is, have a low likelihood of being due to chance

Pves: urodynamic measurement of intravesical pressure, obtained by pressure-sensitive catheter placed into the bladder; reflects both intra-abdominal pressures and pressures resulting from bladder wall stiffness or detrusor contractions

Rectoanal inhibitory reflex (RAIR): reflex relaxation of internal anal sphincter (IAS) in response to rectal distention

"Red flag" bowel symptoms: signs and symptoms associated with colorectal cancer (also known as "alarm symptoms")

Retentive encopresis: fecal soiling caused by stool-withholding behavior

RR (relative risk): compares the risk of an outcome in those with a risk factor (characteristic) and those without it. RR is interpreted the same way as the odds ratio

Sacral nerve stimulation (sacral neuromodulation): stimulation of sacral nerves controlling bladder function and stool elimination using implantable electrodes placed in sacral foramen; used to treat refractory overactive bladder and persistent refractory constipation

Sacral reflex: involves spinal segments S2-S4. It is a motor response that causes contraction of the anal sphincter and pelvic floor muscles induced by stimulation of sensory receptors in the perineum, anus, vulva, clitoris, or penis. The anal wink and bulbocavernosus are sacral reflexes that reflect the integrity of the pudendal nerve and sacral spinal reflex arcs

Sampling reflex: differentiation between gaseous, liquid, and solid rectal contents provided by sensory receptors in anal canal; occurs when internal anal sphincter relaxes briefly in response to rectal distention and permits rectal contents to contact receptors in anal canal

Secretory diarrhea: diarrhea resulting from damage to epithelial cells in intestinal mucosa are damaged by an infectious organism or intestinal toxin; results in abnormal secretion of fluid *into* lumen of bowel and inability to absorb water and electrolytes *from* lumen of bowel

Seminal vesicles: store semen: the bulbourethral glands secrete an alkaline fluid prior to ejaculation that neutralizes the acidity of urine to protect sperm

Septicemia: invasion of the blood stream by virulent microorganisms leading to toxicity and life-threatening systemic inflammatory response syndrome

Simple constipation: transient alteration in stool elimination, most often caused by dietary or environmental factors

Simple cystometrogram (CMG): used as a screening tool to assess bladder sensation and to detect involuntary bladder contractions especially in the frail elderly in settings where urodynamic testing is not practical nor available. It is accomplished by placing a catheter in the bladder and performing a retrograde filling. Capacity is obtained by simple calculation and compliance by watching the meniscus of the column of water

Simple (radical) prostatectomy: removal of the prostate gland and prostatic urethra, with anastomosis of distal urethra to bladder neck

Slow transit constipation: constipation caused by reduced frequency and amplitude of peristaltic contractions in the colon and does not respond well to fiber supplementation or stimulant laxatives

Slow-twitch muscle fibers: muscle fibers that provide sustained tonic contraction; comprise 2/3 of pelvic floor muscle fibers

Sphincteroplasty: surgical repair of damaged sphincter; commonly used to repair sphincter damaged by obstetric trauma

Spina bifida: congenital neural tube defect involving bony defect in vertebral column; most commonly accompanied by myelomeningocele, herniation of the spinal cord through the bony defect

Spinal cord injury: trauma or damage to the spinal cord resulting in loss of motor and/or sensory function

Standardized measurement tools: tools that generate robust data that can be used to guide initial treatment decisions and to evaluate changes in symptoms and the efficacy of treatment

Stimulant laxative: agent that stimulates peristalsis and stool elimination via activation of ganglion cells in the bowel wall

Stimulated defecation: use of peristaltic stimulus to initiate rectal evacuation at time selected by patient; commonly used management approach for patient with neurogenic bowel

Storage symptoms: affect the ability to hold urine in the bladder and are classified into four groups: general (e.g., urinary frequency, nocturia, polyuria); sensory (e.g., urgency, altered bladder filling sensation); urinary incontinence (UI) or involuntary urine loss (e.g., stress UI, urgency UI, mixed UI, overflow UI, enuresis, disability associated UI, insensible UI, sexual arousal incontinence, climacturia); and storage symptom syndrome (i.e., overactive bladder)

Stove-pipe urethra: unable to exert any closure pressure, resulting in continuous urinary leakage

Stress urinary incontinence: involuntary leakage of urine associated with effort or exertion (activities that cause an increase in intra-abdominal pressure)

Stroke: sometimes referred to as cerebrovascular accident is as an acute, focal injury of the central nervous system owing to a vascular cause such as cerebral infarction, intracerebral hemorrhage, or subarachnoid hemorrhage

Superabsorbent polymers (SAPs): molecules that are designed to absorb many times their weight and retain fluid away from the skin used in disposable absorbent products

Suprapubic catheterization: insertion of an indwelling catheter into the bladder through the abdominal wall

Suprasacral level lesions: trauma or disease affecting spinal segments above S2 and below spinal segment C2

Surfactant: a chemical substance dissolved in a liquid that reduces its surface tension, thereby increasing its spreading and wetting properties

Sympathetic nervous system: branch of autonomic nervous system; promotes internal urethral sphincter contraction and bladder wall relaxation; reduces intestinal secretion and motility

Tenesmus: persistent sensation of stool in the rectum and the need to defecate

Terminal detrusor contractions: involuntary detrusor contractions that occur during filling phase of urodynamic study and typically result in complete bladder emptying

Timed voiding: toileting at fixed intervals, such as every 3 hours

TOILETED: mnemonic designed to help clinicians remember the potentially reversible causes of urinary incontinence; several mnemonics exist including

- *TOILETED*—Thin dry urethral epithelium; Obstruction; Infection; Limited mobility; Emotional/psychological issues; Therapeutic medications; Endocrine disorders; Delirium
- *DRIP*— Delirium or Depression, Restricted mobility or Retention, Infection, Pharmaceuticals
- *PRAISED*—Pharmaceuticals/Psychological issues, acute Retention or Restricted mobility, Atrophy of urogenital tissues or Acute pelvic prolapse, Infection, Stool impaction, Excess urine output, Delirium, dietary irritants
- *DIAPPERS*—Delirium or Dietary irritants, Infection, Acute retention or Atrophy, Pharmaceuticals, Psychological, Excess Urine Output, Restricted Mobility, Stool impaction

Toileting programs: an effective treatment strategy for incontinence due to impaired mobility and cognition. There are 3 type of toileting programs:

- *Routine Schedule Toileting (RST)*—a fixed schedule of assisted toileting where there is no attempt to individualize the schedule to conform to normal voiding patterns and there is no attempt made to motivate the individual to remain continent.
- *Prompted Voiding*—behavioral therapy program in which subjects are prompted to toilet and encouraged with social rewards when they void successfully
- *Habit training or PURT (pattern urge response training)*—program involving identification of the individual's toileting patterns via bladder diary, followed by establishment of toileting schedule based on that pattern

Toileting trial: consists of offering toileting assistance to the older adult every 2 hours over a 3-day period and provides valuable information regarding the probable benefit of a toileting program

Trabeculation of the bladder: thickening of the bladder wall caused by overwork of the detrusor

Transanal irrigation: delivery of water into distal colon to stimulate peristalsis and bowel evacuation; water delivered via balloon-tipped catheter to prevent backflow

Transient fecal incontinence: short-term (new-onset) incontinence caused by change in stool consistency or sensory awareness

Transit time studies: diagnostic tool used to objectively differentiate between normal transit and slow transit constipation; utilizes variety of techniques to determine time required for stool to pass through colon and out of anal canal

Transurethral resection of the prostate (TURP): surgical removal of excess prostatic tissue via a resectoscope inserted through the urethra; the gold standard intervention for the treatment of BPH

Transvaginal electrical stimulation: used in treating SUI; causes PFM contraction and increases the number of muscle fibers recruited during rapid contractions

Transvaginal estrogen: topical estrogen in the form of a cream, tablet, ring, or suppository placed in the vagina

Traveler's diarrhea: nonspecific infectious diarrhea, typically bacterial, that occurs when individual travels to area of the world with poor sanitation

Trial without catheterization (TWOC): allowing patients who previously required catheterization due to urinary retention a voiding trial (typically 1 to 3 days) without catheterization while monitoring for recurrent retention

Trigone: triangular-shaped smooth muscle at the base of the bladder

TRUS: transrectal biopsy of the prostate; performed with an ultrasound-guided needle

Upper motor neuron neurogenic bladder: an overactive detrusor that contracts without voluntary control due to an spinal injury or lesion above the sacral cord

Upper urinary tract distress: impaired function of the upper urinary tracts (kidneys, renal pelves, and ureters), associated with neurogenic bladder dysfunction

Urease: enzyme that causes the urea in the urine to hydrolyze to free ammonia, in turn raising the pH and allowing precipitation of minerals such as calcium phosphate and magnesium ammonium phosphate (struvite)

Urethral bulking agents: intra- or periurethral injection to plump up the urethral mucosa; this creates artificial urethral cushions that can improve urethral coaptation and restore continence

Urethral caruncle: cherry red and abnormally prominent (prolapsed) urethral meatus; caused by estrogen deficiency

Urethral hypermobility: distal displacement of urethra in response to increased intra-abdominal pressure

Urethral inserts: a sterile disposable, single-use, intra-urethral device that can be used by women with stress incontinence to prevent leakage

Urethral pressure profile: graphic representation of pressures along length of the urethra; obtained by precise and steady withdrawal of a pressure-sensitive catheter through the urethra

Urethral resistance: the detrusor pressure required to overcome the urethral sphincter mechanism and create urinary flow; measured during urodynamic testing

Urethral sphincter mechanism: conceptualized as containing two components: elements of compression and muscular elements that promote active urethral closure in response to physical exertion; contains periurethral striated muscle and a rhabdosphincter (formerly called the external sphincter)

Urge fecal incontinence: see Fecal incontinence)

Urge inhibition (suppression) strategies: behavioral strategies that patients may be taught to control urgency; include pelvic muscle contractions, controlled breathing, avoidance of sudden activity, and distraction

Urgency: sudden overwhelming desire to void that is difficult to delay and often accompanied by fear of leakage

Urge urinary incontinence: involuntary leakage of urine accompanied by or immediately preceded by a strong urge to void

Urinary bladder: hollow, muscular organ designed to fill with urine at low pressures

Urinary continence: voluntary control of voiding; requires anatomic integrity of the urinary system, neurological control of the detrusor muscle, and an intact urethral sphincter mechanism

Urinary frequency: abnormally frequent voiding, typically defined as diurnal frequency >8

Urinary incontinence: altered ability to store urine effectively and to control the time and place for voiding; involuntary leakage of urine

Urinary retention: incomplete bladder emptying, either due to bladder outlet obstruction or to ineffective bladder contractions

Urinary tract infection (UTI): bacterial infection or invasion of microbial uropathogens occurring in the lower or upper urinary tract or both; can be classified as

- *upper urinary tract* infections (pyelonephritis)
- *lower urinary tract infections* that can be located in the bladder (cystitis) or urethra (urethritis)

- *simple, uncomplicated UTIs* occurring in young, healthy, nonpregnant women with normal anatomy
- *complicated UTI* occurring in patients with factors that increase the risk of bacterial colonization and decrease the efficacy of therapy
- *recurrent (rUTI)*—two or more infections within 6 months of completion of treatment of the initial infection or three or more infections in 12 months with either reinfection with a previously isolated organism or persistence of bacteria

Urodynamic testing: several different tests of lower urinary tract function that, taken together, create a picture of its functional status (ability of bladder to store urine at low pressures and to empty effectively and sphincter's ability to maintain closure during filling and to open for voiding)

Uroflowmetry: measurement of rate of urine flow (mL/second); noninvasive screening tool for voiding dysfunction. Patient voids into commode equipped to measure rate of urine flow

Urosepsis: complex systemic inflammatory host response (SIRS) to a bacterial infection originating from the urogenital tract with potentially life-threatening consequences

Urothelium: inner lining of bladder, comprised primarily of transitional cell epithelium

Urotherapy: conservative-based therapy and treatment of LUT dysfunction that rehabilitates the LUT and encompasses a wide field of health care professionals

Valsalva voiding: use of abdominal muscle contraction to empty the bladder as opposed to bladder contraction often seen in poorly contractile bladders or in bladder outlet obstruction

Vesicoureteral reflux (VUR): condition in which urine flows backward from the bladder to one or both ureters and sometimes to the kidneys; most common in infants, young children, and those who suffer from neurogenic bladder dysfunction

Vesicovaginal fistula (VVF): an abnormal tract that forms between the bladder and vagina, allowing urine to continuously drain into the vagina

Video urodynamics: urodynamic studies utilizing contrast medium for bladder filling and simultaneous use of fluoroscopic imaging

Voiding dysfunction: altered ability to effectively empty the bladder, resulting in some degree of urinary retention

Voiding symptoms: slow and/or interrupted stream, the perception of reduced flow; hesitancy, difficulty in initiating voiding; straining, the need to use Valsalva or abdominal muscles to void; terminal dribble, prolongation of the last phase of voiding; hematuria (blood in the urine); and dysuria, a burning sensation or general discomfort during voiding

Vulvodynia: pelvic pain syndrome characterized by chronic vulvar pain especially characterized by complaints of burning, stinging, irritation, and or rawness

Watchful waiting: conservative approach to management of localized prostate cancer or LUTS. Involves deferral of active treatment

Weight bias: negative attitude toward or beliefs about adiposity that alters the quality of care because of one's size, weight, or body habitus

Weighted vaginal cones: feedback device to assist women to strengthen their PFMs

Wein classification system: classification system for urinary incontinence or voiding dysfunction based on urodynamic findings; classifies lower urinary tract dysfunction as one of the following failure to store because of the bladder: failure to store because of the sphincter, failure to empty because of the bladder, and failure to empty because of the sphincter

WOC nurse: a generic term used for a nurse specializing in the care of an individual with wound, ostomy, or continence issues. A certified WOC nurse may use the CWOCN® credential

Wound, Ostomy and Continence Nurses Society™: WOCN® Society is a professional, international nursing society of health care professionals who are specialists in the care of patients with wound, ostomy, and continence needs

INDEX

Note: Page numbers followed by "*f*" denote figures, page numbers followed by "*t*" denote tables, and those followed by "*b*" denote boxes.